W9-DBM-625

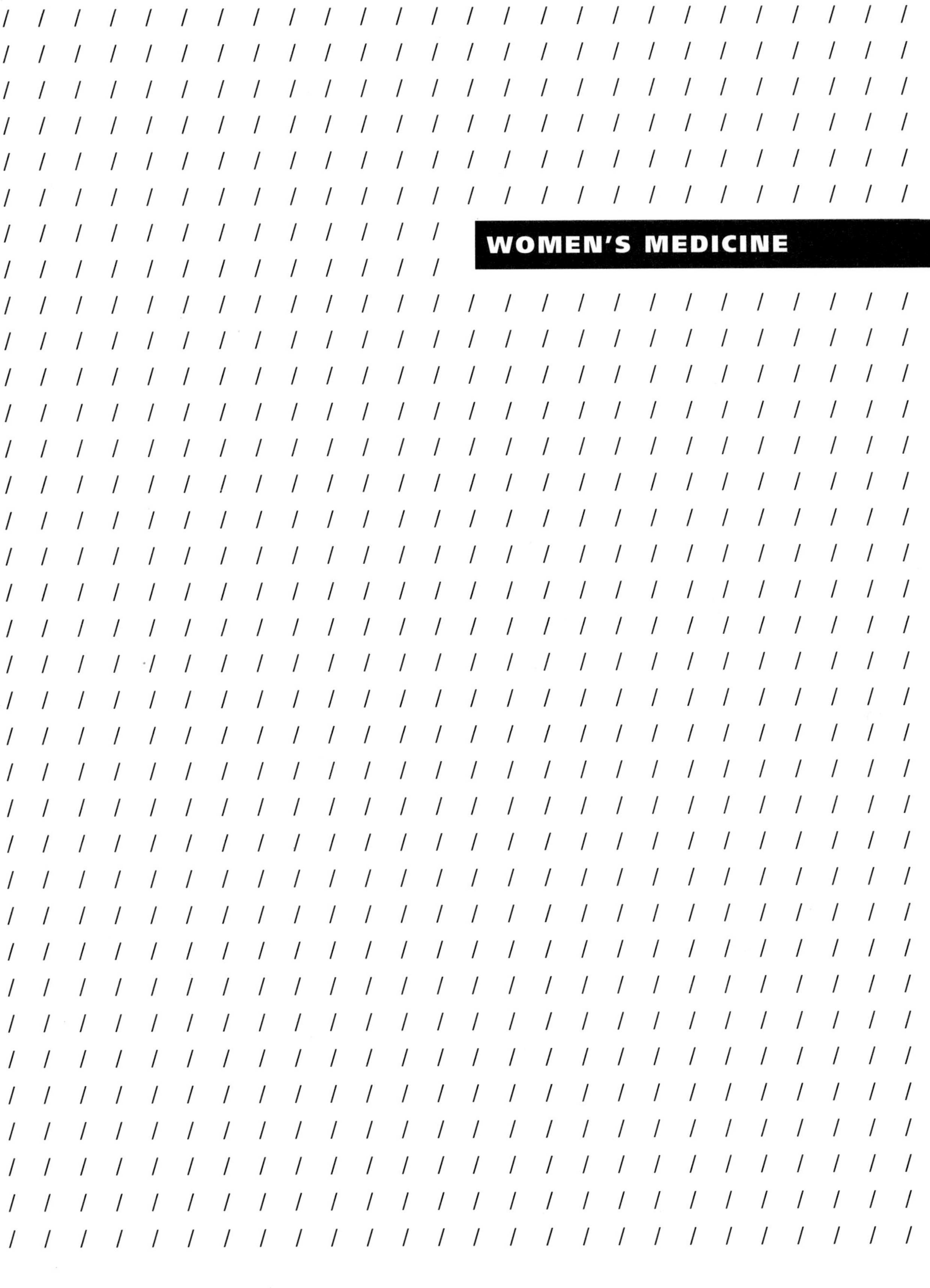

WOMEN'S MEDICINE

This book is dedicated to three physicians who greatly influenced my career: Lindsey D. Campbell, MD (psychiatrist), William C. Croom, Jr., MD (dermatologist), and John Champneys Taylor, MD (obsterician-gynecologist). These men taught me self-insight, dedication, and discipline, which have served me well throughout my career.

A special thanks should be given to Murrill Lynch, my Administrative Associate, for helping to coordinate this manuscript and prepare the text.

Richard E. Blackwell

WOMEN'S MEDICINE

Edited by

Richard E. Blackwell, PhD, MD

Professor of Obstetrics and Gynecology
Department of Obstetrics and Gynecology
Director, Division of Reproductive Biology
and Endocrinology
University of Alabama
Birmingham, Alabama

Blackwell
Science

Blackwell Science
Editorial offices:
238 Main Street, Cambridge, Massachusetts 02142, USA
Osney Mead, Oxford OX2 0EL, England
25 John Street, London WC1N 2BL, England
23 Ainslie Place, Edinburgh EH3 6AJ, Scotland
54 University Street, Carlton, Victoria 3053, Australia
Arnette Blackwell SA, 1 rue de Lille, 75007 Paris, France
Blackwell Wissenschafts-Verlag GmbH
Kurfürstendamm 57, 10707 Berlin, Germany
Feldgasse 13, A-1238 Vienna, Austria

Distributors:

North America
Blackwell Science, Inc.
238 Main Street
Cambridge, Massachusetts 02142
(Telephone orders: 800-215-1000 or 617-876-7000)

Australia
Blackwell Science Pty. Ltd.
54 University Street
Carlton, Victoria 3053
(Telephone orders: 03-347-0300
fax: 03-349-3016)

Outside North America and Australia
Blackwell Science, Ltd.
c/o Marston Book Services, Ltd.
P.O. Box 87
Oxford OX2 0DT
England
(Telephone orders: 44-1865-791155)

Acquisitions: Victoria Reeders
Development: Kathleen Broderick
Production: Paula Card Higginson
Manufacturing: Kathleen Grimes

Printed and bound by Maple-Vail, Binghamton, New York

Printed in the United States of America

96 97 98 99 5 4 3 2 1

Notice: The indications and dosages of all drugs in this book have been recommended in the medical literature and conform to the practices of the general medical community. The medications described do not necessarily have specific approval by the Food and Drug Administration for use in the diseases and dosages for which they are recommended. The package insert for each drug should be consulted for use and dosage as approved by the FDA. Because standards of usage change, it is advisable to keep abreast of revised recommendations, particularly those concerning new drugs.

Library of Congress Cataloging-in-Publication Data

CONTENTS

Contributors ix

Preface xiii

Section One: Wellness and Lifestyle

1. Risk Factors and Screening 3
Diane Bodurka

2. Lifestyle, Diet, Exercise, and Work 12
Karen R. Hammond and Richard E. Blackwell

Section Two: Vascular Diseases

3. Hypertension 23
Herman A. Taylor, Jr.

4. Hyperlipidemia 44
Vera A. Bittner

5. Peripheral Vascular Disease 66
Sriram S. Iyer, Michael Jaff, Gary S. Roubin, and Gerald Dorros

6. Angina Pectoris 83
Larry S. Dean

7. Heart Failure 91
Douglas J. Pearce

8. Mitral Valve Prolapse/Dysautonomia 104
Richard O. Russell, Jr.

Section Three: Pulmonary Diseases

9. Hyperactive Airway Disease 119
Susan M. Harding

10. Chronic Obstructive Pulmonary Disease 139
John I. Kennedy, Jr.

11. Lung Cancer 154
Robert I. Garver, Jr.

12. Community-Acquired Pneumonia 163
Nancy E. Dunlap

Section Four: GI Medicine

13. Bowel Dysfunction 177
Richard E. Blackwell

14. Biliary Tract and Gallbladder Disease 182
William G. Blackard, Jr. and Todd H. Baron

15. Inflammatory Bowel Disease 191
Stephen Holland

Section Five: Hematology

16. Anemia 205
James W. Shine

17. Coagulation Disorders 213
Pradip K. Rustagi

Section Six: Endocrine Disorders

18. Thyroid Disease 239
Elizabeth J.v.B. Stahl, Elizabeth Delionback Ennis, and Robert A. Kreisberg

19. Diabetes Mellitus 264
Christine Heckemeyer

20. Obesity 278
Donald D. Hensrud and Roland L. Weinsier

21. Hyperprolactinemia 292
Richard E. Blackwell and Karen R. Hammond

22. Hirsutism 302
Richard E. Blackwell

Section Seven: Infectious Diseases

23. Anogenital Human Papillomavirus Infections 313
Michael Saccente and Peter G. Pappas

24. Viral Hepatitis and Its Imitators 324
Dirk J. van Leeuwen and Andree Dadrat

25. The Approach to the Patient at Risk for Sexually Transmitted Diseases 339
David M. Ennis

Section Eight: Otolaryngology

26. Nasal and Sinus Disease 357
C. Elliott Morgan

Section Nine: Neurology

27. Chronic Fatigue 373
William Fulcher

28. Headaches 384
Bradley K. Evans

Section Ten: Rheumatology

29. Osteoporosis 401
Jiri Dubovsky

30. Osteoarthritis 421
Gene L. Watterson, Jr. and Larry W. Moreland

31. Rheumatoid Arthritis 435
S. Louis Bridges, Jr.

32. Systemic Lupus Erythematosus 454
W. Winn Chatham

Section Eleven: Dermatology

33. Common Skin Diseases 475
Jane McClure Blaum

34. Skin Cancers 492
Patricia Mercado

Section Twelve: Psychiatry

35. Premenstrual Syndrome 503
Shambhavi Chandraiah

36. Depression 518
Carl A. Houck

37. Alcohol and Drug Addictions 538
Norman D. Huggins

38. Eating Disorders 547
Richard E. Blackwell

39. Sleep Disorders 553
G. Vernon Pegram, Robert L. Yuspeh, Virginia H. Pascual, and Robert C. Doekel

40. Personality Disorders 573
Nathan Smith

41. Anxiety Disorders 586
John L. Shuster

Section Thirteen: Aging

42. Aging 603
Donna M. Bearden, Sherron H. Kell, and Linda G. Jones

Index 619

CONTRIBUTORS

Todd H. Baron, MD
Assistant Professor
Division of Gastroenterology
University of Alabama at Birmingham
Birmingham, Alabama

Donna M. Bearden, MD
Assistant Professor
Department of Gerontology/Geriatric Medicine
University of Alabama at Birmingham
Birmingham, Alabama

Vera A. Bittner, MD, MSPH
Associate Professor of Medicine
Division of Cardiovascular Diseases
University of Alabama at Birmingham
Birmingham, Alabama

William G. Blackard, Jr., MD
Fellow in Gastroenterology
Division of Gastroenterology
University of Alabama at Birmingham
Birmingham, Alabama

Richard E. Blackwell, PhD, MD
Professor of Obstetrics and Gynecology
Department of Obstetrics and Gynecology
Director, Division of Reproductive Biology and Endocrinology
University of Alabama at Birmingham
Birmingham, Alabama

Jane McClure Blaum, MD
Bay Shore Dermatology
Fairhope, Alabama

Diane Bodurka, MD
Fellow in Oncology
Department of Obstetrics and Gynecology
M.D. Anderson Hospital
Houston, Texas

S. Louis Bridges, Jr., MD, PhD
Assistant Professor of Medicine
Division of Clinical Immunology and Rheumatology
University of Alabama at Birmingham
Birmingham, Alabama

Shambhavi Chandraiah, MD
Assistant Professor
Department of Psychiatry
University of Alabama at Birmingham
Birmingham, Alabama

W. Winn Chatham, MD
Assistant Professor
Division of Clinical Immunology and Rheumatology
University of Alabama Arthritis Center
Birmingham, Alabama

Andree Dadrat
Fellow in Gastroenterology
Division of Gastroenterology
University of Alabama at Birmingham
Birmingham, Alabama

Larry S. Dean, MD
Associate Professor
Division of Cardiovascular Diseases
University of Alabama at Birmingham
Birmingham, Alabama

Robert C. Doekel, MD
Sleep Disorders Center of Alabama
Baptist Montclair Hospital
Birmingham, Alabama

Gerald Dorros, MD
Peripheral Vascular Specialist
Milwaukee Heart and Vascular Clinic
Milwaukee, Wisconsin

Jiri Dubovsky, MD
Associate Professor
Division of Endocrinology/Metabolism
University of Alabama at Birmingham
Birmingham, Alabama

Nancy E. Dunlap, MD, PhD
Associate Professor
Division of Pulmonary Diseases
University of Alabama at Birmingham
Birmingham, Alabama

David M. Ennis, MD
Clinical Instructor
Department of Internal Medicine
University of Alabama at Birmingham
Internal Medicine and Transitional Year Education
Baptist Health System, Inc.
Birmingham, Alabama

Elizabeth Delionback Ennis, MD
Instructor in Medicine
Division of Endocrinology/Metabolism
University of Alabama at Birmingham
Birmingham, Alabama

Bradley K. Evans, MD
Associate Professor of Neurology
University of Mabama at Birmingham
Chief of VA Services
Birmingham, Alabama

William Fulcher, MD
Assistant Professor and Director of Residency Program
University of Alamaba at Birmingham
Birmingham, Alabama

Robert I. Garver, Jr., MD
Associate Professor
Division of Pulmonary Diseases
University of Alabama at Birmingham
Birmingham, Alabama

Karen R. Hammond, MSN, CRNP
Division of Reproductive Biology and Endocrinology
University of Alabama at Birmingham
Birmingham, Alabama

Susan M. Harding, MD
Assistant Professor
Division of Pulmonary/Critical Care Medicine
University of Alabama at Birmingham
Birmingham, Alabama

Christine M. Heckemeyer, MD
Associate Professor
Division of Endocrinology/Metabolism
University of Alabama at Birmingham
Birmingham, Alabama

Donald D. Hensrud, MD, MPH
Mayo Clinic
Division of Preventive Medicine
Rochester, Minnesota

Stephen Holland, MD
Assistant Professor
Department of Clinical Pharmacology and Department of Gastroenterology
Peoria, Illinois

Carl A. Houck, MD
Assistant Professor and Medical Director
Pharmacology Consortium
Department of Psychiatry
University of Alabama at Birmingham
Birmingham, Alabama

Norman D. Huggins, MD
Assistant Professor and Medical Director
Department of Psychiatry
University of Alabama at Birmingham
Birmingham, Alabama

Sriram S. Iyer, MD
Assistant Professor
Division of Cardiovascular Diseases
University of Alabama at Birmingham
Birmingham, Alabama

Michael Jaff, MD
Interventional Cardiologist
Milwaukee Heart and Vascular Clinic
Milwaukee, Wisconsin

Linda G. Jones, CRNP, MN
Department of Gerontology/Geriatric Medicine
University of Alabama at Birmingham
Birmingham, Alabama

Sherron H. Kell
Assistant Professor of Medicine
Department of Gerontology/Geriatric Medicine
University of Alabama at Birmingham
Birmingham, Alabama

John I. Kennedy, Jr., MD
Associate Professor
Division of Pulmonary Diseases
University of Alabama at Birmingham
Birmingham, Alabama

Robert A. Kreisberg, MD
Vice Chairman for the Development of Clinical Investigation
Professor
University Consortium for Clinical Research
University of Alabama at Birmingham
Birmingham, Alabama

Dirk J. van Leeuwen, MD
Associate Professor of Medicine
Medical Director
Hepatology and Liver Transplantation
University of Alabama at Birmingham
Birmingham, Alabama

Patricia Mer cado, MD
Assistant Professor
Division of Dermatology
University of Alabama at Birmingham
Birmingham, Alabama

Larry W. Moreland, MD
Assistant Professor
Division of Clinical Immunology and Rheumatology
University of Alabama at Birmingham
Birmingham, Alabama

C. Elliott Morgan, DMD, MD
Assistant Professor
Department of ENT
University of Alabama at Birmingham
Birmingham, Alabama

Peter G. Pappas, MD
Assistant Professor
Division of Infectious Diseases
University of Alabama at Birmingham
Birmingham, Alabama

Virginia H. Pascual, MD
Sleep Disorders Center of Alabama
Baptist Montclair Hospital
Birmingham, Alabama

Douglas J. Pearce, MD
Assistant Professor
Division of Cardiovascular Diseases
University of Alabama at Birmingham
Birmingham, Alabama

G. Vernon Pegram, MD
Administrative Director
Sleep Disorders Center of Alabama
University of Alabama at Birmingham
Birmingham, Alabama

Gary S. Roubin, MD
Professor
Division of Cardiovascular Diseases
University of Alabama at Birmingham
Birmingham, Alabama

Richard O. Russell, Jr., MD
Alabama Heart Institute
Birmingham, Alabama

Pradip K. Rustagi, MD
Associate Professor

Division of Hematology/Oncology
University of Alabama at Birmingham
Birmingham, Alabama

Michael Saccente, MD
Associate in Infectious Diseases
Division of Infectious Diseases
University of Alabama at Birmingham
Birmingham, Alabama

James W. Shine, MD
Assistant Professor
Family/Community Medicine
University of Alabama at Birmingham
Birmingham, Alabama

John L. Shuster, MD
Assistant Professor
Department of Psychiatry
University of Alabama at Birmingham
Birmingham, Alabama

Nathan Smith, MD
Assistant Professor
Department of Psychiatry
University of Alabama at Birmingham
Birmingham, Alabama

Elizabeth J.v.B. Stahl, MD
Endocrinology and Internal Medicine
Birmingham, Alabama

Herman A. Taylor, Jr., MD
Assistant Professor
Division of GI Medicine
University of Alabama at Birmingham
Birmingham, Alabama

Gene L. Watterson, Jr., MD
Fellow in Rheumatology
Division of Clinical Immunology and Rheumatology
University of Alabama at Birmingham
Birmingham, Alabama

Roland L. Weinsier, MD, DrPH
Professor and Chairman
Department of Nutritional Science
University of Alabama at Birmingham
Birmingham, Alabama

Robert L. Yuspeh, PhD
Psychiatric Services
Veterans Affairs Medical Center
Biloxi, Mississippi

PREFACE

Obstetricians and gynecologists have delivered primary care to their patients before this topic became fashionable in the arena of health policy. Frequently obstetricians-gynecologists were the only physicians caring for reproductive-age women, and they worked in consult with internists in the care of postmenopausal patients. Although textbooks of obstetrics frequently deal with medical complications of pregnancy, and the excellent textbooks of internal medicine furnish a compendium of diseases, there were no volumes designed for the practicing obstetrician-gynecologist on the subject of primary care. As a result of this, practicing obstetricians-gynecologists throughout the state of Alabama and surrounding areas were surveyed. Physicians were asked to comment on the types of problems they see most frequently their practice and on which of these required an update. As suspected, the traditional topics of vascular and pulmonary disease, gastrointestinal medicine, hematology, endocrinology, infectious diseases, and rheumatology were mentioned. However, also frequently mentioned was the need for education in a variety of subjects: wellness, lifestyles, risk factors, screening, nutrition, exercise, areas such as ear-nose-throat, evaluating sinusitis and rhinitis, neurology dealing with chronic fatigue syndrome and headache, dermatology dealing with common skin problems, psychiatry dealing with a variety of conditions from alcoholism to eating disorders, and an overview of the aging process. Because of the great diversity of material that had to be covered in the text, it became apparent why this subject had not been approached before. After discussion with the publisher, Blackwell Science, my colleagues and friends in reproductive endocrinology, and Dr. Claude Bennett (then the Chairman of the Department of Medicine at the University of Alabama in Birmingham and coauthor of *Cecil's Textbook of Medicine*, 19th edition), it was decided that a group of physicians from disciplines including obstetrics and gynecology, internal medicine, neurology, otolaryngology, dermatology, and psychiatry, should be assembled to prepare the text, coordinated by a reproductive endocrinologist.

What has been assembled is a text that deals with the specific needs of the practicing obstetrician-gynecologist delivered in what we hope is a user-friendly manner with attention being paid to presentation, diagnostics, appropriate therapy with reference to the pharmacology of drugs, and appropriate referral. It is hoped that this book will serve in the continuation of the education of the obstetrician-gynecologist in the primary care of women.

SECTION ONE

WELLNESS AND LIFESTYLE

CHAPTER 1

RISK FACTORS AND SCREENING

Diane Bodurka

By the year 2000, 12% of the U.S. population will be over the age of 65. Women will comprise 60% of this group. This chapter discusses health risks and screening of women with special attention being paid to the postmenopause age patient. Cardiovascular, central nervous system and metabolic aspects are addressed, as well as cancer prevention and screening.

General Factors

Hypertension

High blood pressure is the major factor responsible for the 500,000 strokes and 175,000 stroke-related deaths that occur annually. Hypertension also contributes to 570,000 cardiac deaths and 1,500,000 heart attacks yearly (1). Box 1.1 illustrates risk factors associated with elevated blood pressure.

Although diastolic blood pressure values have traditionally been used to demonstrate the benefits of blood pressure reduction, recent evidence indicates that systolic elevation may be a more accurate predictor of cardiovascular sequelae of hypertension (2). This principle is especially important in the elderly because isolated systolic elevations occur frequently in this population. The 3-year incidence of cerebrovascular accident was 2.5 times greater in patients with elevated systolic blood pressure as compared to those without in the Chicago Stroke Study (3). In a 2-year follow-up of participants aged 55 to 74 in the Framingham study with elevated systolic blood pressure, the excess risk of cardiovascular death was increased two- to fivefold (4). In a prospective study of 13,740 Dutch women, high systolic blood pressure was found to be a significant predictor of both cardiovascular disease and mortality for women older than 50 years of age; mortality was highest in diabetic women with cardiovascular disease (5).

Recommendations for blood pressure screening are essentially uniform for adults, regardless of age. A blood pressure cuff of the appropriate size should be used. Readings should be taken on multiple occasions to ensure accurate results and to account for blood pressure fluctuations. Hypertension is diagnosed by "an average systolic blood pressure greater than or equal to 160 mm Hg and/or an average diastolic blood pressure greater than or equal to 90 mm Hg on three consecutive visits" (6). Note that when the diastolic blood pressure is less than 90 mm Hg, systolic pressures in the 140 to 160 mm Hg range represent borderline isolated systolic hypertension (6).

The following studies are recommended to detect end-organ damage secondary to hypertension and assist with treatment planning: urinalysis with microscopic studies, serum creatinine, serum potassium, serum uric acid, plasma glucose, serum cholesterol with fractions, electrocardiogram (6).

Lipid Profile

Cardiovascular disease is the leading cause of death of American women, and accounts for almost 500,000 deaths annually. Twice as many women die from cardiovascular disease than from cancer each year (7). Despite recent studies evaluating cardiovascular disease in women, many individuals still believe that cardiovascular disease primarily affects men. Although the number of women afflicted with cardiac disease before menopause is relatively rare, the incidence of cardiovascular disease rises rapidly after menopause, and quickly equals that of men. Women develop coronary heart disease at the same

Box 1.1 Hypertension Increases the Risk of:

- Myocardial infarction
- Cerebrovascular accidents
- Renal failure
- Aortic aneurysms
- Congestive heart failure
- Peripheral vascular disease

Box 1.2 Risk Factors for Coronary Heart Disease

- Family history of premature coronary heart disease (myocardial infarction in parent or sibling <55 yr)
- Cigarette smoking (>10/day)
- Diabetes mellitus
- Severe obesity (>30% ideal body weight)
- History of cerebrovascular disease
- Low HDL level (<35 mg/dL)
- History of occlusive peripheral vascular disease
- Prior myocardial infarction
- Established myocardial ischemia

rate as men, although this occurs 6 to 10 years later (8).

Cholesterol is a lipid, and an important component of cell membranes. It also is a precursor in the biosynthesis of steroid hormones and bile acids. This substance is carried in the blood by molecules that contain lipids and lipoproteins. The major groups of lipoproteins that can be measured in serum include the high-density lipoproteins (HDL), low-density lipoproteins (LDL), and very low-density lipoproteins (VLDL). The HDL usually comprise 20% to 30% of the total cholesterol and are inversely related to the risk of cardiovascular disease. The LDL account for 60% to 70% of the total cholesterol and are responsible for atherogenesis. The VLDL make up the remaining 10% to 15%, and consist mainly of triglycerides. Substantial data support the relationship between the levels of serum total cholesterol and LDL cholesterol and the rate of coronary heart disease (9). Other risk factors for coronary heart disease are listed in Box 1.2 (10).

Blood lipid levels are a significant predictor of coronary heart disease risk. Data from the Framingham Study (11) reveal that atherogenic lipids increase until age 60, then decrease. HDL levels in women of all ages are approximately 10 mg/dL higher than men of equal ages. However, the percent of HDL cholesterol decreases as women become older; this increases the total to HDL cholesterol ratio. Because the risk of coronary heart disease increases as the total to HDL cholesterol ratio increases, women lose protection against coronary heart disease as they age (12).

The total serum cholesterol should be quantified in everyone 20 years of age or older. This should be repeated every 5 years. Samples should not be fasting levels; if the total cholesterol is less than 200 mg/dL, the level should be repeated every 5 years. Risk factors and diet should be discussed with the patient. If the total cholesterol is greater than 240 mg/dL, or if the level is between 200 and 239 mg/dL in patients with definite coronary heart disease, or two other risk factors mentioned in Box 1.2, the lipoprotein fractions should be quantified; additional treatment should be given depending on the results of the lipoprotein analysis. Lastly, if the total cholesterol is between 200 and 239 mg/dL, and the patient has no history of coronary heart disease or other risk factors mentioned in Box 1.2, dietary counseling should be provided (Box 1.3). The total cholesterol should be checked yearly and treated appropriately (10).

It is important to remember that for every 1% increase in the total serum cholesterol, there is a 2% increase in the incidence of coronary heart disease (8).

Central Nervous System

Alzheimer's disease is defined as "... a progressive, degenerative disorder of insidious onset, characterized by memory loss, confusion, and a variety of cognitive disabilities" (13). It most frequently occurs after the age of 60, but may occur as early as 40 years of age. The diagnosis is often difficult to make because Alzheimer's may mimic the symptoms of normal aging in its early stages. Once this disease has progressed, it can be mistaken for other types of dementias. The National Institute on Aging Task Force reported a 10% to 30% incidence of incorrect diagnosis of Alzheimer's in the general medical

Box 1.3 Dietary Counseling

Foods that Raise Blood Cholesterol

- Shellfish
- Organ meats
- Eggs
- Butter
- Hydrogenated fat products
- Beef fat
- Whole milk products
- Natural cheeses
- Coconut, palm, palm kernel oil
- Lard
- Bacon fat

Foods that Lower Blood Cholesterol

- Fruits and vegetables
- Rolled oats and other grains
- Legumes
- Soy milk
- Safflower, sesame, soybean oil
- Corn, soy, cod liver, garlic, olive oil
- Vegetarian diet
- Skim milk products

population (14). The etiology of this disease remains unknown although a genetic component may exist. There are currently no valid tests to detect this disease process other than a postmortem examination of the brain, which confirms the presence of senile plaques and neurofibrillary tangles (13).

The prevalence of dementia increases greatly with age after an individual reaches the age of 65 (15). Although dementia secondary to vascular disease primarily affects men, the incidence of Alzheimer's disease in greater in women (16,17). A recent cohort study of 8877 women revealed that the risk of Alzheimer's disease was less in estrogen users relative to nonusers. The risk of Alzheimer's disease decreased with increased estrogen dose and duration of estrogen use (18).

Glaucoma

Glaucoma includes a group of diseases that increase intraocular pressure to such a degree that visual field defects and degeneration of optic disk occur. Approximately 50,000 Americans are blind secondary to glaucoma (19). The incidence of glaucoma in individuals older than 40 is about 1.5%. This disease is especially common in the black population. In blacks aged 45 to 65, the prevalence is 15 times that of whites in the same age group (20).

Although the management of glaucoma is best left to ophthalmologists, all physicians should make ophthalmoscopy and tonometry a part of the routine physical examination. This is especially important in patients with a family history of glaucoma.

A thorough visual assessment should be performed at least every 10 years beginning at the age of 40. More frequent examinations are indicated when visual defects occur, especially if the change is acute. Eyeglass prescriptions should be evaluated periodically. Cataract surgery consisting of lens extraction is usually performed for the increasingly blurred vision and visual distortion. This improves visual acuity in more than 90% of patients.

Hearing Loss

Gradual progressive hearing loss with age reflects deterioration in the cochlear receptor system with degeneration of hair cells, especially at the base. A patient's quality of life can be improved significantly with the use of hearing aids when indicated by auditory examination. Improvements in the quality of hearing aids, as well as advances in cosmetic appearance of these devices, have increased their acceptance by more individuals, especially elderly women.

Metabolic Factors

Weight

Fat normally makes up about 22% of a woman's body weight, with the remainder consisting of water (55% to 60%), muscle and other lean tissue (10% to 20%), and bone mineral (8% to 10%).

Obesity is seen in 25% to 30% of all adults. Among older people, one third of the men and one half of the women are obese (21). Obesity is commonly defined as greater than 85% of the body mass index (weight kg, height m^2). Obesity is a risk factor for hypertension, diabetes, and increased total cholesterol. This is clearly a major concern in the health care of aging women.

Patients should be weighed at all office visits; weight should be routinely checked during all hospital admissions.

Diabetes

The prevalence of diabetes mellitus increases with age. Approximately 10% of Americans 60 years of age are diabetic; this disease occurs in 20% of Americans 80 years and older. These figures represent a sevenfold increase in the occurrence of diabetes mellitus in the elderly versus individuals 30 to 50 years of age. This group is clearly at increased risk for developing both acute and chronic complications of diabetes (22,23). These patients, as well as those with documented diabetes, are at risk for coronary artery disease (24). Therefore, almost half of all elderly individuals are at risk for complications associated with diabetes (Box 1.4).

Due to the high prevalence of both diabetes and glucose intolerance in elderly women, physicians are obligated to inquire about symptoms and to screen routinely for carbohydrate intolerance. The symptoms of diabetes are polyuria, polydipsia, blurred vision, weight loss, fatigue, neuropathy. If diabetes is suspected, a fasting plasma glucose test should be performed. Diabetes mellitus is diagnosed if the fasting plasma glucose is 140 mg/dL or greater on two separate occasions; the fasting plasma glucose is greater than 116 mg/dL and less than 140 mg/dL, and greater than 200 mg/dL 1 to 2 hours after a meal containing simple carbohydrates (orange juice, chocolate milk, pancake syrup, etc.) on two occasions.

Box 1.4 Complications of Diabetes

- Nephropathy
- Retinopathy
- Neuropathy
- Hypertension
- Angina
- Cerebrovascular insufficiency
- Increased susceptibility to infection

The diagnosis of glucose intolerance is made if the fasting plasma glucose is greater than 116 mg/dL and less than 140 mg/dL, and greater than 140 mg/dL and less than 200 mg/dL 2 hours after a sweet meal (25). Strategies for successful treatment of diabetes and glucose intolerance are presented in Chapter 19. Note that special attention must be paid to the prevention of the most serious complications of diabetic treatment in the elderly—hypoglycemia.

Hypothyroidism

The incidence of hypothyroidism increases as individuals age. In the elderly, the signs and symptoms can often go unnoticed. Special attention should be paid to such complaints as weight loss, increased fatigue, cold intolerance, feelings of depression, and anorexia. A thyroid-stimulating hormone level and T_4 should be measured when a patient presents with any of the above complaints because they may be subtle signs of hypothyroidism and the patient can easily be treated with appropriate hormone replacement.

Osteoarthritis

Osteoarthritis is a joint disease characterized by degeneration and loss of articular cartilage and alterations of subchondral bone. Its pathogenesis is not well understood (26). This disorder may be due to other diseases that cause joint deformity or to repeated joint trauma. However, in many patients, no such associated factor is present. The incidence of osteoarthritis increases with increasing age and occurs with fairly equal frequency in men and women. The patterns of joint involvement, however, differ among the sexes. Osteoarthritis of the hands and kness is more common in women, whereas osteoarthritis of the hips is more common in men. Eighty to 90% of individuals over the age of 40 have radiographic evidence of osteoarthritis, but a large percentage have minimal or no symptoms (26). The severity of the changes increase dramatically with increasing age (27).

Joint pain is the most important symptom of osteoarthritis. Joint stiffness and decreased range of motion may also occur. Elderly patients exhibit symptoms most often. The number of people retiring from the work force annually due to osteoarthritis is more than 5%, second only to cardiovascular disease (28).

Osteoarthritis commonly affects the distal interphalangeal joints, causing bony enlargements called

Heberden's nodes. This disease can also affect the knees, hips, spine, and other joints. Diagnosis is usually made by physical examination, with mild tenderness, pain, and crepitus on motion. Firm swelling may also be present. When the disease becomes advanced, bony enlargement, angulation, and limited motion occur (29). Treatment consists primarily of nonsteroidal anti-inflammatory agents.

Cancer

Cancer prevention is a frequent topic of discussion, especially due to the well-known relationship between certain lifestyle factors and specific types of cancer (Box 1.5). Table 1.1 illustrates the estimated cancer incidence by site as well as cancer deaths by site in women (30).

Lung Cancer

Lung cancer is estimated to be responsible for 13% of all female cancers and 23% of cancer deaths in women in 1994 (30). The majority of the cases are due to smoking. The physician can play an integral part in a patient's decision to stop smoking. Be persistent in your encouragement of smoking cessation.

Colorectal Cancer

Colorectal cancers ranked third in estimated incidence as well as cause of death in women in 1994 (30). Twenty-nine thousand women are expected to die from colorectal cancer this year (30). Many factors appear to increase the risk of colon cancer. These include dietary habits, familial conditions, and a history of or current medical illnesses. High-fiber diets have been associated with lower rates of colon cancer as compared to diets low in fiber content. This is thought to be secondary to an increased transit time of possible carcinogens. Not all studies have agreed with the conclusion, however. A diet with moderate fiber and low saturated fat content is a prudent recommendation for patients to follow. Age, history of colon cancer, history of adenomatous polyps, history of ulcerative colitis,

Table 1.1 1994 Cancer Incidence and Deaths for Women by Site

Incidence	%	Death	%
Melanoma	3	Melanoma	1
Bowel	2	Bowel	1
Breast	32	Breast	18
Lung	13	Lung	23
Colon/rectum	13	Colon	11
Pancreas	2	Pancreas	5
Ovary	4	Ovary	5
Uterus	8	Uterus	4
Urinary	4	Urinary	3
Blood	6	Blood	8
Other	13	Other	21

Reproduced by permission from Boring CC, Squires TS, Tong T, Montgomery S. Cancer statistics, 1994. CA Cancer J Clin 1994;44:7–26.

Box 1.5 Recommendations for Cancer Prevention

1. Stop smoking and the use of all tobacco products. Remind your patients that use of a patch containing nicotine while smoking can cause a fatal myocardial infarction.
2. Use a condom for protection against AIDS when engaging in sexual relations with partners at risk.
3. Take both an estrogen and progestin for hormone replacement if a hysterectomy has not been performed.
4. Drink alcohol in moderation (no more than 1/day).
5. Avoid using carcinogenic drugs.
6. Avoid excessive sun exposure. Use sunscreen with ultraviolet protection.
7. Be aware of possible carcinogens while at work.
8. Eat a diet low in saturated fat and meat. Add fiber, grains, and vegetables to your daily food intake.
9. Exercise regularly. Try to maintain a body mass index less than or equal to 23%.
10. Various cancer screening tests are recommended in the text. Have tests performed at the appropriate time intervals. The goal of the tests is prevention and early detection.

and history of ovarian or uterine cancer are all known risk factors for colon cancer.

The American Cancer Society recommends the following guideline for colorectal cancer screening.

1. Asymptomatic patients with no known risk factors should have a digital rectal examination yearly beginning at 40 years of age, a fecal occult blood test yearly beginning at 50 years of age, and a flexible sigmoidoscopy every 3 to 5 years beginning at 50 years of age.

2. First-degree family members of patients with colorectal cancer diagnosed at or before 55 years of age are recommended to have a colonoscopy or double-contrast barium enema every 5 years beginning at 35 to 40 years of age (31).

Breast Cancer

Breast cancer affects one of every eight American women. Randomized, controlled studies have demonstrated a decrease in death rate among women between the ages of 50 and 69 (32). These is a paucity of data, however, evaluating the efficacy of mammograms in patients 70 years of age and older. The American College of Obstetricians and Gynecologists released the following Screening Guidelines for Mammography in 1994 (33).

1. Mammographic screening should be offered "every 1 to 2 years to women 40 to 49 years old, and annually to women over 50 years old."

2. "There is insufficient data regarding women ages 70 and older to make a definitive recommendation about screening in this age group."

Other recommendations include:

1. All women should be instructed in breast self-examination by the age of 20 years. A good time to introduce the proper technique is at the time of the patient's first pelvic examination. The benefits should be verbally reinforced at the time of each gynecologic examination.

2. All women should have an annual breast examination performed by a physician trained in breast examination. There is not a consensus regarding the time of first examination; however, a breast examination should be performed at the time of yearly pelvic examination, regardless of the patient's age.

3. A baseline mammogram should be performed between the ages of 35 and 40, earlier if risk factors for breast cancer exist (Box 1.6) (34).

Box 1.6 Breast Cancer Risk Factors

- Early menarche
- Late menopause
- Nulliparity
- Term pregnancy after age 30
- Alcohol use >2 drinks/day
- Family history in first- or second-degree relative
- Exposure to ionizing radiation
- Dysplasia on mammogram
- Biopsy-proven proliferative breast disease

Skin Cancers and Melanoma

Sun exposure without ultraviolet light protection is the major risk factor for skin cancer and melanoma. Recommendations for family members with dysplastic nevi or melanoma include: monthly skin self-examination using photographs, professional skin examinations every 3 to 6 months, low tolerance for biopsies of nevi with suspicious changes, avoidance of mid-day sun exposure (10:00 AM to 3:00 PM), avoidance of tanning booths and sunbeds, use of sunscreen with SPF greater than 15, complete avoidance of sunburn, and avoidance of hormonal medications (35).

Gynecologic Malignancies

Cervical Cancer

Cervical cancer is currently the sixth most common cause of cancer mortality in women; however, the prevalence of cervical cancer has dropped dramatically since the advent of the Pap smear (36). More than 50,000 American women are diagnosed with cervical intraepithelia neoplasia every year (36). It is thought that cervical cancer progresses in an orderly fashion through a spectrum of dysplasias before it becomes invasive (37). Invasive cervical cancers have been shown to develop in 30% to 71% of women with untreated carcinoma in situ over a 10-year period (37).

The current recommendation is that all women who have reached the age of 18, or who are or who have been sexually active at any age, have an annual Pap test and pelvic examination. After a woman has had three or more consecutive normal annual examinations, the Pap test may be performed less frequently at the discretion of her physician (38). Although a detailed outcomes analysis regarding the utility of yearly Pap tests for all women has not yet been performed, it is prudent to advise women with high risk factors such as multiple sexual partners, a history of condyloma, patients with human immunodeficiency virus or acquired immunodeficiency syndrome, to have yearly Pap tests. Also, Pap tests should not be ignored in postmenopausal patients because the incidence of cervical cancer in this population is significant.

Ovarian Cancer

Ovarian cancer is the leading cause of mortality due to gynecologic malignancies. The risk of a woman developing ovarian cancer in her lifetime is 1 in 70 (39). Because of a lack of good screening tests, the majority of women present with advanced stage disease and a poor prognosis. The cure rate of individuals who present with early disease is excellent (80% to 90% 5-year survival); however, less than one third of ovarian cancer patients have their disease discovered in these early stages. The patients with advanced disease at the time of presentation have a 5-year survival of 10% to 15% (40).

Despite these somber statistics, screening methods for ovarian cancer remain suboptimal. A combination of CA125 and ultrasound has not been demonstrated to be cost effective for ovarian cancer screening (41).

Conclusion

Once women reach the age of 40, they should undergo an annual physical examination and receive frequent counseling regarding weight control and nutrition, exercise, breast and skin self-examinations, the consumption of alcohol, and smoking. Further, a discussion needs to be carried out regarding sexual practices and injury prevention. The patient should undergo a complete physical examination including measurement of vital signs with emphasis on blood pressure, breast, and pelvic examination. A Pap smear should be obtained annually or every other year if three consecutive Pap smears have been negative. A rectal examination should be carried out and a stool guaiac test performed to rule out occult blood. At about age 40 women should undergo visual examinations every 2 years and have their hearing assessed every 5 years. Tetanus boosters are given every 10 years or after injury. A lipid profile should be carried out every 5 years, and hematocrit and high-sensitivity thyroid-stimulating hormone should generally be performed every 10 years unless otherwise indicated. Baseline mammograms would normally be carried out at age 40 unless the patient has a positive family history and should be repeated every other year between ages of 40 and 50, and each year at age 50 and beyond. Flexible sigmoidoscopy should be carried out every 5 years beginning at age 50 unless there is a strong family history of colon cancer. In this case, screening should be done much earlier.

Using such an algorithm results in adequate screening of the well women, a wise allocation of resources, and at the same time contains the cost of health care. This protocol, when combined with modifications of lifestyle, nutrition, and exercise as discussed in Chapter 2, should facilitate the maintenance of wellness.

REFERENCES

1. Kannell WB, Doyle JT, Ostfeld AM, et al. Optimal resources for primary prevention of atherosclerotic diseases. Atherosclerosis Study Group. Circulation 1984;70:153A–205A.

2. Kannell WB. Some lessons in cardiovascular epidemiology from Framingham. Am J Cardiol 1976;37:269–282.

3. Shekelle RB, Ostfeld AM, Klawana HL Jr. Hypertension and risk of stroke in an elderly population. Stroke 1974;5:71–75.

4. Kannell WB. Implications of Framingham study data for treatment of hypertension: impact of other risk factors. In: Laragh JH, Buhler FR, Seldiin DW, eds. Frontiers in hypertension research. New York: Springer-Verlag, 1981:17–21.

5. Van der Giezev AM, Schopman-Geurts Van Kessel JG, Schouten EG, Slotboom BJ, Kok FJ, Collette HJ. Systolic blood pressure and cardiovascular mortality among 13,740 Dutch women. Prev Med 1990;19:456–465.

6. Special Communication. Statement of hypertension in the elderly. The working group on hypertension in the elderly. JAMA 1986;256:70–74.

7. Walker M, Shaper AG. Follow-up of subjects in prospective studies based in general practice. JA Colol Gen Pract 1984;34:365–370.

8. Castelli WP, Garrison RJ, Wilson PW, Abbott RD, Kalousdian S, Kannell WB. Incidence of coronary heart disease and lipoprotein cholesterol levels, the Framingham Study. JAMA 1986;256:2835–2838.

9. Grundy SM. Cholesterol and coronary heart disease: a new era. JAMA 1986;256:2849–2858.

10. Report of the National Cholesterol Education Program Expert Panel on detection, evaluation, and treatment of high blood cholesterol in adults. Arch Intern Med 1988;148:36–69.

11. Kiely DK, Wolf PA, Cupples LA, Beiser AS, Kannell WB. Physical activity and stroke risk: the Framingham study. Am J Epidemiol 1994;140:608–620.

12. Kannel WB. Metabolic risk factors for coronary heart disease in women: perspective from the Framingham study. Am Heart J 1987;114:413–419.

13. Khachaturin ZS. Diagnosis of Alzheimer's disease. Arch Neurol 1985;42:1097–1104.

14. National Institute on Aging Task Report. Senility reconsidered: treatment responsibilities for mental impairment in the elderly. JAMA 1980;244:259–263.

15. Breitner JCS, Folstein MF. Familial Alzheimer dementia: a prevalent disorder with specific clinical features. Psychol Med 1984;95:80–84.

16. Martin WRW, Adam MJ, Ruth TJ. A study of dopa metabolism in man with positron emission tomography. Neurology 1985;35:110–114.

17. Wooten GF, Ferrari MB. Compound imaging brain dopamine receptors in vivo. Neurology 1985;35:115–118.

18. Paganini-Hill A, Henderson VW. Estrogen deficiency and risk of Alzheimer's disease in women. Am J Epidemiol 1994;140:256–261.

19. Armaly MF. Glaucoma: annual review. Arch Ophthalmol 1975;93:146.

20. Vaughan D, Asbury T. General ophthalmology. Los Altos, CA: Lange Medical Publications, 1986:184.

21. Hamilton EM, Whitney EN, Sizer FS. Nutrition: concepts and controversies. New York: West Publishing, 1985:190.

22. Bennet PH. Diabetes in the elderly: diagnosis and epidemiology. Geriatrics 1984;39:37–41.

23. Lipson LG. Aging. In: Bieglelman PM, Kumar D, eds. Diabetes mellitus for the house officer. Baltimore: Williams & Wilkins, 1986:1984–1985.

24. Jarrett RJ, McCartner P, Keen H. The Bedford survey: ten-year mortality rates in newly diagnosed diabetics, borderline diabetics, and normoglycemic controls, and risk indices for coronary artery disease in borderline diabetics. Diabetologica 1983;22:79–84.

25. Schwartz SL. Management of diabetes mellitus. Durant: Essential Medical Information Systems, Inc. 1991:21.

26. Hamerman D. The biology of osteoarthritis. N Engl J Med 1989;320:1322.

27. Lawrence RC, Hochberg MC, Kelsey JL. Estimates of the prevalence of selected arthritic and musculoskeletal diseases in the United States. J Rheumatol 1989;16:427.

28. Mankin HJ. Clinical feature of osteoarthritis. In: Kelly WN, Harris ED Jr, Ruddy S, et al., eds. Textbook of rheumatology. 3rd ed. Philadelphia: WB Saunders, 1989:1480.

29. Moskowitz RW. Clinical and laboratory findings in osteoarthritis. In: McCarty DJ, ed. Arthritis and allied conditions: a textbook of rheumatology. 11th ed. Philadelphia: Lea & Febiger, 1989:1605.

30. Boring CC, Squires TS, Tong T, Montgomery S. Cancer statistics, 1994. CA Cancer J Clin 1994;44:7–26.

31. DeCosse JJ, Tsioulias GJ, Jacobson JS. Colorectal cancer: detection, treatment and rehabilitation. CA Cancer J Clin 1994;44:27–42.

32. Beghe C, Balducci L, Cohen H. Secondary prevention of breast cancer in the older woman: issues related to screening. Cancer Control 1994;1:3206.

33. The American College of Obstetricians and Gynecologists, Statement on Mammography Screening Guidelines. December, 1994.

34. DeVita VT Jr, Hellman S, Rosenberg SA, eds. Cancer principles & practice of oncology. Philadelphia: JB Lippincott, 1993:1266–1268.

35. Guidelines for melanoma-prone families in primary care and cancer, vol. 14, 6;1994:5.

36. Garfinkle L. Cancer statistics and trends. In: Arthur IH, Fink DJ, Murphy GP, eds. American Cancer

Society textbook of clinical oncology. Atlanta: American Cancer Society, 1991:1–24.

37. Peterson O. Spontaneous course of cervical precancerous conditions. Am J Obstet Gynecol 1956;72:1063–1071.

38. Fink DJ. Change in American Cancer Society checkup guidelines for detection of cervical cancer. CA 1988;38:128.

39. Yancik R, Ries LG, Tayes JW. Ovarian cancer in the elderly: an analysis of surveillance, epidemiology, and end results program data. Am J Obstet Gynecol 1986;154:639.

40. Oram DH, Jacobs IJ, Brady JL, Pyrs-Davies A. Early diagnosis of ovarian cancer. Br J Hosp Med 1990;44:320–324.

41. Piver SM, Recio FO. When is ovarian cancer screening helpful? Contemporary Ob/Gyn 1993;38: 17–32.

CHAPTER 2

LIFESTYLE, DIET, EXERCISE, AND WORK

Karen R. Hammond,
Richard E. Blackwell

Before the turn of the century, women generally died before the onset of menopause. Many factors contributed to this, the foremost being the risk associated with childbirth or complications of hemorrhage or infections after this event. In general, women limited their consumption of tobacco and alcohol, lived in societies with fewer urban stressors, had unified family support systems, and lived in a world that was completing a transition from an agrarian to an industrial pattern. This chapter examines many of these factors that affect both the mental and physical health in the woman and gives the primary care physician an overview of events that influence all of the disease processes that are discussed in the remainder of this text.

Lifestyle and Longevity

In Africa, 50,000 years ago, the mean age of survival was less than 24 years. By 1100 BC, Romans had a mean death age of approximately 35. Contemporary studies indicate that men and women are living longer, men having a life expectancy of 71.2 years and women 78.2 years (1984 National Center for Health Statistics). It should be noted, however, that survival for both men and women to the age of 100 is not uncommon, and it has been estimated that approximately three million survivors are age 100, and that each additional year of longevity reduces the number by approximately 50%. By age 105 only 37,000 of the 3 million would remain alive and by age 110 there would be only three survivors. However, there have been rare reports of individuals who survived to 150 years of age in the midlands of England.

To a great degree, longevity appears to be a function of several things: genetics, improved public health measures, and the avoidance of deleterious life risks. At least 10 modifiable factors could alter mortality rates. These include smoking, sexual habits, alcohol consumption, consumption of animal products, consumption of vegetables and fruits, social support, obesity, exercise, use of automobile seat belts, and the early detection and diagnosis of disease.

The Seventh Day Adventists advocate a lifestyle that includes the use of clean water, pure air, good nutrition, adequate exercise, rest, regularity of life functions, moderation of most activities, and positive mental attitude (1). A review of 7000 members of this denomination has shown that men can increase their longevity by 11 years and women by 3 years by avoiding smoking, restricting alcohol consumption, eating breakfast daily, by not snacking between meals, achieving 7 hours of sleep per night, maintaining normal body weight, and exercising.

Stroke, cancer, and heart disease are the major causes of death in the United States (2). When the Seventh Day Adventists' lifestyle was reviewed to attempt to correlate association of life habits with the occurrence of these entities, individuals who ate meat were found to be three times more likely to die of heart disease than vegetarians, men 55 years of age were at twice the risk of heart attack if they ate meat than if they avoided it, and meat consumption six or more times a week led to twice the incidence of obesity and had an increased death rate from diabetes. Vegetarian Seventh Day Adventists showed lower mortality rates from a number of cancers when compared to meat consumers and were also less likely to experience heart disease and stroke when compared with a controlled population in California. The abstinence from smoking and alcohol use resulted in a decrease in heart disease, cirrhosis of the liver, stroke, and alcohol- and smoking-related cancers.

These findings seem to recommend an active stress-controlled lifestyle that is free from tobacco and involves little or no use of alcohol, features a diet that is relatively high in whole grains, fruit, and vegetables, low in sugars, with less total fat, refined foods, and salt. This, combined with annual physical examination and the use of automobile seat belts, would seem to be a reasonable way for human beings to increase both the length and quality of their lives although many would argue that such a regimented lifestyle distracts from the enjoyment of living (Box 2.1).

Tobacco Abuse

Tobacco accounts for approximately 400,000 deaths each year among Americans. Deaths occur from cancer of the lung, esophagus, oral cavity, pancreas, kidney, and bladder. In addition, deaths occur from cardiovascular disease, pulmonary disease, problems of pregnancy, and burn trauma. Cigarette smoking remains the chief preventable cause of death and illness in the United States. It is responsible for approximately one sixth of all deaths, and although smoking decreased from 40% in 1965 to 29% in 1987, over 50 million Americans continue to smoke, and the incidence of smoking in women has risen at an alarming rate. Accompanying this is a near parallel increase in the occurrence of lung cancer in women (3).

Historically, the Baroness Dudevant (Chopin's mistress in Paris, 1840), was the first woman to wear trousers and smoke in public. After that time, the image of a woman smoking a cigarette became associated with independence, success, and defiance. Tobacco companies capitalized on this image by creating advertising campaigns depicting the glamour of women smoking cigarettes, thus leading to increasing numbers of female smokers. However, the smoking prevalence in men, as mentioned earlier, has declined by 50% since 1965. The prevalence of smoking in women since that time has only diminished by about one third. If this trend continues, the number of female smokers may equal that of their male counterparts early in the next century. Smoking in women has been called "An equal opportunity killer" (4). Smoking was considered by some to be symbolic of emancipation. It became the center of marketing for the tobacco industry. In 1919, Lorilard published images of women smoking its Murad and Helman brands. Thinness became linked to smoking when Lucky Strike encouraged women to "Reach for a Lucky instead of a sweet," in advertisements published in 1928. In fact, Lucky Strike choose green as an original package color because it was the fashion that year. Finally, Phillip Morris has capitalized on its highly successful Virginia Slim brand and its motto, "We've come a long way, baby."

Not only has the tobacco industry aimed its advertising campaign to women in general, but more alarming, to children, adolescents, and young women (5). There has been an abrupt increase in smoking in girls 11 to 17 years of age, and this coincided with the 1967 launch of specific women's cigarette brands. We have glorified supermodels encouraging young women to smoke and lovable cartoon characters such as Joe Camel sell not only cigarettes but also paraphernalia such as T-shirts and ball caps. If this is not deplorable enough, we have the tobacco industry altering the level of nicotine in cigarettes, and the Natural Tobacco Company, Santa Fe, New Mexico, selling the Natural American Spirit, a "Pure, unadulterated leaf" which is now being sold along side tofu and granola in health food stores.

The economic cost of tobacco use is staggering, and probably exceeds $100 billion. The average medical cost to smokers exceeds those of nonsmokers by more than $6000 in a lifetime. It has been reported that three insurance firms owned by tobacco companies charge smokers nearly double the term life insurance premiums because the death age of the smoker is likely to be considerably lower than that of the nonsmoker. It has

Box 2.1 Longevity Risk Factors

Factor	
Smoking	−
Alcohol consumption	−
Sexual habits	−
Consumption of animal products	−
Obesity	−
Consumption of vegetables and fruits	+
Social support	+
Exercise	+
Seat belts	+
Early detection and diagnosis	+

been estimated by the Office of Technology Assessments that smoking in 1990 cost society $2.59/pack of cigarettes. Cigarette smokers are absent from work 6.5 days more per year, have about six more health care visits per year than nonsmokers; dependents of nonsmokers make about four visits more per year to the health care providers than nonsmokers, highlighting the problem of second-hand smoke. The Office of Technology Assessments estimated that loss of productivity from persons disabled by disease contributed to smoking falls in the $47 billion range. It further estimated that the loss of productivity due to passive smoking was estimated to be about $8.6 billion annually. Fire from cigarette smoking is the leading cause of civilian fire deaths in the United States with an estimated 81,000 men, women, and children being killed or injured by fires started by cigarettes in 1983. The National Fire Protection Association lists 187,100 fires caused by smoking material, which resulted in property damage of $552 million (1991).

The benefits of stopping smoking are immediate and undeniable. Although the social consequences have been dealt with in this chapter, specific medical sequelae are discussed in the rest of this text. By making the transition from claiming that smoking is unhealthy to actually quitting is not easy, and the primary care physician can play a pivotal role in encouraging this beneficial change of lifestyle (6–8). The process of education is made more difficult by the finding that since 1965 the sale in women's brand cigarettes had a marginal increase in the patient population who has attended college. However, there has been a disproportional increase in cigarette smoking in women who do not have a college education. Nevertheless, despite this educational discrepancy, 26% of adult women smoke, and it has been estimated that less than 2% will be able to spontaneously quit, whereas, between 20% and 23% may discontinue smoking with a structured program. The smoking status (abstinence of smoking) during the first 2 weeks of nicotine patch therapy, particularly the second week, showed a high correlation with clinical outcome and is a very powerful predictor of smoking cessation (9–11).

The National Cancer Institute has established an eight-step approach for smoking cessation (Box 2.2).

1. Create a smoke-free office. Post no smoking signs. Remove ashtrays. Display nonsmoking material.
2. Select an office smoking cessation coordinator.
3. Ask every patient about smoking. Do you smoke? How much do you smoke? Have you ever tried to stop smoking? Are you interested in a stop smoking program?
4. Establish assessment of the patient's status by short self-administered questionnaire.
5. Place a visual cue on the patient's chart indicating that smoking is a problem and it needs to be addressed.
6. Advise all smokers to stop. Devise the message to accent the role of smoking in the patient's family history of diseases or current disease processes.
7. Assist the patient in a helping to stop smoking program and provide adequate follow-up, which may include self-help materials or the use of nicotine gum or the nicotine patch.
8. Arrange for follow-up visits. Have an office member call the patient with follow-up as a reinforcement to the decision to stop smoking. Establish a secondary self-help plan should the primary effort fail.

The following materials are available for physicians and patients to assist with smoking cessation:

Quit for Good kit from The National Cancer Institute
Office of Consumer Communications
Building 31, Room 10A24
Bethesda, MD 20891

Clinical Opportunities for Smoking Intervention—A Guide for the Busy Physician

Box 2.2 Steps to Smoking Cessation

1. Smoke-free office
2. Establish plan and appoint coordinator
3. Ask patients about smoking
4. Use questionnaire
5. Use visual cue on chart
6. Advise patient to stop
7. Establish cessation plan for patient
8. Follow-up visit

National Heart and Lung Institute
Smoking Education Program
4733 Bethesda Avenue, Suite 530
Bethesda, MD 20814-4820

Smoking in Women, a patient education pamphlet
ACOG Resource Center
Telephone 202-638-6677

How to Quit Cigarettes
American Cancer Society
3340 Peachtree Road NE
Atlanta, GA 30329-4251

Two aids can be used in smoking cessation programs—nicotine gum and the nicotine patch (12,13). In these methods, patients discontinue smoking immediately before the onset of therapy. The nicotine polacrilex gum is supplied in 2-mg doses (one piece), is used every 20 to 30 minutes PRN when one desires a cigarette, with a maximum of 30 pieces in a 24-hour period. One gum is equal to about two cigarettes and the general range of therapy is from 3 to 6 months. Ninety-six pieces of gum are supplied per box, which sells for $25 to $30. Gum should be chewed slowly so that absorption will occur through the buccal mucosa and it is not to be swallowed. Fluid should not be consumed with gum chewing because pH maintenance is necessary for release of the nicotine. The frequency of usage should be tapered over about 3 months. Potential side effects include mouth irritation, heartburn, nausea, sore throat, and palpitations. The gum should not be used in patients who have recently experienced myocardial infarction or are experiencing angina or any life-threatening arrhythmia.

The nicotine transdermal system is supplied in 21-mg patches used daily for 4 to 6 weeks; 14 mg each day is used if the patient has any cardiovascular disease, weighs less than 100 pounds, or smokes less than one half package of cigarettes per day. It is tapered to 14 mg a day over 2 to 4 weeks and it ends with 7 mg daily for 2 to 4 weeks. A box of 12 patches costs $50 to $60, and a box of thirty $100 to $120. Side effects include skin irritation, burning at the application site, edema, headache, vertigo, insomnia, somnolence, abnormal dreams, myalgias, arthralgias, abdominal pain, nausea, dyspepsia, diarrhea, nervousness, anxiety, irritability, and depression. The patch is contraindicated in patients with psoriasis, dermatitis, peptic ulcer disease, renal impairment, hypertension, hyperthyroidism, pheochromocytoma, or insulin-dependent diabetes.

Substance Abuse

Although alcoholism is discussed in Chapter 37, substance abuse in general is a common finding in the primary care practice (14). Ten percent of the American population has a problem with alcoholism and 25% of all families are affected by a member with this disorder. Ten to 20% of patients in a typical practice have a problem with drinking alcohol and some 14% of patients are affected by some type of substance abuse. One to three million Americans use cocaine, 500,000 are addicted to heroin, two million have used heroin occasionally, and 10 million smoke marijuana. Thirty percent of individuals abuse alcohol plus other drugs. Drug use and alcoholism are associated with an increased incidence of crime, trauma, domestic violence, child abuse, and the acquisition of sexually transmitted diseases. Human immunodeficiency virus (HIV) prevalence rates range from 61% of addicts in New York City to 5% in Seattle, Washington. Almost all substance abuse is associated with behavioral abnormalities, diminished motivation, psychomotor retardation, irregular sleep patterns, sexual dysfunction, and depression. Patients should be asked about alcohol intake, particularly in case of marital dysfunction, memory loss, unexplained trauma or accidents, chronic gastric complaints, hypertension, disorders of sleep, psychological disorders, or hypertension (15,16). The Cage questionnaire has a sensitivity of 75% to 90% and a specificity of 85% to 95% for making the diagnosis of alcoholism when two or more questions are answered affirmatively (Box 2.3). If substance

Box 2.3 Cage Questionnaire

1. Have you ever tried to cut down on your drinking?
2. Have you ever been annoyed by criticism about your drinking?
3. Have you ever felt guilty about your drinking?
4. Have you ever had a morning eye opener?

abuse is identified, the patient should be referred to specialty counseling, Alcoholics Anonymous, or Al-Anon. These chapters are usually listed in the local telephone directory.

Drugs such as cocaine are associated with seizure, myocardial infarction, sudden death, cerebral hemorrhage, arrhythmia, and pulmonary edema. Intravenous drugs such as heroin are associated with the transmission of HIV infections, hepatitis, bacterial endocarditis, and pulmonary edema. In addition, addictive substances have a marked effect on reproduction. For instance, smoking adversely affects menstrual cyclicity, oocyte production, and tubal function and in case control studies, women who smoke have an increased risk of infertility and anomalies of the cervical mucus. The active ingredient of marijuana, Δ^9-tetrahydrocannabinol (THC), causes alteration of a variety of endocrine functions and is used by 20% of young adults five or more times per month. THC has been demonstrated to be a potent inhibitor of gonadotropin-releasing hormone and has a deleterious effect on reproduction in both men and women.

However, moderate alcohol consumption has been touted by some as promoting health. Cited are the low rates of cardiac disease in persons in alcohol-consuming countries such as France. This seems to be associated with the intake of red wines specifically, limited to one to two glasses per day. The explanation as to this risk reduction may be the association of alcohol consumption and high-density lipoprotein cholesterol concentrations. Atherosclerosis is associated with hemostatic function, and a cohort study of 8 of the 7526 nurses who drank moderately demonstrated a lower risk of both coronary heart disease and ischemic stroke, but an increased risk of hemorrhagic stroke (17). The intake of moderate amounts of alcohol with evening meals appears to have a beneficial effect on fibrinolytic factors. This is associated with a lower risk of coronary heart disease, a strong increase in plasminogen activator inhibitor activity, and tissue plasminogen activator antigen levels that return to normal within 24 hours. Tissue plasminogen activator activity has been shown to be initially strongly reduced up to 9 hours after moderate alcohol consumption with dinner, but is higher than normal in the morning (18). Both the French and Dutch experiences perhaps speak to the differences in alcohol consumption in Europe and the United States. Whereas Europeans frequently drink wine or beer in family settings and at meals, Americans frequently drink in bars or at parties with an emphasis on achieving an euphoric state rather than as a food enhancer. Europeans might limit their quantity of alcohol intake to one to two drinks; Americans might typically consume considerably more, giving rise to gastrointestinal, neurologic, cardiovascular, and orthopedic dysfunction.

Exercise

Approximately 40% of Americans are sedentary, and only 20% exercise at a level that has any positive effect on their cardiovascular system (19). Exercise is associated with increasing socioeconomic class with the most popular sports being walking, swimming, calisthenics, cycling, and jogging. The positive advantages to exercise would be reduction in coronary heart disease, hypertension, and obesity; decreased non–insulin-dependent diabetes mellitus; reduced anxiety and depression; and prevention of osteoporosis in the postmenopausal woman. On the negative side, soft tissue injuries may occur, with tendinitis and stress fractures leading the list. The primary care physician should encourage the patient to undertake aerobic weight-bearing exercises such as walking two to four times a week for about 30 minutes each session. However, cardiovascular fitness requires 70% to 85% of the maximal heart rate (220 minus age). It is advised that exercise begin at a 50% to 60% maximum heart rate and increase every 2 weeks until a target heart rate is achieved. Exercise should be done in moderation with avoidance of tachycardia, vomiting, nausea, lightheadedness, claudication, confusion, dyspnea, or angina. Exercise should be avoided after large meals or after the consumption of alcohol, and should be avoided in very hot or cold weather. Exercise is associated with a decreased risk of cardiovascular disease and total mortality in men. A dose-related relationship exists with beginning exercise later in life. Exercise appears to be beneficial to individuals over 65 years of age and to be an additive in preventing osteoporosis in women on replacement estrogen therapy (20,21). There also may be some decrease in the incidence of colorectal cancer in individuals who exercise regularly.

The following activities are associated with the calculated calorie consumption. The estimates are based on values calculated per calories burned per minute for a 150-pound person as provided by the President's Council on Physical Fitness and Sports: cycling 174, reading 84, swimming 288, walking 198, golf 324, rollerblading 384, ice skating 384, cross country skiing 690, dancing 210, and basketball 450.

Diet, Nutrition, and Weight Control

The ideal body weight varies with sex, age, and culture. Most tables such as those derived from the U.S. Department of Agriculture or the Metropolitan Life Insurance Company are based on population means. As an example, a woman 5′2″, between the ages of 19 and 34 weighs 104 to 137, whereas over age 35 she weighs 115 to 148. However, at 5′6″, at 19 to 34 years of age, the range increases from 118 to 155, and greater than age 35, from 130 to 167. It has frequently been pointed out that weight does not correlate with fitness. An equation developed by Kidchi and Ghaw allows that for an individual of medium build, add 100 lb for the first 5 feet, 5 lb for each additional inch (22). For a small build subtract 10% and for a large build add 10%. However, one cannot be too preoccupied with absolute body weight because weight does not equate to fitness; however, caloric needs vary with exercises. For instance, basal calories might be estimated by taking the ideal body weight in pounds × 10 + 30% for a sedentary individual, + 50% for one who exercises moderately, + 100% for an individual engaged in strenuous exercise. Caloric intake should be distributed approximately 50% to carbohydrates, 30% to fat, 20% to protein and high fiber, and divided into approximately three meals a day. The Department of Agriculture has developed the food pyramid indicating that the vast majority of our calorie intake should be in the form of grains, cereals, and fiber, followed by vegetables and fruits, with a smaller amount consisting of seafoods and poultry with minimum consumption of eggs, dairy products, and red meat, plus sweets. An Italian version has been proposed that includes the consumption of a significant amount of pasta products at the bottom of the chain and adding two glasses of wine per day. Regardless of the form of diet followed, it certainly appears that excessive dietary fat intake is linked to an increased risk of obesity, coronary artery disease, and certain cancers as demonstrated by the Centers for Disease Control and Prevention in the Third National Health and Nutrition Examination survey (23). The NAHNES 1 study further found that a high body mass index (weight divided by height^2) was a predictor of long-term mortality and disability in older women and that this risk persisted until old age (24). Although some of the increase in body weight appears to be acquired by unavoidable means, the Cardia study suggests that women experience moderate but adverse increases in body weight and fat distribution after the first pregnancy, and that these changes are persistent (25). Total body weight in men increases until about age 55, then declines, whereas in women, the increase tends to extend into their sixties before a decline occurs. The so-called middle-age spread appears to be a product of reduced physical activity and increased food intake and it is not found in less affluent societies.

Sexuality and Contraception

Perhaps at no other time in recent history has the issue of sexuality been brought to the public forefront than with the onset of the epidemic of acquired immunodeficiency syndrome (AIDS). Although both the subject of AIDS and other sexually transmitted diseases (STDs) will be dealt with in other chapters, a discussion of safe sex practice seems appropriate for a discussion of life-styles. Risk factors that seem to predispose individuals to the acquisition of STDs include a history of having some other STD, intercourse with more than one partner in the last year, intercourse with more than one partner in the last month, intercourse with a risky partner (one who has had multiple sexual partners or is bisexual), unprotected vaginal intercourse within the last month, unprotected anal intercourse within the last month, sex after the intake of alcohol or drugs within the last month, and sex in exchange for either drugs or money in the last month (26,27). Combined with these sexual practices is the appalling figure that of the six million pregnancies that occurred in 1987, more than half were unintended and 23% of these occurred among women between 15 and 19 years of age (28). By age 18, 140 pregnancies per 1000 occured in U.S. women, whereas that figure was approximately 50 in England. Also, at age 18, nearly 65 abortions per 1000 were performed as opposed to an average of 25 in most western societies. In 1992, teenage pregnancies cost the U.S. taxpayers approximately $25.1 billion, being distributed among AIDS, the families with dependent children, food stamps, and Medicaid.

Both the increased transmission rate of STDs and the rising occurrence of unwanted pregnancies and prevalence of abortion speak to not only the need for improvement in our educational system but the development and availability of contraception. Many picturesque methods of contraception, such as the use of pessaries made out of a mixture of honey and crocodile dung, the swallowing of 14 live tadpoles, or the eating of uteri of mules, have been described. Methods that are highly efficacious in controlling not only STDs including AIDS, but controlling fertility, have existed since the mid-1800s. The condom, for instance, is used by 17% of individuals using contraception and has a 97% efficacy rate if used in conjunction with contraceptive gels or creams; nonoxynol-9, one of the principle detergent components of contraceptive jellies and creams is efficacious against retarding AIDS infections (29). Barrier methods such as diaphragms, the cervical cap, and vaginal sponges, all use contraceptive gels or creams; therefore, they theoretically should convey similar protection. Likewise, the newly developed Hers condom should offer both anti-STD and contraceptive protection.

Although barrier contraceptives reduce at least in part the risk of STDs, they do not convey to the user the beneficial effects of oral contraceptive agents. Oral contraceptive agents not only inhibit ovulation by suppression of the luteinizing hormone/follicle-stimulating hormone surge, they alter cervical mucus to inhibit the transport of pathogens, interfere with ovum transport, and suppress the endometrium. It is estimated that as many as 50,000 hospital admissions a year are prevented because of the noncontraceptive benefits of oral contraceptive agents (30). Not only do they regulate menstrual dysfunction, they are used to treat endometriosis, reduce excess androgen production, and prevent pregnancy. The risk of hospitalization from pelvic inflammatory disease is reduced by 50% by birth control pill use, and they appear to retard gonococcal infections from progressing. Data from the Oxford Family Planning Study demonstrate that there is a 30% decrease in the incidence of uterine fibroids in oral contraceptive users, the risk of developing both endometrial and ovarian cancer is decreased by one half by oral contraceptive use, and these effects seem to persist long after the pill is discontinued (31). It has been estimated that about 17,000 cases of ovarian cancer are averted every year by the use of oral contraceptive agents in the United States alone (32). Current users of oral contraceptives have a 50% reduction in the incidence of chronic breast cysts and an 85% decrease in the incidence of breast fibroadenomas. Further, the Food and Drug Administration has given approval for the use of oral contraceptive agents through the perimenopause and women can now enjoy pill use if they are nonsmokers up to age 55.

Work Environment

Many factors involving the work environment affect health and longevity. Hearing loss is a subtle loss that is often times not dealt with (33). Hearing loss affects 4% of people under the age of 45 and 29% of people over age 65. It is estimated that 28 million Americans have hearing impairment and 2 million of these are profoundly deaf. Such economic loss of hearing may represent $1.3 billion per year. Acoustic trauma (exposure to noise) produces sensory neural damage. There is individual susceptibility to noise trauma with damage occurring far below the threshold approved by the Occupational Safety and Health Administration. In addition, there may be a synergy with commonly administered medications such as aspirin. Serial audiometry is the only way to detect noise trauma. A clinically useful guideline would be that if noise is significantly loud to be painful or cause tinnitus or a temporary sensation of blocking of the ear, it is likely that prolonged exposure will cause permanent damage. Such exposure is not restricted to the work place because auditory fatigue and permanent hearing deficits can occur from exposure to rock and roll music (34).

Support Network

Since the turn of the century, our nation has become more urban and more ethnic, and many changes have occurred in terms of our values and traditions. We reproduce less frequently and terminate those pregnancies more readily; many of our best educated citizens delay childbearing until they are in the perimenopause. We are less educated as a people, less skilled as a work force, and are becoming increasingly older. We will be forced to survive with decreased senses, slower cognitive function, altered metabolism, and decreased mobility. These constraints will be applied on our aging population in an environment that ever increasingly worships youth. Our aging citizens have had less income and economic and political influence than their younger counterparts and are often forced to live in an environment that is not adapted to accommodate their limitations. They often have inadequate nutrition and live in social isolation.

Along with the aging of the population has occurred an astronomical rise in single-parent families, and for some ethnic groups the abolition of the family unit. Generations are separated not only by geography, but economics, education, and philosophy, and this trend is likely to worsen with business globalization. The end of the social contract between worker and corporation will lead to a more highly mobile and transient work force and further lessen the sense of community and social commitment. Therefore, the primary care physicians will face an older population primarily made up of women, some of whom will be wealthy but many poor, isolated from their children and families. Therefore, many of the stabilizing and health-promoting factors of life such as marriage, family, stable employment, community, friends, and regularity of life pattern may be denied the patients of tomorrow. Fortunately, women's social networking skills are vastly superior to men's and perhaps with the help of those of us who care for them, social change combined with medical progress and an awareness of physiologic well-being, can be brought about that will hopefully improve the quality of life experienced during aging.

REFERENCES

1. Register U. The Seventh-Day Adventist diet and life-style and the risk of major degenerative diseases. In: Morin RJ, ed. Frontiers in longevity research. Springfield, IL: Charles C. Thomas, 1985:74.

2. McGinnis MJ, Foege WH. Actual causes of death in the United States. JAMA 1993;270:2207–2212.

3. MacKenzie TD, Bartecchi CE, Schrier RW. The human costs of tobacco use. N Engl J Med 1994;330: 975–980.

4. Kaufman NJ. Smoking and young women: the physician's role in stopping an equal opportunity killer. JAMA 1994;271:629–630.

5. Pierce JP, Lee L, Gilpin EA. Smoking initiation by adolescent girls, 1994 through 1988. JAMA 1994;271:608–611.

6. Pearse WH. Smoking cessation. Primary Care Update for Ob/Gyns 1994;1:9–11.

7. Benowitz NL. Pharmacologic aspects of cigarette smoking and nicotine addition. N Engl J Med 1988; 319:1318–1330.

8. Greene HL, Goldberg RJ, Ockene JK. Cigarette smoking: the physician's role in cessation and maintenance. J Gen Intern Med 1988;3:75–87.

9. Kottke TE, Battista RN, DeFriese GH, Brekke ML. Attributes of successful smoking cessation interventions in medical practice: a meta-analysis of 39 controlled trials. JAMA 1988;259:2883–2889.

10. Lam W, Sacks HS, Sze PC, Chalmers TC. Meta-analysis of randomized controlled trials of nicotine chewing gum. Lancet 1987;2:27–30.

11. Kenford SL, Fiore MC, Jorenby DE, Smith SS, Wetter D, Baker TB. Predicting smoking cessation: who will quit with and without the nicotine patch. JAMA 1994;271:589–594.

12. Hurt RD, Dale LC, Fredrickson PA, et al. Nicotine patch therapy for smoking cessation combined with physician advice and nurse follow-up. JAMA 1994;271:595–600.

13. Fiore MC, Smith SS, Jorenby DE, Baker TB. The effectiveness of the nicotine patch for smoking cessation. JAMA 1994;271:1940–1948.

14. Coulehan JL, Zettler SM, Black M, McCelland M, Schulberg HC. Recognition of alcoholism and substance abuse in primary care patients. Arch Intern Med 1987;147:349–352.

15. Babor TF, Ritson EB, Hodgson RJ. Alcohol-related problems in the primary health care setting: a review of early intervention strategies. Br J Addict 1986;81:23–46.

16. Cleary PD, Miller M, Bush BT, Warburg M, Delbanco TL, Aronson MD. Prevalence and recognition of alcohol abuse in a primary care population. Am J Med 1988;85:466–470.

17. Stampfer MJ, Colditz GA, Willett WC, Speizer FE, Hennekens CH. A prospective study of moderate alcohol consumption and the risk of coronary heart disease and stroke in women. N Engl J Med 1988;319:267–273.

18. Hendriks HF, Veenstra J, Velthuis-te Wierik EJM, Schaafsma G, Kluft C. Effect of moderate dose of alcohol with evening meal on fibrinolytic factors. Br Med J 1994;308:1003–1006.

19. Harris SS, Caspersen CJ, DeFriese GH, Estes EH. Physical activity counseling for healthy adults as a primary preventive intervention in the clinical setting: report for the U.S. Preventive Services Task Force. JAMA 1989;261:3590–3598.

20. Lowenthal DT, Pollock ML, Graves JE, Scarpace NT. Exercise and aging: prescription for wellness. South Med J 1994(suppl 1):87.

21. Pahor M, Guralnik JM, Salive ME, Chrischilles EA, Brown SL, Wallace RB. Physical activity and risk of severe gastrointestinal hemorrhage in older persons. JAMA 1994;272:595–599.

22. Kitabchi AE, Ghawji M. Diabetes in the nonpregnant patient. Primary Care Update for Ob/Gyns 1994;1:86–94.

23. Launer LJ, Harris T, Rumpel C, Madans J. Body mass index, weight change, and risk of mobility disability in middle-aged and older women. JAMA 1994;271:1093–1098.

24. Nutrition during pregnancy and lactation: an implementation guide. Washington, DC: National Academy of Sciences, 1992.

25. Smith DE, Lewis CE, Caveny MS, Perkins LL, Burke GL, Bild DE. Longitudinal changes in adiposity associated with pregnancy. JAMA 1994;271:1747–1751.

26. Ickovics JR, Morrill AC, Beren SE, Walsh U, Rodin J. Limited effects of HIV counseling and testing for women. JAMA 1994;272:443–448.

27. Lemp GF, Hirozawa AM, Givertz D, et al. Seroprevalence of HIV and risk behaviors among young homosexual and bisexual men. JAMA 1994;272:449–454.

28. Burnhill MS. Adolescent pregnancy rates in the US. Contemporary Ob/Gyn 1994;39:26–30.

29. Rietmeier CAM, Krebs JW, Feorino PM, et al. Condoms as physical and chemical barriers against human immunodeficiency virus. JAMA 1988;259: 1851–1853.

30. Kost K, Forrest JD, Harlap S. Comparing the health risks and benefits of contraceptive choices. Family Plan Perspect 1991;23:54–61.

31. Vessey MP, McPherson K, Johnson B. Mortality among women participating in the Oxford/Family Planning Association Contraceptive Study. Lancet 1977;2:731–733.

32. Rosenberg L, Shapiro S, Slone D, et al. Epithelial ovarian cancer and combination oral contraceptives. JAMA 1982;247:3210–3212.

33. Nadol JR Jr. Hearing loss. N Engl J Med 1993;329:1092–1102.

34. Dey FL. Auditory fatigue and predicted permanent hearing defects from rock-and-roll music. N Engl J Med 1970;282:467–470.

SECTION TWO

VASCULAR DISEASES

CHAPTER 3

HYPERTENSION

Herman A. Taylor, Jr.

Hypertension is one of the most common medical problems encountered by physicians in any specialty. As many as 63 million Americans are affected; among those, 46% are undiagnosed and 67% are untreated (1,2). Given the well-known risks of high blood pressure and the well-established benefit of treatment in preventing these sequelae, it is incumbent on the primary physician to identify cases and initiate appropriate therapy. Except for the forms of hypertension unique to women (i.e., oral contraceptive pill-induced hypertension or pregnancy-related hypertension), the clinical approach to hypertension does not differ between men and women. This chapter reviews the diagnosis and management of hypertension in women, exclusive of hypertension during pregnancy (i.e., pregnancy-induced hypertension or preeclampsia).

Diagnosis

Definition

The diagnosis of hypertension is important because elevated blood pressure places patients at excess risk for morbidity, disability, and death from cardiovascular disease. *Hypertension* can be operationally defined as any blood pressure reading exceeding 140 mm Hg systolic *or* 90 mm Hg diastolic. Higher readings carry greater risk; lower readings imply lesser but still increased risk down to levels as low as 130/80 mm Hg (1). The cut point of 140/90 mm Hg is practical and logical because risk increases substantially above this level and lowering blood pressure by medical intervention to levels much below 140/90 mm Hg does not consistently improve patient outcome (3,4).

Blood pressure is now characterized as either normal, "high normal," or as one of four *stages* of hypertension (Table 3.1). These classifications are important guides to follow-up, prognosis, and treatment. The actual degree of elevation in blood pressure is a critical determinant of the patient's absolute risk for cardiovascular disease. Patients in the "high normal" category are at high risk to develop frank hypertension and therefore should be followed more closely than normotensive persons. Increasingly aggressive follow-up and therapeutic strategies should be undertaken for increasingly severe stages of high blood pressure (Table 3.2).

Detection

Accurate measurement of blood pressure is the essential first step in managing hypertension. A falsely elevated reading may unnecessarily commit the patient to years of pharmacologic therapy (exposing the individual needlessly to side effects and toxicity) and label the patient as having a disorder associated with substantial medical risk (with its attendant psychological and insurance implications). Indeed, as many as 30% of people currently treated for hypertension may not need prescriptions. On the other hand, a reading that is falsely low may allow a patient with a significant health problem to go untreated and thereby face great risk for early mortality or significant morbidity. Millions fall into this latter category.

The proper measurement of blood pressure should proceed as follows:

1. Blood pressures should be measured in both arms while the patient is seated and relaxed. The arm should be supported and the bladder of the cuff should be placed approximately at heart level. The patient should not have smoked or had any caffein-

Table 3.1 Classification of Blood Pressure for Adults

Category	Systolic (mmHg)	Diastolic (mmHg)
Normal	<130	<85
High normal	130–139	85–89
Hypertension*		
Stage 1 (Mild)	140–159	90–99
Stage 2 (Moderate)	160–179	100–109
Stage 3 (Severe)	180–209	110–119
Stage 4 (Very severe)	≥210	≥120

* Not taking antihypertensive drugs and not acutely ill. When systolic and diastolic pressures fall into different categories, the higher category should be selected to classify the individual's blood pressure status.
Source: The fifth report of the Joint National Committee on Detection, Evaluation and Treatment of High Blood Pressure (JNC V). National Institutes of Health. Publication No. 93-1088, 1993.

ated beverage within 30 minutes before the measurement.

2. After resting for approximately 5 minutes, the measurement should be taken. The cuff size is critical: the width of the cuff should be approximately two thirds the length of the upper arm; the length of the cuff should encircle at least 80% of the arm (falsely elevated readings will be obtained from cuffs that are either too narrow or too short).
3. The sphygmomanometer should be the standard mercury, calibrated electronic, or aneroid manometer. Recent (within the last 6 months) calibration is especially important for the aneroid type to ensure accuracy.
4. Two or more readings separated by approximately 2 minutes should be obtained and averaged. If readings vary more than by 5 mm Hg, additional readings should be obtained.
5. Initially, pressure should be taken in both arms. The higher value should be used if the pressures differ.
6. If arm pressure is elevated, take pressure in one leg, particularly in young patients (less than 30 years old).

Table 3.2 Recommendations for Follow-up Based on Initial Set of Blood Pressure Measurements for Adults Age 18 and Older

INITIAL SCREENING BLOOD PRESSURE (MM HG)*		
Systolic	Diastolic	Follow-up Recommended[a]
<130	<85	Recheck in 2 yr
130–139	85–89	Recheck in 1 yr[b]
140–159	90–99	Confirm within 2 mo
160–179	100–109	Evaluate or refer to source of care within 1 mo
180–209	110–119	Evaluate or refer to source of care within 1 week
≥210	≥210	Evaluate or refer to source of care immediately

* If the systolic and diastolic categories are different, follow recommendation for the shorter time follow-up (e.g., 160/85 mm Hg should be evaluated or referred to source of care within 1 mo).
[a] The scheduling of follow-up should be modified by reliable information about past blood pressure measurements, other cardiovascular risk factors, or target organ disease.
[b] Consider providing advice about life-style modifications.
Source: The fifth report of the Joint National Committee on Detection, Evaluation and Treatment of High Blood Pressure (JNC V). National Institutes of Health. Publication No. 93-1088, 1993.

7. The diastolic pressure recorded should be the number corresponding to Korotkoff phase V (i.e., disappearance of sound).

This meticulous approach will allow accurate determination of the patient's blood pressure. The diagnosis of hypertension should ideally be made on the basis of three sets of readings obtained over the course of several weeks (1,5); a single elevated reading usually is not justification for treatment. However, if systolic blood pressure is greater than or equal to 210 mm Hg and/or diastolic blood pressure is 120 mm Hg or greater (stage IV), or if there is evidence of significant target organ damage, immediate treatment may be necessary.

Clinical Evaluation

History

The proper clinical approach to the hypertensive patient demands a carefully obtained history. Several major issues deserve particular attention during the patient interview.

Duration

If known, the age of onset of hypertension gives the clinician a perspective on the duration of illness and the likelihood of target organ damage; this will help focus the subsequent physical examination and laboratory assessment. The history of past therapy for hypertension should also be elicited, noting therapeutic successes or failures and side effects of medications. These data will help guide selection of treatment options for the individual patient.

Target Organ Damage

Target organ damage is damage or compromise of any of the major organ systems affected by hypertension: cardiovascular, cerebrovascular, or renal. Along with the actual degree of blood pressure elevation and the presence of significant coexisting risk factors, the degree of target organ damage is a key parameter in determining the level of aggressiveness with which the clinician should approach the patient. Pertinent questions should focus on symptoms of cardiovascular dysfunction (e.g., chest pain, dyspnea on exertion, claudication), cerebrovascular compromise (e.g., transient weakness or history of stroke), and renal insufficiency (e.g., known past elevation in creatinine or abnormal urinalysis). Data on this aspect of the patient's clinical status will also be obtained in the physical examination and the laboratory assessment (see below).

Cardiovascular Disease Risk Factors

Hypertension is a major risk factor for cardiovascular disease such as myocardial infarction and cerebrovascular accident. Unfortunately, it is often accompanied by the presence of other significant risk factors that greatly amplify risk for the individual patient. Table 3.3 gives a partial list of additional cardiovascular risk factors; the patient should be specifically asked about each of these conditions. The coexistence of hypertension along with one or more of these problems adds a greater urgency to prompt work-up of hypertension and establishment of an appropriate plan of therapy.

Table 3.3 Risk Factors for Cardiovascular Disease

Nonmodifiable	Modifiable
Age	Hypertension
Sex	Cigarette smoking
Family history	Hypercholesterolemia
	Low high-density lipoprotein cholesterol levels
	Diabetes mellitus
	Obesity
	Sedentary life-styles
	Cerebrovascular or occlusive peripheral vascular disease

Exogenous Factors

Ingestion of estrogen (oral contraceptive pills) is a leading cause of curable hypertension in the United States; it is a major cause of hypertension for the population that consults obstetrics-gynecology specialists. (*Note*: With rare exceptions, conjugated or natural estrogens used in postmenopausal or postsurgical estrogen replacement therapy do not have a similar effect on blood pressure; in fact, such treatment may lower blood pressure as well as improve overall cardiovascular risk [6–8]. However, due to exceptional cases of blood pressure elevation, blood pressures of women on estrogen replacement therapy should be monitored more frequently after treatment is begun [9].) Hypertension may be caused by other prescription drugs as well, including steroids, tricyclic antidepressants and monoamine oxidase inhibitors, erythropoietin, cylcosporine, and a variety of sympathomimetic agents. Popular over-the-counter agents such as nasal decongestant and other cold remedies, nonsteroidal anti-inflammatory drugs (NSAIDs), and appetite suppressants can also elevate blood pressure. These nonprescription agents must be asked about specifically during the interview of a patient with elevated blood pressure (Box 3.1).

Inquiry should also be made regarding other exogenous factors such as diet (e.g., high salt intake may

Box 3.1 Agents That May *Raise* Blood Pressure

Oral contraceptive pills
Adrenal steroids
Monoamine oxidase inhibitors
Tricyclic antidepressants
Cyclosporine
Erythropoietin
Sympathomimetics*
Excessive dietary sodium
Excessive alcohol consumption

*Includes certain nasal decongestants, cold remedies, appetite suppressants, and nonsteroidal anti-inflammatory drugs.

raise blood pressure), habits (excess alcohol consumption is associated with elevations in blood pressure), and extreme environmental stressors (e.g., domestic strife, work conditions). Such factors may contribute to high blood pressure and may frustrate attempts to lower blood pressure with therapy.

Physical Examination

The principal aims of the physical examination of the hypertensive patient are to 1) measure the actual degree of blood pressure elevation, 2) uncover evidence of target organ dysfunction, 3) determine overall cardiovascular risk, and 4) determine whether secondary (possibly curable) hypertension exists. We have reviewed the details of accurate measurement of blood pressure above; this section focuses on other aspects of the physical examination.

General Appearance

Height, weight, and distribution of body fat should be noted as a part of the initial evaluation of the hypertensive patient. The presence of significant obesity, especially truncal or abdominal obesity (waist-to-hip ratio greater than 0.85 in women) is a significant risk factor for cardiovascular disease. Because obesity is often found in association with diabetes and dyslipidemia, the obese hypertensive patient may be at extremely high risk for coronary artery disease (10).

Funduscopic Examination

Examination of the optic fundi is traditionally done as part of the initial assessment of the hypertensive patient (Box 3.2). The utility of this examination has been questioned by some, however. One study found that the arteriosclerotic changes (i.e., diffuse narrowing, arteriovenous nicking, sliver wiring, etc) are more closely related to age than blood pressure. This suggests that class I and II retinopathy is a relatively nonspecific finding (11). However, class III and IV retinopathy (exudates, hemorrhages, and papilledema), which may be collectively called the "neuroretinopathy" of hypertension, has been found to correlate strongly with severe (stage IV) hypertension (12). Given the importance of establishing severity of hypertension to guide therapy and prognostication, it is strongly recommended that the funduscopic examination be performed during the initial assessment and yearly thereafter (13).

The room should be darkened for this portion of the examination. If this does not produce sufficient pupillary dilatation, a short-acting mydriatic (e.g., tropicamide 1%) can be used to achieve satisfactory dilatation in the vast majority of patients within 15 minutes after application (14).

Box 3.2 Summary: The Physical Examination

- Accurate blood pressure measurement
- General appearance (especially height and weight, distribution of body fat, skin lesions, alertness, muscle strength)
- Funduscopic examination
- Neck (thyroid, bruits, distended neck veins)
- Heart (especially size, rhythms, gallops, murmurs)
- Abdomen (bruits, enlarged kidneys, masses, abnormal aortic pulsations)
- Extremities (pulses, bruits, edema)

Source: The fifth report of the Joint National Committee on Detection, Evaluation and Treatment of High Blood Pressure (JNC V). National Institutes of Health. Publication No. 93-1088, 1993.

Neck

The thyroid should be assessed for enlargement. Enlargement of the thyroid especially in association with a wide pulse pressure (defined as systolic blood pressure minus diastolic blood pressure) may indicate hyperthyroidism and a potentially curable form of hypertension. Carotid bruits may be present and may provide the first clue of the existence of significant cerebrovascular disease. Distended neck veins may indicate heart failure.

Chest

Auscultation of the lungs may reveal rales reflecting left ventricular dysfunction (either diastolic dysfunction due to impaired compliance of the hypertensive heart of systolic dysfunction due to poor contractile function). Pulmonary rales may be detected in patients with long-standing hypertension or an acute hypertensive emergency.

The heart of most hypertensive patients will appear normal on physical examination; however, this does not diminish the importance of this part of the clinical evaluation. The initial examination is important not only for establishing a useful baseline for further comparison, but also for detecting cardiac dysfunction that may have developed before the patient presented for evaluation. Mild increases in heart rate and a hyperkinetic apex beat are changes often seen early in the hypertensive state. Left ventricular hypertrophy or left ventricular dilatation may be detected by palpation of the anterior chest wall. Auscultation often reveals an S_4 gallop. This early sign of decreased compliance is more sensitive and develops earlier than palpable left ventricular hypertrophy (13). Development of an S_3 gallop is ominous in the context of hypertensive heart disease and may indicate significant left ventricular systolic (contractile) dysfunction.

Abdomen

The abdominal examination is crucial in the initial evaluation of the hypertensive patient because it can yield information on the extent of vascular damage caused by hypertension and may reveal evidence of secondary (potentially curable) hypertension. Careful palpation for organomegaly or masses may reveal an intrarenal cause of hypertension (e.g., polycystic kidneys). A midline pulsatile mass may represent an abdominal aortic aneurysm; auscultation may reveal bruits in the abdomen, flanks, or back. Finding bruits in these locations can provide an important sign of renal vascular disease. (Diastolic bruits are more specific for disease than systolic sounds, especially among the elderly.)

Extremities

Examination of the extremities should include a careful assessment of the peripheral vasculature. The examiner should palpate the femoral and brachial pulsations simultaneously; any significant delay or diminution in the femoral pulse may indicate coarctation of the aorta. This part of the examination is especially important in young patients, who are more likely to have undetected aortic coarctation. The lower extremities should be assessed for the presence of dependent edema.

Neurologic

Deficits in alertness or orientation should be noted. Gross asymmetry of facial or eye movements, gait, strength, or posture should also be recorded. Central nervous system (CNS) compromise in the hypertensive patient may be reflected in dementia (of varying severity) as well as more obvious motor or sensory deficits.

Laboratory Evaluation

Routine Testing

The aim of the laboratory examination is to complement and further objectify findings of the history and physical examination. Estimates of overall cardiovascular risk, quantification of target organ damage, and screening for secondary hypertension are facilitated by laboratory testing. The results of an appropriate set of initial screening tests will guide subsequent work-up and therapy.

Routine evaluation may be limited to a relatively small number of tests (Box 3.3). A complete blood count (CBC) is essential; a low hematocrit may be a sign of renal impairment or hemoglobinopathy. Patients with low white blood cell counts are poor candidates for certain therapeutic agents (e.g., angiotensin-converting enzymes [ACE] inhibitors), which may produce more profound leukopenia. Urinalysis can detect abnormal urinary sediment (consistent with renal parenchymal disease), glycosuria (suggestive of diabetes mellitus), and alkaline urine (frequently seen in patients with primary hyperaldosteronism).

Box 3.3 Routine Laboratory Evaluation

Complete blood count

Chest x-ray

Electrocardiogram

Urinalysis

Blood glucose (fasting preferable)

Cholesterol (total and high-density lipoprotein)

Uric acid

Serum NA^+, K^+, creatinine, blood urea nitrogen

Serum calcium

A growing body of literature has documented the frequent association of hypertension, diabetes mellitus, dyslipidemia, and obesity (the syndrome of insulin resistance, also known as the "deadly quartet" or "syndrome X") (15). Given the high risk of such patients, the hypertensive patient must have blood sugar (preferably fasting) and cholesterol (preferably total cholesterol and high-density lipoprotein [HDL]) determinations as part of the initial screening.

Several serum electrolytes are important to measure. Serum potassium is particularly important for excluding certain secondary forms of hypertension such as hyperaldosteronism and exogenous corticorsteriod excess. Further, periodic testing of potassium will be required if diuretic therapy is initiated for the individual patient. Serum calcium may likewise exclude secondary forms of hypertension because hyperparathyroidism and hypervitaminosis D are both associated with hypertension and are characterized by high calcium levels. Uric acid levels provide an important baseline indicator of a patient's risk for developing hyperuricemia or gout on diuretic therapy. Serum creatinine and blood urea nitrogen (BUN) are essential tests for assessing renal function.

The chest x-ray can be helpful in assessing cardiac size (although left ventricular enlargement may only result in a change in the shape of the cardiac silhouette). The chest x-ray may also reveal evidence of coarctation of the aorta. The electrocardiogram (ECG) is important in evaluating the extent of cardiac involvement. Although ECG criteria for left ventricular hypertrophy are insensitive, they are highly specific and carry profound prognostic implications. Persons with left ventricular hypertrophy have a substantially higher risk of sustaining major cardiovascular events (e.g., myocardial infarction, sudden death, cerebrovascular accidents) than do hypertensive patients without evidence of left ventricular hypertrophy (15–17).

Other Tests

Many other specialized tests are available for evaluation of hypertension. These additional studies are aimed primarily at detecting secondary forms of hypertension and are not routinely necessary. (Less than 5% of all hypertensive individuals have a secondary form of the disease.) If the results of the evaluation as described above suggest the need for further testing, referral to a cardiovascular disease, renal, or endocrine specialist may be necessary. In general, the younger the patient and the higher the blood pressure, the more aggressive should be the search for secondary causes. However, the new appearance of hypertension or the sudden loss of blood pressure control in elderly patients may also represent secondary hypertension. Table 3.4 lists some available tests for specific diagnostic possibilities.

Table 3.4 Testing for Secondary Hypertension

Renovascular disease	Captopril/enalapril renal scan Renal arteriogram
Primary aldosteronism	Serum K^+ Urine K^+ Plasma renin-aldosterone (ratio)
Renal parenchymal disease	Serum creatinine Urinalysis Renal ultrasound
Pheochromocytoma	Urinary catechols Plasma catechols Clonidine suppression test
Cushing's syndrome	Morning plasma cortisol after 1 mg dexamethasone at bedtime
Coarctation	Chest x-ray Aortograms

Treatment of Hypertension

Effective treatment of high blood pressure has been repeatedly shown to substantially reduce morbidity and mortality among hypertensive patients (19–21). The dramatic trend of declining stroke and coronary disease over the last three decades can be attributed in large part to more effective blood pressure control achieved among American patients (Fig 3.1). The treatment of hypertension, when discovered, is of paramount importance. Effective antihypertensive therapy is one of the most productive interventions made by modern physicians.

Lifestyle Modifications

Effective therapy for hypertension should *always* include lifestyle modifications as part of the regimen (Box 3.4). Even if these interventions do not completely normalize blood pressure, they can significantly lower it and thereby reduce the number and dosage of drugs needed for blood pressure control.

Box 3.4 Lifestyle Modifications for Cardiovascular Disease Risk Reduction

- Lose weight (if overweight)
- Limit alcohol intake to 1 oz ethanol per day or less (i.e., 24 oz beer, 8 oz wine, or 2 oz 100-proof whiskey)
- Exercise (aerobic) regularly
- Reduce sodium intake to <100 mmol/day (<2.3 gm sodium or <6 gm sodium chloride)
- Maintain adequate dietary potassium, calcium, and magnesium intake
- For overall cardiovascular health: reduce fat and cholesterol intake stop smoking

Source: The fifth report of the Joint National Committee on Detection, Evaluation and Treatment of High Blood Pressure (JNC V). National Institutes of Health. Publication No. 93-1088, 1993.

Weight Loss and Exercise

In overweight patients with mild (stage I and stage II) hypertension, an effort should be made to lower blood pressure with weight loss and other nonpharmacologic interventions for 3 to 6 months before beginning drug therapy. If drugs are needed, weight loss should still be a priority in the overall management of overweight hypertensive patients. Loss of as little as 10 lb substantially reduces blood pressure and provides significant, measurable reduction in cardiac mass among individuals with left ventricular hypertrophy (22). Increased physical activity is an important adjunct to any weight loss program, enhancing the effects of caloric restriction as well as helping reduce recidivism. Additionally, regular aerobic exercise (e.g., brisk walk-

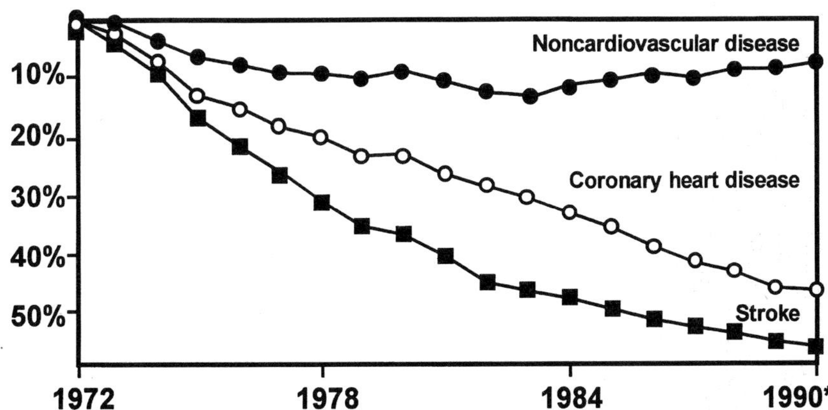

Fig 3.1 Percent decline in age-adjusted mortality rates since 1972. *Provisional data for 1990. *(Source: NCHS data calculated by NHLBI. Adapted from the fifth report of the Joint National Committee on Detection, Evaluation and Treatment of High Blood Pressure (JNC V). National Institutes of Health. Publication No. 93-1088, 1993.)*

ing 30 to 45 minutes three to five times per week) itself can reduce systolic blood pressure in hypertensive patients by as much as 10 mm Hg (23).

Alcohol

Alcohol consumption must be limited to the equivalent of 1 oz or less of ethanol per day; high levels can raise the blood pressure and interfere with effective medical therapy for hypertension. It is important to note, however, that if high chronic alcohol ingestion is stopped abruptly, the subsequent alcohol withdrawal will produce transient hypertension. The pressor effect of the withdrawal state will reverse a few days after consumption is reduced (24).

Restriction of Dietary Sodium

Some patients with stage I hypertension can achieve normal blood pressures with sodium restriction alone. Other patients with more advanced or severe hypertension may be able to take fewer medicines at lower dosage if an effective moderation of salt intake is achievable with appropriate counseling (25).

Other Dietary Factors

Dietary calcium and potassium may be important in protecting against the development of high blood pressure (26,27). Patients should be urged to include ample potassium- and calcium-rich foods in their diets because low potassium and calcium levels have been associated with increases in blood pressure (28). In the case of hypokalemia associated with diuretic therapy, pharmacologic potassium supplementation may be necessary, or an alternative antihypertensive medication can be chosen (e.g., a potassium-sparing diuretic or a nondiuretic agent, see below). Currently, calcium supplementation beyond the recommended daily allowances 20–30 mmol (800–1200 mg) is not suggested as a part of antihypertension therapy because clinical trials of this intervention have yielded equivocal results.

Drug Therapy for Hypertension

Although many patients have encouraging blood pressure responses to life-style modification, most will ultimately require some pharmacologic therapy as well. Among mild hypertensive patients (stage I and stage II), the use of drugs should only be considered after a 3 to 6 month trial of nondrug interventions such as those outlined above. However, among hypertensive patients with more severe blood pressure elevation (stage III and stage IV) or those with evidence of significant target organ damage or a high cardiovascular risk profile, medical therapy should be initiated sooner (see Table 3.2).

The "stepped care" approach to hypertension treatment introduced in the 1970s by the Joint National Committee (JNC) has been supplanted recently. An increasingly wide selection of agents of proven efficacy has allowed a less rigid approach to therapy for hypertension. The modern approach emphasizes the importance of life-style modification and the use of β blockers and diuretics – the two drug classes proven to reduce morbidity and mortality among hypertensive patients.

Currently available data suggest that the pharmacologic approach to hypertension in women should not differ from strategies used in men. Therefore, the following recommendations are equally applicable for hypertensive patients of both genders unless otherwise indicated. Table 3.5 summarizes salient features of the most commonly used antihypertensive agents.

Diuretics

The most frequently prescribed medications for hypertension treatment are the diuretics. Although their popularity has waned slightly in recent years, over 65% of all clinicians still prescribe diuretics as their first-line therapy for high blood pressure. Three subcategories are available in this class: thiazide diuretics, loop diuretics, and potassium-sparing diuretics. Although they act at different sites in the nephron, all diuretics reduce blood pressure by a similar series of hemodynamic effects. First, a significant reduction in extracellular volume and plasma volume occurs after therapy is begun. Lower plasma volume in turn reduces cardiac output. However, with prolonged diuretic therapy, total peripheral resistance decreases and cardiac output returns to pretreatment levels. The clinical result is a significant and sustained reduction in systemic blood pressure (29).

The salutary effects of diuretics can be accompanied by significant side effects, particularly at high doses of the drugs. In some cases, the side effects will require withdrawal of this form of therapy. Metabolic derangements such as hypokalemia, hyperuricemia,

Table 3.5 Antihypertensive Agents

Type of Drug	Trade Name	Usual Dosage Range (Total mg/day)*	Frequency (Once/day unless Otherwise noted)	Mechanisms	Comments
Initial Antihypertensive Agents					
Diuretics					■ For thiazide and loop diuretics, lower doses and dietary counseling should be used to avoid metabolic changes.
Thiazides and related agents				Decreased plasma volume and decreased extracellular fluid volume, and decreased cardiac output initially, followed by decreased total peripheral resistance with normalization of cardiac output. Chronic effects include a slight decrease in extracellular fluid volume.	■ More effective antihypertensive than loop diuretics except in patients with serum creatinine ≥221 μmol/L (2.5 mg/dL). ■ Hydrochlorothiazide or chlorthalidone is generally preferred; were used in most clinical trials.
Bendroflumethiazide	Naturetin	2.5–5			
Benzthiazide	Exna, Aquatag	12.5–50			
Chlorothiazide	Diuril	125–500	twice		
Chlorthalidone	Hygroton	12.5–50			
Cyclothiazide	Anhydron	1.0–2			
Hydrochlorothiazide	[Esidrix, Oretic] [Hydro Diuril]	12.5–50			
Hydroflumethiazide	Saluron	12.5–50			
Indapamide	Lozol	2.5–5			
Methyclothiazide	Enduron	2.5–5			
Metolazone	Zaroxolyn	0.5–5			
Polythiazide	Renese	1.0–4			
Quinethazone	Hydromox	25.0–100			
Trichlormethiazide	Naqua, Metahydrin	1.0–4			
Loop diuretics				See thiazides.	■ Higher doses of loop diuretics may be needed for patients with renal impairment or congestive heart failure. ■ Ethacrynic acid is the only alternative for patients with allergy to thiazide and sulfur-containing diuretics.
Bumetanide	Bumex	0.5–5	twice		
Ethacrynic acid	Edecrin	25.0–100	twice		
Furosemide	Lasix	20.0–320	twice		
Potassium sparing diuretics					■ Weak diuretics. ■ Used mainly in combination with other diuretics to avoid or reverse hypokalemia from other diuretics. ■ Avoid when serum creatinine ≥221 μmol/L (2.5 mg/dL).
Amiloride	Midamor	5–10	once or twice	Increased potassium reabsorption.	
Spironolactone	Aldactone	25–100	twice or thrice	Aldosterone antagonist.	
Triamterene	Dyrenium	50–150	once or twice		

Table 3.5 *Continued*

Type of Drug	Trade Name	Usual Dosage Range (Total mg/day)*	Frequency (Once/day unless Otherwise noted)	Mechanisms	Comments
Potassium sparing diuretics (Continued)					
					▪ May cause hyperkalemia, and this may be exaggerated when combined with ACE inhibitors or potassium supplements.
Combination diuretics					
Amiloride and Hydrochlorothiazide	Moduretic	5/50		See above under component agents.	
Spironolactone and Hydrochlorothiazide	Aldactazide	25/25 50/50	twice (tablets) twice (capsules)		
Triamterene and Hydrochlorothiazide	Dyazide Maxzide	75/50	twice		
Potassium supplement					
	K-Lyte/CL Potassium Gluconate Elixir Slow-K Klorvess	20/25 mEq	once		
Adrenergic inhibitors					
β Blockers					
Atenolol Betaxolol Bisoprolol Metoprolol Metoprolol (extended release)	Tenormin Kerlone Zebeta Lopressor Toprol XL	25–100[a] 5–40 5–20 50–200 50–200	once or twice	Decreased cardiac output and increased total peripheral resistance. Decreased plasma renin activity. Atenolol, betaxolol, bisoprolol, and metoprolol are cardioselective.	▪ Selective agents will also inhibit β_2-receptors in higher doses, e.g., all may aggravate asthma.
Nadolol Propranolol Propranolol (long acting)	Corgard Inderal Inderal LA	20–240[a] 40–240 60–240	twice		
Timolol	Blocadren	20–40	twice		
β Blockers with intrinsic sympathomimetic activity					
Acebutolol	Sectral	200–1200[a]	twice	Acebutolol is cardio-selective.	▪ No clear advantage for agents with intrinsic sympathomimetic activity except in those with bradycardia who must receive a β blocker; they produce fewer or no metabolic side effects.
Carteolol	Cartrol	2.5–10[a]			
Penbutolol	Leratol	20–80[a]			
Pindolol	Visken	10–60[a]	twice		

Table 3.5 *Continued*

Type of Drug	Trade Name	Usual Dosage Range (Total mg/day)*	Frequency (Once/day unless Otherwise noted)	Mechanisms	Comments
α-β Blocker					
Labetalol	Normodyne Trandate	200–1200	twice	Same as β blockers plus α_1-blockade.	▪ Possibly more effective in African Americans than other β blockers. ▪ May cause postural effects, and titration should be based on standing blood pressure.
α_1-Receptor blockers					
Doxazosin	Cardura	1.0–16		Block postsynaptic α_1-receptors and cause vasodilation.	▪ All may cause postural effects, and titration should be based on standing blood pressure.
Prazosin	Minipress	1.0–20	twice or thrice		
Terazosin	Hytrin	1.0–20			
ACE inhibitors					
Benazepril	Lotensin	10.0–40[a]	once or twice	Block formation of angiotensin II, promoting vasodilation and decreased aldosterone. Also increased bradykinin and vasodilatory prostaglandins.	▪ Diuretic doses should be reduced or discontinued before starting ACE inhibitors whenever possible to prevent excessive hypotension.
Captopril	Capoten	12.5–150[a]	twice		
Enalapril	Vasotec	2.5–40[a]	once or twice		
Fosinopril	Monopril	10.0–40	once or twice		
Lisinopril	Prinivil, Zestril	5.0–40[a]	once or twice		
Quinapril	Accupril	5.0–80[a]	once or twice		▪ Reduce dose of those drugs marked "[a]" in patients with serum creatinine ≥221 μmol/L (2.5 mg/dL). ▪ May cause hyperkalemia in patients with renal impairment or in those receiving potassium-sparing agents. ▪ Can cause acute renal failure in patients with severe bilateral renal artery stenosis or severe stenosis in an artery to a solitary kidney.
Ramipril	Altace	1.25–20[a]	once or twice		
Calcium antagonists					
Diltiazem	Cardizem	90–360	thrice	Block the inward movement of calcium ion across cell membranes and cause smooth muscle relaxation.	▪ These agents also block the slow channels in the heart and may reduce sinus rate and produce heart block.
Diltiazem (sustained release)	Cardizem SR	120–360	twice		
Diltiazem (extended released)	Dilacor XR Cardizem CD	180–360			
Verapamil	Isoptin, Calan Verelan	80–480	twice		

Table 3.5 *Continued*

Type of Drug	Trade Name	Usual Dosage Range (Total mg/day)*	Frequency (Once/day unless Otherwise noted)	Mechanisms	Comments
Calcium antagonists (Continued)					
Verapamil (long acting)	Isoptin SR Calan SR Verelan capsules	120–480	once or twice		
Dihydropyridines					■ Dihydropyridines are more potent peripheral vasodilators than diltiazem and verapamil and may cause more dizziness, headache, flushing, peripheral edema, and tachycardia.
Amlodipine	Norvasc	2.5–10			
Felodipine	Plendil	5–20			
Isradipine	DynaCirc	2.5–10	twice		
Nicardipine	Cardene	60–120	thrice		
Nifedipine	Adalat Procardia	30–120	thrice		
Nifedipine (GITS)	Adalat CC Procardia XL	30–90			
Supplemental Antihypertensive Agents					
Centrally acting α_2-agonists					
Clonidine	Catapres	0.1–1.2	twice	Stimulate central α_2-receptors that inhibit efferent sympathetic activity.	■ Clonidine patch is replaced once a week. ■ None of these agents should be withdrawn abruptly. Avoid in nonadherent patients.
Clonidine TTS (patch)[b]	(Catapres patch)	0.1–0.3	once *weekly*		
Guanabenz	Wytensin	4–64	twice		
Guanfacine	Tenex	1–3			
Methyldopa	Aldomet	250–2000	twice		
Peripheral acting adrenergic antagonists					
Guanadrel	Hylorel	10–75	twice	Inhibits catecholamine release from neuronal storage sites.	■ May cause serious orthostatic and exercise-induced hypotension.
Guanethidine	Ismelin	10–100			
Rauwolfia alkaloids					
Rauwolfia root		50–200		Depletion of tissue stores of catecholamines.	
Reserpine	Serapsil, Sandril	0.05[c]–0.25			
Direct vasodilators					
Hydralazine	Apresoline	50–300	twice to four times	Direct smooth muscle vasodilation (primarily arteriolar).	■ Hydralazine is subject to phenotypically determined metabolism (acetylation). ■ For both agents: should treat concomitantly with a diuretic and a β blocker due to fluid retention and reflex tachycardia.
Minoxidil	Loniten	2.5–80	once or twice		

in all patients, life-style modifications should also be advised.

* The lower dose indicated is the preferred initial dose, and the higher dose is the maximum daily dose. Most agents require 2–4 weeks for complete efficacy, and more frequent dosage adjustments are not advised except for severe hypertension. The dosage range may differ slightly from the recommended dosage in the *Physicians' Desk Reference* or package insert.

[a] Indicates drugs that are excreted by the kidney and require dosage reduction in the presence of renal impairment (serum creatinine ≥221 μmol/L [2.5 mg/dL]).

[b] Weekly patch is 1, 2, 3 equivalent to 0.1–0.3 mg/day.

[c] 0.1 mg dose may be given every other day to achieve this dosage.

Sources: The fifth report of the Joint National Committee on Detection, Evaluation and Treatment of High Blood Pressure (JNC V). National Institutes of Health. Publication No. 93-1088, 1993. Scientific American Medicine. New York. 1993.

glucose intolerance (or frank hyperglycemia), hypercholesterolemia, and hypomagnesemia are frequently noted. Many of these biochemical abnormalities are easily managed by using low doses of the drug or with supplementation therapy; however, patients with preexisting metabolic abnormalities (e.g., non–insulin-dependent diabetes mellitus, hyperuricemia/gout, dyslipidemias) may be unsuitable candidates for diuretic therapy. In any event, use of diuretics will require initial and periodic monitoring of serum electrolytes (sodium, potassium, magnesium, calcium), BUN, creatinine, blood glucose, cholesterol, and uric acid.

Maintaining normal potassium levels is especially important. Low serum potassium has been associated with an increase in ventricular ectopy in several studies (30). Also, in the large Multiple Risk Factor Intervention Trial (MRFIT), diuretic therapy in patients with mild hypertension and baseline ECG abnormalities was associated with increased mortality when compared with untreated mild hypertensive patients. Hypokalemia-mediated arrhythmia has been one presumed mechanism of mortality in this mildly hypertensive group (31).

Potassium supplementation during diuretic therapy can be achieved through dietary means (including the use of potassium chloride-based salt substitutes), through pharmacologic supplementation, or with the use of potassium-sparing diuretics. The potassium-sparing diuretics in most common use are combination agents that consist of a thiazide plus a potassium-sparing agent (e.g., amiloride, spironolactone, or triamterene). This category of diuretics may cause hyperkalemia in certain patient subgroups: diabetic patients, those with renal insufficiency, and patients using ACE inhibitor agents. Triamterene-containing drugs may precipitate nephrolithiasis; therefore, these agents should not be chosen for patients with a history of kidney stones. Spironolactone, an aldosterone antagonist, may cause mastodynia or amenorrhea.

The loop diuretics are indicated in hypertensive patients with impaired renal function (creatinine level greater than 2.5 mg/dL) or congestive heart failure. These agents are more costly and often require more frequent dosing than most thiazides but frequently find use in patients with advanced hypertension and target organ damage.

Several commonly used drugs interact in clinically important ways with diuretics. The most notable drug interaction is with the NSAIDs (1). NSAIDs, including over-the-counter aspirin, naproxyn sodium, and ibuprofen, may blunt the effect of diuretic therapy by inhibiting prostaglandin synthesis (32). The lipid-lowering agents cholestyramine and colestipol decrease diuretic absorption. Patients on lithium therapy can experience marked elevations in serum lithium levels after starting diuretics, predisposing them to toxicity. These interactions underscore the importance of a carefully acquired history regarding the patient's use of prescription and nonprescription drugs.

Diuretics as Second-line Therapy

Diuretics can be effective in combination with other antihypertensive agents. Lowering the blood pressure with nondiuretic agents will typically produce a reflex increase in fluid retention and expansion of the intravascular volume, limiting the ultimate effectiveness of the drug. Addition of a diuretic to the original agent will produce a contraction of plasma volume and often a significant lowering of systemic blood pressure beyond levels that were achieved with the original monotherapy. (This effect is least profound when a diuretic is added to a calcium channel blocker because the calcium blockers have an intrinsic mild natriuretic effect).

Use in Special Populations

Diuretics have been reported to be particularly effective among black and elderly hypertensive patients (21,33). Hypertension in these two groups often is of the "low-renin," "volume-dependent" type, and, therefore, is often responsive to agents that contract the plasma volume. Caution must be exercised, however, in using simple demographics to guide therapeutic choices. The specifics of individual patient history, laboratory data, and physical examination may, in fact, make the choice of a diuretic unwise (e.g., in the case of a black patient with non–insulin-dependent diabetes mellitus or the elderly woman with gout).

Summary

Diuretic therapy is an inexpensive and effective mode of hypertension treatment. Low doses (e.g., 12.5 mg or less of thiazide or equivalent) are recommended for initial therapy; doses should not exceed the equivalent of 25 mg thiazide daily. Patients with preexisting metabolic abnormalities (e.g., diabetes mellitus, hypercholesterolemia, gout, hypokalemia) may suffer an exacerbation of the baseline abnormality. If diuretic therapy is chosen for such patients, periodic blood sampling is essential to avoid significant metabolic derangements. Potassium supplementation or choice of a potassium-sparing agent may be necessary to prevent significant and potentially dangerous hypokalemia.

Sympatholytic Agents

β-Adrenergic Blockers

The β blockers are the second most frequently prescribed drugs for hypertension in the United States. Overall, a 15% reduction in a patient's blood pressure can be expected from usual doses of β-blocking drugs. Furthermore, 40% to 60% of all patients with mild to severe hypertension respond to monotherapy with one of the β blockers. The antihypertensive action is seen within a few days of initiating therapy; maximal effects are apparent after 1 to 7 weeks. These drugs appear to be especially efficacious in young patients; they also appear to be relatively more effective as monotherapy for white patients than for black patients (33,34).

The antihypertensive effect of all β blockers appears to be mediated through reduction of cardiac output and impairment of renal renin release. However, ancillary pharmacologic properties—principally "β selectivity," lipid solubility, and intrinsic sympathomimetic activity—may help determine the choice of agent from within the β-blocker class. "β Selective" agents have a very high affinity for β_1 receptors. Selective blockade of these receptors will lower heart rate, decrease contractility and cardiac output, and suppress release of renin from the juxtaglomerular cells of the kidney, without producing bronchospasm or constriction of peripheral arteries (i.e., β_2 receptor-mediated side effects are avoided). It is important to note, however, that the cardioselectivity of these agents may be lost if prescribed doses are too high (e.g., more than 200 mg atenolol or more than 150–200 mg metoprolol every day).

Nonselective agents block β_1 and β_2 receptors. These agents have been extensively studied and proven to reduce morbidity and mortality among hypertensive patients. They are highly useful; however, clinically important side effects (e.g., bradycardia, tiredness, decreased exercise ability, cool extremities) and often seen. These potentially troublesome side effects can be minimized with lower-range dosing. Furthermore, nonselective agents often have attractive features. Propranolol is inexpensive and highly effective; with careful patient selection, significant side effects are infrequent. Nadolol is a nonselective agent that offers once-a-day dosing and low lipid solubility, which may reduce the CNS side effects sometimes seen in patients on β-blocker therapy (see below).

Lipid solubility largely determines the drug's duration of action and propensity to cross the blood–brain barrier. Highly lipid-soluble agents (e.g., propranolol, metoprolol, timolol) are extensively metabolized (up to 70%) on first pass of portal blood through the liver. Also, these agents are more likely to cause CNS side effects (e.g., depression, hallucinations, vivid dreams) because they readily cross the blood–brain barrier. In contrast, the relatively nonlipid-soluble agents tend to have longer duration of action and are less likely to cause CNS side effects. Nadolol and atenolol are examples of this latter group.

The subclass of β blockers with intrinsic sympathomimetic activity have a partial agonist effect on β_1 and β_2 receptors in addition to β-blocking characteristics. Patients taking this type of β blocker (e.g., pindolol, acebutolol) have fewer complaints of fatigue (because cardiac output is preserved) and fewer CNS side effects. There is a less marked rise in triglycerides or fall in HDL levels.

Summary

β-Blocking agents have been a cornerstone of hypertension therapy for over two decades. They are effective in most hypertensive patients requiring pharmacologic therapy. Caution should be exercised in using these drugs in some clinical settings. Asthmatic patients generally should not receive β blockers, although low-dose cardioselective agents may be used if no viable clinical option exist. Peripheral vascular symptoms (e.g., intermittent claudication) may be aggravated by the nonselective agents or with high doses of the β_1-selective drugs; the intrinsic sympathomimetic activity subclass may be useful in this clinical context. Insulin-dependent diabetic patients at risk for hypoglycemic episodes should not, in most cases, receive β-blocker drugs. The response to hypoglycemic episodes is highly dependent on β-adrenergic stimulation of glucose synthesis and secretion, especially in insulin-dependent diabetic patients who cannot secrete glucagon. β-Blocker therapy may cause more intense and more prolonged hypoglycemic episodes. Further, classic warning symptoms of hypoglycemia (palpitations, tremulousness, hunger) are diminished. (Diaphoresis still occurs; diabetic patients taking β blockers should be informed of the importance of this symptom in regard to their blood glucose levels.)

Patients with certain concomitant medical conditions may be especially good candidates for β-blocker therapy. Patients with histories of palpitations or tachycardia in association with hypertension, patients with a history of coronary artery disease (especially after a heart attack), and patients with migraine headaches and glaucoma may all gain special benefit from β-blocker therapy for their hypertension.

α-Adrenergic Blockers

The α-adrenergic receptor blocking drugs terazosin, prazosin, and doxazosin and highly useful agents with generally favorable side effect profiles. They act by blocking α_1 receptors on vascular smooth muscle. The resulting vasodilation causes a fall in total peripheral resistance and subsequently a lower blood pressure. The α blockers are useful first-line agents; they also work well in combination with a number of other drugs for two-drug therapy. Diuretics, ACE inhibitors, and calcium channel blockers all combine well with α blockers.

The α blockers have a generally favorable side effect profile. Unlike many antihypertensive agents that have a negative impact on metabolic risk factors for cardiovascular disease, the α blockers may actually improve HDL and total cholesterol levels (36).

The most troublesome side effects from these agents is the "first-dose hypotension," particularly in patients already taking a diuretic. In volume-contracted patients, administration of an α-adrenergic blocker can result in significant vasodilatation, which predisposes the patient to severe orthostatic hypertension. To lessen this risk, the initial dose should be low (1 mg), diuretics should be stopped 24 to 48 hours before the first dose of the α blocker (5). Prescribing the first dose to be taken at bedtime can also lessen the risk of symptomatic postural hypotension; however, some authors prefer giving the first dose on a day when the patient can remain inactive all day. Thereafter, the regimen can be adjusted to a level that effectively maintains a lower blood pressure.

Central Adrenergic Inhibiting Drugs

These antihypertensive drugs act directly in the CNS as agonists of α_2 receptors. Stimulation of the central α_2 receptors results in a generalized reduction of sympathetic outflow from the CNS. Methyldopa is frequently used by obstetric-gynecology specialists because of its known safety during pregnancy. Aside from this clinical context, however, aldomet has become a rarely used agent because of the availability of new agents with fewer side effects. Aldomet has been associated with hepatic toxicity ranging from minor elevations of hepatic transaminases to hepatic necrosis, positive Coombs test (and rarely hemolytic anemia), and other toxicities.

Clonidine has a similar mode of action to methyldopa but substantially fewer known side effects. It is effective in small doses; a cutaneous route of administration (patch) is available. Clonidine has a much shorter duration of action than methyldopa. Its principle side effects are dry mouth and sedation. The clonidine "rebound" (marked elevation of blood pressure caused by stopping the drug) is widely discussed; however, if the total daily dosage is low, dramatic rises in blood pressure do not occur frequently if doses are missed. An interesting feature of clonidine is its ability to facilitate smoking cessation, probably by blunting the exaggerated sympathetic tone seen in patients withdrawing from nicotine. It, therefore, may have a unique role in smoking hypertensive patients who have decided to quit (37).

Guanabenz is a third central α_2 agonist. Uniquely, it has been shown to lower serum cholesterol levels by approximately 10%. Another theoretical advantage to its use is that it is not associated with fluid retention, which characterizes many other agents that cause vasodilatation. It may, therefore, be particularly useful in patients with hypercholesterolemia because it not only lowers total serum cholesterol, but it is also effective without administration of diuretics (which have the effect of raising serum cholesterol).

Guanfacine hydrochloride is a newer central α agonist. Once daily dosing is a convenience. It does have typical central α-agent side effects although reportedly these are less severe than seen with the older agents.

Peripheral Sympatholytic Agents

Reserpine has been used for the management of hypertension for many years. Although infrequently prescribed today, it remains an effective and inexpensive agent. Significant side effects have led to declining usage; however, low doses (0.05–0.10 mg) in combination with small dose amounts of a thiazide diuretic have resulted in a reduction of the amount of sedation, nasal congestion, and depression seen.

Guanethidine is rarely used. An unacceptable side effect profile (including postural hypertension, diarrhea, and retrograde ejaculation in men) make it an agent of last resort (see Table 3.5). Guanadrel is similar in its pharmacology to guanethidine, but a shorter duration of action reduces the severity and frequency of side effects.

Calcium Channel Blockers

The calcium channel blockers are agents that currently enjoy wide popularity among practicing clinicians. Dosing convenience and minimal toxicity make these drugs highly desirable in managing hypertension, a disease that may require the patient to take pills for 10 to 40 years. Calcium channel blockers are effective in all age groups, but they may be particularly effective in the elderly as monotherapy. Also, they are effective in "low renin" hypertension, a form of hypertension frequently seen in the African American population.

The vasoconstriction that produces hypertension is dependent, at least in part, on the influx of calcium into vascular smooth muscle. The calcium channel blockers act by interfering with calcium ion influx into vascular smooth muscle and producing a marked vasodilatation with subsequent reduction in systemic blood pressure. Two forms of calcium channel blockers exist. The *dihydropyridine* types (nifedipine is the prototype) are highly effective. However, the older short-acting formulations frequently produce symptoms of tachycardia (due to reflux sympathetic stimulation) headache, flushing, and postural hypertension. The newer long-acting formulations have overcome virtually all such side effects. The *non-dihydropyridines* in wide clinical usage are verapamil and diltiazem. Due to their prominent cardiac effects, these drugs should be used with caution in patients with known conduction abnormalities (e.g., heart block) or impaired left ventricular function (e.g., peripartum cardiomyopathy).

Because of their particular efficacy in "low renin" hypertension, calcium channel blockers are touted as being particularly beneficial in black and elderly hypertensive patients, two groups with a high prevalence of salt-sensitive "low renin" hypertension. However, younger patients and non-black patients respond to this class of drugs as well. In patients requiring a second agent, calcium channel blockers work well in combination with ACE inhibitors, β blockers, and clonidine, although other combinations are also acceptable. Unlike other vasodilators, calcium channel blockers do not produce a reflex expansion of intravascular volume and do not require diuretics. In fact, they have been shown to produce a significant saliuresis during early therapy (i.e., 6 to 10 gm loss of salt). Dietary salt restriction therefore may not be required in patients taking calcium channel blockers; some studies even suggest that salt reduction decreases the efficacy of these drugs (38).

Side effects vary significantly among the different drugs in this class. All of these agents can cause nausea, presumably due to their action on smooth muscle function. Verapamil is also a common cause of constipation, limiting its usage in the elderly. Notably, the ankle edema seen with the dihydropyridines and diltiazem can be pronounced and may lead to discontinuation of the drug. Metabolic side effects do not occur with calcium channel blockers.

Angiotensin-Converting Enzyme Inhibitors

The ACE inhibitors are a relatively new class of drugs in wide clinical use. The name of this class describes its chief mode of action—these drugs all inhibit the elaboration of angiotensin II, a potent natural vasoconstrictor, by blocking the final enzymatic step in its production. These are highly effective, well-tolerated agents with favorable metabolic and hemodynamic profiles. These features make them suitable for single or combination therapy for a wide variety of patients. Furthermore, management of conditions that frequently accompany hypertension (e.g., diabetes mellitus, heart failure) may be facilitated by the use of ACE inhibitors.

Captopril and enalapril have been the most widely prescribed agents in this class. Captopril has a rapid onset of action (peak action 30 to 60 minutes) and a short half life 2 hours); standard dosing is 25–50 mg two or three times a day. Enalapril (in doses beginning at 5 mg/day) is a prodrug that requires hepatic conversion to enaliprat, its active form. Peaks in concentration are achieved 4 hours after dosing; half-life allows daily or twice daily dosing schedules. Lisinopril, in starting doses of 5–10 mg/day can be given once daily. Several newer ACE inhibitors (benazipril, fosinopril, quinapril, and ramipril) have identical mechanisms of action as the older drugs although they may differ in duration of action, tissue affinities, and root of administration.

Efficacy of ACE Inhibitors

Overall, 35% to 70% of hypertensive patients respond well to ACE inhibitors as monotherapy (39). This compares favorably to response rates seen with β blockers, calcium channel blockers, and diuretics. Blacks have been found to respond less well as a group to monotherapy with ACE inhibitors, possibly due to the high prevalence of the "low renin" form of hypertension in this ethnic group. The response in any *individual* black patient maybe quite satisfactory, however. Addition of a small dose of diuretic (e.g., 6.25–12.5 mg of thiazide) may greatly enhance the blood pressure lowering produced by the ACE inhibitor. A low dose of each agent will also minimize dose-related adverse effects of the diuretic. Combination tablets (ACE inhibitor plus a thiazide diuretic) are popular and widely available.

Elderly patients frequently have low renin levels as well (renin secretion declines with age). However, these patients tend to respond well to ACE inhibitor therapy (40). ACE inhibitors are generally well tolerated when used properly. The most notable patient complaint is the frequent occurrence of a persistent dry cough. Some clinicians suggest that this complication is more frequently seen among women. Hyperkalemia is a risk in patients with renal insufficiency or those who are given potassium supplementation. Significantly, renal insufficiency or failure can be induced with ACE inhibitor therapy if there is bilateral renal artery stenosis (or a solitary kidney with a stenosed renal artery). In the absence of bilateral artery stenosis, the development of significant ACE inhibitor-induced renal insufficiency is exceedingly rare unless there are diffused intrarenal stenotic lesions. Finally, patients with significant volume contraction (e.g., because of diuretic therapy) may develop azotemia after initiation of ACE inhibitors. Stopping the diuretic for a few days before initiating ACE inhibitor therapy can avoid this problem.

The ACE inhibitors show no adverse affects on lipids, glucose metabolism, uric acid levels, or electrolytes (in euvolemic patients with normal renal function). They are especially appropriate in patients with diabetic nephropathy (delaying the progression of renal dysfunction) (41), congestive heart failure/cardiomyopathy (improving survival in these patients) (42) coronary artery disease (improved survival after myocardial infarction) (43), and other clinical contexts. These agents will likely continue to grow in popularity among primary care physicians, renal and cardiovascular subspecialists alike.

General Guidelines for Treatment

Treatment Strategy

Figure 3.2 summarizes an approach to therapy for hypertension as endorsed by JNC V. Life-style modification is always the first step. When pharmacologic therapy is deemed necessary, several treatment options are available. For stage I and II hypertension patients (the large majority of hypertensives) monotherapy (i.e., treatment with a single drug) should be attempted initially. The drug should be selected with the patient's overall health status in mind (e.g., β blockers should be avoided in asthmatics but may be preferred monotherapy for patients with migraine headaches, etc). The drug should be started at low dosages and continued for 2 to 4 weeks before increasing the dose; this should minimize side effects. If the blood pressure is still elevated 1 to 3 months after initiating therapy, the clinician should either increase the dose, change medications, or add a second or third agent. Dosages should be raised in reasonable increments toward maximum levels at approximately 2-week intervals. Alternatively, a second drug can be added. Two agents with different mechanisms of action often act synergistically and allow very low dosages of both agents to be used effectively. This minimizes the risk of dose-dependent side effects of either drug (e.g., combining ACE inhibitor and low-dose diuretic is much more effective than incremental increases in the dose of the ACE inhibitor alone).

Half of all hypertensive patients will be controlled with monotherapy; another significant portion will

Treatment Algorithm

Lifestyle Modifications:
- Weight reduction
- Moderation of alcohol intake
- Regular physical activity
- Reduction of sodium intake
- Smoking cessation

↓ Inadequate Response* ↓

Continue Lifestyle Modifications

Initial Pharmacological Selection:

- Diuretics or beta-blockers are preferred because a reduction in morbidity and mortality had been demonstrated
- ACE inhibitors, calcium antagonists, alpha$_1$-receptor blockers, and the alpha-beta blocker have not been tested nor shown to reduce morbidity and mortality

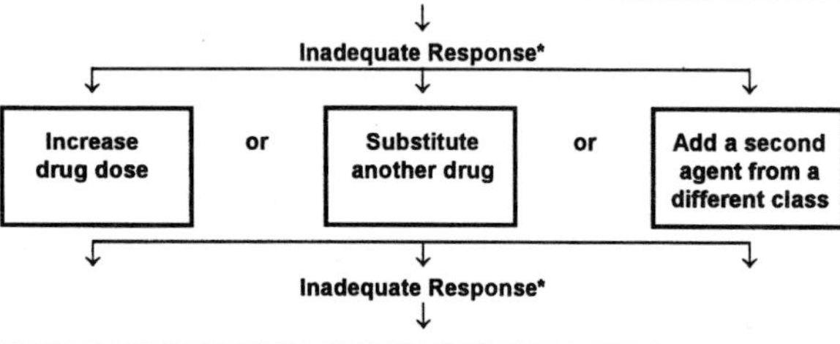

Add a second or third agent and/or diuretic if not already prescribed

Fig 3.2 Treatment algorithm. * Response means achieved goal blood pressure or patient is making considerable progress toward this goal. *(Adapted from the fifth report of the Joint National Committee on Detection, Evaluation and Treatment of High Blood Pressure (JNC V). National Institutes of Health. Publication No. 93-1088, 1993.)*

have adequate blood pressure lowering with two drugs. If patients continue to have elevated blood pressure after an adequate trial of two or more drugs (up to a total of 4 to 6 months), referral should be made to a clinician with special interest in hypertension.

Patients with stages III or IV hypertension require the same general approach. However, a second or third drug may be added after a shorter time interval in this group; in some cases, initial therapy may require two drugs. If the diastolic blood pressure is greater than 120 mm Hg, prompt consultation is recommended.

Special Populations

Many individual patient characteristics may guide choice of specific agents. Some special categories of patients are briefly considered here.

1. Elderly. Most people in the United States over age 60 have elevated blood pressure. Often, the elderly have isolated systolic hypertension, a form of hypertension that has been conclusively proven to be a significant risk for morbidity death in this age group. Guidelines for the management of isolated systolic hypertension are as follows: systolic blood pressure greater than 180 mm Hg should be lowered to less than 160 mm Hg; systolic blood pressures between 160 and 179 mm Hg should be lowered by at least 20 mm Hg. Drugs should be started at the lowest therapeutic dose and increased gingerly in this age group. Furthermore, because the elderly are especially prone to dehydration or orthostatic blood pressure changes, labetalol, α_1 blockers (often chosen in older men with prostatism), and diuretics should be used with caution.

2. Black patients. Calcium channel blockers and diuretics may be more effective monotherapy than β blockers and ACE inhibitors among these patients. However, other common comorbid conditions (diabetes, congestive heart failure, coronary artery disease) may make ACE inhibitor or β-blocker therapy treatments of choice for a given individual black hypertensive patient.

3. Dilated cardiomyopathy. Because the ACE inhibitors have been shown to improve survival in patients with significant left ventricular systolic dysfunction (ejection fraction 35% or less) of any etiology. Also, risk of death after acute myocardial infarction is reduced among patients who are maintained on ACE inhibitor therapy when the ejection fraction is less than 40%. Therefore, the ACE inhibitors are drugs of choice for hypertensive patients with left ventricular dysfunction.

4. Patients with preexisting metabolic abnormalities. Patients with hyperuricemia may develop gout while taking diuretics. Similarly, borderline diabetic or obese patients with latent glucose intolerance may develop hyperglycemia on diuretic therapy. Significant peripheral vascular disease, reversible airways disease (asthma), and other disorders may worsen with β-blocker therapy. (See Table 3.5 for other examples of metabolic side effects of various antihypertensive agents.)

Table 3.6 Classification of Hypertension in the Young by Age Group

	High Normal 90–94th Percentile (mm Hg)	Significant Hypertension 95–99th Percentile (mm Hg)	Severe Hypertension >99th Percentile (mm Hg)
Children (13–15 yr)	SBP 130–135 DBP 80–85	SBP 136–143 DBP 86–91	SBP ⩾ 144 DBP ⩾ 92
Adolescents (16–18 yr)	SBP 136–141 DBP 84–91	SBP 142–149 DBP 92–97	SBP ⩾ 150 DBP ⩾ 98

DBP, diastolic blood pressure; SBP, systolic blood pressure
Source: Report of the Second Task Force on Blood Pressure Control in Children—1987. Pediatrics 1987;79:1–25.

5. Adolescents, The obstetrics-gynecology specialist may be the first person diagnosing hypertension in a young female patient. Initial therapy should concentrate on life-style modification (particularly weight loss in obese children, exercise, review of diet, and a search for addictive habits such as alcohol or cocaine use). Laboratory testing should generally be the same as for adults. However, secondary hypertension is relatively more frequent among children; therefore, consultation with the pediatrician and further testing may be required. Drug therapy should generally be reserved for children or adolescents whose blood pressure is above the 99th percentile (Table 3.6). If target organ damage is present, the threshold for drug therapy should be lower.

Acknowledgements

The authors would like to thank Ms. Selina Todd for her expert preparation of the text.

REFERENCES

1. Fifth report of the Joint National Committee on Detection, Evaluation, and Treatment of High Blood Pressure. The U.S. Department of Health and Human Services. Public Health Service, National Institutes of Health. NIH Publication No. 93-1088, 1993.

2. 1993 Heart and stroke facts. Dallas: American Heart Association, 1993.

3. Fletcher AE, Bulpitt CJ. How far should blood pressure be lowered? N Engl J Med 1992;326:251–254.

4. Farnett L, Mulrow CD, Linn WD, Lucey CR, Tuley MR. The J-curve phenomenon and the treatment of hypertension. Is there a point beyond which pressure reduction is dangerous? JAMA 1991;265:489–495.

5. Kaplan NM. Clinical hypertension. 5th ed. Baltimore: Williams & Wilkins, 1990.

6. Woods JW. Oral contraceptives and hypertension. 1988;11(suppl II):II-11–15.

7. Layde PM, Beral V, Kay CR. Further analyses of mortality in oral contraceptive users. Royal College of General Practitioners' Oral Contraceptive Study. Lancet 1981;1:541–546.

8. Lim KG, Isles CG, Hodsman GP, Lever AF, Robertson JWK. Malignant hypertension in women of childbearing age and its relation to the contraceptive pill. B Med J 1987;294:1057–1059.

9. Wren BG, Routledge DA. Blood pressure changes: oestrogens in climacteric women. Med J Aust 1981;2:528–531.

10. Despre's J-P, Moorjani S, Lupien PJ, Tremblay A, Nadeau N, Bouchard C. Regional distribution of body fat, plasma lipoproteins, and cardiovascular disease. Arteriosclerosis 1990;10:497–511.

11. van Buchem FSP, v.d. Heuvel-Aghina JWMTh, v.d. Heuvel JEA. Acta Med Scand 1964;176:539–548.

12. Harnish A, Pearce ML. Evolution of hypertensive retinal vascular disease: correlation between clinical and postmortem observations. Medicine 1973;52:483–533.

13. Schouten EG, Vandenbroucke JP, van der Heide-Wessel C, van der Heide RM. Retinopathy as an independent indicator of all-causes mortality. Int J Epidemiol 1986;15:234–236.

14. Steinmann WC, Millstein ME, Sinclair SH. Pupillary dilation with tropicamide 1% for funduscopic screening. A study of duration of action. Ann Intern Med 1987;107:181–184.

15. National High Blood Pressure Education Program. Working group report on the heart in hypertension. U.S. Department of Health and Human Services. Public Health Service, National Institutes of Health. National Heart, Lung, and Blood Institute. NIH Publication No. 91-3033, 1991.

16. Working Group on Hypertension in Diabetes. Statement on hypertension in diabetes mellitus. Final report. Arch Intern Med 1987;147:830–842.

17. Levy D, Garrison RJ, Savage DD, Kannel WB, Castelli WP. Prognostic implications of echocardiographically determined left ventricular mass in The Framingham Heart Study. N Engl J Med 1990:322:1561–1566.

18. Casale PN, Devereux RB, Milner M, et al. Value of echocardiographic measurement of left ventricular mass in predicting cardiovascular morbid events in hypertensive men. Ann Intern Med 1986;105:173–178.

19. Cooper RS, Simmons BE, Castaner A, Santhanam V, Ghali J, Mar M. Left ventricular hypertrophy is associated with worst survival independent of ventricular function and number of coronary arteries severely narrowed. Am J Cardiol 1990;65:441–445.

20. Hypertension Detection and Follow-Up Program Cooperative Group. Five-year findings of the hypertension detection and follow-up program. II. Mortality by race-sex, and age. JAMA 1979;242:2572–2577.

21. SHEP Cooperative Research Group. Prevention of stroke by antihypertensive drug treatment in older persons with isolated systolic hypertension. Final results of the Systolic Hypertension in the Elderly Program (SHEP). JAMA 1991;265:3255–3264.

22. MacMahon SW, Wilcken DE, Macdonald GJ. The effect of weight reduction on left ventricular mass. A randomized controlled trial in young, overweight hypertensive patients. N Engl J Med 1986;314:334–339.

23. Hypertension Detection and Follow-up Program Cooperative Group. Persistence of reduction in blood pressure and mortality of participants in the Hypertension Detection and Follow-up Program. JAMA 1988;259:2113–2122.

24. Maheswaran R, Gill JS, Davies P, Beevers DG. High blood pressure due to alcohol. A rapidly reversible effect. Hypertension 1991;17:787–792.

25. Beard TC, Cooke HM, Gray WR, Barge R. Randomized controlled trial of a no-add-sodium diet for mild hypertension. Lancet 1982;2:455–458.

26. Intersalt Cooperative Research Group. Intersalt: an international study of electrolyte excretion and blood pressure. Results for 24 hour urinary sodium and potassium excretion. Br Med J 1988;297:319–328.

27. Hamet P, Mongeau E, Lambert J, et al. Interactions among calcium, sodium, and alcohol intake as determinants of blood pressure. Hypertension 1991;17 (suppl I):I-150–154.

28. Cutler JA, Brittain E. Calcium and blood pressure. An epidemiologic perspective. Am J Hypertens 1990; 3:137S–146S.

29. Shah S, Khatri I, Freis ED. Mechanism of antihypertensive effect of thiazide diuretics. Am Heart J 1978;95:611–618.

30. Kaplan, NM. Our appropriate concern about hypokalemia. Am J Med 1984;77:1–4.

31. The Multiple Risk Factor Intervention Trial Research Group. Exercise electrocardiogram and coronary heart disease mortality in the Multiple Risk Factor Intervention Trial. Am J Cardiol 1985;55:16–24.

32. Gurwitz JH, Avorn J, Bohn RI, et al. Initiation of antihypertensive treatment during nonsteroidal anti-inflammatory drug therapy. JAMA 1994;272:781–786.

33. Veterans Administration Cooperative Study Group on Antihypertensive Agents. Comparison of propranolol and hydrochlorothiazide for the initial treatment of hypertension. I. Results of short-term titration with emphasis on racial differences in response. II. Results of long-term therapy. JAMA 1982;248:1996–2003, 2003–2011.

34. Hall WD, Kong W. Hypertension in blacks: nonpharmacologic and pharmacologic therapy. In: Saunders E, ed. Cardiovascular diseases in blacks. Cardiovascular Clinics. Philadelphia: FA Davis.

35. Day JL, Metcalfe J, Simpson N, Lowenthal L. Adrenergic mehanisms in the control of plasma lipids in man. Am J Med 1984;76:94–96.

36. Hansson L, Dahlof B. What are we really achieving with long-term antihypertensive drug therapy? In: Laragh J, Brenner B, eds. Hypertension: pathophysiology, diagnosis, and treatment. New York: Raven Press, 1990.

37. Glassman AH, Stetner F, Walsh BT, et al. Heavy smokers, smoking cessation, and clonidine. Results of a double-blind, randomized trial. JAMA 1988;259:2863–2866.

38. MacGregor GA, Pevahouse JB, Cappuccio FP, Markandu ND. Nifedipine, diuretics and sodium balance. J Hypertens 1987;suppl 4:S127–S131.

39. Williams GH. Converting-enzyme inhibitors in the treatment of hypertension. N Engl J Med 1988;319:1517–1525.

40. Reid JL, Macdonald NJ, Lees KR, Elliott HL. Angiotensin-converting enzyme inhibitors in the elderly. Am Heart J 1989;117:751–755.

41. Lewis EJ, Hunsicker LG, Bain RP, Rohde RD, et al. The effect of angiotensin-converting-enzyme inhibition on diabetic nephropathy. N Engl J Med 1993;329:1456–1462.

42. SOLVD Investigators. Effect of enalapril on survival in patients with reduced left-ventricular ejection fractions and congestive heart failure. N Engl J Med 1991; 325:303–310.

43. Pfeffer MA, Braunwald E, Moyé LA, et al. Effect of captopril on mortality and morbidity in patients with left-ventricular dysfunction after myocardial infarction: results of the survival and ventricular enlargement trial. N Engl J Med 1992;327:669–677.

CHAPTER 4

HYPERLIPIDEMIA

Vera A. Bittner

Cardiovascular disease is the most common cause of death among men and women of all ethnic groups in the United States. Over 50% of all female deaths are due to cardiovascular disease (1) and women currently incur approximately 58% of the yearly health care costs related to cardiovascular disease (2). Age-adjusted cardiovascular disease death rates are higher among black women than among white women (1). Mortality rates and prevalence of cardiovascular disease increase with age and disability rates are high. It is estimated that one in three women over the age of 65 has some form of cardiovascular disease and over half the women over the age of 75 who have coronary heart disease (CHD) are disabled from their disease (2). The public health impact of cardiovascular disease in women will increase in the future as the population demographics continue to change due to aging of the population and the longer life expectancy among women. By the beginning of the next century, it is estimated that women will outnumber men by 2 : 1 in the age group over 65 and 3: 1 in the age group over 85 (3).

Epidemiologic studies, investigations of genetic disorders, animal studies, and clinical intervention trials support a direct relationship between hypercholesterolemia and subsequent CHD in men and women. In the United States, mean total and low-density lipoprotein (LDL-C) cholesterol levels among adults have declined 6% to 8% since 1960 across all gender and race subgroups, whereas high-density lipoprotein (HDL-C) and very low-density lipoprotein (VLDL-C) cholesterol levels have remained unchanged (4). Despite this decline, 19% of adult men and 20% of adult women have hypercholesterolemia (total cholesterol above 240 mg/dL) (4). Based on 1990 population data and current guidelines for the management of hypercholesterolemia, it has been estimated that as many as 52 million Americans would be candidates for dietary therapy and 12.7 million might be candidates for drug therapy (5). Familiarity with the diagnosis and management of hyperlipidemia is thus essential for all primary care practitioners and subspecialists in cardiovascular disease and endocrinology.

Lipoprotein Composition and Metabolism

Lipoproteins are heterogeneous globular particles of differing size and composition that transport lipid constituents through the circulation (Fig 4.1) (6). They consist of a hydrophic core of cholesteryl ester and triglyceride (TG) and a hydrophilic shell of phospholipids, free cholesterol, and apoproteins. Physical characteristics of chylomicrons, VLDL, intermediate-density lipoproteins (IDL), LDL, HDL, and lipoprotein (a) (Lp[a]) are shown in Table 4.1.

Exogenous Pathway

Chylomicrons are large triglyceride-rich particles that are synthesized in the intestine and transport dietary TG and cholesterol through the body. In the circulation, they are hydrolyzed by lipoprotein lipase to progressively smaller and progressively cholesterol-enriched chylomicron remnants that are then removed from the circulation by hepatic receptors. Chylomicrons deliver fatty acids to peripheral tissues and cholesterol to the liver. After a meal, chylomicrons are cleared rapidly from the circulation. In some patients, however, clearance of chylomicrons may be abnormally slow resulting in prolonged postprandial hypertriglyceridemia. Although not universally accepted, many investigators believe that high levels of

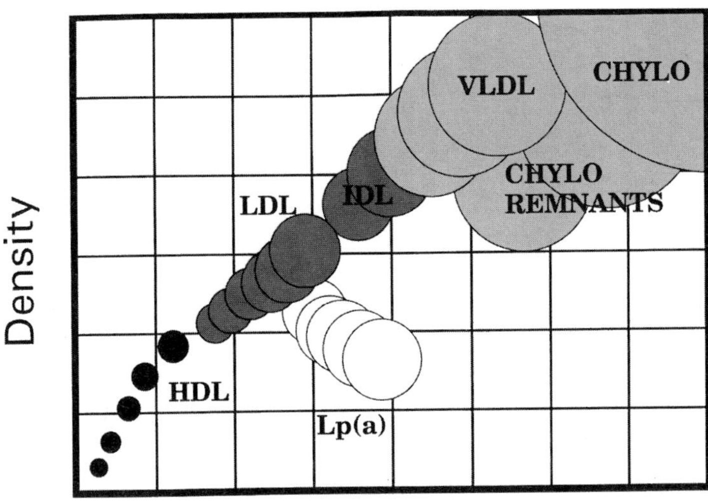

Fig 4.1 Schematic representation of lipoprotein particles. Particles are depicted by size and density. Chylomicrons are the largest and least dense particles and HDL the smallest and densest. Each class of particle has several subclasses. Chylo, chylomicron; HDL, high-density lipoprotein; IDL, intermediate-density lipoprotein; LDL, low-density lipoprotein; Lp(a), lipoprotein (a); VLDL, very low-density lipoprotein. *(Reproduced by permission from Segrest JP, Brouillette CG, Harvey SC, Anantharamaiah GM. The amphipathic alpha-helix: a multifunctional structural motif in plasma apolipoproteins. In: Anfinsen CB, Edsall JT, Richards FM, Eisenberg DS, eds. Advances in protein chemistry. San Diego: Academic Press, 1994:305.)*

Table 4.1 Characteristics of Major Lipoproteins

LIPOPROTEIN (SIZE)	MAJOR APOPROTEIN	MAJOR LIPID COMPONENTS (%)		DENSITY (GM/ML)	FLOTATION RATE (SF AT 1.063)	ELECTROPHORETIC MOBILITY
		C/CE	TG			
CM (75–1200 nm)	B-48, C, E	4	90	<0.98	⩾400	Origin
VLDL (30–80 nm)	B-100, C, E	18	60	0.98–1.006	20–400	Prebeta
IDL (25–35 nm)	B-100, C, E	36	30	1.006–1.019	12–20	Broad beta
LDL (15–25 nm)	B-100	51	5	1.019–1.063	0–12	Beta
HDL (5–12 nm)	A, C, D, E	23	7	1.063–1.21	–	Alpha
Lp(a) (25 nm)	(a)	42	3	1.05–1.12	–	Prebeta

C, cholesterol; CE, cholesteryl ester; CM, chylomicron; Sf, Svedberg units; VLDL, very low-density lipoprotein; IDL, intermediate-density lipoprotein; LDL, low-density lipoprotein; HDL, high-density lipoprotein; Lp(a) = lipoprotein (a), Adapted by permission from Oberman A, Kreisberg RA, Henkin Y. Principles and management of lipid disorders. A primary care approach. Baltimore: Williams & Wilkins, 1992:89.

postprandial triglyceride-rich lipoproteins are atherogenic (7).

Endogenous Pathway

Very low-density lipoprotein particles are triglyceride-rich particles of variable size that are synthesized in the liver and hydrolyzed by lipoprotein lipase on the surface of capillary endothelial cells to form IDL. The IDL particles are either taken up by the liver or metabolized further to form the cholesterol-rich LDL particles. About two thirds of LDL particles are removed by the specific LDL receptor, which recognizes apoproteins B-100 and E; the remainder is removed by scavenger receptors and other nonspecific pathways. LDL is believed to be the major atherogenic particle, and current therapeutic guidelines specifically target this lipoprotein. Several subspecies of LDL that vary in density have been recognized. Dense subspecies tend to predominate in persons with hypertriglyceridemia and are believed to be particularly atherogenic (pattern B) (8).

Levels of HDL are inversely related to CHD risk and are believed to play a role in reverse cholesterol transport although the precise pathway has not been elucidated. It is hypothesized that HDL particles are synthesized by the liver and intestine and secreted into the circulation as phospholipid discs ready to accept free cholesterol from peripheral tissues. This free cholesterol is then esterified in HDL by lecithin-cholesterol-acyltransferase, transferred to circulating IDL, LDL, and VLDL, and then transported to the liver. Women have higher HDL-C levels than men and have higher levels of HDL particles that contain only apo-AI; levels of HDL particles that contain apo-AI and apo-AII are comparable in both genders.

Lipoprotein (a) (Lp[a]) is a unique lipoprotein that consists of an LDL particle whose apoprotein B-100 is covalently linked to apoprotein (a), a glycoprotein with homology to plasminogen. Blood concentrations are largely genetically determined and blacks tend to have higher levels than whites. Recent studies suggest that hormones and in particular estrogen can also influence Lp(a) concentrations (9). In some but not all studies, high levels of Lp(a) are associated with increased risk of premature CHD, possibly because of interference with the fibrinolytic system.

Measurement of Lipoproteins and Phenotypic Classification of Lipid Disorders

The clinical management of dyslipidemias is currently based on measurement of cholesterol content in total serum and in the HDL fraction as well as measurement of fasting serum TG. If the TG value is below 400 mg/dL, VLDL-C can be estimated by dividing the TG value by 5 and LDL-C is then calculated by the Friedewald equation (LDL-C = total cholesterol − HDL-C − TG/5; all values in mg/dL). For TG above 400 mg/dL, LDL-C has to be determined by ultracentrifugation in a specialized laboratory. Assays of apolipoproteins, Lp(a), LDL subclass patterns, etc also generally require access to a specialized laboratory.

Biologic and analytic factors affect the accuracy and reproducibility of these measurements. To minimize this variability, the National Cholesterol Education Program (NCEP) has developed detailed recommendations for improving cholesterol measurement (10). Physicians should seek out laboratories that participate regularly in standardization programs and preferably those that standardize their assays against one of the member laboratories in the National Reference Method Laboratory Network established by the Centers for Disease Control and Prevention and the National Institutes of Health. Lipid values vary diurnally and seasonally and are generally not representative of the patient's usual baseline during an acute illness, after trauma or surgery, during periods of weight loss or unusual dietary intake, or during pregnancy. After myocardial infarction, it may take as long as 3 months before lipid values return to baseline. Similarly, the NCEP recommends that lipid measurements after pregnancy be deferred for 3 to 4 months after delivery. Vigorous exercise immediately before venipuncture can lower TG values. Posture during venipuncture, duration of venous occlusion, and the use of anticoagulants also affect the lipid measurements. It is, therefore, recommended that venipuncture be performed after the patient has been sitting for 5 minutes and tourniquet use should be as brief as possible; collection of blood in tubes without ethylenediametetraacetic acid (EDTA) is preferred. To avoid patient misclassification, therapeutic decisions should be based on a minimum of two separate lipoprotein determinations.

The Frederickson classification divides dyslipidemias into six phenotypes designated I, IIa, IIb, III, IV, and V based on the lipoprotein present in excess (Table 4.2). Because each phenotype represents heterogenous primary or secondary disorders of lipoprotein metabolism and because the classification does not address disorders of HDL metabolism, it has been deemphasized in the recent literature. The classification remains useful, however, when discussing choice of pharmacologic agents in the treatment of dyslipidemias and phenotypic categories are still frequently used as patient enrollment criteria for clinical studies.

Because apoproteins determine the metabolic fate of lipoprotein particles and apoprotein measurements reflect the number of lipoprotein particles, assessment of apoprotein levels adds additional information to conventional lipid measurements and could provide a more precise assessment of CHD risk than measurements of cholesterol and TG levels. Measurement of apoproteins, however, is poorly standardized. Furthermore, prospective epidemiologic data assessing the relationship between apoproteins and CHD is limited and, to date, there is a dearth of studies to document benefits of intervention. At this time, apoprotein measurement remains a research tool.

Primary Lipid Disorders

This section reviews inherited disorders that are frequently encountered by the primary care practitioner, with particular emphasis on those associated with increased risk of CHD development or development of pancreatitis. Interested readers are referred to detailed recent reviews for a more in-depth discussion of the topic (11–13).

Familial Hypercholesterolemia and Familial Polygenic Hypercholesterolemia

Familial hypercholesterolemia is an autosomal codominantly inherited disorder characterized by delayed clearance and high levels of LDL (phenotype IIa) due to lack of expression of LDL receptors or expression of defective LDL receptors. The heterozygous state occurs with a frequency of approximately 1 : 500 in the population. Affected individuals generally develop arcus senilis and tendon xanthomas, have LDL-C levels above 250 mg/dL with generally normal levels of HDL-C and TG, and develop premature CHD with an average age of onset of 45 years among men and 55 years among women. The clinical diagnosis is considered established in families with two or more family members with LDL-C above the 90th percentile and the presence of tendon xanthomas in the kindred. Homozygotes have LDL-C above 500 mg/dL, often decreased HDL-C, and develop CHD during childhood or adolescence. Although heterozygotes can be treated with standard pharmaceutical agents, homozygotes require LDL-apheresis or liver transplantation; gene therapy remains in the experimental stage.

In familial polygenic hypercholesterolmia, affected individuals have LDL-C values above the 90th per-

Table 4.2 Frederickson Classification of Dyslipidemias

PHENOTYPE	LIPOPROTEIN IN EXCESS	TYPICAL LIPID RANGE (MG/DL)	
		Cholesterol	Triglyceride
I	CM	300–500	5000–6000
IIA	LDL	250–800	<250
IIB	LDL, VLDL	240–350	250–500
III	beta-VLDL, IDL	300–450	300–1000
IV	VLDL	200–240	300–700
V	CM, VLDL	200–1000	2000–6000

Abbreviations as in Table 4.1.
Adapted by permission from Oberman A, Kreisberg RA, Henkin Y. Principles and management of lipid disorders. A primary care approach. Baltimore: Williams & Wilkins, 1992:138.

centile (i.e., the heterozygous familial hypercholesterolemia phenotype) and are predisposed to premature CHD, but they and their relatives lack the characteristic tendon xanthomas. The disorder is believed to be polygenic and, in some series, is twice as common as heterozygous familial hypercholesterolemia; a precise metabolic or genetic defect has not been identified.

Familial Combined Hyperlipidemia

Familial combined hyperlipidemia is believed to be due to overproduction of apo B-100, but the mode of inheritance and the precise metabolic defect are unknown. The condition is associated with premature development of CHD and it is estimated that 10% to 14% of individuals with premature CHD manifest the disorder. Affected family members express hypercholesterolemia, hypertriglyceridemia, or both, often associated with decreased HDL-C levels (phenotypes IIa, IIb, IV). Phenotypes can vary over time in the same individual. Clinically, familial combined hyperlipidemia is diagnosed when two or more family members have LDL-C, TG levels, or both above the 90th percentile and when both high LDL-C and TG levels are present in the same kindred. Familial hyperapobetalipoproteinemia is probably a variant and accounts for about 5% of patients with premature CHD. It is characterized by apo B values above the 90th percentile in two or more family members without other lipid abnormalities in the kindred.

TIII Hyperlipidemia (Familial Dysbetalipoproteinemia)

Type III hyperlipidemia is characterized by delayed catabolism of VLDL remnants and the accumulation of abnormally cholesterol-enriched beta-VLDL particles (VLDL-C/VLDL-TG ratio of greater than 0.3). Patients with type III hyperlipidemia are homozygous for apo E2, an isoform of apoprotein E, which has less affinity for the LDL receptor. Hyperlipidemia is only expressed if a second disorder of lipoprotein metabolism is present, either one of the primary dyslipidemias or the secondary dyslipidemias due to obesity or diabetes. Affected patients have characteristic tuberous or palmar xanthomas and are at risk for premature CHD; it is estimated that 0.5% of patients with premature CHD have familial dysbetalipoproteinemia.

Familial Hypoalphalipoproteinemia

Familial hypoalphalipoproteinemia is observed in about 4% of patients with premature CHD and is characterized by HDL-C levels below the 10th percentile in two or more family members. Low HDL-C levels often compound other primary or secondary dyslipidemias and increase CHD risk further in affected individuals. As many as 30% of patients hospitalized with acute myocardial infarction have low HDL-C levels. Although low HDL-C is in general associated with increased CHD risk, some uncommon primary disorders of HDL metabolism such as fish eye disease or Tangier disease do not show this association. Why some disorders with low HDL-C predispose to premature CHD and others do not is as yet poorly understood.

Familial Dyslipidemia

Familial dyslipidemia is a common disorder characterized by TG levels above the 90th percentile and HDL-C levels below the 10th percentile in at least two family members. Metabolically, affected patients have increased hepatic TG secretion and increased HDL catabolism, but the precise defect and mode of inheritance are unknown. Patients often manifest signs of insulin resistance, frank diabetes, male pattern obesity, and hypertension. Some authors have suggested that as many as 5% to 15% of patients with premature CHD have this disorder.

Familial Hypertriglyceridemia

Familial hypertriglyceridemia is inherited in autosomal dominant fashion, is present in about 1% to 2% of the population, and may account for as many as 15% to 25% of those with increased VLDL levels and hypertriglyceridemia. HDL-C is generally reduced and total cholesterol levels are relatively normal. In contrast to familial combined hyperlipidemia, apo B and apo AI levels are normal in familial hypertriglyceridemia, indicating that the number of VLDL and HDL particles is normal and that the VLDL particles are abnormally TG enriched; only 10% of these large VLDL particles are converted to LDL particles during metabolism. Family screening is necessary to distinguish the condition from the more common secondary hypertriglyceridemias. CHD risk is significantly lower in this disorder than in familial combined hyperlipidemia.

Some patients may develop hyperchylomicronemia, pancreatitis, and eruptive xanthomas.

Hyperchylomicronemia Syndrome

Primary forms of hyperchylomicronemia due to lipoprotein lipase deficiency and apoprotein C-II deficiency are rare. Homozygous lipoprotein lipase deficiency (phenotype I) occurs in 1 in 1 million persons and manifests in infancy and early childhood. Affected individuals are at risk for pancreatitis. Characteristic physical findings include lipemia retinalis, eruptive xanthomas, hepatosplenomegaly, and lymphadenopathy. The heterozygous state occurs in 1 in 500 persons; many do not exhibit any lipoprotein abnormality and are asymptomatic.

When primary abnormalities of TG metabolism are compounded by secondary disorders (e.g., diabetes, alcohol or medication effects), patients may present with striking hypertriglyceridemia of several thousand mg/dL due to elevated VLDL and chylomicron levels (phenotype V) and a syndrome of abdominal pain, eruptive xanthomas, depression, memory loss, and shortness of breath. Lipemia retinalis, eruptive xanthomas, and hepatosplenomegaly may be present on physical examination and spurious hyponatremia and hypoxemia will be evident on laboratory evaluations.

Secondary Dyslipidemias

Secondary dyslipidemias are acquired hyperlipidemias caused by an underlying disorder that leads to alterations in lipoprotein metabolism (11,14). Phenotypically, secondary dyslipidemias can appear as hypercholesterolemia, hypertriglyceridemia, or both (Table 4.3). They may occur in isolation or can further exacerbate lipoprotein abnormalities in patients with inherited lipid disorders. The acquired lipid alterations carry the same risks of CHD, extracardiac atherosclerosis, and pancreatitis as those caused by inherited abnormalities in lipoprotein metabolism. Identification of secondary dyslipidemias before initiation of standard lipid-lowering therapy is important

Table 4.3 Causes of Secondary Dyslipidemias

Hypercholesterolemia	Hypertriglyceridemia	Combined Hyperlipidemia
Common Disorders		
Hypothyroidism Nephrotic syndrome Obstructive liver disease	Diabetes Obesity Alcohol Chronic renal failure	Hypothyroidism Nephrotic syndrome Chronic renal failure
Uncommon Disorders		
Pregnancy Anorexia nervosa	Myocardial infarction Acute infection Connective tissue diseases Nephrotic syndrome Pregnancy Bulimia	Acromegaly Liver disease
Medications		
Thiazide diuretics Retinoids Glucocorticoids Cyclosporine Progestins Androgens	β Blockers Retinoids Oral estrogens	Thiazide diuretics Glucocorticoids Retinoids

Adapted by permission from Oberman A, Kreisberg RA, Henkin Y. Principles and management of lipid disorders. A primary care approach. Baltimore: Williams & Wilkins, 1992:155.

(Table 4.4) because many of the lipoprotein abnormalities will resolve or at least improve with treatment of the underlying disorder.

Obesity, Insulin Resistance, and Diabetes Mellitus

Obesity is an important contributor to dyslipidemia in men and women (15,16). Obese individuals overproduce VLDL particles and have higher total, non–HDL-C, LDL-C, and TG levels and lower HDL-C levels than their nonobese counterparts. Hypertriglyceridemia and low HDL-C are particularly pronounced in central obesity, which is associated with insulin resistance, hypertension, and increased CHD risk in both genders (Reaven's syndrome) (17,18).

Lipid abnormalities are common in patients with non–insulin-dependent diabetes mellitus (NIDDM) (19,20). Characteristically, these individuals have elevated VLDL levels, hypertriglyceridemia, and low HDL-C. Total cholesterol and LDL-C tend to be normal, but LDL particles tend to be smaller and denser and thus presumably more atherogenic (8). Cholesteryl-ester enrichment of VLDL and IDL may further increase atherogenicity. When renal failure or nephrotic syndrome complicate NIDDM, lipoprotein changes become even more complex (see below). Hypertriglyceridemia in NIDDM tends to improve with better glycemic control. Oral hypoglycemics are generally ineffective in improving HDL-C levels. Insulin therapy, especially when combined with weight loss, may restore HDL-C levels to normal. In contrast to NIDDM, lipid abnormalities in uncontrolled insulin-dependent diabetes (IDDM) tend to respond promptly to insulin therapy and IDDM patients with good diabetic control tend to have lipid levels similar to age- and sex-matched controls.

Table 4.4 Identification of Common Secondary Dyslipidemias

General history and physical	Signs and symptoms of Thyroid disease Diabetes mellitus Liver disease Renal disease
	Medication history
	Body weight normalized for height (body mass index) Distribution of body fat (waist-hip ratio)
Dietary assessment	Fat intake Cholesterol intake Calorie intake Alcohol consumption
Laboratory evaluation	Fasting glucose Glycosylated hemoglobin in diabetics Liver function tests Blood urea nitrogen, creatinine Urinalysis for protein Thyroid function tests

Alcohol and Liver Disease

Consumption of alcohol in moderate quantities is associated with decreased CHD risk in men and women, presumably related to an increase in HDL-C levels (21,22). In the liver, alcohol competes with fatty acid oxidation, increases fatty acid incorporation into TG, and results in increased VLDL secretion into the plasma. In patients with primary or secondary defects in TG clearance, alcohol, even when consumed in low doses, may thus lead to severe hypertriglyceridemia and the chylomicronemia syndrome.

The liver has a central role in both synthesis and catabolism of lipoproteins. Depending on the type of liver injury, hepatic dysfunction results in a variety of abnormal lipoprotein phenotypes. Acute hepatocellular disease is associated with hypertriglyceridemia and decreased HDL-C, both intra- and extrahepatic cholestatic liver disease are characterized by the secretion of an abnormal lipoprotein (LP-X), and advanced chronic liver disease that is often accompanied by poor nutritional status results in low levels of all endogenous lipoproteins due to impaired synthesis and secretion.

Thyroid Disease

Lipoprotein abnormalities are common in hypothyroidism, even in the absence of overt clinical symptoms (23). Patients may present with hypercholesterolemia, combined elevations in TG and cholesterol, or with remnant accumulation mimicking type III hyperlipidemia. Receptor-mediated LDL catabolism is decreased and decreased activity of lipoprotein lipase results in decreased clearance of VLDL particles. Supplementation with thyroid hormone leads to normalization of lipoprotein metabolism.

Hyperthyroidism results in hypocholesterolemia due to enhanced LDL catabolism and decreased levels of HDL-C and apoprotein A-I. Triglyceride levels tend to be normal or slightly increased because increased synthesis of VLDL-C tends to offset the increased activity of lipoprotein lipase.

Chronic Renal Disease and Nephrotic Syndrome

When creatinine clearance decreases below 20 mL/min, patients tend to develop hypertriglyceridemia due to decreased activity of lipoprotein lipase and, secondarily, lower levels of HDL-C and appear to be at increased CHD risk. Patients with nephrotic syndrome have increased levels of LDL-C, often accompanied by elevated VLDL-C levels and low HDL-C. Overproduction of apolipoprotein B-100, decreased VLDL clearance, and loss of apoproteins in the urine have been documented. Glucocorticoid therapy may further exacerbate the dyslipidemia.

The lipoprotein abnormalities associated with nephrotic syndrome resolve after institution of dialysis and after renal transplantation. In contrast, the hypertriglyceridemia associated with chronic renal failure is not affected by dialysis but resolves after renal transplantation. After renal transplantation, however, many patients develop secondary lipoprotein abnormalities due to immunosuppressive therapy with glucocorticoids and cyclosporine.

Autoimmune Disease

Hypercholesterolemia, hypertriglyceridemia, or both may be seen in patients with multiple myeloma when antibodies bind to and modify enzymes or receptors involved in lipoprotein metabolism. Autoimmune dyslipidemia has also been described in patients with systemic lupus erythematosus, idiopathic thrombocytopenic purpura, and Graves' disease.

Drug-Induced Dyslipidemia

Many drugs can alter plasma lipoprotein levels unfavorably (24). Most studies are short in duration and it is thus often unclear whether changes in serum lipids persist with long-term use. Whether any of the drug-induced lipoprotein alterations are associated with increased CHD risk has not been determined.

Antihypertensives

Thiazide-type diuretics may increase TG and VLDL-C levels by as much as 50% (on average 25%) and LDL-C by 15% without significant changes in HDL-C levels. Lipid-altering effects of loop diuretics are less pronounced and some of the newer diuretics such as indapamide may be lipid neutral. Nonselective β blockers without intrinsic sympathomimetic activity increase serum TG and VLDL-C levels by 20% to 50% and decrease HDL-C by approximately 15%; LDL-C is generally not affected. The HDL-C lowering effect is less pronounced with β_1-selective blockers and β blockers with intrinsic sympathomimetic activity may raise HDL-C by up to 9% with only minor changes in TG levels. Despite the apparent "adverse" lipid effects, both nonselective and selective β blockers have been shown to significantly decrease mortality after myocardial infarction and may inhibit atheroma formation and plaque rupture (25,26). Calcium channel blockers and angiotensin-converting enzyme inhibitors are generally lipid neutral, whereas some postsynaptic α blockers appear to result in slight reductions in TG and increases in HDL-C.

Sex Hormones

Oral estrogens decrease LDL-C and total cholesterol and increase HDL-C and TG. The magnitude of the effects is related to the dose of estrogen administered. Most epidemiologic studies show a significant decrease in CHD risk among women who receive postmenopausal oral estrogen therapy (27). This reduction in risk is at least in part mediated by the rise in HDL-C levels. Transdermal estrogens have a lesser impact on hepatic protein synthesis and levels of serum lipoproteins and thus provide a good therapeutic alternative for hypertriglyceridemic women who cannot tolerate the oral formulation. Whether transdermal estrogens decrease cardiovascular risk in postmenopausal women is as yet unclear.

Progestins tend to lower HDL-C levels, but the magnitude of HDL-C lowering varies. Androgenic progestins such as levonorgestrel cause more pronounced HDL-C lowering and C-19 progestins in general tend to have more pronounced metabolic effects than C-21 progestins such as medroxyprogesterone acetate. The net effect of estrogen/progestin combination therapy depends on the relative doses of each and the type of progestin used. Newer oral contraceptive formulations tend to cause only minor changes in lipoproteins and a recent large epidemiologic study suggests that addition of a progestin to postmenopausal estrogen replacement therapy does not adversely affect cardiovascular risk factors and may even ameliorate estrogen's adverse effects on clotting factors (28).

Anabolic Steroids

Androgens are used therapeutically in the treatment of endometriosis and a variety of other disorders and are often abused by athletes who desire increased strength and muscle mass. These agents cause profound reductions in HDL-C and increases in LDL-C, changes that are likely to be pro-atherogenic when sustained over long time periods.

Immunosuppressives

Corticosteroid therapy in transplant recipients is associated with elevations in total cholesterol, LDL-C, HDL-C, and TG. Similar changes have been observed in steroid-treated patients in remission from connective tissue disease, rheumatoid arthritis, and asthma, more prominently in women than in men. Cyclosporin A increases LDL-C, apoprotein B, total cholesterol, and TG without significant changes in HDL-C. Concomitant use of this agent with lovastatin has been linked to an increased incidence of rhabdomyolysis.

Other Drugs

Phenothiazines have been implicated in HDL-C reduction and increases in total cholesterol, but data are sketchy. Anticonvulsants and in particular phenytoin (Dilantin) appear to have significant HDL-C raising properties without affecting LDL-C levels significantly. Retinoids are synthetic vitamin A analogues used most commonly in the treatment of acne. Isotretinoin in particular has been associated with elevations in total cholesterol, LDL-C, VLDL-C, and TG and decreases in HDL-C. These changes are believed to be potentially atherogenic; pancreatitis due to retinoid-induced hypertriglyceridemia has also been described.

Lipids and Coronary Heart Disease—Gender Differences

The cause and effect relationship between hypercholesterolemia and CHD in both genders is no longer debated (29). Data from cross-cultural studies, from longitudinal follow-up studies, and from intervention trials in the United States and elsewhere support a continuous and direct association between CHD and total cholesterol levels beginning at approximately 150 mg/dL (30). In the Framinghman study 30-year follow-up, total cholesterol was a strong predictor of CHD in men and women up to the age of 94 years (31). Although data from Framingham and many observational studies show a close relationship between LDL-C levels and CHD risk in all races, in both genders, and in all age groups (32,33), LDL-C appears to be a less potent predictor of CHD in women compared to men (34,35). The inverse relationship between HDL-C levels and risk of CHD is seen in all age groups, both genders, and in different ethnic groups and appears to be stronger in women than in men (34–36). In the Lipid Research Clinics follow-up study, for example, women with an HDL-C of less than 50 mg/dL had a 2.71-fold increase in risk of cardiovascular death compared to women with an HDL-C above 50 mg/dL (35). In the elderly, HDL-C is also a better predictor of CHD than LDL-C (37). Interventions that lower LDL-C or increase HDL-C or both result in clinical benefit in both women and men (see below).

The role of TG in atherogenesis remains controversial, but there is increasing evidence that triglyceride-rich lipoproteins are directly atherogenic in certain individuals and in others could be linked to CHD by their metabolic consequences including increased HDL catabolism and hypercoagulability (7,38). Most epidemiologic studies document a strong univariate relationship between TG levels and CHD in both sexes, but TG levels are often no longer significant in multivariate analyses that include other lipid risk factors and in particular HDL-C. The appropriateness of studying these highly statistically correlated and metabolically linked lipid parameters in multivariate models has been questioned (38). The relationship between hypertriglyceridemia and CHD appears to be stronger in women than men. In the 1993 report from the LRC follow-up study, for example, TG levels above 200 mg/dL in women were strongly associated with cardiovascular death (35). Increased susceptibility to the atherogenic effects of VLDL and TG elevation in association with low HDL-C levels may also explain the disproportionate elevation in CHD risk among diabetic women compared to diabetic men (20,39).

During pregnancy, total cholesterol, LDL-C, HDL-C, and TG increase. After pregnancy, HDL-C levels drop below baseline and parous women tend to have lower HDL-C levels than nulliparous women (40). This may in part explain data from Framingham and the National Health and Nutrition Examination Epidemiologic Follow-Up Study, which show an increase in CHD risk with increasing parity (41). Natural or surgical menopause increases CHD risk among women independent of age (42). This increase in risk appears to be in part mediated by unfavorable changes in lipoprotein levels. Total cholesterol, LDL-C, apoprotein B, and TG levels increase; HDL-C decreases slightly or does not change (43–45). The metabolic risk factor profile improves markedly with hormone replacement therapy (28).

Clinical Trials and the Risks and Benefits of Cholesterol Lowering

In published randomized trials, CHD incidence is reduced on average by 2.5% for every 1% lowering of cholesterol (46). Secondary prevention trials and angiographic trials of lipid lowering show consistent and significant reductions in CHD morbidity and mortality and favorable alterations in the natural history of coronary artery disease progression (47). Pooled data from angiographic trials where LDL-C levels were decreased by approximately 40% and HDL-C levels increased by up to 40% suggest a 36% reduction in coronary lesion progression and an over twofold increase in coronary lesion regression in the treated group (48). Women benefit to a similar degree as men (49). Although many of these short-term angiographic trials show no difference in clinical end points, lesion changes observed during the trials are independent predictors of future clinical events and thus reasonable surrogate end points (50).

Although there is a general consensus that benefits of cholesterol lowering outweigh potential risks in patients with established CHD, the relationships between "naturally" low cholesterol levels and mortality and cholesterol lowering as primary prevention of CHD and mortality continue to be the subject of vigorous debate. Epidemiologic studies to date have not been designed to specifically assess the relationship between naturally low cholesterol levels and noncardiovascular mortality. Interpretation of existing studies is problematic because of methodologic problems: definitions of "low cholesterol" vary; risk estimates are often confounded by smoking, alcohol use, and subclinical disease; different etiologies of hypocholesterolemia are not considered individually; and outcomes are so broadly defined that an assessment of cause and effect becomes difficult. In "healthy" populations, there is no association between low cholesterol and increased mortality: on the contrary, there is a direct relationship between cholesterol levels and total mortality (51,52). Recent reviews have concluded that the association between "naturally" low cholesterol and noncardiovascular mortality is unlikely to be causal (51,53).

In primary prevention trials, cholesterol lowering by diet or drugs or both lowered CHD incidence, but total mortality was not altered and analyses of pooled data showed an increase in noncardiovascular mortality in the treated group (54). Although the reduction in CHD mortality is related to the degree of cholesterol reduction, a dose-response relationship is not apparent for non-CHD mortality and the adverse effect on noncardiovascular mortality seems to be largely confined to drug trials (55). These data suggest that the observed increase in non-CHD mortality is not causally related to cholesterol lowering, but rather represents an adverse effect of the therapeutic agents used. The revised NCEP guidelines thus recommend an emphasis on lifestyle modifications and a generally more cautious approach to drug use in primary prevention patients (56).

Approach to the Patient

Guidelines for screening, diagnosis, and management of patients with high blood cholesterol have recently been updated (56). This section summarizes these recommendations and attempts to provide the reader with a systematic approach to the patient.

Screening, Diagnosis, Risk Assessment, and Determination of Treatment Goals

Total and HDL-C should be measured every 5 years in all adults over the age of 20. These measurements can be made in the nonfasting state, but a fasting sample that also includes a determination of TG is preferable. Only with the latter can LDL-C be estimated. Screening should not be performed during an acute illness and any treatment decisions should be based on at least two separate lipoprotein determinations.

Although the relationship between hypercholesterolemia and CHD is continuous and graded, a classification system with somewhat arbitrary cut-off points based on CHD risk has been developed to guide subsequent therapy. A total cholesterol level less than 200 mg/dL is considered desirable, a level between 200 and 239 mg/dL borderline, and a level above 240 mg/dL high. An individual with a total cholesterol value of 240 mg/dL has approximately twice the risk of CHD as an individual with a total cholesterol level of 200 mg/dL and risk rises steeply above this cut point. For HDL-C, a cut point of 35 mg/dL was chosen for men and women—those with HDL-C levels below this value are considered at risk. Women have higher HDL-C levels than men and many investigators believe that a cut point of 45 mg/dL would have been more appropriate for women based on the available epidemiologic data.

Patients with desirable total cholesterol and HDL-C levels should be provided with educational materials on the diet recommended for the general population, advised to be rescreened in 5 years, and receive counseling regarding smoking cessation, weight normalization or maintenance, physical activity, and treatment of other CHD risk factors as appropriate.

For those with borderline or abnormal total cholesterol and HDL-C values, subsequent management is based on LDL-C levels and an assessment of CHD risk. Patients with established CHD or extracardiac atherosclerosis are at highest risk for CHD events and are treated most vigorously. Among primary prevention patients, intensity of therapy is determined by the presence or absence of several risk factors for CHD (Table 4.5). In contrast to the 1988 guidelines, male gender is now only a risk factor for those 45 years and older. For women, the age cutoff is 10 years later; postmenopausal women not on hormone replacement therapy are also considered at higher risk. Although somewhat controversial, HDL-C above 60 mg/dL has been designated as a "negative" risk factor. Obesity and physical inactivity, although not considered in the NCEP risk stratification algorithm, are nevertheless targets for nonpharmacologic intervention. LDL-C cut points for the initiation of diet and drug therapy and LDL-C treatment goals are summarized in Table 4.6. Before beginning nonpharmacologic or drug therapy, all patients should be evaluated for the presence of secondary dyslipidemias that might require specific therapy for the underlying disorder (see above). Screening of family members will aid in the diagnosis of inherited lipoprotein disorders and may uncover additional persons in need of lipid-lowering therapy.

Table 4.5 Risk Factors for CHD Other than LDL Cholesterol

Positive Risk Factors
Age: Male ⩾45 yr Female ⩾55 yr or premature menopause without ERT
Family history of premature CHD: Definite MI or sudden death before age 55 in male first-degree relatives or before age 65 in female first-degree relatives
Current cigarette smoking
Hypertension
Diabetes mellitus
Low HDL cholesterol (<35 mg/dL)
Negative Risk Factor
High HDL cholesterol (⩾60 mg/dL)
Other Risk Factors
Obesity (BMI >27 kg/m^2)
Visceral obesity (WHR) (⩾0.9 in men, ⩾0.8 in women)
Sedentary lifestyle

BMI, body mass index; ERT, estrogen replacement therapy; HDL, high-density lipoprotein; MI, myocardial infarction; WHR, waist-hip ratio.

Source: Expert Panel on Detection, Evaluation, and Treatment of High Blood Cholesterol in Adults. Second report of the Expert Panel on Detection, Evaluation, and Treatment of High Blood Cholesterol in Adults. NIH Publication No. 93-3095, September 1993.

Table 4.6 LDL Treatment Goals According to CHD Risk

Patient Category*	Initiation Level	LDL Goal
Dietary Therapy		
Primary Prevention		
No CHD, <2 RF	⩾160 mg/dL (4.1 mmol/L)	<160 mg/dL (4.1 mmol/L)
No CHD, ⩾2 RF	⩾130 mg/dL (3.4 mmol/L)	<130 mg/dL (3.4 mmol/L)
Secondary Prevention		
CHD	>100 mg/dL (2.6 mmol/L)	⩽100 mg/dL (2.6 mmol/L)
Drug Therapy		
Primary Prevention		
No CHD, <2 RF	⩾190 mg/dL (4.9 mmol/L)	<160 mg/dL (4.1 mmol/L)
No CHD, ⩾2 RF	⩾160 mg/dL (4.1 mmol/L)	<130 mg/dL (3.4 mmol/L)
Secondary Prevention		
CHD	⩾130 mg/dL (3.4 mmol/L)	⩽100 mg/dL (2.6 mmol/L)

*Note that CHD in the context of this table refers to established CHD and CHD risk equivalents, i.e., other atherosclerotic disease.

CHD, coronary heart disease; LDL, low-density lipoprotein; RF, risk factor.

Source: Expert Panel on Detection, Evaluation, and Treatment of High Blood Cholesterol in Adults. Second report of the Expert Panel on Detection, Evaluation, and Treatment of High Blood Cholesterol in Adults. NIH Publication No. 93-3095, September 1993.

Nondrug Therapies of Lipid Disorders

High intake of saturated fat and cholesterol and calorie consumption in excess of caloric expenditure are the major dietary factors that contribute to hypercholesterolemia. Although nonpharmacologic therapy aims to reduce LDL-C levels, weight loss, increase in physical activity, and modification of fat intake may also reduce CHD risk by other means. Weight loss and increase in physical activity decrease fasting VLDL-C and TG levels, improve postprandial lipoprotein metabolism, tend to increase HDL-C levels, and will often improve blood pressure and glucose tolerance in both genders (7,56). Regression of coronary lesions has been demonstrated with diet and vigorous exercise (57,58). Decreased saturated fat and cholesterol intake and increased consumption of fruits, vegetables, grain products, and fish increase the supply of substances such as dietary fibers, antioxidants, and polyunsaturated fatty acids, which may lower CHD risk independent of LDL-C levels (56).

The initial step in dietary therapy is the assessment of the patient's current eating habits. For those with high saturated fat and cholesterol intake, dietary treatment begins with a step I diet; patients already on a diet equivalent to step I and patients with established CHD should be instructed in a step II diet (Table 4.7). A simple dietary assessment tool, data on food composition, sample menus for men and women of varying ethnic backgrounds, and practical guidelines for the initiation of weight reduction therapy and an exercise program are provided in the NCEP update (56). Responses to dietary therapy are individually variable and depend on the baseline diet, the degree of adherence to the prescribed diet, and differences in inherent biologic responsiveness to dietary modification. Women may have a somewhat smaller response than men (59). On average, men and women on a typical American diet should expect a 5% to 7% decrease in total cholesterol on the step I diet and an additional 3% to 7% reduction on the step II diet; those on a high-

Table 4.7 Dietary Treatment of Hypercholesterolemia

Nutrient	RECOMMENDED INTAKE	
	Step I Diet	Step II Diet
Total fat	≤30% of total calories	≤30% of total calories
Saturated fatty acids	8–10% of total calories	<7% of total calories
Polyunsaturated fatty acids	Up to 10% of total calories	Up to 10% of total calories
Monounsaturated fatty acids	Up to 15% of total calories	Up to 15% of total calories
Carbohydrates	≥55% of total calories	≥55% of total calories
Protein	Approximately 15% of total calories	Approximately 15% of total calories
Cholesterol	<300 mg/day	<200 mg/day
Total calories	To achieve and maintain desirable body weight	To achieve and maintain desirable body weight

Source: Expert Panel on Detection, Evaluation, and Treatment of High Blood Cholesterol in Adults. Second report of the Expert Panel on Detection, Evaluation, and Treatment of High Blood Cholesterol in Adults. NIH Publication No. 93-3095, September 1993.

fat diet typical of the 1960s, may experience a cholesterol reduction of up to 25% with intensive dietary therapy.

Repeat cholesterol determinations to assess the results of dietary therapy should be performed after 4 to 6 weeks and at 3 months. Adherence to the diet should be assessed at each follow-up visit and further dietary instruction provided. For "low risk" primary prevention patients, dietary therapy should be continued for at least 6 months; at that time, drug therapy should be considered for those who have not lowered their LDL-C below 190 mg/dL. For "high risk" primary prevention patients who do not achieve their LDL-C goal of less than 130 mg/dL after 6 months of dietary therapy, drug therapy should be considered for those whose other risk factors are difficult to modify and for those with particularly high LDL-C levels. A multifaceted approach that addresses not only the hyperlipidemia but all other risk factors is essential in these patients to minimize CHD risk. For secondary prevention patients, drug therapy should be considered if the goal of therapy has not been reached after 6 to 12 weeks of dietary therapy. The decision to proceed with drug therapy in patients who achieve an LDL-C between 100 and 129 mg/dL with dietary therapy alone should be individualized.

Pharmacologic Therapy of Lipid Disorders

Drug therapy should be used in addition to and not as a substitute for dietary therapy and lifestyle modifications. In most patients, drug therapy should be considered a lifetime commitment although discontinuation of medication may be possible in selected patients who are able to decrease their CHD risk over time by close adherence to lifestyle changes. LDL-C levels for initiation of drug therapy and LDL-C treatment goals are detailed in Table 4.6 for patient subsets stratified by CHD risk. Among young adult primary prevention patients without other risk factors for CHD, who are thus at low risk of developing CHD over the next decade, the level of LDL-C elevation after dietary therapy is an important factor in the decision to initiate drug therapy. Drug therapy for individuals with LDL-C above 220 mg/dL is generally considered appropriate; the choice is less clear for those with LDL-C between 190 and 220 mg/dL, but many investigators believe that therapy with the relatively safe bile acid sequestrants is justified even in the absence of other risk factors (56).

Many, if not most, hyperlipidemic patients with CHD will require drug therapy to achieve the more aggressive LDL-C goal of less than 100 mg/dL. Choice of individual agents is determined by the underlying lipoprotein phenotype, the efficacy and safety of the agent, its anticipated side effect profile, and its cost. Drug therapy should only be initiated if there is a reasonable expectation of benefit; patients with coexistent medical conditions that significantly limit survival may not be candidates for pharmacologic lipid lowering. Table 4.8 provides an overview of lipid-lowering agents described in more detail in the next section and

Table 4.8 Lipid-Lowering Drugs

DRUG	DOSE RANGE	EFFECT ON LIPIDS IN %*			MECHANISM	SIDE EFFECTS/ PRECAUTIONS
		LDL-C	HDL-C	TG		
Bile Acid Sequesrants						
Cholestyramine Colestipol	4–24 gm 5–30 gm	−10 to −30	+3 to +5	+15	Promote bile acid excretion, stimulate LDL receptors	GI symptoms; alters absorption of other drugs; increases TG level
Nicotinic Acid						
Regular Release Sustained Release[a]	1–6 gm 1–2 gm	−10 to −30	+15 to +40	−20 to −50	Decreases VLDL synthesis	Abnormal liver function; hyperglycemia; increases serum uric acid; heartburn; flushing; dry skin; peptic ulcer
Fibric Acid Derivatives[b]						
Gemfibrozil	1200 mg	−10 to −15	+10 to +15	−20 to −50	Decrease VLDL synthesis; stimulate lipoprotein lipase action	May increase LDL-C; increases lithogenicity of bile; myositis; GI distress; interacts with anti-coagulants; increased toxicity in patients with renal failure
HMG CoA Reductase Inhibitors						
Lovastatin Pravastatin Simvastatin Fluvastatin	10–80 mg 10–40 mg 5–40 mg 20–40 mg	−20 to −40	+5 to +15	−10 to −20	Inhibit cholesterol synthesis; induce LDL-receptor expression	Abnormal liver function; myositis; mild GI distress
Probucol						
	500 mg twice daily	−25	−10	0	Antioxidant; enhances non-LDL receptor-mediated removal of LDL	GI distress; prolonged QT interval; decreases HDL-C
Estrogen						
Premarin Micronized estradiol	0.625 mg 2 mg	−15	+15	variable increase	Increases VLDL production; increases LDL-receptor mediated removal of LDL; increases synthesis of Apo A-I	Endometrial hyperplasia; endometrial cancer; ? breast cancer

* There is marked individual variability and effects depend on the initial lipoprotein profile.
[a] Safety of sustained release niacin is not established.
[b] Clofibrate, another fibric acid derivative, is also available in the U.S., but is not widely used because of concerns about increased mortality.
GI, gastrointestinal; TG, triglyceride.

Table 4.9 Choice of Drugs by Lipoprotein Phenotype

Lipoprotein Phenotype	Choices of Single Drug Therapy	Choices for Combination Drug Therapy*
Type IIa	Resins Niacin Statins Estrogen in women	Resin with statin Resin with niacin Niacin with statin[a] Resin, niacin, and statin
Type IIb	Niacin Gemfibrozil Statins	If TG controlled: Niacin with resin Gemfibrozil with resin Statin with resin If TG still elevated: Niacin with statin[a] Niacin with gemfibrozil Gemfibrozil with statin[b]
Type III	Gemfibrozil Niacin Statins	Niacin with statin[a] Niacin with gemfibrozil Gemfibrozil with statin[b]
Type IV and V	Gemfibrozil Niacin Fish oil	Gemfibrozil with niacin
Isolated Low HDL	To increase HDL-C: Niacin Estrogen in women To decrease LDL-C: Niacin Statins Resin Estrogen in women	Statin with niacin[a] Statin with gemfibrozil[b] For patients with high normal TG: Niacin with gemfibrozil

* In women with LDL-C elevation or low HDL-C, estrogen should also be considered provided that the patients are not hypertriglyceridemic.
[a] Combination may be associated with increased risk of myopathy.
[b] Combination not approved by the Food and Drug Administration because of increased risk of myositis. May be used in selected cases only with careful monitoring.

Table 4.9 lists drugs of choice for specific lipoprotein phenotypes.

Follow-up LDL-C levels and chemistries tailored to the side effect profile of the lipid-lowering drug used should be measured after the patient has been on a stable dose of drug for about 6 weeks and again at about 12 weeks. Efficacy of drug therapy should be judged by the mean of these two determinations and doses of drugs titrated where appropriate. During the first year, follow-up at 3-month intervals is recommended by the NCEP; after that, follow-up intervals can be lengthened to 4 to 6 months if there is no evidence of toxicity. Adherence to lifestyle modification and to the drug treatment regimen should be encouraged at each follow-up visit.

Bile Acid Sequestrants

The bile acid sequestrants, cholestyramine and colestipol, are not absorbed from the gastrointestinal tract. They lower LDL-C by binding bile acids in the intestine. This interrupts the enterohepatic circulation of cholesterol, secondarily upregulates LDL receptors, and results in increased LDL clearance from the plasma. Sequestrants have a long-term safety record and have been shown to decrease clinical CHD risk and lesion progression (60–62). These agents may be particularly well suited for the treatment of young patients who require drug therapy but are otherwise at low risk. Adherence to these drugs is a problem because of unpleasant taste and frequent gastrointestinal side effects. Even low doses of these agents (8 gm cholestyramine or 10 gm colestipol daily in single or divided doses), however, cause 10% to 20% decreases in LDL-C; up to 30% LDL-C lowering can be achieved with doses up to 24 gm cholestyramine or equivalent. Bile acid sequestrants may increase hepatic VLDL production and are thus contraindicated in patients with untreated hypertriglyceridemia. Because both cholestyramine and colestipol can interfere with the absorption of other medications such as digitoxin, warfarin, thyroxine, thiazide diuretics, statins, and β blockers (and potentially many others), patients should be instructed to take other medications either 1 hour before or 4 hours after the sequestrant. A sample instructions sheet for patients detailing the use of resins is provided in the NCEP guidelines (56).

Niacin

Niacin (but not nicotinamide) at a dose of 1–6 gm reduces production of VLDL particles in the liver and lowers total cholesterol, LDL-C, and TG levels and increases HDL-C. In some cases, niacin may also significantly lower Lp(a) levels. Niacin is available in crystalline and sustained-release preparations. Clinical trials and angiographic regression studies have demonstrated the long-term safety and efficacy of crystalline niacin (62,63) although a number of adverse effects (flushing, hepatotoxicity, hyperglycemia, hyperuricemia and gout, skin changes, and gastrointestinal complaints) limit its use. The incidence of flushing can be decreased by gradual dose titration and premedication with aspirin or an antihistamine. A sample patient instruction sheet is included in the NCEP guidelines (56). Some patients may only be able to take the sustained-release form of niacin but should not exceed a dose of 2 gm and should be carefully monitored for hepatotoxicity, which is seen more frequently than with crystalline niacin preparations (64).

Reductase Inhibitors

Four hydroxymethylglutaryl coenzyme A (HMG CoA) reductase inhibitors are currently on the market—lovastatin, pravastatin, simvastatin, and fluvastatin. All four agents are generally given as a single dose in the evening; when lovastatin, pravastatin, and fluvastatin are used at higher doses, twice-a-day administration may achieve slightly higher efficacy. These agents are potent LDL-C-lowering drugs and work by inhibiting the rate-limiting enzyme of cholesterol synthesis, HMG CoA reductase, which results in upregulation of LDL receptors and enhanced LDL clearance from plasma. Statins also increase HDL-C by 5% to 15% and lower TG by up to 20%. Fluvastatin is the least and simvastatin the most potent of these drugs. Two angiographic regression trials have demonstrated the efficacy of lovastatin in limiting progression of coronary lesions and trials with the other agents are in progress (62,65). These agents are easy to administer and generally well tolerated, but side effects increase in a dose-dependent fashion. Most of the LDL-C lowering effect is achieved at low to moderate doses. If LDL-C goals are not achieved at these doses, combination therapy with a resin or niacin may be more efficacious and better tolerated than monotherapy at maximal doses of the reductase inhibitor. The most common side effects are gastrointestinal including dyspepsia, flatus, constipation, and abdominal discomfort. Significant transaminase elevations occur at higher doses in 1% to 2% of users but have aslo been observed with lower-dose therapy. Myopathy (myalgia and creatine kinase values more than 10 times normal) has been described with all statins; rhabdomyolysis with acute renal failure occurs rarely but is more likely when statins are used in combination with cyclosporine, gemfibrozil, erythromycin, and possibly niacin (56). In some patients, muscle complaints may occur in the absence of significant creatine kinase elevations and, if persistent, may require discontinuation of the drug. Creatine kinase measurements are highly variable and elevations are particularly likely after exercise. When asymptomatic and mild, these creatine kinase elevations should not lead to discontinuation of drug therapy. Statins may potentiate the effect of oral anticoagulants. They are contraindicated in pregnancy and should not be used by nursing mothers.

Fibric Acid Derivatives

Clofibrate and gemfibrozil are the two fibric acid derivatives currently marketed in the United States.

Both agents increase activity of lipoprotein lipase, which enhances VLDL catabolism, causes pronounced decreases in TG levels, and, secondarily, increases HDL-C. In patients with hypertriglyceridemia, LDL-C may paradoxically increase during fibrate therapy because of increased conversion of VLDL to LDL. In patients with high LDL-C levels, both fibrates cause modest LDL-C reductions. Although clofibrate decreased CHD events in the World Health Organization trial, total mortality was increased in this study (66). Most clinicians, therefore, prefer to use gemfibrozil, which decreased fatal and nonfatal myocardial infarctions in the Helsinki Heart Study, a primary prevention trial in men with dyslipidemia (67). The drug was most effective in the subgroup of men who had an LDL/HDL ratio greater than 5 and TG levels above 200 mg/dL (68). To date there is no secondary prevention trial using gemfibrozil. Although fibrates are generally well tolerated, they increase the lithogenicity of bile and may increase the likelihood of developing gallstones. Gemfibrozil in combination with lovastatin has been associated with myopathy and rhabdomyolysis; patients on combination therapy should be monitored carefully. Gemfibrozil also potentiates oral anticoagulants and may worsen renal dysfunction in patients with preexisting chronic renal insufficiency.

Other Agents

The role of probucol in lipid-lowering therapy is currently undefined (56). Despite its only modest LDL-C-lowering effects and despite reductions in HDL-C up to 20% to 30%, probucol has been reported to cause regression of xanthomas in patients with severe hypercholesterolemia. Its mechanism of action is unclear, but it may retard oxidative modification of LDL particles and may thus interfere with uptake of these particles by macrophages and with foam cell formation in atherosclerotic lesions. Probucol is generally well tolerated. Gastrointestinal side effects are most common. Prolongation of the QT interval by probucol has been associated with life-threatening ventricular arrhythmias. The drug is, therefore, contraindicated in patients with long QT syndrome and in those who receive other medications that cause QT prolongation and are thus predisposed to ventricular arrhythmias.

Although vitamins C and E have appeal as potential antioxidants and although epidemiologic studies suggest a reduction in CHD risk among men and women who use vitamin E supplements (69,70), the long-term safety and efficacy of this therapy have not been established. It is thus premature to recommend routine use of vitamins C and E in this setting.

Fish oil may be used as primary or adjunctive therapy in severe hypertriglyceridemia that is refractory to treatment with niacin or fibrates or in situations where side effects to these agents preclude their use. The long-term safety of fish oil use has not been established.

Hormone Replacement Therapy

Oral estrogen given at a dose of 0.625 mg Premarin or 2 mg micronized estradiol daily lowers LDL-C approximately 15% and increases HDL-C up to 15% in postmenopausal women. Because of the epidemiologic data cited above, the NCEP has tentatively endorsed estrogen therapy as a modality of lipid lowering among postmenopausal women. The apparent benefits of estrogen replacement therapy have to be balanced against the increased risks of endometrial hyperplasia, endometrial cancer, and possibly breast cancer. Oral estrogens are contraindicated in women with uncontrolled hypertriglyceridemia. Although addition of progestins may counteract some of the beneficial effects of estrogen on the lipoprotein profile, combination therapy appears to result in an overall favorable risk factor profile (28). Whether this improvement in the risk factor profile with combined estrogen/progestin therapy translates into protection from CHD is as yet unclear.

Combination Therapy

Options for combination therapy are detailed in Table 4.9. Although side effects of lipid-lowering drugs tend to be dose dependent, most of the lipid-lowering effects are generally achieved at low to moderate doses of these agents. Combining drugs with different mechanisms of action at submaximal doses of each thus improves both efficacy and safety and often results in cost savings when compared to drug monotherapy at maximal doses. Because resins are not absorbed, they can be safely added to statins, niacin, and gemfibrozil without enhancing toxicity provided that the patient is no longer hypertriglyceridemic. Combining statins with niacin or gemfibrozil may increase the potential for hepatotoxicity and myopathy. Patients on combination therapy with these agents require careful follow-up.

Special Issues

Treatment of Dyslipidemia in the Elderly

A high percentage of older individuals have high cholesterol levels (71). Although hypercholesterolemia remains a predictor of CHD in the elderly, the relative risk for any given level of LDL-C and HDL-C is lower in older than in younger individuals (30,31,33). Because the absolute risk of CHD is high in this age group, however, the CHD risk attributable to lipoprotein abnormalities is also higher than in young and middle-aged persons. The elderly as a group would thus be expected to benefit from lipid-lowering therapy. There is significant heterogeneity in functional status among the elderly, however, and lipid-lowering therapy should only be considered for those who are not otherwise severely disabled and whose prognosis is not significantly limited by other factors (56). Dietary therapy, weight loss, and regular physical activity are the mainstay of therapy for both primary and secondary prevention. Dietary therapy must be individualized and great care taken not to precipitate malnutrition. Drug therapy with cholestyramine, niacin, and gemfibrozil in the elderly may be associated with a higher incidence of side effects than in younger patients (56). Statins at low doses appear to be well tolerated. In a randomized pilot study of lovastatin therapy in the elderly, 20 mg lovastatin lowered total cholesterol by 17%, LDL-C by 24%, and TG by 4.4% and increased HDL-C by 7%; results with the 40-mg dose were only marginally better (71). Side effects were infrequent in both groups. Age alone should not preclude attempts at aggressive secondary prevention, but patients should be carefully selected.

Treatment of Diabetic Patients

Diabetes is a strong risk factor for CHD, particularly among women (39). In the NCEP guidelines, diabetes enters into the determination of treatment goals as one of several risk factors for CHD. In contrast, a 1989 consensus panel of the Amercian Diabetes Association suggested that diabetic patients require special consideration (20). The panel recommended that all diabetic adults undergo yearly fasting lipoprotein determinations and suggested that therapy be tailored to achieve an LDL-C less than 130 mg/dL. Others have recommended a more stringent LDL-C goal of less than 100 mg/dL for diabetic patients (19). Because VLDL levels also correlate with CHD risk, the same investigators further suggested that the combined fraction of VLDL-C plus LDL-C ("non–HDL-C") be targeted for therapy and recommended an ideal goal of under 130 mg/dL for non–HDL-C (19). The use of bile acid-binding resins is often limited in diabetic patients because of hypertriglyceridemia and niacin is at least relatively contraindicated because it worsens glucose control. Gemfibrozil is a reasonable choice for diabetic patients with significant hypertriglyceridemia and low HDL-C and statins appear to be the drugs of choice for those who have hypercholesterolemia with only modest hypertriglyceridemia.

Isolated Low High-Density Lipoprotein

Low HDL-C in the absence of frank hypercholesterolemia or hypertriglyceridemia is commonly seen in patients with CHD (12). To date it is unclear whether raising HDL-C reduces CHD risk, but meta-analyses of angiographic trials suggest an association between changes in HDL-C and regression of coronary lesions. Many patients with isolated low HDL-C have other risk factors for CHD that tend to lower HDL levels, such as obesity, smoking, physical inactivity, and diabetes. Modification of these risk factors should be a treatment priority. Drug treatment is aimed toward lowering LDL-C to less than 100 mg/dL and to increase HDL-C. Niacin may accomplish both and is the drug of choice in many patients. In some patients, statins may be required to achieve the LDL-C goal. In patients with high normal TG, niacin alone or in combination with gemfibrozil is a reasonable choice. In women, HDL-C may be favorably modified by the addition of estrogens. Alcohol consumption at low to moderate doses may increase HDL-C, but the risks of addiction should be carefully weighed against the anticipated benefits. In primary prevention patients with low HDL-C as their sole risk factor, drug treatment is currently not recommended by the NCEP (56).

Approach to Hypertriglyceridemia

Severe hypertriglyceridemia (TG above 1000 mg/dL)

and chylomicronemia predispose to pancreatitis. Nonpharmacologic treatment consists of dietary fat restriction, avoidance of alcohol and triglyceride-raising drugs (see above), and treatment of underlying disorders such as obesity and diabetes. Drug therapy should be initiated with the goal of lowering TG to below 500 mg/dL. Gemfibrozil and niacin are the drugs of choice in these disorders.

It is clear that hypertriglyceridemic patients with familial combined hyperlipidemia, type III hyperlipidemia, diabetes, central obesity, or a family history of premature CHD are at increased risk for CHD, whereas familial hypertriglyceridemia does not appear to predispose to CHD (38,56). There is currently no agreement on whether this increase in risk is due to direct atherogenicity of triglyceride-rich lipoproteins, to low HDL-C levels that occur as a consequence of hypertriglyceridemia, or both. Although no trial has been designed to specifically evaluate the effect of TG lowering on CHD risk, results from the Helsinki Heart Trial (68) and the Stockholm Ischemic Heart Disease Study (72) suggest that treatment of hypertriglyceridemia is beneficial in primary and secondary prevention of CHD. In the Helsinki Heart Trial, individuals with an LDL/HDL–cholesterol ratio greater than 5 and TG above 200 mg/dL had a more than three-fold increase in risk of cardiac events compared with those who had a high LDL/HDL ratio and lower TG and benefit with treatment was most pronounced in the high TG subgroup. In the Stockholm study, the reduction in 5-year mortality from ischemic heart disease was proportional to the degree of TG lowering.

As in severe hypertriglyceridemia, hygienic measures as outlined above are the primary forms of therapy for patients with more moderate TG elevations. For those perceived to be at high risk for CHD, drug therapy aims to reduce LDL-C, to increase HDL-C, and to reduce potentially atherogenic VLDL and chylomicron remnants. Nicotinic acid and gemfibrozil are the drugs of choice. Statins are a reasonable alternative in patients with mild TG elevations.

REFERENCES

1. Heart and stroke facts. 1994 statistical supplement. Dallas: American Heart Association, 1993:1–22.

2. Eaker ED, Chesebro JH, Sacks FM, Wenger NK, Whisnant JP, Winston M. Cardiovascular disease in women. AHA medical/scientific statement. Circulation 1993;88:1999–2009.

3. Day JC. Population projections of the United States by age, sex, race, and Hispanic origin: 1993 to 2050. In: U.S. Bureau of the Census: current population reports. Washington, DC: U.S. Government Printing Office, 1993:25–1104.

4. Johnson CL, Rifkind BM, Sempos CT, et al. Declining serum total cholesterol levels among US adults. The National Health and Nutrition Examination Surveys. JAMA 1993;269:3002–3008.

5. Sempos CT, Cleeman JI, Carroll MD, et al. Prevalence of high blood cholesterol among US adults. An update based on guidelines from the second report of the National Cholesterol Education Program Adult Treatment Panel. JAMA 1993;269:3009–3014.

6. Segrest JP, Brouillette CG, Harvey SC, Anantharamaiah GM. The amphipathic alpha-helix: a multifunctional structural motif in plasma apolipoproteins. In: Anfinsen CB, Edsall JT, Richards FM, Eisenberg DS, eds. Advances in protein chemistry, vol. 45. San Diego: Academic Press, 1994:

7. Bittner V. Atherogenicity of postprandial lipoproteins and coronary heart disease. The Endocrinologist 1994;4(5):359–372.

8. Austin MA, Breslow JL, Hennekens CH, Buring JE, Willett WC, Krauss RM. Low-density lipoprotein subclass patterns and risk of myocardial infarction. JAMA 1988;260:1917–1921.

9. Sacks FM, McPherson R, Walsh BW. Effect of postmenopausal estrogen replacement on plasma Lp(a) lipoprotein concentrations. Arch Intern Med 1994;154:1106–1110.

10. The Laboratory Standardization Panel of the National Cholesterol Education Program. Recommendations for improving cholesterol measurement. NIH Publication No. 90–2964, 1990:1–63.

11. Oberman A, Kreisberg RA, Henkin Y. Principles and management of lipid disorders. A primary care approach. Baltimore: Williams & Wilkins, 1992:1–323.

12. Schaefer EJ, Genest JJ Jr, Ordovas JM, Salem DN, Wilson PWF. Familial lipoprotein disorders and premature coronary artery disease. Curr Opin Lipidol 1993;4:288–298.

13. Schonfeld G. The genetic dyslipoproteinemias—nosology update 1990. Atherosclerosis 1990;81:81–93.

14. Chait A, Brunzell JD. Acquired hyperlipidemia (secondary dyslipoproteinemias). Endocrinol Metab Clin North Am 1990;19:259–278.

15. Denke MA, Sempos CT, Grundy SM. Excess body weight. An underrecognized contributor to high blood

cholesterol levels in white American men. Arch Intern Med 1993;153:1093–1103.

16. Denke MA, Sempos CT, Grundy SM. Excess body weight. An underrecognized contributor to dyslipidemia in white American women. Arch Intern Med 1993;154:401–410.

17. Reaven GM. Insulin resistance and compensatory hyperinsulinemia: role in hypertension, dyslipidemia, and coronary heart disease. Am Heart J 1991;121:1283–1288.

18. DeFronzo RA, Ferrannini E. Insulin resistance. A multifaceted syndrome responsible for NIDDM, obesity, hypertension, dyslipidemia, and atherosclerotic cardiovascular disease. Diabetes Care 1991;14:173–194.

19. Garg A, Grundy SM. Management of dyslipidemia in NIDDM. Diabetes Care 1990;13:153–169.

20. Dunn FL. Management of hyperlipidemia in diabetes mellitus. Endocrinol Metab Clin North Am 1992;21:395–414.

21. Langer RD, Criqui MH, Reed DM. Lipoproteins and blood pressure as biological pathways for effect of moderate alcohol consumption on coronary heart disease. Circulation 1992;85:910–915.

22. Garg R, Wagener DK, Madans JH. Alcohol consumption and risk of ischemic heart disease in women. Arch Intern Med 1993;153:1211–1216.

23. Oettgen P, Ginsburg GS, Horowitz GL, Pasternak RC. Frequency of hypothyroidism in adults with serum total cholesterol levels >200 mg/dl. Am J Cardiol 1994;73:955–957.

24. Henkin Y, Como JA, Oberman A. Secondary dyslipidemia. Inadvertent effects of drugs in clinical practice. JAMA 1992;267:961–968.

25. Byington RP, Worthy J, Craven T, Furberg CD. Propranolol-induced lipid changes and their prognostic significance after a myocardial infarction: the Beta-Blocker Heart Attack Trial Experience. Am J Cardiol 1990;65:1287–1291.

26. Cruickshank JM. Beta-blockers, plasma lipids, and coronary heart disease. Circulation 1990;82(suppl II):60–65.

27. Grady D, Rubin SM, Petitti DB, et al. Hormone therapy to prevent disease and prolong life in postmenopausal women. Ann Intern Med 1992;177:1016–1037.

28. Nabulsi AA, Folsom AR, White A, et al. Association of hormone-replacement therapy with various cardiovascular risk factors in postmenopausal women. N Engl J Med 1993;328:1069–1075.

29. Bittner V, Oberman A. Epidemiology of coronary heart disease. In: Roubin GS, Califf RM, O'Neill WW, Phillips III HR, Stack RS, eds. Interventional cardiovascular medicine. Principles and practice. New York: Churchill Livingstone, 1994:147–164.

30. Stamler J, Wentworth D, Neaton JD, et al. Is the relationship between serum cholesterol and risk of premature death from coronary heart disease continuous and graded? Findings in 356,222 primary screenees of the Multiple Risk Factor Intervention Trial (MRFIT). JAMA 1986;256:2823–2828.

31. Anderson KM, Castelli WP, Levy DL. Cholesterol and mortality: 30 years of follow-up from the Framingham study. JAMA 1987;257:2176–2180.

32. Castelli WP, Garrison RJ, Wilson PW, et al. Incidence of coronary heart disease and lipoprotein cholesterol levels. The Framingham Study. JAMA 1986;256:2835–2838.

33. Denke MA, Grundy SM. Hypercholesterolemia in elderly persons: resolving the treatment dilemma. Ann Intern Med 1990;112:780–792.

34. Brunner D, Weisbort J, Meshulam N, et al. Relation of serum total cholesterol and high density lipoprotein cholesterol percentage to the incidence of definite coronary events: twenty-year follow-up of the Donolo-Tel Aviv Prospective Coronary Artery Disease Study. Am J Cardiol 1987;59:1271–1276.

35. Bass KM, Newschaffer CJ, Klag MJ, Bush TL. Plasma lipoprotein levels as predictors of cardiovascular death in women. Arch Intern Med 1993;153:2209–2216.

36. Gordon DJ, Rifkind BM. High density lipoprotein – the clinical implications of recent studies. N Engl J Med 1989;321:1311–1316.

37. Gordon T, Castelli WP, Hjortland MC, Kannel WB, Dawber TR. High density lipoprotein as a protective factor against coronary heart disease. The Framingham Study. Am J Med 1977;62:707–714.

38. Austin M. Plasma triglyceride and coronary heart disease. Arterioscler Thromb 1991;11:2–14.

39. Lerner DJ, Kannel WB. Patterns of coronary heart disease morbidity and mortality in the sexes: a 26-year follow-up of the Framingham population. Am Heart J 1986;111:383–390.

40. Van Stiphout WAHJ, Hofman A, de Bruijn AM. Serum lipids in young women before, during, and after pregnancy. Am J Epidemiol 1987;126:922–928.

41. Ness RB, Harris T, Cobb J, et al. Number of pregnancies and the subsequent risk of cardiovascular disease. N Engl J Med 1993;328:1528–1533.

42. Kannel WB, Hjortland MC, McNamara PM, Gordon T. Menopause and risk of cardiovascular disease. The Framingham Study. Ann Intern Med 1976;85:447–452.

43. van Beresteijn ECH, Korevaar JC, Huijbregts PCW, Schouten EG, Burema J, Kok FJ. Perimenopausal increase in serum cholesterol: a 10-year longitudinal study. Am J Epidemiol 1993;137:383–392.

44. Matthews KA, Meilahn E, Kuller LH, Kelsey SF, Caggiula AW, Wing RR. Menopause and risk factors for coronary heart disease. N Engl J Med 1989;321: 641–646.

45. Bonithon-Kopp C, Scarabin PY, Darne B, Malmejac A, Guize L. Menopause-related changes in lipoproteins and some other cardiovascular risk factors. Int J Epidemiol 1990;19:42–48.

46. Holme I. An analysis of randomized trials evaluating the effect of cholesterol reduction on total mortality and coronary heart disease incidence. Circulation 1990;82:1916–1924.

47. LaRosa JC. Cholesterol lowering, low cholesterol, and mortality. Am J Cardiol 1993;72:776–786.

48. Vos J, de Feyter PJ, Simoons ML, Tijssen JGP, Deckers JW. Retardation and arrest of progression or regression of coronary artery disease: a review. Prog Cardiovasc Dis 1993;35:435–454.

49. Kane JP, Malloy MJ, Ports TA, et al. Regression of coronary atherosclerosis during treatment of familial hypercholesterolemia with combined drug regimens. JAMA 1990;264:3007–3012.

50. Waters D, Craven TE, Lesperance J. Prognostic significance of progression of coronary atherosclerosis. Circulation 1993;87:1067–1075.

51. Stamler J, Stamler R, Brown WV, et al. Serum cholesterol. Doing the right thing. Circulation 1993;88:1954–1960.

52. Klag MJ, Ford DE, Mead LA, et al. Serum cholesterol in young men and subsequent cardiovascular disease. N Engl J Med 1993;328:313–318.

53. Meilahn EN, Ferrell RE. 'Naturally occurring' low blood cholesterol and excess mortality. Coron Artery Dis 1993;4:843–853.

54. Muldoon MF, Manuck SB, Matthews KA. Lowering cholesterol concentrations and mortality: a quantitative review of primary prevention trials. Br Med J 1990;301:309–314.

55. Smith GD, Song F, Sheldon TA. Cholesterol lowering and mortality: the importance of considering initial level of risk. Br Med J 1993;306:1367–1373.

56. Expert Panel on Detection, Evaluation, and Treatment of High Blood Cholesterol in Adults. Second report of the Expert Panel on Detection, Evaluation, and Treatment of High Blood Cholesterol in Adults. NIH Publication No. 93-3095, September 1993:O-1–R-32.

57. Ornish D, Brown SE, Scherwitz LW, et al. Can lifestyle changes reverse coronary heart disease: the Lifestyle Heart Trial. Lancet 1990;336:129–133.

58. Hambrecht R, Niebauer J, Marburger C, et al. Various intensities of leisure time physical activity in patients with coronary artery disease: effects on cardiorespiratory fitness and progression of coronary atherosclerotic lesions. J Am Coll Cardiol 1993;22:468–477.

59. Boyd NF, Cousins M, Beaton M, Kriukov V, Lockwood G, Tritchler D. Quantitative changes in dietary fat intake and serum cholesterol in women: results from a randomized, controlled trial. Am J Nutr 1990;52:470–476.

60. Lipid Research Clinics Program. The Lipid Research Clinics Coronary Primary Prevention Trial results. I. Reduction in incidence of coronary heart disease. JAMA 1984;251:351–364.

61. Blankenhorn DH, Nessim SA, Johnson RL, et al. Beneficial effects of combined colestipol-niacin therapy on coronary atherosclerosis and coronary venous bypass grafts. JAMA 1987;257:3233–3240.

62. Brown G, Albers JJ, Fisher LD, et al. Regression of coronary artery disease as a result of intensive lipid-lowering therapy in men with high levels of apolipoprotein B. N Engl J Med 1990;323:1289–1298.

63. Canner PL, Berge KG, Wenger NK, et al. Fifteen year mortality in Coronary Drug Project patients: long-term benefit with niacin. J Am Coll Cardiol 1986;8:1245–1255.

64. McKenney JM, Proctor JD, Harris S, Chinchili VM. A comparison of the efficacy and toxic effects of sustained- vs immediate-release niacin in hypercholesterolemic patients. JAMA 1994;271:672–677.

65. Blankenhorn DH, Azen SP, Kramsch DM, et al. Coronary angiographic changes with lovastatin therapy. The Monitored Atherosclerosis Regression Study (MARS). Ann Intern Med 1993;119:969–976.

66. Committee of Principal Investigators World Health Organization. W.H.O. cooperative trial on primary prevention of ischaemic heart disease using clofibrate to lower serum cholesterol: mortality follow-up. Lancet 1980;2:379–385.

67. Frick MH, Elo O, Haapa K, et al. Helsinki Heart Study: a primary-prevention trial with gemfibrozil in middle-aged men with dyslipidemia. Safety of treatment, changes in risk factors, and incidence of coronary heart disease. N Engl J Med 1987;317:1237–1245.

68. Manninen V, Tenkanen L, Koskinen P, et al. Joint effects of serum triglyceride and LDL cholesterol and HDL cholesterol concentrations in coronary heart disease risk in the Helsinki Heart Study: implications for treatment. Circulation 1992;85:37–45.

69. Stampfer MJ, Hennekens CH, Manson JAE, et al. Vitamin E consumption and the risk of coronary disease in women. N Engl J Med 1993;328:1444–1449.

70. Rimm EB, Stampfer MJ, Ascherio A, et al. Vitamin E consumption and the risk of coronary disease in men. N Engl J Med 1993;328:1450–1456.

71. LaRosa JC, Applegate W, Crouse JR, et al. Cholesterol lowering in the elderly. Results of the Cholesterol Reduction in Seniors Program (CRISP) Pilot Study. Arch Intern Med 1994;154:529–539.

72. Carlson LA, Rosenhamer G. Reduction of mortality in the Stockholm ischaemic heart disease secondary prevention study by combined treatment with clofibrate and nicotinic acid. Acta Med Scand 1988;223:404–418.

CHAPTER 5

PERIPHERAL VASCULAR DISEASE

Sriram S. Iyer, Michael Jaff,
Gary S. Roubin, Gerald Dorros

Among the diseases afflicting women, cardiovascular aliments account for greater mortality than do cancer, diabetes, and accidents combined (1). Atherosclerotic peripheral vascular (arterial) disease accounts for a significant portion of the morbidity and subsequent mortality from cardiovascular diseases and venous thromboembolic disease is a not uncommon, potentially lethal, disorder. Although peripheral vascular disease occurs predominantly in men, women are not exempt from this problem. On the basis of large population studies (e.g., Framingham study) and other observational data, certain unique features of this condition in women have been recognized. Significant vascular disease whether in the coronary, cerebrovascular, or peripheral distribution is distinctly unusual in the premenopausal nondiabetic, nonsmoking individual. This observation is perhaps related to protective hormonal factors, the latter having a favorable effect on the serum concentrations of high-density lipoprotein (HDL) cholesterol and triglycerides (2). More recently, the effects of estrogen and progesterone on lipoprotein (a) (Lp[a]) have been reported. Lp(a), a unique, cholesterol-rich plasma lipoprotein with structural homology to plasminogen, is considered to be one of the most atherogenic and thrombogenic molecules studied. Compared to a control group, postmenopausal women treated with estrogen and progesterone showed a 50% decrease in Lp(a) levels after 6 months of treatment (3).

Atherosclerotic disease involves the lower extremities much more often than the upper extremities. Hence, if the vascular problem involves the upper extremities and hands, the clinician should look for nonatherosclerotic causes (e.g., arteritis). Broadly, occlusive arterial disease can be divided into acute and chronic categories. Causes of acute arterial occlusion include embolic occlusion, luminal compression by dissection flaps, such as progressive central aortic dissection extending into the subclavian artery, trauma, etc. Features suggesting that the cause of occlusive peripheral arterial disease may be an uncommon type include: 1) its occurrence in patients under age 40; 2) digits of the upper extremity are involved; 3) acute presentation; and 4) vascular disease in the nondiabetic, nonsmoking premenopausal woman (4). The most common cause of chronic occlusive arterial disease is atherosclerosis (arteriosclerosis obliterans). This chapter reviews the clinical approach to and the management of women with atherosclerotic disease affecting the peripheral arterial vessels and also briefly comments on venous thromboembolic disease and venous varicosities.

Accelerated Atherosclerosis in Premenopausal Women—The Risk Factors of Diabetes Mellitus and Tobacco Abuse

The protective hormonal effects alluded to above are offset by diabetes mellitus and cigarette smoking. Reporting from the Framingham data and using carotid bruits and absent pedal pulses as future markers of cerebral and peripheral vascular disease, Abbott and colleagues noted that diabetic women younger than 60 years had a higher incidence of carotid bruits (×2.7) and absent pedal pulses (×2.0) when compared to their nondiabetic counterparts (5). Further, women may be more susceptible to the vascular complications of long-standing diabetes especially in the below-knee distribution. Orchard and colleagues reported a 30% incidence of lower extremity peripheral vascular disease in women with long-standing (over 30 years), insulin-dependent diabetes mellitus compared to a 11% incidence in men. Interestingly, there was no difference in the incidence of atherosclerosis in the cerebral or coronary distributions (6).

Tobacco use is an independent risk factor for atherosclerosis, across the board, for all age groups, in both genders. The vast majority of patients with atherosclerotic vascular disease are either current smokers or have a history of tobacco use. Smokers have a higher incidence of claudication (approximately twice that of nonsmokers in both genders) and the risk of stroke in women who smoke is substantially higher (7).

On the basis of the vascular distribution involved, peripheral vascular disease can be subdivided into three broad groups—lower extremity disease, brachiocephalic disease, and abdominal aortic disease.

Group I: Lower Extremity Disease

This includes lesions involving the distal (infrarenal) abdominal aorta, aortoiliac, iliofemoral, femoral, popliteal, and tibioperoneal arteries. The atherosclerotic lesions may be focal, segmental, or diffuse. Diffuse vascular involvement, particularly of the tibial and peroneal arteries (below-knee vessels), is a situation frequently encountered in the patient with long-standing diabetes and presents a difficult therapeutic problem. Such diffusely diseased vessels are not suitable targets for vascular grafting and have a high frequency of restenosis after percutaneous interventional techniques. The symptomatic status of the patient with stenotic vascular disease of the lower extremities is influenced not only by the degree of stenosis severity but also by the adequacy of the collateral circulation. The latter depends on the integrity of the profunda (deep) femoris system.

The classic presentation in this group is *intermittent claudication*, the symptomatic hallmark of occlusive peripheral vascular disease. Intermittent claudication or leg pain after walking is usually described as an aching, squeezing pain in the major muscle groups of the legs. The discomfort only occurs with walking and is relieved by rest. Patients report a consistent pain-free walking distance (the claudication distance) before the onset of discomfort. The muscle groups involved reflect vessel stenosis or occlusion one segment proximal. Patients most frequently report pain; at times they complain of a "tight sensation," "feeling of tiredness," "unable to walk," or "paresthesia" in the legs. Although these latter symptoms maybe the result of arterial insufficiency, the more atypical the symptoms, the greater should be the search for nonvascular causes. The nonvascular causes arise from muscular and skeletal problems and include joint disorders, neurogenic causes, intrinsic muscle diseases, and lumbosacral spine syndromes. A careful history and clinical examination can help the physician establish the correct diagnosis.

Pseudoclaudication, symptoms attributable to lumbar canal stenosis, manifests more as paresthesia as opposed to pain. Like vascular claudication, symptoms are brought on by walking; however, unlike classic vascular claudication, the symptoms of pseudoclaudication persist with standing still but are usually relieved by lying down. This is because symptoms of lumbar canal stenosis are attributable to lumbar spine extension, a situation that persists with standing and walking but relieved by sitting, which flexes the lumbar spine. Whereas claudication distances (at least over the short term) are usually constant, pseudoclaudication occurs at varying distances and when questioned patients frequently offer a history of arthritic disorders or spine trauma.

The location of the claudication distress in the lower extremity is of some value in localizing the occlusive arterial disease because the latter is always proximal to the level of the discomfort, although not necessarily immediately proximal. Thus, stenosis or occlusion at the level of the popliteal artery usually results in claudication of the calf muscles and of the foot and patients usually do not complain of thigh, hip, or buttock pain. Stenosis of the distal abdominal aorta and especially of the iliac and femoral arteries can cause claudication discomfort not only in the calf but also in the thigh, hip, and buttock. Rest pain is usually the result of severe peripheral vascular disease with inadequate collaterals and typically involves the arch of the foot and toes. The pain is much worse at night and patients report improvement by placing the limbs in a dependent position, often resulting in them sleeping with their ischemic limb hanging over the side of the bed in an effort to get some relief. This may lead to dependent edema, which can initially confuse the diagnosis with acute deep vein thrombosis. Rest pain is generally aggravated by limb elevation and exposure to cold.

Ischemic ulcerations (Fig 5.1) classically occur in the most distal portions of the foot (toes, heel) or over areas of bony prominences. The lesions are usually severely painful and often the triggering event is trauma. Because ischemic tissue heals poorly after skin and tissue breakdown, even minimal trauma can result in terrible ischemic ulcerations. Regardless of the location, ischemic ulcers appear dry and pale, enlarge over time, and usually have discrete ulcer edges. Gangrene is the further deterioration of tissue viability as a result of inadequate arterial supply causing necrosis classically in distal areas of the foot. The syndrome of atheroembolism-embolic occlusion of the arterioles supplying the dermis as well as the digital arteries by atheromatous debris from atherosclerotic plaque gives rise to a classic picture that consists of livedo reticularis and blue toes (Fig 5.2) and at times hypertension and renal insufficiency, the latter resulting from embolization of the renal arteries (8,9). Etiology of "ischemic-appearing" ulcerations in less common locations include vasculitis, atherosclerosis with superimposed trauma, and insect bites (brown recluse spider).

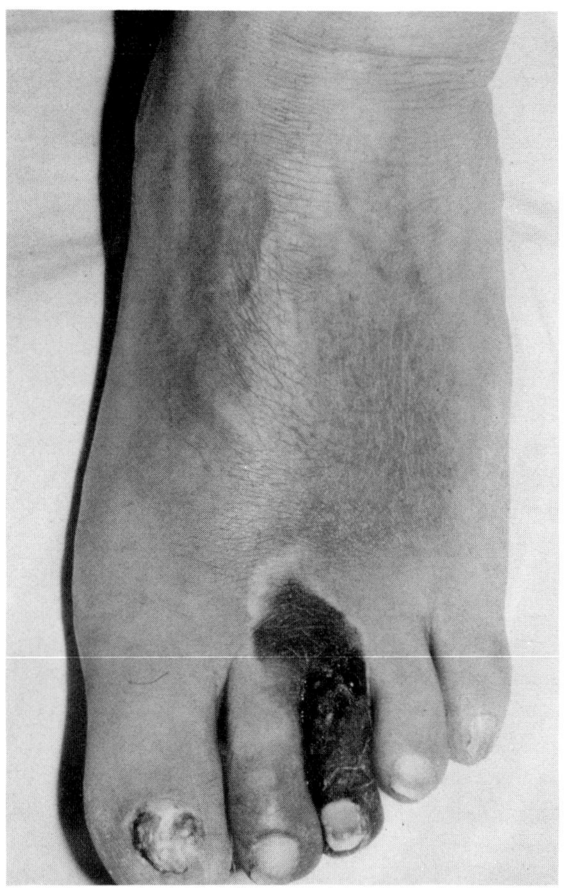

Fig 5.1 Left foot. Gangrene of left third toe, cyanosis of left second toe. Superficial thrombophlebitis on dorsum of left foot. Diagnosis: thromboangiitis obliterans (Burger's disease).

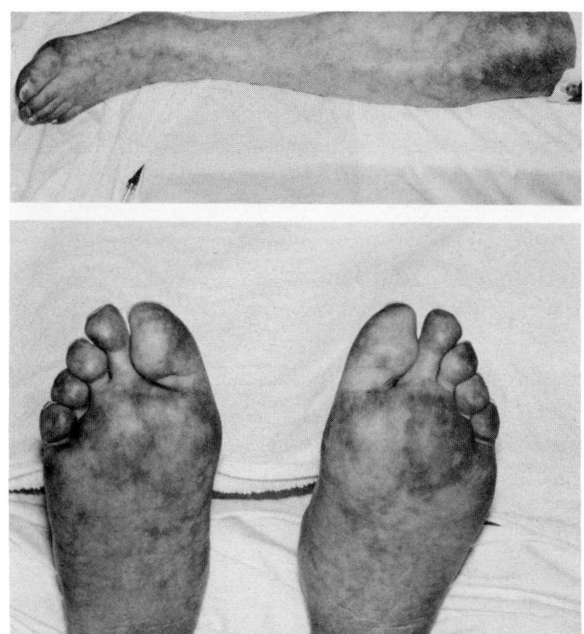

Fig 5.2 Atheroembolic disease of lower extremities after cardiac catheterization.

Clinical Evaluation

The diagnosis of peripheral vascular disease is relatively easy in the symptomatic patient and often can be deduced from the history. Patients with milder forms of peripheral vascular disease are often asymptomatic. A careful clinical examination as outlined in the following paragraphs will be helpful in arriving at the diagnosis. After the clinician obtains a detailed history, the examination begins with an evaluation of the peripheral pulses beginning with the carotids and following through with the axillary, brachials, radials, abdominal aorta, femorals, popliteals, and pedal pulses. The examiner notes the presence or absence, the amplitude, and the symmetry of the pulses and records the findings with the patient at rest. The examiner should next auscultate the larger arteries (carotids, subclavian, abdominal aorta, femorals, and popliteals) to detect bruits. The presence of a bruit indicates that there is turbulence of flow and often there is a stenosis proximal to the site of the bruit. Most often systolic in timing, at times the bruit extends into diastole and is indicative of a stenosis severe enough to produce a gradient throughout the cardiac cycle. Next, the examiner performs elevation and dependency tests. The elevation tests are based on the time it takes for the development of pallor after elevating the extremity at an angle of 60° for 1 minute. The rapidity with which the pallor develops has been graded (Table 5.1). (*Note*: even grade 1 pallor indicates a significant degree of occlusive arterial disease.) Next, the examiner should observe the patient with the extremity hanging down and note the time it takes for the color to return and for venous filling to be complete. As shown in Table 5.2, the longer it takes for color to return and for venous filling to be complete the more severe the ischemia. Finally, palpable pedal pulses that disappear after moderate exercise likely suggest proximal arterial disease (10). Development of bruits over the femoral and popliteal arteries after exercise may be the result of arterial stenosis that is not severe enough to produce a bruit at rest (11). Other examination findings including loss of hair, dry skin, dystrophic nails, coolness of feet, and cyanotic toes are nonspecific and usually not of any major help in the diagnosis of occlusive peripheral vascular disease.

Table 5.1 Grading of Elevation Pallor

Grade of Pallor	Duration of Elevation
0	No pallor in 60 sec
1	Definite pallor in 60 sec
2	Definite pallor in <60 sec
3	Definite pallor in <30 sec
4	Pallor on the level

Reproduced by permission from Spittell JA. Recognition and management of chronic atherosclerotic occlusive peripheral arterial disease. Mod Concepts Cardiovasc Dis 1981;50:19–23.

Table 5.2 Color Return (CR) and Venous Filling Time (VFT)

Condition	Time for CT (Sec)	VFT (Sec)
Normal	10	15
Moderate ischemia	15–20	20–30
Severe ischemia	>40	>40

Reproduced by permission from Spittell JA. Recognition and management of chronic atherosclerotic occlusive peripheral arterial disease. Mod Concepts Cardiovasc Dis 1981;50:19–23.

Noninvasive Evaluation

Noninvasive tests can be performed to document the presence of occlusive peripheral vascular disease, localize the site of obstruction, and help add an element of reproducible objectivity to the evaluation.

Ankle Brachial Index

The ankle brachial index is a simple, inexpensive, and reproducible method of assessing the overall severity of peripheral vascular disease. The brachial artery systolic blood pressure is obtained with a handheld Doppler monitor. A sphygmomanometer cuff is then placed around the distal calf and is inflated above the brachial systolic pressure. The handheld Doppler is then placed over each pedal artery (dorsalis pedis and posterior tibial). The first Doppler signal heard as the cuff pressure is released is the pressure in that vessel. An index is then obtained by dividing the pedal pressure by the brachial pressure. An index of 0.95 or greater is normal; an index of 0.5 or less indicates severe peripheral vascular disease. Generally, indices below this level will not heal ischemic ulcers and these patients are more likely to have rest pain and are at high risk for gangrene and limb loss. In women with a low ankle brachial index, the relative risk of mortality from all causes in general and those from cardiovascular disease in particular ranges from 1.9 to 4.0 (12–14). The assessment of the ankle brachial index before and after exercise enhances the detection of occlusive arterial disease because the difference in systolic pressure between the ankle and the arm is magnified after exercise. Other methods of evaluation include segmental pressure analysis (Fig 5.3) (the blood pressure cuff is placed at different levels in the leg), Doppler or pulse volume wave form analysis to assess levels of disease, and color duplex ultrasonography, which offers specific identification of level of obstruction and severity of disease.

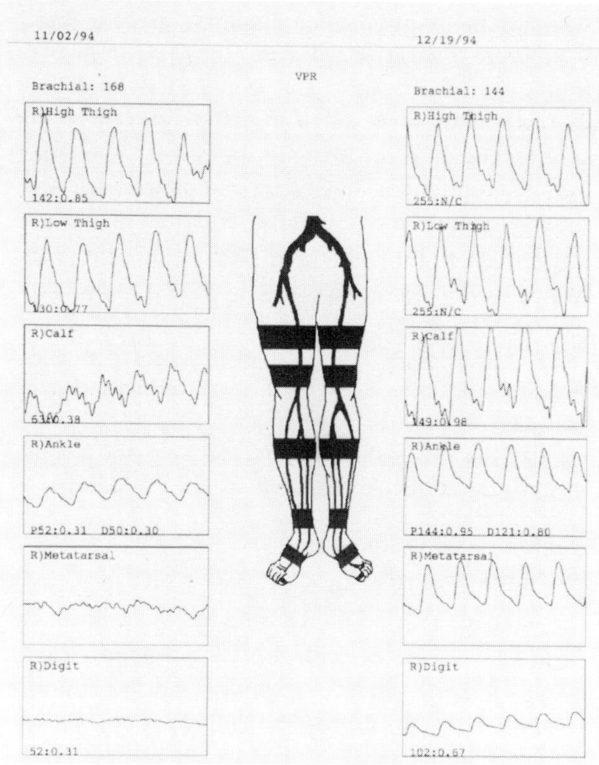

Fig 5.3 Segmental pressures and pulse volume recordings. 11/02/94—thrombosed right femoral-popliteal bypass graft; 12/19/94—status after thrombolytic therapy and stent placement.

Transcutaneous Oximetry

Transcutaneous oximetry is a noninvasive, indirect measurement of local blood flow. It uses the polarographic technique. Two electrodes are placed on the skin—one acts as a sensor, the other is a reference point. Oxygen diffusion from the tissues and skin to the membrane causes a chemical reaction, which ultimately generates an electric current. This current allows for an indirect measurement of transcutaneous oximetry pressures ($TcPo_2$). In practice, transcutaneous oximetry is determined on the chest (below the clavicle) and then compared to values obtained on the involved limb. A significantly lower limb $TcPo_2$ suggests arterial disease as the cause for diminished transcutaneous oximetry. Limitations of transcutaneous oximetry are related to variable skin properties, including capillary density, the presence of edema, skin thickness, diseases of the skin, and overall cellular metabolism at this level. Often, the initial transcutaneous oximetry measurement is compared to a second measurement during inhalation of 100% oxygen. This has been thought to more accurately predict limb healing when considering lower extremity amputations. Despite some widely varying values in relation to wound healing, $TcPo_2$ levels less than 20 mmHg suggest a bad prognosis, whereas values greater than 40 mm Hg correlate with more hopeful probabilities of wound healing.

Magnetic Resonance Angiography

It is to be anticipated that as much of the therapeutic work in managing patients with vascular disease moves from the surgical suite to the percutaneous route, in a parallel fashion much of the diagnostic work may move from the invasive to the noninvasive laboratory. A rapidly developing method for assessing the cerebral and peripheral vasculature is magnetic resonance angiography (MRA). Medical magnetic resonance imaging (MRI) uses a strong external magnetic field, rapidly switching gradients of local magnetic field strength and pulses of radiofrequency energy to produce high-resolution images of soft tissues and vascular anatomy. MRI is noninvasive, requires no contrast injection, and provides detailed information regarding flow in normal and diseased vascular segments. Patients with peripheral vascular disease can be evaluated using MRA. Figure 5.4 is an example of noninvasive iliofemoral MRA in a patient with unilateral high-grade focal stenosis. A recent report by Owen and colleagues suggests that MRA may be more sensitive than invasive contrast angiography in detecting peripheral runoff vessels in patients with severe peripheral arterial occlusive disease (15). We can expect many more developments in magnetic resonance methods and the interested reader is referred to several recent reviews that describe the clinical usefulness of cardiovascular MRI in general and MRA in particular (16,17).

Management of Lower Extremity Peripheral Vascular Disease

General Principles

Irrespective of the location of the atherosclerotic vascular disease and regardless of the type of intervention performed, risk factor modification is an important tenet of management. Controlling hypertension and

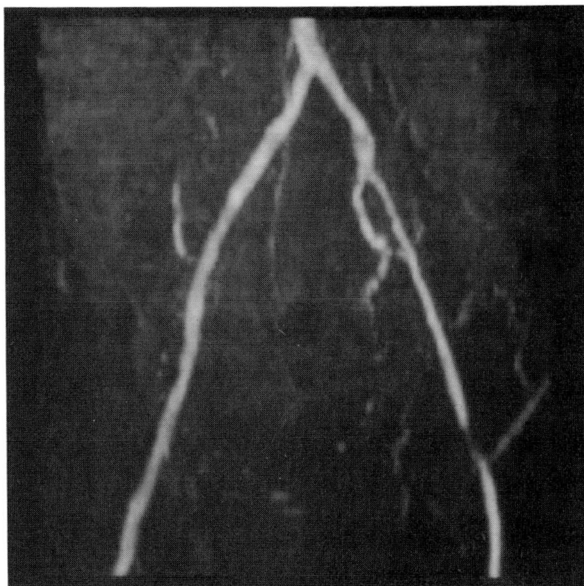

Fig 5.4 Noninvasive iliofemoral magnetic resonance angiography in a patient with high-grade focal left iliac stenosis.

diabetes mellitus, attaining ideal body weight, and stopping tobacco use are of paramount importance. The risk of atherosclerosis decreases soon after cessation of tobacco use and continues to decline over the next 10 to 15 years (18,19). Patients who continue to smoke can expect progression of symptoms (intermittent claudication advancing to rest pain) and have a higher incidence of limb and graft loss (20). Aggressive treatment of hyperlipidemia is recommended beginning with diet therapy and progressing to the various lipid-lowering drugs. If not otherwise contraindicated, use of postmenopausal hormonal replacement therapy must be considered given the high incidence of atherosclerotic coronary artery disease in patients with peripheral vascular disease. A 40% to 50% decrease in risk of significant coronary disease has been shown with the use of estrogen therapy (21). In addition, estrogen has a favorable impact on lipids—increasing HDL and lowering low-density lipoproteins (LDL) and total cholesterol (22). Based on a history of angina pectoris, prior myocardial infarction, transient ischemic attack, or stroke, other noninvasive tests should be performed.

Because peripheral arterial disease is a marker for coronary atherosclerosis and confers a 25% increase in mortality in comparison to similiar patients without peripheral vascular disease (23,24), all patients with documented peripheral vascular disease should undergo assessment to confirm the presence or rule out significant coronary artery disease. The presence of a carotid bruit on examination should prompt carotid duplex ultrasonograpy. If physical examination suggests presence of abdominal aortic or peripheral arterial aneurysms ultrasound, computed tomography (CT) scan, or MRI studies should be requested.

Laboratory assessment of renal function, hemogoblin/hematocrit, platelet counts, coagulation tests (prothrombin time, partial thromboplastin time), lipid profile (total cholesterol, HDL, triglycerides), and glucose should be obtained at the same time as the referral to the noninvasive vascular laboratory is planned.

Specific Recommendations

Local Care: The need for fastidious *skin and foot care* cannot be overstated. The importance of soft well-fitting footwear and avoidance of trauma to the ischemic limb needs to be repeatedly emphasized.

Medications: Although *thrombolytic* treatment (frequently prolonged local infusion of urokinase) is at times useful as part of the strategy in treating acute limb ischemia or graft occlusion, lytic therapy, in general, does not have an established role in the management of patients with stable chronic limb ischemia.

If drug tolerance is not an issue, *aspirin and antiplatelet agents* should be used in all patients with peripheral vascular disease because of their beneficial effects on coronary and cerebrovascular disease as well as their ability to improve patency rates after surgical bypass and native vessel endovascular therapy (25).

Pentoxiphylline (Trental) is a methylxanthine that inhibits cyclic adenosine monophosphate phosphodiesterase and increases deformability of the erythrocytes, permitting them to negotiate vessels with reduced caliber. Other purported beneficial effects include relaxation of vascular smooth muscle tone and reduction of blood viscosity. The medication is expensive and clinical response is variable. The recommended oral dose is 400 mg three times a day perferably taken with meals to reduce gastrointestinal side effects.

Walking Program: In patients whose claudication is not considered severe, exercise training should be prescribed to increase initial claudication distances and maximize walking distances. A regular walking program can have a significant benefit and has been shown to improve exercise performance (26,27).

Reestablishing Pulsatile Flow: Despite the conservative measures listed above, if patients report severe or lifestyle limiting claudication or if rest pain, nonhealing ischemic ulceration, or gangrene is present, an attempt at restoring pulsatile blood flow should be made. At this point arteriography is perfomed. This study must include the abdominal aorta, iliac, femoral, and popliteal arteries and below-knee tibial vessels. Risks of angiography include local vascular complications (hematoma, pseudoaneurysm formation), worsening of limb ischemia (as a result of distal embolization), and contrast-induced acute tubular necrosis with acute renal insufficiency. Although these complications are uncommon, their occurrence has prompted interest in MRA as a noninvasive method of assessing peripheral vascular disease (15,28). Treatment options include vascular surgery (endarterectomy, bypass procedures using prosthetic materials as well as in situ venous grafts and microvascular techniques) and percutaneous nonsurgical interventional therapy (balloon angioplasty). The introduction of vascular stents has revolutionized the practice of percutaneous interventional therapy (Fig 5.5). The most appropriate therapy—surgery versus percutaneous intervention—should be individualized, and the clinician, interventionist, and vascular surgeon should be jointly involved in the decision-making process.

Group II: Brachiocephalic Disease

Subclavian Artery Stenosis/Occlusion

Although some of these patients can be asymptomatic, the condition can be suspected and noninvasive workup (ultrasound Doppler, MRA) can be initiated on the basis of unequal pulses or blood pressure readings in the upper extremities. Frequently patients complain of pain or a feeling of tiredness after using the extremity in question. If the stenosis or occlusion is proximal to the origin of the vertebral artery, use of the arm can result in reversed flow in the vertebral artery and set up the scenario for vertebral artery steal. Based on the adequacy of the opposite vertebral artery, such steal may result in symptoms of vertebrobasilar insufficiency. Percutaneous balloon angioplasty with or without vascular stenting can effectively treat this condition (Fig 5.5). Finally, establishing the diagnosis of subclavian disease is important, particularly when the ipsilateral internal mammary artery is being considered for coronary artery bypass surgery or has been used for that purpose (29) (Fig 5.6).

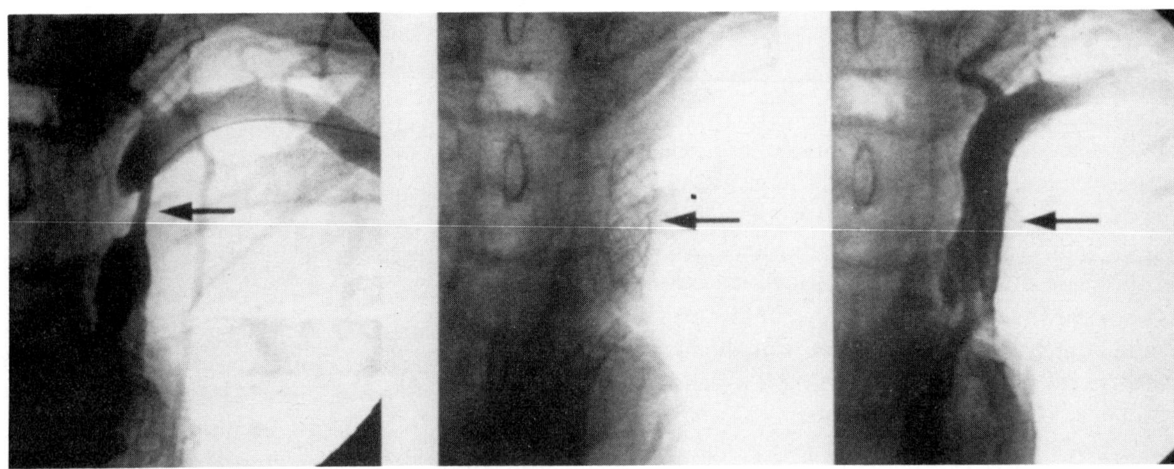

Fig 5.5 Subclavian stenosis. Woman, aged 63, with symptoms of left upper extremity claudication.

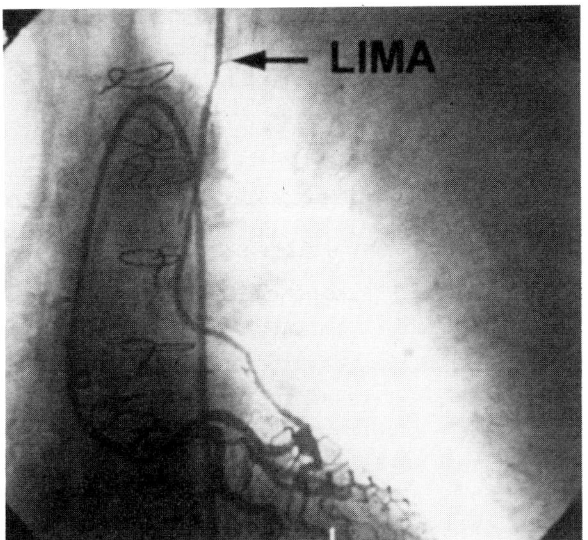

Fig 5.6 Woman, aged 72, with symptoms of angina, dizziness, and left upper extremity claudication. The subclavian was occluded at its origin and could not be recanalized by percutaneous techniques. The left main coronary artery had an ostial stenosis that was successfully angioplastied and stented. (Arrow shows Retrograde filling of LIMA from native left coronarly injections.)

Carotid Disease

Stroke is the third leading cause of death and the sixth leading cause of decreased life expectancy in adult women in the United States (30). Etiologic and risk factors vary and depend on the age of the subject. Whereas use of oral contraceptives containing high doses of estrogens and valvular heart disease (especially rheumatic mitral stenosis and atrial fibrillation) are risk factors in younger women, in the older population the usual risk factors for atherosclerotic vascular disease, namely hypertension, diabetes mellitus, tobacco abuse, and obesity, are important. Hypertension is by far the single most important risk factor for stroke irrespective of gender (31–35) and the contribution of systolic hypertension should not be overlooked (36,37). Atrial fibrillation as a result of both valvular and nonvalvular disease increases the risk of stroke and underlies the basis for recommending antiplatelets or anticoagulants to these patients.

Noninvasive Techniques for Diagnosis

Carotid Duplex Ultrasonography

This has become the noninvasive diagnostic test of choice to evaluate patients for possible carotid arterio-

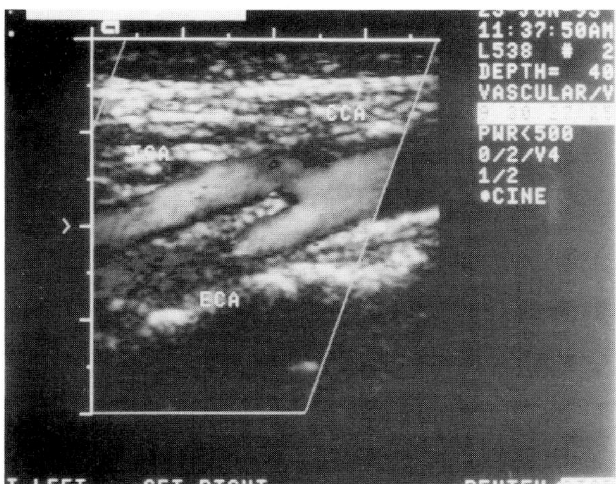

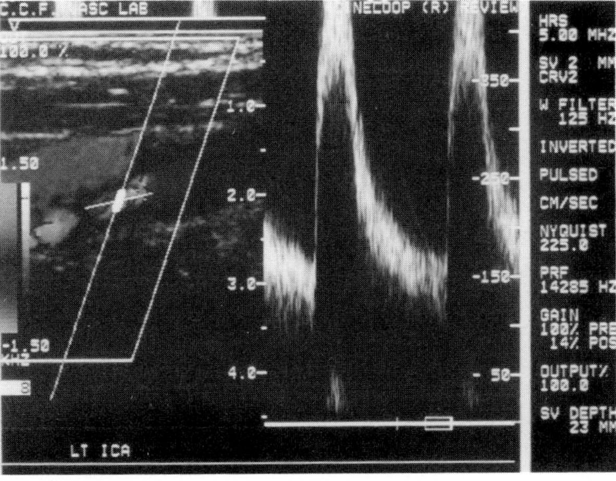

Fig 5.7 Carotid ultrasonography. *Left*: Normal carotid bifurcation with enhancement. *Right*: Carotid duplex ultrasound demonstrates severe proximal left internal carotid artery stenosis. *Note*: Marked elevation in peak systolic and end diastolic velocities.

sclerosis (Fig 5.7). In several comparative trials with arteriography, it has been proven to be reliable in detecting moderate to severe carotid artery stenosis due to atherosclerosis or other pathophysiologic conditions. The gray scale imaging allows characterization of intimal thickening and assessment of plaque morphology. Focused Doppler analysis can determine degrees of stenosis based on changes in the velocity shifts, in addition to characterization of Doppler wave form morphology. The addition of color imaging has shortened examination times and allowed the ultrasonographer to assess laminar versus turbulent blood flow. Limitations include the inability to visualize segments of the internal carotid artery distal to the angle of the mandible. The origin of the common carotid artery is often difficult to visualize, as well. There may be a future role for MRA because this technology offers a noninvasive method of assessing not only the origin of the common carotid artery, but the intracranial circulation as well.

Magnetic Resonance Angiography

Both the intracranial and extracranial cerebral vasculature can be visualized using MRA, affording a comprehensive assessment of patients with known or suspected cerebral vascular disease. Already several major medical centers are willing to perform carotid revascularization procedures with information obtained noninvasively by the combination of carotid ultrasound and MRA. The ability to acquire reliable information noninvasively in this patient population is particularly relevant given the fact that there is a nontrivial risk of permanent neurologic complications associated with diagnostic cerebral angiography (38).

Management of Brachiocephalic Disease

Medical Management

Aspirin: The value of aspirin in reducing the risk of a future stroke or transient ischemic attack (TIA) in women has been controversial. The Canadian cooperative study of antiplatelet therapy was among the first to address the issue of whether aspirin could reduce the risk of a subsequent stroke in patients with prior TIAs (39). No significant reductions in stroke rates were shown in men or women. When the combined end point of stroke or death from any reason (including myocardial infarction) was used, a beneficial effect was demonstrated in men only. More recently, the European Stroke Prevention Study (ESPS) showed benefit for both men and women treated with aspirin and dipyridamole in an attempt to reduce future stroke or TIAs (40).

Ticlopidine: The value of ticlopidine as a secondary prevention measure and stroke prevention has been evaluated in two large randomized prospective trials, the Canadian Aspirin Ticlopidine Study (CATS) and the Ticlopidine Aspirin Stroke Study (TASS). In the CATS study, 1053 patients with a recent (1 week to 4 month) stroke were randomized to receive ticlopidine 250 mg PO twice daily or placebo (41). In TASS, 3069 patients with a recent neurologic event (TIA or minor stroke) were randomized to receive either aspirin (1300 mg/day) or ticlopidine (250 mg PO twice daily) (42). The CATS study showed that ticlopidine significantly reduced the subsequent occurrence of nonfatal stroke, nonfatal myocardial infarction, or vascular death and the benefits were seen regardless of gender.

The TASS study showed that ticlopidine was more effective than aspirin and again benefited both men and women. Several subgroup analyses of this study have been performed and as with any subgroup analysis, because of the smaller numbers, caution should be exercised when interpreting the results. Still, certain trends emerged and it appears ticlopidine seems to be particularly suitable in female patients (especially in their first year after a TIA or minor stroke), in African American patients, in both male and female patients at risk for recurrent stroke, and in patients who cannot tolerate aspirin (43–45).

Important side effects of ticlopidine include neutropenia seen in 2% to 3% of the patients, which occasionally (less than 1%) may be severe (absolute neutrophil counts less than 450 cells/μL). Hence, leukocyte counts should be monitored every 2 weeks for the first 3 months of therapy. The disorder is reversible when the medication is stopped. Other side effects of ticlopidine include diarrhea and skin rash. These side effects may clear up with reduction of the dose although in some cases the medication may need to be discontinued. All the side effects of ticlopidine can be easily diagnosed and managed if patients are closely clinically monitored along with periodic estimation of complete blood cell counts.

Anticoagulants: Because atrial fibrillation increases the risk of a cardiac source of embolus (and hence that of an embolic stroke) and atrial fibrillation is not an uncommon disorder particularly in the elderly population, a number of clinical trials examining the benefit of aspirin or coumadin in reducing the risk of an embolic stroke in this patient population have been reported (46–49). Both aspirin and coumadin have been shown to reduce the risk of future TIAs or strokes in patients regardless of gender. Patients with valvular atrial fibrillation benefit more, but treatment may be indicated in patients with nonvalvular atrial fibrillation. Although the yearly risk of stroke in untreated patients is approximately 5% to 6%, certain features increasing the risk of stroke in these patients have been recognized. These include a history of hypertension, congestive heart failure especially in the preceding 3 months, and prior TIA or stroke. Thus, young patients without any of the above risk factors have a stroke risk of approximately 2.5%/yr. The presence of one risk factor increases the risk to about 7.2%/yr and that of two or three risk factors to 17.6%/yr (47). These figures are important to keep in mind when discussing the value of initiating aspirin versus anticoagulant treatment in patients with atrial fibrillation and help place in perspective the risks and benefits of treatment versus no treatment. Although coumadin is more effective than aspirin in its potential for stroke reduction, the risk of hemorrhagic stroke in patients receiving anticoagulants cannot be ignored. Data from the Stroke Prevention and Atrial Fibrillation II Study (SPAF II) (50) are helpful in drawing up some guidelines as to which patients benefit more from coumadin compared to aspirin. In general, younger patients *without* clinical evidence of congestive heart failure, systolic hypertension (greater than 160 mm Hg) and prior TIA or stroke or thromboembolism can be effectively treated with aspirin. The majority of patients less than 65 or 70 years old will probably fall in this category. The remaining 25% to 30% of patients who have risk factors in this age group will need coumadin. The risk of hemorrhagic stroke in this group is low and is generally outweighed by the benefit of continuing treatment to prevent an embolic stroke. In the elderly group, besides the above risk factors, female gender is an additional risk factor. The majority of patients in this group usually have one or more of the above risk factors listed and consideration should be given for coumadin treatment if otherwise appropriate. Of course, the risk of hemorrhagic stroke is more in the elderly population, but the clinician needs to balance that risk against the benefit accrued from preventing an embolic stroke in patients with atrial fibrillation. The above recommendations will probably change as data from ongoing clinical studies (e.g., SPAF III) become available. Until such time the above guidelines should serve as rough rules of thumb when addressing the issue of anticoagulation in patients with nonvalvular atrial fibrillation.

Surgical Management: Carotid Endarterectomy

Symptomatic Patients: The interim results of two large prospective randomized trials, the North American Symptomatic Carotid Endarterectomy Trial (NASCET) and the European Carotid Surgical Trial (ECST) were published in 1991 (51–53). These trials involved a large number (659 in NASCET and 778 in ECST) of symptomatic, generally healthy, patients and randomized them to either best medical treatment including aspirin and risk factor modification or best medical treatment plus carotid endarterectomy. Based on follow-up periods ranging from 24 to 30 months the following conclusions can be drawn:

1. For patients with carotid diameter stenosis 70% or greater, endarterectomy significantly reduces the risk of stroke.
2. There is no difference between medically and surgically treated patients when stenosis severity is less than 30%.
3. The value of carotid endarterectomy for patients with 30% to 69% stenosis remains unknown.

Certain important points need to be stressed:

1. Surgeons in the NASCET trial were preselected to minimize the trial's complication rates. In NASCET, participating surgeons were required to have a perioperative stroke and death rate of 6% or less for at least 50 consecutive endarterectomies in the preceding 2 years. The stroke and death rate in the NASCET trial was 5.8%. The ECST, which did not preselect surgeons, had a complication rate of 7.5%.
2. Patient selection plays an important role and *high-risk surgical patients were excluded from the NASCET study.*
3. The NASCET results were not stratified based on gender; the ECST did not find any significant differ-

ence in the results between male and female patients.

Asymptomatic Patients: The Asymptomatic Carotid Atherosclerosis Study (ACAS), a randomized prospective clinical trial, enrolled patients if they were 40 to 79 years of age, had a life expectancy of at least 5 years and at least 60% carotid stenosis near the bifurcation of the common or internal carotid artery. The primary question proposed to be answered by this study was: among patients with severe but asymptomatic carotid stenosis does carotid endarterectomy (despite a perioperative risk of any stroke or death from any cause) reduce the overall 5-year rate of fatal and nonfatal ipsilateral carotid stroke? In addition to aspirin and risk factor modification half the patients were randomized to surgery. Surgeons had to meet a perioperative complications rate of 3% or less (54,55).

In September 1994, the investigators released the results when the trial reached statistical significance and on the advice of the study's data monitoring committee. The trial, conducted in 39 U.S. and Canadian centers, randomized 1662 patients—828 to surgery and 834 to medical management only. There were more men (2:1) and the study found that carotid endarterectomy is beneficial with a significant absolute reduction of 5.8% in the risk of the primary end point within 5 years. The overall relative risk reduction was 55%. Whereas men had a 69% relative risk reduction, women had only a 16% relative risk reduction. The reason for this difference is unknown at the present time.

Pecutaneous Intervention

Balloon angioplasty is rapidly emerging as an effective, minimally invasive, technique for treating extracranial (cervical) carotid stenosis (Fig 5.8). The University of Alabama at Birmingham has pioneered the technique and practice of elective stenting of carotid vessels following balloon angioplasty (56). Initial, short-term results are extremely encouraging and follow-up studies are underway to determine the long-term outcome of these patients.

Fibromuscular dysplasia, an idiopathic condition affecting medium- and small-sized arteries occurs almost exclusively in young and middle-aged white women. Although fibromuscular dysplasia can affect different arteries (e.g., renal, carotids, subclavian, celiac, mesenteric, etc) cerviocephalic involvement accounts for roughly a third of all cases of the disorder (57,58). The usual site of involvement in the internal carotid artery is at or above the level of the second cervical vertebrae, making surgical access difficult and at times impossible. Frequently, both carotids are involved. Patients are often asymptomatic. Symptomatic presentations include headaches, complaints of a "swooshing" sound in the ear (pulsatile tinnitus), TIAs, or stroke. Arterial dissection is a known complication and cephalad extension of the dissection can

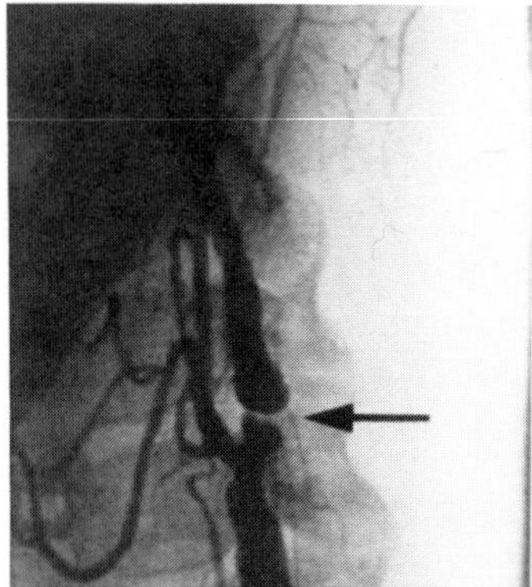

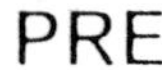

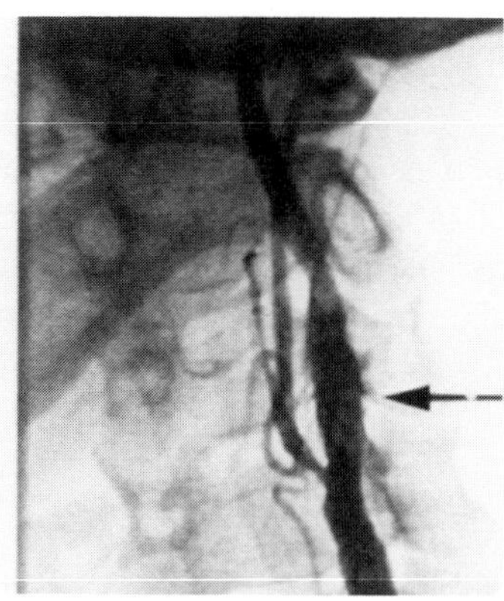

Fig 5.8 Percutaneous balloon carotid followed by stenting (primary carotid stenting).

result in subarachnoid or intracerebral (parenchymal) bleed. Angiography reveals the typical "string of beads" appearance although other appearances have been described. Optimal treatment is unknown; medical treatment includes use of antiplatelets and angicoagulants. Surgical options include endarterectomy with dilatation, excision with primary or patch repair, and external carotid-internal carotid bypass. Percutaneous balloon angioplasty has been successful, aided more recently by deployment of intravascular stents (Fig 5.9).

Group III: Abdominal Aortic Disease

Abdominal aortic aneurysms are distinctly unusual in women and are usually seen in older subjects (59). In a large multicenter study involving more than 600 patients only one fifth of the patients were women (60). Interestingly, a family history of abdominal aortic aneurysms was more commonly noted among the women in this series compared to the men. There were no significant differences in major postoperative complications between men and women (61). Currently, a few centers around the world are investigating the use of stent graft devices as a method of nonsurgical treatment of aneurysms (62–64) and their initial results are encouraging. Both the technique and the devices will undoubtedly undergo revisions and modifications so that in the future this less invasive technique with reduced morbidity should become available as a viable option for treatment of abdominal aortic aneurysms.

One particular type of *discrete atherosclerotic disease* involving the infrarenal abdominal aorta has been reported almost exclusively in women (65). The patient is usually a middle-aged nondiabetic woman with a history of chronic heavy smoking. Angiographically, the lesions appear as discrete stenosis in the distal abdominal aorta; the rest of the vascular tree, although small in caliber, usually does not have significant stenosis. Although limited endarterectomy has been successful, the problem can be treated with percutaneous balloon angioplasty and placement of a vascular stent (Fig 5.10).

Chronic mesenteric ischemia presents as severe postprandial epigastric pain (abdominal angina) and weight loss, both from fear of eating and also from coexistent malabsorption syndromes. The clinical syndrome appears only when two or more mesenteric vessels are involved. Further, clinical presentation is usually late in the natural history of the disease and it is not unusual to see significant angiographic disease without clinical sequalae. Mesenteric angiography

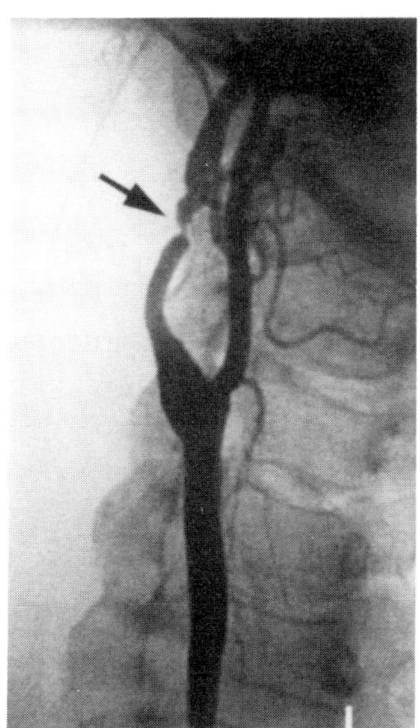

PRE

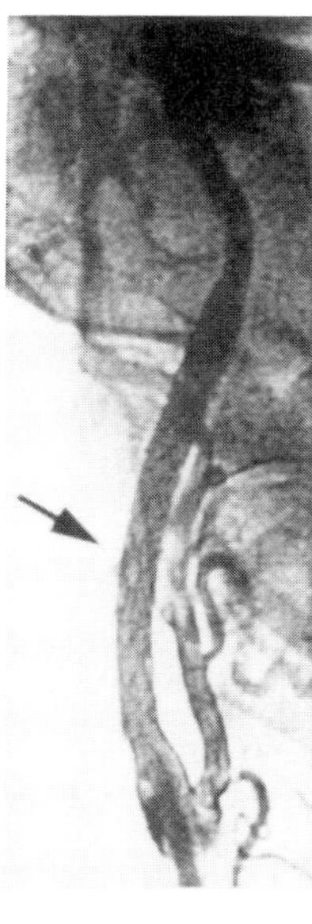

POST STENT

Fig 5.9 Fibromuscular dysplasia. Woman, aged 53, with bilateral asymptomatic carotid bruits. Angiography showed bilateral high-grade internal carotid stenosis. Both sides were successfully angioplastied and stented.

should be considered in patients with chronic postprandial pain (66). Although successful surgical series have been reported (67,68), mortality and morbidity are high because of comorbid conditions such as coronary and cerebrovascular disease, advanced age, and diabetes. Successful treatment using percutaneous balloon angioplasty techniques for releasing stenosis in superior mesentric and celiae arteries with or without use of stents has been reported (69–71) (Fig 5.11).

Venous Thromboembolic Disease

Venous thromboembolic disease is a common but frequently misdiagnosed and inappropriately treated disorder. Although the true incidence is unknown, autopsy data have suggested almost 40% of deaths in one hospital in 1987 had evidence of deep venous thrombosis, and, on review of hospital records, 9.4% of these deaths were related to a fatal pulmonary embolism (72). Many patient groups have underlying factors that increase the risk for development of venous thromboembolic disease. These include increasing age, pregnancy, prolonged immobility, surgery, trauma, concomitant malignancy, serious medical illness, obesity, and oral contraceptives. Orthopedic and pelvic surgical procedures are associated with the highest incidence of postoperative venous thromboembolic disease.

Patient symptoms of unilateral leg pain and edema are not helpful as diagnostic criteria for the condition. Physical examination often reveals a normal leg appearance despite a large proximal deep venous thrombosis. In addition, small muscular calf vein thrombi may cause severe leg pain and edema. Therefore, physical findings and symptoms are absent in 50% of cases and should not be used as criteria for diagnosis or therapy (Fig 5.12). An objective examination must be performed to establish the presence or absence of venous thromboembolic disease. Practical options include impedance plethysmography, compression duplex ultrasonography, ascending contrast venography, and perhaps magnetic resonance venography (73). Despite the reputation of contrast venography as the "gold standard" diagnostic test, duplex ultrasonography offers many advantages without compromising accuracy (74).

Once established, the treatment is either anticoagulation, thrombolytic therapy, inferior vena cava filter placement, or in the case of isolated calf vein thrombosis, serial duplex ultrasonography to detect propagation of thrombus. Types of anticoagulation include standard unfractionated heparin (intravenous or sub-

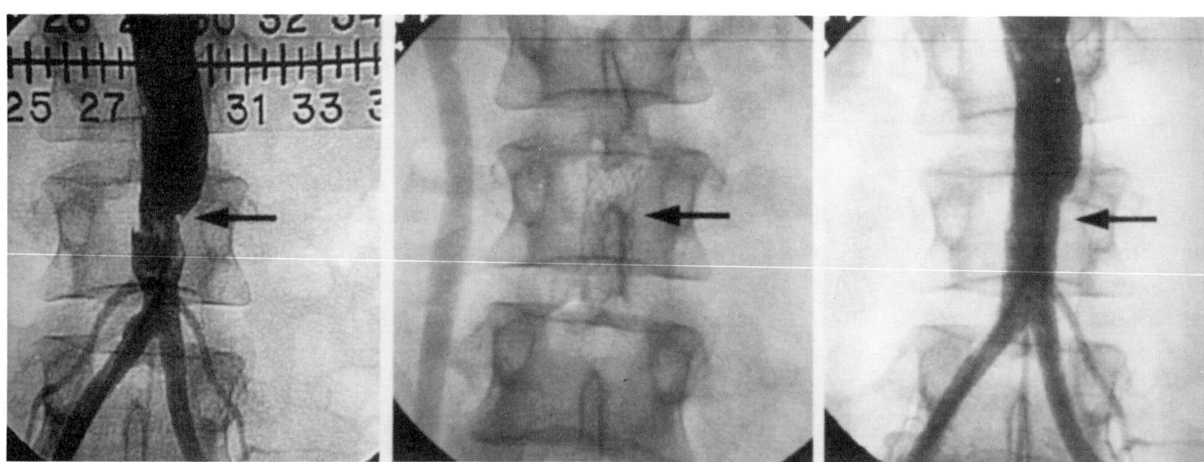

Fig 5.10 Discrete abdominal aortic stenosis. Woman, aged 46, a heavy chronic smoker, presented with bilateral hip, buttock, and upper thigh claudication. The rest of the lower extremity vasculature did not have any significant stenosis. Follow-up angiography at 3 months showed persistent patency.

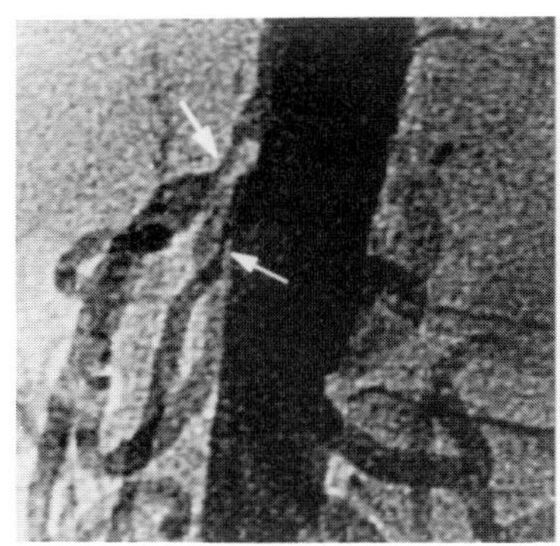

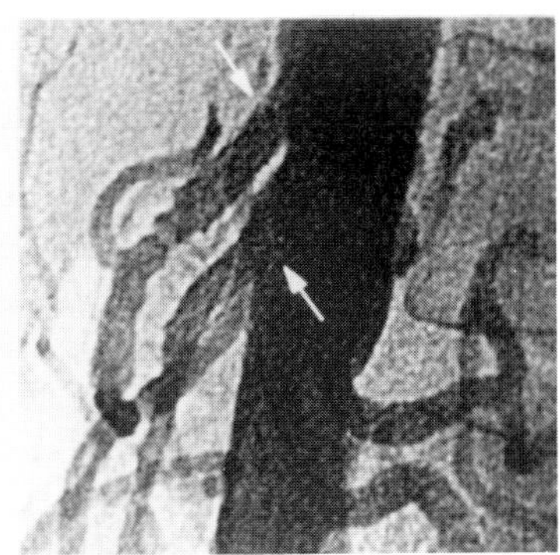

Fig 5.11 Celiac and superior mesenteric balloon angioplasty and stenting. Woman, aged 75, presented with severe post-prandial abdominal pain, weight loss, and diarrhea. She had had balloon angioplasty (without stenting) of these stenoses 3 months before this procedure. She was admitted because of recurrent symptoms.

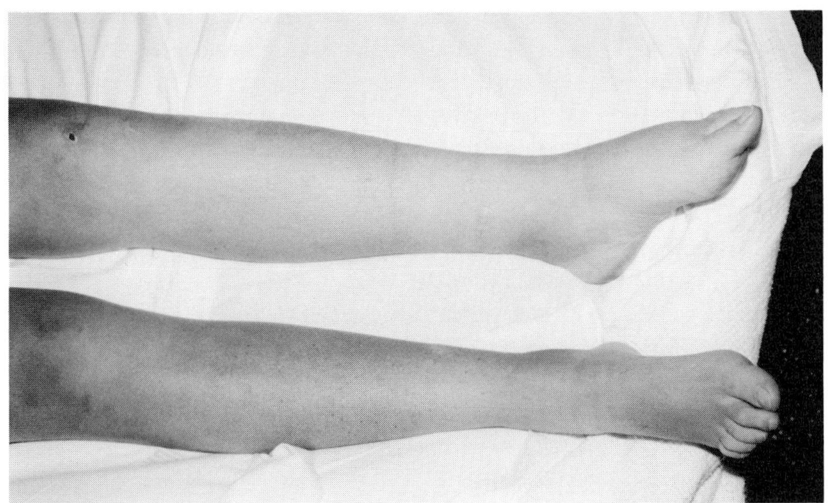

Fig 5.12 Lower extremities. *Left*: Lymphedema due to multiple left pelvic surgeries for renal transplantation. *Note*: Edema on dorsum of left foot. *Right*: Leg demonstrates erythrocyanotic hue. Patient has iliofemoral deep venous thrombosis.

cutaneous) (75), oral anticoagulants (76), or low molecular weight heparin (77). The duration of oral anticoagulation should extend for 3 to 6 months (78).

Recurrent events require investigation for underlying etiologies, as well as a prolonged course of anticoagulation (79). Thrombolytic therapy is an underutilized, but often effective treatment for acute venous thromboembolism, preventing chronic venous insufficiency and perhaps chronic thrombembolic pulmonary hypertension (80,81). Vena caval filters are useful in patients who cannot receive anticoagulation due to prohibitive risk of hemorrhage (82).

Venous varicosities, or dilated incompetent veins, are common with an estimated prevalence of 2.25% (0.8% in men; 3.5% in women) (83). These occur as a result of valvular defects, vein wall weakness, increased venous pressure, and incompetent perforating veins. These veins can cause pain, superficial thrombophlebitis, ulceration, or stasis pigmentation and may predispose to deep vein thrombosis. They can be treated with surgical excision (stripping), injection venous sclerotherapy, and external compression stockings (84).

REFERENCES

1. Eaker ED, Chesebro JH, Sacks FM, et al. Cardiovascular disease in women. Circulation 1993;88:1999–2009.

2. Matthews KA, Meilahn E, Kuller LH, et al. Menopause and risk factors for coronary heart disease. N Engl J Med 1989;321:641–646.

3. Soma MR, Osnago-Gadda I, Pasletti R, et al. The lowering of lipoprotein (a) induced by estrogen plus progesterone replacement therapy in postmenopausal women. Arch Intern Med 1993;153:1462–1468.

4. Spittell JA Jr. Some uncommon types of occlusive peripheral vascular disease. Curr Probl Cardiol 1983; 8:6.

5. Abbott RD, Brand FN, Kannel WB. Epidemiology of some peripheral arterial findings in diabetic men and women: experience from the Framingham Study. Am J Med 1990;88:376–381.

6. Orchard TJ, Dorman JS, Maser RE, et al. Prevalence of complications in IDDM by sex and duration. Diabetes 1990;39:1116–1124.

7. Krupski WD. The peripheral vascular consequences of smoking. Ann Vasc Surg 1991;5:291–304.

8. Kazmier FJ, Sheps SS, Bernatz PE, et al. Livedo reticularis and digital infarcts: a syndrome due to cholesterol emboli arising from atheromatous abdominal aortic aneurysms. Vasc Dis 1966;3:12–24.

9. Carvajal JA, Anderson R, Weiss L, et al. Atheroembolism. Arch Intern Med 1967;119:593–599.

10. DeWeese JA, Leather R, Porter J. Practice guidelines: lower extremity revascularization. J Vasc Surg 1993;18:280–293.

11. Carter SA. Arterial auscultation in peripheral vascular disease. JAMA 1981;246:1682–1686.

12. Vogt MT, Cauley JA, Newman AB, et al. Decreased ankle/arm blood pressure index and mortality in elderly women. JAMA 1993;270:465–469.

13. Vogt MT, McKenna M, Wolfson SK, Kuller LH. The relationship between ankle-brachial index, other atherosclerotic disease, diabetes, smoking and mortality in older men and women. Atherosclerosis 1993;101:191–202.

14. Vogt MT, McKenna M, Anderson SJ, et al. The relationship between ankle-arm index and mortality in older men and women. J Am Geriatr Soc 1993;41:532–530.

15. Owen RS, Carpenter JP, Baum RA, Perloff LJ, Cope C. Magnetic resonance imaging of angiographically occult runoff vessels in peripheral vascular disease. N Engl J Med 1992;326:1577–1581.

16. Blackwell GG, Pohost GM. The clinical usefulness of cardiovascular magnetic resonance imaging. Curr Probl Cardiol 1994;3:117–176.

17. Edelman RR. MR angiography: present and future. AJR Am J Roentgenol 1993;161:1–11.

18. Witteman JCM, Grobbee DE, Valkenburg HA, et al. Cigarette smoking and the development and progression of aortic atherosclerosis: a 9 year population-based followup study in women. Circulation 1993;88(part 1):2156–2162.

19. Kawachl I, Colditz GA, Stampfer MJ, et al. Smoking cessation and time course of decreased risks of coronary heart disease in middle-aged women. Arch Intern Med 1994;154:169–175.

20. McDaniel MD, Cromwell, JL. Basic data related to the natural history of intermittent claudication. Ann Vasc Surg 1989;3:273–277.

21. Stampfer MJ, Colditz GA. Estrogen replacement therapy and coronary heart disease: a quantitative assessment of the epidemiologic evidence. Prev Med 1991;20:47–63.

22. Belchetz PC. Hormonal treatment of postmenopausal women. N Engl J Med 1994;330:1062–1071.

23. Eagle KA, Rihal CS, Foster ED, et al. Long-term survival in patients with coronary artery disease: importance of peripheral vascular disease. J Am Coll Cardiol 1994;23:1091–1095.

24. Hertzer NR, Beven EG, Young JR, et al. Coronary artery disease in peripheral vascular patients. Ann Surg 1984;199:223–233.

25. Patrono C. Aspirin as an antiplatelet drug. N Engl J Med 1994;330:1287–1295.

26. Hiatt WR, Reginstenner JG, Hargarten ME, et al. Benefit of exercise conditioning for patient with peripheral arterial disease. Circulation 1990;81:602–609.

27. Ernst EE, Matria A. Exercise for intermittent claudication. Cardiology Board Review 1988;5:82.

28. Carpenter JP, Owen RS, Baum RA, et al. Magnetic resonance angiography of peripheral runoff vessels. J Vasc Surg 1992;16:807–815.

29. Valentine RJ, Fry RE, Wheelan KR, et al. Coronary-subclavian steal from reversed flow in an internal mammary artery used for coronary bypass. Am J Cardiol 1987;59(6):719–720.

30. Hershey LA. Stroke prevention in women. Am J Med 1991;90:288–292.

31. Wolfe PA, Kannel WB, Verter J. Current status and risk factors for stroke. Neurol Clin 1983;1:317–348.

32. Klaz MJ, Whelton PK, Seidler AJ. Decline in U.S. stroke mortality: demographic trends and antihypertensive therapy. Stroke 1989;20:14–21.

33. Folsom AR, Prineas RJ, Kaye SA, Munger RG.

Incidence of hypertension and stroke in relation to body fat distribution and other risk factors in women. Stroke 1990;21:701–706.

34. Barnett HJ. Stroke in women. Can J Cardiol 1990;6(suppl B):11B–17B.

35. Medical Research Council Working Party. MRC trial of treatment of mild hypertension: principal results. Br Med J 1985;291:97–104.

36. Kannel WB, Wolf PA, McGee DL, et al. Systolic blood pressure, arterial rigidity, and risks of stroke. JAMA 1981;245:1225–1229.

37. Shekelle RB, Ostfeld AM, Klawans HL. Hypertension and risk of stroke in an elderly population. Stroke 1974;5:71–75.

38. Cohen M, Biller J, Saver JL. Advances in the management of carotid disease. Curr Probl Cardiol 1994;8:473–532.

39. The Canadian Cooperative Study Group. A randomized trial of aspirin and sulfinpyrazone in threatened stroke. N Engl J Med 1978;299:53–59.

40. Sivenius J, Riekkinen PJ, Smets P, et al. The European Stroke Prevention Study: results by arterial distribution. Ann Neurol 1991;29:596–600.

41. Gent M, Blakely JA, Easton JD, et al. The Canadian American Ticlopidine Study (CATS) in thromboembolic stroke. Lancet 1989;1:1215–1220.

42. Hass WK, Easton JD, Adams HP Jr, et al. A randomized trial comparing ticlopidine hydrochloride with aspirin for the prevention of stroke in high-risk patients. N Engl J Med 1989;321:501–507.

43. Harbison JW. Ticlopidine versus aspirin for the prevention of recurrent stroke. Analysis of patients with minor stroke from the Ticlopidine Aspirin Stroke Study. Stroke 1992;23:1723–1727.

44. Grotta JC, Norris JW, Kamm B. Prevention of stroke with ticlopidine: who benefits most? Neurology 1992;42:111–115.

45. Weisbery LA. The efficacy and safty of ticlopidine and aspirin in non-whites: analysis of a patient subgroup from the Ticlopidine Aspirin Stroke Study. Neurology 1993;43:27–31.

46. Petersen P, Boysen G, Godtfredsen J, et al. Placebo-controlled, randomised trial of warfarin and aspirin for prevention of thromboembolic complications in chronic atrial fibrillation: the Copenhagen AFASAK Study. Lancet 1989;1:175–179.

47. Stroke Prevention in Atrial Fibrillation Investigators. Stroke Prevention in Atrial Fibrillation Study: final results. Circulation 1991;84:527–539.

48. Ezekowitz MD, Bridgers SL, James KE, et al. Warfarin in the prevention of stroke associated with nonrheumatic atrial fibrillation. N Engl J Med 1992;327:1406–1412.

49. The Boston Area Anti-coagulation Trial for Atrial Fibrillation Investigators. The effect of low-dose warfarin on the risk of stroke in patients with nonrheumatic atrial fibrillation. N Engl J Med 1990;323:1505–1511.

50. Warfarin compared to aspirin for prevention of thromboembolism in atrial fibrillation. Stroke Prevention in Atrial Fibrillation II Study. Lancet 1994;343:687–691.

51. North American Symptomatic Carotid Endarterectomy Trial Collaborators: Beneficial effect of carotid endarterectomy in symptomatic patients with high grade carotid stenosis. N Engl J Med 1991;325:443–445.

52. European Carotid Surgery Trialists' Collaborative Group: MRC European Carotid Surgery Trial: Interim results of symptomatic patients with severe (70–99%) or with mild (0–29%) carotid stenosis. Lancet 1991;337: 1235–1243.

54. The Asymptomatic Carotid Atherosclerosis Study Group. Study designed for randomized prospective trial of carotid endarterectomy for asymptomatic atherosclerosis. Stroke 1989;20:844–849.

55. Moore WS, Vescera CL, Robertson JT, Baker H, et al. Selection process for participating surgeons in the Asymptomatic Carotid Atherosclerosis Study (ACAS). Stroke 1991;22:1353–1357.

56. Yadav SS, Roubin GS, Iyer SS, et al. Application of lessons learned from cardiac interventional techniques to carotid angioplasty (PTA). J Am Coll Cardiol 1995;25(suppl A):380A.

57. Mettinger KL, Ericson K. Fibromuscular dysplasia of the brain: observation on angiographic, clinical and genetic characteristics. Stroke 1982;13:46–52.

58. Sandrok BA. Fibromuscular dysplasia of the internal carotid artery. Neurol Clin 1983;1:17–26.

59. Bickerstaff LK, Hollier LH, VanPeenen JH, et al. Abdominal aortic aneurysms: the changing natural history. J Vasc Surg 1984;1:6–12.

60. Johnston KW, Scobie TK. Multicenter prospective study of nonruptured abdominal aortic aneurysms. I. Population and operative management. J Vasc Surg 1988;7:69–81.

61. Johnston KW. Multicenter prospective study of nonruptured abdominal aortic aneurysm. Part II. Varia-

bles predicting morbidity and mortality. J Vasc Surg 1989;9:437–447.

62. Diethrich EB, Papazogluo CO, Rodriguez-Lopez J, Lopez-Galarza L. Endoluminal grafts for percutaneous aneurysm exclusion and intraluminal bypass. Circulation 1994;90(4.2):1–206.

63. Dake MD, Semba CP, Mitchel RS, Zarins CK, Miller DC. Transluminally placed endovascular stent/grafts for the treatment of abdominal aortic and non-aortic aneurysms. Circulation 1994;90(4.2):1–206.

64. Rutz CE, Zhang HP, Douglas JT, Zuppan CW. Use of a new endovascular device to treat abdominal aortic aneurysm. Circulation 1994;90(4.2):1–387.

65. Jernigan WR, Fallat ME, Hatfield DR. Hypoplastic aortoiliac syndrome: an entity peculiar to women. Surgery 1983;94:752–757.

66. Jardine DL, Fitzpatrick MA, Troughton WD. Small bowel ischemia in Fabry's disease. Gastroenterol Hepatol 1994;9:201–214.

67. Calderon M, Ruce JT, Gregonic ID, Jacobs MJ, et al. Long term results of the surgical management of symptomatic chronic intestinal ischemia. J Cardiovasc Surg 1992;33:723–728.

68. McCollum CH, Graham MJ, DeBakey ME. Chronic mesenteric arterial insufficiency: result of revascularization in 33 cases. South Med J 1976;69:1266–1268.

69. Constans J, Grelet P, Baste JC, et al. Endoluminal angioplasty of the superior mesenteric artery in the treatment of intestinal angina. J Chir (Pairs) 1992;129:384–386.

70. Wilms G, Baert AL. Transluminal angioplasty of superior mesenteric artery and celiae trunk. Ann Radiol (Paris) 1986;29:535–558.

71. Finch IJ. Use of the Palmaz stent in ostial celiac artery stenosis. J Vasc Intervl Radiol 1992;3:633–635.

72. Lindblad B, Sternby NH, Berquist D. Incidence of venous thromboembolism verified by necropsy over 30 years. Br Med J 1991;302:709–711.

73. Sprintizer CE, Sternby NH, Berquist D. Detection of deep venous thrombosis by magnetic resonance imaging. Chest 1993;104:54–60.

74. White RH, McGahan JP, Daschbach MM, Hartling RO. Diagnosis of deep-vein thrombus using duplex ultrasound. Ann Intern Med 1989;111:297–304.

75. Homines DW, Bura A, Mazzolal L, et al. Subcutaneous heparin compared with continuous intravenous heparin administration in the initial treatment of deep vein thrombosis. A meta-analysis. Ann Intern Med 1992;116:279–284.

76. Brandjes DPM, Heljboer J, Buller HR, et al. Acenocoumarol and heparin compared with acenocoumarol alone in the intital treatment of proximal vein thrombosis. N Engl J Med 1992;327:1485–1489.

77. Simanneau G, Charbonnier B, Decousus H, et al. Subcutaneous low-molecular-weight heparin compared with continuous intravenous unfractionated heparin in the treatment of proximal deep vein thrombosis. Arch Intern Med 1993;153:1541–1546.

78. Research Committee of the British Thorac Society. Optimum duration of anticoagulation for deep vein thrombosis and pulmonary embolism. Lancet 1992;340:873–876.

79. Prandoni P, Lensin AWA, Buller HR, et al. Deep vein thrombosis and the incidence of subsequent symptomatic cancer. N Engl J Med 1992;327:1128–1133.

80. Goldhaber SZ. Thrombolysis in venous thromboembolism. An international perspective. Chest 1990;97(suppl):1765–1815.

81. Goldhaber SZ. Recent advances in the diagnosis and lytic therapy of pulmonary embolism. Chest 1991;99(suppl):1735–1795.

82. Becker DM, Philbrick JT, Selby JB. Inferior vena cava filters. Indications, safety, effectiveness. Arch Intern Med 1992;152:1985–1994.

83. U.S. Department of Health, Education and Welfare. National health survey 1935–1936. Washington, DC: 1938.

84. Srother IG, Bryson A, Alexander S. Treatment of varicose veins by compression sclerotherapy. Br J Surg 1974;61:387–393.

CHAPTER 6

ANGINA PECTORIS

Larry S. Dean

Chest pain or chest discomfort is one of the more common patient complaints. It is a frequent complaint of women although the incidence of structural coronary disease as an etiology appears to be less until the later decades of life (1,2). Angina pectoris, the clinical symptom produced by myocardial ischemia, must be differentiated from other causes of chest discomfort. Obviously, the diagnosis of angina pectoris and its prognostic implications will have a substantial impact on the patient. Therefore, the diagnosis of angina pectoris and the differentiation from other types of chest pain or discomfort is of great importance.

It has been generally held that incidence of coronary artery disease is less in women than in men. Long-term studies such as the Framingham study (2) have shown that although the incidence of clinical coronary disease varies between men and women depending on age, by the seventh to eighth decade of life the incidences are similar (1). Cardiovascular death remains the most common killer in women as it is in men and therefore the appropriate evaluation and treatment of angina pectoris are of great importance to the practicing physician.

It the Framingham study angina pectoris was about twice as common as the initial presentation of cardiovascular disease in women than in men (3). Although the prognosis of angina in women appears to be better than men with fewer women having myocardial infarction in follow-up (4), subsequent evaluation (2) has shown that the incidence of obstructive coronary disease in women is less than that in men until later in life. Therefore, in the Framingham study many of the women with typical angina by history probably did not have significant coronary disease. The pathologic process responsible for the presentation of angina pectoris in women with normal or minimally diseased coronary arteries remains unknown.

Clinical Presentation

Angina pectoris or chest discomfort is typically located in the substernal area. It is described as either a heaviness, a severe pressure, or as severe pain. The discomfort typically radiates into the left side of the neck and left arm along the medial aspect. It less frequently presents as intrascapular discomfort, jaw pain, or isolated left arm pain. It is important when obtaining the history from the patient that the word chest pain not be used. A better term is chest discomfort. Many patients will adamantly deny that they have chest pain but when asked if they have chest discomfort will describe the symptoms typical of angina.

Angina is usually precipitated by exertion or other physical activity. The amount of activity required to produce angina will vary and many patients will complain of angina after eating and exercising or with extremes of temperature. Angina usually builds to a crescendo over 2 to 5 minutes and then will resolve over the next 5 to 10 minutes. The total duration therefore is approximately 10 to 15 minutes. Angina is not abrupt in its onset or cessation. The use of sublingual nitroglycerin or cessation of activity will usually bring relief of the symptoms over a short period of time. Vasospastic or Prinzmetal's angina classically occurs in the early morning hours, is nonexertional, is associated with ST segment elevation during pain on a standard electrocardiogram (ECG), and responds rapidly to nitroglycerin.

Angina can either be stable, in other words predictable, or unstable. Unstable angina has various definitions. The more common are: 1) recent onset (<30

Box 6.1 Chest Pain: A Common Clinical Complaint

A. Angina pectoris

B. Gastrointestinal source
   1. Esophageal spasm
   2. Gastritis
   3. Esophageal reflux
   4. Peptic ulcer disease
   5. Cholecystitis

C. Pulmonary source
   1. Pulmonary embolus/infarction
   2. Pleurisy

D. Great vessel/aortic disease
   1. Aortic dissection
   2. Aortic aneurysm

E. Musculoskeletal source

F. Miscellaneous
   1. Aortic stenosis
   2. Idiopathic hypertrophic subaortic stenosis
   3. Mitral stenosis
   4. Pericarditis
   5. Severe anemia

days); 2) angina at rest, which is sometimes nocturnal; and 3) an accelerating pattern of either frequency, duration, or severity. The prognostic impact of unstable angina will be discussed shortly.

Unfortunately many other causes of chest discomfort must be distinguished from angina pectoris. Some of the more common etiologies are outlined in Box 6.1. One of the more difficult to differentiate from angina is esophageal spasm. The lower esophageal sphincter is comprised of smooth muscle cells and therefore responds to nitroglycerin in a fashion similar to that seen in angina pectoris. Many of these patients will present with chest discomfort that is virtually indistinguishable from typical angina. The use of sublingual nitroglycerin in these patients as a diagnostic test has limitations because the discomfort will resolve after its use. However, esophageal spasm is not precipitated by exertion or other physical activities. It may, however, be worsened with certain foods or emotional stress, or may be seen in patients with other gastrointestinal symptoms as such as esophageal reflux. A history of reflux-type symptoms including regurgitation of brackish material into the throat or undigested food into the mouth should always be elicited in patients with the complaint of chest discomfort. The chest discomfort associated with pulmonary emboli is typically pleuritic and may be associated with other symptoms such as hemoptysis. Aortic dissection can also be confused with angina pectoris because it has similar quality and location. However, the radiation of the discomfort is usually into the intrascapular area from the anterior chest and the discomfort does not typically radiate into the left arm. It is also described as a tearing type of sensation and is severe in most patients. Musculoskeletal discomfort is usually exacerbated by moving the offending part or it is positional. The symptoms of pericarditis usually have a pleuritic component and the pain is improved in the sitting position; it worsens when the patient lies flat.

It is reasonable to conclude that chest discomfort that has various locations, is described as sharp and shooting lasting a few seconds, and is made worse or better by changes in position or respiration usually does not represent angina pectoris. It is always important when eliciting the history of chest discomfort that the location, duration, radiation, and any alleviating or exacerbating factors be inquired of the patient. Otherwise, unnecessary and expensive additional procedures may be undertaken when the diagnosis of noncardiac chest pain could be made more simply by an adequate history.

Pathophysiology

Angina pectoris is the symptom associated with myocardial ischemia. It is transient as noted and is typically due to a problem of supply or demand of oxygenated blood. In patients with obstructive coronary disease the problem is both one of supply and demand because an obstruction of greater than approximately 70% will produce symptoms of angina with exercise. The supply of oxygenated blood is diminished because of the coronary obstruction and with exercise the myocardial oxygen demand increases, thereby resulting in the clinical manifestations of angina. In addition to an obstructive coronary stenosis it is also possible to have a vasospastic component either in an angiographically normal coronary artery or more commonly at the site of minimal to moderate coronary obstruction. This produces a dynamic alteration in coronary blood flow. In a small group of patients with classic exertional angina the epicardial coronary arteries are angiographically normal. These patients usually have evidence of myocardial ischemia on radionuclide studies despite normal coronary arteriograms. The pathologic abnormality is felt to be due to microvascular arterial disease and has been commonly termed syndrome X. These patients uniformly respond to vasodilator drugs such as nitroglycerin or calcium channel antagonists.

There are other situations in which supply is not adversely affected but demand is increased. This is commonly seen in patients with left ventricular hypertrophy either due to hypertension or idiopathic hypertrophic subaortic stenosis, a form of asymmetric septal hypertrophy of the myocardium. Patients with significant valvular heart disease and especially those with aortic stenosis and in some patients with mitral stenosis typical symptoms of angina can be present without significant obstructive coronary disease. Patients with profound anemia, especially those with significant coronary obstruction, or if the anemia is severe enough, mild to moderate coronary obstruction can also present with angina. It is important to exclude the other possible causes of angina most of which can be excluded after a thorough cardiovascular history and physical examination.

Natural History

The natural history of this disease depends on the presence or absence of obstructive coronary disease and the pattern of angina. Although patients with mild to moderate coronary disease are at increased risk for cardiovascular events over the general population, patients with severe three-vessel coronary disease, especially those with left main and proximal left anterior descending disease, seem to be at increased risk for subsequent cardiovascular events (5,6). This is especially true in patients with multivessel coronary disease and poor left ventricular function (7). However, most patients do not present for evaluation with prior coronary or cardiac anatomy known and therefore the history becomes extremely important in predicting the prognosis. Patients with unstable angina, as previously defined, clearly have an increased incidence of subsequent cardiovascular events in the first year after presentation. Patients who have an unstable pattern of angina, presence of ECG changes with chest discomfort and those who fail to respond to medical therapy within 48 hours of presentation have the highest risk of subsequent events (8).

Evaluation of the Patient with Suspected Angina Pectoris

History

It is important to elucidate any history of chest discomfort and to completely define the nature of the discomfort, its location, and alleviating and precipitating factors. An adequate history will also typically allow one to exclude the other causes of chest discomfort in a particular patient (see Box 6.1). It is also important while taking the history that specific questions regarding cardiovascular risk factors be asked of patients. These include a history of diabetes mellitus, cigarette smoking and its extent, hypertension, and premature coronary disease in the family. A family history of premature coronary disease has been defined as the development of a cardiovascular event in a first-degree relative who is less than 55 years of age if a man and less than 65 years of age if a woman (9). It is also important to elicit the history of hypercholesterolemia or other lipid abnormality because the prognosis once the diagnosis has been established is clearly affected by the presence of an abnormal lipid profile and the likelihood of coronary artery disease is increased in these patients. The prevalence of coronary artery disease varies by gender and the history obtained can be important in determining the pretest likelihood of the disease and therefore the extent of the evaluation of a patient complaining of chest pain (Table 6.1).

Table 6.1 Prevalence of Coronary Artery Disease in Asymptomatic Subjects and in Patients with Different Chest Pain Syndromes

Pain Syndrome	Men	Women
Asymptomatic, age <50yr	0.04	0.007
Asymptomatic, age >50yr	0.11	0.05
Nonanginal chest pain	0.22	0.05
Atypical angina	0.67	0.35
Typical exertional angina	0.88	0.58

Source: Sox HC Jr. Noninvasive testing in coronary artery disease. Selection of procedures and interpretation of results. Postgrad Med 1983;74:319–336.

Physical Examination

A thorough cardiovascular examination should be performed on any patient who presents with the chief complaint of chest discomfort. In most patients presenting with the complaint of angina pectoris the physical examination will not be particularly remarkable unless the patient is having chest discomfort at the time of examination. However, the presence of xanthelasma and arterial bruits would be of interest because xanthelasma is associated with hyperlipidemia and peripheral vascular disease is associated with coronary disease; the presence of these entities would increase concern when evaluating a patient with the complaint of chest discomfort. When examining a patient it is also important to carefully examine the symmetry of the arterial pulses because peripheral vascular disease or aortic dissection could be manifested as asymmetry of the peripheral pulses. It is important to document the presence or absence a pericardial friction rub because this would be more consistent with the diagnosis of pericarditis. Likewise, the presence of a pleural rub would lend more credence to a diagnosis of either pneumonia with pleuritis or perhaps pulmonary embolus as a possible etiology. Manual palpation of the chest wall, usually at the site of maximal discomfort, may also elicit worsened discomfort and make the diagnosis of chest wall pain more likely.

If a patient is examined during an episode of chest discomfort, then additional physical findings are sometimes present and again would make one more strongly favor a diagnosis of angina over other possible causes of chest discomfort. During examination of a patient with chest discomfort, the presence of a new murmur of mitral regurgitation suggesting papillary muscle dysfunction would be a strong indication of probable coronary disease. The development of a transient S_3 or transient pulmonary edema lends strong credence to the diagnosis as well. Some patients with significant coronary disease who are examined during episodes of chest discomfort will also be noted to be hypotensive and the general appearance could be one of profuse sweating, increased anxiety or agitation, and a generally ashen appearance.

Laboratory Evaluation

Standard 12-lead ECGs may or may not show an abnormality. The absence of ECG changes in a patient with the complaint of chest discomfort does not exclude coronary disease as a possible etiology. Likewise the presence of ECG changes does not necessarily imply that coronary disease is present because other abnormalities including hypertension, pulmonary embolus, esophageal spasm, and mitral valve prolapse can produce ECG ST-T wave changes. The use of digitalis is also associated with ECG changes that would be consistent with ischemia. In patients having pain at the time of examination ECG changes of ST depression or elevation (Prinzmetal's angina) or ST-T wave changes that resolve with resolution of chest discomfort are strong indicators of coronary disease. Likewise, the development of transient atrioventricular (AV) conduction abnormalities during chest pain is of concern. An echocardiogram obtained during an episode of chest discomfort that shows a segmental wall motion abnormality that reverses with cessation of discomfort likewise strongly predicts the presence of coronary disease.

Routine laboratory evaluation including creatine phosphokinase and its isoenzymes is usually not helpful in the diagnosis of angina and is typically not useful in excluding the possibility of ischemic heart disease. In patients in whom the diagnosis of angina has been made or in patients with known ischemic heart disease it is quite important that some assessment of the lipid profile be assessed. At a minimum, the total cholesterol and low-density and high-density lipoprotein (LDL, HDL) levels should be obtained.

The formal evaluation of a patient suspected of having angina pectoris should include a stress exercise treadmill test. The incidence of false-positive results from stress treadmill testing in women is higher than in men because the pretest probability of the disease being present is lower for a given age (Table 6.2) (10). The addition of a radionuclide such as thallium or sesta-MIBI increases the sensitivity and specificity of the test both in women and men (11). False-positive stress radionuclide studies still occur and are most commonly due to technical factors including breast or diaphragmatic attenuation of the radionuclide. The use of stress radionuclide ventriculography is not useful in women because the typical increase in ejection fraction of at least five percentage points with exercise is not seen in women despite the absence of coronary disease (12). The early data on the use of stress echocardiography shows that it appears to have a sen-

Table 6.2 Test Performance of the Exercise ECG in Patients with Various Chest Pain Syndromes

Pain Syndrome	True-Positive Rate (Men/Women)	False-Positive Rate (Men/Women)
Nonanginal chest pain	0.46/0.22	0.21/0.19
Atypical angina	0.72/0.67	0.20/0.31
Typical exertional angina	0.84/0.80	0.29/0.43

Source: Sox HC Jr. Noninvasive testing in coronary artery disease. Selection of procedures and interpretation of results. Postgrad Med 1983;74:319–336.

sitivity and specificity for the diagnosis of ischemic heart disease, which is similar between men and women (13). Therefore, after a careful cardiovascular history, physical examination, and stress treadmill testing, the likelihood of coronary artery disease being present can be easily estimated (Table 6.3) and the need for more extensive evaluation including coronary arteriography can be determined.

Medical Therapy of Ischemic Heart Disease and Angina

A number of medications and groups of medications can be used in the treatment of patients with angina pectoris or its symptoms. Special care in dosing is important in elderly patients because they are many times more prone to side effects and respond generally to lower doses of medication.

Nitrates

Nitroglycerin is extremely effective in the treatment of angina pectoris. When given sublingually it produces a rapid systemic vasodilation that decreases afterload and preload, thereby decreasing myocardial oxygen demand. It is a potent vasodilator of the epicardial coronary tree and improves collateral circulation. It is typically given in a dose of 0.4–0.8 mg and usually it has an effect within 5 to 15 minutes. Patients should be instructed to take multiple doses if necessary; however, if pain persists despite three doses at 5-minute intervals they should be instructed to seek care with their physician immediately. Unfortunately, it has a relatively short plasma half-life and therefore cannot be used for chronic therapy. Nitroglycerin is also available in a paste form for cutaneous dosing at 4- to 6-hour intervals.

Other longer-acting nitrate preparations are avail-

Table 6.3 Probability of Coronary Artery Disease Depending on History, Exercise ECG Findings, and Myocardial Scintiscan Results in Patients with Various Chest Pain Syndromes

	HISTORY	POSITIVE RESULTS		NEGATIVE RESULTS	
		Exercise ECG	Scan	Exercise ECG	Scan
Men					
Nonanginal chest pain	0.22	0.38	0.74	0.16	0.08
Atypical angina	0.67	0.88	0.95	0.42	0.38
Typical exertional angina	0.88	0.96	0.99	0.62	0.69
Women					
Nonanginal chest pain	0.05	0.06	0.35	0.05	0.02
Atypical angina	0.35	0.54	0.85	0.20	0.14
Typical exertional angina	0.58	0.72	0.93	0.33	0.29

Source: Sox HC Jr. Noninvasive testing in coronary artery disease. Selection of procedures and interpretation of results. Postgrad Med 1983;74:319–336.

able and can be given either orally or transcutaneously. The nitrate patch can be used, but nitrate tolerance develops rapidly if the patch is kept in place for 24 hours. The patient should be instructed to remove the patch at bedtime to allow a nitrate-free period and to minimize the development of nitrate tolerance. Nitrates can also be given orally as a sustained-released preparation but should be dosed at 8:00 AM and 2:00 PM to avoid a constant nitrate level and the development of nitrate tolerance.

Common side effects of nitrates include headache, flushing, and dizziness. Patients taking sublingual nitroglycerin should be warned that significant hypotension can develop and they should be instructed to take the medication while sitting or lying down if possible. The flushing and headache commonly associated with oral preparations of nitroglycerin are sometimes diminished with repetitive dosing or if the medications are taken with food in the stomach. The headache can sometimes be improved by the use of an analgesic before dosing.

β-Adrenergic Blockade

β-Adrenergic blockers are important in the management of patients with angina. They decrease myocardial oxygen demand by decreasing heart rate, contractility, and afterload by diminishing systemic blood pressure. These medications are helpful in reducing the increase in contractility and heart rate seen with exercise. Numerous β-adrenergic blockers are available. Compliance has probably improved with the use of once daily dosing of the long-acting β-adrenergic blocker such as atenolol (Tenormin).

Common side effects include fatigue and listlessness, bad dreams, decrease in libido, and symptomatic bradycardia. These drugs should be avoided or used with caution in patients with insulin-dependent diabetes and in patients with significant broncospastic pulmonary disease. They should likewise be avoided in patients with severe peripheral vascular disease and in patients with significant AV conduction abnormalities. This includes patients with second-degree AV block. There is a relative contraindication to the use of β-adrenergic blockade in patients with documented vasospastic or Prinzmetal's angina because theoretically these agents could provoke episodes of vasospasm. β-Adrenergic blockade should be used cautiously in patients with known left ventricular dysfunction because many of these patients will have worsened symptoms or develop frank congestive heart failure when given these medications.

Calcium Channel Antagonists

Calcium channel antagonists were initially developed for the treatment of vasospastic or Prinzmetal's angina but have found wide use in the treatment of symptomatic ischemic heart disease. A number of calcium channel antagonists are available and their cardiovascular effects are primarily due to vasodilation, the relief of any vasospastic component in the coronary tree, and, with some agents, changes in contractility. Some are stronger vasodilator agents than others (e.g., amlodipine versus verapamil) and the effect on the individual will depend on patient factors as well as the agent chosen. Care should be taken in using calcium channel blockers that have significant negative inotropic effects such as verapamil. The use of such agents may worsen congestive heart failure and, like β-adrenergic blockade agents, can worsen AV conduction. Side effects of agents that are primarily vasodilators such as nifedipine include the development of significant peripheral edema. Although this is cosmetic and does not imply any specific pathology, the patient should be warned of this potential side effect so as not to become alarmed if significant edema develops.

A calcium channel antagonist of the vasodilator group can be combined with a β-adrenergic blocker to potentiate the antiangina effect. However, care should be exercised because the patient response may be variable. If the calcium channel antagonist is the type that produces a decrease in AV node conduction (e.g., verapamil or diltiazem), significant bradycardia may develop. This seems to be especially common in elderly patients.

Additional side effects include the development of cutaneous rashes. These resolve with cessation of the medication. Typically, if patients develop a rash to one calcium channel antagonist they will develop similar rashes to others although occasionally a calcium channel antagonist can be found that does not produce a rash in a patient with such a history.

Aspirin

The use of aspirin in a dose of 160–325 mg/day has been shown to have a positive impact on cardiovascular mortality and cardiovascular events in patients with ischemic heart disease (14). Although the data involved follow-up in men only, unless there is a specific contraindication, all patients, including women, with known ischemic heart disease should be treated routinely with aspirin. The use of enteric-coated preparations is possible in patients with gastrointestinal side effects to uncoated aspirin. However, the absorption of these preparations varies. The use of other antiplatelet agents such as ticlopidine have not undergone the extensive epidemiologic studies that have been performed with aspirin and therefore their use in place of aspirin cannot be condoned.

Antihyperlipidemic Agents

In patients who have documented coronary disease there is solid evidence (15,16) that aggressive lowering of lipids is effective in decreasing progression of the disease and improving survival at follow-up. The most recent National Cholesterol Education Program recommendations (17) are that patients with known coronary disease be treated initially with diet in an attempt to control the total cholesterol and LDL. In patients in whom aggressive dietary modification is not effective a number of antihyperlipidemic medications can be used to lower total cholesterol and LDL (see Chapter 4).

The Treatment of Unstable Angina

In general patients with unstable angina should be hospitalized for more aggressive management of their symptoms. The medications used for the treatment of unstable angina are similar to those used for the treatment of chronic angina. In addition patients should be treated with intravenous heparin, which has been shown to decrease subsequent events and mortality in the hospital (18). In patients who have unstable symptoms despite aggressive medical treatment more aggressive management of their coronary disease such as coronary artery bypass grafting or percutaneous transluminal coronary angioplasty should be considered.

When Should a Patient with Angina Be Referred to a Subspecialist?

Many patients with angina can be treated quite effectively by primary care physicians. Patients with chronic, stable angina who are either intolerant of medications or desire to take as few medications as possible can be referred to a cardiologist for evaluation of possible revascularization, which would include percutaneous transluminal coronary angioplasty or bypass graft surgery. Patients with progression of symptoms while on medical therapy or patients who have unstable angina should be referred to a cardiologist for additional evaluation and therapy.

Patients who have markedly positive exercise stress treadmill tests, specifically, those who develop profound ST segment depression early in exercise, those who do not reach stage two on a standard Bruce protocol treadmill test, and those with multiple radionuclide perfusion defects, should be referred to a cardiologist.

Patients with known coronary disease should have a preoperative evaluation before any planned substantial surgical procedure. Additional evaluation including treadmill stress testing or potential cardiac catheterization maybe warranted before the surgical procedure.

Conclusions

The development of chest discomfort in any patient should be of concern and, as has been recently recognized through epidemiologic studies, this is likewise the case with women as well. Although the incidence of coronary heart disease in women at a given age is less than that found in men, by the seventh to eighth decade in life it is equally prevalent. It remains the number one cause of death in women and actually exceeds the death rate in men. In addition, the prognosis in women after the first myocardial infarction appears to be worse than that found in men and therefore the appropriate diagnosis and treatment of women with ischemic heart disease is paramount. The practicing primary gynecologist should be well equipped to treat these patients with referral of appropriate patients to subspecialists as discussed.

REFERENCES

1. Lerner DJ, Kannel WB. Patterns of coronary heart disease morbidity and mortality in the sexes: a 26 year follow-up of the Framingham population. Am Heart J 1986;111:383–390.

2. Chaitman BR, Bourassa MG, Davis K, et al. Angiographic prevalence of high risk of coronary artery disease

in patient subsets (CASS). Circulation 1981;64:360–367.

3. Kannel WB, Dawber TR, Kagan A, et al. Factors of risk in the development of coronary heart disease–six year follow-up experience. The Framingham study. Ann Intern Med 1961;55:33–50.

4. Kannel WB, Feinleib M. Natural history of angina pectoris in the Framingham study: prognosis and survival. Am J Cardiol 1972;29:154–163.

5. Ellis S, Alderman EL, Cain K, et al. Morphology of left anterior descending coronary territory lesions as a predictor of anterior myocardial infarction: A CASS registry study. J Am Coll Cardiol 1989;13:1481–1491.

6. Taylor HA, Deumite NJ, Chaitman BR, et al. Asymptomatic left main coronary artery disease in the Coronary Artery Surgery Study (CASS) registry. Circulation 1989;79:1171–1179.

7. Mock MB, Fisher LD, Holmes DR, et al. Comparison of effects of medical and surgical therapy on survival in severe angina pectoris and two-vessel coronary artery disease with and without left ventricular dysfunction: a coronary artery surgery study registry study. Am J Cardiol 1988;61:1198–1203.

8. Roberts KB, Califf RM, Harrell FE, et al. The prognosis for patients with new-onset angina who have undergone cardiac catheterization. Circulation 1983;68:970–978.

9. Rissanen AM. Familial occurrence of coronary heart disease: effect of age at diagnosis. Am J Cardiol 1979;44:60–66.

10. Weiner DA, Ryan TJ, McCabe CH, et al. Correlations among history of angina, ST segment response, and prevalence of coronary artery disease in the Coronary Artery Surgery Study (CASS). N Engl J Med 1979;301:230–235.

11. Hung J, Chaitman BR, Lam J, et al. Non-invasive diagnostic test choices for the evaluation of coronary artery disease in women: a multi-variate comparison of cardiac fluoroscopy, exercise electrocardiography and exercise thallium myocardial perfusion scintigraphy. J Am Coll Cardiol 1984;4:8–16.

12. Gibbons RJ, Lee KL, Cobb F, Jones RH. Ejection fraction in response to exercise in patients with chest pain and normal coronary arteriograms. Circulation 1981;64:952–957.

13. Sawada SG, Ryan T, Fineberg NS, et al. Exercise echocardiographic detection of coronary artery disease in women. J Am Coll Cardiol 1989;14:1440–1447.

14. Ridker PM, Manson JE, Gaziano JM, et al. Low dose aspirin therapy for chronic stable angina. A randomized clinical trial. Ann Intern Med 1991;114: 835–839.

15. Kane JP, Malloy MJ, Ports TA, et al. Regression of coronary atherosclerosis during treatment of familial hypercholesterolemia with combined drug regiments. JAMA 1990;264:3007–3012.

16. Miettine NM, Karvonen MJ, Turpeinen O, et al. Effect of cholesterol lowering on mortality from coronary heart disease and other causes. Lancet 1972;2:835–838.

17. National Cholesterol Education Program. Second report of the Expert Panel on Detection, Evaluation, and Treatment of High Blood Cholesterol in Adults (Adult Treatment Panel 2). Circulation 1994;89:1333–1445.

18. Theroux P, Ouimet H, McCans J, et al. Aspirin, heparin, or both to treat unstable angina. N Engl J Med 1988;319:1105.

19. Sox HC Jr. Noninvasive testing in coronary artery disease. Selection of procedures and interpretation of results. Postgrad Med 1983;74:319–336.

CHAPTER 7

HEART FAILURE

Douglas J. Pearce

Cardiovascular disease remains the number one killer in North America. Although the incidence of other causes of cardiovascular death have steadily declined over the last decade, the incidence of heart failure is rising. It is estimated that over three million Americans have heart failure, with approximately 400,000 new cases diagnosed each year. Annually, heart failure accounts for nearly one million hospital admissions and 200,000 deaths. Additionally, over $8 billion is spent each year in the United States to care for these patients (1).

As the incidence of heart failure has been increasing the etiology has been changing. Fifty years ago the most common causes of heart failure were hypertensive heart disease and valvular heart disease. Today, heart failure is most frequently secondary to ischemic heart disease. Overall, the prognosis of patients with congestive heart failure remains poor. In fact, there has been no significant change over the 40 year period from 1948 to 1988 (2).

Definition

Left ventricular dysfunction remains central to the pathophysiology of congestive heart failure. However, heart failure is perhaps best defined as a clinical syndrome, characterized by dyspnea and fatigue, and modulated by the compensatory neurohumoral mechanisms that promote fluid retention (1).

Causes of Heart Failure

The causes of heart failure are protean and are listed in Box 7.1. In the United States the most common cause of heart failure is ischemic heart disease. This may be seen in the form of impaired ventricular contraction and relaxation due to ongoing ischemia (acute or chronic) or manifest as chronic left ventricular enlargement with systolic dysfunction after loss of myocardium from infarction.

Systolic Versus Diastolic Ventricular Dysfunction

Patients with left ventricular dysfunction can usually be classified as having either primarily systolic or diastolic dysfunction. Although admittedly many, if not most, patients demonstrate aspects of both, this classification system aids in our understanding of the pathophysiology, treatment options, and prognosis.

Systolic Dysfunction

Irrespective of etiology, when myocardial contractile function begins to fail and cardiac output is reduced, a complex series of compensatory mechanisms come into play. These mechanisms principally surround the activation of neurohormonal systems designed to increase the inotropic stimulation to the heart and to increase plasma volume through salt and water retention. Activation of the sympathetic nervous system results in an increase in circulating plasma catecholamines as well as activation of the renin–angiotensin–aldosterone system (3,4). Combined, these adaptive mechanisms restore blood pressure and cardiac output by augmenting myocardial contractility, increasing ventricular preload, and increasing peripheral vascular resistance (5,6). The most important method for augmenting myocardial contractility and improving cardiac output is the Frank-Starling mechanism. As can be seen from the Frank-Starling curve in Figure 7-1, an increase in left ventricular end-diastolic volume caused by fluid retention results, at

Box 7.1 Causes of Heart Failure

Primary abnormality of myocardial cells
- Cardiomyopathy and myocarditis

Secondary abnormality of myocardial cells
- Due to prolonged exposure to a hemodynamic burden (i.e., aortic regurgitation, hypertensive heart disease, primary or secondary pulmonary hypertension)
- Due to reduced O_2 delivery (ischemia)

Structural abnormalities
- Valvular heart disease
- Congenital heart disease
- Pericardial disease
- Coronary artery disease (ischemia, myocardial infarction, left ventricular aneurysm)
- Intracavity outflow obstruction

High-output states

Precipitating causes
- Increased salt intake
- Inappropriate reduction of a drug regimen
- Excess exertion or emotion
- Arrhythmias
- Systemic infection
- Onset of high-output states: anemia, hyperthyroidism, pregnancy
- Pulmonary embolism
- Increased fluid load
- Renal failure
- Myocardial ischemia
- Cardiac depressants (e.g., disopyramide)

Adapted by permission from Kloner RA, ed. The guide to cardiology, 2nd ed. Greenwich, CT: LeJacq Communications, 1990:362.

least to a point, in improved ventricular performance. Patients with impaired systolic function operate along curve B, which is depressed. Activation of the neurohumoral systems described above, along with increased production of arginine vasopressin (antidiuretic hormone), results in an expansion of plasma volume and, at least initially, a restoration of ventricular function. As part of the compensatory process the myocardium may hypertrophy and the ventricle enlarge (8). Unfortunately, as the myocardium continues to fail the compensatory mechanisms can no longer keep up, and may in fact become detrimental. Additional fluid retention eventually results in elevated pulmonary pressures and pulmonary and peripheral edema. The increase in systemic vascular resistance further compromises cardiac output and tissue perfusion.

The prognosis of patients with heart failure from systolic left ventricular dysfunction is poor. Median survival following the diagnosis of heart failure is 1.66 years for men and 3.17 years for women (2). For patients with New York Heart Association class IV symptoms, and a VO_2max of less than 10 mL/min per kg, the mortality rate exceeds 50% (9).

Diastolic Dysfunction

Patients with systolic dysfunction often have a component of diastolic dysfunction. However, for some patients with heart failure, impaired ventricular relaxation is the primary problem (10).

When patients present with signs and symptoms of heart failure but normal or near normal ventricular function (ejection fraction >0.45), significant diastolic dysfunction should be considered. Failure of proper ventricular relaxation results in elevated ventricular diastolic pressure, which in turn causes an increase in atrial pressure and subsequent pulmonary or systemic congestion. Intermittent episodes of ischemia can cause diastolic dysfunction and "flash" pulmonary edema, even though systolic function is preserved. Other common causes of diastolic dysfunction include

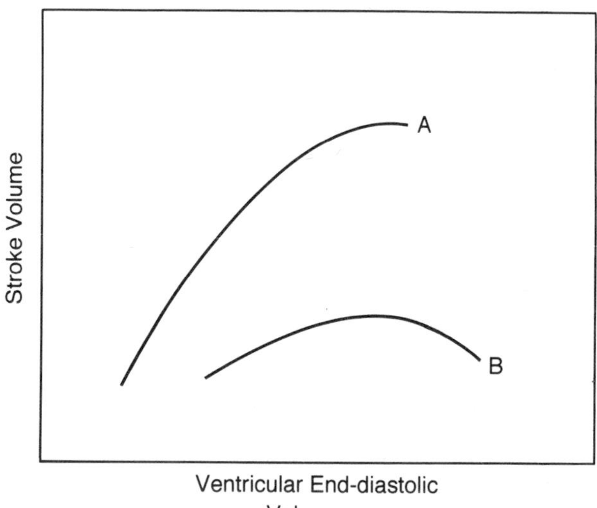

Fig 7.1 Frank-Starling curve for cardiac output.

the stiff ventricles of hypertrophic and restrictive cardiomyopathies (11–15).

Patients with heart failure primarily on the basis of diastolic dysfunction generally have a better prognosis than those with systolic dysfunction. In the V-HeFT-I trial, patients with heart failure and a left ventricular ejection fraction (LVEF) of at least 0.45 had an annual mortality rate of 8.0%. This is in comparison to 19.0% in those whose LVEF was less than 0.45 (16). However, patients with diastolic dysfunction remain at risk for ischemic events and disease progression. Close follow-up is required (17). Despite their better prognosis, patients with predominately diastolic dysfunction demonstrate poor exercise tolerance. This impairment in exercise ability is at least partially due to failure of the Frank-Starling mechanism to increase cardiac output during exercise by increasing ventricular filling (18).

Clinical Forms of Heart Failure

Forward Versus Backward Heart Failure

The classification of patients as suffering predominantly from either forward or backward heart failure is somewhat artificial. The concept behind backward failure is that as end-diastolic ventricular volume and pressure rise, pressure increases in the venous system proximal to the failing ventricle. The increase in venous pressure in turn results in transudation of fluid into the systemic or pulmonary interstitium, which in turn is responsible for the signs and symptoms of heart failure. In contrast, the forward failure hypothesis dictates that the signs and symptoms of heart failure are due to reduced forward output to the brain, vital organs, and skeletal muscles. Neurohormonal activation with sodium and water retention follows. In reality, most patients suffer from symptoms of both. As noted above, even patients with diastolic dysfunction and a normal LVEF may demonstrate evidence of inadequate organ perfusion due to a reduction in cardiac output, resulting from impaired ventricular filling (18).

Right-Sided Versus Left-Sided Heart Failure

The most common cause of right-sided heart failure is left-sided heart failure. Most patients with long-standing heart failure have signs and symptoms of biventricular failure. Nevertheless, it is not uncommon for patients to present with signs and symptoms of excess fluid primarily "backed up" behind one ventricle or the other. For example, patients with pathology principally affecting the right ventricle, such as primary pulmonary hypertension or pulmonary hypertension secondary to recurrent pulmonary emboli, may present with peripheral edema, congestive hepatomegaly, and ascites. However, a hallmark of heart failure, poor exercise tolerance, remains a prominent symptom. When the right ventricle fails, left ventricle filling is inadequate, leading to poor cardiac output and impaired exercise tolerance. In fact, inadequate left ventricle filling due to right ventricular failure is an important cause of impaired exercise tolerance even in patients with poor left ventricular systolic function (19).

Patients with primary left ventricular pathology may initially present with signs or symptoms of pulmonary congestion and impaired exercise tolerance. However, given adequate time, fluid retention results in peripheral edema, and the elevated left ventricular end-diastolic pressure transmitted to the pulmonary vasculature eventually results in right ventricular failure. Additionally, irrespective of the ventricle initially involved, the myocytes of the contralateral ventricle eventually develop biochemical and structural changes (20–22).

High-Output Versus Low-Output Heart Failure

The majority of patients presenting with heart failure have low or low-normal cardiac output. However, heart failure may also develop in patients in whom the cardiac output is high normal or high. High-output heart failure may be seen with pregnancy, hyperthyroidism, arteriovenous fistula, Paget's disease, anemia, and beriberi. The pathophysiology of high-output heart failure is complex, but essentially results from the mechanical and bioenergetic burden placed on the heart by pumping large volumes of blood over a long period of time. In the case of severe anemia, the myocardium is further compromised by impaired oxygen delivery to the myocytes. Generally, some underlying cardiac pathology is necessary for the increase in circulatory demand to result in heart failure (23). In the case of thyrotoxicosis, there may be direct metabolic effects that further impair cardiac function (24). In fact, hyperthyroidism in children has been reported to cause heart failure in the absence of underlying heart disease (25).

Acute Versus Chronic Heart Failure

The majority of patients with heart failure seen in clinical practice have had progressive symptoms over weeks to months, with concomitant neurohormonal changes. Occasionally, rupture of a mitral valve papillary muscle or perforation of the interventricular septum will occur after a myocardial infarction. This results in almost instantaneous pulmonary edema, frequently with reduced cardiac output and hypotension. Nonetheless, the basic therapeutic concepts of diruesis and afterload reduction are the same as with chronic heart failure.

Clinical Manifestations of Heart Failure

Signs and Symptoms

Right-Sided Heart Failure

The signs and symptoms of right-sided failure are predominantly those of systemic venous congestion. These include peripheral edema, hepatic congestion with right upper quadrant pain (secondary to stretching the hepatic capsule), ascites, and a sense of abdominal fullness. Although rales and pulmonary edema would be unexpected in right-sided heart failure, poor exercise tolerance is universal (26).

Left-Sided Heart Failure

The principle symptoms of left-sided heart failure are poor exercise tolerance, dyspnea on exertion, orthopnea, paroxysmal nocturnal dyspnea, and fatigue. As the disease progresses, patients may complain of dyspnea at rest and impaired mentation. Nocturia is frequently seen in patients with heart failure. It is largely due to diuresis of previously dependent fluid after the lower extremities are elevated.

Impaired exercise tolerance and dyspnea are hallmarks of heart failure. Impaired exercise tolerance results from inadequate perfusion of skeletal muscles but is in part due to the dyspnea itself (27). As the left ventricle begins to fail, pulmonary pressures rise. This results in engorgement of the pulmonary vasculature and interstitial pulmonary edema. The compliance of the lungs is reduced resulting in a restrictive ventilatory defect. Initially, dyspnea may be seen only during periods of exercise, but as ventricular dysfunction progresses, interstitial pulmonary fluid increases and pulmonary compliance decreases. Dyspnea is eventually seen with even minimal activity. If unchecked, alveolar edema results in severe dyspnea even at rest.

Orthopnea, an increase in dyspnea when recumbent, results from a further increase in pulmonary hydrostatic pressure as fluid is redistributed from the lower extremities and abdomen. A severe form of orthopnea, paroxysmal nocturnal dyspnea, may be seen when recumbency results in interstitial pulmonary edema. Patients with paroxysmal nocturnal dyspnea complain of wakening at night with severe dyspnea and coughing. Wheezing, often called cardiac asthma, frequently accompanies paroxysmal nocturnal dyspnea and is secondary to bronchial spasm. Whereas patients with orthopnea may obtain relief by simply adding an extra pillow or hanging their legs over the side of the bed, patients with paroxysmal nocturnal dyspnea have more severe symptoms requiring additional diuretics or oxygen for relief.

The New York Heart Association has devised a functional classification for assessing the severity of cardiovascular disease based on the amount of exertion required to illicit symptoms. This classification is useful for following the patient and assessing the effect of therapy.

- Class I: Patients with cardiac disease, but without resulting limitation of physical activity. Ordinary physical activity does not cause undue fatigue, palpitation, dyspnea, or anginal pain.
- Class II: Patients with cardiac disease resulting in slight limitation of physical activity. They are comfortable at rest. Ordinary physical activity results in fatigue, palpitation, dyspnea, or anginal pain.
- Class III: Patients with cardiac disease resulting in marked limitation of physical activity. They are comfortable at rest. Less than ordinary physical activity causes fatigue, palpitation, dyspnea, or anginal pain.
- Class IV: Patients with cardiac disease resulting in inability to carry on any physical activity without discomfort. Symptoms of cardiac insufficiency or of the anginal syndrome may be present even at

rest. If any physical activity is undertaken, discomfort is increased (28).

Physical Examination

The physical findings of left ventricular failure depend on the severity of the heart failure. With mild to moderate heart failure, the patient may appear normal at rest but develops breathlessness with activity. Resting tachycardia is not infrequent and suggests severe ventricular dysfunction. The blood pressure may range from hypotensive to hypertensive. When heart failure becomes severe, the patient may be pale with cool cyanotic extremities. The cardiac examination frequently reveals evidence of left ventricular hypertrophy and dilatation with the presence of a precordial heave and displacement of apical impulse laterally. Although the S_1 is generally normal, the P_2 is frequently accentuated secondary to high pulmonary pressures. An S_3 and an S_4 are often heard, although neither is a specific sign for heart failure.

Despite severe impairment of left ventricular function and elevated pulmonary pressures, the lungs may remain clear. This is primarily due to enhanced lymphatic drainage. However, the majority of patients will eventually develop bilateral rales, initially at the bases, with progression toward the apices as their failure worsens. Pleural effusions are also a common finding. If the effusion is unilateral, it is most commonly found on the right. The murmurs of mitral and tricuspid regurgitation are often heard. Even when the pathology principally involves the left ventricle, systemic venous pressures are frequently elevated resulting in jugular venous distention and hepatojugular reflux (increase in jugular venous distention during gentle abdominal compression over the liver). As left ventricular function declines, Cheyne-Stokes respirations and pulsus alternans may be seen.

Patients with severe chronic heart failure frequently develop cardiac cachexia with anorexia and weight loss (29). With severe congestion of the viscera (particularly in right-sided failure), a protein-loosening enteropathy may develop further compromising nutritional status and exacerbating ascites and peripheral edema (30).

Laboratory Findings and Heart Failure

The chest radiograph frequently reveals cardiomegaly with a cardiothoracic ratio greater than 0.5. The lung fields may demonstrate pulmonary venous congestion and interstitial edema. Pleural effusions may be present, and as noted above, if unilateral are more common on the right.

The electrocardiogram, while without specific findings for heart failure, may demonstrate evidence of prior infarction, chamber enlargement, or hypertrophy.

Two-dimensional echocardiography with Doppler flow studies is invaluable for assessing the patient with congestive heart failure. Regional and global ventricular function can be assessed as well as ascertaining valvular structure and competence.

Although echocardiography is valuable for estimating ventricular function, radionuclide ventriculography has less user variability and is probably the best test for serial evaluations.

Eventually most patients with heart failure will undergo right and left heart catheterization, which provides information on cardiac output, left and right heart pressures, and coronary anatomy. This information is useful for planning and modifying treatment strategies.

In mild to moderate heart failure, blood chemistries are usually normal. As cardiac output declines, the blood urea nitrogen level may rise. With salt restriction and diuretic use, hyponatremia may develop. A serum sodium level of 134 mEq/L or less is a particularly poor prognostic sign (31). Additionally, hepatic congestion frequently leads to elevations in aspartate aminotransferase, alanine aminotransferase, and bilirubin levels.

Differential Diagnosis of Heart Failure

Clearly, not all pulmonary edema is cardiac in etiology. The differential diagnosis of noncardiogenic pulmonary edema is shown in Box 7.2. Additionally, the numerous pulmonary causes of dyspnea (chronic obstructive pulmonary disease, pulmonary fibrosis, pulmonary embolism, etc) must be excluded. The lower extremity edema of heart failure is generally bilateral, but other causes of lower extremity edema such as venostasis disease, lymphatic etiologies, and renal failure need exclusion.

Ascites is a frequent finding in hepatic cirrhosis. However, cirrhotic patients generally do not have ele-

Box 7.2 Noncardiac Causes of Pulmonary Edema

Decreased plasma oncotic pressure: hypoalbuminemia due to renal, hepatic disease, nutritional cause, or protein-losing enteropathy

Altered alveolar-capillary membrane permeability (often referred to as adult respiratory distress syndrome [ARDS])
- Pneumonia: viral, bacterial, parasite, aspiration
- Inhaled toxins: smoke, nitrogen dioxide, phosgene
- Circulating toxins: bacterial endotoxins, snake venom
- Radiation pneumonitis
- Endogenous vasoactive substances: kinins, histamines
- Disseminated intravascular coagulation
- Uremia
- Immunologic reactions: hypersensitivity pneumonitis
- Associated with drowning

Lymphatic insufficiency: carcinomatosis, fibrosing lymphangitis

Unknown or not well understood
- Narcotic overdose: heroin
- High altitude pulmonary edema
- Neurogenic: subarachnoid hemorrhage, central nervous system trauma
- Eclampsia
- Postcardiopulmonary bypass
- Postcardioversion
- Postanesthesia

Adapted by permission from Kloner RA, ed. The guide to cardiology, 2nd ed. Greenwich, CT: LeJacq Communications, 1990:364.

vated jugular venous pressure nor the presence of hepatojugular reflux.

Treatment of Heart Failure

The primary goals in the management of heart failure are to improve quality of life and to reduce mortality. Braunwald and Grossman have divided the treatment of heart failure into three components: 1) removal of the precipitating cause, 2) correction of the underlying cause, and 3) control of the congestive heart failure state (23). The first step is to determine if there is an acute precipitating cause such as anemia or severe hypertension that can be treated. The second step is to determine if there is a reversible underlying cause. For instance, patients with severe ischemic heart disease may benefit from revascularization. Patients with aortic or mitral valvular disease may benefit from surgical replacement or valvular repair. And in case of alcoholic cardiomyopathy, abstinence results in improvement in a significant number of patients (32–35). The third step, treatment, is discussed in detail below.

Treatment of Acute Pulmonary Edema

Acute pulmonary edema is a life-threatening medical emergency. Initial treatment efforts are targeted at improving oxygenation and reducing pulmonary hydrostatic pressure.

Oxygen should be administered at high concentrations (unless carbon dioxide retention is known to be a major concern) and the effect monitored by arterial blood gas determinations followed by continuous transcutaneous oxygen saturation monitoring.

Intravenous morphine (2–5 mg) results in preload reduction and reduces anxiety. Uncommonly this may result in respiratory depression, so naloxone should be available.

Intravenous furosemide (40–80 mg) has a rapid venodilating effect, thus reducing preload even before a diuresis ensues.

Unless the patient is already taking digitalis, it should be administered IV. The initial dose is 0.25–0.50 mg digoxin, with additional 0.25-mg doses every 6 hours to a total of 1.0 mg. Digitalis is particularly helpful in patients with atrial fibrillation with a rapid ventricular response.

Nitroglycerin results in additional preload reduction and may further reduce ischemia. Patients who are not hypotensive should receive sublingual nitroglycerin, followed by an IV infusion of 10–20 μg/min up to 200 μg / min.

Patients who remain hypertensive after the above can be treated with IV nitroprusside (0.5–8.0 μg/kg per minute) for further afterload reduction. However, IV nitroprusside has been reported to cause coronary steal and should probably be avoided in acute ischemic syndromes. Hypertensive patients may also be treated with the IV angiotensin-converting enzyme (ACE) inhibitor, enalaprilat. The dose is 1.25 mg IV every 6 hours. Enalaprilat should be avoided in renal insufficiency and pregnancy.

Additionally, patients with bronchial constriction may benefit from IV aminophylline. Aminophylline also increases renal blood flow augmenting diuresis.

Finally, maintaining the patient in an upright position, if possible, will further reduce preload.

Treatment of Chronic Heart Failure

Irrespective of the etiology, patients with chronic heart failure benefit from salt restriction and avoidance of stressful physical exertion. Once stabilized, a program of low level aerobic exercise is safe, improves functional capacity, and promotes a sense of well-being. Additionally, patients benefit from a reduction in emotional and environmental stress (36). Obese patients should be strongly encouraged to lose weight in an effort to reduce cardiac workload.

Once reversible underlying causes have been addressed, and the patient continues to have class II or greater heart failure symptoms, pharmacologic intervention is indicated. Based on the results of large scale clinical trials conducted over the last decade, standard therapy of patients with heart failure secondary to systolic dysfunction includes the use of a vasodilator (preferably an ACE inhibitor), diuretics, and digoxin. In specific cases, the use of nitrates, or β blockers may be beneficial.

Vasodilators

Hydralazine and ACE inhibitors are the vasodilators proved to be effective in decreasing symptoms and improving mortality in patients with systolic dysfunction. The V-HeFT-I trial randomized 642 men with moderately severe heart failure, already receiving digoxin and a diuretic, to placebo, prazosin, or a combination of hydralazine and isorbide dinitrate (37). Although no benefit was obtained from receiving prazosin, the hydralazine/isorbide dinitrate group had a 34% decrease in 2-year mortality when compared to placebo.

The ACE inhibitors demonstrate both venous and arterial dilating properties. Several studies have demonstrated that they are effective in reducing both the symptoms and the mortality of heart failure (38–41). The V-HeFT II study compared the effects of enalapril with those of hydralazine and isorbide dinitrate. Mortality at 2 years was 28% lower in the group receiving enalapril (42). Thus, unless there are clear contraindications, ACE inhibitors are considered to be the vasodilator of choice in heart failure.

Although it is generally agreed that an ACE inhibitor should be first-line therapy in heart failure secondary to left ventricular systolic dysfunction, the exact timing of initiation of therapy is less clear. The SOLVD study had both a treatment and a prevention arm. The prevention arm randomized 4228 patients who had an LVEF of 0.35 or less and were not receiving heart failure drug therapy to placebo or enalapril. The majority of the patients randomized were in New York Heart Association functional class I. Treatment with enalapril slowed or reversed left ventricular dilatation in these patients (43). Over a 3-year period, treatment with enalapril reduced the development of heart failure by 37% and reduced hospitalization for heart failure by 36% (44). Based on this information, patients with asymptomatic left ventricular dysfunction and an LVEF of 0.35 or less should probably be begun on ACE inhibitor therapy.

Unfortunately, not all vasodilators have proven to be equally efficacious in heart failure. The Prospective Randomized Flosequinon Longevity Evaluation (PROFILE) study of the drug flosequinon and the Flolan International Randomized Survival Trial (FIRST) evaluation of the drug flolan both resulted in higher mortality in the treatment groups (45).

Finally, most calcium channel blockers are poorly tolerated in heart failure. However, the highly vasoselective dihydropyridine calcium channel blockers, felodipine and amlodipine, are presently being investigated for use as vasodilators in the management of this disease (46).

Diuretics

Patients with congestive symptoms and peripheral edema should be treated with diuretics. When heart failure is mild, almost any diuretic can be used. In fact, overdiuresis can be a greater problem than underdiuresis. Thiazide diuretics reduce the reabsorption of sodium, and thus water, in the distal tubule. These drugs are effective in mild heart failure as long as the glomerular filtration rate remains above 30 to 50 mL/min. Hypokalemia, particularly dangerous in the presence of digitalis toxicity, may result from thiazide diuretics. Although patients taking ACE inhibitors may not require potassium supplementation, potassium levels should be followed closely. Indapamide, a thiazide diuretic reported to be lipid neutral, may be of particular advantage in patients with atherosclerosis. Metolazone also works in the distal convoluted tubules. However, it has been reported to be more effective than the thiazides in the presence of moderate renal failure. Spironolactone, triamterene, and amiloride also act in the distal tubal. These agents are primarily used in combination with the thiazide diuretics to reduce potassium loss. Some evidence indicates that spironolactone may exert an antifibrotic effect on the myocardium. If additional research proves this to be true, spironolactone may have a special role in the management of heart failure (47). One of the "loop" diuretics, furosemide, bumetanide, toresamide, or ethacrynic acid, is almost universally necessary in moderate to severe heart failure. These agents act in the thick ascending limb of Henle's loop and are extremely potent. Patients need to be observed closely for overdiuresis, hypokalemia, and hyponatremia.

Patients with severe heart failure who fail to respond to high doses of loop diuretics are generally treated with the combination of a loop diuretic and a thiazide. Most frequently, metolazone (2.5–10.0 mg) is added to a loop diuretic. A marked increase in diuresis is often seen, and the patient must be closely monitored for overdiuresis and hypokalemia.

Digitalis

Digitalis has been used for the treatment of heart failure for over 200 years. To date, no study has been completed demonstrating the effect of digitalis on mortality in heart failure. Nonetheless, the use of digitalis in heart failure remains a standard of care. Digitalis exerts a positive inotropic effect on the heart by inhibition of the sodium potassium ATPace pump which results in an increase in intracellular sodium concentration, which in turn leads to an increase in calcium influx via the sodium–calcium exchange mechanism. Digoxin also modulates the neurohormonal aspects of heart failure, an effect that may prove to be its most clinically important (48).

Two recent trials, the Prospective Randomized Study of Ventricular Failure and the Efficacy of Digoxin (PROVED), and the Randomized Assessment of Digoxin on Inhibitors of the Angiotensin-Converting Enzyme (RADIANCE), demonstrated that withdrawal of digoxin in patients with New York Heart Association class II to III heart failure was associated with a worsening of heart failure symptoms and significant deterioration in exercise performance. Furthermore, neither study demonstrated an increase in adverse events due to treatment with digitalis (49,50).

Pending the results of a placebo-controlled mortality study by the Digitalis Investigative Group, cautious analysis of the data on the use of digoxin in heart failure support the addition of digoxin to a treatment with an ACE inhibitor and a diuretic, particularly in patients who remain symptomatic.

Nondigitalis Inotropes

Because myocardial contractility is impaired in patients with systolic dysfunction and heart failure, the use of positive inotropic agents seems intuitive. Over the years, numerous positive inotropic agents have been developed that have been effective in improving hemodynamics. However, the use of these agents has not been associated with a long-term benefit and may actually increase mortality (51–55). The Prospective Randomized Milrinone Survival Evaluation (PROMISE), a study of the phosphodiesterase III inhibitor, milrinone, was terminated prematurely due to excess mortality in the treatment group (56). Finally, a new positive inotropic agent, vesnarinone, which possesses some type III antiarrhythmic properties, is presently under investigation and shows some promise (57).

Nitrates

Patients with symptoms of congestive heart failure despite therapy with vasodilators, diuretics, and digitalis may benefit from the addition of nitrates (58,59). Nitrates further reduce preload and may have a positive effect on ischemia. If a long-acting preparation is used, a nitrate-free interval of 10 to 12 hours should be used to avoid tolerance (60). If the patient's symptoms are primarily dyspnea on exertion, the nitrate-free interval should be scheduled during the hours of sleep. Conversely, if the patient suffers from paroxysmal nocturnal dyspnea and orthopnea, the nitrates should be administered at night with a nitrate-free interval during the waking hours. Effective regimens include isorbide dinitrate LA at 8:00 AM and 2:00 PM (if daytime dosing is used) or the use of a transdermal nitroglycerin patch, placed on at 8:00 AM and removed at 8:00 PM.

β Blockers

Although the use of β blockers in patients with congestive heart failure secondary to systolic dysfunction seems paradoxical, there is increasing evidence of benefit. Used with caution, β blockers may improve ventricular function, increase exercise tolerance, and decrease mortality (61,62). The exact mechanism(s) behind the beneficial effect of β blockers is unclear, but protection from sympathetic overstimulation is believed to be important (63). The initiation of β blockers in patients with impaired left ventricular systolic function should be with very low doses, frequent monitoring, and cautious titration.

Calcium Channel Blockers

The use of calcium channel blockers in patients with systolic dysfunction has generally not resulted in improvement and in some cases has led to deterioration (64). The highly vasoselective dihydropyridine calcium channel blockers, amlodipine and felodipine, are undergoing investigation as vasodilators in patients with impaired left ventricular function (46). It is hoped that they will have a role in patients who are unable to tolerate ACE inhibitors or hydralazine, but their routine use at this time is discouraged.

Intravenous Therapy

Patients with severe heart failure despite optimal oral therapy should be admitted for IV diuretics and inotropic therapy. A 48- to 72-hour infusion of one of the IV inotropes, dobutamine, amrinone, or milrinone, frequently results in a diuresis and significant improvement in hemodynamics (65–69). This beneficial effect may be maintained for several weeks (70,71). Finally, patients who are end stage may derive some short-term benefit from a continuous ambulatory infusion of dobutamine. Although the effect of this therapy on mortality is unclear, it may allow the patient a few more weeks or months at home with his or her family.

Cardiac Transplantation

On December 7, 1967, Dr. Christiaan Barnard performed the first successful human cardiac transplantation. Presently, the 1-year survival rate is 80% with a 5-year survival rate of 60% (72). Unfortunately, the use of cardiac transplantation is restricted by the limited donor pool and high cost (73). In general, patients with end-stage heart failure who are physiologically age 65 or younger, have preserved organ function, and the absence of other terminal disease, should be referred for cardiac transplant evaluation (74).

Treatment of Patients with Heart Failure due to Diastolic Dysfunction

The primary therapeutic goals of the treatment of patients with diastolic dysfunction are the same as for those with systolic dysfunction, namely, to improve the quality of life and decrease mortality. As with systolic dysfunction, precipitating and underlying causes should be sought and treated. Congestive symptoms are treated with cautious diuresis. Diastolic function can be improved by decreasing the heart rate to increase the diastolic filling time. This is done through the use of β blockers or the use of heart rate-lowering calcium channel blockers such as verapamil. Atrioventricular (AV) synchrony is important for optimal diastolic filling. Attempts should be made to maintain the patient in sinus rhythm and a dual-chamber (AV sequential) pacemaker considered if necessary. Recent data suggest that permanent pacing may be particularly effective in patients with hypertrophic cardiomyopathy and outflow tract obstruction (75,76).

Issues of Particular Importance to Women

Peripartum Cardiomyopathy

Peripartum cardiomyopathy is generally defined as left ventricular systolic dysfunction occurring during the final 3 months of pregnancy or within the first 6 months postpartum in women without a prior history of heart disease (77). Whether or not peripartum cardiomyopathy is a specific entity or is representative of idiopathic dilated cardiomyopathy occurring during the peripartum remains debatable. The incidence of peripartum cardiomyopathy is about 1 in 1300 to 1 in 4000 deliveries. The incidence appears to be greater in women who are over 30 years of age, pregnant with twins, or black (78). The etiology of peripartum cardiomyopathy is unknown. Several potential mechanisms have been postulated including toxemia, nutritional deficiency, hormonal effects, myocarditis, and a maternal immunologic response to fetal antigens (78,79). A recent study demonstrated a high incidence of myocarditis on endomyocardial biopsy (80). However, other studies have been less conclusive (81).

The clinical presentation of peripartum cardiomyopathy is of systolic left ventricular dysfunction and congestive heart failure. Patients frequently complain of increasing dyspnea on exertion, paroxysmal nocturnal dyspnea, orthopnea, and peripheral edema.

Despite our lack of a clear etiology and definitive treatment, the prognosis of peripartum cardiomyopathy is somewhat better than other forms of idiopathic dilated cardiomyopathy. Approximately 50% of patients demonstrate a return to near normal, or normal, ventricular function within 6 months of diagnosis. Unfortunately, the remaining 50% generally deteriorate. Mortality in this group is high (81,82).

Treatment of peripartum cardiomyopathy with diuretics, digitalis, and oxygen if needed is similar to other forms of dilated cardiomyopathy. Hydralazine is the preferred afterload reducing agent and appears to be safe in pregnancy (83). ACE inhibitors, generally the afterload reducing agents of choice for the management of heart failure, should be avoided. They have resulted in a number of complications including risk of early delivery, low birth weight, and neonatal renal failure (84). The role of immunosuppressive therapy remains controversial. However, immunosuppressive therapy may have a role in a clearly deteriorating patients (80,85). Patients unable to be managed on medical therapy should be considered for cardiac transplantation.

Finally, patients with peripartum cardiomyopathy are at increased risk of recurrence with subsequent pregnancies, unless ventricular size and function have returned to normal (86,87). Even if cardiac size and function have normalized, cardiac function should be closely followed during subsequent pregnancies.

Prognosis

Despite improved understanding of the pathophysiology as well as enhanced medical management, the prognosis of heart failure has not substantially changed over the last 40 years (2). Data from the Framingham study demonstrate a median survival of 1.7 years for men and 3.2 years for women following the diagnosis of heart failure. Irrespective of etiology, older patients have a worse prognosis. However, at least for men, patients with ischemic heart disease (a potentially reversible cause) have a somewhat better prognosis compared with those in whom the etiology is valvular or idiopathic. Overall, the 5-year survival rate is 25% for men and 38% for women (2). It is hoped that earlier initiation of ACE inhibitors, before the onset of symptoms, will improve survival (44,88).

Patients with heart failure but preserved left ventricular systolic function (diastolic dysfunction) have a significantly better prognosis (16).

REFERENCES

1. Garg R, Packer M, Pitt B, Yusuf S. Heart failure in the 1990s: evolution of a major public health problem in cardiovascular medicine. J Am Coll Cardiol 1993;22 (suppl A):3A–5A.

2. Ho KK, Anderson KM, Kannel WB, et al. Survival after the onset of congestive heart failure in Framingham heart study subjects. Circulation 1993;88:107–115.

3. Garr MD, McDonald KM, Francis GS. Neurohormonal activation and its relationship to the early stages of left ventricular dysfunction. Heart Failure 1992;8:167–176.

4. Packer M. The neurohormonal hypothesis: a theory to explain the mechanism of disease progression in heart failure. J Am Coll Cardiol 1992;20:248–254.

5. Cohn JN. Abnormalities of peripheral sympathetic nervous system control in congestive heart failure. Circulation 1990;82(suppl I):I-59–I-67.

6. Wei CM, Lerman A, Rodeheffer RJ, et al. Endothelin in human congestive heart failure. Circulation 1994;89:1580–1586.

7. Moalic JM, Charlemagne D, Mansier P, et al. Cardiac hypertrophy and failure – a disease of adaptation. Circulation 1993;87(suppl IV):IV-21–IV-26.

8. Gaudron P, Eilles C, Ertl G, Kochsiek K. Adaptation to cardiac dysfunction after myocardial infarction. Circulation 1993;87(suppl IV):IV-83–IV-89.

9. Szlachcic J, Massie B, Kramer B, et al. Correlates and prognostic implication of exercise capacity in chronic congestive heart failure. Am J Cardiol 1985;55:1037–1042.

10. Dougherty AH, Naccarelli GV, Gray EL, et al. Congestive heart failure with normal systolic function. Am J Cardiol 1984;54:778–782.

11. Litwin SE, Grossman W. Diastolic dysfunction as a cause of heart failure. J Am Coll Cardiol 1993;22(suppl A):49A–55A.

12. Stauffer JC, Gaasch WH. Recognition and treatment of left ventricular diastolic dysfunction. Prog Cardiovasc Dis 1990;32:319–332.

13. Grossman W. Diastolic dysfunction and congestive heart failure. Circulation 1990;81(suppl III):III-1–III-7.

14. Bonow RO, Udelson JE. Left ventricular diastolic dysfunction as a cause of congestive heart failure. Ann Intern Med 1992;117:501–510.

15. Gassch WH. Diagnosis and treatment of heart failure based on left ventricular systolic or diastolic dysfunction. JAMA 1994;271:1276–1280.

16. Cohn JN, Johnson G, Veterans Administration Cooperative Study Group. Heart failure with normal ejection fraction. Circulation 1990;81(suppl III):48–53.

17. Setaro J, Soufer R, Remetz M, et al. Long-term outcome in patients with congestive heart failure and intact systolic left ventricular performance. Am J Cardiol 1992;69:1212–1216.

18. Kitzman DW, Higginbotham MB, Cobb FR, et al. Exercise intolerance in patients with heart failure and preserved left ventricular systolic function: Failure of the Frank-Starling mechanism. J Am Coll Cardiol 1991;17:1065–1072.

19. Baker BJ, Wilen MM, Boyd CM, et al. Relation of right ventricular ejection fraction to exercise capacity in chronic left ventricular failure. Am J Cardiol 1984;54:596–599.

20. Chidsey CA, Kaiser GA, Sonnenblick EH, et al. Cardiac norepinephrine stores in experimental heart failure in the dog. J Clin Invest 1964;43:2386–2393.

21. Spann JF, Chidsey CA, Pool PE, et al. Mechanism of norepinephrine depletion in experimental heart failure produced by aortic constriction in the guinea pig. Circ Res 1965;17:312–321.

22. Chandler BM, Sonnenblick EH, Spann JF, et al. Association of depressed myofibrillar adenosine triphosphate and reduced contractility in experimental heart failure. Circ Res 1967;21:717–725.

23. Braunwald E, Grossman W. Clinical aspects of heart failure. In: Braunwald E, ed. Heart disease. 4th ed. Philadelphia: WB Saunders, 1992:458–462.

24. Polikar RP, Burger AG, Scherrer U, Nicod P. The thyroid and the heart. Circulation 1993;87:1435–1441.

25. Cavallo A, Joseph CJ, Casta A. Cardiac complications in juvenile hyperthyroidism. Am J Dis Child 1984;138:479–482.

26. Palevsky HI, Fishman AP. Chronic cor pulmonale. JAMA 1990;263:2347–2353.

27. Wilson JR, Mancini DM. Factors contributing to the exercise limitation of heart failure. J Am Coll Cardiol 1993;22(suppl A):93A–8A.

28. Goldman L, Hashimoto B, Cook E, Loscalzo A. Comparative reproducibility and validity of systems for assessing cardiovascular functional class: advantages of a new specific activity scale. Circulation 1981;6:1227–1234.

29. Levine B, Kalman J, Mayer L, et al. Elevated circulating levels of tumor necrosis factor in severe chronic heart failure. N Engl J Med 1990;323:236–241.

30. Strober W, Cohen LS, Waldmann TA, Braunwald E. Tricuspid regurgitation: a newly recognized cause of protein-losing enteropathy, lymphocytopenia and immunologic deficiency. Am J Med 1968;44:842–850.

31. Saxon LA, Stevenson WG, Middlekauff HR, et al. Predicting death from progressive heart failure secondary to ischemic or idiopathic dilated cardiomyopathy. Am J Cardiol 1993;72:62–65.

32. Milgaard H, Kristensen BO, Baandrup U. Importance of abstention from alcohol in alcoholic heart disease. Int J Cardiol 1990;26:373–375.

33. Schwartz L, Sample KA, Wigle ED. Severe alcoholic cardiomyopathy reversed with abstention from alcohol. Am J Cardiol 1975;36:963–966.

34. Baudet M, Rigaud M, Rocha P, et al. Reversibility of alcoholic cardiomyopathy with abstention from alcohol. Cardiology 1979;64:317–324.

35. Hung J, Harris PJ, Kelly DT, et al. Improvement of left ventricular function in alcoholic cardiomyopathy documented by serial gated cardiac pool scanning. Aust N Z J Med 1979;9:420–422.

36. Pashkow FJ, Squires RW. Rehabilitation of cardiologically complex patients. In: Pashlow FJ, Dafoe WA, eds. Clinical cardiac rehabilitation: a cardiologist's guide. Baltimore: Williams & Wilkins, 1993:143–163.

37. Cohn JN, Archibald D, Johnson G, VA Cooperative Study Group. Effects of vasodilator therapy on peak exercise oxygen consumption in heart failure. V-HeFT. Circulation 1987;76(suppl IV):IV-443.

38. The CONSENSUS Trial Study Group. Effects of enalapril on mortality in severe congestive heart

failure: results of the Cooperative North Scandinavian Enalapril Survival Study (CONSENSUS). N Engl J Med 1987;316:1429–1435.

39. The SOLVD Investigators. Studies of left ventricular dysfunction (SOLVD): rationale, design, and methods: two trials that evaluate the effect of enalapril in patients with reduced ejection fraction. Am J Cardiol 1990;66:315–322.

40. Pfeffer MA, Braunwald E, Moye LA, et al. Effect of captopril on mortality and morbidity in patients with left ventricular dysfunction after myocardial infarction: results of the survival and ventricular enlargement trial. N Engl J Med 1992:327:669–677.

41. Acute Infarction Ramipril Efficacy (AIRE) Study Investigators. Effect of ramipril on mortality and morbidity of survivors of acute myocardial infarction with clinical evidence of heart failure. Lancet 1993;342:821–827.

42. Cohn JN, Johnson G, Ziesche S, et al. A comparison of enalapril with hydralazine-isosorbide dinitrate in the treatment of chronic congestive heart failure. N Engl J Med 1991;325:303–310.

43. Konstam MA, Kronenberg MW, Rousseau MF, et al. Effects on the angiotensin converting enzyme inhibitor enalapril on the long term progression of left ventricular dilatation in patients with asymptomatic systolic dysfunction. Circulation 1993;88:2277–2283.

44. Effect of enalapril on mortality and the development of heart failure in asymptomatic patients with reduced left ventricular ejection fractions. N Engl J Med 1992;327:685–691.

45. Annual Scientific Session of the American College of Cardiology, Atlanta, GA, March, 1994.

46. Conti CR. Use of calcium antagonists to treat heart failure. Clin Cardiol 1994;17:101–102.

47. Brilla CG, Matsubara LS, Weber KT. Antifibrotic effects of spironolactone in preventing myocardial fibrosis in systemic arterial hypertension. Am J Cardiol 1993;71:12A–16A.

48. Gheorghiade M, Ferguson D. Digoxin: a neurohormonal modulator in heart failure? Circulation 1991;84(suppl 5):2182–2186.

49. Uretsky BF, Young JB, Shahidi FE, et al. Randomized study assessing the effect of digoxin withdrawal in patients with mild to moderate chronic congestive heart failure: results of the proved trial. J Am Coll Cardiol 1993;22:955–962.

50. Packer M, Gheorghiade M, Young J, et al. Withdrawal of digoxin from patients with chronic heart failure treated with angiotensin-converting-enzyme inhibitors. N Engl J Med 1993;329:1–7.

51. Benotti JR, Grossman W, Braunwald E, et al. Hemodynamic assessment of amrinone: a new inotropic agent. N Engl J Med 1978;299:1373–1377.

52. Baim DS, McDowell AV, Cherniles J, et al. Evaluation of a new bipyridine inotropic agent—milrinone—in patients with severe congestive heart failure. N Engl J Med 1983;309:748–756.

53. Weber KT, Janicki JS, Jain MC. Enoximone (MDL 17043) for stable, chronic heart failure secondary to ischemic or idiopathic cardiomyopathy. Am J Cardiol 1986;58:589–595.

54. Massie B, Bourassa M, DiBianco R, et al. Long-term oral administration of amrinone for congestive heart failure: lack of efficacy in a multicenter controlled trial. Circulation 1985;71:963–971.

55. Uretsky BF, Jessup M, Konstam MA, et al. Multicenter trial of oral enoximone in patients with moderate to moderately severe congestive heart failure: lack of benefit compared with placebo. Circulation 1990;82:774–780.

56. Packer M, Carver JR, Rodeheffer RJ, et al. Effect of oral milrinone on mortality in severe chronic heart failure. N Engl J Med 1991;325:1468–1475.

57. Feldman AM, Bristow MR, Parmley WW, et al. Effects of vesnarinone on morbidity and mortality in patients with heart failure. N Engl J Med 1993;329:149–155.

58. Leier CV, Huss P, Magorien RD, Unverferth DV. Improved exercise capacity and differing arterial and venous tolerance during chronic isosorbide dinitrate therapy for congestive heart failure. Circulation 1983;67:817–822.

59. Mehra A, Ostrzega E, Shotan A, et al. Persistent hemodynamic improvement with short-term nitrate therapy in patients with chronic congestive heart failure already treated with captopril. Am J Cardiol 1992;70:1310–1314.

60. Parmeley WW. Pathophysiology and current therapy of congestive heart failure. J Am Coll Cardiol 1989;13:771–785.

61. Fisher ML, Gottlieb SS, Plotnick GD, et al. Beneficial effects of metoprolol in heart failure associated with coronary artery disease: a randomized trial. J Am Coll Cardiol 1994;23:943–950.

62. Andersson B, Hamm C, Persson S, et al. Improved exercise hemodynamic status in dilated cardiomyopathy after beta-adrenergic blockade treatment. J Am Coll Cardiol 1994;23:1397–1404.

63. Eichhorn EJ. The paradox of β-adrenergic blockade for the management of congestive heart failure. Am J Med 1992;92:527–537.

64. Elkayam U, Amin J, Mehra A, et al. A prospective, randomized, double-blind, crossover study to compare the efficacy and safety of chronic nifedipine therapy with that of isosorbide dinitrate and their combination in the treatment of chronic congestive heart failure. Circulation 1990;82:1954–1961.

65. Thomas RL, Watson D, Marshall LE. Review of intermittent dobutamine infusions for congestive cardiomyopathy. Pharmacotherapy 1987;7:47–53.

66. Krell MJ, Kline EM, Bates ER, et al. Intermittent, ambulatory dobutamine infusions in patients with severe congestive heart failure. Am Heart J 1986;112:787–791.

67. Applefeld MM, Newman KA, Grove WR, et al. Intermittent, continuous outpatient dobutamine infusion in the management of congestive heart failure. Am J Cardiol 1983;51:455–458.

68. Roth S, Gordon M. Intermittent intravenous amrinone infusion: a potentially cost effective mode of treatment of patients with refractory heart failure. Can J Cardiol 1993;9:231–237.

69. Anderson JL. Hemodynamic and clinical benefits with intravenous milrinone in severe chronic heart failure: results of a multicenter study in the United States. Am Heart J 1991;121:1956–1964.

70. Unverferth DV, Magorien RD, Lewis RP, Leler CV. Long term benefit of dobutamine in patients with congestive cardiomyopathy. Am Heart J 1980;100:622–630.

71. Unverferth DV, Magorien RD, Altschuld R, Kollbash AJ, Lewis RP, Leler CV. The hemodynamic and metabolic advantages gained by a three-day infusion of dobutamine in patients with congestive cardiomyopathy. Am Heart J 1983;106:29–34.

72. McGregor C. Cardiac transplantation: surgical considerations and early postoperative management. Mayo Clin Proc 1992;67:577–585.

73. Stevenson LW, Warner SL, Steimle AE, et al. The impending crisis awaiting cardiac transplantation: modeling a solution based on selection. Circulation 1994;89:450–457.

74. O'Connell JB, Bourge RC, Costanzo-Nordin MR, et al. Cardiac transplantation: recipient selection, donor procurement, and medical follow up. Circulation 1992;86:1061–1079.

75. Fananapazir L, Cannon R, Tripodi D, Panza J. Impact of dual-chamber permanent pacing in patients with obstructive hypertrophic cardiomyopathy with symptoms refractory to verapamil and β-adrenergic blocker therapy. Circulation 1992;85:2149–2161.

76. McAreavey D, Fananapazir L. Altered cardiac hemodynamic and electrical state in normal sinus rhythm after chronic dual-chamber pacing for relief of left ventricular outflow obstruction in hypertrophic cardiomyopathy. Am J Cardiol 1992;70:651–656.

77. Demakis JG, Rahimtoola SH, Sutton GC, et al. Natural course of peripartum cardiomyopathy. Circulation 1971;44:1053–1061.

78. Homans DC. Current concepts: peripartum cardiomyopathy. N Engl J Med 1985;312:1432–1437.

79. Lee W, Cotton D. Peripartum cardiomyopathy: current concepts and clinical management. Clin Obstet Gynecol 1989;32:54–67.

80. Midei MG, DeMent SH, Feldman AM. Peripartum myocarditis and cardiomyopathy. Circulation 1990;81:922–928.

81. O'Connel JB, Costanzo-Nordin MR, Subramanian R, et al. Peripartum cardiomyopathy: clinical, hemodynamic, histologic and prognostic characteristics. J Am Coll Cardiol 1986;8:52–56.

82. Carvalho A, Brandao A, Martinez E, et al. Prognosis in peripartum cardiomyopathy. Am J Cardiol 1989;64:540–544.

83. Elkayam U. Pregnancy and cardiovascular disease. In: Braunwald E, ed. Heart disease. 4th ed. Philadelphia: WB Saunders, 1992:1798–1799.

84. Are ACE inhibitors safe in pregnancy? Lancet 1989;2:482–483.

85. Baughman KL, Herskowitz A, Feldman AM, Hutchins GM. Peripartum cardiomyopathy with myocarditis: who to treat. Circulation 1989;80:(suppl II):II-320.

86. Demakis JG, Rahimtoola SH, Sutton AC. Natural course of peripartum cardiomyopathy. Circulation 1971; 44:1053–1061.

87. Sutton M, Cole P, Saltzman D, Goldhaber S. Risks of cardiac dysfunction in peripartum cardiomyopathy (PPCM) with subsequent pregnancy. Circulation 1989;80:(suppl II):II-320.

88. Cody RJ. Comparing angiotensin-converting enzyme inhibitor trial results in patients with acute myocardial infarction. Arch Intern Med 1994;154:2029–2036.

CHAPTER 8

MITRAL VALVE PROLAPSE/DYSAUTONOMIA

Richard O. Russell, Jr.

The designation or diagnosis of mitral valve prolapse has functioned as a keyhole through which physicians (as well as patients and sometimes their families) have been able to see a fascinating panoramic vista of common but vague and poorly understood symptoms. We have come to recognize that there is far more to the medical problem than a tiny seemingly insignificant movement of the mitral leaflets. A plethora of symptoms and characteristics occur with such regularity, though the symptoms may be many and varied among patients and fluctuate in severity within a given patient, that persons with this problem are almost unconsciously recognized, so much so, that some physicians might choose to shun them.

Although an echocardiogram has been used to make the diagnosis because of the 1 to 2 mm movement of the posterior leaflet of the mitral valve toward the left atrium, the collage of symptoms is so characteristic that, in actuality, this leaflet movement or prolapse is not a sine qua non for the syndrome. Because no better name for the syndrome has emerged, even though the term dysautonomia or neuroendocrine disorder has been suggested, the constellation of symptoms still hails by the term mitral valve prolapse syndrome.

The Concept

A general concept is emerging that the prolapse of the mitral valve is simply a marker, and not even an absolutely necessary marker, of the syndrome. Many of the symptoms noted by the patient result from a temporarily disordered or overactive, hypersensitized autonomic nervous system. The symptoms are often not constant and continuous over time but many come at times with such disconcerting intensity that the patient relates it as nearly cataclysmic or the symptoms may vary in intensity over some days, weeks, or months ebbing and flowing with no apparent association.

What becomes so frustrating and almost maddening to patients is that no organic or specific cause can be found to explain the symptoms and patients are told "You're fine! You just need to get your life together" or some similar implication. All the while patients know they're feeling *something*, that it is truly *there*. They almost always feel that there *is* something wrong and that they have "something bad" and the doctor is not finding it. In a sense, they're correct. They do have something—something that may be wrecking their life or at least their sense of well-being. They have the mitral valve prolapse syndrome. They rarely see the association of their symptoms to the stresses in their life or the burdens under which they labor often with grinding frustration and dissatisfaction.

The intrinsic physical findings, that is, not related to sympathetic or vagal overdrive, may be the prolapse of the section of the mitral valve, giving rise to a systolic click, and the presence of spinal variations, such as mild scoliosis, straight dorsal spine, or variations in rib or sternal anatomy (often subtle) that has led to a preliminary hypothesis that there may be some probably minor molecular biologic variation resulting in some protein abnormality. (The tissues of the mitral valve, sternum, rib, vertebrae, or connecting tissue are all partly protein.) This resulting molecular biologic variation may then allow the total multifold symptoms. Presently our diagnostic and scientific techniques may be inadequate to precisely determine what this variation is. It may not be possible to determine it until we can understand the human genome.

It is of more than incidental interest that the mitral valve undergoes embryologic differentiation and also that the vertebral column and the thoracic cage develop their shape and form through chondrification during the sixth week of fetal life, and the affected tissues are embryologically derived from mesenchymal cell origins (1).

History

The mitral valve prolapse syndrome/dysautonomia moves clinicians back to the listener-counselor role. The syndrome demands that clinicians spend time in concerned listening to patients to truly hear what they are saying, to hear the plea for understanding of their sufferings and tribulations. Only in this way can physicians gain the insight into patients immersed in all that is having an impact on their life at that time. Only in this way can the physicians discern the multiple variations, yet the recurrent patterns and similarities of the varied symptoms, and makeup of these patients.

Patients often voice no understanding or suspicion that what is going on in their life, the stresses, the pressures, relates to their symptoms. This is particularly true in the younger decades. Often by the forties and beyond, patients suspect that the events going on and their reaction to them, may be playing a role in their symptoms. By their sixties, patients may have a strong inkling of the relationship of their symptoms to their life pressures. However, almost invariably at every age, patients have the strong fear that something bad or not yet discovered is going on with them. One hears this constantly. "Do you think we've missed something? Do you think something else is going on? There must be something wrong. I just know it." In fact this questioning, lingering doubt is almost universally prevalent and is part of the anxiety and hyperconcern with their health and the compelling need to relate in minute detail every feeling and symptom in chronological order.

It has seemed to us that the syndrome or some fragment of it is so prevalent and that we are so accustomed to it, we do not recognize it for what it is. Human beings, in fact all mammals, have an active autonomic nervous system. Witness how we ourselves have felt before a dreaded examination or encounter, before a major talk to a large audience, or when we are frightened by an unexpected noise in the night or upon becoming suddenly very angry. Our pulse rate and blood pressure may rise, often with a feeling of our heart pounding; our urinary frequency may increase; our gastrointestinal tract surges into turmoil; our hands get cool and sweaty; our mouth gets dry and when frightened or cold; the hair stands up on the nape of our neck or our arms.

It is as though patients with this syndrome have a hypersensitive response or exaggerated expression of normal feelings. This heightened awareness of feelings in their body and awareness of or sensitivity to everything in their external environment (smells, temperature, sounds) is also a characteristic part of the syndrome.

The prevalence and commonality of the events of our autonomic nervous system is such that we overlook it or give it no cognizance. In a sense, it is like the air. "I don't see it, how do I know it is there?" One may think of the oft present symptoms according to systems of the body. *Cardiovascular symptoms* include chest pain, nonspecific, not following any rules of our learned causes of pain, variable from place to place in the chest and from time to time and in intensity in the same patients and may be dissimilar between patients. It seems as chimeric as the patients themselves. It may be described as a pain or a tightness, sharp, dull, "not a pain" or "I can't describe it."

Patients may describe their symptoms as "very aware of my heart"; "I can see it through my shirt/blouse," pounding, fluttering, racing, rapid, forceful, extra heartbeat, skipped heartbeat, or "that kerboom." Peripheral vascular symptoms are cold hands and feet, sweaty hands, sweaty feet, excess sweating under many circumstances.

Anxiety, and less frequently panic attacks (if they are willing to admit it), are common. They may feel detached or out of their body, often depressed, sometimes especially in the morning after arising "until I have my coffee"; "jitters or jittery"; "I feel all ajitter inside." Similarly, symptoms of agoraphobia are prevalent: "I avoid public places"; "avoid driving" (especially on freeways); "avoid supermarkets." "I want to stay home more"; "I can't go anyplace without somebody with me"; "I want somebody with me all the time"; "I'm afraid I'll lose control."

Among the most prevalent are symptoms of *fatigue*, "I'm just so tired"; "I'm tired all the time"; "I get up tired"; "Do you think it's my thyroid?"; "I have no energy"; "I used to have so much energy"; "I'm short of breath with everything I do"; "I can't exercise because I get so tired." Elements of poor sleeping, depression, and anxiety may play a role in this fatigue. Fatigue is so common that one wonders if the nosocomial term chronic fatigue syndrome is not related or a part of this overall medical condition.

Gastrointestinal symptoms include diarrhea, constipation, alternating diarrhea and constipation, abdominal symptoms related to meals, symptoms before meals, after meals, relieved by meals, bloating, and cramping. "Food goes right through me"; "I have to go to the bathroom every time I eat"; "I'm afraid to go out to eat because of these symptoms"; "I crave chocolates"; "I crave sweets"; hyperactivity or emotional outbursts after sweets; or "I have a lump in my throat—right here" (pointing); "I have difficulty swallowing." We've even heard husbands say, "I'm not going to let you have sweets any more."

Grouped among symptoms related to the *central nervous system* are dizziness, dizziness on arising, unsteadiness, "I feel the floor is uneven"; "I feel the floor is mushy or soft"; tingling of left arm; inability to concentrate; "I can't remember things"; headache often described as "migraine headache" or fainting.

Sleep symptoms are prevalent: difficulty falling asleep, difficulty staying asleep, "I wake up after a couple of hours and my mind is racing"; "I think of all these things when I wake up." These symptoms are so common that repair of faulty sleep should be a key effort. Faulty sleep may contribute to the fatigue so often experienced.

Premenstrual symptoms are almost universal in women. Premenstrual syndrome seems to be an integral part of the overall syndrome—premenstrual bloating, moodiness, emotional swings, depression, anxiety, and painful tender breasts. Fibrocystic mastitis or disease seems highly prevalent along with breast tenderness in women with mitral valve prolapse syndrome/dysautonomia.

Other problems include an increased incidence of allergies or frequent respiratory infection for a season or two, marked sensitivity to medication so that a fraction of any given tablet may be effective (this is so frequent that one doubts if it is psychological). Soreness all over the body or feeling of knots under the skin (perhaps small lipomas or fibromyomas) and the apparent increased incidence of fibromyalgia (fibromyositis) are present.

Patients, especially women, are often quite creative, artistic, or talented (in any field), often highly intelligent, highly motivated, "driven," often perfectionistic, and often "worriers." Often other members of the family will have a makeup similar to the patient and the patient will recognize this, because this syndrome, or a proclivity for it, often runs in families (i.e., is genetic). Whereas some patients will have had symptoms at various times in their lives, others can remember an event in their lives after which symptoms started. Symptoms may be precipitated or brought to awareness by an illness, an operation, a fall, an accident or after a period of prolonged (perhaps onerous) personal stress. It seems as though the background or diathesis to have the syndrome is congenital (and probably present before birth) and that certain life events unmask the symptoms and allow them to come to the fore. One illustrative example is a patient who had her first problems during her late twenties when she was trying to complete her doctorate. Symptoms then disappeared until her early forties when at full career and with her own family, she had to care for an invalid and aging relative. After discussion she saw clearly the relationship of her symptoms to the events in her life.

After listening to the history (it is important to "hear" through the history into what is being said), it is often instructive to ask "What's going on in your life now?"

Thus the underlying proclivity is probably present throughout the person's lifetime only to be unmasked or brought to the fore at any given time by life events.

Empathic listening to the history with the cataloging of symptoms will probably take considerable time, longer than allocated or anticipated. However, the therapeutic benefit of relating it to an "empathic someone" who listens is often highly regarded by the patient who later may express, "I've never had anyone listen to me (or to my problems)." That fact alone, the telling of the history often serves to elucidate to the patient the totality of the situation and the symptoms.

Physical Examination

No invariable physical features allow diagnosis of mitral valve prolapse syndrome/dysautonomia. Although certain findings may often be present, the absence of them does not negate the diagnosis. For example, the systolic click may frequently be absent or missed on auscultation. It may be present on one occasion but not on another. The diagnosis of the syndrome is a *clinical* diagnosis and is not dependent on one or more diagnostic physical findings.

On inspection the patient is often thin and gracile, but not always. One clinician indicated that many of the female patients were "attractive or alluring." Men, too, may be thin. However, individuals with the syndrome may be overweight. The thinness may be related to the sensitive gastrointestinal tract (a function of the dysautonomia) and thus the patients eat sparingly.

Often the hands and feet may be cool to examination (or this fact may be pointed out by history from the patient or significant other). On occasion the hands may be quite moist from perspiration.

Often the blood pressure is labile, being high while being examined but low normal when taken elsewhere. It may be consistently high (and this needs to be treated) or low. Historically patients may indicate they have "low blood pressure." The pulse may be fast, often 90 to 120/min at rest during which time the patient indicates he or she is not tense or "nervous." (The labile blood pressure and tachycardia are doubtless related to the dysautonomia.) Rarely sinus bradycardia may be present and even more rarely bradycardia with conduction problems may require a pacemaker.

The midsystolic click is usually single but three to four may be heard. If the click is heard, squatting may make the click move further from the S_1 (due to greater filling of the ventricle and later closure of the mitral valve) and standing may make the click move closer to the S_1 (as less filling makes the ventricle smaller and the mitral valve closes earlier).

Often there are costosternal abnormalities such as pectus excavatum, dorsal excavatum (less commonly), or minor variations of the sternum such as minor excavation inferiorly hardly noticeable by the patient. Concomitantly, either alone or in combination with sternal variation, there are variations anteriorly in the upper ribs or costochondral structures frequently asymmetrical (i.e., costochondral structures are more prominent on one side).

There may be scoliosis or kyphoscoliosis, often so minor as to never be noticed by the patient or even by a parent. Probably patients with so-called "straight back syndrome" fall into the overall category of what is presently called mitral valve prolapse syndrome/dysautonomia. Perhaps the backache experienced by patients with this syndrome is related to the scoliosis with its accompanying muscular tension.

The patients may have temporomandibular joint imbalance (TMJ syndrome). This may be diagnosed clinically by placing an index finger in each external auditory canal (which is just external to the TMJ) and observing with examiner's eyes at the level of the fingers in the canals. An imbalance may be obvious; usually the left is lower than the right. (This finding may help explain headache or backache.) The cause of symptoms related to TMJ displacement is not clear but may be related to muscular tension imbalance, which may involve the paraspinal muscles as well as head, neck, and jaw muscles.

Women may have chronic cystic mastitis with increased lumpiness and thickness of the breast tissue. The tenderness is increased premenstrually. There may have been one or more breast biopsies by history with negative pathologic findings.

Differential Diagnosis

One view, and a reasonable hypothesis, is that mitral valve prolapse syndrome/dysautonomia is inclusive, that is, it is an umbrella diagnosis. It incorporates or is associated with the diagnosis of hypoglycemia, premenstrual syndrome, migraine headaches, irritable bowel syndrome, hyperkinetic heart syndrome, neurocardiogenic or vasovagal fainting, neuroendocrine syndrome, syncope, "nervous heart," vasoregulatory asthenia (neurocirculatory asthenia), straight back syndrome, kyphoscoliotic heart disease (when scolosis is advanced), and perhaps even chronic fatigue syndrome. We have recognized each of these conditions in patients with the mitral valve prolapse/dysautonomia syndrome. The underlying constitutional makeup of these patients could be likened to a golf ball with its many dimples analagous to the constitutional makeup and the many symptoms, not necessarily all present in any individual or at any given time.

Almost certainly we do not have the best name for this syndrome as the plethora of names indicates because our understanding of its pathophysiology is incomplete. There are intrinsic variations in each person and the socioenvironmental and neuroendocrine ("hormonal") nuances at play at any given time in any given person can hardly be known.

Laboratory Evaluation

There are no tests to diagnose the syndrome. The finding of prolapse of the mitral valve on echocardiography is confirmatory, but the absence of it does not invalidate the diagnosis. Similarly one may see prolapse of the tricuspid valve.

There are no characteristic hematologic or chemical tests. A 5-hour glucose tolerance test may confirm hypoglycemia. It seems that the rapidity of the fall of blood sugar at 3 or 4 or 5 hours is as important as the depth of the drop in these patients. A mammogram in view of the cystic mastitis is probably indicated.

Two general philosophies obtain in patients with this syndrome. The first is to explain the symptoms to the patients so that they may gain some understanding of why they feel the way they do. The second is to be certain nothing else is going on. To satisfy the second need various laboratory investigations may be indicated. It is reasonable to perform a complete blood count, chemical profile including thyroid function studies, electrocardiogram if the patient is over age 35 or if there are cardiovascular symptoms, a chest x-ray and probably an exercise test to emphasize that it is not only appropriate but safe to exercise.

It is important to review the laboratory findings with the patient, emphasizing those that are normal and planning follow-up for any abnormalities. Formal autonomic nervous system testing with sophisticated experimental techniques has been somewhat disappointing with regard to its diagnostic capabilities in our experience. Perhaps these are not sensitive enough and do not measure the proper responses.

Treatment

Treatment begins with taking the history, with allowing the time for the patient to explain the way she (or he) feels. Empathic, attentive listening is crucial in helping the patient begin to feel better.

There are five areas of therapy plus the concept of the condition that are important to incorporate for improvement of patients with mitral valve prolapse syndrome/dysautonomia. First is exercise. Some form of exercise is vitally important. Walking is almost always available and easy and should be done three to five times a week for 20 to 30 minutes or longer at a session. This may be done indoors or outside. Alternative forms of exercise might include jogging, aerobics, swimming, or use of machine aids including bicycling. The critical factors are the persistence of the habit over time.

Second is the avoidance of caffeine. Caffeine is in coffee and tea (unless decaffeinated), colas ("brown drinks"), certain lemon-lime sodas (unless specified otherwise), and chocolate. Caffeine stimulates the release of catecholamines and thus creates biochemical stress.

Third is a high fluid intake of up to eight 8-ounce glasses (2 quarts) of fluid a day. Water is ideal but other fluids (noncaffeniated, low calorie) are acceptable. This is to maintain intravascular volume by supporting general hydration. Patients with this syndrome seem sensitive to volume shifts and become symptomatic easily with light-headedness and dizziness. (However, all dizziness is probably not dehydration.) One rule of procedure is an ounce of fluid per degree of temperature Fahrenheit when the temperature is over about 65°F.

Fourth is the avoidance of sweets—especially sweet snacks. Appropriate eating of three meals a day is important. The patient should not skip meals. The induced hyperglycemia of a sweet snack is followed by a fall, occasionally rapid, in blood glucose with accompanying symptoms of hypoglycemia. The physiologic response to hypoglycemia is, in part, the elaboration of adrenalin, which has the potential to aggravate symptoms of hyperadrenergic dysautonomia. Often a close family member will notice that the patient gets very "hyper" on sweets and will advise the loved one to avoid sweets. If the patient should feel hungry between meals or before bed, an appropriate snack is fruit, cut raw vegetables, popcorn, or something with protein in it to counteract the possible falling blood glucose level. It does not seem always necessary to obtain a 5-hour glucose tolerance test to document hypoglycemia, but the physician can advise this simple plan for combating possible relative hypoglycemia.

Fifth, and final, is the use of medications. Pharmacologic therapy alone has a poor chance of correcting the symptoms without the first four adjunctive therapies. Although there is no standard therapeutic program, the physician should attempt to assess whether the patient is hyperadrenergic (palpitations, heart pounding). If so, β blockers in low doses are usually helpful. It is anticipated that these will blunt the effects of adrenalin. β blockers that have been most useful are atenolol at 25 mg or 12.5 mg once or twice a day, betaxolol 5 mg or less daily, nadalol at 40 mg or 20 mg daily, all orally. Although most patients can tolerate small doses of β blockers some will relate that they cannot take β blockers at all. It is wisest to listen to this protestation and respect it. However a few of this latter subgroup are willing to try a very small dose of β blockers and may be able to tolerate it. However, a few cannot tolerate them at all and will get marked hypotension or bradycardia or profound weakness often requiring bed rest in a normally vigorous, active person. Fortunately the duration of these symptoms is short lived, a matter of hours. This intolerance should alert the clinician to other possibilities of therapy.

An alternative medication that may help when β blockers prove unsuccessful are small doses of diltiazem 15 mg twice daily initially.

The patient may indeed not be hyperadrenergic but have predominantly hyperparasympathetic (hypervagal) dysautonomia or more commonly have mixed symptoms. The symptom complex may vary at different times as well. In patients who are predominantly hypervagal, β blockers are poorly tolerated. Some of the patients may respond to Donnatal, which probably has both central and peripheral actions.

Patients who are hypervagal may have gastrointestinal symptoms and postural hypotension and light-headedness on standing. Donnatal, 1 tablet before each meal and bedtime or just thrice or twice daily, may be helpful. In patients with postural hypotension extra salt intake or flurohydrocortisone 0.1 mg or 0.05 mg daily may be helpful. However, the patient may "escape" from the fluorohydrocortisone in a few days.

With gastric symptoms such as gastric distress, bloating, discomfort, fullness, cramping, Donnatal before meals and at bedtime or twice a day before breakfast and supper may help. A combination of phenobarbital in the small dose of 16 mg, hyoscyamine, atropine and scopolamine, Donnatal probably has central as well as local gastrointestinal effects. On occasion, the small dose of 15 mg phenobarbital one to three times a day may be helpful. One tends to think of gastrointestinal symptoms with excess sweating and postural hypotension as vagal or hypervagal symptoms. Additionally an H_2-receptor antagonist such as cimetidine 400 mg at bedtime, ranitidine 150 mg twice daily or 300 mg at bedtime, famotidine 20 mg at bedtime, nizatidine 300 mg daily at bedtime or 150 mg twice daily may be helpful. Metoclopramide 5–10 mg before meals and at bedtime or once or twice a day is helpful with low-grade nausea, which is often present.

Patients with colonic symptoms of excess gas, cramping, and hypermolity or softening of stool are often helped by increased fiber as tolerated, dicyclomine, an antispasmodic, anticholinergic (antimuscarinic), 10–20 mg two to four times daily and a scheduled bowel action daily at appointed times.

Marked anxiety and panic are frequent problems in patients with mitral valve prolapse syndrome/dysautonomia. Symptoms may include generalized anxiety, feelings of foreboding and doom for themselves and their environment, palpitations, dyspnea, feelings of inability to get a deep breath, headache, inability to concentrate, sweating, and cold moist hands and feet. These symptoms may be accompanied by agoraphobia, fear of the marketplace, fear of being alone but more frequently fear of going outside of home alone, fear of driving or flying, avoidance of public places, fear of driving on expressways, or fear of supermarkets. Although patients with these symptoms may need psychiatric help, it is important for the primary physician to hear and understand the patient. Often an empathic understanding, use of clonazepam 0.25–1.0 mg at bedtime with a small amount of clonazepam 0.25–0.5 mg in the morning may be helpful. Alprazolam 0.25–0.5 mg one to three times a day is helpful in the short term but has significant dependency problems. Lorazepam 0.5 mg once or twice daily or 1.0 mg at bedtime may be helpful. Also encouraging the patient to make small trips alone or gradually undertake new challenges is important as well. Each new, small challenge overcome serves as a springboard to further forays out of the protected environment. Appropriate praise from the physician should accompany these gains and improvements.

Dizziness, light-headedness, instability, a feeling of a "crazy head," though all characteristic of some patients with mitral valve prolapse syndrome/dysautonomia have been some of the most recalcitrant of symptoms, fluctuating without apparent cause and difficult to treat and eradicate. As patients improve in other ways and as their confidence grows in their ability to cope with their symptoms, this symptom often improves. Occasionally meclizine 25 mg or 12.5 mg two to four times daily is helpful symptomatically.

A hallmark of patients with the mitral valve prolapse/dysautonomia syndrome is the sensitivity (not allergy) to practically all medication. Small, sometimes apparently unbelievably small, doses of medication are effective. The small doses could be, and probably are, having a pharmacologic effect, not just a placebo effect. Perhaps this is because of the marked sensitivity to pharmacologic agents such patients have. Similarly intolerance and even allergy to medicines occur frequently. It is probably wisest to heed the histories these patients give of their symptoms. We have a relatively poor understanding of the cellular and subcellular effects of many medications and this is particularly true in this set of patients.

Inability to sleep properly, usually consisting of falling asleep easily, but awakening in a relatively few hours with mind racing and turning over all manner of events in their lives is by far the most common sleep complaint. Trouble falling asleep, awaking very tried, and restive, and unsatisfactory sleep are also noted with some frequency. Probably the most helpful medication for this symptom has been clonazepam 0.5 mg or perhaps 0.25 mg before bedtime. Less commonly lorazepam 0.5–1.0 mg before bedtime is helpful for allowing restful sleep and is better tolerated. Often with the sleep problem repaired, the patient has made a great stride in overcoming the symptom complex and the life stress problems seem more manageable.

Other clinical observations in patients with mitral valve prolapse syndrome/dysautonomia are that they are highly sensitive to sensations inside as well as outside their body. They are acutely aware of their heartbeat or premature heartbeats and of gastrointestinal variations. Similarly they are very aware and sensitive to external stimuli, to sounds and smells and often touch. This sensitivity applies to medications as well. They may be quite artistic or creative, may be very intelligent and may be perfectionistic. Occasionally moody, patients may become depressed and this may need therapy. The central nervous system neuronal uptake inhibitors of serotonin fluoxetine (Prozac) 20 mg a day or every other day or sertraline (Zoloft) at 50 mg daily or on alternate days have been most helpful in assisting patients regain a sense of self-esteem and self-control. This may occur in a few days but may take place gradually over 2 to 6 weeks. When after therapy, a particular body system remains especially symptomatic such as cardiac or cardiovascular, gastrointestinal, or central nervous system with depression or panic-anxiety, it is appropriate to refer the patient to an empathic specialist with an understanding and appreciation of the syndrome. As cardiologists, perhaps we have viewed the syndrome as cardiovasculocentric, and the concept of a wagon-wheel with spokes (various other body systems with the system specialists) has been a helpful concept (Fig 8.1).

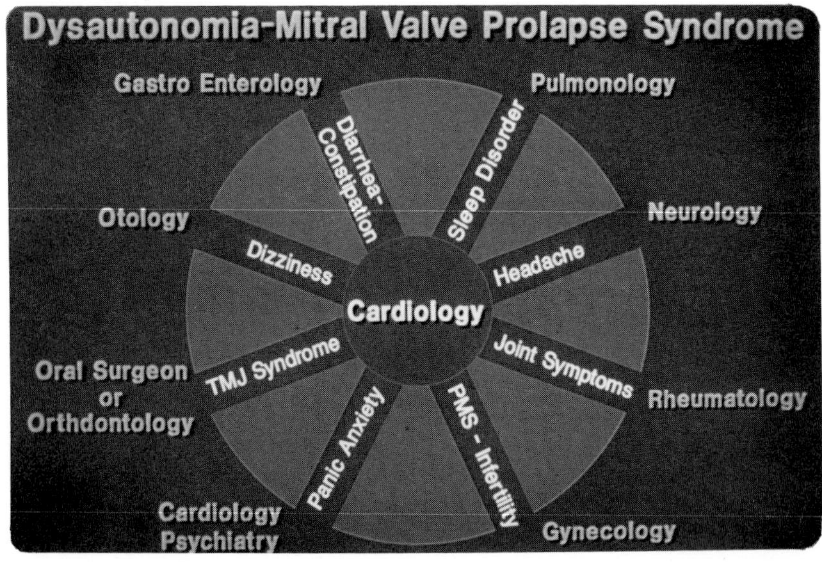

Fig 8.1 "Spoke-wheel" diagram indicates the many subsystems and corresponding subspecialists who may evaluate patients with mitral valve prolapse syndrome/dysautonomia.

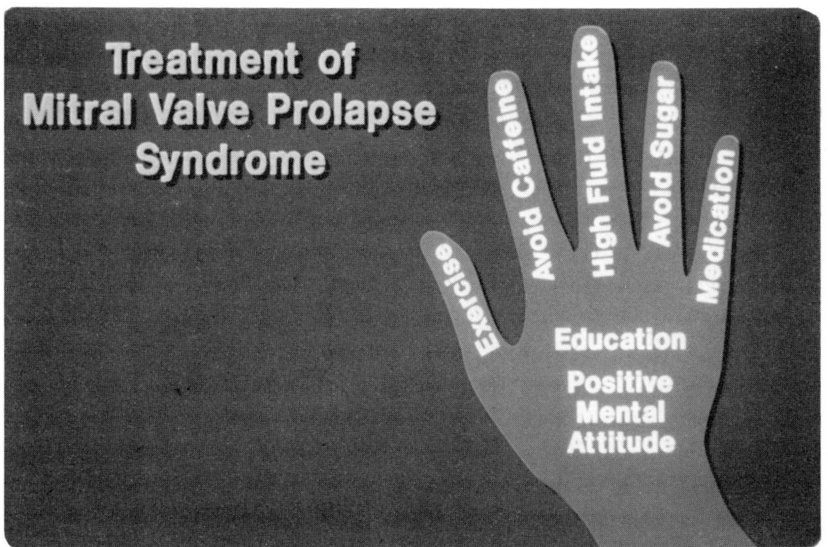

Fig 8.2 Open hand used as a teaching tool to represent the essentials of therapy for mitral valve prolapse syndrome/ dysautonomia.

It is important for patients to understand that this total symptom complex of mitral valve prolapse syndrome/dysautonomia is not a "pill problem." It requires the total approach of appropriate exercise, avoidance of caffeine and sweets, high fluid intake, an understanding of what is going on, and why they feel as they do. Medications are adjunctive, albeit important, therapy. With the total approach described, in a sense, the patient is his or her own best doctor or therapist. This can be demonstrated using the open hand as a teaching tool with the thumb representing exercise, the index finger, avoidance of caffeine, the middle (high) finger, the high fluid intake, the fourth finger, the avoidance of sweets plus appropriate eating and the fifth finger, the smallest representing medication. The palm of the hand represents understanding and positive mental attitude (Fig 8.2). This part of the hand pulls it all together for a good impact, the closed fist. Alternatively a wheel of therapy illustrating the continuous and interdependent facets of treatment surrounding the central portion of learning about and understanding the syndrome has been useful (Fig 8.3).

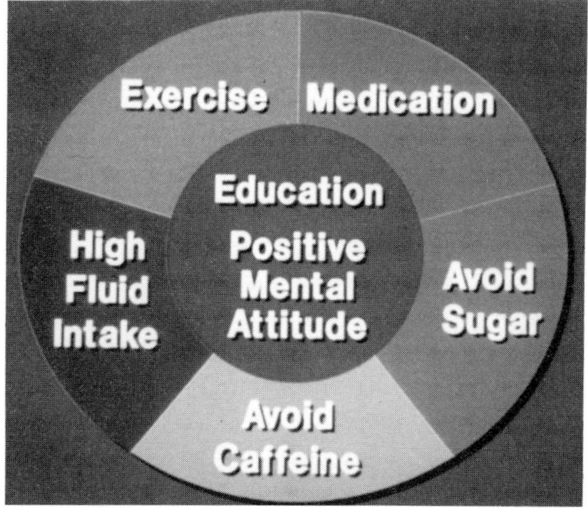

Fig 8.3 Wheel of therapy of mitral valve prolapse syndrome/dysautonomia.

Hypothesis

It has seemed apparent that while seeing mitral valve prolapse on echocardiogram or left ventricular angiogram or hearing the systolic click or mid-late systolic murmur, though confirmatory of its presence, the absence of detecting the small movement of the mitral valve does not invalidate the diagnosis of mitral valve prolapse syndrome despite the name of the syndrome. Another name for the syndrome would probably be better and perhaps one will emerge as understanding of it improves. Clearly the prolapse of the mitral valve is only one finding in a multisystem syndrome and not the cause of all the other characteristic features.

This recognition led to the formation of an hypothesis that the mitral valve prolapse/dysautonomia syndrome can be diagnosed by symptoms alone without the need for determining prolapse of the mitral valve.

To study this question we asked two groups of patients to answer a questionnaire. The first group,

group A, consisted of 171 patients who had mitral valve prolapse on echocardiogram. These patients had at least a 2.0 mm systolic prolapse of the mitral valve on echocardiogram taken in the parasternal long axis view. A control group, group B, consisted of a group of first-year psychology graduate students and also a group of individuals attending a health fair representing the population as a whole.

The questionnaire was a list of symptoms frequently mentioned by patients. These symptoms were arranged by body systems. Both groups ranked separately the severity and frequency of the 40 selected symptoms on a 4-point scale. The separate scores were then surveyed (Fig 8.4).

The symptom list is presented in Box 8.1.

SYMPTOMS OF PATIENTS WITH MITRAL VALVE PROLAPSE SYNDROME / DYSAUTONOMIA: RANKING OF SYMPTOMS

Severity	Frequency
0 = None	0 = Never
1 = Annoying	1 = Less than once a week
2 = Uncomfortable	2 = One to six times a week
3 = Limits regular activity	3 = Daily

For each patient, the severity and frequency were summed
Example:

Chest Pain Severity = 1
Chest Pain Frequency = 2

Chest Pain This Patient = 3

Fig 8.4 Method of scoring severity and frequency of symptoms in patients with mitral valve prolapse syndrome/dysautonomia. The scores are then summed.

Box 8.1 Symptom List Used in Questionnaire

Group 1 Chest Pain
- Chest pain
- Chest tightness

Group 2 Other Cardiac
- Awareness of heartbeat
- Rapid heartbeat
- Fluttering in chest
- Forceful heartbeat
- Skipped heartbeat
- Extra heartbeat

Group 3 Panic or Anxiety
- Feeling detached/depressed
- Shakes or jitters
- Panic or anxiety
- Losing control
- Avoid public places or crowds
- Avoid driving
- Avoid supermarkets

Group 4 Fatigue
- Lack of energy
- Fatigue
- Shortness of breath
- Low exercise tolerance

Group 5 Gastrointestinal
- Diarrhea
- Constipation
- Abdominal cramping
- Symptoms worse after meals
- Symptoms worse before meals
- Symptoms relieved by meals

Group 6 Central Nervous System
- Dizziness on arising
- Dizziness
- Inability to concentrate
- Memory problems
- Migraine
- Fainting

Group 7 Sleep Disorders
- Symptoms at night
- Difficulty going to sleep
- Difficulty staying asleep

Group 8 Premenstrual
- Painful breasts
- Premenstrual bloating
- Premenstrual anxiety
- Premenstrual depression

Group 9 Other
- Craving sweets
- Cold hands and feet
- Allergies
- Difficulty with upper body
- Lump in throat
- Difficulty swallowing
- Excessive sweating
- Inability to sweat

For 34 of 40 symptoms, the average scores for individuals with mitral valve prolapse on echocardiogram (who scored themselves) were statistically higher than a group of controls, some of whom may, by chance, have had mitral valve prolapse. ($p < .01$ for averaged individual scorings). The total averaged self-scores for mitral valve prolapse individuals was 82.94 ± 34.97 (SD), whereas for the control group it was 37.73 ± 23.82 ($p < .001$). This is illustrated in Table 8.1 and Fig 8.5.

Table 8.1 Ranked Symptoms Comparison

Symptom	Control	MVP	F Value
1. Lack of energy	2.07 (1.77)*	4.19 (1.77)	$p < .0001$
2. Fatigue	1.84 (1.78)	4.10 (1.79)	$p < .0001$
3. Awareness of heartbeat	1.15 (1.38)	3.24 (1.58)	$p < .0001$
4. Rapid heartbeat	1.26 (1.48)	2.84 (1.63)	$p < .0001$
5. Cold hands or feet	1.54 (1.74)	2.70 (1.88)	$p < .0001$
6. Shortness of breath	0.81 (1.27)	2.69 (1.86)	$p < .0001$
7. Low exercise tolerance	0.81 (1.44)	2.69 (2.24)	$p < .0001$
8. Craving sweets	1.84 (1.55)	2.60 (1.78)	$p < .0002$
9. Premenstrual bloating	1.72 (2.00)	2.59 (2.15)	$p < .0112$
10. Chest pain	0.69 (1.21)	2.58 (1.61)	$p < .0001$
11. Panic or anxiety attacks	0.84 (1.38)	2.55 (2.13)	$p < .0001$
12. Premenstrual anxiety	1.17 (1.68)	2.50 (2.35)	$p < .0001$
13. Difficulty concentrating	1.63 (1.55)	2.49 (2.09)	$p < .0008$
14. Fluttering in chest	0.59 (1.10)	2.44 (1.61)	$p < .0001$
15. Premenstrual depression	1.13 (1.77)	2.33 (2.31)	$p < .0001$
16. Dizziness when rising	1.47 (1.47)	2.32 (1.71)	$p < .0001$
17. Shakes or jitters	0.81 (1.30)	2.28 (1.96)	$p < .0001$
18. Forceful heartbeat	0.53 (1.09)	2.27 (1.83)	$p < .0001$
19. Dizziness	0.84 (1.18)	2.27 (1.79)	$p < .0001$
20. Tightness in chest	0.47 (0.95)	2.25 (1.85)	$p < .0001$
21. Difficulty with memory	1.20 (1.46)*	2.14 (2.02)	$p < .0001$
22. Allergies	1.40 (1.82)	2.09 (2.05)	$p < .0041$
23. Difficulty going to sleep	1.64 (1.74)	2.07 (1.95)	$p < .0007$
24. Difficulty staying asleep	0.82 (1.40)	1.96 (2.00)	$p < .0001$
25. Migraines	1.02 (1.55)	1.82 (2.00)	$p < .0001$
26. Painful breasts	0.96 (1.48)	1.75 (1.61)	$p < .0005$
27. Skipped heartbeat	0.28 (0.85)	1.75 (1.77)	$p < .0001$
28. Difficulty with upper body	0.23 (0.73)	1.64 (2.20)	$p < .0001$
29. Constipation	1.16 (1.36)	1.63 (1.75)	$p < .0194$
30. Abdominal cramps	1.44 (1.61)	1.60 (1.74)	$p < .0860$
31. Extra heartbeat	0.23 (0.72)	1.58 (1.78)	$p < .0001$
32. Avoid public places	0.62 (0.89)	1.53 (2.05)	$p < .0001$
33. Lump in throat	0.42 (0.89)	1.37 (1.81)	$p < .0001$
34. Diarrhea	1.02 (1.29)	1.25 (1.44)	$p < .2235$
35. Difficulty swallowing	0.38 (0.97)	1.23 (1.74)	$p < .0001$
36. Excessive sweating	0.68 (1.28)	1.19 (1.72)	$p < .0079$
37. Avoid driving	0.42 (1.06)	0.92 (1.79)	$p < .0334$
38. Avoid supermarkets	0.24 (0.79)	0.82 (1.67)	$p < .0005$
39. Inability to sweat	0.20 (0.75)	0.37 (1.05)	$p < .4025$
40. Fainting	0.18 (0.65)	0.31 (0.88)	$p < .0031$

*Mean (SD)

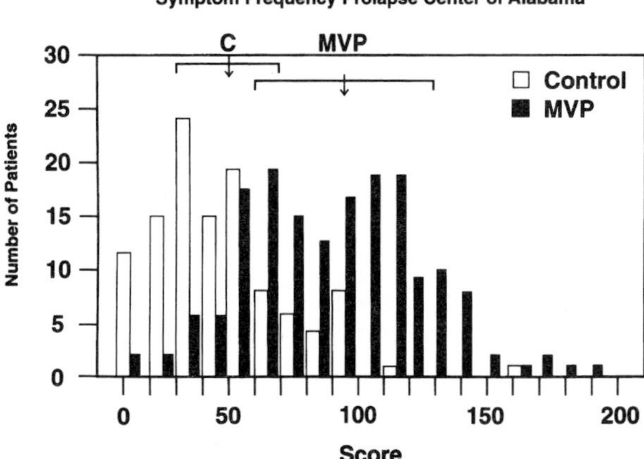

Fig 8.5 Summed scores for symptoms in normals and in patients with mitral valve prolapse syndrome/ dysautonomia.

The conclusion drawn was that by symptoms alone the diagnosis of mitral valve prolapse syndrome/dysautonomia can be made. This is a clinical diagnosis not requiring prolapse of the mitral valve to confirm or deny that diagnosis.

Because the tissue of the mitral valve is constituted by protein and the bony skeleton similarly is constituted by protein matrix, it seems reasonable to hypothesize that there may be a congenital biochemical or molecular biologic variation in individuals with this structural makeup to allow for the prolapse of the mitral valve and the rib-sternal and usually mild scoliotic variation and similarly the biobehavioral characteristics found in this syndrome.

Supportive evidence is available from other lines of investigation than the clinical bedside analysis. In patients with mitral valve prolapse syndrome baseline β-adrenergic receptor coupling on neutrophils was elevated compared to normal controls. Symptomatic mitral valve prolapse patients were desensitized by a 4-hour isoproterenol infusion, whereas sensitivity in normals did not change. This study demonstrated both physiologic and pharmacologic β-adrenergic hypersensitivity in vivo directly corresponding to biochemical supercoupling in patients with mitral valve prolapse syndrome (2).

With careful evaluation of change in heart rate and symptoms with tilting and with the Valsalva maneuver and hand grip in evaluating autonomic dysfunction and the brain–heart connection in patients with the mitral valve prolapse syndrome, Coghlan found marked fluctuations in heart rate (teleologically, apparently seeking the proper level) with autonomic dysregulation. The implication was that the "clumsy circulation" was getting and giving inappropriate messages in what appeared to be "faulty central processing and integration of afferent information" (3). Gaffney and Blomquist (4) emphasize the marked heterogeneity of the mitral valve prolapse syndrome/dysautonomia syndrome and hypothesize that the common denominator for symptoms is the pathophysiology that includes the self-sustaining triad of chronic adrenergic activity, vasoconstriction, and hypovolemia. In such patients, they point out that symptoms such as palpitations, cold hands and feet, weakness, and poor exercise tolerance are direct manifestations of an abnormal hemodynamic state rather than the cardiovascular manifestations of chronic anxiety. The postural decrease in stroke volume requires baroreflex-mediated adrenergic activation to maintain normal cerebral blood flow in upright body position during normal daily activities (4).

In patients with mitral valve prolapse syndrome/ dysautonomia norepinephrine levels were higher than in controls and remained so over a span of 6 years. Some patients with the syndrome had higher levels of atrial natriuretic factor, higher systolic blood pressure, and faster heart rate and significantly lower blood volume than those with normal values of atrial natriuretic factors. There was an inverse relationship between atrial natriuretic factor and blood volume and similarly an inverse relationship between plasma volume and plasma norepinephrine (5). Platelets from patients with mitral valve prolapse syndrome/ dysautonomia had higher platelet factor 4, higher β-thromboglobulin, and higher fibrinopeptide A, all indicating proclivity for platelet aggregation. In hyperadrenergic patients platelet aggregation was significantly elevated and in patients with both click and murmur, aggregation with increased 40% to 60% with collagen and with adenosine diphosphate over those with click alone (5).

Approximately 10% of patients with redundant mitral valve leaflets identified echocardiographically had sudden death, infective endocarditis, or a cerebral embolic event, whereas in patients with nonredundant valves only about 1% had such complications (6).

Patients with mitral valve prolapse syndrome/dysautonomia have an intriguing and protean variety of metabolic, neuroendocrine, and structural dysfunctions and abnormalities that characterize them as far more complex than "nervous, anxious women."

REFERENCES

1. Rosenberg CA, Derman GH, Crabb WC, Buda AJ. Hypomastia and mitral valve prolapse. Evidence of a linked embryologic and mesenchymal dysplasia. N Engl J Med 1983;309:1230–1232.

2. Davies AO, Mares A, Pool JL, Taylor AA. Mitral valve prolapse with symptoms of beta-adrenergic hypersensitivity. Am J Med 1987;82:193–201.

3. Coghlan HC. Autonomic dysfunction in the mitral valve prolapse syndrome: the brain heart connection and interaction. In: Boudoulas H, Wooley CF, eds. Mitral valve prolapse and the mitral valve prolapse syndrome. Mt. Kisco, NY: Futura Publishing, 1988:389–426.

4. Gaffney FA, Blomquist CG. Mitral valve prolapse and autonomic nervous system dysfunction: a pathophysiological link. In: Bordoulas H, Wooley CF, eds. Mitral valve prolapse and the mitral valve prolapse syndrome. Mt. Kisco, NY: Futura Publishing, 1988:427–443.

5. Pasternac A, Latour JG, Leger-Gauthier C, et al. Stability of hyperadrenergic state, atrial natriuretic factor and platelet abnormalities in mitral valve prolapse syndrome. In: Bordoulas H, Wooley CF, eds. Mitral valve prolapse and the mitral valve prolapse syndrome. Mt. Kisco, NY: Futura Publishing, 1988:445–463.

6. Nishimura RA, McGoon MD, Shub C, et al. Echocardiographically documented mitral valve prolapse. Long-term follow-up of 237 patients. N Engl J Med 1985;313:1305–1309.

SECTION THREE

PULMONARY DISEASES

CHAPTER 9

HYPERACTIVE AIRWAY DISEASE

Susan M. Harding

Asthma is a clinical syndrome characterized by airway hyperresponsiveness resulting in episodic narrowing of the tracheobronchial tree and airflow obstruction. Many stimuli ignite airway narrowing. This chapter reviews the epidemiology, pathophysiology, diagnosis, and therapy of asthma. It also reviews special clinical considerations including asthma during pregnancy, exercise-induced asthma, nocturnal asthma, and emergency room management of asthma.

Asthma Definition

In 1991, the National Asthma Education Program Expert Panel Report (NAEP) defined asthma as a lung disease with the following characteristics: airway obstruction, airway inflammation and airway hyperresponsiveness to a variety of stimuli (1). The International Consensus Report on Diagnosis and Management of Asthma defined asthma as "a chronic inflammatory disorder of the airways in which many cells play a role, including mast cells and eosinophils. In susceptible individuals this inflammation causes symptoms which are usually associated with widespread but variable airflow obstruction that is often reversible either spontaneously or with treatment, and causes an associated increase in airway responsiveness to a variety of stimuli" (2).

Airflow obstruction is responsible for the clinical manifestations of asthma such as wheezing, dyspnea, and cough. Airway narrowing is caused by a combination of bronchial smooth muscle contraction, mucosal edema, and mucous secretion. Airway inflammation plays a key role in airway narrowing. After an initial stimulus, there is release of inflammatory mediators leading to migration of eosinophils and neutrophils to the bronchial mucosa. This leads to the further release of mediators, bronchial epithelial injury, and airway edema.

The NAEP defined airway hyperresponsiveness as "an exaggerated bronchoconstriction response to many physical, chemical and pharmacological agents" (1). Airway hyperresponsiveness can be measured by standard inhalation challenge testing with methacholine or histamine. The level of airway hyperresponsiveness usually correlates with asthma severity and medication requirements.

Asthma is a heterogenous disorder with clinical variations ranging from an occasional attack of bronchospasm after exercise to severe chronic airflow obstruction leading to disability or even death.

Epidemiology of Asthma

Asthma is a common disease, affecting 5% of the American population or 10 to 15 million people. Below age 10, boys are affected approximately 1.5 times more often than girls; however, after age 10, the onset of disease is slightly higher in girls. Overall, at least half of asthmatics are women (3).

The economic impact of asthma is a major one. In 1988, asthma-related health care expenditures exceeded *$4 billion* in the United States. American women working outside the home lost $211 million in wages and women working in the home lost an additional $406 million of indirect costs related to asthma. The total estimated cost of asthma, including health care expenditures, lost wages, and indirect costs, in 1988 was $6.2 billion (4).

The prevalence of asthma in the United States has increased 29% from 1980 to 1987 (5). Of even more concern is that despite improved medical therapy, the

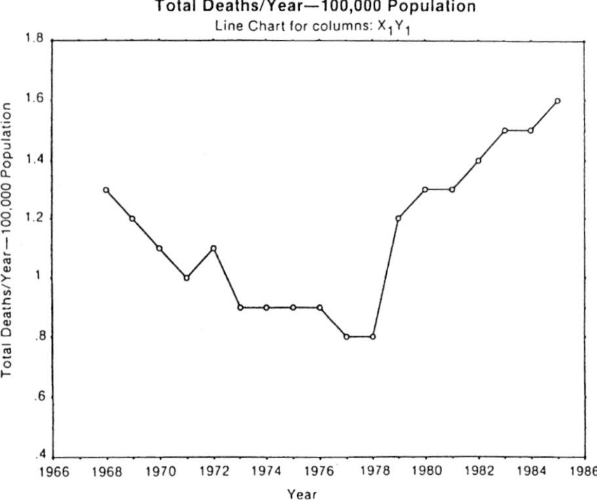

Fig 9.1 **Deaths from asthma per 100,000 population in the United States, 1968–1984.** *(Reproduced by permission from Robin ED. Death from bronchial asthma. Chest 1988;93:614–618.)*

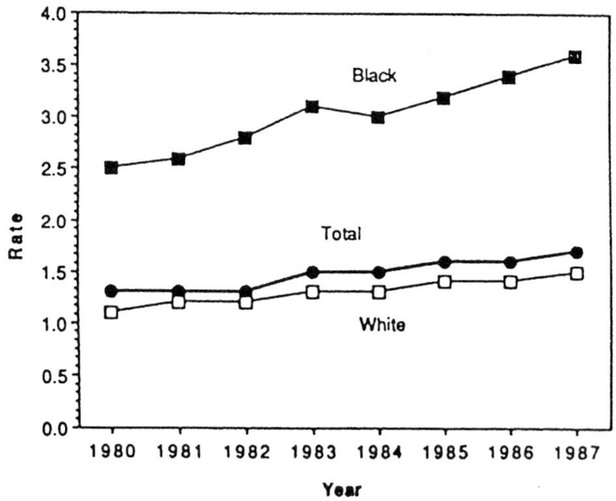

Fig 9.2 **Age-adjusted death rates per 100,000 persons for asthma as the cause of death by race and year–United States, 1980–1987.** *(Source: Fulwood R, Parker S, Hurd SS. Asthma–United States, 1980–1987. MMWR 1990;39:493–497.)*

Box 9.1 Risk Factors for Asthma-Related Death

- Prior intubation or admission to an intensive care unit for asthma
- Two or more hospitalizations for asthma within the past year or an emergency room visit within the past month
- Current or recent use of systemic corticosteroids
- History of syncope or hypoxic seizure related to asthma
- Psychiatric illness, especially depression
- Race (black)
- Lack of education
- Poverty
- Inadequate access to health care
- Over 65 years of age

asthma mortality rate is rising. The overall death rate from asthma in the United States increased 31% from 1980 to 1987 from 2891 deaths in 1980 to 4360 in 1987 (Fig 9.1). Death rates were generally higher in older age groups, with the highest rate being in those over 65 years old (7.9/100,000 in 1987). Blacks had a death rate almost three times higher than whites as shown in Figure 9.2 (6). Risk factors associated with asthma mortality include prior intubation for asthma, admission to an intensive care unit for asthma, at least two hospitalizations for asthma during the past year, emergency room visit for asthma within the past month, use of systemic corticosteroids or recent steroid withdrawal, past history of asthma-related syncope or hypoxic seizure, and serious psychosocial problems (Box 9.1).

Pathophysiology

The pathophysiology of asthma is complex. There is a reduction in small-airway diameter due to bronchial smooth muscle spasm, mucosal edema, mucosal inflammation, and increased mucous secretion. This leads to an increase in airway resistance and airflow obstruction. These points are illustrated in Figure 9.3, which shows a bronchiole from a person who died of asthma. Note that there is bronchial smooth muscle hyperplasia with inflammatory cells present in the airway lumen. The basement membrane is thickened and the epithelium contains a large number of mucous-secreting goblet cells.

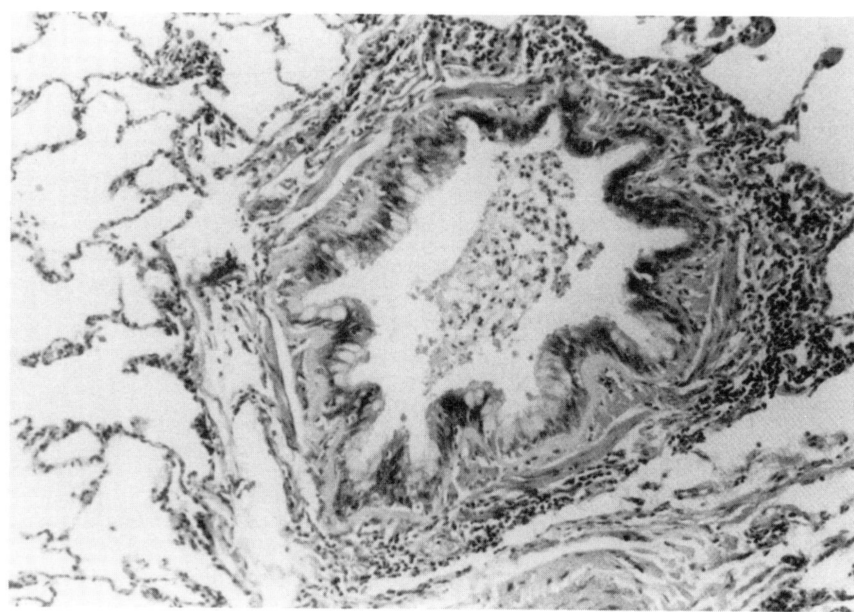

Fig 9.3 Histologic section of a bronchiole from a patient who died of asthma. *(Reproduced by permission from Hogg JC, James AL, Pare PD. Evidence for inflammation in asthma. Am Rev Respir Dis 1991;143:S40.)*

Many triggers exacerbate asthma including allergens such as house dust mites, pollens, animal danders; foods, including milk, nuts, or eggs; physical agents such as exercise, hyperventilation, (especially of cold air), strong odors or aerosols; air pollution, including cigarette smoke; medications and food additives such as aspirin, nonsteroidal anti-inflammatory agents, monosodium glutamate, food dyes, and β blockers. Other triggers include occupational chemicals, gastroesophageal reflux, emotional factors, and respiratory tract infections (1,7,8).

Once an individual is exposed to an exacerbating factor, such as a specific allergen, there is an immediate (within 1 hour) bronchoconstrictor response. This immediate asthmatic response is shown as a decrease in forced expiratory volume at 1 second (FEV_1) illustrated in Figure 9.4. After 1 to 2 hours, airflow obstruction improves spontaneously. Over the next few hours, there is a late phase asthmatic response with progressive deterioration in airflow related to immune events. It is important to understand the early and late asthmatic responses because different bronchodilators are effective during different phases of the asthmatic response. A patient sent home an hour ago may return with more severe airflow obstruction. Bronchial hyperresponsiveness after an allergen exposure will remain for days or even weeks.

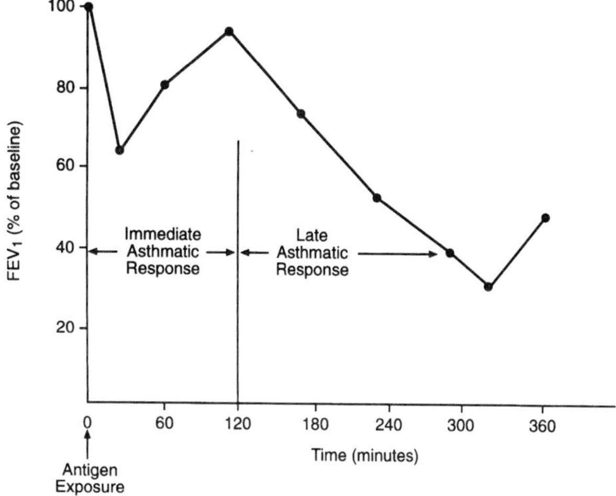

Fig 9.4 Pulmonary function response in an asthmatic exposed to an allergen over time. After allergen exposure, there is an immediate decrease in forced expiratory volume at 1 second (FEV_1). After 2 hours, there is a late phase response that causes more severe and prolonged airflow obstruction.

Clinical Presentation

History

"Asthma" was derived from the Greek word for panting or breathlessness. Other classic symptoms of asthma include episodes of cough and wheezing alternating with periods of improvement or even remission. Patients often describe tightness or congestion in their chest without chest pain. Initially, the cough may be nonproductive; however, frequently it becomes productive and may appear purulent. Other pertinent points in the history include a family history of asthma or atopy, age of onset of symptoms, frequency and severity of asthma symptoms, and whether there is any seasonal variation in symptoms.

Of prime importance is determining what triggers an asthma attack in individual patients. Specific questions include occupational exposures or hobbies, changes in the environment at home or work, and animal contacts, especially cats. Does the patient have symptoms of gastroesophageal reflux including indigestion or regurgitation? Are symptoms worse at night? Does the patient awaken during sleep with bronchospasm? Does exercise trigger an attack? Ask about weather changes and nonspecific irritants such as cigarette smoke and strong odors. Does the patient have a history of atopy, allergic rhinitis, or urticaria? What therapies in the past, including pharmacologic and immunologic have been successful? Does the patient require chronic corticosteroids? Was the patient ever admitted to the hospital or the intensive care unit for asthma? Are there risk factors for asthma mortality present? Does the patient have a history of nasal polyps or sinusitis? Ask about medication usage including over-the-counter agents such as aspirin and NSAIDs. Ask about tobacco use. The history is useful in both determining asthma severity and ascertaining what triggers are responsible for worsened symptoms.

Differential Diagnosis

All that wheezes is not asthma. The differential diagnosis of asthma is extensive (Box 9.2). Asthma can usually be differentiated by historical clues, physical examination findings, chest radiography, and laboratory and pulmonary function studies, which are available to most clinicians. One important clue that asthma may not be the cause of the patient's wheezing is that the patient fails to improve clinically despite aggressive bronchodilator therapy.

Laryngeal and tracheal abnormalities can be differentiated from asthma in that lung sounds are harsher in character and more prominent during inspiration. Stridor can sometimes be elicited by rapid inspiratory–expiratory movements. Pulmonary function studies, specifically the flow–volume loop, will show a fixed inspiratory and expiratory flow rate with laryn-

Box 9.2 Differential Diagnosis of Wheezing

Large-Airway Obstruction

- Thermal or chemical injury to the airways
- Laryngospasm
- Vocal cord paralysis
- Functional vocal cord dysfunction (emotional laryngeal wheezing)
- Foreign body in large airways
- Benign tracheal stenosis including tracheomalacia and postintubation lesions
- Broncholithiasis
- Extrinsic tracheal compression
- Tracheal tumors

Mediator-Mediated Wheezing

- Angioneurotic laryngeal edema
- Carcinoid syndrome
- Mastocytosis
- Anaphylaxis
- Pulmonary thromboembolism

Eosinophilic Syndromes

- Parasitic infestations
- Chronic eosinophilic pneumonia
- Churg-Strauss syndrome
- Hypereosinophilic syndrome

Left Ventricular Cardiac Dysfunction

Chronic Aspiration Syndrome

Other Forms of Obstructive Pulmonary Disease

- Chronic bronchitis and emphysema
- α_1-Antitrypsin deficiency
- Bronchiectasis
- Cystic fibrosis
- Bronchiolitis

geal or tracheal abnormalities as displayed in Fig 9.5. Patients with a foreign body or tumor in a large airway may have a localized wheeze.

Patients with wheezing related to the release of inflammatory mediators often have historical clues such as skin flushing with carcinoid syndrome or mastocytosis. Acute reactions after an allergen exposure may be present as in anaphylaxis. Pulmonary embolism should be investigated with a ventilation perfusion scan if pleuritic chest pain or clinical suspicion is present. Eosinophilic syndromes can be differentiated by the presence of parenchymal radiographic abnormalities in the setting of eosinophilia. Left ventricular cardiac dysfunction or cardiac wheezing often be presents with physical findings of rales, a left ventricular S_3 or other findings of cardiac dysfunction. Chest radiograph in left ventricular dysfunction shows evidence of cardiomegaly, pulmonary edema, or cephalization of pulmonary veins consistent with pulmonary venous congestion.

Other forms of obstructive pulmonary disease may be difficult to differentiate from asthma. Patients with chronic bronchitis and emphysema often give a history of smoking. Chronic bronchitics have daily sputum production, especially in the morning. Patients with emphysema may show loss of normal pulmonary parenchyma with bullae formation on the chest radiograph. Patients with bronchiectasis often have copious sputum production and chest radiograph abnormalities with a history of recurrent pneumonias.

In summary, clues that wheezing in the patient may not be caused by asthma include evidence of parenchymal pulmonary disease on chest radiograph, atypical history for asthma, presence of a localized wheeze, harsh wheezes versus a musical wheeze, inspiratory noises, and the patient's lack of improvement with bronchodilators.

Physical Findings

Physical findings of bronchospasm may be absent between asthma exacerbations. Examination of the eyes, ears, nose, and throat may reveal otitis media, conjunctivitis, rhinitis, nasal polyps, or sinusitis reflecting an allergic component. During mild exacerbations of asthma, wheezing may be heard only during forced expiration. With more severe impairment, wheezing is

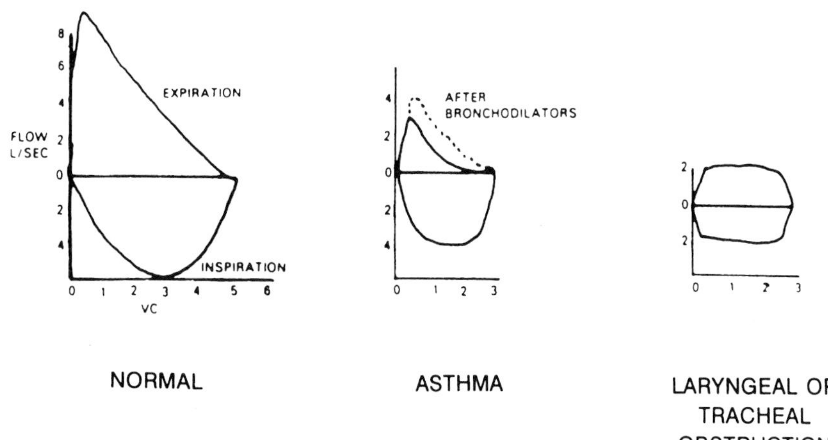

Fig 9.5 Flow–volume loop from a normal individual, a patient with asthma, and a patient with tracheal stenosis (fixed extrathoracic obstruction). Flow is in liters per second, volume in liters. The normal individual has no airflow limitation during inspiration or expiration. The asthmatic shows airflow limitation during expiration, which improves with bronchodilators (*dotted line*). The patient with tracheal stenosis has airflow limitation both during inspiration and expiration (note flattening of the curve, almost to a square box).

heard during both inspiration and expiration and is associated with a prolonged expiratory phase. As respiratory failure ensues, muscle fatigue leads to minimal air movement and the absence of wheezing. Patients may use accessory muscles of respiration including the sternocleidomastoids, which contract during inspiration. The presence of altered mental status signifies a severe attack with respiratory failure and the need for intensive therapy including ventilatory support.

Vital signs during an asthma attack include a rapid respiratory rate, often 25 to 40 breaths per minute, and tachycardia. The presence of pulsus paradoxus, an inspiratory decline in systolic blood pressure greater than 10 mm Hg, often signifies a severe attack.

Laboratory Findings

Objective measurements of airflow obstruction and its variability are critical to both establishing a diagnosis and determining the severity of asthma, which is used to guide therapy. Spirometry includes the forced vital capacity (FVC), FEV_1, FEV_1/FVC, maximum forced mid-expiratory flow rate ($FEF_{25-75\%}$), and peak expiratory flow rate (PEF) (Fig 9.6). The hallmark of airflow obstruction is a decrease in FEV_1/FVC ratio below 69%. This reflects large-airway obstruction (9). With less severe impairment, there is a decrease in FEF 25–75% or PEF. Patient symptoms may not be reliable indicators of airflow obstruction. It is not uncommon for asthmatics to say that their asthma is under adequate control and find their PEF severely reduced. Patients can be taught how to monitor PEF with a portable mini-peak expiratory flow rate meter. If then PEF are reduced, asthmatic patients can alter their therapy or contact their physician.

There are many methods to measure airway reactivity. One method is to perform spirometry before and after giving an inhaled bronchodilator such as albuterol. Both a 12% improvement in FEV_1 and an absolute improvement of 200 mL are required to show that there is a significant response to bronchodilator therapy (9). When a patient's symptoms suggest a diagnosis of asthma, but spirometry and the response to bronchodilators are normal, then bronchial challenge testing can be performed. A positive methacholine challenge test can establish the diagnosis of asthma (10,11). The bronchial challenge test is performed measuring FEV_1 before and after inhaling increasing concentrations of methacholine aerosol (Fig 9.7). The concentration of methacholine which produces a 20% decrease in FEV_1 is called the PC_{20} (provocative concentration–20%). A PC_{20} less than

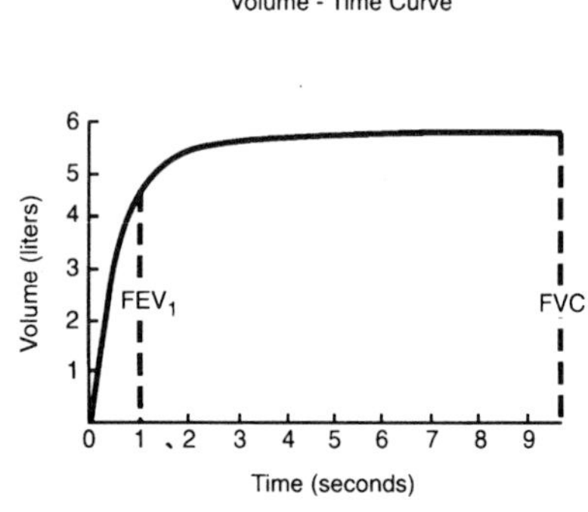

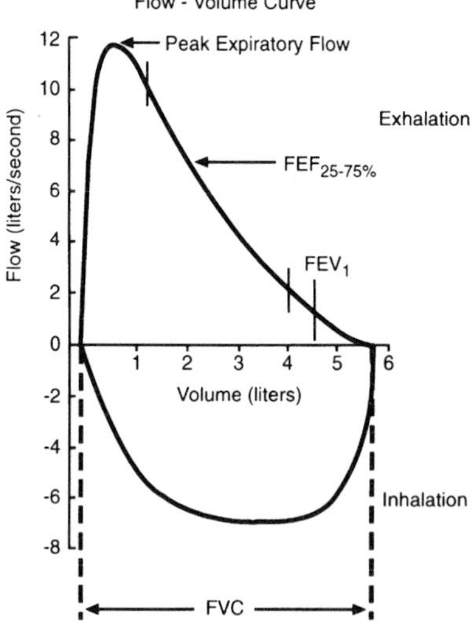

Fig 9.6 Spirometry showing both the volume–time curve and the flow–volume curve for a normal individual. FEV_1, forced expiratory volume at 1 second; FVC, forced vital capacity; $FEF_{25-75\%}$, mean forced expiratory flow during the middle half of the FVC.

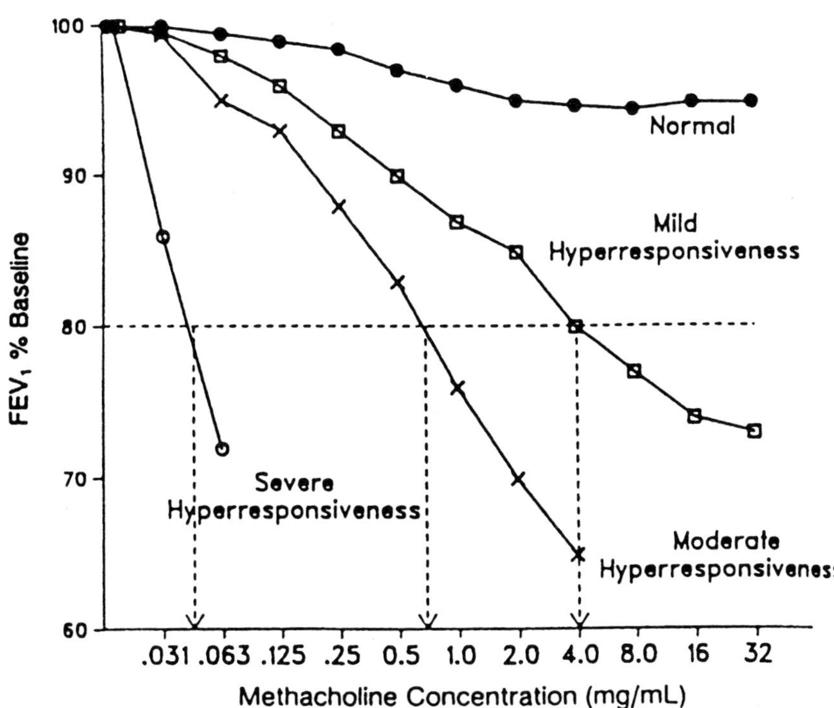

Fig 9.7 Methacholine challenge test to assess airway hyperresponsiveness. Normal subjects rarely experience a 20% decrease in FEV_1 (PC_{20}). With increasing severity of asthma, the PC_{20} (***vertical arrows***) decreases. *(Reproduced by permission from Kelley WN et al. Textbook of internal medicine: asthma. 2nd edition. Philadelphia: JB Lippincott, 1992:1710.)*

2 mg/mL is consistent with severe airway hyperresponsiveness, one of the diagnostic criteria for asthma. A PC_{20} between 2 and 8 mg/mL is very suggestive of asthma and a PC_{20} of 16 mg/mL or more virtually rules out asthma. Other inhalation challenge tests used include histamine and cold air challenge tests. Exercise challenge tests can be performed in patients with suspected exercise-induced asthma.

Chest radiographs are done to rule out infiltrates or pneumothorax, which may complicate asthma. They may also be used to rule out other causes of bronchospasm. During acute attacks, chest radiographs show hyperinflation. There may be evidence of bronchial wall thickening.

Arterial blood gas determinations are helpful in determining the severity of an acute attack and to rule out respiratory failure. The Pao_2 may be normal; however, it falls in a linear pattern as FEV_1 decreases. The $Paco_2$ will be mildly reduced (30 to 35 mm Hg) until respiratory failure ensues. As the FEV_1 approaches 1 liter, the $Paco_2$ normalizes (40 mm Hg) which signifies a severe attack and respiratory failure. If airflow worsens, hypercapnia and respiratory acidosis develop and the patient will most likely require mechanical ventilatory support.

Other laboratory findings commonly found in asthmatic patients include eosinophilia and increased serum IgE levels. Asthmatic sputum is thick and may be white or green. Sputum microscopy reveals numerous eosinophils, Charcot-Leyden crystals (degenerated eosinophils), Curschmann's spirals, and Creola bodies (clumps of epithelial cells). The electrocardiogram adds little to the diagnosis or routine management. Other tests such as allergy testing or evaluating for gastroesophageal reflux are indicated if clinical suspicion is present.

Asthma Severity

To establish a treatment regimen, it is important to determine if a patient has mild, moderate, or severe asthma. It is also important to determine if the patient has risk factors associated with asthma mortality. Asthma severity has been characterized by both the National Asthma Education Program and the International Consensus Report on Diagnosis and Management of Asthma (1,2). Severity is based on clinical characteristics and lung function.

Patients with chronic mild asthma have intermittent, brief (<1 hour) symptoms of wheezing, coughing, or dyspnea occurring up to twice a week. Patients are asymptomatic between asthma exacerbations. They may experience brief (<1/2 hour) asthma symptoms with activity. They also have infrequent (<twice a month) nocturnal symptoms of coughing or wheezing. Pulmonary function tests reveal that PEF are greater than 80% predicted at baseline. PEF variability (the difference between morning and nighttime PEF) is less than 20% and the PEF normalizes with bronchodilators.

Moderate asthmatic patients are characterized by frequent symptoms (> one or two times a week). Exacerbations affect sleep and activity level and may last for several days. Patients occasionally seek emergency room care. Symptoms often require daily inhaled β agonists. Pulmonary function studies including PEF or FEV_1 are 60% to 80% of predicted at baseline. PEF variability is between 20% and 30%. The PEF may normalize after bronchodilator use.

Chronic severe asthmatic patients should be managed by a pulmonologist or an allergist. Patients have almost continuous symptoms with very limited activity, frequent exacerbations, and nocturnal symptoms. They require occasional hospitalization and emergency room treatment. They may have had a previous life-threatening exacerbation of asthma. Pulmonary function is often less than 60% predicted at baseline. Their PEF variability is greater than 30%. Their peak PEF or FEV_1 may not normalize despite optimal therapy.

Therapy

Nonpharmacologic Measures

Trigger Avoidance

Successful asthma management depends on a variety of medications as well as other nonpharmacologic measures (1,2,12,13). It is important to treat the patient with optimal medications while evaluating possible triggers that exacerbate asthma, including allergic and nonallergic irritants. Important nonpharmacologic measures include environmental management to control allergens and irritants.

One way to avoid outdoor allergens including ragweed, grass, pollens, and molds is to stay indoors with closed windows in an air conditioned environment. Patients should stay indoors especially during the midday and afternoon when pollen and mold counts are highest. Prominent indoor allergens consist primarily of house dust components including dust mites and indoor molds. If animals are present, attempts should be made to remove them from the house or at least keep them out of the allergic person's bedroom. Central heating and cooling system ducts must also be sealed to this bedroom.

House dust mites depend on atmospheric moisture and human dander for survival. They appear to have a significant role in allergic asthma. High levels of mite antigen are found in dust from mattresses, pillows, carpeting, upholstered furniture, bedcovers, clothes, and soft toys. Methods to control house dust mites include encasing the mattress and pillow in an airtight cover and weekly washing of pillows and bedding in hot water (130°F). Avoid sleeping or lying on upholstered furniture. Consider removing carpets and replacing them with hardwood or tile floors. It is also desirable to reduce indoor humidity to less than 50%. Consider using chemical agents to kill mites. Many asthmatic individuals are allergic to cockroach allergens and roach control may have a significant benefit.

Indoor molds may also cause a problem. Bathrooms, kitchens, and basements require adequate ventilation and frequent cleaning. Dehumidifiers with humidity levels set less than 50%, but above 25%, may be helpful. An air conditioner allows the windows to stay closed and reduces indoor humidity. Indoor air cleaning devices are useful, especially the high-efficiency particulate air filters, which can be used within central heating and cooling systems or as free-standing units. Patients should not use a vacuum cleaner because this mobilizes many allergens. Alternatively, they may want to use a mask. Humidifiers are potentially harmful and may harbor mold spores. It is important to avoid inhaled irritants such as tobacco smoke, smoke from wood burning stoves, strong odors, sprays, and air pollutants.

Immunotherapy may be helpful when avoiding allergens and irritants is impossible. Immunotherapy should be administered by a specialist who has facilities and trained personnel to manage anaphylaxis.

Patient Education

Patient education is an extremely powerful tool in helping patients gain confidence in controlling their asthma and improving their quality of life. Asthma education should commence when asthma therapy is started. There should be a partnership between the physician, nurses, and others in the health care system and the patient. It is helpful to have written guidelines for patients including instructions about their medications and signs of asthma deterioration. Instruction on how to perform PEF measurements should be given. Educate the patient on what to do in the event of an acute asthma attack and understand when they should seek further help and emergency care. They must be knowledgeable of their own asthma triggers and how to avoid them. Teach all patients how to use their inhalers correctly with an extension tube. It is crucial that the physician and other caretakers be sensitive to the patients' needs.

Poor patient compliance is often related to problems with inhaler devices, awkward regimens, side effects from medications, medication cost, and availability of medical care. Some patients cannot afford medications and may not openly discuss this with you. Ask patients how they plan to pay for the medications. Inhalers cost up to $40 each and if they use three or four different inhalers, monthly medication costs can exceed $100.

It is essential to educate patients about the hazards of smoking. If the patient is a smoker or is exposed to passive smoke, smoking cessation should be encouraged. There are various programs available, some of which include the use of nicotine patches. All programs provide additional psychological support, which is beneficial during this difficult time. The outcome is excellent if the patient is motivated.

Pharmacologic Agents

Therapy for asthma appears complicated at first glance. It is important to individualize therapy based on asthma severity. A combination of medications should be used that will reverse the early phase response as well as the late phase response. Reduction in bronchial hyperresponsiveness is also a goal. This section briefly outlines the pharmacologic agents available and discusses medications that affect each asthma phase. Finally, we discuss step-care therapy in the management of mild, moderate, and severe asthma.

Asthma medications can be divided into those with a primary bronchodilator effect and those with anti-inflammatory effects (1,2,12–15). Medications that have a primary bronchodilator effect include β_2 agonists, theophylline, and anticholinergic drugs. Anti-inflammatory agents used in the therapy of asthma include corticosteroids, cromolyn sodium, and nedocromil sodium. Table 9.1 reviews asthma medication dosages and formulations available. Table 9.2 reviews each class of medication and shows in which phase of asthma each has therapeutic efficacy.

β_2-Adrenergic Agonists

β_2-Adrenergic agonists are by far the most effective bronchodilators. Activation of β-adrenergic receptors on airway smooth muscle leads to activation of adenyl cyclase, which leads to an increased intracellular cyclic adenosine monophosplate (AMP) resulting in relaxation of bronchial smooth muscle. There is no indication for administration of nonselective β_2-adrenergic agonists, such as isoproterenol. These agents are associated with a high incidence of cardiovascular side effects due to β_1-adrenergic receptor stimulation. Fortunately, there are many inhaled selective β_2-adrenergic agonists including albuterol, terbutaline, fenoterol, bitolterol, metaproterenol, and pirbuterol. These selective β_2-adrenergic agonists have a rapid onset of action, within minutes, and are effective for 3 to 6 hours. Recently, a longer-acting β_2-adrenergic agonist, salmeterol, has been approved by the Food and Drug Administration (FDA) and is effective for 12 hours. Salmeterol may be particularly useful in treating nocturnal asthma. Inhaled β_2-adrenergic agonists are indicated for short-term relief of acute bronchoconstriction and are the treatment of choice for an acute exacerbation of asthma. They may also be helpful in preventing bronchoconstriction induced by exercise or other stimuli.

β_2-Adrenergic agonists are available in inhaled and oral forms. However, when taken orally there is an increased incidence of systemic side effects. Oral β_2-adrenergic agents may be more useful in the prevention of nocturnal asthma.

Significant side effects of inhaled β_2-adrenergic agonists are rare. Side effects are more common when medications are given by nebulizer or orally and include tremor, tachycardia, and palpitations. With continued administration these side effects may diminish as tolerance develops. At higher doses, hypokalemia may occur. Patients with significant coronary artery disease have had episodes of angina and

Table 9.1 Medications for Asthma

BRONCHODILATORS	
β_2 Agonists	
Inhaled metered-dose inhaler (MDI)	
albuterol	2 puffs every 4–6 hr
metaproterenol	2 puffs every 4–6 hr
terbutaline (Brethaire)	2 puffs every 4–6 hr
bitolterol (Tornalate)	2 puffs every 4–8 hr
pirbuterol (Maxair)	2 puffs every 4–8 hr
salmeterol (Serevent)	2 puffs every 12 hr
Dry powder inhaler	
albuterol (Ventolin)	1 capsule every 4–6 hr
Nebulized solution	
albuterol	2.5 mg 0.5 mL 0.5% solution in 2 ml NS every 4–6 hr
metaproterenol	15 mg 0.3 mL 5% solution in 2 ml NS every 4–6 hr
Oral medication	
albuterol	2–4 mg every 6 hr 4 mg sustained-release every 12 hr
metaproterenol	10–20 mg every 6 hr
terbutaline	2.5 or 5 mg every 6 hr
Subcutaneous	
epinephrine	0.3 mg SQ
terbutaline	0.25 mg SQ
Ipratropium bromide (Atrovent)	
Inhaled MDI	
Ipratropium bromide	2 puffs every 6–8 hr
Nebulized solution	0.5 mg unit dose every 6–8 hr
Methylxanthines	
IV	
aminophylline	loading dose 0.6 mg/kg lean body weight (if not previously on it) then 0.1–0.6 mg/kg per hr by continuous infusion (many factors alter metabolism) keep level 5–15 μg/mL
Oral	
theophylline	sustained-release (total dose aminophylline for 24 hr × 0.80) divided for twice daily dosing

ANTI-INFLAMMATORY AGENTS	
Corticosteroids	
Inhaled MDI	
beclomethasone (Beclovent, Vanceril)	42 μg/puff, 2–4 puffs twice to four times daily
triamcinolone (Azmacort)	100 μg/puff, 2–4 puffs twice a day to four times a day
flunisolide (Aerobid)	250 μg/puff, 2–4 puffs twice daily
Oral	
prednisone	Dosing should be individualized
prednisolone	and tapered at the discretion of
methylprednisolone	the physician.
IV	
methylprednisolone	40–125 mg IV every 6–8 hr
Cromolyn sodium (Intal)	
Inhaled MDI	800 μg/puff, 2 puffs two to four times daily
Nebulized solution	20 mg/mL; 1 ampule two to four times daily
Dry powder capsule with inhaler (Spinhaler)	20 mg/capsule, 1 capsule two to four times daily
Nedocromil sodium (Tilade)	
Inhaled MDI	1.75 mg/puff, 2 puffs four times a day
Experimental anti-inflammatory drugs	
methotrexate	
gold salts	
cyclosporin A	
dapsone	
colchicine	
troleandomycin	
chloroquine	
5-lipoxygenase inhibitor	
leukotriene synthesis inhibitor	
leukotriene D_4 antagonist	

Table 9.2 Action of Asthma Medications

Medication	Improves Early Asthma Phase Response	Improves Late Asthma Phase Response	Reduces Bronchial Hyperresponsiveness
β_2-Adrenergic agents	+	0	0
Theophylline	+/−	+	0
Anticholinergic drugs	+	0	0
Corticosteroids	0	+	+
Cromolyn sodium and Nedocromil sodium	+	+	+

acute cardiac ischemia with the use of β_2-adrenergic agonists.

Theophylline

Theophylline has been used in asthma therapy for more than 50 years. Initially it was thought that it caused bronchodilatation by inhibiting production of phosphodiesterase, thus increasing intracellular cyclic AMP. This is not true, however, because the concentration of theophylline needed to inhibit phosphodiesterase greatly exceeds the optimal therapeutic range.

Theophylline is a less effective bronchodilator than β_2-adrenergic agents although it is synergistic with β-adrenergic agents. Slow-release preparations may be useful in preventing symptoms in nocturnal asthma.

Because of the high incidence of unwanted side effects and the narrow therapeutic window, theophylline levels should be monitored. The therapeutic range is from 10–20 μg/mL. The NAEP experts recommend a more conservative approach and suggest that levels be between 5 and 15 μg/mL. Several factors affect serum theophylline levels. Box 9.3 reviews factors that alter theophylline clearance.

Theophylline has many toxic side effects. Cardiac arrhythmias and seizures may occur even when drug concentrations are in the therapeutic range. Other common side effects include nausea and headache.

Anticholinergic Drugs

Cholinergic antagonists, primarily atropine, have been used for many years in asthma therapy. However, systemic side effects limit their use. The introduction of

Box 9.3 Factors Affecting Theophylline Blood Levels

- **Conditions Increasing Theophylline Levels**

Older age (>50 yr)
Obesity
Liver disease
Pulmonary edema
Febrile illness
Chronic obstructive pulmonary disease
Acute viral infections
High-carbohydrate, low-protein diet
Influenza A vaccine
Drugs: caffeine
β blockers
erythromycin
allopurinol
cimetidine
oral contraceptives
ciprofloxacin (other quinolones)
troleandomycin

- **Conditions Decreasing Theophylline Levels**

Young age (<16 yr)
Cigarette or marijuana smoking
High-protein diet or charcoal-broiled meat
Alcohol
Cystic fibrosis
Drugs: phenobarbital
phenytoin
rifampin
carbamazepine
isoproterenol

quaternary derivatives such as ipratropium bromide, which are not absorbed systemically, are more attractive bronchodilators. Anticholinergic agents block muscarinic receptors in airway smooth muscle and inhibit vagal cholinergic tone, resulting in bronchodilitation. Anticholinergic agents provide varying degrees of protection against bronchoconstrictor challenges. They are not particularly effective against allergen challenges. Anticholinergic agents are less effective than β-adrenergic agonists in the treatment of acute asthma. Anticholinergics are usually used in combination with other bronchodilators. The onset of action is slower than β_2-adrenergic agonists with peak activity in approximately 1 hour. The bronchodilator effect can last up to 8 hours. Because ipratropium bromide is poorly absorbed, there are very few side effects.

Anti-inflammatory Drugs

Chronic inflammation is central to the pathogenesis of asthma. Anti-inflammatory agents used in asthma therapy include inhaled corticosteroids, oral corticosteriods, cromolyn sodium, and nedocromil sodium. Inhaled steroids should become first-line therapy for chronic asthma. Corticosteroids act on various components of the inflammatory response. They inhibit release of mediators from macrophages and eosinophils. With inhaled corticosteroids, there is a gradual reduction in bronchial hyperresponsiveness. Full therapeutic response takes up to 3 months.

Inhaled corticosteroids include beclomethasone, triamcinolone, and flunisolide. All are active locally and can control asthma without systemic effects or adrenal suppression. Inhaled corticosteroids should be part of all regimens for moderate or severe asthma.

Oral corticosteroids such as prednisone, prednisolone, or methylprednisolone are still necessary to control asthma during severe acute exacerbations and to treat patients with severe asthma. A single dose in the morning is associated with fewer side effects. Alternate day dosing may also improve side effects; however, this may not control asthma. Short courses of orally administered corticosteroids are indicated for exacerbations of asthma.

Side effects are rare with low doses of inhaled corticosteroids, up to 400 μg/day but become more frequent with higher doses. Side effects from inhaled corticosteroids include oral pharyngeal candidiasis and dysphonia. These effects are less common if a large volume spacer is used and patients wash their mouths out after use. Orally administered corticosteroids cause many well known side effects including osteoporosis, weight gain, hypertension, diabetes, myopathy, psychiatric disturbances, skin fragility, and cataracts. Because of the many side effects of oral corticosteroids, patients should be educated and understand the risk-benefit ratio. Every attempt should be made to keep the patient on the lowest dose required to control asthma.

Cromolyn sodium is given by inhalation. Its mechanism of action is still unknown. Cromolyn protects against various indirect bronchoconstrictor stimuli including exercise. Nedocromil sodium is chemically unrelated to cromolyn but has a similar clinical profile.

It appears that both cromolyn and nedocromil inhibit the immediate response to allergens and exercise as well as prevent the late response and improve bronchial hyperresponsiveness. Side effects are minimal with cromolyn or nedocromil and they are very well tolerated.

Stepwise Approach to Pharmacologic Therapy Determined by Asthma Severity

The International Consensus Report in 1992 and the NAEP Expert Panel Report recommend that aggressive asthma therapy include both bronchodilator and anti-inflammatory agents. Both recommend a stepwise approach to pharmacologic therapy based on whether the patient has mild, moderate, or severe asthma (1,2). Figure 9.8 reviews this stepwise approach. Chronic management of patients with mild asthma includes the use of an inhaled β_2 agonist PRN for bronchospasm. They may also use inhaled cromolyn sodium or β_2 agonists before exercise or exposure to a specific allergen.

Patients with moderate asthma should add an inhaled anti-inflammatory agent daily such as nedocromil sodium, cromolyn sodium, or an inhaled corticosteroid 200–500 μg/day. If necessary, increase the inhaled corticosteroid to 400–700 μg/day. For breakthrough bronchospasm, patients should use an inhaled β_2 agonist as needed, not to exceed three to four times a day. Patients with more severe moderate asthma should use high-dose inhaled corticosteroids using 800–1000 μg/day. The addition of sustained-

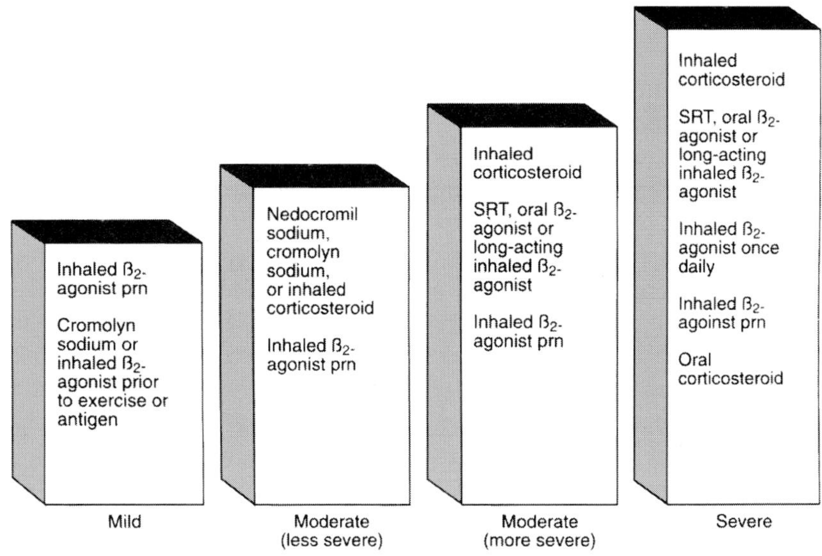

Fig 9.8 Stepwise approach to asthma therapy. Therapeutic regimen recommended by the International Consensus Report based on asthma severity. *(Reproduced by permission from International Consensus Report on Diagnosis and Management of Asthma. AL Sheffer Chair. U.S. Department of Health Services, National Institutes of Health, Publication No. 92-3091, March 1992:34.)*

release theophylline or oral β_2 agonist should be considered.

Patients with severe asthma should use high-dose inhaled corticosteroids 800–1000 μg/day along with a slow-release theophylline derivative and an oral β_2 agonist with or without a long-acting inhaled β_2 agonist once per day. Patients with continued symptoms should be on oral corticosteroids and an inhaled β_2 agonist up to three to four times per day. Once asthma control is reached and sustained, attempt to reduce therapy. While doing this, it is vital to monitor PEF.

It is essential that all patients learn how to use an inhaler correctly with an extension tube. An extension tube improves the delivery of the medication to the airways.

Special Considerations

Pregnant Asthmatic Patients

Seven percent of women of childbearing age have asthma. Asthma occurs in approximately 1% of pregnancies. Asthma complications occur more often in adolescent pregnancies than in older gravidas. Physicians taking care of women should have a clear understanding about the treatment of pregnant asthmatic patients.

Physiologic Effects

Many physiologic and anatomic changes occur in the respiratory system during pregnancy (16–18). Changes to the airway mucosa include hyperemia, edema, and mucous secretion. These changes are more pronounced during the third trimester. Hormonal changes that affect airway reactivity include an increase in cortisol levels. Prostaglandin E_2, a bronchodilator, remains constant until the third trimester. Prostacyclin, a bronchodilator, increases throughout pregnancy. Prostaglandin $F_{2\alpha}$, a potent bronchoconstrictor, increases throughout pregnancy. Another bronchodilator, cyclic AMP, increases during the first and third trimesters. Cyclic glucose monophosphate increases during the first trimester. The clinical relevance of these hormonal and mediator changes is purely speculative in terms of bronchomotor tone.

Respiratory muscle and thoracic cage dimensions change during pregnancy. The diaphragm elevates by 4 cm. The anterior posterior diameter of the chest increases by 2 cm. This broadens the subcostal angle leading to a 5- to 7-cm increase in chest circumference. Diaphragmatic function remains normal.

Pulmonary function tests are also affected. There are decreases in residual volume of up to 20%, and functional residual capacity of up to 25% by the sixth month. Total lung capacity and vital capacity are unchanged. By the end of the first trimester there is an increase in minute ventilation by 48% related to an increase in tidal volume and a minor increase in respiratory rate. Progesterone is responsible for this increase. There is no significant change in FEV_1 or lung compliance during pregnancy.

Maternal gas exchange is also altered. Because of alveolar hyperventilation, chronic respiratory alkalosis with renal compensation is present. $Paco_2$ ranges from 27 to 32 mm Hg and Pao_2 from 106 to 108 mm Hg with a serum bicarbonate level of 18 to 21 mEq/L.

Fetal oxygen transport is achieved by flow gradients across the placenta with the chorionic villi providing a large surface area for diffusion. The fetus exists in a hypoxic environment with minimal oxygen storage and has minimal reserve to tolerate maternal hypoxia. The umbilical vein has a Pao_2 of 26 to 32 mm Hg with an oxygen saturation of up to 90%. If the mother has an acute asthma attack and her Pao_2 goes from 91 to 65 mm Hg, the umbilical vein Pao_2 goes from 32 to 26 mm Hg, resulting in a marked decrease in oxygen content with potentially devastating effects on the fetus.

Because of the poor efficiency of fetal oxygenation, fetal hemoglobin is structured somewhat differently so that the fetal oxygen hemoglobin curve is shifted to the left. Fetal hemoglobin is less responsive to the effects of 2,3-diphosphoglycerate, and fetal hemoglobin level is increased to 16.5 gm/dL. For these reasons, fetal hemoglobin has a higher oxygen affinity than maternal hemoglobin.

Maternal hypocarbia associated with hyperventilation during an acute asthma attack results in a marked reduction in fetal oxygenation. Maternal hypocarbia shifts the maternal hemoglobin oxygen disassociation curve to the left. Hypocarbia causes uterine artery vasoconstriction. Elevated serum catacholamines also decrease uterine blood flow. Fetal cardiac output decreases because of the mechanical effects of hyperventilation.

Juniper and colleagues examined airway responsiveness in mild asthmatic patients (19). They noted an improvement in airway responsiveness during pregnancy, which peaked in the second trimester. Within 1 month postpartum, airway responsiveness returned to the preconception state (Fig 9.9). Patients with the most airway hyperresponsiveness showed the greatest improvement in airway responsiveness during pregnancy. They also noticed a reduction in medication usage.

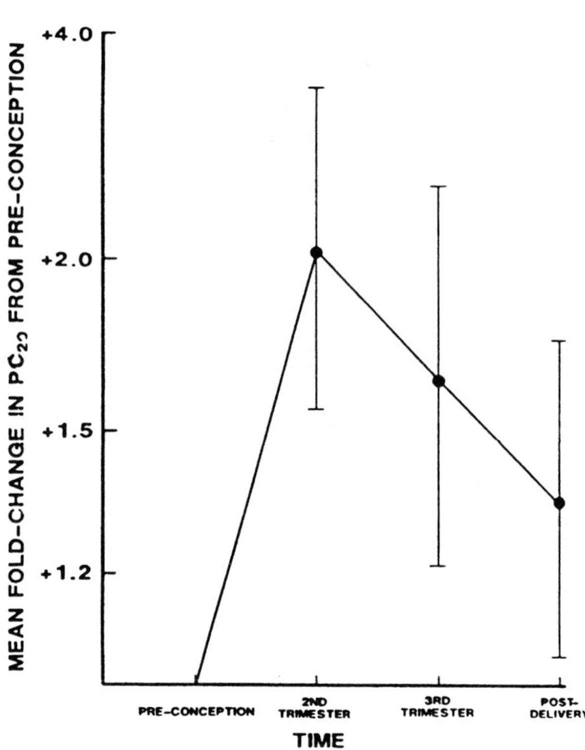

Fig 9.9 Airway responsiveness before, during, and after pregnancy expressed as fold change in PC_{20} from preconception. The error bars represent the standard deviation of within-subject change. There is a twofold improvement in airway reactivity that peaks during the second trimester. *(Reproduced by permission from Juniper EF, Daniel EE, Roberts RS, et al. Improvement in airway responsiveness and asthma severity during pregnancy. A prospective study. Am Rev Respir Dis 1989;140:926.)*

The Effect of Pregnancy on Asthma

Gluck and Gluck studied 47 patients in a prospective study of pregnant asthmatic women and noticed asthma improvement in 13%, no significant change in 43%, and worsening symptoms in 43% (20). Patients with mild asthma tended to improve and patients with severe asthma grew worse. Exacerbations tended to occur at the end of the second trimester. Another study by Schatz and colleagues examining 366 pregnancies noted that 28% of the patients improved, 33% had no significant change, 35% worsened, and 4% were uncertain (21). The tendency for asthma to worsen was more common between the 29th and 36th weeks of gestation. Asthma seemed to improve during the last 4 weeks of pregnancy and attacks during labor were rare. Turner and coworkers reviewed nine earlier studies between 1953 and 1976 and of 1054 pregnancies there was asthma improvement in 29%, no change in 49%, and asthma deterioration in 22% (22). In summary, patients with severe asthma are likely to worsen and those with mild asthma improve. Individuals are likely to repeat the same clinical pattern with each pregnancy. There are no large studies using current medication strategies looking at asthma outcome during pregnancy.

Fetal Outcome in Pregnant Asthmatic Patients

Schatz and associates studied 330 mild asthmatic patients and found no difference in fetal outcome compared to normal controls (21). In 1986, Fitzsimmons, and colleagues studied 56 pregnant severe asthmatic women taking corticosteroids and noted no deaths; however, there was an increase preterm labor and growth retardation compared to normal controls (23). Patients had normal fetal outcome if they did not have status asthmaticus during their pregnancy. In 1970, Gordon and coworkers studied 277 pregnancies and noted no increase in prematurity when compared to 30,000 normal controls (24). They noted a 5.8% perinatal death rate with 81% of these deaths being in blacks. Apter and associates examined 28 adolescent gravidas with severe asthma and noted no maternal deaths or growth retardation. One noncompliant mother with multiple episodes of status asthmaticus had a child with cerebral palsy (25). The Kaiser-Permanente Asthma Pregnancy Study noted a relationship between low birth weight and intrauterine growth retardation with decline in maternal pulmonary function (26).

Of importance, concerning fetal outcome, is that blacks have twice the number of low birth weight infants than whites and perinatal mortality is increased in severely uncontrolled asthmatic patients. Also, intrauterine growth retardation is found in moderately uncontrolled asthmatic women as well as in cigarette smokers. In one study, prematurity was noted in patients taking chronic theophylline therapy, in those who smoked cigarettes during their pregnancy, and in those who had uterine muscle hyperactivity.

Modern data show that mothers with asthma have normal fetal outcome if their asthma is under control. Poor asthma control leads to poor fetal outcome. Infants from asthmatic mothers may have a higher incidence of low weight births. It is extremely important to treat asthma aggressively during pregnancy.

Management of Asthma During Pregnancy

The goals of therapy are to maintain normal pulmonary function and control symptoms. It is important to avoid acute exacerbations of asthma because this has severe impact on fetal oxygenation. It is also important to avoid adverse effects from asthma medications. If these goals are maintained and the patient does not have severe attacks of asthma during the pregnancy, then the risk of perinatal morbidity is similar to patients without asthma. The general treatment principles of pregnant asthmatic patients are similar to those previously outlined. You should use both pharmacologic and nonpharmacologic therapies. It is important that pregnant asthmatics monitor PEF to detect deterioration of asthma before clinical symptoms. It is crucial to avoid or control asthma triggers. This includes environmental control measures such as avoiding specific irritants and allergens that may increase airway inflammation, hyperresponsiveness, and worsen airflow obstruction. Tobacco smokers should be educated about the hazards of smoking during pregnancy because smoking has a significant negative impact on fetal growth. Motivate these women to participate in an active smoking cessation program. Eliminating all exposure to tobacco smoke, including passive smoke, is essential for pregnant women. It is necessary to avoid food additives such as sulfites. β-Blocking drugs and drugs containing aspirin can exacerbate airflow obstruction and should be avoided.

It is safe to continue immunotherapy during pregnancy if the patient was receiving immunotherapy before conception. Usually immunotherapy is not started nor antigen doses increased during pregnancy because of the possibility of anaphylaxis. Influenza vaccine is recommended for all patients with moderate to severe asthma and should be given every year. Because influenza vaccine is a killed virus vaccine there is no fetal risk.

Pharmacologic therapy of asthma during pregnancy is similar to the management of nonpregnant asthmatic patients. Many practitioners remain reluctant to prescribe aggressive medication therapy for fear of litigation in the event of an untold perinatal outcome. The National Heart, Lung and Blood Institute organized a working group on asthma and pregnancy (27). The Executive Summary recommended that a patient–physician partnership be formed that allows ongoing communication about the benefits and risks of various treatment approaches. These discussions should acknowledge the fact that no drug is absolutely safe but uncontrolled asthma is far more dangerous to the fetus than any of the recommended medications. Asthma should be aggressively treated during pregnancy with every effort made to avoid acute exacerbations. Boxes 9.4 and 9.5 review asthma medications that are safe and those that are not safe to use during pregnancy.

The FDA has established drug safety guidelines during pregnancy. Class A drugs have undergone controlled studies that fail to reveal increased risk in human beings. Class B drugs show no reported adverse affects in animal or human studies. Class C drugs show adverse effects in animal studies but not in human studies. Class D drugs are found to have adverse affects in human beings. Class E drugs are contraindicated during pregnancy. Many asthma medications are not classified. Classifications may change from year to year, so it is worthwhile to check your *Physician's Desk Reference* for changes.

β_2-Agonist agents have been used safely during pregnancy. Albuterol and terbutaline are the two most frequently used. However, albuterol may be tocolytic in high doses. Less is known about fenoterol and isoproterenol, and it is recommended that these agents not be used because albuterol has excellent therapeutic efficacy. Avoid metaproterenol because it has been found to be teratogenic in mice. Congenital malformations were increased in mothers who received epinephrine during pregnancy. Avoid using systemic β_2 agonists during labor because they prolong labor. In a study of 259 women taking inhaled β_2 agonists, there was no difference in fetal outcome compared to normal controls.

Inhaled corticosteroids are also safe to use during pregnancy. Beclomethasone is safe and frequently used during pregnancy (28). The National Institute of Health Executive Summary on Management of

Box 9.4 Asthma Medications Safely Used During Pregnancy

β_2 Agonists	albuterol terbutaline
Methylxanthines	aminophylline theophylline
Inhaled corticosteroids	beclomethasone
Inhaled anticholinergics	ipratropium bromide
Inhaled cromolyn	cromolyn sodium
Oral anti-inflammatory agents	hydrocortisone methylprednisolone prednisone prednisolone
Antibiotics	ampicillin erythromycin

Box 9.5 Asthma Medications to Avoid During Pregnancy

β_2 Agonists	metaproterenol epinephrine
Corticosteroids	dexamethasone
Expectorants	iodide containing
Antibiotics	ciprofloxacin sulfonamides tetracycline chloramphenicol trimethoprim

Asthma During Pregnancy recommended beclomethasone because of its widespread experience (27). Less well studied agents include triamcinolone (Azmacort) and flunisolide (Aerobid). If a patient has moderate to severe asthma or an acute exacerbation of asthma, it is important to add oral corticosteroids. Human studies show no adverse effects from oral corticosteroids. Prednisone and methylprednisolone cross the placenta poorly. However, one animal study performed in mice showed congenital malformations (cleft palate) with high-dose corticosteroids. It is important to watch for neonatal adrenal insufficiency. Oral corticosteroids used safely in pregnant women include hydrocortisone, methylprednisolone, prednisone, and prednisolone. Dexamethasone should not be used because it crosses the placenta and is teratogenic in mice.

Methylxanthines have been safely used although they cross the placenta and may cause tachycardia in neonates. Because methylxanthines prolong labor by inhibiting uterine contractions, they should not be used in high doses during labor. One study noted no ill effects in pregnancy outcome in 117 women taking theophylline and 76 women taking aminophylline. Pharmacokinetics of methylxanthines during pregnancy are complicated and levels should be monitored.

Other medications safely used during pregnancy include inhaled cromolyn sodium and ipratropium bromide. Ipratropium bromide is poorly absorbed and studies show that there is no increased risk of congenital malformations. Disodium cromoglycate is poorly absorbed and, when given in very large doses, does not cause teratogenic affects in animals; 296 women taking disodium cromoglycate during pregnancy had no ill effects.

Expectorants with iodide can cause fetal goiter and should be avoided. Avoidance of decongestants is also recommended.

Antibiotics are occasionally used in asthma therapy. Antibiotics safe to use during pregnancy include ampicillin, penicillin, and erythromycin. Antibiotics to avoid include ciprofloxacin, which results in fetal arthropathy; sulfa drugs, which cause hyperbilirubinemia; tetracycline, which inhibits bone growth; and chloramphenicol, which leads to gray baby syndrome.

It is extremely important to keep asthma under good control. With careful selection of drugs there should be no significant teratogenic effects. You may consider prescribing only nonteratogenic drugs to women of childbearing age because 50% of pregnancies are unplanned. Remember, treat asthma attacks aggressively.

During labor and delivery avoid IV aminophylline. Oxytocin has no effect on bronchial smooth muscle. Conversely, prostaglandin $F_{2\alpha}$ and prostaglandin E_2 can cause severe bronchospasm. Spinal, epidural, or caudal anesthesia is preferred. Terbutaline may also inhibit labor. Severe asthma attacks during labor are rare and patients should require no specific intervention during labor if their asthma is under good control. Consider using stress doses of hydrocortisone if patients are taking systemic corticosteroids. Hydrocortisone is chosen because it crosses the placenta rapidly so the fetus is also treated.

After delivery, airway reactivity returns to the prepregnant state within 3 months. It is important to encourage breast-feeding. Monitor theophylline levels. The patient should avoid using tetracycline, sulfa drugs, iodide, and chloramphenicol while breastfeeding.

With aggressive pharmacologic and nonpharmacologic therapy, the pregnant asthmatic patient should have a normal fetal outcome. If there are any questions about the management of a pregnant asthmatic woman consider referring her to an allergist or a pulmonologist.

Exercise-Induced Asthma

With more women performing extremely well in numerous athletic events, it is necessary to discuss exercise-induced asthma, which affects approximately 80% of all patients with asthma. Classically it begins 8 to 15 minutes after exercise has stopped. Heat loss due to hyperventilation plays a role. Bronchospasm is often worse in low temperatures and low humidity. Airway cooling followed by abrupt rewarming when exercise is concluded contributes to acute bronchoconstriction. Other possible factors leading to bronchoconstriction are water loss and hyperventilation. Probably a combination of factors contributes to the physiologic events of exercise-induced asthma. There is also evidence of airway inflammation in these patients (29).

Diagnosis often comes directly from the history. Many patients, especially those without a known history of asthma, may relate breathlessness to "being out of shape." Many people ignore these symptoms. When airway function testing is performed in elite athletes before and after exercise, a significant percentage will have a marked decrease in airflow without symptoms. Exercise testing using a stationary bicycle or treadmill can be performed in many pulmonary function laboratories. Patients perform continuous exercise at a target heart rate, usually 70% to 80% of the predicted maximum, for at least 6 minutes. Spirometry is measured before, immediately after exercise, and at frequent intervals over the subsequent 30 to 60 minutes. A 12% to 15% drop in FEV_1 will make the diagnosis of exercise-induced asthma.

At the 1994 Winter Olympics, up to 80% of the athletes used an inhaled β_2 agonist. With therapy, athletes with exercise-induced asthma can perform well at the international level. One well known athlete with asthma is Jackie Joyner-Kersee, three time Olympian, gold medal winner and world record holder of the heptathalon. Fortunately, exercise-induced asthma is treatable and should not keep anyone from engaging in athletics.

Inhaled β_2 agonists 15 to 20 minutes before exercise are useful in controlling exercised-induced asthma. Inhaled cromolyn is also useful; however, when compared with a β_2 agonist, the latter proves superior in preventing the condition. Therefore, a β_2 agonist should be tried first. If both inhaled agents are used, amelioration of exercise-induced asthma is seen in approximately 90% of patients. Other medications shown to have some effect include theophylline, oral β_2 agonists, calcium channel blockers, nedocromil sodium, and even furosemide. Nonpharmacologic measures may also be beneficial and should not be overlooked. Wearing a scarf over the nose and mouth in cold weather can be helpful. A warm-up period and a cool-down period are also recommended. Exposure to pollutants including ozone should be avoided. In a metropolitan area, ozone levels peak during rush hour traffic, especially during the late afternoon. With these simple measures, most will be able to enjoy the multiple physical and psychological benefits of daily exercise.

Nocturnal Asthma

Nocturnal or early morning wheezing is common in asthmatic patients. Turner-Warwick found that 74% of asthmatics awakened at least once a week, and 64% reported awakening at least three times a week with wheezing (30). Many asthma deaths occur during the early morning hours. Patients with nocturnal symptoms have poor quality sleep, which may have a significant negative impact on their quality of life.

The mechanism of nocturnal bronchospasm is complex. There is diurnal variation of cyclic AMP, cortisol, and epinephrine levels. There is decreased peak expiratory flow rates at 4 AM. Plasma histamine levels also rise at 4 AM. Vagal tone is increased at night. Other factors include allergen exposure (dust mites in bedding), diminished mucociliary clearance, and airway cooling during sleep (31–36).

Whatever the mechanism, nocturnal symptoms peak between 2:00 and 6:00 AM and treatment should be timed to provide maximum medication levels between these hours (37). Inhaled salmeterol (Serevent) has bronchodilator action for 12 hours and can be used. Another treatment option is to take an oral β_2 agonist (albuterol or terbutaline) before going to sleep. Long-acting theophylline preparations given once a day should be given at 7 PM. Inhaled anticholinergics such as ipratropium bromide (Atrovent) may be helpful. If patients have frequent nocturnal awakenings, they should be taking inhaled corticosteroids. Prednisone dosing at 3 PM may be helpful.

Asthma in the Emergency Room

When a patient with asthma presents for acute emergency care, objective measurements of airflow are essential. Many emergency rooms use FEV_1 or PEF to monitor patients. History and physical examination are also essential. Arterial blood gases should be obtained if the patient appears to be in significant distress. A chest x-ray should be obtained to rule out the possibility of pneumothorax or acute parenchymal disease. The patient should be given an inhaled β_2 agonist immediately along with three doses over the next 60 to 90 minutes. PEF or FEV_1 should be monitored after the first dose. An alternative is SQ β_2 agonists. A pulse oximeter should be placed on the patient. If there is any question about oxygenation, supplemental oxygen should be given. Early consideration of systemic corticosteroids, such as methylprednisolone 125 mg IV, should be given if the patient does not respond immediately to bronchodilators or the patient is already taking oral corticosteroids. It is extremely important to monitor patients frequently. If there is a good clinical response with resolution of bronchospasm, and the FEV_1 is greater than 70% baseline, then the patient can be discharged with close medical follow-up on oral corticosteroids.

If there is an incomplete response with an FEV_1 of less than 70%, then the patient should remain in the emergency room and admission considered. If a poorer response is obtained, or the FEV_1 is less than 40% or PEF is less than 40%, patients should be admitted. If the patient develops respiratory failure, signified by extreme distress, impaired consciousness, with PEF of less than 25%, or a $Paco_2$ of 40 mm Hg or higher, the patient should be admitted to the intensive care unit. Treatment should begin with systemic corticosteroids, frequent inhaled β_2 agonists, and consideration for possible intubation and mechanical ventilation. Pulmonary and critical care specialists should be called immediately for this patient. If the patient has risk factors for asthma mortality, strong consideration for admission should be considered early. If there is any question about the patient's response, it is better to err on the side of hospital admission. Once in the hospital, begin IV aminophylline, inhaled β_2 agonists, IV methylprednisolone and continue to monitor clinical response and airway function (1,2).

REFERENCES

1. National Asthma Education Program Expert Panel Report. Executive Summary: Guidelines for the diagnosis and management of asthma. AL Sheffer Chair. U.S. Department of Health and Human Services, Public Health Service, National Institutes of Health Publication No. 91-3042A, June 1991.
2. International Consensus Report on Diagnosis and Management of Asthma. AL Sheffer Chair. U.S. Department of Health Service, National Institutes of Health Publication No. 92-3091, March 1992.
3. McFadden ER Jr, Gilbert IA. Medical progress. Asthma. N Engl J Med 1992;327:1928–1937.
4. Weiss KB, Gergen PJ, Hodgson TA. An economic evaluation of asthma in the United States. N Engl J Med 1992;326:862–866.
5. Robin ED. Death from bronchial asthma. Chest 1988;93:614–618.
6. Fulwood R, Parker S, Hurd SS. Asthma—United States, 1980–1987. MMWR 1990;39:493–497.
7. Shephard RJ. Environmental tobacco smoke and asthma. Chest 1993;103:330–331.
8. Chan-Yeung M, Lam S. State of art: occupational asthma. Am Rev Respir Dis 1986;133:686–703.
9. Crapo RO. Current concepts. Pulmonary function testing. N Engl J Med 1994;331:25–30.
10. Perpina M, Pellicer C, de Diego A, et al. Diagnostic value of the bronchial provocation test with methacholine in asthma. Chest 1993;104:149–154.
11. Sekizawa K, Sasaki H, Shimizo Y, Takishima T. Dose-response effects of methacholine in normal and asthmatic subjects. Am Rev Respir Dis 1986;133: 593–599.
12. Kemp JP. Approaches to asthma management. Arch Intern Med 1993;153:805–812.
13. Barnes PJ. Drug therapy. A new approach to the treatment of asthma. N Engl J Med 1989;321:1517–1527.
14. Reiss TF, Ahmad M. Asthma current strategies for treatment. Cleve Clin J Med 1991;58:161–169.
15. The Medical Letter. Drugs for ambulatory asthma. Med Lett Drugs Ther 1991;33:9–12.
16. Elkus R, Popovich J Jr. Respiratory physiology in pregnancy. Clin Chest Med 1992;13:555–565.
17. Weinberger ST, Weiss ST, Cohen WR, et al. Pregnancy and the lung. Am Rev Respir Dis 1980;121:559–581.
18. Greenberger PA. Asthma in pregnancy. Clin Chest Med 1992;13:597–606.
19. Juniper EF, Daniel EE, Roberts RS, et al. Improvement in airway responsiveness and asthma severity during pregnancy. A prospective study. Am Rev Respir Dis 1989;140:924–931.
20. Gluck JC, Gluck PA. The effects of pregnancy on asthma: a prospective study. Ann Allergy 1976;37:164–168.
21. Schatz M, Harden K, Forsythe A, et al. The course of asthma during pregnancy, postpartum and successive pregnancies: a prospective analysis. J Allergy Clin Immunol 1988;81:509–517.
22. Turner ES, Greenberger PA, Patterson R. Management of the pregnant asthmatic patient. Ann Intern Med 1980;93:905–918.
23. Fitzsimmons R, Greenberger PA, Patterson R. Outcome of pregnancy in women requiring corticosteroids for severe asthma. J Allergy Clin Immunol 1986;78:349–353.
24. Gordon M, Niswander KR, Berendes H, Kantor AG. Fetal morbidity following potentially anoxygenic

obstetric conditions. VII. Bronchial asthma. Am J Obstet Gynecol 1970;106:421–429.

25. Apter AJ, Greenberger PA, Patterson R. Outcomes of pregnancy in adolescents with severe asthma. Arch Intern Med 1989;149:2571–2575.

26. Schatz M, Zeiger RS, Hoffman CP, Kaiser-Permanente Asthma and Pregnancy Group. Intrauterine growth is related to gestational pulmonary function in pregnant asthmatic women. Chest 1990;98:389–392.

27. Working Group on Asthma and Pregnancy of the National Asthma Education Program. Executive summary: management of asthma during pregnancy. AT Luskin Chair. National Institutes of Health. National Heart, Lung and Blood Institute. NIH Publication No. 93-3279A, March 1993.

28. Greenberger PA, Patterson R. Beclomethasone diproprionate for severe asthma during pregnancy. Ann Intern Med 1983;98:478–480.

29. McFadden ER Jr. Current concepts. Exercise induced asthma. N Engl J Med 1994;330:1362–1367.

30. Turner-Warwick M. Epidemiology of nocturnal asthma. Am J Med 1988;85(suppl 1B):6–8.

31. McFadden ER Jr. Circadian rhythms. Am J Med 1988;85(suppl 1B):2–5.

32. Barnes P, Fitzgerald G, Brown M, Dollery C. Nocturnal asthma and changes in circulating epinephrine, histamine and cortisol. N Engl J Med 1980;303:263–267.

33. Busse WW. Pathogenesis and pathophysiology of nocturnal asthma. Am J Med 1988;85(suppl 1B):24–29.

34. Martin RJ, Cicutto LC, Ballard RD. Factors related to the nocturnal worsening of asthma. Am Rev Respir Dis 1990;141:33–38.

35. Ballard RD, Saathoft MC, Patel DK, et al. Effect of sleep on nocturnal bronchoconstriction and ventilatory patterns in asthmatics. J Appl Physiol 1989;67:243–249.

36. Barnes PJ. Inflammatory mechanisms and nocturnal asthma. Am J Med 1988;85(suppl 1B):64–70.

37. Martin RJ, Cicutto LC, Ballard RD, et al. Circadian variations in theophylline concentrations and the treatment of nocturnal asthma. Am Rev Respir Dis 1989;139:475–478.

CHAPTER 10

CHRONIC OBSTRUCTIVE PULMONARY DISEASE

John I. Kennedy, Jr.

Chronic obstructive pulmonary disease (COPD) is a term that has been used to describe a group of disorders characterized by obstruction of airflow. The currently accepted use of this term is in the description of chronic bronchitis, emphysema, or small-airways disease, entities that often coexist in the same patient. In contrast to asthma, COPD is associated with physiologic impairment that is not completely reversible. In the overwhelming majority of cases COPD is directly attributable to a history of cigarette smoking.

Most patients with COPD manifest a combination of chronic bronchitis and emphysema. To fully understand this syndrome, precise definitions of these components are required (1). Chronic bronchitis is defined in historical terms. The presence of cough with sputum production on most days during 3 or more months of 2 consecutive years identifies the presence of chronic bronchitis. Emphysema, the dilation and destruction of distal airspaces within the lungs, is most strictly identified by histopathology. In practice, however, tissue samples are rarely available for examination in patients with COPD. When advanced, emphysema may be appreciated by the presence of bullae on chest x-rays. Impairment of diffusing capacity is a more sensitive, though nonspecific, indicator of the presence of emphysema.

The disease is a major public health problem in the United States. It is currently the fifth leading cause of mortality (2,3), and death rates from COPD have been rising in recent years (3,4). The slower rate of decline in smoking among women in the United States makes it likely that COPD will remain an important and increasingly frequent health problem among women for many years to come (5).

Presentation

Patients with COPD typically present for medical attention in the fifth or sixth decades of life. Those for whom symptoms of chronic bronchitis dominate may present as early as age 30. A history of cigarette smoking is usual, and the absence of such a history should provoke consideration of alternative diagnoses. Cough and dyspnea are the most common symptoms reported. Symptoms are most often gradual in onset with steady progression over time. Dyspnea usually begins with exertion and progresses, with increasing functional limitation over several to many years. Often it is not until exercise capacity has become severely limited, or symptoms have precipitously increased as a result of a superimposed acute infection, that patients seek medical attention. Wheezing is also common and may lead to confusion about the diagnosis of COPD versus asthma. Orthopnea is reasonably common in patients with COPD, but nocturnal exacerbations of symptoms are unusual. Sleep-disordered breathing and nocturnal hypoxemia can occur in association with COPD (6,7). Weight loss occurs in some patients with advanced disease, typically in those where emphysema is the predominant pathology (8,9). As with any chronic illness, depression is a common occurrence in patients with COPD (10). Cognitive dysfunction may also result as a manifestation of impaired gas exchange (11).

Although chronic bronchitis and emphysema typically coexist in an individual patient, a relative dominance of one or the other may lead to one of two classic clinical syndromes. Patients in whom emphysema predominates manifest a constellation of symptoms and signs that has led them to be labeled as "pink puffers." A different group of clinical findings causes

Table 10.1 Features Characterizing the Two Major Clinical Types of COPD

	Emphysema Predominant ("Pink Puffer")	Bronchitis Predominant ("Blue Bloater")
Age at onset	Usually 40–50 yr	30–40 yr
Dyspnea	Prominent, early onset	Late onset
Sputum	Scant	Copious
Body habitus	Thin, barrel chest	Heavier, edema common
Chest x-ray	Hyperinflation, oligemia, bullae often present	Prominent bronchovascular markings
Pulmonary function testing	↓ FEV_1 ↑ TLC ↑↑ RV ↓ D_LCO	↓ FEV_1 Other findings variable
Pao_2 (resting)	Normal or slightly low	Often very low
$Paco_2$	Normal or low	Elevated
Cyanosis	Unusual	Common
Cor pulmonale	Unusual	Common

D_LCO, diffusing capacity for carbon monoxide; FEV_1, forced expiratory volume in 1 second; RV, residual volume; TLC, total lung capacity

the group of patients with a predominance of chronic bronchitis to be referred to as "blue bloaters." Some of the characteristics that distinguish these two groups are outlined in Table 10.1. Although experienced clinicians will find these two prototypes familiar, it is important to recognize that most patients fall somewhere along a spectrum between the two extremes and manifest symptoms and findings of both.

Differential Diagnosis

The clinical syndrome of cough, dyspnea, and airflow obstruction may suggest a number of diagnostic possibilities in addition to COPD (Box 10.1). The primary condition that must be differentiated from COPD is asthma. Asthma is characterized by frequent variations in pulmonary function resulting from exposures to triggering agents. In contrast to COPD, the intervals between such exacerbations in asthmatic patients are associated with normal, or near-normal, function. Although some variations in function may occur, COPD is usually associated with persistent symptoms and physiologic derangement. In addition, the level of airway reactivity and response to bronchodilator therapy are both generally more pronounced in asthma than in COPD. The long-term trends in these two diseases are also significantly disparate. Patients with COPD have continued, progressive decline in pulmonary function over time at a rate exceeding that of normals. Asthma is typically not associated with a decline in function over time.

Localized obstruction of a large airway may sometimes mimic COPD. The clinician must be alert for the finding of a localized wheeze, suggesting a fixed anatomic lesion. The chest x-ray will often reveal a mass lesion in such cases, but bronchoscopic inspection of airways may be required. Fixed or variable obstructing lesions involving the proximal trachea or larynx may sometimes produce sounds that are transmitted to the peripheral chest and misinterpreted as wheezing. In such cases, careful auscultation over the trachea may alert the physician to the proper diagnosis. Alternatively, the finding of a pattern of variable extrathoracic obstruction, or fixed obstruction, on a flow–volume loop may target the investigation to the proximal large airways.

A variety of disorders characterized by excessive mucous production and expectoration may be con-

Box 10.1 Differential Diagnosis of COPD

Disease	Distinguishing Feature/Test
Asthma	Variable course over time; normal function at times
Large-airway obstruction	Flow–volume loop
Bronchiectasis	Computed tomography of the chest
α_1-Antitrypsin deficiency	α_1-Antitrypsin level
Cystic fibrosis	Sweat chloride (? DNA analysis)
Lymphangio-leimyomatosus	Extrapulmonary disease, chylous effusions, lung biopsy or other histopathology

fused with COPD. Severe purulent bronchitis may be slow to resolve on occasion and lead to a question about the presence of COPD. Bronchiectasis is now less common than in the past but may be confused with chronic bronchitis. Computed tomography of the chest has essentially replaced bronchography for the identification of bronchiectasis.

In younger patients who present with findings suggestive of COPD, alternative diagnoses should always be considered. Two relatively common genetic disorders, cystic fibrosis and α_1-antiprotease deficiency, may occasionally mimic COPD. Cystic fibrosis is the most common genetic disorder affecting the respiratory tract. Although cystic fibrosis has historically been a disease of children, more affected individuals are now living to adulthood. In addition, the diagnosis of relatively mild cystic fibrosis in an adult is no longer an extreme rarity. The presence of symptoms in a young adult, fibrocystic changes on chest x-ray, or culture of *Pseudomonas* species from sputum should raise the consideration of cystic fibrosis. α_1-Antiprotease deficiency typically presents as early onset emphysema. Clues to considering this diagnosis should be the presence of emphysema before age 40, emphysema in the absence of a history of smoking, and a basilar predominance of emphysema.

Many authors use the term asthmatic bronchitis to describe a subset of patients with chronic airflow limitation. This group typically experiences the onset of symptoms during middle age or later. The syndrome is typified by cough, sputum production, and periods of worsened function. Many of these patients are nonsmokers or never-smokers. Their course is associated with more fluctuation in function than is characteristic of COPD, but, unlike asthma, pulmonary physiology typically does not return to normal between exacerbations. Also, in contrast to patients with asthma, those with asthmatic bronchitis often experience progressive decline in function over time. Asthmatic bronchitis is a more difficult entity to define, and, as a result, has been omitted from many discussion of chronic airways diseases. From the standpoint of implementation of therapy, making the distinction between asthmatic bronchitis and other chronic diseases of airways is of minor importance.

Another rare disease, lymphangioleiomyomatosus, may occasionally be confused with COPD. Lymphangioleiomyomatosus is a disease of reproductive age women, which may affect multiple organs, but the most common target is the lungs. It produces diffuse pulmonary disease, typically with interstitial or fibrocystic changes on chest x-rays. Cough and dyspnea are common, and hyperinflation with obstructive physiology may lead to confusion of this disorder with COPD. Spontaneous pneumothorax and chylous pleural effusions are reasonably common in lymphangioleiomyomatosus.

Pathogenesis

Cigarette smoking is the primary agent associated with the development of COPD in the overwhelming majority of cases (12–14). However, not all smokers develop chronic bronchitis or emphysema, and the reasons for the variability in occurrence of disease are not entirely evident. Host factors, such as a propensity to develop hyperreactive airways, or immunologic factors may be important.

The inhalation of smoke or other irritants may contribute to the development of COPD through a variety of mechanisms. Inhalation of toxic substances may directly stimulate mucous hypersecretion within airways. Smoke interferes with ciliary function leading to impaired clearance of secretions from the airways.

Smoke-induced alterations in the function of alveolar macrophages, and possibly other cells, result in impaired host defense and increased susceptibility to infection. Stimulation of neutrophils with subsequent elaboration of proteases can result in an "autodigestion" of lung with disruption of the alveolar architecture. Histologic changes in the lung of patients with COPD are identified in three different compartments: the large airways, small (peripheral) airways, and parenchyma.

The earliest identifiable changes seen in lungs of smokers is inflammation within respiratory bronchioles, characterized by a prominent infiltration by macrophages (15). Goblet cell metaplasia may also be present (16). Excess mucous production results and may produce impaction within small airways. Focal obstruction of small airways may also result from localized surfactant deficiency secondary to Clara cell destruction (17).

Within the larger airways, the primary pathologic change is mucous gland hyperplasia. This process can be quantitated using of the thickness of the mucous glands relative to the thickness of the bronchial wall, a parameter known as the Reid index (18). Smooth muscle hyperplasia may also be seen in the large airways (19).

The final pathologic feature of COPD is emphysema. The American Thoracic Society has defined emphysema as "a condition of the lung characterized by abnormal permanent enlargement of the airspaces distal to the terminal bronchiole, accompanied by destruction of their walls, and without obvious fibrosis" (1). Three categories of emphysema are reported (20). Centrilobular and panlobular (panacinar) emphysema both appear to be associated with COPD. The third form, distal acinar or paraseptal emphysema, is thought to be associated with spontaneous pneumothorax. The protease–antiprotease hypothesis continues to dominate thinking about the pathogenesis of emphysema (21). This hypothesis contends that normal lung is protected by maintenance of an appropriate balance between injurious proteases and protective antiproteases. Support for this hypothesis came first from the observation of emphysema in subjects with who are homozygous for deficiency of α_1-antitrypsin (α_1-protease inhibitor) (22,23). Constituents of cigarette smoke activate macrophages to secrete chemoattractants, which recruit neutrophils to lung. The neutrophils in return are stimulated to secrete proteases such as elastase, resulting in digestion of the abundant elastin in lung. Stimulated macrophages may also elaborate elastase-like metalloproteases and other potentially injurious agents, such as cysteine proteinases and cathepsins.

Work-Up

Physical Findings

The relative predominance of chronic bronchitis and emphysema in a given patient has a significant influence on the findings at clinical examination. Individuals with a predominance of emphysema fit the clinical characterization of "pink puffers." They often experience significant weight loss and typically are thin (24). Cyanosis is uncommon in these patients. The chest is hyperinflated and the anteroposterior diameter is increased, yielding the classic "barrel chest" configuration. The diaphragms are often displaced inferiorly and have limited excursion. Auscultation reveals a relatively quiet chest; the breath sounds may be severely diminished, and wheezing, if present, is usually heard only late in exhalation. When disease is advanced, or during exacerbations, there may be significant use of accessory muscles of respiration. Occasionally, the severe downward displacement of the diaphragm may result in inward motion of the lower thorax with inspiration (Hoover's sign) reflecting the inefficient position of the diaphragm (25).

Patients with a predominance of chronic bronchitis rarely exhibit significant weight loss. Cyanosis and edema are common, producing the stereotypical pattern of the "blue bloater." The chest is often noisy, with prominent wheezing. Signs of hyperinflation are less prominent than with emphysema. In severe disease, the full syndrome of cor pulmonale may be manifest, with dilated neck veins, hepatic enlargement, and peripheral edema (26). Again, emphysema and chronic bronchitis coexist in most patients, and the findings may be a combination of those associated with these two extremes.

Radiographic Findings

The spectrum of radiographic findings is broad (27). Early disease may be associated with a near-normal chest x-ray or evidenced only by mild hyperinflation.

Signs of emphysema include inferior displacement of the diaphragms, oligemia, and hyperlucency. In some cases, well defined bullae are visible. These bullae occur predominantly in the upper lung fields, except in cases of α_1-antitrypsin deficiency, where basilar bullae are typical. Chronic bronchitis may be manifest radiographically as an increase in bronchovascular markings, typically most prominent in the bases. Computed tomography of the chest appears to be more sensitive than plain x-rays for the identification of emphysema but is rarely indicated for this purpose alone.

Pulmonary Function Testing

Physiologic testing is an important component of the initial evaluation of patients with known or suspected COPD. It also provides a means for objective and quantitative assessment of exacerbations, disease progression, and response to therapy. The characteristic pattern is that of an obstructive ventilatory defect. However, extensive abnormalities are required to produce a reduction in the forced expiratory volume in 1 second (FEV_1) (28,29). More sensitive tests, such as closing volume and frequency dependence of dynamic compliance, may identify abnormalities of small airways earlier in the course of disease, but these are not routinely used clinically (30,31).

When emphysema and hyperinflation predominate, there is usually a significant increase in total lung capacity and residual volume, and the ratio of residual volume to total lung capacity is often increased. Reduction in single breath diffusion capacity for carbon monoxide (D_LCO) is characteristic of emphysema.

Gas exchange abnormalities are common. With pure emphysema, hypoxemia at rest is unusual, but it may occur with exercise or more advanced disease.

Preoperative Assessment

Pulmonary complications of surgical procedures remain an important problem. Postoperative pain can result in decrease in cough and sighing, which, in turn, can promote the development of microatelectasis and impaired clearance of secretions (32). Narcotics administered for control of pain can likewise abrogate these important reflexes, and the use of these drugs necessitates the use of measures to countermand these untoward effects (33,34). Thoracic and upper abdominal procedures are associated with the greatest risk of postoperative pulmonary complications, whereas other procedures are associated with much less risk. Lower abdominal procedures typically produce a reduction in vital capacity of 25% to 30% and are associated with only a mild transient decrease in $Pa{O_2}$. Upper abdominal procedures result in important changes in lung volumes and breathing patterns (35). These changes occur through a variety of mechanisms including diaphragmatic dysfunction, a decline in functional residual capacity, microatelectasis with subsequent ventilation–perfusion mismatching and impaired mucous transport.

In any patient requiring an operative procedure, some thought must be given to the relative risk of postoperative pulmonary complications. Both pulmonary and nonpulmonary risk factors for postoperative complications have been identified (32). Among the nonpulmonary risk factors are age (36), obesity (37), type and duration of anesthesia and type of surgery (32,35). Age greater than 60 has been associated with increased complications of surgery, particularly of thoracotomy (36). The presence of COPD or other known pulmonary disease is a clear risk factor for postoperative pulmonary complications. Parameters that have been suggested as indicators for increased pulmonary risk in patients with COPD include a maximum breathing capacity of less than 50% of predicted value, FEV_1 less than 2 liters and $Pa{CO_2}$ greater than 45 (32). Severe dyspnea with climbing a single 19-step flight of stairs (i.e., stair test) has also been suggested as a marker for increased risk. In cases where pulmonary hypertension or increased pulmonary vascular resistance are prominent physiologic manifestations of disease, pulmonary artery balloon occlusion may help identify increased risks associated with pulmonary resection (38). A pulmonary artery pressure of greater than 30 mm Hg in association with occlusion of the right or left main pulmonary artery has been associated with increased risk. Unfortunately, pulmonary function testing does not allow for a graded or graduated assessment of the degree of risk for postoperative pulmonary complications.

Identifications of patients who require further evaluation and possible prophylactic treatment is critical (32) (Box 10.2). A history of heavy smoking (i,e., more than 20 pack-years) or chronic cough should provoke preoperative pulmonary assessment. Patients sched-

Box 10.2 Indicators of the Need for Preoperative Pulmonary Assessment

History of heavy smoking (>20 pack-years)
Thoracic or upper abdominal procedure
Obesity
Age > 60 yr
Known COPD or other lung disease

uled for thoracic or upper abdominal procedures should also be screened. Obesity or age greater than 60 years should also trigger preoperative evaluations. All patients with COPD or any other identified pulmonary disease should undergo preoperative assessment and at least limited intervention.

Spirometry should be performed in all patients who are identified as candidates for preoperative pulmonary assessment. This provides a means for both defining increased risk and objectively assessing the response to subsequent intervention. If abnormalities of spirometry are seen, arterial blood gases, and possibly complete pulmonary function testing with lung volumes and diffusing capacity, are warranted. In selected cases, particularly in subjects being considered for thoracic procedures, assessment of regional lung function may be warranted. This assessment may be done with quantitative perfusion lung scanning (39) or balloon occlusion of the pulmonary artery (38). Such evaluation of regional lung function should most often be done with consultative assistance. When abnormalities of pulmonary mechanics are identified, the clinician must seek to fully characterize them and identify ways in which the abnormalities might be improved. Once lung function has been optimized, it is critical to reassess pulmonary function and to examine the balance between the need for the procedure and the associated perioperative risks.

In patients with COPD (or other pulmonary disorders) who require operative intervention, pulmonary function should be maximized before surgery. One of the most important measures is smoking cessation for patients who have continued to smoke (40). Many patients appear to benefit from preoperative intensification of medical therapy, and many clinicians advocate hospitalization before surgery for this purpose. Inhaled bronchodilators and systemic methylxanthines are commonly used. Preoperative education regarding interventions that will be used after surgery to prevent pulmonary complications is also advisable.

After surgery, a variety of interventions may reduce the risk of pulmonary complications. A number of lung expansion maneuvers have been used. Deep-breathing exercises and incentive spirometry are among the simplest of these. Incentive spirometry is routinely used every 2 hours for the first several days after surgery (41). Chest physiotherapy has been widely used as well. Its utility, in general, appears to be greatest in subjects who have prominent cough and sputum production (42). Its usefulness in other circumstances is less clear, and it is a moderately expensive modality. Continuous positive airway pressure may help to prevent atelectasis in some subjects (43), but it involves the use of occlusive masks and is often poorly tolerated. Intermittent positive pressure breathing has no clear role in the routine postoperative management of patients with COPD and may be potentially harmful in some subjects with enhanced pulmonary compliance due to emphysema. Judicious use of analgesics is an important component of postoperative care. Narcotics or other analgesics should be used in sufficient doses to allow the patient to inhale deeply and cough effectively (34). Early ambulation (44,45) and timely removal of nasogastric tubes are also important adjuncts in the scheme to prevent postoperative pulmonary complications (46).

Treatment of COPD

Smoking Cessation

Perhaps the most important therapy for patients with COPD is to promote smoking cessation. Indeed, assessment of smoking status and intervention is an important component of all primary care. There are many benefits to smoking cessation. Cough, sputum production, dyspnea, and wheezing all typically improve within 1 month of smoking cessation (47). Populations of smokers who have been followed after discontinuing smoking have shown that the overall level of symptoms declines to that of nonsmokers over a period of about 6 years (48). Patients who quit smoking also evidence a lower rate of respiratory infection than current smokers (49). Some patients will have a demonstrable improvement in a respiratory function

(FEV_1 increase of 75 to 150 mL) after smoking cessation, and stopping smoking is associated with a return in the rate of decline of FEV_1 over time to that of nonsmokers (approximately 20 mL/yr) (50).

Physician involvement in the process of smoking cessation is vitally important. A minority of physicians actually assess smoking status of patients they encounter (51). The process of smoking cessation has been categorized into four stages: 1) precontemplation, 2) contemplation, 3) action, and 4) maintenance. The physician should assess not only the current smoking status, but also the patient's stage relative to quitting. Physician advice instructing the patient to quit smoking has a powerful influence on the probability of smoking cessation, increasing the rates of successful quitting by double or more (52,53).

In addition to providing a directive for smoking cessation, a physician must also provide advice regarding the methodology. This advice may come in the form of a referral to a smoking cessation program or clinic or through direct assistance. Tools used to assist patients with smoking cessation include setting a date for quitting, having the patient sign a contract for smoking cessation, providing written materials, and arranging for follow-up visits. The physician should assess the level of nicotine dependence and consider whether nicotine replacement therapy is warranted. Persons who smoke more than a pack a day, patients who smoke immediately on arising in the morning, and those who have experienced strong urges to smoke during previous efforts at quitting should be considered for nicotine replacement therapy. Nicotine replacement is currently available in the form of nicotine gum or nicotine transdermal patches. The technique of chewing the gum is vitally important to its optimal effectiveness and tolerance. Although some patients find the gum intolerable, nicotine patches have a high level of patient acceptance. Several commercial products are available using different dosing regimens.

Transdermal clonidine may be effective as an adjunct to a smoking cessation program for selected patients (54). The results with clonidine have been variable, and side effects have been relatively common. Women appear to be better candidates than men for clonidine therapy.

A final component of smoking cessation effort should be prevention of relapse. The timely scheduling of follow-up visits is an important component of this effort. The patient and physician need to be aware that there is a high relapse rate among first-time quitters, and this does not preclude a successful subsequent attempt at smoking cessation.

Pharmacologic Therapy

A number of general principles should serve as guides for the use of pharmacologic agents in the treatment of patients with COPD (55). The major goals of such treatment should be to improve the reversible components of physiologic abnormalities and to relieve symptoms. Many of the potentially useful agents have important adverse effects. These effects may occur with increased frequency in patients with COPD compared to those with asthma because such patients are generally older and more likely to have other coexistent diseases. Thus, the use of any drug in this setting must be undertaken with careful attention to balancing the therapeutic effects against toxicity. In general, it is appropriate to begin with one agent and assess the response to its use. If toxicity occurs, or no response is demonstrated, then that agent can be discontinued and another one substituted. Alternatively, if the response to a given agent is one of limited improvement, an additional agent may be added and evaluated in a similar fashion. This sequential approach is in many ways analogous to the "stepped care" that was used in treatment of hypertension for many years.

Bronchodilators

Sympathomimetic agents are a major component of the available bronchodilator drugs (56). Short-acting catecholamines, such as epinephrine, have been used extensively for many years. A large number of relatively selective β_2-agonist drugs are now available and are the mainstay of this category of agents. β_2-Agonist drugs differ in regard to their relative potency and pharmacokinetics, but are otherwise essentially interchangeable with regard to clinical effectiveness.

Acute inhalation challenge with β-agonist drugs is sometimes used to assess the degree of "reversibility" relative to "fixed obstruction" in patients with COPD. However, the lack of demonstrable acute response to inhalation of β-adrenergic agonists drugs does not always predict lack of clinical benefit (57).

The toxicity of β-agonist agents can be significant

(58,59). Advancing age and coexistent underlying disease may increase the probability of intolerable side effects. The most common problems related to the sympathomimetic agents are tachycardia and arrhythmias. The presence of underlying cardiovascular disease is an important factor increasing susceptibility to these effects. In addition, the hypokalemia sometimes produced by use of β-agonist drugs may lower the threshold at which cardiovascular side effects occur (60,61). Tremor and nervousness are also common problems with these agents.

Several potential routes for delivery of sympathomimetic agents are available. In most adult patients, the preferred route of delivery is via a metered-dose inhaler. Metered-dose inhalers are, however, moderately difficult to use, and technique varies enormously among treated patients (62). The use of spacer devices can be an important means to improve delivery of drug to the lungs by metered-dose inhalers (63). Some patients with COPD will be unable to use metered-dose inhalers effectively, and delivery of drugs with nebulizer devices is appropriate in such patients. The clinician must recognize that the standard doses of most β-agonists drugs delivered by nebulizer are significantly larger than those delivered by two or three puffs from a metered-dose inhaler. Several studies have shown that in hospitalized patients metered-dose inhaler delivery is as effective as nebulized delivery, at substantially lower costs (64–66).

Oral preparations of β agonists are also available. In general, the balance between therapeutic effects and toxicity is less favorable with this route than with aerosol delivery (56). However, oral medication is more acceptable to some patients than aerosolized medication. In addition, sustained-release preparations are now available and may provide smoother delivery of drug and reduced toxicity relative to other preparations. The sustained-release preparations offer the potential for maintaining prolonged therapy through the night for patients with nocturnal symptoms.

Parental delivery of sympathomimetics has a limited role. As with oral therapy, toxicity is significantly more frequent than with inhalation therapy. Epinephrine and terbutaline are available for SQ injection. Although these agents are widely used in this form for the treatment of asthma, the advancing age of patients with COPD, and the prevalence of coexistent cardiovascular disease, make SQ delivery of these drugs less appealing in patients with COPD (63).

Anticholinergic Therapy

Anticholinergic agents can be an important part of treatment of patients with COPD. Increased cholinergic tone is known to be associated with bronchoconstriction. More than a century ago atropine was shown to be effective in treatment of asthma (67). Nebulized solutions of atropine have been used successfully in treating patients with COPD, but side effects such as blurred vision, tachycardia, and mucosal drying occur, particularly with higher doses (68). The use of atropine has been largely supplanted by the availability of another anticholinergic agent, ipratropium bromide (69,70). It is devoid of most of the adverse affects of atropine and has been demonstrated to be a highly effective bronchodilator in patients with COPD. Ipratropium bromide is currently available both in metered-dose inhaler form as well as a solution for nebulizer. It is most commonly used on a scheduled basis for maintenance therapy in patients with COPD. Because of its relatively paucity of adverse effects, many experts advise its use as the first agent in the treatment with patients with COPD. The onset of action of ipratropium bromide is delayed for approximately 15 to 20 minutes after its inhalation. This has led some to recommend use of other bronchodilators as primary therapy for acute exacerbations. However, at least one study has suggested that anticholinergic and β-adrenergic agents are equivalent for the treatment of acute exacerbations of COPD (71).

Methylxanthines

Although methylxanthine preparations have quite a long history of use in the treatment of obstructive lung disease, the use of these preparations continues to generate great controversy. Theophylline was found to be present in tea leaves as early as 1888, and it was recognized for its bronchodilator properties in 1922 (56). Coffee was appreciated to be a bronchodilator as early as 1786. Interest in caffeine for this purpose waned but has enjoyed a modest resurgence in recent years (72,73).

Despite the long history of use, the exact mechanism of action of methylxanthines such as theophylline remains unclear (56). Theophylline lowers cyclic AMP levels through its inhibition of phosphodiesterase, but recent data have demonstrated that this mechanism does not appear to be responsible for the clinical effects observed. Other actions of theophylline have been identified and put forward as potential mechanisms for its clinical effects. Among these are its effects on calcium ion movement among cellular compartments, antagonism of adenosine action, and inhibition of prostaglarndin E_2. Some, or all, of these effects may be clinically relevant, or other mechanisms may underlie the drug's effectiveness.

Although the mechanism of effect may be unclear, theophylline has a number of actions that make it a potentially useful agent in patients with COPD. Theophylline clearly has bronchodilator properties, but it is often difficult to demonstrate improvement in FEV_1 as a result of theophylline treatment in patients with COPD. Patients who fail to evidence rise in FEV_1 with theophylline therapy, but who report subjective improvement, may have physiologic evidence of increased lung volumes and a reduction in air trapping (74,75). In addition to its bronchodilatory properties, theophylline also increases respiratory muscle strength (76,77). This appears to result not only through alterations in the tension-developing properties of muscle, but through increase in blood flow to the diaphragm, and possibly recruitment of other muscles to respiratory efforts. A subjective decline in dyspnea is frequently associated with theophylline therapy (78), and mucociliary clearance can be shown to improve (79,80). Theophylline increases central respiratory drive, which may be a useful effect in "blue bloaters" (81,82). Although tremendous attention is often paid to the deleterious cardiovascular effects of theophylline, it also has a potential for salutary effects on the circulatory system. Theophylline is a pulmonary vasodilator and, therefore, reduces right ventricular afterload (83). In patients with significant right ventricular impairment, this may be a valuable effect. Theophylline is also a positive inotropic agent, and in conjunction with a reduction in ventricular afterload may significantly enhance overall cardiac function.

Theophylline preparations have a number of important toxicities that have been well publicized (82,84,85). Sleep disturbance, anxiety, and tremulousness are among the most common adverse effects. Tachycardia, palpitations, and arrhythmias are also relatively common. However, life-threatening arrhythmias appear to be relatively uncommon in the absence of serum levels that exceed the therapeutic range. At high serum levels, the risk for arrhythmias and for seizures becomes significant. Theophylline-induced seizures are difficult to manage, and patients who manifest this level of toxicity have a significant risk of death. Unfortunately the "therapeutic window" for theophylline is relatively narrow. This is especially true in patients with COPD because of their advanced age and high prevalence of coexistent cardiovascular disease. Optimum serum levels for theophylline in patients with COPD appear to be in the range of 8 to 12 μg/mL.

A wide variety of preparations of theophylline are available. The advent of sustained-released preparations has made dosing simpler, and most patients can achieve therapeutic levels with twice daily dosing. Once daily preparations are available and may achieve satisfactory results in some patients. However, patients with rapid gastrointestinal transit times of patients who are rapid metabolizers of theophylline may not have predictable theophylline levels with once daily treatment (56).

Corticosteroids

As with theophylline preparations, the use of corticosteroids in COPD has been associated with significant controversy. The role of inflammation in the pathogenesis of airway diseases has received tremendous attention in recent years. This has heightened the interest in use of anti-inflammatory agents, such as corticosteroids. While the utility of corticosteroid therapy has been reasonably well demonstrated in severe asthma, the value of steroids in COPD continues to be debated.

A large number of studies with conflicting results have been published on the topic of steroid treatment in COPD, but reasonable consensus has emerged that at least some patients with COPD appear to benefit from corticosteroid treatment (86,87). Factors that may possibly identify a higher probability of effectiveness of steroids in COPD include the presence of wheezing, a variable history of airflow obstruction over time, and a history of atopy. In patients with COPD who have been stabilized on an optimal regimen of other drugs, but who have had less than satisfactory response, a trial of corticosteroid therapy may be warranted (55). If elected, such a trial should involve administration of relatively high doses (e.g., 40 mg prednisone daily) over a 2-week period with an objective assessment of response to therapy (i.e., physiologic testing). If a positive response is obtained, then an effort should be made to taper steroids to the lowest possible dose and to consider alternate day therapy. Inhaled corticosteroids may be of benefit in some patients with COPD (88), but their exact role remains unclear.

Adverse effects of systemic corticosteroid therapy are numerous (56). One must weigh the potential for these effects strongly against the probability of benefit in each patient. Side effects increase with larger doses and longer duration of therapy. Among the more common problems are weight gain, glucose intolerance, skin changes (thinning and purpura), cataracts, gastrointestinal bleeding, serious infections, and osteoporosis.

Antibiotics

Antibiotic medications are widely used in the treatment of exacerbations of COPD. Despite this, evidence to support their utility is relatively weak (56). The lower airways of patients with COPD are commonly colonized, and organisms such as *Streptococcus pneumoniae*, *Haemophilus influenzae*, and *Branhamella catarrhalis* can frequently be identified. These organisms appear to be among the most important bacteria associated with exacerbations of chronic bronchitis, but it is likely that viral infections are significantly more common precipitators of acute deteriorations. Based on current information, it is reasonable to use antibiotics as a component of the management of acute exacerbations of COPD for patients who exhibit increased sputum purulence as a major symptom (89). Trimethoprim-sulfamethoxazole, ampicillin, tetracycline, or erythromycin are all reasonable and inexpensive choices for therapy. Treatment should be given for at least 10 days, and some evidence suggests that longer therapy, up to 20 days, may be appropriate.

Mucolytics

Although viscid secretions from the lower respiratory tract are a vexing problem for many patients with COPD, management strategies directed at this symptom have had limited utility (90). It seems intuitive that maintaining adequate hydration would be prudent and potentially beneficial, yet evidence of this is lacking. Similarly, aerosols have not been clearly demonstrated to improve mucous clearance (56). Iodide preparations have been extensively used for improving mucous clearance. Of these, iodinated glycerol is probably the best tolerated. Limited data suggest that this preparation may be of some benefit (91). Acetylcystine is sometimes used by nebulization for its mucolytic properties, but can occasionally provoke bronchospasm. A promising new potential therapy is deoxyribonuclease (DNase). Recombinant human DNase has been used successfully in cystic fibrosis (92,93), and trials are underway to examine its effectiveness in COPD.

Oxygen

Oxygen is an important component of therapy for many patients with COPD. The potential need for oxygen therapy should be considered in virtually all patients with significant COPD, and criteria for use of this therapy should be assessed. Unfortunately, oxygen therapy is expensive and somewhat burdensome to the patient. Therefore, guidelines for its use have been established (94,95). In general, long-term oxygen therapy is recommended for patients with Pa_{O_2} less than 55 mm Hg. Oxygen is also recommended for those who show evidence of secondary end-organ dysfunction resulting from hypoxemia, such as secondary erythrocytosis, cognitive impairment, or cor pulmonale, which responds to oxygen therapy. Patients who exhibit significant exercise desaturation may be candidates for oxygen supplementation during exercise. The need for chronic oxygen therapy should be periodically reassessed, and particularly reassessed after optimal medical therapy has been in place for 2 to 3 months. A variety of supply systems are available. Most patients receive long-term oxygen therapy via nasal cannulae, but devices that conserve oxygen are also available. In addition, some patients may prefer transtracheal oxygen delivery.

Lung Transplantation

Lung transplantation has proven to be successful in carefully selected patients with end-stage COPD (96,97). Single-lung transplantation is preferred over double-lung transplantation for most COPD patients. Functional capacity is improved, but long-term follow-up data are limited.

Prophylactic Measures

It is critical to consider preventive measures whenever possible in managing patients with COPD. Influenza infection can have devastating sequelae in these patients. Therefore, it is important to ensure that all COPD patients receive annual influenza vaccination unless there is a contraindication (98,99). Use of amantadine should be considered in those who have been exposed to influenza A. The efficacy of pneumococcal vaccine in these patients has been disputed, but it remains a general recommendation that patients with COPD be vaccinated against pneumococcal disease (98,99).

Rehabilitation

Rehabilitation, when feasible, is certainly a desirable goal in the management of patients with COPD who have important functional limitation. A rehabilitation program can take a variety of forms ranging from the physician's recommendation for walking or other simple exercise to an elaborate, multidisciplinary team approach (100). Most pulmonary rehabilitation programs involve exercise as the major component, but the more elaborate programs have many facets. In addition to improving exercise tolerance, the potential benefits gained include an enhanced sense of well-being and psychosocial support. Pulmonary rehabilitation has not been demonstrated to improve pulmonary function per se, but can enhance exercise capability.

A variety of components may be included in a pulmonary rehabilitation program. Exercise conditioning is among the most important of these. Exercise training has been shown to improve maximal oxygen consumption in patients with COPD (101). Some have advocated respiratory muscle training using inspiratory resistive loading (102). It has been demonstrated that such training programs can enhance respiratory muscle strength, but it is unclear how to identify the patients who are most likely to show benefit from this approach (103). In contrast, patients with chronic respiratory muscle fatigue or hypercapnia may benefit from intermittent respiratory muscle rest (104,105). The availability of noninvasive ventilation through nasal masks has made this therapeutic approach more practical. Although periodic rest for the respiratory musculature appears to have a sound basis in principle, long-term benefit has not yet been demonstrated. Finally, nutritional supplementation may be an important adjunct to rehabilitation programs in patients who are significantly malnourished (106).

Natural History/Prognosis

The course of COPD can be highly variable, and it is difficult to render an accurate prognosis in individual circumstances. Many factors relate to the variability of natural history including the access to medical care and responsiveness to therapy. Reports of outcomes in patients with COPD also provide disparate assessments because of problems with the definition of disease (107). Identifying well defined, homogeneous populations of patients is difficult.

All adults exhibit progressive decline in pulmonary function with time. In normal adults, FEV_1 decreases by 20 to 30 mL/yr. Patients with COPD exhibit an accelerated decline in FEV_1, in the range of 40 to 80 mL/yr (108,109). Patients who continue to smoke are among those with more rapid rate of decline in lung function. Age and postbronchodilator FEV_1 appear to be the best predictors of outcome. In one series, subjects with an FEV_1 less than 30% predicted value had a 60% survival in 3 years (110). Other factors associated with a less favorable prognosis included malnutrition and progressive weight loss (9), continued smoking (111), and the presence of cor pulmonale (112).

Although it is difficult to predict longevity, some assessment of the expected level of functioning can be made based on a simple spirometry. As a general rule of thumb, it is relatively uncommon for patients to present for medical attention until the FEV_1 has fallen below 2 liters. Dyspnea with moderate levels of exertion typically occurs when the FEV_1 falls below 1.5 liters. Patients with an FEV_1 of less than 1 liter are usually restricted to a relatively sedentary lifestyle, and those with an FEV_1 less than 500 mL have profound limitation of exercise capacity.

Many patients with COPD can be adequately managed in a primary care setting. However, a variety of circumstances should provoke consideration of obtaining consultative assistance. Patients in whom the diagnosis remains uncertain should be evaluated by a pulmonary specialist. In addition, patients with known or suspected α_1-antiprotease deficiency should be referred for consultation. The requirement for more than one or two chronic medications or a need for chronic oxygen therapy should also provoke more thorough evaluation. Patients who requrie hospitalization or emergency department visits for respiratory difficulties are similarly candidates for referral. Finally, patients who require preoperative pulmonary assessment should usually receive that assessment in collaboration with a consultant.

REFERENCES

1. American Thoracic Society. Standards for the diagnosis and care of patients with chronic obstructive pulmonary disease (COPD) and asthma. Am Rev Respir Dis 1987;136:225–244.
2. Redline S. The epidemiology of COPD. In: Cherniack NS, ed. Chronic obstructive pulmonary disease. Philadelphia: WB Saunders, 1991:225–234.
3. Feinleib M, Rosenberg H, Collins J, et al. Trends in COPD morbidity and mortality in the United States. Am Rev Respir Dis 1989;140:S9–S18.
4. Task Force Report. Epidemiology of respiratory diseases. National Institutes of Health Publication No. 82-2019, 1981:153.
5. Fiore MC. Trends in cigarette smoking in the United States. The epidemiology of tobacco use. Med Clin N Am 1992;76:289–303.
6. Wynne JW, Block AJ, Hemenway I, et al. Disordered breathing during sleep in patients with chronic obstructive pulmonary disease. Chest 1978;73:301–305.
7. Fletcher EC, Levin DC. Cardiopulmonary hemodynamics during sleep in subjects with chronic obstructive pulmonary disease. Chest 1984;85:6–14.
8. Braun SR, Keim NL, Dixon RM, et al. The prevalence and determinants of nutritional changes in chronic obstructive pulmonary disease. Chest 1984;86:558–563.
9. Wilson DO, Rogers RM, Wright EC, et al. Body weight in chronic obstructive pulmonary disease. The National Institutes of Health Intermittent Positive Pressure Breathing Trial. Am Rev Respir Dis 1989;139:1435–1438.
10. Light RW, Merrill EJ, Despars JA, et al. Prevalence of depression and anxiety in patients with COPD. Relationship to functional capacity. Chest 1985;87:35–38.
11. Grant I, Heaton R, McSweeney J, et al. Neuropsychologic findings in hypoxemic chronic obstructive pulmonary disease. Arch Intern Med 1982;142:1470–1476.
12. Ferris BG, Higgens IT, Higgins MW, et al. Chronic non-specific respiratory disease, Berlin, New Hampshire, 1961–67: a cross-sectional study. Am Rev Respir Dis 1971;104:232.
13. United States Public Health Service. The health consequences of smoking. Chronic obstructive lung disease. A report of the Surgeon General. Rockville, MD: U.S. Government Printing Office, Department of Health and Human Services Publication No. 84-50205, 1984.
14. Lebowitz MD, Knudson RJ, Burrows B. Tucson epidemiologic study of obstructive lung diseases. I. Methodology and prevalence of disease. Am J Epidemiol 1975;102:137.
15. Niewoehner D, Kleinerman J, Rick D. Pathologic changes in the peripheral airways of young cigarette smokers. N Engl J Med 1974;291:755–758.
16. Karpick R, Pratt P, Asmundsson T, et al. Pathologic findings in respiratory failure. Ann Intern Med 1970;72:189–197.
17. Dunnill M, Massarella G, Anderson J. A comparison of the quantitative anatomy of the bronchi in normal subjects, in status asthmaticus, in chronic bronchitis and in emphysema. Thorax 1969;24:176–179.
18. Reid L. Measurement of the bronchial mucus gland layer: a diagnostic yardstick in chronic bronchitis. Thorax 1960;15:132–141.
19. Hassain S, Heard B. Hyperplasia of bronchial muscle in chronic bronchitis. J Pathol 1970;101:171–184.
20. Snider GL. Emphysema: the first two centuries—and beyond. A historical overview, with suggestions for future research, part 1. Am Rev Respir Dis 1992;146:1334–1344.
21. Snider GL. Emphysema: the first two centuries—and beyond. A historical overview, with suggestions for future research, part 2. Am Rev Respir Dis 1992;146:1615–1622.
22. Laurel CB, Ericksson S. The electrophoretic alpha-1-globulin pattern of serum alpha-1-antitrypsin deficiency. Scand J Clin Lab Invest 1963;15:132–140.
23. Ericksson S. Pulmonary emphysema and alpha$_1$-antitrypsin deficiency. Acta Med Scand 1964;175:197–205.
24. Openbrier D, Irwin M, Rogers R, et al. Nutritional status and lung function in patients with emphysema and chronic bronchitis. Chest 1983;83:17–22.
25. Gilmartin JJ, Gibson GJ. Mechanisms of paradoxical rib cage motion in patients with chronic obstructive

pulmonary disease. Am Rev Respir Dis 1986;134:683–687.

26. Wiedemann HP, Matthay RA. Cor pulmonale in chronic obstructive pulmonary disease. Circulatory pathophysiology and management. Clin Chest Med 1990;11:523–545.

27. Clausen JL. The diagnosis of emphysema, chronic bronchitis, and asthma. Clin Chest Med 1990;11:405–416.

28. Hale K, Ewing S, Gosnell B, et al. Lung disease in long-term cigarette smokers with and without chronic airflow obstruction. Am Rev Respir Dis 1984;130:716–721.

29. Nagai A, West W, Thurlbeck W. The National Institutes of Health Intermittent Positive Pressure Breathing Trial: pathology studies. II. Correlation between morphologic findings, clinical findings, and evidence of expiratory air-flow obstruction. Am Rev Respir Dis 1985;132:946–953.

30. Buist A, Ross B. Quantitative analysis of the alveolar plateau in the diagnosis of early airway obstruction. Am Rev Respir Dis 1973;108:1078–1087.

31. Wright JL, Cagle P, Churg A, et al. Diseases of the small airways. Am Rev Respir Dis 1992;146:240–262.

32. Tisi GM. Preoperative evaluation of pulmonary function. Validity, indications, and benefits. Am Rev Respir Dis 1979;119:293–310.

33. Egbert LD, Bendixen HH. Effect of morphine on breathing pattern. JAMA 1964;188:485–488.

34. Bromage PR. Spirometry in assessment of analgesia after abdominal surgery. Br Med J 1955;2:589–593.

35. Latimer RG, Dickman M, Day WC, et al. Ventilatory patterns and pulmonary complications after upper abdominal surgery determined by preoperative and postoperative computerized spirometry and blood gas analysis. Am J Surg 1971;122:622–632.

36. Boushy SF, Billig DM, North LB, et al. Clinical course related to preoperative and postoperative pulmonary function in patients with bronchogenic carcinoma. Chest 1971;59:383–391.

37. Pasulka PS, Bistrian BR, Benotti PN, et al. The risks of surgery in obese patients. Ann Intern Med 1986;104:540–546.

38. Olsen GN, Block AJ, Swenson EW, et al. Pulmonary function evaluation of the lung resection candidate: a prospective study. Am Rev Respir Dis 1975;111:379–387.

39. Wagner HN. The use of radioisotope techniques for the evaluation of patients with pulmonary disease. Am Rev Respir Dis 1976;113:203–218.

40. Warner MA, Offord KP, Warner ME, et al. Role of preoperative cessation of smoking and other factors in postoperative pulmonary complications: a blinded prospective study of coronary artery bypass patients. Mayo Clin Proc 1989;64:609–616.

41. Celli BR, Rodriguez KS, Snider GL. A controlled trial of intermittent positive pressure breathing, incentive spirometry, and deep breathing exercises in preventing pulmonary complications after abdominal surgery. Am Rev Respir Dis 1984;130:12–15.

42. Kiriloff LH, Owens GR, Rogers RM, et al. Does chest physical therapy work? Chest 1985;88:436–444.

43. Stock MC, Downs JB, Gauer PK, et al. Prevention of postoperative pulmonary complications with CPAP, incentive spirometry, and conservative therapy. Chest 1985;87:151–157.

44. Anscombe AR, Buxton RS. Effect of abdominal operations on total lung capacity and its subdivisions. Br Med J 1958;2:84–87.

45. Meyers JR, Lembeck L, O'Kane H, et al. Changes in functional residual capacity of the lung after operation. Arch Surg 1975;110:576–583.

46. Mitchell C, Garrahy P, Peake P. Postoperative respiratory morbidity: identification and risk factors. Aust N Z J Surg 1982;52:203–209.

47. Buist AS, Sexton GJ, Nagy JM, Ross B. The effect of smoking cessation and modification of lung function. Am Rev Respir Dis 1976;114:115–122.

48. Comstock GW, Brownlow WJ, Stone RW, et al. Cigarette smoking and changes in respiratory findings. Arch Environ Health 1970;21:50–57.

49. Hammond EC. Evidence on the effects of giving up cigarette smoking. Am J Public Health 1965;55:682–691.

50. United States Public Health Service. The health benefits of smoking cessation. A report of the Surgeon General. Rockville, MD: U.S. Government Printing Office, Department of Health and Human Services Publication No. 90-8416, 1990.

51. Eraker SA, Beker MH, Streicher VJ, et al. Smoking behavior cessation techniques, and the health decision model. Am J Med 1985;78:817–823.

52. Russell MAH, Wilson C, Taylor C, et al. Effect of general practitioners' advice against smoking. Br Med J 1979;2:231–235.

53. Wilson D, Wood G, Johnston N, et al. Randomized clinical trial of supportive follow-up for cigarette smoking in a family practice. Can Med J 1982;126:127–129.

54. Covey LS, Glassman AH. A meta-analysis of double-blind placebo-controlled trials of clonidine for smoking cessation. Br J Addict 1991;86:991–998.

55. Ferguson GT, Cherniack RM. Management of chronic obstructive pulmonary disease. N Engl J Med 1993;328:1017–1022.

56. Ziment I. Pharmacologic therapy in obstructive airway disease. Clin Chest Med 1990;11:461–486.

57. Bellamy D, Hutchinson DCS. The effects of salbutamol aerosol on lung function in patients with pulmonary emphysema. Br J Dis Chest 1981;75:190–196.

58. Ziment I. Cardiovascular side effects in patients requiring bronchodilator therapy. Cardiovasc Rev Rep 1984;5:443–452.

59. Sly RM, Jenne JW, Cohn J. Toxicity of beta-adrenergic drugs. In: Jenne JW, Murphy S, eds. Drug therapy for asthma. Research and clinical practice. New York: Marcel Dekker, 1987:953–996.

60. Gelmont DM, Balmes JR, Yee A. Hypokalemia induced by inhaled bronchodilators. Chest 1988;94:763–766.

61. Martelli A, Otero C, Gil B, Gonzalez S. Fenoterol and serum potassium. Lancet 1989;1(8648):1197.

62. Rand CS, Tashkin D, Wise RA, et al. How acurate are cannister weighing and self-reports as measures of metered-dose inhaler compliance in a clinical trial? Am Rev Respir Dis 1989;139:A16.

63. Noseda A, Yernault JC. Sympathomimetics in acute severe asthma: inhaled or parenteral, nebullizer or spacer? Eur Respir J 1989;2:377–382.

64. Morley TF, Marozsan E, Zappasodi SJ, et al. Comparison of beta-adrenergic agents delivered by nebulized vs metered dose inhaler with InspirEase in hospitalized asthmatic patients. Chest 1988;94:1205–1210.

65. Saltzman GA, Steele MT, Pribble JP, et al. Aerosolized metaproterenol in the treatment of asthmatics with severe airflow obstruction. Comparison of two delivery methods. Chest 1989;95:1017–1020.

66. Summer W, Elston R, Tharpe L, et al. Aerosol bronchodilator delivery methods. Relative impact on pulmonary function and cost of respiratory care. Arch Intern Med 1989;149:618–623.

67. Courty MA. Treatment of asthma. Edin Med J 1959;5:665.

68. Gross NJ, Skorodin MS. Anticholinergic, antimuscarinic bronchodilators. Am Rev Respir Dis 1984;129:856–870.

69. Gross NJ, Petty TL, Friedman M, et al. Dose response to ipratropium as a nebulized solution in patients with chronic obstructive pulmonary disease. Am Rev Respir Dis 1989;139:1185–1191.

70. Chapman KR. The role of anticholinergic bronchodilators in adult asthma and chronic obstructive pulmonary disease. Lung 1990;168(suppl):295–303.

71. Karpel JP. Bronchodilator responses to anticholinergic and beta-adrenergic agents in acute and stable COPD. Chest 1991;99:871–876.

72. Gong H, Simmons MS, Tashkin DP, Hui KK, Lee EY. Bronchodilator effects of caffeine in coffee. A dose-response study of asthmatic subjects. Chest 1986;89:335–342.

73. Bukowskyj M, Nakatsu K. The bronchodilator effect of caffeine in adult asthmatics. Am Rev Respir Dis 1987;135:173–175.

74. Chrystyn H, Mulley BA, Peake MD. Dose response relation to oral theophylline in severe chronic obstructive airways disease. Br Med J 1988;297:1506–1510.

75. Peake MD, Chrystyn J, Mulley BA. Response to oral theophylline in severe chronic obstructive airways disease. Br Med J 1989;298:523–524.

76. Aubier M, De Troyer A, Sampson M, et al. Aminophylline improves diaphragmatic contractility. N Engl J Med 1981;305:249–252.

77. Aubier M, Murciano D, Viires N, et al. Diaphragmatic contractility enhanced by aminophylline: role of extracellular calcium. J Appl Physiol 1983;54:460–464.

78. Mahler DA. The role of theophylline in the treatment of dyspnea in COPD. Chest 1987;92:2S–6S.

79. Ziment I. Theophylline and mucociliary clearance. Chest 1987;92:38S–43S.

80. Wanner A. Effects of methylxanthines on airway mucociliary function. Am J Med 1985;79(6A):16–21.

81. Hill NS. The use of theophylline in "irreversible" chronic obstructive pulmonary disease. Arch Intern Med 1988;148:2579–2584.

82. Sharp JT. Theophylline in chronic obstructive pulmonary disease. J Allergy Clin Immunol 1986;78:800–805.

83. Matthay RA, Berger HJ. Cardiovascular function in cor pulmonale. Clin Chest Med 1983;4:269–295.

84. Skinner MH. Adverse reactions and interactions with theophylline. Drug Safety 1990;5:275–285.

85. Ziment I, Au JP. Making the best use of aminophylline in the ICU. J Crit Illness 1986;1:21–32.

86. Stoller JK, Gerbarg ZB, Feinstein AR. Corticosteroids in stable chronic obstructive pulmonary disease. J Gen Intern Med 1987;2:29–35.

87. Callahan CM, Dittus RS, Katz BP. Oral corticosteroid therapy for patients with stable chronic obstructive pulmonary disease. A meta-analysis. Ann Intern Med 1991;114:216–223.

88. Kerstjens HAM, Brand PLP, Mughes MD, et al. A comparision of bronchodilator therapy with or without inhaled corticosteroid therapy for obstructive airways disease. N Engl J Med 1992;327:1413–1419.

89. Anthonisen NR, Manfreda J, Warren CPW, et al. Antibiotic therapy in exacerbations of chronic obstructive pulmonary disease. Ann Intern Med 1987;106:196–204.

90. Wanner A. The role of mucus in chronic obstructive pulmonary disease. Chest 1990;97:11S–15S.

91. Petty TL. The National Mucolytic Study. Results of a randomized, double-blind, placebo-controlled study of iodinated glycerol in chronic obstructive bronchitis. Chest 1990;97:75–83.

92. Ramsey BW, Astley SJ, Aitken ML, et al. Efficacy and safety of short-term administration of aerosolized recombinant human deoxyribonuclease in patients with cystic fibrosis. Am Rev Respir Dis 1993;148:145–151.

93. Fuchs HJ, Borowitz DS, Christiansen DH, et al. Effect of aerosolized recombinant human DNase on exacerbations of respiratory symptoms and on pulmonary function in patients with cystic fibrosis. The Pulmozyme Study Group. N Engl J Med 1994;331:637–642.

94. Anthonisen NR, Block AJ, Kvale P, Petty TL. O_2 therapy. Am Rev Respir Dis 1987;136:235–236.

95. Neff TA, Conway WA, Lakshminarayan S. Indications for oxygen therapy. Chest 1984;86:239–240.

96. Mal H, Andreassian B, Pamela F, et al. Unilateral lung transplantation in end-stage pulmonary emphysema. Am Rev Respir Dis 1989;140:797–802.

97. Trulock EP, Cooper JD, Kaiser LR, et al. The Washington University-Barnes Hospital experience with lung transplantation. JAMA 1991;266:1943–1946.

98. Gardner P, Schaffner W. Immunization of adults. N Engl J Med 1993;328:1252–1258.

99. American College of Physicians Task Force on Adult Immunization, Infectious Disease Society of America. Guide for adult immunization. 3rd ed. Philadelphia: American College of Physicians, 1994.

100. Hodgkin JE. Pulmonary rehabilitation. Clin Chest Med 1990;11:447–460.

101. Casaburi R, Patessio A, Ioli F, et al. Reductions in exercise lactic acidosis and ventilation as a result of exercise training in patients with obstructive lung disease. Am Rev Respir Dis 1991;143:9–18.

102. Larson JL, Kim MJ, Sharp JT, Larson DA. Inspiratory muscle training with a pressure threshold breathing device in patients with chronic obstructive pulmonary disease. Am Rev Respir Dis 1988;138:689–696.

103. Smith K, Cook D, Guyatt GH, et al. Respiratory muscle training in chronic airflow limitation: a meta-analysis. Am Rev Respir Dis 1992;145:533–539.

104. Fernandez E, Weiner P, Meltzer E, et al. Sustained improvement in gas exchange after negative pressure ventilation for 8 hours per day on 2 successive days in chronic airflow limitation. Am Rev Respir Dis 1991;144:390–394.

105. Ambrosino N, Nava S, Bertone P, et al. Physiologic evaluation of pressure support ventilation by nasal mask in patients with stable COPD. Chest 1992;101:385–391.

106. Donahoe M, Rogers RM. Nutritional assessment and support in chronic obstructive pulmonary disease. Clin Chest Med 1990;11:487–504.

107. Hodgkin JE. Prognosis in chronic obstructive pulmonary disease. Clin Chest Med 1990;11:555–569.

108. Van der Lende R, Kok TJ, Peset Rerg R, et al. Decreases in VC and FEV_1 with time: indicators for the effects of smoking and air pollution. Bull Eur Physiopathol Respir 1981;36:752–759.

109. Xu X, Dockery DW, Ware JH, et al. Effects of cigarette smoking on rate of loss of pulmonary function in adults: a longitudinal assessment. Am Rev Respir Dis 1992;146:1345–1348.

110. Traver GA, Cline MG, Burrows B. Predictors of mortality in chronic obstructive pulmonary disease. Am Rev Respir Dis 1979;119:895–902.

111. Kanner RE, Renzetti AD, Stanish WM, et al. Predictors of survival in subjects with chronic airflow limitation. Am J Med 1983;74:249–255.

112. France AJ, Prescott RJ, Biernacki W, et al. Does right ventricular function predict survival in patients with chronic obstructive lung disease? Thorax 1988;43:621–626.

CHAPTER 11

LUNG CANCER

Robert I. Garver. Jr.

Lung cancer has recently surpassed breast cancer as the leading cause of cancer death in women (Fig 11.1). The reason for the rapid rise in lung cancer among women is widely believed to be the consequence of increased tobacco use by women. Furthermore, one recent epidemiologic study has suggested that women may have a higher cigarette smoking-associated lung cancer risk than men when controlled for a comparable level of smoking (1). Because lung cancer is a major cause of death and morbidity in women, it is important for the primary care physician to consider this diagnosis in the appropriate clinical setting.

Presentation

Lung cancer can present with a wide range of nonspecific symptoms and signs (Box 11.1). The typical symptomatic individual will have some combination of complaints related to the respiratory system, including chest pain, dyspnea, cough, sputum production, hemoptysis, and recurrent pneumonias. Complaints that are less clearly localized to the chest include weight loss, fevers, anorexia, joint or bone pains, neurologic changes, and psychiatric disturbances, among others. The presence of physical signs most frequently heralds the presence of advanced disease, which can be categorized as those directly referable to the chest, such as local wheezes, or more generalized signs, such as weight loss. In many cases, the cancer is incidentally identified in a chest x-ray obtained for other reasons.

When to Look for Lung Cancer

At some point in time, many patients will complain of at least one symptom that can be associated with lung cancer. Because most of these complaints will be secondary to benign etiologies, it is important to have good criteria for identifying individuals in whom further investigation is warranted.

The medical history can greatly assist in identifying individuals who warrant further investigation for possible lung cancer (Box 11.2). A long duration of cigarette smoking is the single greatest risk factor for the development of bronchogenic carcinoma (2). Ex-smokers need to remain tobacco free for 15 years before their risk decreases to that of the nonsmoking control population. Among cigarette smokers, those who develop chronic obstructive pulmonary disease (COPD) have an increased risk over a smoking history-matched population without COPD (3). As is widely publicized, the lung cancer risk in individuals with asbestosis is much higher in those who smoke compared to nonsmokers (4). Other important risk factors include a family history of lung cancer in a first-degree relative and a history of a head or neck cancer. In the absence of any risk factors, lung cancer remains a relatively uncommon malignancy. Conversely, among the population at risk, the possibility of lung cancer needs to be carefully considered if any of the symptoms or signs previously mentioned develop.

Specific features of the symptoms can also be helpful in identifying those patients requiring further evaluation. Some symptoms that are of particular concern are those of long duration (>2 to 3 months), those that cannot be explained by a benign diagnosis (e.g., hemoptysis in the absence of an acute bronchitis), or any potential lung cancer complaint in combination with a history of unintentional weight loss.

The physical examination is most commonly unrevealing except in advanced cases of the disease. Local-

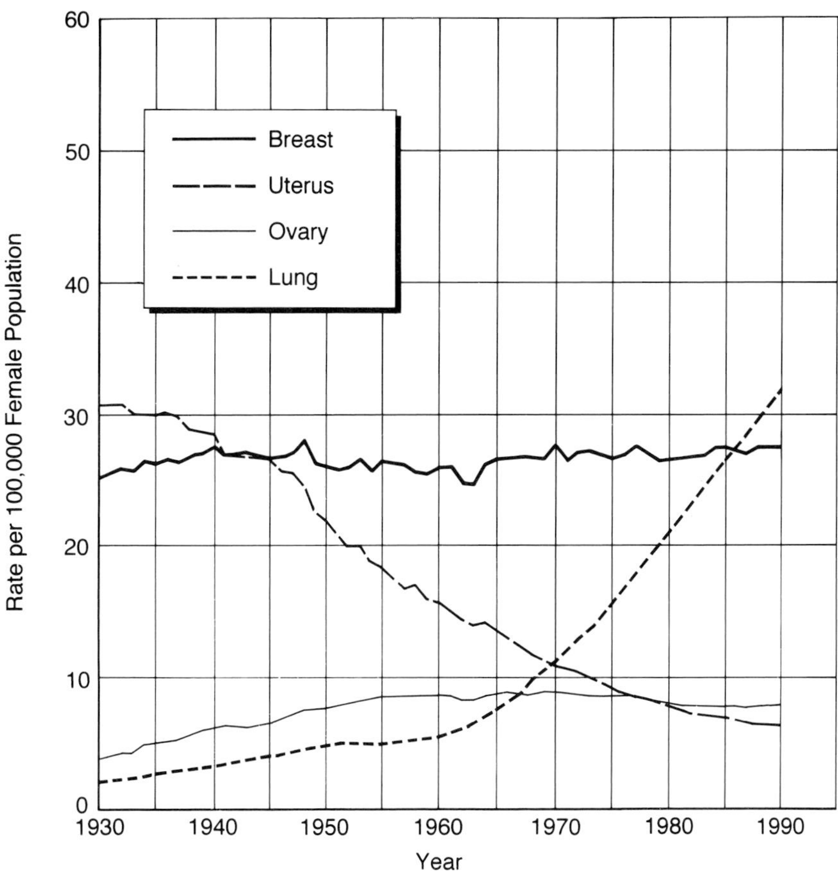

Fig 11.1 Cancer death rates for several common malignancies in women. Ordinate: age-adjusted rate per 100,000 (age adjusted to the 1970 US standard population); abscissa: year rates were determined. *(Source: Adapted from Boring CC, Squires TS, Jong J, Montgomery S. Cancer statistics, 1994. CA Cancer J Clin 1994;44:7–26.)*

izing chest sounds may be appreciated, or a pleural effusion detected by percussing the chest cavity. Cervical and supraclavicular nodes should be carefully palpated, and aspirated if enlarged in the potential lung cancer patient. In women, a careful examination of the breasts and pelvic region is helpful as a first step toward excluding metastatic disease to the chest from those organs. A good neurologic examination is also important early in the evaluation, because the requirement for a head computed tomography (CT) scan is most often based on the presence or absence of neurologic symptoms and signs.

Lung Cancer Screening

Although populations at risk for lung cancer have been clearly delineated, currently available technology has not provided an effective screening strategy (5). Large scale clinical studies have investigated the utility of frequent chest x-rays and sputum cytology examinations for increasing the detection of surgically amenable lung cancers. The most recent large scale study was limited to cigarette smoking men (>1 pack a day) over the age of 45. Although a larger percentage of resectable cancers was detected in the group receiving frequent sputum and chest x-ray examinations compared to the control population, the mortality rates were not significantly improved in the experimental group. Based on this type of data, the American Cancer Society does *not* recommend sputum cytology or chest x-rays as screening tests for high-risk patients. It is important to emphasize, however, that the clinician caring for a high-risk individual should have a low threshold for obtaining a chest x-ray as part

Box 11.1 Symptoms and Signs of Lung Cancer

Local

- Increased cough
- Increased sputum
- Increased dyspnea
- Chest/scapula pain
- Hemoptysis
- Localized chest sounds
- Recurrent pneumonias
- Pneumonia that does not clear
- Cervical/supraclavicular adenopathy
- Dysphagia
- Hoarseness
- Congestive heart failure/pericardial involvement

Distant

- Weight loss
- Fever
- Psychiatric disturbances
- Endocrinopathies: SIADH, hypercalcemia, hypercortisolism
- Bone pains
- Neurologic deficits: central and peripheral nervous system
- SVC syndrome
- Horner's syndrome
- Ulnar pain

SIADH, syndrome of inappropriate antiduiretic hormone; SVC, superior vena cava

Box 11.2 Lung Cancer Risk Factors

- Current smoker
- Ex-smoker <15 yr
- Chronic obstructive pulmonary disease
- Exposures: asbestos, others
- Positive family history
- History of head/neck cancer

of the evaluation for any complaints that might be associated with lung cancer, as described in the previous sections.

Lung Cancer: Two Major Types

Lung cancer is pathologically and biologically divided into two broad types: non–small cell lung cancer (NSCLC) and small cell lung cancer (SCLC) (6).

Three fourths of all lung cancers are NSCLC. This category includes adenocarcinoma, squamous and large cell carcinomas, among other less common variants. All of the subtypes share several common features (7). First, they are all believed to be derived from respiratory epithelial cells based on morphology and on immunohistochemical and genetic analyses, which demonstrate the presence of differentiated features present in the normal respiratory epithelial cells. Second, this group of lung cancers tends to be relatively slow growing with metastasis outside of the chest occurring late in the disease course. Third, this group of lung cancers usually does not respond well to chemotherapeutic agents.

The other 25% of lung cancers are SCLC. Often called "oat cell carcinoma," these cancers usually demonstrate immunohistochemical signs of neuroendocrine differentiation thought to reflect their origin from neuroendocrine cells present within normal respiratory epithelium. These are aggressive, rapidly growing cancers that metastasize widely early in the disease course (8). SCLC are very responsive to chemotherapy, initially.

Pathogenesis

A growing body of evidence suggests that lung cancer is the consequence of accumulated, somatic mutations in genes responsible for modulating cellular growth (9). Proto-oncogenes are normal genes that generally promote cell division. In lung cancer, as well as in many other carcinomas, sizable fractions of patient tumor specimens have been shown to contain mutations of proto-oncogenes. Mutated proto-oncogenes are referred to as "oncogenes," or alternatively as "activated" proto-oncogenes. The *ras* and *myc* proto-oncogenes have been shown to be commonly activated in lung cancer. Another large class of genes mutated in lung cancer tissues are the "antioncogenes." These are normal genes that generally inhibit cell division and growth. Mutations that inactivate the growth inhibitory function of antioncogenes contribute to the uncontrolled growth of the malignant cells. The p53 antioncogene is one example of an antioncogene frequently mutated in lung cancer.

On a more macroscopic level, it has been well documented that lung cancers frequently arise from scarred or fibrotic areas of the chest. It is possible that the scarred areas contain some cells with mutations in proto-oncogenes or antioncogenes that lead to abnormal but not invasive growth (i.e., causing the scar). In any case, it is important for the clinician to be wary of dismissing a chest x-ray abnormality as inconsequential based on a previous history of an abnormality *without* directly comparing the films. The failure to directly compare chest x-rays to previous abnormal films can and does lead to inappropriate evaluations and missed opportunities for potentially curative resections.

Initial Evaluation of the Patient with Suspected Lung Cancer

Although the complete staging and diagnosis usually requires the skills of a pulmonologist or thoracic surgeon, the primary care practitioner can initiate important aspects of the evaluation. Among laboratory findings, an abnormal chest x-ray is the most common finding that should prompt concern. A pleural effusion should almost always be pursued with a diagnostic thoracentesis, the exceptions being cases where an effusion has been recently evaluated, or clearly in association with worsening congestive heart failure that resolves or greatly decreases with treatment of the heart failure (Fig 11.2). If malignancy or tuberculosis is a strong consideration, many pulmonologists or thoracic surgeons advocate obtaining a pleural biopsy at the time of the thoracentesis to increase the diagnostic

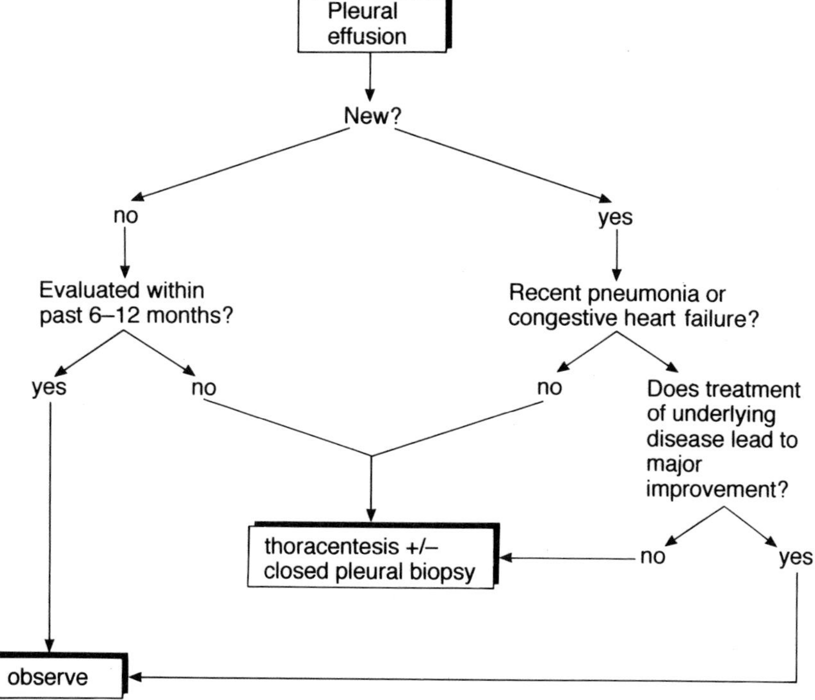

Fig 11.2 Algorithm for evaluation of a pleural effusion.

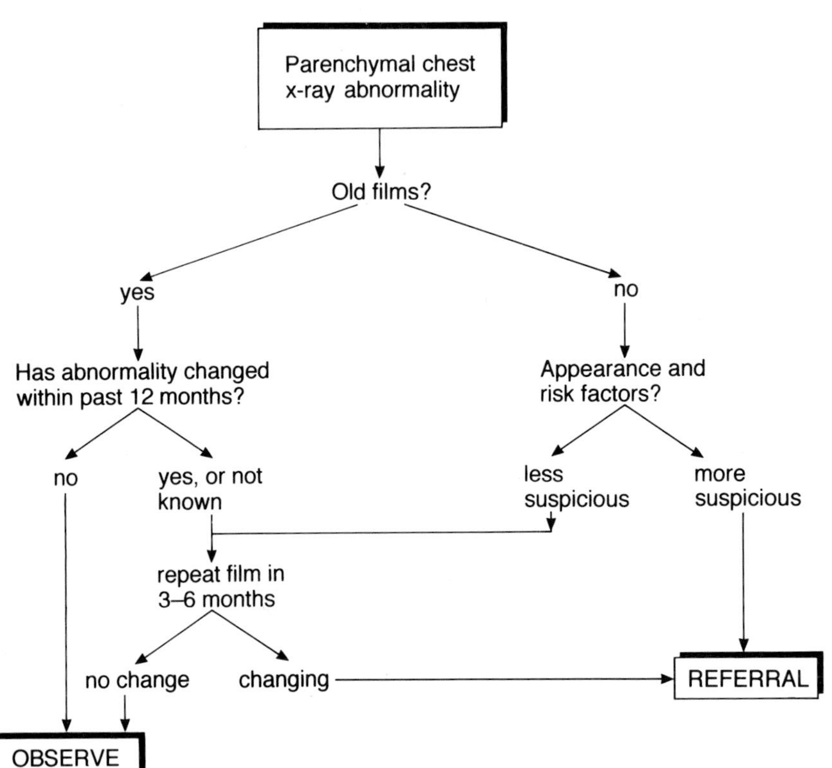

Fig 11.3 Algorithm for evaluation of a parenchymal lung abnormality.

yield. The aspirated fluid should be sent for pH (blood gas syringe on ice), cell counts and differential (tube with anticoagulant), protein and glucose measurements, cytopathology, and culture. Other studies are sometimes helpful, but in general the studies just described will be most useful in the vast majority of cases. The pleural biopsy, if obtained, should also be sent for culture and pathologic evaluation.

Parenchymal chest x-ray abnormalities do not always require immediate intervention (Fig 11.3). A parenchymal abnormality, for the purposes of this discussion, includes changes that could be caused by malignancy, such as noncalcified nodules, infiltrates not clearly associated with pneumonia, scars, lobar atelectasis, or adenopathy. The first step in the evaluation of a parenchymal abnormality should include the direct comparison with an old film by a qualified chest x-ray reader. It is not sufficient to rely on an old chest x-ray report that mentions the same abnormality because a change in the size, shape, or character of the lesion may only be appreciated by direct comparison to the old film, that is, lung cancers frequently arise from long-standing abnormalities within the lung. If old films are not available, the approach depends in large part on the probability of malignancy based on radiographic appearance and risk factors. For example, an 8-cm mass in the chest of a long-time smoker is lung cancer until proven otherwise. On the other hand, apical scarring may represent nothing more than the residua of healed granulomatous infection. Once an abnormality is found to be changing, or is highly suspicious for malignancy, the patient should be referred for further evaluation.

A frequently overlooked aspect of the early evaluation in the suspected lung cancer patient is an objective assessment of pulmonary physiologic function (10). It may seem inappropriate for the primary care practitioner to consider this apsect. However, the subsequent evaluation and referral are different for individuals who are "physiologically inoperable" compared to those who could withstand a resection if indicated. In this context, it clearly is a waste of time and money to initiate an extensive staging evaluation to rule out metastatic disease if the individual is not a surgical candidate. In addition, one would not send a physiologically inoperable patient to a thoracic surgeon for the initial referral. The most widely accepted physiologic variable used for the determination of operability is the forced expiratory volume in 1 second (FEV_1). This measurement should be obtained from a formal pulmonary physiology laboratory by a well trained technician rather than from office spirometry administered by less experienced personnel. The specific numerical values of FEV_1 used to determine operability may vary slightly among thoracic surgeons and the overall health of the patient. In general, an FEV_1 of less than 1 liter will disqualify a patient from further operative consideration; those individuals with an FEV_1 of greater than 1.5 liters will qualify for pulmonary resection. The operability of those patients falling between 1 and 1.5 liters frequently depends on the extent of resection required, the overall health of the patient, and the practice style of the surgeon.

Obtaining a chest CT scan is another test that frequently can be ordered by the primary care physician to facilitate the subsequent evaluation. The scan ordered should be with and without contrast for the evaluation of a chest mass. The area scanned should include the thorax, liver, and adrenals to evaluate the primary lesion, look for other lesions that may have been missed on the plain films, assess the mediastinal structures and lymph nodes, and rule out metastatic lesions in the liver or adrenals. There is no evidence that the more expensive magnetic resonance imaging scans, or thin-section "high-resolution" CT scans are in any way superior to standard CT scans for evaluating the potential lung cancer patient. On the other hand, this expensive test should be reserved for patients with a chest x-ray lesion that is highly suspicious for lung cancer. As a general rule, the CT scan should not be used during the initial evaluation of a diffuse infiltrate, a focal pneumonitis, or to simply look for abnormalities in the presence of a completely normal chest x-ray.

Staging and Diagnosis of the Suspected Lung Cancer

The final staging and tissue diagnosis of the lung cancer patient should be left to the pulmonologist or thoracic surgeon, depending on the local standard of practice. Commonly, a bronchoscopy is performed both for the purpose of obtaining tissue and to examine the airways for tumor invasion as a component of the staging process. Because the diagnostic yield of bronchoscopy diminishes significantly for small or peripheral lesions, transthoracic needle aspiration is often used to obtain tissue for diagnosis. The results of the tissue diagnosis and bronchoscopic evaluation dictate the remainder of the staging work-up. The subsequent evaluation varies for SCLC and NSCLC (11).

For NSCLC, the evaluation after tissue diagnosis is geared toward identifying patients who are potentially eligible for surgery. The staging system most widely used is a TNM-based categorization divided into stages I to IV, although it should be noted that stage III is subdivided into IIIa and IIIb (12). The definition of the T, N, and M categories with stage definitions is included in Table 11.3. The decision to search for metastatic disease is highly predicated on symptoms and signs. In patients without any bony or neurologic symptoms, the incidence of bone or cranial metastases is so low that bone and head CT scans are not required. Bone marrow examinations are not part of the routine staging process either because bone marrow infiltration is also very unusual.

Staging for SCLC is different than that for NSCLC. Although the TNM system used for NSCLC can be used, more commonly the disease extent is defined as "limited" or "extensive." Although this staging system does not define an operable category, the chemotherapy regimens used may differ, particularly in the context of experimental protocols. Due to the very common metastases to brain and bone marrow, these patients commonly receive head CT scans and bone marrow examinations routinely, even in the absence of any symptoms or signs referable to those areas.

Lung Cancer Treatments

Non-small Cell Cancer

It is widely accepted that stage I and II disease should be surgically resected with intent to cure in physiologically eligible patients. The most common surgery performed is a lobectomy with nodal dissection. Wedge resections can be done in appropriately selected patients with outcomes comparable to a lobectomy. The removal of an entire lung may be dictated by tumor location or extent, but obviously can only be performed in patients capable of withstanding the loss of half their pulmonary capacity. Stage IIIa patients are a borderline group for whom surgery may improve outcome, but the patients need to be carefully selected by a combination of overall functional status, location of the N2 nodes, and tissue type, among other variables. Among stage IIIa patients, limited data suggest that neoadjuvant chemotherapy may improve outcome.

Stages IIIb and IV are not curable by resection, but can be palliated by either chemotherapy or radiotherapy. Because NSCLC is usually so poorly responsive to chemotherapy, external beam radiotherapy is generally the preferred treatment. The indications for irradiating the chest disease vary slightly among radiation oncologists. Although there is general agreement that disease associated with postobstruction pneumonitis or pain should be irradiated, some would advocate irradiating unsymptomatic disease that is close to vital structures. Brachytherapy is a form of radiation therapy analogous to that used in pelvic oncology. A catheter is placed via the bronchoscope through the malignant region, after which radioactive pellets are instilled into the catheter and subsequently retrieved at the conclusion of the session. This therapy is advocated as a lung-sparing form of radiation therapy for patients with local, symptomatic lesions through which a catheter can be threaded. However, there have not been any data demonstrating that this expensive and invasive form of therapy improves outcome compared to more conventional therapies.

Because inoperable lung cancer outcome is so poor with conventional therapies, lung cancer is an obvious target for experimental therapies. Few data suggest that newer chemotherapeutic agents will have any significant impact on this difficult problem. The few cases of lung cancer reported to have been treated with the lymphokine-activated killer cell-based therapies were also not very encouraging. At this time, gene therapy approaches that direct therapeutic gene expression to the cancer cells may offer new hope.

Small Cell Lung Cancer

This aggressive cancer is amenable to surgical resection only in the rare case that presents as a solitary nodule without any nodal or other metastatic disease. The vast majority of SCLC cases present with disease that is best treated with chemotherapy, frequently in combination with radiation therapy. The chemotherapy regimens produce complete remissions in the majority of patients with limited disease and a significant percentage of patients with extensive disease. Because central nervous system recurrences are common, the use of prophylactic total cranial irradiation has been advocated, although its use is controver-

Table 11.1 Lung Cancer Staging

T	T1	<3 cm, within lung tissue, distal to mainstem bronchus
	T2	>3 cm, or any size with a) visceral pleura invasion, b) lobar atelectasis, c) mainstem bronchus >2 cm from carina
	T3	Any size with invasion of chest wall, diaphragm, mediastinal pleura/pericardium, mainstem bronchus within 2 cm of carina
	T4	Any size with invasion of mediastinum, heart, great vessels, trachea, esophagus, vertebral bodies, carina, or malignant pleural effusion
N	N0	No nodes
	N1	Peribronchial or ipsilateral hilar
	N2	Ipsilateral mediastinal or subcarinal
	N3	Contralateral mediastinal or hilar, any scalene or supraclavicular nodes
M	M0	No mets
	M1	Mets present
	Stage I	T1/T2–N0–M0
	Stage II	T1/T2–N1–M0
	Stage IIIA	T3–N0/N1–M0
		T1/T2/T3–N2–M0
	Stage IIIB	any T–N3–M0
		T4–any N–M0
	Stage IV	any T or any N = M1

sial. Unfortunately, the vast majority of patients will relapse within 2 years and ultimately die from the cancer. As a chemosensitive cancer, there is more interest in continuing to explore new combinations of chemotherapy in hopes of increasing the number of patients with cures.

Care of the Lung Cancer Patient After Treatment

Although immediate complications of surgical, chemical, or radiation therapies are frequently dealt with by the specialist administering that therapy, the more chronic sequelae of lung cancer therapies frequently fall within the primary care domain. The most common problems are discussed in the following sections.

Dyspnea

One of the most common complaints is dyspnea related to the surgical resection, radiation therapy, or residual tumor. Furthermore, many lung cancer patients have underlying lung disease from years of tobacco abuse that further exacerbates the physiologic lung impairment associated with therapy. It is often helpful to obtain posttreatment spirometry, arterial blood gases (room air), and a chest x-ray as a baseline for future evaluation of increased dyspnea or other new pulmonary symptoms.

In the patient with obstructive impairment, inhaled albuterol plus ipatropium bromide plus inhaled steroids may provide significant symptomatic relief. In general, most patients report the greatest relief with albuterol. One cost-effective way to initiate this therapy is to start with albuterol alone and subsequently add the ipatropium or the inhaled steroids and ask the patient to subjectively evaluate the value of the additional inhalers after a 2- to 3-week trial period. Oral steroids may be helpful in patients with very severe COPD in a dosage range of 20–30 mg prednisone daily. The use of theophylline compounds may or may not be helpful in this population—a therapeutic trial can be useful to make this determination in specific patients. Many of these patients are relatively hypoxic, but supplemental oxygen therapy is conventionally reserved for only those patients qualifying for Medicare reimbursement ($Po_2 \leq 55$ or O_2 saturation $<90\%$ at room air).

In patients complaining of increased dyspnea after the immediate posttreatment stage, the differential diagnosis should include the following: worsened obstructive impairment from progression or exacerbation of underlying COPD, infection (bronchitis versus pneumonitis), recurrent or increased tumor growth, pleural effusion, cardiac decompensation, or pulmonary embolism. The history, physical examination, and chest x-ray should comprise the initial evaluation to identify the most likely etiology among the differential possibilities.

Cough

Cough is a common problem with causes similar to those of dyspnea. Cough associated with COPD is obviously treated like the dyspnea of COPD. The cough associated with persistent or recurrent endobronchial tumor can be a major symptomatic problem for the patient because it may interfere with all daily living activities. In these cases, oral codeine in doses of 30 to 60 mg every 6 hours is helpful. Patients with endobronchial disease after undergoing therapy have a very limited life span, so concerns about the potential addictive nature of codeine use in this setting should not lead one to withhold this helpful medication in this population.

Hemoptysis

The onset of hemoptysis is frequently an ominous sign of endobronchial recurrence or progression although a bronchitis or pneumonitis not associated with malignancy is sometimes the etiology. The primary care practitioner should first assess the severity of the hemoptysis by crudely quantifying the volume of blood being produced. Patients coughing up bright red blood throughout the day in volumes that cumulatively are estimated to be more than several tablespoons should be evaluated promptly by a specialist for further evaluation because a catastrophic episode may be imminent. Depending on the particular clinical situation, the specialist may localize the bleeding by bronchoscopy to assist in future mangement or initiate local therapy to the lesion responsible for the bleeding. The exception, of course, is a terminal patient for whom running doses of codeine at 60 mg every 4 to 6 hours can be helpful. Smaller amounts of hemoptysis, such as streaking or spotting within sputum at low frequency, can be more leisurely assessed.

Chest Pain

Persistent chest pain at the incision site of thoractomy patients is not uncommon although the majority of these patients eventually experience a gradual diminution in the discomfort. In some patients, however, the pain can be severe and debilitating requiring chronic pain relief measures, such as nerve blocks. New chest pain should be investigated with a chest x-ray to rule out a chest wall recurrence that might be amenable to radiation therapy. Depending on the character of the pain, other causes should be considered in the appropriate setting, such as cardiac ischemia or pulmonary embolism.

Summary and Conclusions

Lung cancer is a common malignancy in women and requires a multidisciplinary approach for diagnosis and management. The primary care provider is frequently called on to perform the initial evaluation of symptoms or signs that may represent lung cancer. Results of the primary care evaluation should determine the subsequent evaluation, which can include observation or referral for invasive diagnostic, staging, and therapeutic procedures.

Primary care providers also care for lung cancer patients after treatment. This population may require medical therapies for relief of pulmonary physiologic impairment, vigilance for symptoms and signs that may herald recurrence, and often palliative measures for relief of symptoms associated with the terminal course of the disease.

REFERENCES

1. Risch HA, Howe GR, Jain M, et al. Are female smokers at higher risk for lung cancer than male smokers? Am J Epidemiol 1993;138:281 - 293.
2. Garfinkel L, Silverberg E. Lung cancer and smoking trends in the United States over the past 25 years. CA Cancer J Clin 1991;41:137-145.
3. Tockman MS, Anthonisen NR, Wright EC, et al. Airways obstruction and the risk for lung cancer. Ann Intern Med 1987;106:512-518.
4. Sellers TA, Balley-Wilson JE, Eiston RC, et al. Evidence for mendelian inheritance in the pathogenesis of lung cancer. J Natl Cancer Inst 1990;82:1272-1279.
5. Szabo E, Birrer MJ, Mulshine, JL. Early detection of lung cancer. Semin Oncol 1993;20:374-382.
6. Sobin LH. The World Health Organization's histological classification of lung tumors: a comparison of the first and second editions. Cancer Detect Prev 1982;5:391-406.
7. Ihde DC, Minna JD. Non-small cell lung cancer. Part I: Biology, diagnosis, and staging. Curr Probl Cancer 1991;15:61-104.
8. Cook RM, Miller YE, Bunn PA Jr. Small cell lung cancer: etiology, biology, clinical features, staging and treatment. Curr Probl Cancer 1993;17:69-141.
9. Kratzke RA, Shimizu E. Oncogenes in human lung cancer. Cancer Treat Res 1992;63:61-85.
10. Dunn WF, Scanlon PD. Preoperative pulmonary function testing for patients with lung cancer. Mayo Clin Proc 1993;68:371-377.
11. Patel AM, Dunn WF, Trastek VF. Staging systems of lung cancer. Mayo Clin Proc 1993;68:475-482.
12. Mountain CF. A new international staging system for lung cancer. Chest 1986;89:225S-233S.
13. Boring CC, Squires TS, Tong T, Montgomery S. Cancer statistics, 1994. CA Cancer J Clin 1994;44:7-26.

CHAPTER 12

COMMUNITY-ACQUIRED PNEUMONIA

Nancy E. Dunlap

Community-acquired pneumonia is a common medical problem that physicians manage in both the ambulatory and hospital settings. In the outpatient setting, the mortality rate of pneumonia remains low, in the range of 1% to 5%. However, among patients who require hospitalization, the mortality rate approaches 25% (1–7). Historically, community-acquired pneumonias have been divided into "typical" and "atypical" patterns. The prototype of the "typical" pneumonia is *Streptococcus pneumoniae* infection with the clinical presentation of cough, fever, chills, dyspnea, pleuritic chest pain, sputum production, or altered mental status (2). "Atypical" pneumonias have been characterized by a gradual onset, viral prodrome, absence of rigors, nonproductive cough, lower degree of fever, diarrhea, and absence of pleurisy. Although the clinical findings associated with "typical" or "atypical" pneumonias may be more prevalent in groups of patients with certain pathogens, there is significant overlap in clinical findings between the groups. Therefore, for a given patient, these findings are not helpful in determining the etiology of pneumonia. In the discussion to follow, no distinction will be made between "typical" and "atypical" pneumonias. Instead, patients will be categorized according to the likelihood of acquiring pneumonia with certain pathogens. Thus, classification of patients according to the initial, empiric therapy will be presented.

In this chapter, we provide an approach to the initial evaluation and treatment of community-acquired pneumonia in both the clinic and the hospital. Because the risks of pneumonia increase with advancing age and comorbidities, factors that should influence the decision whether to hospitalize are presented. Guidelines for hospital discharge and follow-up are also discussed. This presentation does not address pneumonia in immunocompromised individuals such as those with human immunodeficiency virus infection. Considerations for patients who develop pneumonia during pregnancy are discussed separately.

Presentation

Pneumonia is a microbial infection of the terminal airways and alveoli of the lungs. Organisms that typically cause pneumonia include aerobic and anaerobic bacteria, mycobacteria, mycoplasma, viruses, and fungi. Patients with pneumonia frequently present with a prodromal upper respiratory infection and the sudden onset of chills followed by fever. A painful cough, fatigue and apprehension, and failure of antipyretic medication to provide relief are also common. Young adults usually have the more classic symptoms of a lower respiratory tract infection, whereas infants and the elderly may have nonspecific symptoms that make diagnosis more difficult. Altered mental status may be the only symptom of pneumonia in the elderly. Elderly or severely ill patients may have an unimpressive amount of cough, scant sputum production, little evidence of respiratory symptoms, and a deceptive absence of fever. Because of this, pneumonia should be included in any differential diagnosis in elderly or ill patients with nonspecific findings.

In any evaluation of a patient with pneumonia, a concientious medical history and physical examination are essential to categorize patients into treatment groups. Knowledge of coexisting medical problems is necessary to determine the relative risks of pneumonia in any given patient. The presence of chronic obstructive pulmonary disease (COPD), diabetes mellitus, or chronic renal or liver disease will increase the morbidity or mortality for a patient with pneumonia (Table 12.1). Historical information can give clues as to the etiologic agent causing infection. For example, if the patient has episodes of unconsciousness or difficulty swallowing, aspiration pneumonia with anaerobic organisms is more likely. If other members of the family have similar illnesses, *Mycoplasma pneumoniae*, *Chlamydia pneumoniae*, or viruses are more likely pathogens. It is also vital to know if the patient is allergic to certain antibiotics so that those drugs will be avoided. Antibiotic doses may also need to be altered in renal or hepatic failure.

Physical Findings

The most common signs associated with community-acquired pneumonia include tachycardia and tachypnea (2). Significant tachypnea, hypotension, or high temperatures (see Table12.1) suggest serious disease and may prompt hospitalization. Splinting during breathing may suggest pleuritic chest pain and one can frequently gauge the discomfort the patient is experiencing by merely observing the patient breathe. Cyanosis of the skin or nailbeds should be sought because hypoxemia may occur in these patients, necessitating the need for supplemental oxygen therapy. Clubbing of the nailbeds may give a clue to underlying lung disease. Dehydration is common in elderly patients with pneumonia and thus the appearance of the skin and mucous membranes can help assess fluid status. Assessment of oral hygiene, condition of the teeth and gingiva, and adequacy of the gag reflex could all point to a likely aspiration syndrome and anaerobic infection.

Auscultation and percussion of the chest may reveal rales, egophony, increased fremitus, and typical signs of lung consolidation, which affirm the existence and location of the pneumonia. Wheezing or rhonchi may be heard, thus prompting the institution of bronchodilator therapy. Areas of decreased breath sounds and dullness to percussion may localize a parapneumonic effusion that needs prompt evaluation in the setting of acute pneumonia. Because acute endocarditis can complicate pneumonia, auscultation of the heart to identify new cardiac murmurs and a search for signs of distal emboli are important. Illicit drug users have an increased risk for right-sided endocarditis and thus examination of the skin for needle tracts may be indicated.

Upper abdominal tenderness is occasionally present in patients with pneumonia and may cause confusion as to its etiology. The abdominal tenderness associated with pneumonia reflects diaphragmatic

Table 12.1 Risk Factors Associated with Morbidity/Mortality in Community-Acquired Pneumonia

Clinical Features	Physical Findings	Laboratory Findings
Age >65 yr	High respiratory rate (>30/min)	Extremes of white blood cells (<4 or >30 × 10^6/mL)
Coexisting illness		
COPD	Low blood pressure (systolic <90 mm Hg)	Hypoxemia (Pao_2 <60 mm Hg)
Diabetes mellitus		
Chronic renal disease		
Liver disease	High temperature (>38.3°C or 101°F)	Hypercarbia ($Paco_2$ >50 mm Hg)
Altered mental status		
Alcohol abuse/malnutrition		
Absence of spleen	Extrapulmonary sites of infection	Extensive disease (>1 lobe involvement, cavity, pleural effusion, rapid progression of disease)
Recent hospitalization		
		Anemia (Hematocrit <30%; hemoglobin <9 gm/dL) Sepsis

irritation resulting from inflamed pleural surfaces and is not an indication of abdominal pathology. Mental status changes may occur, particularly in the elderly, as a result of fever or infection. However, because meningitis can occasionally complicate pneumonias, especially those caused by gram-negative bacilli, this diagnosis must be sought. A thorough neurologic examination, therefore, should be part of the initial evaluation of pneumonia.

Laboratory

To treat patients with pneumonia with the most specific antibiotics, it would be optimal to identify the agent causing pneumonia. Many of the tests discussed below are directed toward that end. However, in over half of all patients with community-acquired pneumonia, the pathogen is never identified (1–3).

Sputum Gram Stain and Culture

There is debate over the value of a sputum Gram stain in determining the etiologic agent in pneumonia (8). Some authorities believe that a properly performed Gram stain of expectorated sputum is useful in the initial evaluation of patients with pneumonia (8–10). The commonly used criterion is to examine and culture a sputum sample only if it has more than 25 neutrophils and fewer than 5 squamous epithelial cells per low power field. Obtaining a good sputum specimen in some patients may be difficult. Inducing sputum with inhalation of a warmed saline aerosol can be helpful in obtaining a useful specimen. However, attempts to obtain lung secretions by passing a small rubber catheter through the nose or mouth rarely get beyond the vocal cords and is not recommended.

The usefulness of Gram stains to determine the etiologic agents in community-acquired pneumonias is uncertain (8). But there are instances when an adequate sputum sample shows a predominance of organisms and can be used to guide therapy. Also, direct staining of sputum for determining pneumonia caused by *Mycobacterium* species, endemic fungi, *Pneumocystis carinii*, and *Legionella* species may be diagnositc, but these tests must be suspected and ordered specifically.

Routine bacterial culture of sputum often demonstrate pathogenic organisms, but the sensitivity and specificity of this test is poor (8). Even when sputum cultures are positive, it is frequently difficult to determine the specific pathogen in community-acquired pneumonia. Because bacteria colonize the oropharynx, isolation of an organism normally found in the oropharynx is not tantamount to infection by that organism (2). Unless one is confident that the agent cultured is the pathogen, it is best to continue broad antibiotic coverage. Only when organisms are not common respiratory flora such as *Mycobacterium* species, endemic fungi, and *Legionella* species are sputum cultures routinely diagnositc. Sputum should not be sent for anaerobic culture because contaminating pharyngeal organisms may produce misleading results. Viral cultures are not useful in the inital evaluation of patients with community-acquired pneumonia and should not be routinely performed (1,8).

Invasive Diagnostic Procedures

Most patients with community-acquired pneumonia do not require invasive diagnostic tests in their initial management unless a patient is severely ill. When properly performed, bronchoscopy with protected brush catheters or bronchoalveolar lavage with or without balloon protection may give useful culture information, but they are most sensitive when performed before the administration of any antibiotics (6,11–14). These bronchoscopy procedures carry less risk and are usually more acceptable to patients than transtracheal or direct lung aspiration.

Blood Tests

Routine laboratory tests, although not useful in determining the etiology of pneumonia, may be helpful in identifying risk factors that may indicate the need for hospitalization. When determining whether a patient should be hospitalized with pneumonia, a complete blood count (CBC) and arterial blood gas may be useful. Extremely high or low white blood cell (WBC) counts suggest overwhelming infection, whereas anemia may signal chronic disease. Hypoxemia or hypercapnea suggests pulmonary compromise. If renal disease, diabetes, or hepatic dysfunction is in question, blood chemistries should be obtained. All tests do not necessarily need to be obtained on everyone, but selected results will help identify risk factors for morbidity and mortality from pneumonia (see Table 12.1).

Hospitalized patients should have two sets of blood cultures collected before initation of antibiotic therapy. Blood cultures can identify the etiologic agent causing pneumonia. In *S. pneumoniae* pneumonia, blood cultures are positive in 10% to 25% of patients (3). Patients with pleural effusion should have a diagnostic thoracentesis to ensure that an empyema is not present. Pleural fluid examination should include WBC and differential and measurement of lactate dehydrogenase (LDH) and protein. An empyema will be exudative ($LDH_{pleural}/LDH_{serum} > 0.6$; $protein_{pleural}/protein_{serum} > 0.5$ or $LDH_{pleural} > 200$ IU/L) and grossly purulent. Microorganisms can frequently be seen on stained smear and usually grow from cultures, especially anaerobic cultures. A low pleural fluid pH (<7.10) is suggestive of empyema and may be helpful in evaluation.

Serologic testing and cold agglutinin measurements are not useful in the initial evaluation of patients with community-acquired pneumonia and should not be routinely performed. However, acute and convalescent serologic testing may occasionally be useful for the retrospective confirmation of a suspected diagnosis.

Radiology

A standard posteroanterior and lateral chest x-ray should be obtained in patients whose symptoms and physical examination suggest the possiblity of pneumonia. This test is useful in distinguishing pneumonia from other causes of fever and cough. Radiographic findings may suggest specific etiologies of disease such as lung abscess or tuberculosis, or coexisting processes such as bronchial obstruction and pleural effusions. Radiography is also useful for evaluating the extent of disease (i.e., multilobar involvement) and may prompt the decision to hospitalize the patient.

Specific radiographic features, however, are not useful in differentiating the pathogens causing the pneumonia. Although certain microbes, such as *M. pneumoniae*, *C. pneumoniae*, and viruses are more likely to produce a diffuse, interstitial pattern on chest x-ray, these findings are not sensitive nor specific enough in any given patient to direct therapy (5). Thus the chest x-ray should be used to identify the presence of a pulmonary infiltrate and to define the extent of disease.

Differential Diagnosis

The symptoms of pneumonia, fever, cough, and pulmonary infiltrates on chest x-ray can occur in diseases other than pneumonia. Lung abscess may occur as the result of aspiration of anaerobic bacteria or a foreign body. The onset of symptoms in lung abscess may be abrupt as in some types of pneumonia. A history of epilepsy, alcoholic intoxication, esophageal dysmotility, or neurologic disease may predispose to aspiration. The development of cavitation is typically accompanied by expectoration of large amounts of foul-smelling sputum.

Atelectasis may mimic pneumonia and occurs most often in bedridden patients or after surgery when respiratory motion is limited and when the cough reflex is depressed. These are also the clinical settings where pneumonia is common. The diagnosis of atelectasis is facilitated by noting decreased volume of the affected hemithorax on chest radiograph. Occasionally, the volume loss will be sufficient to cause shifting of the mediastinum toward the affected side.

Pulmonary embolus with infarction is especially frequent in patients with congestive heart failure and surgical procedures. It may be asymptomatic or may present many of the features of pneumonia, though true chills are rare. Septic pulmonary infarcts may be complicated by abscess and caviation and, in women, suggest the diagnosis of septic abortion or peripheral sepsis.

Congestive heart failure can cause dyspnea, acute pulmonary edema, and occasionally, hemoptysis. Pleural effusions may occur, particularly in association with biventricular failure. Fever is not commonly associated with congestive heart failure.

Obstructing bronchogenic carcinoma can result in atelectasis or postobstructive pneumonia. Frequently, if infection does occur distal to the obstruction, there is a delay in the resolution of radiographic abnormalities. Bronchoscopy may be useful to identify the lesion if an obstruction is suspected.

Bronchiolitis obliterans and organizing pneumonia (BOOP) is a descriptive term for a fibrosing inflammatory process that occludes the lumens of small airways. Clinically, BOOP may present with cough, dyspnea, and malaise. There may be a history of recent respiratory tract infection or exposure to toxic fumes. The WBC count is often elevated and the chest radiograph may show scattered large or small nodular densities, or areas of consolidation. Lung biopsy may be necessary to distinguish this noninfectious process from pneumonia (15).

Wegener's granulomatosis is a necrotizing granulomatous inflammation of the lung associated with vasculitis. Upper airway involvement is usually present to aid in the diagnosis. Cough, hemoptysis, chest pain, and fever may occur. Chest radiographs typically show multiple nodular densities with occasional cavitation (15).

Eosinophilic pneumonia is a proliferative disorder of histiocytes and is histologically identical to the group of disorders termed histiocytosis X (15). Patients with eosinophilic granuloma commonly present with cough or dyspnea, but symptoms may be minimum or absent. Chest radiographs typically show nodular or cystic lesions. Lung biopsy is needed to diagnose this disorder.

Pathophysiology

Microbial pathogens that cause pneumonia reach the pulmonary alveoli by four routes: 1) the inhalation or airborne organisms, 2) aspiration of oropharyngeal contents, 3) direct extention from contiguous sites, and 4) hematogenous spread from infected sites elsewhere in the body. Organisms that cause community-acquired pneumonia usually fall into the first two categories and therefore this discussion will focus on those pathogens.

The organisms that can cause pneumonia through inhalation tend to be very virulent because low numbers of organisms can cause disease. *M. pneumoniae*, *C. pneumoniae*, *Legionella pneumophilia*, endemic fungi, and viruses are examples of microbes that cause infection by this route. Because low numbers of organisms cause disease, it is uncommon to identify the microbes on Gram stain. Clinically, there is usually a persistent cough associated with these infections, but only scant amounts of sputum may be produced. The chest radiograph in these patients has a tendency to have a more diffuse, interstial pattern, but this finding cannot be relied on to direct therapy (6).

Pneumonia resulting from aspiration occurs with organisms that are present in the upper airway. The oropharynx is normally colonized by a mixture of aerobic and microaerophilic bacteria as well as by anaerobic organisms. The normal oral flora can include *S. pneumoniae* and *Haemophilus influenzae*. Conspicuously absent from the group of bacteria that normally colonize the oropharynx are the enteric gram-negative bacilli. Normal individuals are not colonized by these gram-negative bacteria, but patients with serious illness of any type may harbor these organisms in their oropharynx. The likelihood that a given individual will have upper airway colonization by these bacteria is directly related to how ill the person is and how long he or she has been ill. Thus the risk of gram-negative organisms causing pneumonia increases with age and coexisting illness.

It is often difficult to assign a specific etiologic agent as causing community-acquired pneumonia. This is particularly true with the pathogens that cause disease through inhalation because these organisms tend not to grow well on typical bacterial culture media. Acute and convalescent serology is usually needed to retrospectively assign a specific pathogen. It is almost as difficult to determine the pathogen in pneumonias resulting from aspiration. Although a sputum culture may be positive for oropharyngeal bacteria, determining which agent is responsible for disease may be difficult. The following criteria, however, may be useful in assigning a specific bacterial pathogen in community-acquired pneumonia (16):

1. Positive blood culture for a pulmonary pathogen without another apparent source
2. A positive pleural fluid culture for a pulmonary pathogen
3. Heavy or moderate growth of a predominant bacterial pathogen on sputum culture

Because it is rare to have a definite etiology of community-acquired pneumonia, particularly within the first 48 hours, an empiric approach to initial antimicrobial therapy is usually necessary. In an attempt to develop a rational framework for such therapy, the Canadian Community Acquired Pneumonia Consensus Conference Group and American Thoracic Society both issued statements in 1993 on the guidelines for the managing adults with community-acquired pneumonia (8,17). These statements were compiled after analyzing available clinical studies to identify the most common pathogens associated with community-acquired pneumonia. Patients were grouped into categories based on age and coexisting illnesses. Based on the most likely organisms to cause infection in each of these groups, empiric antibiotic therapy was suggested. Patients are divided into four groups based on age, presence of comorbidity, need for hospitalization, or presence of severe pneumonia. A compilation of recommendations from these two statements appears below.

Less than 60 Years of Age and No Comorbidity

The most common pathogens in otherwise healthy outpatients with pneumonia who were 60 years of age or less were found to be *S. pneumoniae*, *M. pneumoniae*, respiratory viruses, *C. pneumoniae*, and *H. influenzae*. Miscellaneous pathogens included *Legionella* species, *Staphylococcus aureus*, *Mycoplasma tuberculosis*, endemic fungi, and gram-negative bacilli. The mortality of patients within this group is estimated to be 1% to 5% (8). Table 12.2 shows empiric antibiotic therapy as determined by these suspected organisms.

Patients over 60 Years of Age or with Comorbidities

Pathogens among outpatients greater than 60 years of age or with a comorbidity such as COPD, diabetes mellitus, renal insufficiency, congestive heart failure, and chronic liver disease included *S. pneumoniae*, respiratory viruses, *H. influenzae*, aerobic gram-negative bacilli, and *S. aureus*. Diabetic patients and patients who have recently recovered from influenza are at increased risk for *S. aureus* pneumonia. Less common pathogens include *Moraxella catarrhalis*, *Legionella* species, *Mycobacterium* species, and endemic fungi. Mortality within this group remains low, but many patients may require hospitalization (8). Table 12.3 shows empiric therapy suggestions for this group of patients.

Patients Requiring Hospitalization with Community-Acquired Pneumonia

Previous studies have documented great geographic variability in hospital admission rates for adult community-acquired pneumonia, suggesting inconsistent criteria for hospitalization (16,18). There are no firm guidelines for when patients should be admitted to the hospital, but several well known risk factors increase a patient's risk of complications or mortality. When these risk factors are present, especially if multiple risk factors coexist, then hospitalization should be strongly considered (8). The decision to hospitalize should not be viewed as a commitment to long-term hospital care, but rather the opportunity to observe the patient's initial response to therapy. Mortality rates reported for

Table 12.2 Treatment of Pneumonia in Patients Less than 60 Years of Age with No Coexisting Illnesses

Suspected Organisms	Empiric Treatment
Streptococcus pneumoniae	Macrolide
Mycoplasma pneumoniae	Erythromycin 500 mg four times daily
Chlamydia pneumoniae	Azithromycin 500 mg on day 1 then 250 daily on days 2–5*
Haemophilus influenzae	Clarithromycin 250 mg twice a day*
Respiratory viruses	
Miscellaneous	Tetracycline[a]
Mycobacterium tuberculosis	
Staphylococcus aureus	
Legionella pneumophilia	
Endemic fungi	
Aerobic gram-negative bacilli	

* Should be considered in smokers to cover *H. influenzae* and when erythromycin is not tolerated.
[a] Many isolates of *S. pneumoniae* are not sensitive.

Table 12.3 Treatment of Pneumonia in Patients over 60 Years of Age or with Coexisting Illness

Suspected Organisms	Empiric Treatment
Streptococcus pneumoniae	Cephalosporin–2nd generation
Haemophilus influenzae	Cefuroxime 250 mg twice daily
Staphylococcus aureus	
Aerobic gram-negative bacilli	Trimethoprim-sulfamethoxazole
Respiratory viruses	Bactrim 1 DS tablet twice daily
Miscellaneous	Penicillin + β-lactamase inhibitor
Mycobacterium tuberculosis	Augmentin 250 mg three times a day
Moraxella catarrhalis	
Legionella species	+ Macrolide*
Endemic fungi	

*If *Legionella* is a concern (dosing in Table 12.2).

hospitalized patients with pneumonia ranged from 5% to 25%, and most of the deaths occurred within the first 7 days (1,7). Specific risk factors that suggest the need for hospitalization are shown in Table 12.1.

Pathogens common among patients with risk factors that require hospitalization include *S. pneumoniae*, *H. influenzae*, anaerobes, *Legionella* species, *S. aureus*, *C. pneumoniae*, and respiratory viruses. Less common in this setting are *M. pneumoniae*, *M. catarrhalis*, *M. tuberculosis*, and endemic fungi. The clinical symptoms of tuberculosis can be similar to those of severe pneumonia and should be considered in any patient admitted to the hospital with pneumonia (7). Alcoholism, neurologic disorders that may interfere with airway protection, and abnormalities of deglutition or esophageal motility predispose patients to aspiration.

Patients with Severe Community-Acquired Pneumonia

Severe community-acquired pneumonia is practically defined as having severe respiratory or hemodynamic complications. *S. pneumoniae* and *L. pneumophilia* are the most frequent causes of severe community-acquired pneumonia with *M. pneumoniae* being the third most common cause in some series (6). Mortality for severe community-acquired pneumonia is approximately 20% overall (5,19). Mortality is increased in those over 60 years of age and in patients with underlying illnesses (6). If severe pneumonia is suspected, admission to the intensive care unit should be considered. The following are indications of severe pneumonia (8).

1. Respiratory rate greater than 30/min
2. Respiratory failure defined by a $Pa{O_2}$/fraction of inspired oxygen ratio less than 250 mm Hg
3. Requirement of mechanical ventilation
4. Bilateral or multilobar involvement as seen on chest radiograph
5. An increase in infiltrate on chest radiography by 50% at 48 hours
6. Hypotension as defined by systolic blood pressure less than 90 mm Hg
7. Requirement of vasopressors for more than 4 hours
8. Oliguria (urine output <20 mL/hr) or acute renal failure

Treatment

In managing patients with community-acquired pneumonia, three principles should be followed.

1. Obtain all necessary specimens for appropriate bacteriologic cultures before antimicrobial therapy is begun so that there is a reasonable chance for determining pathologic agent.

2. Ensure that the drug therapy is as specific as possible, yet sufficiently broad to cover the common yet unsuspected microorganisms.

3. Tailor or change the antimicrobial coverage in several days if diagnostic tests identify the pathogen and drug susceptibilities.

Empiric treatment for suspected bacterial pneumonia should be directed against the most likely pathogens and should be started promptly after appropriate cultures are obtained. In all cases, knowledge of local epidemiology and resistance patterns should be used to modify the empiric treatment guidelines presented in Tables 12.2 through 12.5 where appropriate. Doses of antibiotics may need to be altered in individual patients. In choosing any antimicrobial, once the issues of efficacy and toxicity have been addressed, cost should then be considered.

Renal and hepatic metabolism are the main routes for elimination of the antimicrobial agents, and thus drug dosages may need to be changed if kidney or liver disease is present. Measurement of serum drug levels when available is especially helpful in these patients.

In addition to antimicrobial therapy, patients who require hospitalization require other forms of therapy. Adequate hydration in all patients is essential. Oxygen should be administered if hypoxemia ($Pa{O_2} <$ 60 mm Hg or O_2 saturation <90%) is present. Occasionally, intubation and mechanical ventilation are required. Antitussives are unnecessary unless persistent coughing exhausts the patient. Control of pleuritic pain may be achieved with anti-inflammatory agents, analgesics, or an intercostal nerve block. Bronchodilators are of significant help if bronchoconstriction is present. However, vibropercussion, postural drainage, mucolytic agents, or intermittent positive pressure breathing have not been shown to be beneficial in acute bacterial pneumonia in nonimmunocompromised hosts (20–22).

Duration of Therapy

There is surprisingly little information available in the literature to guide the duration of therapy (8). Generally, bacterial infections, such as *S. pneumoniae* pneumonia, should be treated for approximately 7 to 10 days. Pneumonia with *M. pneumoniae* and *C. pneumoniae* may need therapy for 10 to 14 days. Immunocompetent patients with *Legionella* pneumonia should be treated for 14 days of therapy; immunocompromised patients will need longer therapy. The severity of illness and comorbidities may require lengthening of antibiotic therapy. For outpatient treatment of pneumonia, some type of follow-up at 2 to 3 days is important.

Shorter courses of therapy may become available with the newer antibiotic agents. Azithromycin has an extremely long half-life and remains in the tissues longer. As a result, the treatment of pneumonia with

Table 12.4 Treatment of Pneumonia in Hospitalized Patients

Suspected Organisms	Empiric Treatment
Streptococcus pneumoniae	Cephalosporin – 2nd or 3rd generation*
Haemophilus influenzae	Cefuroxime 1.5 gm IV every 8 hr
Anaerobic bacteria	Cefotaxime 1–2 gm IV every 4–6 hr
Legionella species	Ceftriaxone 1–2 gm IV every 12–24 hr
Staphylococcus aureus	
Chlamydia pneumoniae	β-lactam/β-lactamase inhibitor
Respiratory viruses	Ticarcillin-clavulanate 3.1 gm IV every 4–8 hr
Miscellaneous	+ Macrolide[a]
Mycobacterium tuberculosis	
Mycoplasma pneumoniae	
Endemic fungi	
Moraxella catarrhalis	

* In penicillin allergic patients, trimethoprim-sulfamethoxazole plus a macrolide can be used.
[a] If *Legionella* is a concern (increase dose to 4.0 gm/day). Rifampicin (10 mg/kg/per day with maximum of 600 mg/day) may be added.

Table 12.5 Treatment of Severely Ill Hospitalized Patients with Community-Acquired Pneumonia

Suspected Organisms	Empiric Treatment
Streptococcus pneumoniae *Haemophilus influenzae* Anaerobic bacteria Aerobic gram-negative bacilli *Legionella* species *Staphylococcus aureus* *Chlamydia pneumoniae* Respiratory viruses Miscellaneous *Mycobacterium tuberculosis* *Mycoplasma pneumoniae* Endemic fungi *Moraxella catarrhalis*	Cephalosporin–3rd generation* Cefotaxime 1 gm IV every 8 hr Ceftriaxone 1 gm IV every 12 hr Imipenem-cilastatin 500 mg IV every 6 hr + Aminoglycoside[a] Gentamicin 3–5 mg/kg/per day (every 8 hr) Tobramycin 3–5 mg/kg/per day (every 8 hr) + Macrolide[b] Vancomycin 1 gm every 12 hr[c]

* In penicillin allergic patients, ciprofloxacin 750 mg PO twice a day or 400 mg IV every 12 hr can be used.
[a] Due to high mortality associated with *Pseudomonas aeruginosa* infections, and aminoglycoside should be added at least for the first few days of therapy.
[b] Rifampicin may be added if *Legionella* species suspected.
[c] Vancomycin should be added if methacillin-resistant *S. aureus* is possible.

azithromycin may be shortened to 5 days (23,24). However, the serum levels of azithromycin achieved are not high enough to treat bacteremic patients. Thus, azithromycin should not be used when bacteremia is suspected or in patients who require hospitalization for their pneumonia.

In hospitalized patients receiving IV therapy, the conversion to oral therapy is somewhat arbitrary. A reasonable guideline is to begin oral therapy once the patient's clinical condition has stabilized and fever has resolved (8).

It is essential to follow the patient's response to therapy and be alerted to complications or clinical deterioration. When effective antimicrobial therapy is initiated, some improvement in clinical condition is expected within the first 72 hours (8). Fever may persist for up to a week, but usually resolves within the first 4 days (25). Leukocytosis usually resolves by the fourth day (8). It is not uncommon for the chest radiograph to worsen initially after therapy is started, with progression of the infiltrate or development of a pleural effusion (8). If clinical improvement is noted, mild worsening in the infiltrate or development of a small effusion has little significance and it is acceptable to watch the condition closely for continued improvement. However, if radiographic deterioration occurs in the absence of clinical improvement or in association with severe community-acquired pneumonia, this is highly predictive of mortality (6). Inadequate antimicrobial therapy or other complications need to be considered.

Resolution of Radiographic Abnormalities

Chest radiograph abnormalities clear slowly and only 60% of patients with *S. pneumoniae* pneumonia will have normal chest x-rays at 4 weeks (26). In general, the older the patient and the more preexisting conditions that are present, the slower the chest radiograph will resolve. A chest radiograph should be obtained approximately 6 weeks after discharge from the hospital to evaluate the rate of resolution. Infiltrates persisting for more than 3 months should be referred for possible bronchoscopy.

If the patient is not improving or clinically deteriorating, a repeat chest radiograph should be obtained to determine presence of pleural effusion. If an effusion is present, pleural fluid should be sampled, analyzed, and cultured to rule out an empyema. The presence of an empyema requires chest tube drainage. Other possible causes for the lack of clinical improvement include:

1. Inadequate antimicrobial selection
2. Unusual pathogens
3. Noninfectious causes of illness

Secondary bacterial infection following a viral pneumonia or superinfection occurring after broad-spectrum antimicrobial therapy may cause fever and worsening of the patient's condition; thus reculturing sputum and blood is necessary when patients do not respond to empiric therapy. Accumulation of secretions or a mucous plug can obstruct an airway, leading to partial collapse of a lung lobe or segment. Vigorous postural drainage and endotracheal suctions may remove secretions and help re-expand the lung portion. Bronchoscopy may be useful for identifying unusual organisms and drug-resistant pathogens, although the identification of usual pathogens in patients receiving antibiotics is rarely possible (12). Bronchoscopy, even in the presence of antibiotics, may be helpful in identifying *Legionella* species, *M. tuberculosis*, *P. carinii*, and anaerobes (12). Bronchoscopy is also useful in detecting bronchial obstruction that may be seen in bronchogenic carcinoma or aspiration of foreign objects.

Patients who remain ill despite antimicrobial therapy may have complications of pneumonia. Metastatic infections that must be considered in the setting of pneumonia include meningitis, arthritis, endocarditis, pericarditis, peritonitis, and empyema. If the patient has developed sepsis syndrome from pneumonia, the chest radiograph and clinical course may deteriorate as a result of adult respiratory distress syndrome. If a patient remains ill or deteriorates clinically, computed tomography scanning of the chest may reveal the presence of unsuspected collections of pleural fluid, multiple lung nodules, or cavitation within a lung infiltrate. Ventilation–perfusion scanning or pulmonary arteriogram should be considered if the patient is at risk of pulmonary embolus. Although the use of serologic testing is not indicated routinely, in patients who fail to respond to antibiotics, serologic tests for *Legionella* species, *M. pneumoniae*, viral agents, and endemic fungi may be useful at this point. If all diagnostic tests are unrevealing and the patient is clinically deteriorating, then open-lung biopsy may be indicated.

Drug allergy causing mild blood eosinophilia and lingering fever is a frequent and often unsuspected complication that requires discontinuation or substitution in the antibiotic regimen. This complication should be considered if fever persists after clinical and radiologic improvement.

Pneumonia in Pregnancy

Pneumonia is uncommon in the pregnant patient, occurring at an incidence of less than 1% (20). However, pneumonia in pregnancy is of significant concern because respiratory failure in these patients approaches 20% (27). Pregnant patients with coexistent disease such as COPD, multiple sclerosis, myasthenia gravis, or asthma are at increased risk for pneumonia.

The diagnosis of pneumonia in pregnancy is based on history and physical findings and corroborated by chest radiograph as in the nonpregnant patient. The onset of infection and the pathogens encountered in community-acquired pneumonia are also similar. However, there is an increased problem of developing aspiration pneumonia in pregnancy (20). Because of the physiologic changes that the gastrointestinal tract undergoes in pregnancy, gastric emptying is delayed and the gastroesophageal sphincter tone is decreased, which leads to an increased risk of aspiration. The most likely time for aspiration is at the time of induction or when emerging from general anesthesia. Limiting oral intake to essential medications once labor has begun or aspiration of stomach contents via a nasogastric tube has been advocated to minimize the risk of aspiration during delivery. Once aspiration has occurred, there is usually a delay of 6 to 8 hours before the occurrence of bronchospasm, tachycardia, tachypnea, and the appearance of a new radiographic infiltrate.

It is important that prompt and effective therapy be instituted in pregnant patients with pneumonia from any cause to reduce the maternal and perinatal morbidity. Treatment is supportive, with oxygen and mechanical ventilation, if needed. Because of the characteristics of the oxygen dissociation curve of hemoglobin, relatively little change in the amount of oxygen delivered to the fetus will occur until the oxygen saturation of hemoglobin drops below 90% (Pa_{O_2} approximately 60 mm Hg). It seems reasonable, therefore, to attempt to maintain an oxygen tension at greater than 60 to 70 mm Hg. Hypercapnia is generally

Box 12.1 Antimicrobial Agents to Avoid Using in Pregnant Patients

Ciprofloxacin
Ofloxacin
Doxycycline
Tetracycline
Trimethoprim-sulfamethoxazole
(at term)

not a significant problem unless respiratory muscle fatigue or other underlying disease plays a role in decreasing the ability of the patient to ventilate adequately.

Treatment with antibiotics is similar in pregnant patients, but many antimicrobials should be avoided (Box 12.1). Although no antibiotic is known to be completely safe in pregnancy, the penicillins and cephalosporins are used most often. Tetracycline and the quinolones are specifically contraindicated in pregnancy, and the sulfonamides and aminoglycosides should be used cautiously. Dosages of most antimicrobials should be increased to compensate for an increased maternal volume of distribution in pregnancy. Additionally, most antibiotics will appear in breast milk and should be used with caution in patients who are breast-feeding.

In pregnancy particularly, pulmonary embolism must be in the differential diagnosis of pneumonia. Factors predisposing to pulmonary embolism in pregnancy include venous stasis, immobilization, and a state of hypercoagulability. Pulmonary embolism complicates approximately 1 in every 2000 pregnancies, causing approximately one quarter to one half of all obstetric morbidity and mortality.

REFERENCES

1. Bates JH, Campbell GD, Barron AL, et al. Microbial etiology of acute pneumonia in hospitalized patients. Chest 1992;101:1005–1012.

2. Fang D, Fine M, Orloff J, et al. New and emerging etiologies for community-acquired pneumonia with implication for therapy; a prospective multicenter study of 359 cases. Medicine 1990;69:307–316.

3. Marrie TJ, Durant H, Yates L. Community-acquired pneumonia requiring hospitalization: 5-year prospective study. Rev Infect Dis 1989;11:586–599.

4. Woodhead MA, MacFarlane JT, McCracken JS, et al. Prospective study of the aetiology and outcome of pneumonia in the community. Lancet 1987;1:671–674.

5. Ortqvist A, Sterner G, Nilsson JA. Severe community-acquired pneumonia: factors influencing need of intensive care treatment and prognosis. Scand J Infect Dis 1985;17:377–386.

6. Torres A, Serra-Battles J, Ferrer A, et al. Severe community-acquired pneumonia: epidemiology and prognostic factors. Am Rev Respir Dis 1991;144:312–318.

7. Pachon J, Prados MD, Capote F, et al. Severe community-acquired pneumonia: etiology, prognosis, and treatment. Am Rev Respir Dis 1990;142:369–373.

8. Society AT. Guidelines for the initial management of adults with community-acquired pneumonia: diagnosis, assessment of severity, and intial antimicrobial therapy. Am Rev Respir Dis 1993;148: 1418–1426.

9. Rein MF, Gwaltney JM Jr, O'Brein WM, et al. Accuracy of Gram's stain in identifying pneumonocci in sputum. JAMA 1978;239:2671–2673.

10. Boerner DF, Zwadyk P. The value of the sputum Gram's stain in community-acquired pneumonia. JAMA 1982;247:642–645.

11. Torres A, Puig del la Bellacasa J, Xaubet A. Diagnostic value of quantitative cultures of bronchoalveolar lavage and telescoping plugged catheters in mechanically ventilated patients with pneumonia. Am Rev Respir Dis 1989;85:499–506.

12. Ortqvist A, Kalin M, Lejdebron L, Lundberg B. Diagnostic fiberoptic bronchoscopy and protected brush culture in patients with community-acquired pneumonia. Chest 1990;97:576–582.

13. Venkatesan P. Gladman J, MacFarlane JT. A hospital study of community-acquired pneumonia. Etiology, prognosis, and treatment. Thorax 1990;45:254–258.

14. Zavala D, Schoell JC. Ultrathin needle aspiration of the lung in infections and malignant diseases. Am Rev Respir Dis 1981;123:125–131.

15. Katzenstein A-LA, Askin FB. Surgical pathology of non-neoplastic lung disease. In: Bennington JL, ed. Major problems in pathology; vol. 13. Philadelphia: WB Saunders, 1982.

16. Fine MJ, Smith DN, Singer DE. Hospitalization decision in patients with community-acquired pneumo-

nia: a prospective cohort study. Am J Med 1990;89:713–721.

17. Mandell LA, Niederman M, Group TCCAPCC. Antimicrobial treatment of community acquired pneumonia in adults: a conference report. Can J Infect Dis 1993;4:25–28.

18. Wennberg JE, McPherson K, Caper P. Will payment based on diagnostic related groups control hospital costs? N Engl J Med 1984;311:295–300.

19. Ruiz-Santana S, Garcia A, Esteban E. ICU pneumonias: a multi-institutional study. Crit Care Med 1987;15:930–932.

20. Maccato M. Respiratory insufficiency due to pneumonia in pregnancy. Obstet Gynecol Clin North Am 1991;18:289–299.

21. Britton S, Bejstedt M, Bedin L. Chest physiotherapy in primary pneumonia. Br Med J 1985;290:1703–1704.

22. Rossing TH. Supportive measures in the treatment of pneumonia. In: Pennington JE, ed. Respiratory infections: diagnosis and management, 2nd ed. New York: Raven Press, 1988:455–460.

23. Schonwald S, Gunjaca M, Kolacny-Babic L, et al. A comparison of azithromycin and erythromycin in the treatment of atypical pneumonias. J Antimicrob Chemother 1990;25(suppl A):123–126.

24. Kinasewitz G. Wood RG. Azithromycin versus cefaclor in the treatment of acute bacterial pneumonia. Eur J Clin Microbiol Infect Dis 1991;10:872–877.

25. Lehtomaki K. Clinical diagnosis of pneumococcal, adenoviral, mycoplasmal and mixed pneumonias in young men. Eur Respir J 1988;1:324–329.

26. Jay SJ, Hohanson WG, Pierce AK. The radiologic resolution of *Streptococcus pneumoniae* pneumonia. N Engl J Med 1975;293:798–801.

27. Madinger NE, Greenspoon JS, Ellrodt AG. Pneumonia during pregnancy: has modern technology improved maternal and fetal outcome? Am J Obstet Gynecol 1989;161:657–662.

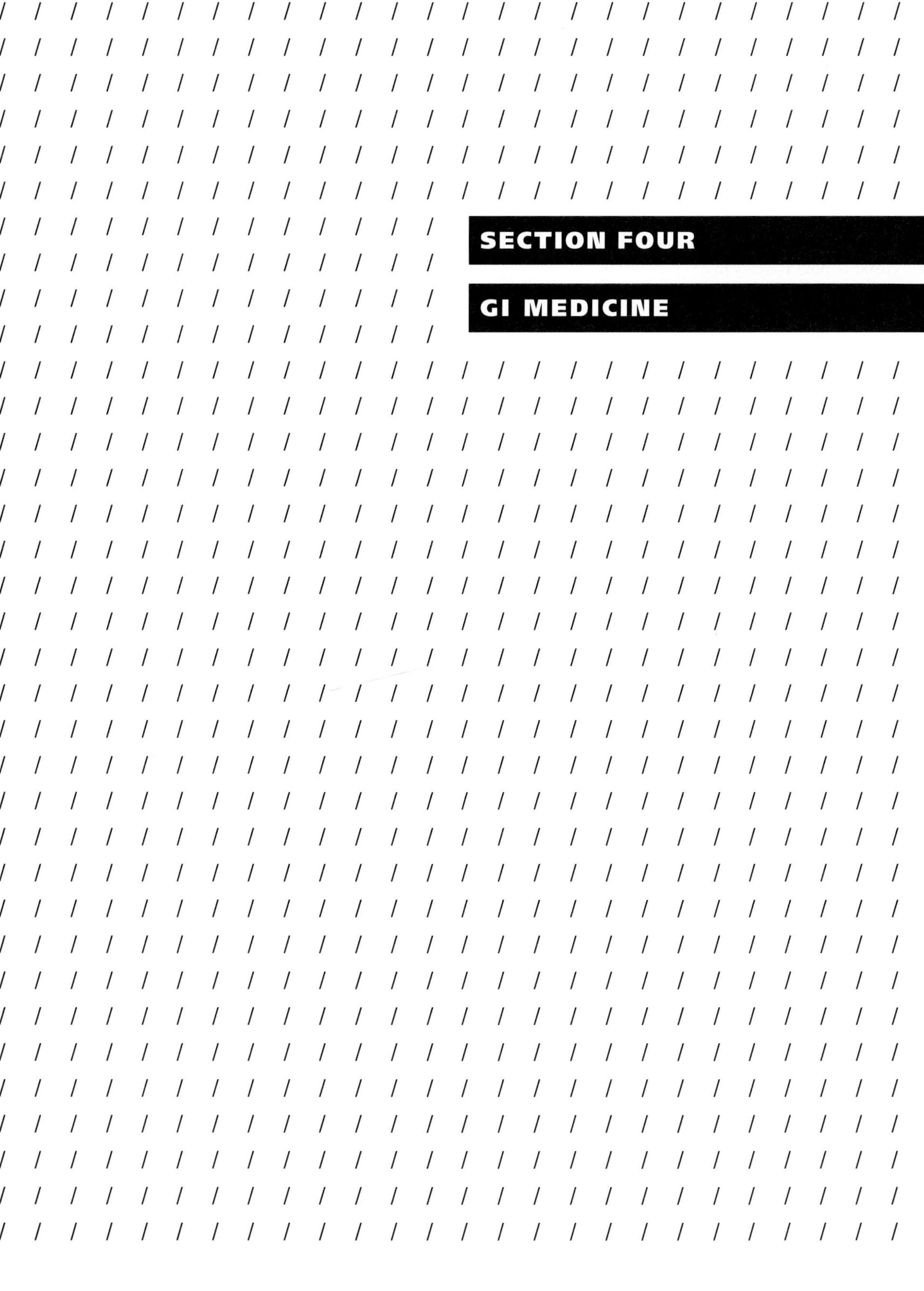

SECTION FOUR

GI MEDICINE

CHAPTER 13

BOWEL DYSFUNCTION

Richard E. Blackwell

The primary care physician is often faced with a patient who presents with complaints of abdominal pain, bloating, diarrhea, constipation, and other associated symptoms that may be of a cyclic, intermittent, or continuous nature. At times these patients will have been subjected to a variety of different therapies and now may be chronically medicated, compounding and masking the primary issues. Further, these patients may be under a great deal of stress, practice continuous or intermittent weight control through altered eating habits, and consume large quantities of liquids containing sugar substitutes (1,2). There is a definite sex difference in disease prevalence with women having greater instances of spastic colon, constipation, diverticulitis, chronic ileitis and colitis, cholecystitis, and gallstones. All of these entities will be considered in this or other chapters. Further, because women are unique carriers of endometriosis and function in a fluctuating milieu of sex steroids, a systematic discussion of this general topic will be carried out with reference to chronic pain syndromes and endometriosis as it affects bowel function.

Diarrhea

Diarrhea is one of the most common presenting symptoms in any society and the average adult generally has one or more episodes per year. These attacks generally last less than 2 days, are associated with three or more loose stools, and may be accompanied by discomfort, bloating, urgency, or fecal incontinence (3). Diarrhea is usually associated with either increased intestinal fluid secretion, increased bowel motility, or decreased fluid absorption. Any mechanism that would alter small (80%) or large (19%) bowel absorption can produce diarrhea.

Causes of Diarrhea

The etiology of diarrhea can be classified under the following headings: infection, inflammation, malabsorption, endocrine dysfunction, disorders of motility, and drug intake. The most common causes of acute diarrhea would be infection with rota virus, common traveler's diarrhea with enterotoxigenic *Escherichia coli*, *Salmonella*, *Shigella*, or *Campylobacter jejune*. These organisms produce mucosal inflammation with rota virus and *E. coli* being noninvasive, *Salmonella*, *Shigella*, *E. coli* and *Campylobacter* being invasive. If unprocessed or contaminated water has been consumed, one must be concerned with small bowel-initiated diarrhea caused by *Vibro cholerae* or *Giardia lamblia*, or large bowel invasive infection with *Entamoeba histolytica*. Sexually transmitted diseases from *Chlamydia trachomatis* or *Neisseria gonorrhoeae* may infect the rectum, resulting in invasion of tissue and diarrhea. Finally, food poisoning (toxin ingestion) occurs with *Staphylococcus aureus* infections, *Bacillus cereus*, *Clostridium perfringens* and *Clostridium botulinum* infections. Rarely, the invasion of small bowel with mycobacteria and tuberculosis can result in either acute or chronic diarrhea; however, these individuals, like those who present with tuberculosis pelvic inflammatory disease, have a pulmonary etiology.

A number of drugs commonly cause diarrhea including alcohol, lactulose, various laxatives, magnesium-containing antacids, and commonly consumed nonsteroidal anti-inflammatory drugs. In addition, various antibiotics, digitalis, colchicine, quinidine, theophylline, various bile salts, and prostaglandins released during normal menstruation can cause either chronic or acute diarrhea.

Inflammatory bowel disease such as ulcerative colitis or Crohn's disease, motility disorders such as the irritable bowel syndrome, the narcotic bowel, and postvagotomy and postgastrectomy syndromes can result in diarrhea.

Malabsorption can result from bacterial overgrowth, radiation enteritis, enteric fistulas, ileal resections, short bowel syndrome, disaccharidase deficiency, and pancreatic insufficiency.

Finally, various endocrine disorders such as diabetic neuropathies of the bowel, hyper- and hypothyroidism, Zollinger-Ellison syndrome, and carcinoids can be responsible for the occurrence of diarrhea (4–7).

Evaluation of Diarrhea

During the history and physical, questions should be directed at stool volume and frequency; the duration of diarrhea; whether fever, weight loss, or dehydration accompanies the syndrome; and whether blood is detected in the stool. Questions should be directed at foreign travel; whether alcohol or diet drinks are consumed; whether the diarrhea occurs cyclically with menstruation; and whether patients have an accompanying history of bowel surgery, inflammatory bowel disease, or endocrine disorders. In general, if the diarrhea is of an acute nature with no blood in the stool it will be self-limited. If blood is present, the stool should be evaluated for white and red blood cells (8). Also, stool cultures, stool for ova and parasite, and perhaps sigmoidoscopy should be performed (9).

In the case of chronic diarrhea in patients with no obvious etiology, the stool should be evaluated for ova and parasites and the patient should be referred for gastrointestinal evaluation and perhaps sigmoidoscopy (Plate 1A,B) (10).

Management of Diarrhea

Acute diarrhea can usually be treated by adequate rehydration and avoidance of the usual diet. Replacement fluids include products like Gatorade, decaffeinated soft drinks, and various types of soups and broths. In addition, over-the-counter diarrhea agents such as Kallin, Imodium AD, or Pepto-Bismol may be used. For the more severe forms of diarrhea with some element of dehydration, the oral intake of compounds that contain sugar or amino acids will enhance absorption of water through the small intestine. Solutions are available such as Pedialyte and Rehydralite. Not infrequently, rehydration has to be carried out by parenteral means. Antidiarrheal agents include the opioids, which act on the mu and possibly lambda receptors of enteric neurons. This increases gastrointestinal contraction but disrupts aboral peristaltic movements, therefore increasing transit time. They should be avoided in patients with ulcerative colitis, colitis, and amoebic dysentery; they can induce toxic megacolon. The mainstay of antidiarrheal therapy consists of diphenoxylate, usually combined with atropine; Lomotil (diphenoxylate 2.5 mg and atropine sulfate 25 μg) administered in doses ranging from 5–20 mg/day should usually stop moderate diarrhea. Loperamide (Imodium) is available in 2-mg capsules or in liquid form 1 mg/5 mL. This is administered in doses of 4–8 mg/day with a maximum of 16 mg/day. This compound is a piperidine opioid, which is primarily secreted in the feces.

For infections of the gastrointestinal tract causing diarrhea, the following antimicrobials are recommended: erythromycin 250 mg PO four times a day for 5 days for *C. jejune* and metronidazole 250 mg PO four times a day for 7 days for *Clostridium difficile*. Trimethomprim-sulfamethoxazole 160–800 mg PO twice daily for 5 days may be used for treatment of either *Salmonella* or *Shigellosis*. Tetracycline 250 mg PO four times a day for 5 to 7 days may be used to treat for *V. cholera*. Metronidazole 250 PO three times a day for 7 days eradicates *G. lamblia*, and quinacrine 100 mg PO three times a day for 5 days is effective against *E. histolytica*.

Factitious Diarrhea

At times, the diagnosis of diarrhea will be unclear and the treatment results unpredictable (11). The clinician should consider the possibility of factitious diarrhea. In this situation patients have been known to dilute their stool samples. This is detected by measuring stool osmolality, which is usually found to be considerably lower than plasma. The diagnosis is usually confirmed by the finding of normal stool osmolality when defecation is supervised and when colonic content is sampled endoscopically. Individuals who present with factitious diarrhea often exhibit many of the clinical characteristics found in variance of Munchausen's syndrome. In general, they undergo extensive evaluation, have been treated with potentially harmful therapies, and insist that they have not diluted their stool samples. Confronted with analytic findings, they request no further therapy.

Constipation

Constipation affects 1 in every 50 individuals. It is generally defined by the rule of threes: more than three stools a day is diarrhea and fewer than three stools per week is constipation. It is more common in women, it affects whites less than nonwhites, and occurs more frequently in individuals over age 65.

Etiology of Constipation

Although the lack of fiber might be suspected as the cause for constipation, the following will result in this condition: certain medications; metabolic and endocrine disorders; various neurologic disorders such as Parkinson's disease; stroke; multiple sclerosis; syphilis; and gastrointestinal disorders such as obstruction, irritable bowel syndrome, diverticular disease, rectocele, rectal prolapse, and anal stenosis or fissure (12).

Medications

The following medications are associated with constipation: analgesics—particularly those containing opiates, iron or heavy metals, calcium channel blockers, verapamil, barium sulfate, various antacids, antiparkinson agents, antihypertensives, anticonvulsives, anticholinergics, and antidepressants.

Metabolic Disorders

Diabetes and hypothyroidism are perhaps the most common endocrinopathies associated with constipation. Some 80% of patients with diabetes have either autonomic or peripheral neuropathy. In addition, hypothyroidism can be associated with the formation of megacolon.

Neurological Disorders

Disorders of bowel function are frequently associated with diseases of the central nervous system. Ten percent of patients with Parkinson's disease have constipation and about 40% of those with multiple sclerosis have bowel dysfunction as well. In addition, neurologic and bowel diseases often meet in the neuromuscular disorders that can affect the myenteric plexus causing constipation and Hirschsprung's disease in which there is an absence of ganglion cells in the distal colon.

Gastrointestinal Disorders

In the patient over 40 years of age with a history of the recent onset of constipation associated with hematochezia, a family history of colon or rectal cancer, and weight loss, one must consider colon carcinoma (Plate 2) (13–15). Further, 50% of patients over age 65 with diverticular disease present with constipation and the most common gastrointestinal disorder associated with constipation is the irritable bowel syndrome with a marked predilection toward women under the age of 35. These individuals have a disorder of gastric motility, pass hard stools, and have bloating and abdominal pain. Half the women who present with this symptom complex have a problem with somatization, anxiety disorders, and depression.

Evaluation of Constipation

The history and physical should focus on dietary habits and drug intake along with family history of endocrine or neurologic disorders and cancer. Anorectal and perineal examinations should be carried out to rule out enterocele, rectocele, rectal prolapse, anal fissures, or hemorrhoids. Rectal examination should be carried out in an attempt to detect rectal masses. It is suggested that a Hemoccult, complete blood count, and tyroid-stimulating hormone be determined as well and in selective patients evaluation of electrolytes, serum calcium, and a fasting blood glucose. Severe forms of constipation should have further examination including a barium enema and flexible sigmoidoscopy.

Treatment of Constipation

Following a negative evaluation it is suggested that treatment be focused in several areas; dietary fiber should be increased to a level of 20 to 30 gm/day. This would be about the equivalent of 1 cup of bran cereal or 2 tablespoonsful of psyllium for a month. In addition, patients should increase the intake of fruits, vegetables, soy, pectin, cellulose or corn; dairy products such as cheese, ice cream and milk should be avoided, and fluid intake should be substantially increased. Bowel habit training should be begun in that patients should schedule time for bowel movements, generally after food intake. Patients who do not respond to this initial management should be referred to a subspecialist for evaluation with barium enema, sigmoidoscopy, perhaps anorectal manometry, electromyography, and perhaps rectal biopsy.

Functional Bowel Disease and Chronic Pain

There is frequently association between vague abdominal pain, bloating, and bowel dysfunction. These disorders have a psychological overtone and frequently occur in young women practicing weight control. It is estimated that 40% to 50% of acute abdominal pain is nonspecific and one might suspect that gas or stool passing through the intestine rapidly might be the etiology of this pain. Irritable bowel syndrome is certainly the most common cause of chronic abdominal pain, which generally is located to the hypogastric and periumbilical area and may be associated with constipation, change in consistency of stool, bloating, and intermittent constipation (16,17). Although depression can be associated with irritable bowel syndrome, it may be associated with a variety of other conditions including endometriosis.

The association of endometriosis with bowel symptoms deserves special comment because this condition also often is unrecognized and goes undiagnosed. The patients with endometriosis involving either the small or large bowel, uterosacral ligaments or cul-de-sac, will frequently present with either constipation or diarrhea that is cyclic in nature (Plates 3 and 4). In general, it follows the typical presentation of endometriosis with the onset occurring just before menses and ending as flow decreases. At times implants on the colon may cause chronic constipation as well. In the patient who presents with bowel complaints, particularly in association with interior thigh pain, accompanying menstruation, or cyclic dysuria that cannot be attributed to a urinary tract infection, endometriosis should be suspected and ruled out with diagnostic laparoscopy. Frequently these patients are approached with sigmoidoscopy, which almost invariably is reported as being negative. This usually follows the detection of blood in the stool with Hemoccult examination. However, it is suggested that care be taken in interpreting the Hemoccult results and that it be repeated after the patient has been cautioned not to eat red meats for several days or take iron supplements. In addition, when carrying out a rectovaginal examination after bimanual examination, gloves should be changed to avoid transferring menses to the Hemoccult card.

The failure to diagnose and adequately treat irritable bowel syndrome associated with endometriosis or not can often lead to the development of chronic pain syndrome (18,19). These individuals generally take multiple medications including analgesics, anxiolytics, and hypnotics. They will frequently have undergone multiple surgical procedures; will show signs of drug dependence, depression, inappropriate affect, inappropriate limitation of activity; and will invariably have seen a large number of physicians previously. These patients will have a history of both eating disturbances, either stringent appetite control or gorging, and generally have problems with insomnia. These patients have a marginal pain tolerance and have adopted the sick role. At times this is reinforced by friends and family as well as the medical system and patients derive positive reinforcement and secondary gain from these experiences. The best approach to dealing with these patients is a careful history and physical examination and review of previous tests. If the evaluations have been appropriate and no evidence of serious disease is detected, little is to be gained by further diagnostics. It should be emphasized that the work-up of these patients, however difficult, should be thorough and if need be, extensive. However, once a diagnosis is established, sedative, hypnotic, and narcotic treatment should be withdrawn even if inpatient detoxification is necessary. They may be treated with a tricyclic antidepressant such as amitriptyline to facilitate sleep. Both the patient and her family members should be involved in psychological counseling. She should be part of a pain management program. An exercise program and an adequate diet should be prescribed. Physical therapy and transcutaneous electrical stimulation may also be used as adjunct therapy. The ultimate goal of this form of therapy should be to *eliminate* the *sick role* and restore the patient to both psychological and physical function. This may or may not involve resolution of the pain, but assist the patient in placing it into proper perspective.

REFERENCES

1. Oster JR, Materson BJ, Rogers AI. Laxative abuse syndrome. Am J Gastroenterol 1980;74:451–458.

2. Fine KD, Santa Ana CA, Fordtran JS. Diagnosis of magnesium-induced diarrhea. N Engl J Med 1991;324:1012–1017.

3. Afzalpurkar RG, Schiller LR, Little KH, et al. The self-limited nature of chronic idiopathic diarrhea. N Engl J Med 1992;327:1849–1852.

4. Toskes PP. Malabsorption. In: Wyngaarden JB, Smith LH Jr, Bennett JC, eds. Cecil texbook of medicine. Philadelphia: WB Saunders, 1988:687–699.

5. Powell DW. Approach to the patient with diarrhea. In: Kelley WN, DeVita VT, Dupont HL, et al., eds. Textbook of internal medicine. 2nd ed. Philadelphia: JB Lippincott, 1992:620–628.

6. Brownlee HJ, ed. Symposium on management of acute nonspecific diarrhea. Am J Med 1990;88(6A):1S–37S.

7. Fine KD, Krejs GJ, Fordtran JS. Diarrhea. In: Sleisenger MH, Fordtran JS, eds. Gastrointestinal disease: pathophysiology/diagnosis/management. 5th ed.; vol. 2. Philadelphia: WB Saunders, 1993:1043–1072.

8. Knight KK, Fielding JE, Battista RN. Occult blood screening for colorectal cancer. JAMA 1989;261:587–593.

9. DuBois D, Binder L, Nelson B. Usefulness of the stool Wright's stain in the emergency department. J Emerg Med 1988;6:483–486.

10. Selby JV, Friedman GD. Sigmoidoscopy in the periodic health examination of asymptomatic adults. JAMA 1989;261:595–601.

11. Topazian M, Binder HJ. Brief report: factitious diarrhea detected by measurement of stool osmolality. N Engl J Med 1994;330:1418–1419.

12. Johanson JF, Sonnenberg A, Koch TR. Clinical epidemiology of chronic constipation. J Clin Gastroenterol 1989;11:525–536.

13. Clayman CB. Mass screening for colorectal cancer: are we ready yet? JAMA 1989;261:609.

14. Eddy DM. Screening for colorectal cancer. Ann Intern Med 1990;113:373–384.

15. Frame PS. Screening flexible sigmoidoscopy: is it worthwhile? An opposing view. J Fam Pract 1987;25:604–607.

16. Freidman G. Treatment of the irritable syndrome. Gastroenterol Clin North Am 1991;20:325–334.

17. Klein KB. Controlled treatment trials in the irritable bowel syndrome: a critique. Gastroenterology 1988;95:232–241.

18. Bonica JJ. General considerations of choronic pain. In: Bonica JJ, ed. The management of pain. Philadelphia: Lea & Febiger, 1990:180–196.

19. Cardenas DD, Eagan KJ. Management of chronic pain. In: Kottle FJ, Stillwell GK, Lehmann JF, eds. Krusen's handbook of physical medicine and rehabilitation. 4th ed. Philadelphia: WB Saunders, 1990:1162–1168.

CHAPTER 14

BILIARY TRACT AND GALLBLADDER DISEASE

William G. Blackard, Jr.,
Todd H. Baron

Although gallstone disease is the most common disorder affecting the biliary system, a number of other disorders also affect the biliary tract (Box 14.1). Gallstones commonly affect women during their reproductive years, whereas other diseases involving the biliary tree occur over a broader age range. Numerous diagnostic tests are available to evaluate biliary diseases, and it is important for the clinician to understand their limitations and benefits to efficiently diagnose and treat patients with these disorders. A large variety of treatment modalities are also available depending on the diagnosis; however, endoscopic retrograde cholangiopancreatography (ERCP), because it can be both diagnostic and therapeutic, is becoming the preferred procedure for biliary disease.

Gallstone Disease

Gallstones are the most prevalent disease involving the biliary system. Approximately 20 million Americans have gallstones, resulting in more than 500,000 cholecystectomies each year in the United States, and the majority of these patients are women, because approximately 35% of women have developed gallstones by the age of 75.

Asymptomatic Cholelithiasis

The majority of patients with gallstones are asymptomatic. Several studies have demonstrated that patients with asymptomatic cholelithiasis remain without symptoms for prolonged periods of time (1). The incidence of new-onset biliary colic is approximately 15% at 10 years and 18% at 20 years from diagnosis. Complications of gallstones (see below) rarely occur without a previous attack of pain.

Symptomatic Cholelithiasis

Biliary Colic

The most common presentation of symptomatic gallstones is biliary colic. It is important to be able to recognize the pain of biliary colic because abdominal pain or nonspecific symptoms ascribed to gallstones may subject the patient to surgical therapy without gratifying results (Box 14.2). Conversely, biliary colic should not be dismissed when the location of the pain is not in the right upper quadrant. Biliary colic is a visceral pain resulting from transient obstruction of the cystic duct by a stone. Thus, the pain is most commonly located in the epigastrium and less frequently in the right upper quadrant, left upper quadrant, precordium, and lower abdomen. The pain, not truly colic, is episodic and severe. It may be precipitated by a large meal, but, contrary to popular belief, high-fat meals do not necessarily precipitate an attack. In fact, no specific type of food reproducibly creates an episode of colic. The pain has a sudden onset, rapidly worsens, reaching a steady plateau and lasting up to 3 hours. Pain may radiate to the interscapular region or right shoulder. Accompanying symptoms may include nausea, vomiting, and sweating. The interval between attacks is variable and may be weeks, months, or years.

Acute Cholecystitis

When obstruction of the cystic duct by stones is prolonged, acute inflammation of the gallbladder occurs. The pain of acute cholecystitis generally lasts longer that 3 hours and localizes to the right upper quadrant because the parietal peritoneum is irritated by the inflammatory process. Associated fever, nausea, and vomiting are common.

Box 14.1 Diseases Affecting the Biliary System

Gallstone diseases
- Biliary colic
- Acute cholecystitis

Common bile duct stones
- Cholangitis
- Pancreatitis

Primary sclerosing cholangitis

Bile duct tumors
- Gallbladder
- Cholangiocarcinoma
- Metastatic disease

Box 14.2 Symptoms Not Attributable to Gallstone Disease

Belching
Bloating
Fatty food intolerance
Chronic pain

Common Bile Duct Stones

Gallstones passing into the common bile duct from the gallbladder may pass spontaneously into the duodenum or remain in the common bile duct. These stones may obstruct the flow of bile into the duodenum resulting in jaundice and infection of the biliary tree (cholangitis). Obstruction to the flow of pancreatic secretions may also occur because the pancreatic duct exits the duodenum through a common channel with the bile duct (Fig 14.1). This results in gallstone pancreatitis, the most common cause of pancreatitis (2).

Differential Diagnosis

The clinical symptoms of biliary tract disorders are not highly specific and may be difficult to distinguish from a number of other disorders. Other disease processes that should be considered when a patient presents with "biliary colic" include peptic ulcer disease, gastroesophageal reflux disease, nephrolithiasis, irritable bowel syndrome, cardiac disorders, and acute intermittent porphyria.

Similarly, the differential diagnosis in a patient presenting with acute cholecystitis is quite broad, including other intra-abdominal infections or inflammatory processes such as acute appendicitis, acute pancreatitis, and perforated peptic ulcer.

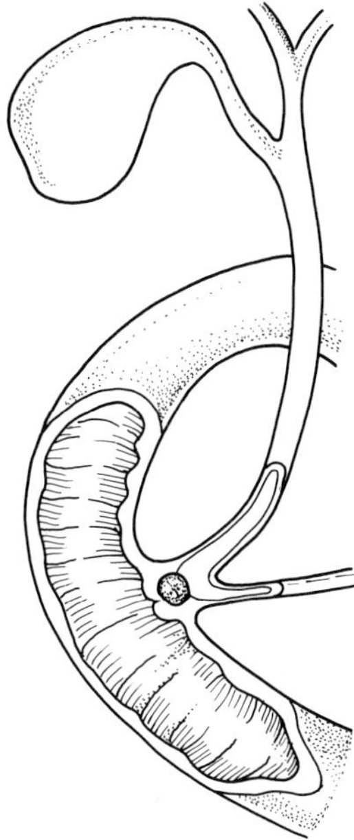

Fig 14.1 Obstruction to the common channel of the common bile duct and the pancreatic duct.

Pancreatitis should be suspected in any patient presenting with abdominal pain associated with nausea and vomiting. The pain of pancreatitis is typically epigastric in nature and boring in quality; it characteristically radiates straight through to the back. When gallstones are the etiology of pancreatitis, there is usually no history or minimal history of alcohol use. Additionally, a history of previous biliary colic can usually be elicited. Finally, abnormalities in the liver profile such as hyperbilirubinemia, elevated transaminases, and alkaline phosphatase are seen. The differential diagnosis of pancreatitis includes a perforated viscus, bowel obstruction, mesentery ischemia/infarction, and cholecystitis and cholangitis.

Pathogenesis of Gallstones

In the United States and other western countries, cholesterol is the predominate component in over 75% of gallstones (3). These stones result from supersaturation of bile with cholesterol and crystal formation. Crystals in turn develop into stones. Causes of cholesterol-saturated bile include an increase in cholesterol secretion, a decrease in bile secretion, or both. Increased cholesterol secretion is seen in advancing age, obesity, and estrogen replacement. Decreased bile acid secretion is seen in terminal ileal diseases (Crohn's disease) and prolonged fasting (total parenteral nutrition).

Noncholesterol stones, which consist of calcium salts of bilirubin, are classified as black or brown pigment stones. Black pigment stones are more common in patients with cirrhosis or chronic hemolytic conditions such as thalassemia and sickle cell disease. Brown pigment stones commonly originate in the bile duct, are associated with infection, and usually are seen in Asians.

Pregnancy promotes the development of cholesterol gallstones by increasing cholesterol saturation of bile secondary to estrogens and decreasing gallbladder emptying due to progesterone (4). Ultrasound studies have demonstrated increased fasting and residual gallbladder volumes beginning late in the first trimester and increasing linearly throughout the second trimester. Additionally, there is a decreased gallbladder emptying response to cholecystokinin during pregnancy. Progesterone also contributes to this decrease in gallbladder emptying as it decreases gallbladder smooth muscle contractility in animals (5).

Diagnostic Evaluation

The physical examination in patients with biliary colic is rarely revealing. In patients with acute cholecystitis, fever and abdominal tenderness are the predominant physical findings. Tenderness in the right upper quadrant with respiratory arrest during palpation of the right upper quadrant (Murphy's sign) may be seen. Jaundice may occur with or without associated common bile duct stones. Charcot's triad is the constellation of findings classically seen with cholangitis and consists of fever, right upper quadrant pain, and jaundice.

Patients with acute pancreatitis appear ill. Fever, abdominal tenderness (diffuse or localized to the epigastrium), and diminished or absent bowel sounds are commonly seen. With severe attacks, hypotension and tachycardia may be noted. Jaundice may occur, especially in the setting of gallstone-induced pancreatitis.

Laboratory findings in patients with uncomplicated cholelithiasis and biliary colic are normal. When acute cholecystitis is present, there is usually an elevated white blood cell count with immature forms in the differential ("left shift"). Mild elevations of the serum transaminases and alkaline phosphatase may be seen. If cholangitis is present, the bilirubin is usually between 2 and 10 mg/dL with a mildly elevated alkaline phosphatase level. The laboratory studies in patients with acute pancreatitis usually reveal an elevated hematocrit and white blood cell count with a left shift. Hyperglycemia, hypoalbuminemia, and hypocalcemia may also occur. Most patients with acute pancreatitis have elevated serum amylase and lipase concentrations. Because a mildly elevated amylase is seen in a variety of other conditions, one must be careful not to make the diagnosis only on this basis. Marked elevations of amylase (>1000 mg/dL), however, are usually diagnostic of pancreatitis.

Radiologic Studies

Ultrasonography is the method of choice to detect cholelithiasis and is highly specific if an echogenic shadow is seen. Ultrasonography is also useful in suggesting concomitant choledocholithiasis when bile duct dilatation is seen. Although the ultrasound may be suggestive of acute cholecystitis when a thickened gallbladder wall is seen, it is not specific because this finding can be seen in a variety of other conditions. The advantages of ultrasound include its rapidity, portability, and lack of ionizing radiation. The main disadvantage is its operator dependence.

Nuclear cholescintigraphy is most useful in evaluating patients with acute cholecystitis. It is performed by injecting a technetium 99m isotope that is bound to one of several iminodiacetic acids (hepatic iminodiacetic acid or HIDA), which are excreted into the bile ducts. Gamma rays emitted by the tracer produce images of the bile ducts and gallbladder. Failure of the tracer to enter the gallbladder suggests obstruction of the cystic duct, as seen in acute cholecystitis. Cholescintigraphy has a sensitivity of approximately 95% for acute cholecystitis in the appropriate clinical setting. The disadvantage of nuclear medicine scanning is its lack of structural information and radiation exposure. It should not be used in the pregnant patient.

The oral cholecystogram (OCG) has largely been replaced by ultrasound, but it is useful in the evaluation of the patency of the cystic duct, which is crucial in the patient in whom nonoperative treatment of gallstones is contemplated. The OCG is an iodinated contrast agent given orally the day before imaging. The contrast agent is absorbed from the intestinal mucosa, taken up by the liver, conjugated, and secreted into bile. It is concentrated in the gallbladder, allowing visualization of stones or sludge. Visualization of the gallbladder depends on patency of the cystic duct and a functional gallbladder, both of which should be present for the patient in whom oral dissolution therapy is chosen (see below).

Endoscopic retrograde cholangiopancreatography has become a valuable diagnostic and therapeutic modality in patients with biliary disease. The procedure is performed under conscious sedation. After passage of the side-viewing endoscope into the duodenum (Fig 14.2), the bile duct is cannulated endoscopically, radiopaque contrast is injected into the biliary system, and radiographs are obtained. This has the highest sensitivity for the detection of common bile duct stones. ERCP has dramatically reduced the need for surgical exploration of the common bile duct by either demonstrating absence of stones or allowing stones to be removed endoscopically. Endoscopic removal is performed by enlarging the common bile duct opening with electrocautery and retrieving stones using balloons or baskets. ERCP has played a greater role in the era of laparoscopic cholecystectomy and continues to be the treatment of choice in the management of postcholecystectomy common bile duct stones. In patients with obstructing bile duct stones and cholangitis, emergent ERCP has a lower morbidity and mortality than surgery (6). In patients with *severe* acute gallstone pancreatitis, urgent ERCP with stone removal from the common bile duct reduces the morbidity and mortality compared to conservative therapy (7). ERCP appears to be safe during pregnancy and allows nonoperative management of patients who present with common bile duct stones as their only presentation of gallstone disease (8).

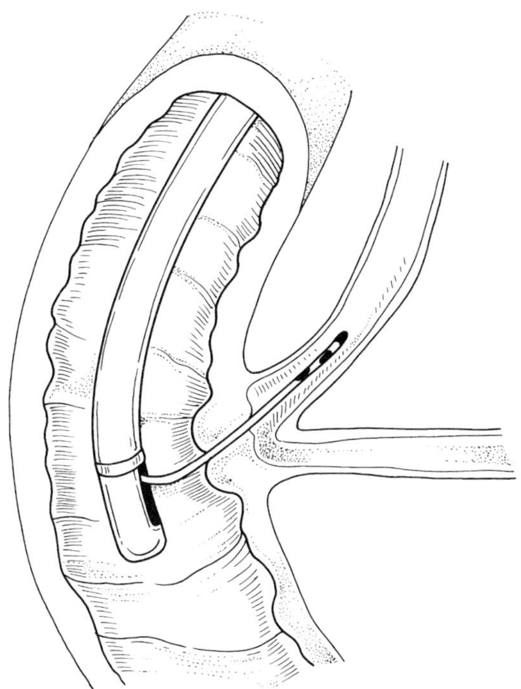

Fig 14.2 Side-viewing endoscope with bile duct cannulated endoscopically.

Percutaneous transhepatic cholangiography (PTC) is performed by passing a needle transcutaneously into the hepatic parenchyma under fluoroscopic or ultrasonographic guidance. Radiopaque contrast is injected to define the biliary tree. Access to the biliary tree can be used for biliary drainage, if necessary. The success rate is greater than 90% when the biliary system is dilated, but falls to 70% (25% to 75%) when the ducts are not dilated. Contraindications include a significant coagulopathy and ascites. In general, the risks of PTC are greater than those of ERCP.

Therapy of Gallstones

Operative Management

Traditional cholecystectomy ("open") has been performed since 1882. It is curative but accompanied by a morbidity rate of 10% to 30% and a mortality rate of 0.1% to 0.6%. Both percentages increase if common bile duct exploration is performed with advancing age or if performed after a biliary complication has occurred (9). Pregnancy is a relative contraindication to open cholecystectomy (see below). The first reported series of laparoscopic cholecystectomies occurred in 1987. The procedure is performed through four abdominal incisions of less than 1 cm each, allowing introduction of surgical instruments. Advantages of laparoscopic cholecystectomy include minimal to no hospitalization, earlier return to work, and excellent cosmetic results. Bile duct injuries occur at a slightly higher rate than open cholecystectomy (10). Relative contraindications are previous upper abdominal surgery and acute cholecystitis, although some authors suggest that laparoscopic cholecystectomy is the procedure of choice in the latter setting (11).

Nonoperative Management

Nonoperative management of gallstones is seldom used, especially with the advent of laparoscopic cholecystectomy. Oral dissolution therapy involves the administration of bile acids. The two agents are ursodeoxycholic (Actigall) and chenodeoxycholic acid (chenodiol or CDC). Ursodeoxycholic acid is almost exclusively used because it is well tolerated without significant adverse effects or toxic reactions; however, its safety during pregnancy has not been established. The effectiveness of oral dissolution therapy depends on the chemical composition of the stones and gallbladder function. Pigment stones or calcified stones respond poorly, if at all, to oral dissolution therapy, whereas floating stones found on OCG suggest a high cholesterol content and portend a successful outcome with bile acid therapy. Unfortunately, only approximately 20% of patients are candidates for oral dissolution therapy. Complete dissolution occurs in up to two thirds of patients after 2 years of therapy. Recurrence of stones is a major drawback and occurs at a rate of 10% a year over 5 years after discontinuing therapy. Additionally, the annual cost of medications is well over $2000. Other costs include laboratory testing, imaging, and physician fees.

Extracorporeal shock wave lithotripsy uses acoustic shock waves to fragment stones into small pieces. After the addition of oral dissolution therapy, these stones either dissolve or pass into the duodenum uneventfully. A more detailed discussion of this therapy is superfluous because this therapy has not been approved by the Food and Drug Administration and has become obsolete in the United States.

Overall Management Strategy of Gallstones

The natural history of asymptomatic gallstones usually involves a benign course. Prolonged follow-up of patients with asymptomatic cholelithiasis suggests that the probability of biliary pain, complications, and death attributable to gallstones is small. Patients with a single episode of biliary colic may never experience recurrent symptoms. Thus, a watch and wait strategy may be appropriate. The rate to develop a biliary complication in these patients is 1% to 2% a year (1). Thus, these patients should not be treated. There are exceptions to this recommendation, however. Certain populations have a high risk for the development of gallbladder cancer in the setting of asymptomatic cholelithiasis, and prophylactic cholecystectomy should be performed in these patients. These exceptions include patients with calcified ("porcelain") gallbladders and Pima Indians. In general, patients with symptomatic cholelithiasis should undergo operative therapy to prevent recurrent attacks and reduce pain.

Acute cholecystitis is best managed with operative intervention. In patients presenting with choledocholithiasis, the common bile duct should be cleared of stones by ERCP followed by laparoscopic cholecystectomy in operative candidates. Poor operative candidates may do well with endoscopic treatment of the bile duct stones alone (6). Endoscopic treatment is the therapy of choice for common bile duct stones presenting in the postcholecystectomy patient.

Gallstones and Pregnancy

Epidemiologic and clinical studies suggest that pregnancy increases the risk of cholesterol gallstone formation. The prevalence of cholelithiasis in asymptomatic pregnant women ranges from 4.5% to 12% (12). Biliary colic has been observed in up to 30% of pregnant women, and thus cholecystectomy is the second most common nonobstetric surgical procedure performed during pregnancy. The treatment of gallstone disease during pregnancy is primarily conservative. Patients presenting with biliary colic should be managed expectantly. Acute cholecystitis complicating pregnancy will usually subside without complications if managed conservatively. The clinician must be careful to consider acute appendicitis in the differential diagnosis of acute cholecystitis because the appendix is displaced toward the right upper quadrant as pregnancy advances. Surgical intervention is required in approximately one third of the patients with acute cholecystitis during pregnancy. Generally, patients are managed medically throughout the first trimester if possible. If symptoms do not resolve, surgery can be performed safely in the second trimester because the uterus is not enlarged enough to impinge on the operating field and the peak for spontaneous abortion has passed (13). During the second trimester, the operative morbidity is no greater for the pregnant patient than for the nonpregnant woman undergoing an uncomplicated cholecystectomy. Recently, laparoscopic cholecystectomy has been performed safely and effectively during pregnancy for both acute cholecystitis and intractable biliary colic (14). Potential benefits of laparoscopic cholecystectomy compared to standard surgery include a marked decrease in wound disruptions and ventral hernias and a decreased risk of pulmonary thromboembolism associated with immobilization after surgery. Undoubtedly, the use of laparoscopic cholecystectomy will increase as the overall experience with this technique improves.

Choledocholithiasis and its attendant complications of cholangitis and pancreatitis are best managed by ERCP. When cholecystectomy is combined with common bile duct exploration in the setting of obstructive jaundice or gallstone pancreatitis, a maternal mortality rate of up to 15% and fetal mortality rate of up to 60% may be seen (15). Successful endoscopic management of choledocholithiasis during pregnancy has been reported by a number of authors (16). Radiation exposure to the fetus can be minimized to a safe level by shielding the fetus with lead aprons, using ultrasound guidance rather than fluoroscopy, and capturing fluoroscopic images on a videotape, which avoids the need for "spot radiographs."

Postcholecystectomy Syndrome

The postcholecystectomy syndrome refers to a wide variety of complaints after successful cholecystectomy. The clinician must attempt to identify if these complaints are 1) secondary to definite gastrointestinal disorders unrelated to the operation, which was performed for symptoms erroneously ascribed to the gallbladder; 2) "functional gastrointestinal symptoms," in which a specific entity cannot be found; or 3) are of biliary tract origin, and these include retained common bile duct stones or other organic biliary diseases, as well as sphincter of Oddi dysfunction. Many of these patients will require referral to an internist or gastroenterologist.

A careful history and physical, laboratory studies (particularly liver function studies), and a limited number of diagnostic tests may allow the clinician to classify the patient into one of the categories mentioned above. ERCP has played an increasing role in diagnosing and treating postcholecystectomy diseases confined to the biliary tree. An example of this is sphincter of Oddi dysfunction. The sphincter of Oddi is composed of smooth muscle fibers encircling the distal bile duct and pancreatic duct as they enter the duodenum. The sphincter controls the flow of bile and pancreatic secretions. Disorders of the sphincter of Oddi can be suspected on the basis of clinical features. The majority of these patients are women, often middle-aged, and abdominal pain is the most common presenting feature. The pain frequently occurs postprandially, is sharp, and radiates from the epigastrium or right upper quadrant to the scapula or back. Most patients have undergone cholecystectomy without evidence of cholelithiasis. Laboratory studies may reveal modest, transient elevation in liver function test results. The "gold standard" for the diagnosis of sphincter of Oddi dysfunction rests on sphincter of Oddi manometry, which is performed during ERCP. Elevated basal sphincter pressure is diagnostic and allows one to predict which patients respond to endoscopic or surgical ablation of the sphincter (17). Medical therapy for the treatment of sphincter of Oddi dysfunction is disappointing.

Primary Sclerosing Cholangitis

Primary sclerosing cholangitis (PSC) is a relatively rare disease of unknown etiology characterized by diffuse fibrosis of both the extrahepatic and intrahepatic bile ducts. PSC is primarily a disease of young men. The clinical presentation is that of progressive weakness, jaundice, pruritus, and right upper quadrant pain present for months to years before diagnosis. The natural history of the disease involves the slow progression to cirrhosis, portal hypertension, and hepatic failure.

Although physical examination can be unremarkable, jaundice or hepatosplenomegaly should lead to consideration of PSC. Laboratory abnormalities include an alkaline phosphatase elevated two to five times normal, which is out of proportion to the increase in the bilirubin. Although there are no known immunologic markers for PSC, recent evidence indicates that peripheral antineutrophil cytoplasmic antibody and antinuclear antibody may be helpful in making this diagnosis (Vierling JM, personal communication, 1994).

Primary sclerosing cholangitis is associated with several autoimmune diseases including thyroiditis, type I diabetes mellitus, chronic pancreatitis, and others. The most common association, however, is with inflammatory bowel disease and specifically ulcerative colitis. Between 50% and 75% of patients with PSC have ulcerative colitis, and usually the diagnosis of inflammatory bowel disease precedes the diagnosis of PSC by several years. Unfortunately, colectomy, which is curative for ulcerative colitis, does not seem to have a protective effect on the development of PSC and, therefore, prophylactic colectomy is not recommended. Thus, in the presence of inflammatory bowel disease in any young to middle-aged patient with an elevated alkaline phosphatase, the diagnosis of PSC must be considered.

Differential Diagnosis

The differential diagnosis of PSC includes diseases causing hepatic cholestasis. Some of the disease processes that are mistakenly diagnosed include chronic active hepatitis secondary to drugs, alcohol, viruses, or autoimmune processes; Wilson's disease; and primary biliary cirrhosis (PBC). The most important distinction is between PBC and PSC. PBC occurs most commonly in middle-aged women, whereas PSC is predominantly a disease of men. A positive antimitochondrial antibody titer is seen in 95% of patients with PBC and is absent in PSC. Liver biopsy can be diagnostic of PBC; however, in PSC, cholangiography is most important in establishing the diagnosis. A distinction must also be made between PSC and secondary sclerosing cholangitis, which may occur as a consequence of biliary surgery, choledocholithiasis, or cholangiocarcinoma. Until recent years, PSC was a diagnosis of exclusion with history, laboratory data, and liver biopsy all contributing to a patient's evaluation. Although liver biopsy is suggestive, it is not definitively diagnostic. Cholangiography has become the preferred diagnostic procedure with the advent and advancement of ERCP techniques. Characteristic findings on cholangiogram are diffuse, multifocal strictures involving both the intrahepatic and extrahepatic ducts.

Pathogenesis

The etiology of PSC is unknown although many factors have been postulated as contributing to the progression of the disease. Three of the more popular theories include copper overload, viral infection, and genetic-immunologic predisposition. Although copper overload is potentially toxic to hepatocytes, this phenomena is more likely related to chronic cholestasis rather than being an initiating event. Infection of the biliary system with various viruses and bacteria has also been considered; however, data supporting this hypothesis have been inconsistent. The theory that currently has the most support involves an genetic-immunologic pathogenesis. The increased frequency of HLA B8 and DR3 alleles noted in patients with PSC combined with the association of PSC with diseases of altered immune function such as ulcerative colitis and type I diabetes mellitus has resulted in the widespread experimental trials with immunosuppressive agents. All of these trials have met with only limited success.

Management

The treatment of PSC involves three goals: 1) management of symptomatic cholestasis, 2) management of complications, and 3) retardation and reversal of the disease process (18). The first two goals are frequently achieved; however, the final goal has been problematic because of incomplete delineation of the pathologic process.

Symptoms of cholestasis include pruritus, vitamin deficiency, and steatorrhea. Pruritus can be controlled with cholestyramine with the addition of activated charcoal capsules for difficult cases. If this is unsuccessful, phenobarbital at bedtime, which theoretically increases bile flow, can be tried. PSC patients are also susceptible to fat-soluble vitamin deficiencies and replacement may be necessary. Finally, steatorrhea can be controlled by restricting dietary fat.

Complications of PSC include cholangitis and cirrhosis. Cholangitis commonly occurs after surgical manipulation of the biliary system. Treatment of cholangitis includes broad-spectrum antibiotics. When cirrhosis occurs, the complications such as esophageal varices, encephalopathy, and ascites are managed using established medical standards.

Attempts to retard or reverse the pathologic process have been aimed at possible etiologic factors. Currently two forms of medical therapy are being considered: immunosuppressive agents and bile acid therapy. Immunosuppressive drugs such as steroids, azathioprine, and methotrexate are still being tried in small groups of patients with limited success. Randomized controlled studies are awaited. Bile acids, and specifically ursodeoxycholic acid, have also been used to improve symptoms as well as to improve the biochemical profile. The theory behind this is that the hydrophobic bile acids are hepatotoxic. The use of ursodeoxycholic acid increases the "hydrophilicity of the bile acid pool" and, thus, decreases the proportion of hydrophobic bile acids (2). Although the above therapeutic measures can improve symptoms and laboratory abnormalities associated with PSC, unfortunately, no specific treatment has been identified that is curative, and, therefore, liver transplantation is the only option for patients who advance to hepatic failure.

Bile Duct Tumors

Gallbladder Cancer

Gallbladder cancer is not a tumor unique to women; however, it is seen three times more commonly in women than men because of its association with gallstones (1). Numerous studies have demonstrated that approximately 80% of patients with gallbladder cancer have evidence of gallstones (1). Gallbladder carcinoma is the fifth most common malignancy of the gastrointestinal tract. The highest prevalence of gallbladder cancer occurs in American Indians, Hispanic American women, and Latin American women. It is a disease of the elderly, commonly occurring after age 65. The pathophysiology of gallbladder carcinoma is unclear, but it may be related to chronic inflammation of the gallbladder mucosa by stones.

The presentation of gallbladder cancer is similar to that of gallstones, primarily mimicking biliary colic or cholecystitis. Jaundice, hepatomegaly, a palpable abdominal mass, and ascites are common physical findings. The predominant laboratory findings are liver function abnormalities with direct hyperbilirubinemia and an elevated alkaline phosphatase representing bile duct obstruction. The most helpful diagnostic imaging studies are ultrasonography and computed tomography (CT) scanning.

Definitive treatment for gallbladder cancer is surgical resection. Unfortunately, only 20% of patients will have resectable disease at the time of operation. The prognosis is poor, with a median survival of 5.2 months after surgery. Chemotherapy is of little benefit. Palliative treatment of jaundice due to bile duct obstruction can be achieved by placement of biliary endoprosthesis by endoscopic (ERCP) or percutaneous methods. Limited tumors, such as those found incidentally at cholecystectomy, have a favorable prognosis.

Bile Duct Carcinoma (Cholangiocarcinoma)

Cancer of the bile ducts is less common than gallbladder cancer and occurs equally in men and women. The association with stone disease is much lower, and the age at presentation is younger. Patients with chronic ulcerative colitis and associated PSC are at increased risk for development of bile duct cancer. The incidence of bile duct tumors is higher in Asian populations, and this occurs because in these areas of the world, infestation of the biliary system with liver flukes is common.

Clinical manifestations of bile duct cancer are nonspecific and include nausea, vomiting, weight loss, and anorexia. Painless jaundice is commonly seen. Laboratory abnormalities are indicative of obstruction to the biliary system with an elevated bilirubin and alkaline phosphatase. Ultrasonography and CT scanning are suggestive diagnostic studies, demonstrating dilated bile ducts above the level of obstruction. Definitive diagnosis requires cholangiography, either endoscopic (ERCP), or percutaneous (PTC). This allows one to determine the extent of the lesion and collect material for cytology.

Several treatment modalities exist for managing bile duct cancer; optimal therapy requires a multidisciplinary team approach in a center experienced with this disease. Surgical resection for cure should be undertaken for anatomically resectable lesions. Palliative therapy for nonoperative candidates includes endoscopic or percutaneous management of biliary obstruction and radiation therapy. Chemotherapy has not provided significantly prolonged survival.

Metastatic malignancies may also involve the liver or biliary system. The most common primary tumors to metastasize to the biliary system are stomach, colon, lung, and breast. Jaundice can occur secondary to extensive hepatic parenchymal metastasis or from obstruction to the bile duct. Notably, there is a significant difference in morbidity and mortality associated with these two patterns because patients with lymph node metastasis and resulting bile duct obstruction have a significantly better prognosis (19). Although at this advanced stage of disease, no curative therapy is available, the majority of patients with metastatic disease benefit from palliative therapy of their obstructive jaundice via biliary decompression. ERCP with stent placement (most often "permanent" metal stents) is successful in these situations with less morbidity and mortality than that associated with percutaneous or surgical decompression. The only limitation to the use of ERCP occurs if the obstruction is at the level of the bifurcation of the common hepatic duct or above. In this situation, two stents are required to maintain adequate drainage, and although technically feasible, the procedure is considerably more difficult with a higher rate of complications.

REFERENCES

1. American College of Physicians. Guidelines for the treatment of gallstones. Ann Intern Med 1993;119:620–622.

2. Yamada T, Alpers DH, Owyang C, et al., eds. Textbook of gastroenterology. Philadelphia: JB Lipincott, 1991:1966–1984.

3. Johnston DE, Kaplan MM. Pathogenesis and treatment of gallstones. N Engl J Med 1993;328:412–421.

4. Parkman HP, Baron TH, Richter JE, Fisher RS. Gastrointestinal motility disorders in pregnancy. In: Karlstadt RG, Surawicz CM, Croit IRU, eds. Gastrointestinal disorders during pregnancy. American Journal of Gastroonterology, 1994.

5. Ryan JP. Effect of pregnancy on gallbladder contractility in the guinea pig. Gastroenterology 1984;87:674–678.

6. Lai ECS, Mok FPT, Tan ESY, et al. Endoscopic biliary drainage for severe acute cholangitis. N Engl J Med 1992;326:1582–1586.

7. Neoptolemos JP, London NJ, James D, Carr-Locke DL, Bailey IA, Fossard DP. Controlled trial of urgent endoscopic retrograde cholangiopancreatography and endoscopic sphincterotomy versus conservative treatment for acute pancreatitis due to gallstones. Lancet 1988:979–983.

8. Ingoldby CJH, el-Saadi J, Hall RI, Denyer ME. Late results of endoscopic sphincterotomy for bile duct stones in elderly patients with gallbladders in situ. Gut 1989; 30:1129–1131.

9. Plaisier PW, van der Hul RL, Terpstra OT, Bruining HA. Current treatment modalities for symptomatic gallstones. Am J Gastroenterol 1993;88:633–639.

10. The Southern Surgeons Club. A prospective analysis of 1518 laparoscopic cholecystectomies. N Engl J Med 1991;324:1073–1078.

11. Weisen SM, Unger SW, Barkin JS, et al. Laparoscopic cholecystectomy: the procedure of choice for acute cholecystitis. Am J Gastroenterol 1993;88:334–337.

12. Valdivesio V, Covarrubias C, Siegal F, et al. Pregnancy and cholelithiasis: pathogenesis and natural course of gallstones diagnosed early in puerperium. Hepatology 1993;17:1–4.

13. Hill LM, Johnson CE, Lee RA. Cholecystectomy in pregnancy. Obstet Gynecol 1975;46:291–293.

14. Morrell DG, Mullins JR, Harrison PB. Laparoscopic cholecystectomy during pregnancy in symptomatic patients. Surgery 1992;112:856–859.

15. Kammerer VS. Non-obstetric surgery during pregnancy. Med Clin North Am 1979;63:1157–1164.

16. Axelrad AM, Fleischer DE, Strack LL, Benjamin SB, Al-Kawas FH. Performance of ERCP for symptomatic choledocholithiasis during pregnancy: techniques to increase safety and improve patient management. Am J Gastroenterol 1994;89:109–112.

17. Geenen JE, Hogan WJ, Dodds WJ, Toouli J, Venu RP. The efficacy of endoscopic sphincterotomy in post-cholecystectomy patients with sphincter of Oddi dysfunction. Results of a 4 year prospective study. N Engl J Med 1989;320:82–87.

18. Zakim D, Boyer TD, eds. Hepatology: a textbook of liver disease. Philadelphia: WB Saunders, 1990.

19. Marsh WH, Cunningham JT. Endoscopic stent placement for obstructive jaundice secondary to metastatic malignancy. Am J Gastroenterol 1992;87:985–989.

CHAPTER 15

INFLAMMATORY BOWEL DISEASE

Stephen Holland

Idiopathic inflammatory bowel disease refers to two chronic inflammatory diseases of the gut, Crohn's disease and ulcerative colitis. The goal for this chapter is to give physicians working with women with inflammatory bowel disease familiarity with issues relating to diagnosis and treatment of idiopathic inflammatory bowel disease in women. This should allow an understanding of the diagnostic and treatment plans that a gastroenterologist may recommend for patients with inflammatory bowel disease and provide a conceptual framework that will improve communications among physicians treating these challenging patients. Some aspects of inflammatory bowel disease, such as epidemiology and histology, have not been covered. These aspects are well described in standard textbooks of internal medicine.

Etiology

Crohn's disease and ulcerative colitis do not have a known etiology, but general theories about the cause or causes of each tend to fall into two groups—autoimmune or infectious. These two groups are not mutually exclusive. Certainly rheumatic fever is an example of an inflammatory disease that can be regarded as both infectious and autoimmune. Inflammatory bowel diseases might some day be understood well enough that the distinction between an autoimmune or infectious etiology is similarly moot.

Bacterial Hypothesis

Because of the granulomatous inflammation found in histologic sections, an infectious etiology for Crohn's disease has been considered since the disease was first described. Subsequently an extensive search for a Crohn's pathogen was undertaken. No convincing data for a mycobacterial etiology came forth, and it seems that most positive studies found only commensal mycobacteria. Although recently there has been some resurgence of interest in the tuberculosis hypothesis driven by more sophisticated and sensitive methods of detection, there are at present insufficient data to be convinced that a mycobacteria is important in the etiology of Crohn's disease.

Although there is little enthusiasm for the slow or indolent infection hypothesis, a body of literature describes the inflammatory characteristics of bacterial cell products. Bacteria make a number of products such as lipopolysaccharide, lipoteichoic acids, peptidoglycan-polysaccharides, heat shock proteins, and f-met-leu-phe. Whether any of these factors are primary in the etiology of Crohn's disease or are secondary factors that perpetuate the disease is not known.

With ulcerative colitis limited to the mucosa, no history of potential pathogens, and recent evidence that depriving the colon of luminal contents may be a factor in the development of ulcerative colitis, there is little interest in a bacterial hypothesis for ulcerative colitis. This does not mean, however, that luminal factors will not turn out to be important in the etiology of ulcerative colitis, for reasons just mentioned.

Autoimmune Hypothesis

The idea of an autoimmune etiology for inflammatory bowel disease is attractive. Aside from the obvious issue that inflammatory bowel disease is by its nature an inflammatory disease, there is a rich body of literature on the nature of regulation of the normal immune response. It is also now understood that immune regulation of mucosal tissues such as the gut, the genitourinary system, the breast and salivary glands, and the pulmonary system, is separate from the systemic immune system. It is as important for the mucosal immune system to not respond to all the benign antigens that it comes into contact with day to day as it is for it to respond to pathogens that find mucosal surfaces the most convenient portal of entry to the body. The appreciation that the immune system is potentially lethal to the host if it is not well regulated, and the more recent appreciation that the mucosal immune system has special autoregulatory pathways, has spawned a rich body of literature regarding what role an abnormal immune response plays in inflammatory bowel disease.

Nutritional Hypothesis

Recent studies have demonstrated the importance of luminal nutrients in the maintenance of normal enterocyte homeostasis. Energy requirements of colonic epithelial cells are met mostly by luminal short chain fatty acids (acetate, butyrate, propionate) that are produced by bacterial fermentation of dietary fiber. In a human model of ulcerative colitis, patients with inflammation of Hartman's pouches can be treated with instillation of short chain fatty acids directly into the pouch. Recently, short chain fatty acids have been shown to be effective in treatment of distal ulcerative colitis. It appears that the anti-inflammatory effect is due to improved nutrition of colonic epithelial cells. Although pouchitis is a model for ulcerative colitis in human beings, it is not clear why patients with ulcerative colitis develop inflammation. The effective treatment of pouchitis just shows that the provision of nutrients alleviates the inflammation, but it does not prove that the etiology of the pouchitis is a nutritional deficiency. For example, if the etiology were microvascular compromise then colonocytes would be nutritionally deprived, and short chain fatty acids would work by providing missing caloric requirements.

Small bowel epithelial cells depend on glycine for their energy requirements. In patients with pouchitis of Koch's pouches, glycine instillation can be effective.

Genetic Predisposition

Twin studies have demonstrated the strength of the genetic component for both ulcerative colitis and Crohn's disease. While the lifetime risk for a sibling developing inflammatory bowel disease is 8%, there is an 84% concordance rate for Crohn's disease and a 36% concordance rate for ulcerative colitis in identical twins. The pattern of inheritance in large families is not a simple single gene pattern. Occasional families have both ulcerative colitis and Crohn's disease found within them, but there has never been a case of identical twins where one had Crohn's disease and the other ulcerative colitis.

Smoking, Oral Contraceptives, and Nonsteroidal Anti-inflammatory Drugs

Several factors have been found that seem to have some importance in relation to either risk of developing inflammatory bowel disease or in aggravating inflammation in patients with inflammatory bowel disease. The major identified factors are smoking, oral contraceptive pills, nonsteroidal anti-inflammatory drugs (NSAIDs), and sugar consumption in Crohn's disease, and smoking in ulcerative colitis. There factors have been found through epidemiologic research. Few studies have been published to determine whether modification of these factors will change the natural history of inflammatory bowel disease or if they are just markers associated with inflammatory bowel disease. There are sufficient anecdotal reports, case series, and a few controlled trials, however, to suggest that modifying these factors might be helpful. It is not yet clear what effect modification of these factors would have on large numbers of patients with inflammatory bowel disease, but these factors may provide clues to the etiology of Crohn's disease and ulcerative colitis.

Smoking history is an intriguing factor because it has a positive association with Crohn's disease, but a negative association with ulcerative colitis. Moreover, a number of patients can date the onset of their ulcerative colitis to shortly after they stopped smoking. Only recently was a controlled trial performed on this subject, but rather than use smoking, nicotine patches were used. This trial demonstrated that nicotine had a mild symptomatic benefit, but there was no evidence of histologic improvement. Given that nicotine administration cannot really be blinded, it is hard to tell whether the symptomatic effect was even real. With cigarette smoke being a complex mixture, it is not known if cigarette usage would be beneficial in ulcerative colitis.

Oral contraceptive use has been studied over the years with retrospective case controlled trials with conflicting results. Most recently, larger studies and better methodology have shown that oral contraceptive pills cause a small increase in the risk of developing Crohn's disease, perhaps a 2.5-fold risk over a control population of women. None of these reports quantified estrogen dosage. A few scattered reports in the literature describe an acute onset of an inflammatory bowel disease-like illness in women taking oral contraceptive pills or estrogen. The varying estrogen content of contraceptives and regional differences in prescribing patterns may explain some differences in the rate of association of Crohn's disease and oral contraceptive pill use, and would predict that the strength of the association will decrease with time. Because the estrogen-associated inflammatory disease resolved when estrogens were stopped and the duration estrogens were used before the onset of the Crohn's-like syndrome could be quite long, it is prudent to stop oral contraceptive pills when a patient presents with inflammatory bowel disease. However, no evidence shows that the severity of disease is worsened by oral contraceptive pills, so the use of oral contraceptive pills in a woman with inflammatory bowel disease can be considered.

The NSAIDs are another interesting class of compounds. There is fair evidence that some patients with Crohn's disease develop flares of disease when they take NSAIDs, but there is no evidence of worsening on NSAIDs in patients with ulcerative colitis. This difference may be another clue to the differences in pathogenesis between Crohn's disease and ulcerative colitis.

Diagnosis

Crohn's Disease

A diagnosis of Crohn's disease is generally made by observing narrowing of the terminal ileum on small bowel follow-through or air contrast barium enema x-ray studies. Patients come to these diagnostic tests due to symptoms of chronic diarrhea, symptoms consistent with obstruction, findings of a right lower quadrant mass or tenderness, abdominal pain, weight loss, anorexia, or evidence of an enterocutaneous fistula or intra-abdominal fistula between intestine and reproductive organ or any other abdominal organ. Enterocutaneous fistulas can be small and a careful examination should be made for them, especially in the perineum. Rarely, Crohn's disease will involve the vulva with just erythema or with granulomatous disease without direct connection by enterocutaneous fistula.

The frequent case where Crohn's disease runs an indolent course explains the common situation where Crohn's disease is initially thought to be irritable bowel syndrome. Early in the course of Crohn's disease there may be diarrhea and abdominal pain without changes detectable on small bowel follow-through, and distinguishing Crohn's disease from irritable bowel syndrome may be impossible. Irritable bowel syndrome and inflammatory bowel disease are discussed later.

Crohn's disease can also present as an acute abdomen. In this setting, the diagnosis may be made at laparotomy. Gross surgical features such as mesenteric fat wrapping, ileal inflammation, and inflammation of multiple segments of the gut may be found. Often the diagnosis is not apparent until examination of the surgical biopsies shows changes compatible with Crohn's disease. Although perforation of the intestine due to Crohn's disease may precipitate an acute abdomen, severe inflammation without perforation may, by itself, cause the clinical picture of an acute abdomen.

Some cases of Crohn's disease only involve the colon. Usually there are features such as rectal sparing, granulomatous changes on biopsy, transmural inflammatory involvement, or the presence of fistulas that show the colitis is Crohn's disease, but in about 20% of cases the distinction between Crohn's colitis and ulcerative colitis cannot be made until distinctive features eventually manifest themselves. The distinction is important because colectomy will cure ulcerative colitis but not Crohn's disease. Because ulcerative colitis is characterized by continuous involvement from the rectum proximally, areas of intervening normal colon strongly suggest Crohn's disease. Areas of sparing, however, need to be shown normal by biopsy to truly establish the existence of intervening normal mucosa.

Early in the evaluation of a patient with findings consistent with Crohn's disease a wide variety of diagnoses are in the differential, such as pelvic inflammatory disease, ectopic pregnancy, ovarian disease, endometriosis, ileal carcinoid, appendiceal diseases, cecal carcinoma, diverticulitis, lymphoma, lymphoid hyperplasia, and radiation enteritis. Diseases that should be considered in the differential diagnosis depend, of course, on the particulars of each case. The differential diagnosis of Crohn's disease also includes tuberculous enteritis and *Yersinia* enteritis. *Yersinia* produces a self-limited illness that will resolve with no inflammatory sequelae. Serologic studies or a subsequent small bowel follow-through after 3 months can be useful. Tuberculosis will be lethal if not diagnosed.

Ulcerative Colitis

The diagnosis of ulcerative colitis is made by a combination of the symptoms of chronic or intermittent diarrhea with or without gross blood with findings on sigmoidoscopy consistent with ulcerative colitis, and with stool studies negative for *Salmonella*, *Shigella*, *Campylobacter*, or *Entamoeba histolytica*. The typical presentation is an acute onset of bloody diarrhea with crampy abdominal pain. Sigmoidoscopy typically demonstrates mucosal friability or gross bleeding and pus exudation in a continuous and diffuse pattern from the rectum to some proximal extent. Fistulas are strong evidence against ulcerative colitis although occasionally rectovaginal fistulas form with severe disease.

Unlike in Crohn's disease, barium contrast x-ray studies are not important in the initial diagnosis of ulcerative colitis. These studies are contraindicated early in the course of an acute colitis due to the risk of perforation, as well as the interference such studies cause for endoscopy or angiographic studies. The risk of perforation is great enough that initial sigmoidoscopy should be limited to confirm the presence of typical findings consistent with ulcerative colitis in the rectum and not to define the proximal extent of disease. Plain film studies can be useful in determining the proximal extent of disease if thumbprinting is prominent. After the acute episode subsides an air contrast barium enema is useful to exclude Crohn's disease.

As mentioned earlier, it is important to exclude infectious causes of colitis. No endoscopic features reliably distinguish ulcerative colitis from infectious causes of diffuse colitis other than in pseudomembranous colitis. Biopsies should be done to look for features such as crypt abscesses, distortion of the crypt architecture, and organisms that can be found histologically. A history of anal intercourse should expand the differential to include gonorrhea, chlamydia, and herpes colitis, and a history of radiation therapy, as for example with endometrial cancer, would expand the differential to include radiation proctitis. It is not uncommon for an acute colitis to resolve with no further sequelae. Presumably these are cases of infectious colitis where the organism cannot be cultured.

Evaluation of Clinical Status

Several systems exist for the characterization of disease activity in ulcerative colitis and Crohn's disease. Standard scoring systems that reflect a consensus opinion on what features in Crohn's disease and ulcerative colitis are important in grading disease severity and activity exist and should be used by those caring for patients with inflammatory bowel disease. Use of these systems helps to standardize the observations and documentation for patients with inflammatory bowel disease; however, no studies relate the clinical features elicited with any scoring system to suggest initial treatment of patients, other than to suggest that more severe disease needs more aggressive therapy.

The most widely accepted system for grading the activity of ulcerative colitis is the Truelove and Witts scale. In this system the clinician notes whether the following clinical features are present: diarrhea with visible blood or more than six bowel movements per day; mean evening temperature over 37.5°C (99.5°F) or over 37.7°C (100°F) for 2 of 4 days; mean pulse greater 90/min; hemoglobin at 75% or less of normal; erythrocyte sedimentation rate over 30 mm/hr; and the presence of guarding, spasm, rebound, or tenderness on light palpation.

There are a number of scoring systems for Crohn's disease, which attests to the lack of satisfaction with any one system. Most systems that have been well studied include measures of pain, fever, abdominal tenderness, number of bowel movements per day, presence of a mass, presence of wasting or other measure of nutritional status, hemoglobin level, subjective opinion of well-being, quantification of use of antidiarrheal drugs, and presence of perianal disease, fistula, or other complications. In the absence of a well accepted system for grading the severity of Crohn's disease, noting the above features will allow the clinician to capture most data needed for most scales of disease activity. If not universally used, the Crohn's Disease Activity Index was the measure used in one of the largest studies of the response of Crohn's disease to steroids in active disease and for maintenance. The variables listed above include those in this activity index.

Symptomatic Flares

One of the issues that makes treating patients with inflammatory bowel disease a challenge is that not all episodes of worsening symptoms are due to worsening inflammation. Worsening symptoms may represent intermittent obstruction of a fibrotic stricture, bacterial overgrowth, or an intercurrent illness. As can be seen from the following discussion, patients with Crohn's disease have a richer variety of noninflammatory causes for recurrent symptoms than do patients with ulcerative colitis.

Fixed Obstructions and Symptomatic Flares

A feature in some cases of Crohn's disease is the development of fixed obstructions. These are areas of narrowing due to fibrosis that develops after inflammation subsides. Being fibrotic, they will not respond to steroids. They are prone to obstruction if undigested food of sufficient size impacts them. These lesions are detectable with a small bowel follow-through. Patients with known fixed obstructions are advised to avoid foods such as raw vegetables, nuts, popcorn, or bulk laxatives. When obstructions due to food impaction develop, conservative management with nasogastric suction is generally effective. If symptoms are mild enough, the use of enteral feedings at home with a product such as Ensure until symptoms abate can be successful. Resection of fixed obstructions is called for when episodes of symptoms are sufficiently frequent. Although there is no absolute rule on the number of episodes of obstruction to warrant a resection, three episodes a year requiring hospitalization is a reasonable number to use. Ulcerative colitis is not generally a stricturing disease. Management of patients with ulcerative colitis with strictures is discussed in the section on malignancy.

Bacterial Overgrowth

Patients with Crohn's with strictures can develop diarrhea if bacterial overgrowth develops in an area of stasis due to a fixed obstruction. A short course of tetracycline is usually effective. If patients develop frequent episodes of symptoms due to bacterial overgrowth, a host of options are available, such as repeat courses of antibiotics as needed, chronic antibiotic administration, or monthly antibiotic administration, as the situation dictates.

Irritable Bowel Syndrome and Inflammatory Bowel Disease

Patients with Crohn's disease frequently have coexisting irritable bowel syndrome because irritable bowel syndrome is such a common disease. Initially, Crohn's disease may present as irritable bowel syndrome, only later to be diagnosed when inflammatory lesions become apparent. In patients with both irritable bowel syndrome and Crohn's disease or ulcerative colitis it is not always possible to distinguish between the symptoms due to irritable bowel syndrome and those due to inflammatory bowel disease because the symptoms in irritable bowel syndrome can be identical to those found in inflammatory bowel disease. Irritable bowel syndrome occasionally is so severe that bright red blood per rectum develops, thought to be due to some degree of mucosal ischemia. Differentiation between irritable bowel syndrome and active inflammatory bowel disease as a cause of bright red blood per rectum should be possible endoscopically.

Mesalamine Intolerance

One drug reaction that causes symptoms similar to a flare of inflammatory bowel disease is acute intolerance to mesalamine. This is discussed further in the treatment section.

Inflammation

Although recurrence of inflammation commonly is the cause of worsening symptoms, it has been listed late in this section to impress on the reader the need to consider noninflammatory causes of worsening of symptoms. Recurrence of inflammation can cause bleeding, pain, diarrhea, or obstruction in Crohn's disease or ulcerative colitis, though in ulcerative colitis bleeding is usually present when inflammation recurs. Whether an obstructive lesion in Crohn's disease is inflammatory or fibrotic is assessed by endoscopy with biopsy, response to steroids, and appearance over time with small bowel follow-through x-ray studies. Additionally, the use of an indium-labeled leukocyte nuclear medicine scan can be helpful because inflammatory lesions will trap leukocytes and light up, whereas fibrotic strictures will not. With the dangerous side effects that can develop with steroids or other immunosupressants, recurrent inflammation should be demonstrated before a course of medical treatment to suppress inflammation is undertaken. On the other hand, delay in starting anti-inflammatory treatment when indicated should also be avoided lest complications such as fistula formation, nutritional depletion, perforation, or exsanguination develop.

Malignancy in Inflammatory Bowel Disease

Patients with ulcerative colitis have an increased risk of cancer of the colon compared to the normal population. The risk increases with severity, duration, and extent of disease, with a risk of colon cancer of 5% at 20 years in patients with moderate and severe disease; patients with mild proctitis may have little increased risk. Longitudinal studies have demonstrated that there is little increased risk for ulcerative colitis-related malignancies until 8 to 10 years after the onset of disease. One peculiarity of ulcerative colitis-related malignancies is that they are often flat lesions that can be difficult to find with air contrast barium enema. Also, there is fair evidence that high-grade dysplasia develops before a malignancy. Therefore, current recommendations are to start periodic surveillance colonoscopies in patients with ulcerative colitis after 8 to 10 years of disease duration.

In screening colonoscopy, done every 1 to 3 years depending on institutional habits, biopsies are taken every 10 cm, and submitted to pathology in separate containers for each level. These are then evaluated for dysplasia. Although conceptually straightforward, in practice the results of the biopsies can lead to great consternation. Areas of inflammation will have changes that resemble high-grade dysplasia, and if the pathologist cannot determine if underlying dysplasia is present in an area with active inflammation, colonoscopy may need to be repeated after intensification of medical therapy. Grading dysplasia is also not as objective a skill as one would wish although agreement among pathologists over high-grade dysplasia is more common that it is for low-grade dysplasia. Because a recommendation for a major operation should be made if high-grade dysplasia is found, some recommend that a repeat colonoscopy be made after a few weeks to repeat biopsies in the area of concern. When high-grade dysplasia is found, there is a 30% to 40% risk that colon cancer is present somewhere in the colon. If low-grade dysplasia is found, there may be a 10% chance of cancer, but with greater difficulty for a pathologist to establish what is low-grade dysplasia, there is more reason to consider repeating biopsies.

Although patients with ulcerative colitis can develop rather severe inflammation, it is less common for strictures to develop, and a carcinoma may be found within such strictures. Therefore, a colon stricture in a patient with ulcerative colitis is cause for close colonoscopic surveillance with biopsies. Dysplasia within a stricture is an indication for colectomy, as is a tight stricture that does not allow passage of an endoscope for surveillance.

In patients with Crohn's disease the risk of colon cancer is about 1%. It is usually found in areas of involvement but is not related to duration or severity as it is in ulcerative colitis. In addition to colon cancer risk, patients with Crohn's disease are also at risk for small bowel malignancies in areas of involvement, with approximately a sixfold increased risk compared to controls. Also, there seems to be a greater risk for carcinoma in bypassed areas of gut. Unfortunately, strictures from carcinoma cannot be radiographically distinguished from strictures that can develop in areas of active Crohn's, and are rarely diagnosed preoperatively or at the time of laparotomy. It is usually the pathologist who discovers the carcinoma in the resected specimen.

Due to the lower absolute risk of cancer in Crohn's disease compared to ulcerative colitis, and the lack of the problem of carcinomas developing without an associated mass, a routine, regular program of surveillance in patients without stricturing disease of the colon is not justified. When colonic strictures are present they should be evaluated periodically with colonoscopy. A stricture that arises without evidence of activity of Crohn's disease should be viewed the same as a stricture arising in someone without Crohn's disease, which means, of course, as if it were malignant.

Complications of Inflammatory Bowel Disease

Approximately 20% of women with Crohn's disease will develop perineal complications. Half of those will develop rectovaginal fistulas. Occasionally patients with ulcerative colitis will develop a rectovaginal fistula. Medical therapy includes the use of metronidazole, usually with steroids and occasionally with immunosupressants such as azathioprine, 6-mercaptopurine, or cyclosporin A. Response will be variable. A surgical approach is often effective in fistulas for both ulcerative colitis and Crohn's disease patients. Medical therapy should be tried at first to close fistulas, but a prolonged course may make an eventual surgical approach difficult due to chronic inflammatory changes. The surgical approach to high vaginal fistulas is usually transabdominal. A modified transvaginal approach is usually successful in low to mid-rectovaginal fistulas if attention is paid to excision of the fistula, interposition of levator ani muscles, and advancement of the vaginal flap.

Rarely patients will develop vulvar granulomatous disease or abscess in association with Crohn's disease. This can occur without vaginal involvement. Case reports have usually described onset of resolution after starting metronidazole, although sulfasalazine was effective in maintaining remission in one patient.

Patients with Crohn's disease and ulcerative colitis can develop a number of other complications such as erythema nodosum, pyoderma gangrenosum, iritis, episcleritis, arthritis, and hepatic lesions such as fatty liver, pericholangitis, and sclerosing cholangitis. Carcinoma complicating inflammatory bowel disease is discussed in the section on malignancy.

Treatment of Inflammatory Bowel Disease

The treatments described in this section are directed at the treatment of inflammation in cases of inflammatory bowel disease. Treatment of symptoms due to obstruction, bacterial overgrowth, and other noninflammtory problems in inflammatory bowel disease are discussed in the section on symptomatic flares.

Steroids

Corticosteroids are the initial treatment of severe Crohn's disease and ulcerative colitis. Moderate to severe disease is treated with high doses, generally 60 mg prednisone a day. Treatment can be prolonged, but responses usually are seen in days in patients treated in hospital with IV steroids. In ulcerative colitis and Crohn's disease cases of severe inflammation are generally treated with 60 mg prednisone orally per day in a single or divided dose, and treatment is continued until symptoms abate. After inflammation is under control, the dose is tapered. Tapering should be done slowly, over months, because more rapid tapering the dose can be associated with early recurrence. Side effects of steroid use are well known, including salt retention, cushingoid changes, emotional changes, improved appetite, and an increased sense of well-being, as well as less common but more dangerous complications such as osteoporosis, cataracts, glaucoma, and others. In long-term use and during pregnancy, calcium administration and vitamin D supplementation are used, but the degree of benefit from supplementation is unknown. Corticosteroids are safe to use during pregnancy and while nursing.

Topical steroids given as enemas are useful for ulcerative colitis and Crohn's disease in the rectum, sigmoid, and sometimes descending colon. Hydrocortisone enemas may cause systemic effects, but a poorly absorbed steroid such as betamethasone will have few systemic effects. Newer steroids that are metabolized by erythrocytes are becoming available and likewise have no systemic effects.

5-Aminosalicylic Drugs

Drugs that deliver mesalamine (5-aminosalicylic acid, 5-ASA) to the gut lumen have been used in ulcerative colitis and Crohn's disease for years. The prototype of this type of drug is sulfasalazine, which is 5-ASA covalently linked to the antibiotic sulfapyridine. Sulfasalazine is poorly absorbed in the small intestine. Bacteria cleave the azo bond that holds the two molecules together, providing local delivery to the colon and terminal ileum. 5-ASA is the anti-inflammatory moiety, probably working by decreasing prostaglandin synthesis by inhibiting cyclooxygenase. Sulfasalazine has classically been used in ulcerative colitis but is also useful in Crohn's disease with colonic involvement. Sulfasalazine decreases the likelihood of flares of ulcerative colitis in a dose-related fashion. Patients are encouraged to take up to 4 gm/day and up to 6 gm/day if flares continue. Sulfasalazine is not uncommonly stopped due to allergic reactions to the sulfa component of sulfasalazine, often manifest as a rash. Other common side effects include anorexia, headache, nausea, vomiting, and gastric distress. These side effects are more common with a daily dose above 4 gm. In men there is also a reversible effect on sperm production, which can be manifest as infertility. Women can use sulfasalazine while pregnant and while breastfeeding. In contrast to its protective effect in ulcerative colitis, sulfasalazine has been shown to not reduce the risk of recurrences in Crohn's disease. In Crohn's disease, the dose of sulfasalazine is chosen for its effect on inflammation with no effort made to push the dose to minimize recurrences. In comparison to other drugs that deliver 5-ASA to the colon, sulfasalazine has a significant price advantage.

Olsalazine (Dipentum) is another poorly absorbed prodrug like sulfasalazine. It is two 5-ASA molecules joined by an azo bond. When cleaved by bacteria it releases two 5-ASA molecules. Because it does not contain sulfapyridine, it has fewer side effects than sulfasalazine. Olsalazine causes diarrhea in 16% of patients, severe enough to cause 70% to stop taking the drug. Because the drug has similar release kinetics compared with sulfasalazine, it is expected that it will have similar therapeutic actions.

Mesalamine can also be delivered by controlled-release preparations. 5-ASA is well absorbed by the small intestine, so delivery to distal small intestine and to large intestine requires either a poorly absorbed prodrug as with sulfasalazine and olsalazine, or a special formulation to control delivery to various levels in the intestine. Asacol is mesalamine compounded such that it is released in the terminal ileum and colon. Pentasa is compounded to release mesalamine in the small intestine and colon. Doses that deliver equivalent amounts of mesalamine on a molar basis to the colon as sulfasalazine have similar efficacy to sulfasalazine. Compounds that deliver mesalamine to the small intestine have particular use in treating small intestinal Crohn's disease.

The safety of mesalamine in pregnancy has not been established but is assumed on the basis of the safety of sulfasalazine. However, sulfasalazine delivers little 5-ASA systemically, so if there is a dose-related toxicity to 5-ASA it could become apparent with the higher systemic absorption found in the timed-release compounds.

Mesalamine Intolerance

Any drug that delivers 5-ASA can cause an acute intolerance syndrome. This rare syndrome presents as acute abdominal pain and diarrhea, often bloody, sometimes accompanied by fever, headache, or rash. It is easily confused with a flare of the underlying disease and must be recognized by its onset within a few days of administration of a 5-ASA drug. Enthusiasm for rechallenge to confirm the intolerance should by tempered by the possibility of death precipitated by rechallenge with 5-ASA. Sensitivity to one 5-ASA compound implies sensitivity to all.

Antibiotics

As an adjunct for treatment of severe ulcerative colitis or Crohn's disease, broad-spectrum IV antibiotics are used during in-hospital treatment to protect against bacteria translocating across damaged mucosa. Antibiotics probably also have a role in primary therapy of mild to moderate Crohn's disease.

Although few papers exist in the literature on the use of antibiotics as primary therapy in Crohn's disease, antibiotics alone can be effective in the treatment of mild to moderate Crohn's disease. The mechanism of action may be to decrease luminal bacteria, consistent with the bacterial hypothesis for Crohn's disease. Antibiotics that have been found to be useful include ampicillin, metronidazole, tetracycline, cefaclor, clindamycin, and erythromycin. If effective, patients with mild to moderate inflammation started on a single agent can expect improvement in 5 to 7 days. After a response, patients are kept on the antibiotic for about a month after signs and symptoms have resolved. Some patients will need to be tried on several antibiotics until one is found that works in them. Patients who respond to antibiotics may get antibiotics for flares using the same antibiotic or changing antibiotic with each episode, or may be kept on antibiotics chronically, on either the same antibiotic or rotating to a different antibiotic every month. Anecdotal reports include evidence of resolution of obstructions with time.

Metronidazole has a special role in the treatment of patients with Crohn's disease. It is the antibiotic of choice in combination with steroids for the treatment of enteric and cutaneous fistulas. It is also the antibiotic most commonly reported to be of benefit in anecdotal reports of treatment of cutaneous manifestations of Crohn's disease such as in rare cases of Crohn's disease of the vulva.

Immunosuppressives

Azathioprine and its metabolite, 6-mercaptopurine, have been gaining increasing favor in the treatment of ulcerative colitis and Crohn's disease. They have been found to be especially useful in cases where disease is resistant to steroids. In 70% of such patients a positive response, such as elimination of steroids, a decrease in dose, or closure of persistent fistulas, is seen. The average time to response is delayed out to an average of 3 months and up to 6 months in some patients. 6-Mercaptopurine should see increasing use in the future as experience is gained with this drug and if it continues to have a low rate of toxicity.

Cyclosporin A has also been used in inflammtory bowel disease, mostly in patients with Crohn's disease. Its onset of action is about 2 weeks, but further studies are needed to determine its role in treatment.

Defined Diets and Total Parenteral Nutrition

Elimination of solid foods is effective in decreasing symptoms from obstruction in Crohn's disease. Placing a patient on total parenteral nutrition or enteral feedings also has been reported to decrease inflammation, perhaps by decreasing luminal antigen load. It is not entirely clear whether the salutary effect is due to a direct anti-inflammatory effect or to improved nutrition. In any case, enteral formulas have a useful role during pregnancy in patients with Crohn's disease, where alone or in combination with steroids they can help control disease sufficiently to delay surgery or obviate the need for immunosuppressives.

Pregnancy and Inflammatory Bowel Disease

Effect of Inflammatory Bowel Disease on Pregnancy

For most patients with inflammatory bowel disease pregnancy will result in a healthy child. Studies have shown that treatment of inflammatory bowel disease is well tolerated by the fetus and almost the full armamentarium of treatments can be safely used in treatment of patients with inflammatory bowel disease. The effect on the fetus is mostly due to the activity of disease during pregnancy. Premature delivery or infants small for gestational age result in about 50% of cases where disease is active but in only about 15% of cases where disease is inactive. Overall, patients with Crohn's disease have a threefold greater rate of premature delivery compared to controls. Patients with ulcerative colitis probably have no increased risk of premature delivery. Markers of maternal status such as weight gain and hemoglobin levels are no different in patients with quiescent disease and controls, and normal maternal weight gain during pregnancy is no protection against having an infant that is small for gestational age. Overall, inflammatory bowel disease alone is not a reason to terminate a pregnancy.

Effect of Pregnancy on Inflammatory Bowel Disease

For both ulcerative colitis and Crohn's disease pregnancy has no significant effect on the course of disease. There is no worsening of disease by pregnancy and, unfortunately, no improvement brought on by pregnancy either. Additionally, pregnancy does not affect relapse rate of inflammatory bowel disease.

Treatment of Inflammatory Bowel Disease During Pregnancy

Treatment of inflammatory bowel disease in pregnant women is similar to treatment in nonpregnant patients. Treatment with steroids and sulfasalazine has been shown to be safe. Folic acid supplementation may be more important in the patient on sulfasalazine because the drug inhibits folic acid uptake. Sulfasalazine is safe to take while nursing. The sulfa moiety released from sulfasalazine does not displace bilirubin very well and is present in insufficient quantities in breast milk to cause kernicteris. Mesalamine (5-ASA) is probably safe to take during pregnancy. There have been case reports of successful pregnancies despite the concomitant administration of azathioprine and 6-mercaptopurine, but current advice is to avoid these drugs during pregnancy because they are known teratogens in animals. Metronidazole has been shown to be safe during pregnancy in a large study that documented fetal complications when metronidazole was taken during the first trimester. Opinion varies widely, however, on whether one should be concerned about its use during pregnancy. A reasonable recommendation would be to use metronidazole in any trimester if there is a clear indication such as perineal disease or fistula, but to avoid it during pregnancy otherwise. Tetracycline, useful for treating bacterial over-growth and for managing mild to moderate Crohn's disease, is contraindicated in pregnancy due to its effect on tooth development.

There are no special issues related to surgery for inflammatory bowel disease during pregnancy other than the usual issues arising regarding surgery during pregnancy. Because a number of effective medical treatments are available for Crohn's disease and ulcerative colitis, the patient can be treated medically to optimize the time at which surgery is performed, with the goal of bringing the patient to 32 weeks' gestation.

Pregnancy After Surgery

Pregnancy after surgery for inflammatory bowel disease does not present any special considerations. The presence of an ileostomy or an ileoanal anastamosis does not affect pregnancy adversely, except that there is increased nighttime stool frequency. The rate of incontinence is not increased over that of controls.

Inflammatory Bowel Disease and Sexual Function

Sexual function in patients with inflammatory bowel disease has not been well studied. Issues important to women include fertility and sexual function. Women with inflammatory bowel disease have a lower number of pregnancies than controls. This seems to be due to patient choice rather than to lesser fecundity. Sexual function in women is often reduced, as measured by rate of intercourse. In the occasional patient with infertility and a spouse with inflammatory bowel disease, decreased spermatogenesis from sulfasalazine should be considered. Rate of sexual intercourse is often decreased because of pain, diarrhea, or fear of incontinence. Dyspareunia is often present but does not seem to be as important a determinant of decreased rate of intercourse.

Colectomy has a variable effect of sexual function. Usually colectomy provides functional improvement that is associated with improved self-image. However, after proctocolectomy about one half of patients have a vaginal discharge, two thirds of which are due to the horizontal vagina syndrome. In this syndrome the vagina does not drain normal secretions well and dyspareunia is often present due to postoperative anatomic changes as well as chronic vaginitis. The incidence of horizontal vagina syndrome is lower when an ileoanal anastamosis is performed. Vaginal reconstruction is possible and is very effective in relieving dyspareunia.

There is little to recommend a Koch pouch over an ileoanal anastamosis. Patients with either report similar rates of several measures of sexual function including copulation frequency and orgasm rate. In women who have had a conventional Brooke ileostomy, both the Koch pouch and ileoanal anastamosis provide superior feelings of self-image and result in improved ability to date.

GENERAL SUGGESTED READINGS

Bayless TM, ed. Current management of inflammatory bowel disease. Philadelphia: BC Decker, 1989.

Korelitz BI. Inflammatory bowel disease in pregnancy. In: Gastrointestinal and liver problems in pregnancy. Gastroenterol Clin North Am 1992;21:827–834.

SUGGESTED READINGS RELATED TO INFLAMMATORY BOWEL DISEASE IN WOMEN

Baird DD, Narendranathan M, Sandler RS. Increased risk of preterm birth for women with inflammatory bowel disease. Gastroenterology 1990;99:987–994.

Bauer JJ, Sher ME, Jaffin H, et al. Transvaginal approach for repair of rectovaginal fistulae complicating Crohn's disease. Ann Surg 1991;213:151–158.

Bohe MG, Ekelund GR, Genell SN, et al. Surgery for fulminating colitis during pregnancy. Dis Colon Rectum 1983;26:119–122.

Bonfils S, Hervoir P, Girodet J, et al. Acute spontaneously recovering ulcerating colitis (ARUC). Report of 6 cases. Am J Dig Dis 1977;22:429–436.

Cappell MS, Friedman D, Mikhail N. Endometriosis of the terminal ileum simulating the clinical, roentgenographic, and surgical findings in Crohn's disease. Am J Gastroenterol 1991;86:1057–1062.

Fedorkow DM, Persaud D, Nimrod CA. Inflammatory bowel disease: a controlled study of late pregnancy outcome. Am J Obstet Gynecol 1989;160:998–1001.

Froines EJ, Palmer DL. Surgical therapy for rectovaginal fistulas in ulcerative colitis. Dis Colon Rectum 1991;34:925–930.

Jarnerot G, Into-Malmberg MB, Esbjorner E. Placental transfer of sulphasalazine and sulphapyridine and some of its metabolites. Scand J Gastroenterol 1981;16:693–697.

Katschinski B, Fingerle D, Scherbaum B, Goebell H. Oral contraceptive use and cigarette smoking in Crohn's disease. Dig Dis Sci 1993;38:1596–1600.

Kingsland CR, Alderman B. Crohn's disease of the vulva. J R Soc Med 1991;84:236–237.

Metcalf AM, Dozois RR, Kelly KA. Sexual function in women after proctocolectomy. Ann Surg 1986;204:624–627.

Mogadam M, Dobbins WO 3d, Korelitz BI, Ahmed SW. Pregnancy in inflammatory bowel disease: effect of sulfasalazine and corticosteroids on fetal outcome. Gastroenterology 1981;80:72–76.

Moody G, Probert CS, Srivastava EM, et al. Sexual dysfunction amongst women with Crohn's disease: a hidden problem. Digestion 1992;52:179–183.

Nelson H, Dozois RR, Kelly KA, et al. The effect of pregnancy and delivery on the ileal pouch-anal anastomosis functions. Dis Colon Rectum 1989;32:384–388.

Radcliffe AG, Ritchie JK, Hawley PR, et al. Anovaginal and rectovaginal fistulas in Crohn's disease. Dis Colon Rectum 1988;31:94–99.

Schade RR, Van Thiel DH, Gavaler JS. Chronic idiopathic ulcerative colitis. Pregnancy and fetal outcome. Dig Dis Sci 1984;29:614–619.

Scott NA, Nair A, Hughes LE. Anovaginal and rectovaginal fistula in patients with Crohn's disease. Br J Surg 1992;79:1379–1380.

Sjodahl R, Nystrom PO, Olaison G. Surgical treatment of dorsocaudal dislocation of the vagina after excision of the rectum. The Kylberg operation. Dis Colon Rectum 1990;33:762–764.

Snabes MC, Samaniego J, Poindexter AN. Hysterosalpingographic diagnosis of Crohn's disease. A case report. J Reprod Med 1992;37:285–288.

Swinson CM, Perry J, Lumb M, Levi AJ. Role of sulphasalazine in the aetiology of folate deficiency in ulcerative colitis. Gut 1981;22:456–461.

Tedesco FJ, Volpicelli NA, Moore FS. Estrogen- and progesterone-associated colitis: a disorder with clinical and endoscopic features mimicking Crohn's colitis. Gastrointest Endosc 1982;28:247–249.

Tuffnell D, Buchan PC. Crohn's disease of the vulva in childhood. Br J Clin Pract 1991;45:159–160.

Veloso FT, Cardoso V, Fraga J, et al. Spontaneous umbilical fistula in Crohn's disease. J Clin Gastroenterol 1989;11:197–200.

Wakefield AJ, Sawyerr AM, Hudson M, et al. Smoking, the oral contraceptive pill, and Crohn's disease. Dig Dis Sci 1991;36(8):1147–1150.

Werlin SL, Esterly NB, Oechler H. Crohn's disease presenting as unilateral labial hypertrophy. J Am Acad Dermatol 1992;27:893–895.

Wikland M, Jansson I, Asztely M, et al. Gynaecological problems related to anatomical changes after conventional proctocolectomy and ileostomy. Int J Colorectal Dis 1990;5:49–52.

Woolfson K, Cohen Z, McLeod RS. Crohn's disease and pregnancy. Dis Colon Rectum 1990;33:869–873.

SECTION FIVE

HEMATOLOGY

CHAPTER 16

ANEMIA

James W. Shine

Anemia is a common problem in a primary care practice. It provides a diagnostic challenge for the physician because it is a nonspecific finding. Anemia is a condition rather than a disease in itself. Thus it does not qualify as a diagnosis and the underlying cause must always be sought. There are over a hundred causes of anemia. Too often the busy physician is tempted to prescribe iron or vitamins without a thorough investigation. Even if this effectively treats an iron deficiency, colon cancer or other pathology may be the underlying cause. Therefore an orderly approach to this condition is important.

Definition

Anemia is normally defined as a decreased concentration of hemoglobin in the blood because it is easy to measure and reproduce. Although a decrease in the red blood cell (RBC) mass may be a more exact definition, it is difficult to measure the mass. Thus the patient's volume status must always be considered lest a significant anemia be masked by dehydration (hemoconcentration) or a mild anemia be exaggerated by overhydration (hemodilution).

Presentation

The presentation of anemia varies from an emergency in acute blood loss to asymptomatic in mild iron deficiency. This variability in the spectrum of presentation depends on the abruptness of onset, the severity, and the ability of the cardiopulmonary system to compensate. When the onset is gradual, few symptoms are noted until the hemoglobin concentration is 8 gm/dL or lower. Initially, dyspnea and mild fatigue occur with strenuous exercise. Later on, tachycardia and a high-output systolic murmur may be noted. High-output cardiac failure occurs in the most severe cases or in patients with underlying cardiac disease. Pallor will be best noted in the mucous membranes of the mouth, lips, conjunctivae, nailbeds, and palmar skin crease. Elements of a thorough history are listed in Table 16.1.

Pathophysiology and Classification

The pathophysiology of anemia is actually quite simple. There are three basic mechanisms: 1) blood loss, 2) destruction of RBCs (hemolysis), and 3) decreased production of RBCs. Although the causes of anemia could be categorized by these mechanisms, the usual classification is by RBC morphology as described by Wintrobe. This classification system is based on RBC size and hemoglobin content as determined from RBC indices and the peripheral blood smear. The automated complete blood count (CBC) provides an electronically measured mean corpuscular volume (MCV), an RBC count, and hemoglobin concentration. In addition, many electronic counters calculate a red cell distribution width (RDW), which is a measure of the variation in size of RBCs. Based on the MCV (normal range is 78 to 98 femtoliters in adults), anemia can be classified as microcytic, normocytic, or macrocytic. This is accurate as long as the RBC population is homogeneous. The RDW (normal range 11.5% to 14.5%) is a calculated index that quantifies the amount of variation in the size of RBCs. Elevation of the RDW suggests anisocytosis (variability of RBC size). Thus when the RDW is elevated, the MCV is less reliable and examination of the peripheral blood smear becomes even more important in classifying the anemia.

Table 16.1 History of the Patient with Anemia

Family history	Blood disorders, autoimmune disorders (thyroid)
Occupational, social, and travel history	Infectious or toxic exposure (lead exposure, alcohol use, malaria exposure)
Dietary history	Vegetarian diet associated with B_{12} deficiency (vegan diet), cravings for a certain food or pica associated with iron deficiency
Drug history	Prescription and over-the-counter agents
Review of symptoms	
Sore tongue or dysphagia	Iron, folate, or B_{12} deficiency
Abdominal pain	Lead poisoning, porphyria, paroxysmal nocturnal hemoglobin (dark urine in last two disorders)
Systemic symptoms	Weight loss, fever, or night sweats suggest an underlying systemic illness, such as a malignancy or chronic infection
Menstrual history	Amount of blood loss
Neurologic symptoms	Paresthesia, weakness or peripheral neuropathy suggests vitamin deficiency, lead poisoning, amyloidosis, or vasculitides

Adapted from Samuels-Reid JH. Anemia. Monograph, Edition No. 150, Home Study Self-Assessment Program. Kansas City, MO: American Academy of Family Physicians, November 1991.

Abnormal RBC morphology is best determined by examination of the peripheral blood smear. The normal RBC is similar in size to the nucleus of a small lymphocyte. The hemoglobin content is estimated by observing the RBC central pallor. Normally, the central pallor has a diameter about one third that of the entire cell. When the central pallor takes up more area, the RBC is considered hypochromic. Other terms used in microscopy are listed in Table 16.2.

Other tests of importance include the serum ferritin, which gives an estimate of the body's iron stores. A low serum ferritin level is diagnostic of iron deficiency. In general, it is a more useful measure of iron status than serum iron or total iron-binding capacity (TIBC), which can be acute phase reactants. In certain situations, however, a spuriously normal or elevated serum ferritin level results in a false-negative test. This usually occurs when iron deficiency coexists with another condition (cancer, infection, inflammation, liver disease). Thus a low serum ferritin level is specific for iron deficiency, but a normal or elevated value is less reliable. The ultimate test of iron stores is a bone marrow biopsy.

The reticulocyte count provides an assessment of bone marrow function. Reticulocytes are newly formed, immature erythrocytes. The count is usually reported as a percentage of RBCs, and it constitutes 1% of RBCs. Theoretically this percentage can increase either because there are more reticulocytes in circulation or because there are fewer mature cells. Therefore, the corrected reticulocyte count equals:

$$\begin{array}{c}\text{Corrected}\\ \text{reticulocyte}\\ \text{count}\end{array} = \begin{array}{c}\text{Reticulocyte}\\ \text{count (\%)}\end{array} \times \frac{\text{Patient's hematocrit}}{\text{Normal hematocrit (45)}}$$

A low corrected reticuloctye count indicates the bone marrow is not producing RBCs appropriately. An elevated corrected reticulocyte count indicates increased erythropoiesis as would be expected in patients with bleeding or hemolysis.

Differential Diagnosis of Anemia

Microcytic Hypochromic Anemia

This is by far the most common type of anemia and especially in a practice limited to women. The algorithm in Figure 16.1 shows the work-up and differential diagnosis for this type of anemia.

Table 16.2 Terms Used to Describe Erythrocyte Morphology

Anisocytosis	Variation in RBC size; suggests early deficiency in iron, vitamin B_{12}, or folic acid
Microcytosis	RBCs smaller than normal; iron deficiency, thalassemia
Macrocytosis	RBCs larger than normal; vitamin B_{12} folate deficiency, liver disease, alcoholism, hypothyroidism, hemolysis
Spherocytosis	Small globular RBC without the usual central pallor; hereditary spherocytosis, hemolytic anemia
Schistocyte	Fragment of an RBC; mechanical hemolytic anemia
Target cell	Abnormally thin RBC with a dark center and a peripheral ring of hemoglobin; hemoglobinopathies, liver disease
Burr cell	Spiculed RBC; uremia
Basophilic stippling	Spotted appearance inside RBC; thalassemia, sideroblastic anemia, heavy metal poisoning

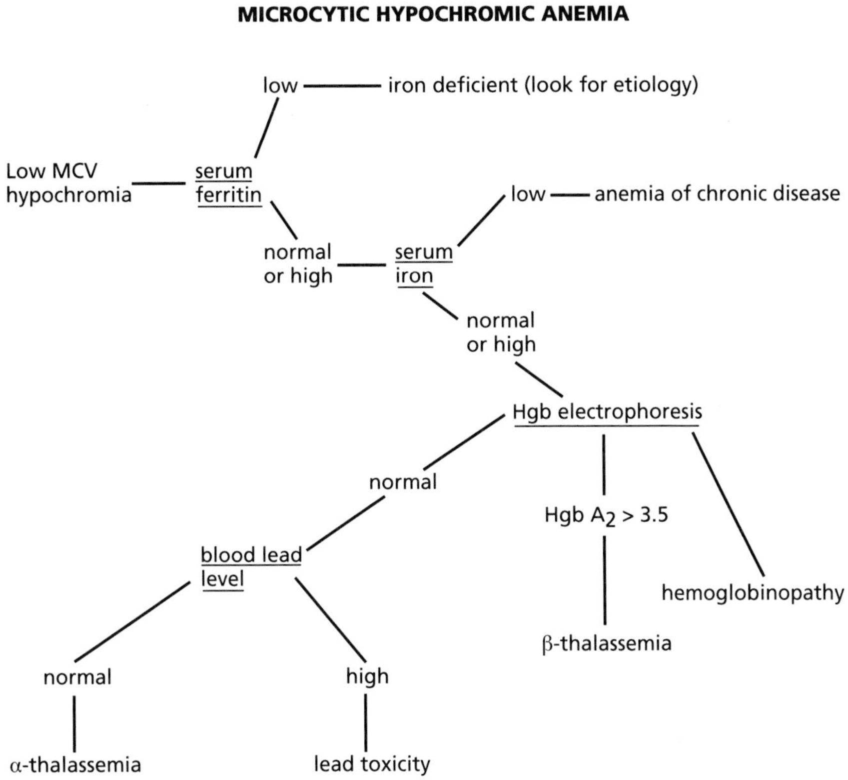

Fig 16.1 Algorithm with differential for microcytic hypochromic anemia.

Iron Deficiency Anemia

The overwhelming majority of microcytic anemia can be classified as iron deficiency anemia. Its prevalence in women is especially high because of menstruation and low iron intake. Women lose 2 mg iron per day (twice as much as men). To replace this with diet alone, a woman would have to eat over 3000 kcal/day (6 mg iron/1000 kcal with 10% absorption rate). Thus,

Table 16.3 Laboratory Values in Iron Deficiency Anemia

Hematocrit	42	42	35	27	19
MCV	92	88	82	75	68
MCHC (32–36 mg/dL)	33	33	33	31	29
SI (65–175 mg/dL)	70	60	35	20	20
TIBC (250–375 mg/dL)	300	300	300	400	450
Serum ferritin (10–200 mg/mL)	60	30	5	3	1
Peripheral smear	Normal	Normal	Normal	1 + Poikilocytosis 1 + Hypochromic	4 + Hypochronic 4 + Hypochromic
Bone marrow Iron stores	Present	Absent	Absent	Absent	Absent

MCHC, mean corpuscular hemoglobin concentration; MCV, mean corpuscular volume; SI, serum iron; TIBC, total iron-binding capacity

even in normal situations, a positive iron balance is difficult for women to achieve. Iron deficiency anemia is a dynamic process so the laboratory diagnosis depends on the degree of iron lost. Normal adults have 3 to 4 gm of iron in stores and anemia may not be detectable until 1 gm is lost. Initially the bone marrow stores will be depleted, followed by a decrease in serum ferritin, which is the first measurable sign of iron deficiency (other than bone marrow biopsy). Then serum iron concentration decreases while TIBC increases; hemoglobin levels decrease and when hemoglobin levels fall below 9 gm/dL a microcytosis will be evident. Table 16.3 shows the spectrum of laboratory values at different stages of iron deficiency anemia. In addition to these changes, the RDW is elevated and the RBC count is decreased.

Once iron deficiency anemia is discovered a cause must be sought. The most common cause is chronic blood loss. The likely etiology of blood loss differs in menstruating and postmenopausal women. In the menstruating patient the etiology is usually due to menstrual irregularities. In the postmenopausal patient the source is more commonly the gastrointestinal tract. Box 16.1 lists underlying causes of iron deficiency anemia.

The ultimate treatment involves identifying and eliminating the cause while replacing the lost iron. Ferrous sulfate ($FeSO_4$) is the most appropriate source of iron (20% elemental iron). The usual dose of elemental iron is 6 mg/kg per day up to 200 mg/day. Ideally this should be taken on an empty stomach with juice containing vitamin C. Vitamin C increases absorption of iron. Side effects are usually gastrointestinal related (constipation, cramping, diarrhea, black stool) and occur in 25% of patients. Tolerance improves if the dose is gradually increased (e.g., 325 mg $FeSO_4$ daily for 1 week, then twice daily for 1 week, then three times a day). Occasionally a lower dose must be used or given with food, which will increase the duration of treatment. Other forms of iron include $FeSO_4$ elixir (44 mg elemental iron per 5 mL) and ferrous glucon-

Box 16.1 Underlying Causes of Iron Deficiency Anemia

Most Common Causes

- Menorrhagia
- Peptic ulcer disease
- Gastrointestinal cancer
- Diverticulosis
- Ulcerative colitis
- Gastritis from nonsteroidal anti-inflammatory drugs
- Hookworms

Less Common Causes

- Hereditary hemorrhagic telangiectasia
- Pulmonary hemosiderosis
- Self-induced bleeding

Iatrogenic Causes

- Blood loss in surgery
- Frequent phlebotomy

ate. Enteric-coated forms and combinations with vitamin C increase cost without significantly increasing efficacy. The response to treatment is first noted in a reticulocytosis, which is maximal 5 to 10 days into therapy. The hemoglobin increases within a week and the anemia is corrected with repletion of iron stores as early as 2 months. Failure to respond indicates malabsorption of iron (as in celiac sprue), continued blood loss, or nonadherence usually secondary to intolerance of side effects.

Thalassemia

Thalassemia is a relatively common cause of microcytosis. It is a disorder of globin chain synthesis that leads to a compensatory overproduction of the unaffected globin chains. These excess chains tend to aggregate and precipitate causing premature RBC hemolysis. Normal adult hemoglobin consists of four heme groups and four globin chains—two each of two different chain types (Table 16.4). The homozygous form, thalassemia major, is devastating but uncommon. The heterozygous form, thalassemia minor, is much more common especially in certain groups. β-Thalassemia is most common in people of Mediterranean origin (Greek, Italian, Northern African) whereas α-thalassemia is more common in blacks, affecting more than 5% of that population. Southeast Asians are also carriers of α-thalassemia. Thalassemia minor is normally asymptomatic and would not be clinically significant if it were not frequently mistaken for iron deficiency anemia. Patients with thalassemia minor are subjected to repeated trials of inappropriate iron therapy and work-up for iron deficiency. Thalassemia minor is usually detected by a routine CBC, which reveals a moderate microcytosis (low MCV) with a mild anemia. In addition, if the RDW and RBC count are normal, this should alert the physician to the possibility of thalassemia instead of iron deficiency anemia where the RDW is elevated and the RBC count is decreased. The peripheral smear often shows stripping of RBCs. β-Thalassemia is confirmed by hemoglobin electrophoresis, which reveals an elevated hemoglobin A_2 (3.75% to 6.5% instead of the normal 2%). α-Thalassemia is more difficult to confirm; there is no relative change in hemoglobin electrophoresis because each hemoglobin molecule has two α-globin chains. However, if the laboratory work is consistent with thalassemia but the hemoglobin electrophoresis is normal, α-thalassemia can be confirmed by noting similar changes in family members. The diagnosis of thalassemia is important to avoid inappropriate iron therapy but also to provide genetic counseling. If both partners carry the thalassemia trait, there is a 25% chance of having a child with homozygous and therefore fatal disease. Also, because sickle thalassemia and hemoglobin C-thalassemia can be severe, partners who carry these traits should be made aware of the 25% risk their offspring carry of developing disease.

Table 16.4 Normal Adult Hemoglobin

Hgb A	$\alpha_2\beta_2$	97%
Hgb A_2	$\alpha_2\delta_2$	2%
Hgb F	$\alpha_2\gamma_2$	1%

Hemoglobinopathies

The homozygous state of hemoglobinopathies is usually recognized early in life. The heterozygous state, however, is usually asymptomatic and may be discovered through routine testing. Microcytosis is common and distinct morphologic changes such as the sickle cell may be noted. Diagnosis is confirmed by hemoglobin electrophoresis. Hemoglobins S and C are common in blacks and people of Mediterranean origin. Hemoglobin E is found in 10% of southeast Asians. Hemoglobin D is common in parts of India.

Anemia of Chronic Disease

Although normally the anemia of chronic disease is normocytic normochromic, it occasionally is microcytic hypochromic, necessitating its differentiation from iron deficiency anemia. If the serum ferritin is normal or increased and the serum iron is low, anemia of chronic disease is likely. Occasionally, iron deficiency anemia may coexist with anemia of chronic disease and a trial of iron therapy is necessary.

Lead Toxicity

Lead poisoning is most common in children; however adults are at risk from occupational exposure. If suspected, a blood lead level should be examined.

Normocytic Normochronic Anemia

The differential diagnosis of normocytic normochromic anemia is aided by the corrected reticulocyte count, which distinguishes two broad categories:

1. A low or normal corrected reticulocyte count reflects poor bone marrow function and decreased RBC production.
2. An elevated corrected reticulocyte count reflects normal bone marrow function implying increased RBC loss or destruction.

Figure 16.2 is an algorithm showing the differential diagnosis of normocytic normochromic anemia.

Decreased Red Blood Cell Production

Primary bone marrow disease is often accompanied by leukopenia and thrombcytopenia. A bone marrow biopsy and aspiration are indicated in these cases. Secondary bone marrow hypoplasia should be suspected when no other signs of bone marrow dysfunction are present (no leukopenia or thrombcytopenia). In addition if one of the disorders listed on Figure 16.2 under secondary bone marrow hypoplasia is present, it will be the likely etiology. Drugs that can cause anemia are listed in Table 16.5.

Increased Red Blood Cell Loss or Destruction

Again, a high corrected reticulocyte count is indicative of this. The causes are acute blood loss, which is usually apparent, hypersplenism that becomes hematologically significant only when the spleen is three times normal size (seen in portal hypertension, chronic infections, or myeloproliferative disorders), and in hemolytic anemia. Hemolytic anemia can be further defined by reviewing the peripheral smear and checking a Coombs' test if the smear is normal. Table 16.6 lists the different types of hemolytic anemia. Finally, a microcytic and macrocytic anemia can combine to present as a normocytic anemia (e.g., coexistent iron and folate deficiencies). The peripheral smear usually reveals signs of a dual diagnosis.

Macrocytic Anemia

By reviewing a peripheral smear, macrocytic anemia can be divided into megaloblastic and nonmegaloblas-

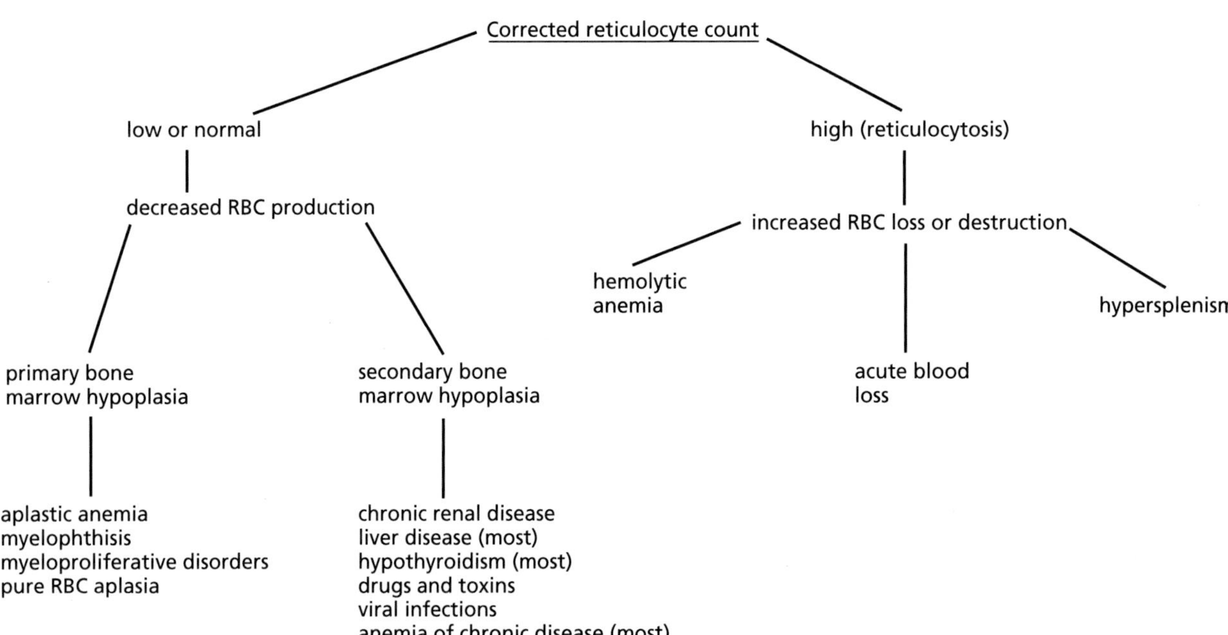

Fig 16.2 Algorithm with differential for normocytic normochromic anemia.

Table 16.5 Drugs Than Can Cause Anemia

Drugs Causing Marrow Hypoplasia Aplasia
Antineoplastic drugs
Antimetabolites: 6-mercaptopurine, azathioprine, 5-fluorouracil, hydroxyuria, cytosine arabinoside
Alkylating agents: cyclophosphamide, chlorambucil, busulfan, melphalan
Antimicrobial drugs: chloramphenicol, quinacrine, streptoymycin, sulfas
Anticonvulsant drugs: trimethadione, phenytoin, primidone, carbamazepine
Anti-inflammatory drugs: phenylbutazone, gold salts, aspirin, colchicine
Oral hypoglycemics: chlorpropamide, tolbutamide
Tranquilizers: chlordiazepoxide, meprobamate
Major tranquilizers/antiemetics: chlorpromazine (Thorazine), prochlorperazine (Compazine)
Antihistamines: chlorpheniramine, tripelennamine
Miscellaneous: alcohol, acetaxolamide, potassium perchlorate
Drugs Causing Hemolytic Anemia
In glucose-6-phosphate dehydrogenase deficiency
Antimicrobial drugs: sulfas, primaquine, quinacrine, nitrofurantoin, nalidixic acid
Others: acetanilid, phenazopyridine (Pyridium)
In immune hemolytic anemia
Penicillin, sulfas, quinine, quinidine, methyldopa, para-aminosalicylic acid, mefenamic acid (Ponstel), levodopa
Folate antagonists
Methotrexate, pyrimethamine, trimethoprim, triamterene
Porphyrin/heme synthesis antagonists
Alcohol, izoniazid
Drugs Causing Gastrointestinal Blood Loss
Aspirin, nonsteroidal anti-inflammatory agents, alcohol

Table 16.6 Hemolytic Disorders

Congenital
Hemoglobinopathies (sickle cell anemia, etc.)
Disorders of RBC membrane
Spherocytosis
Elliptocytosis
RBC enzyme deficiencies
Glucose-6-phosphate dehydrogenase deficiency
Acquired
Mechanical hemolysis
Prosthetic heart valves
Disseminated intravascular coagulation
Thrombotic thrombocytopenic purpura
Hemolytic uremic syndrome
Immune Mediated
Autoimmune hemolysis
Drug-induced hemolysis
Paroxysmal nocturnal hemoglobinuria
Erythroblastosis fetalis

tic anemia. Megaloblastic anemia is characterized by hypersegmented neutrophils and oval macrocytes. Nonmegaloblastic anemia does not show these features.

Megaloblastic Anemia

Once the macrocytic anemia is defined as megaloblastic, a thorough history and physical as well as B_{12} and RBC folate level will help differentiate the cause. Underlying causes are listed in Box 16.2. When megaloblastic anemia is not associated with B_{12} or folate deficiency, it is usually caused by drug interaction. Table 16.5 lists the antimetabolite and folate antagonists most commonly encountered.

Nonmegaloblastic Anemia

If the peripheral smear does not reveal hypersegmented neutrophils and oval macrocytes, a nonmegaloblastic anemia is present. A corrected reticulocyte count will help differentiate the causes. A reticulocytosis naturally causes an increase in MCV because the larger, more immature RBC is forced into circulation. The

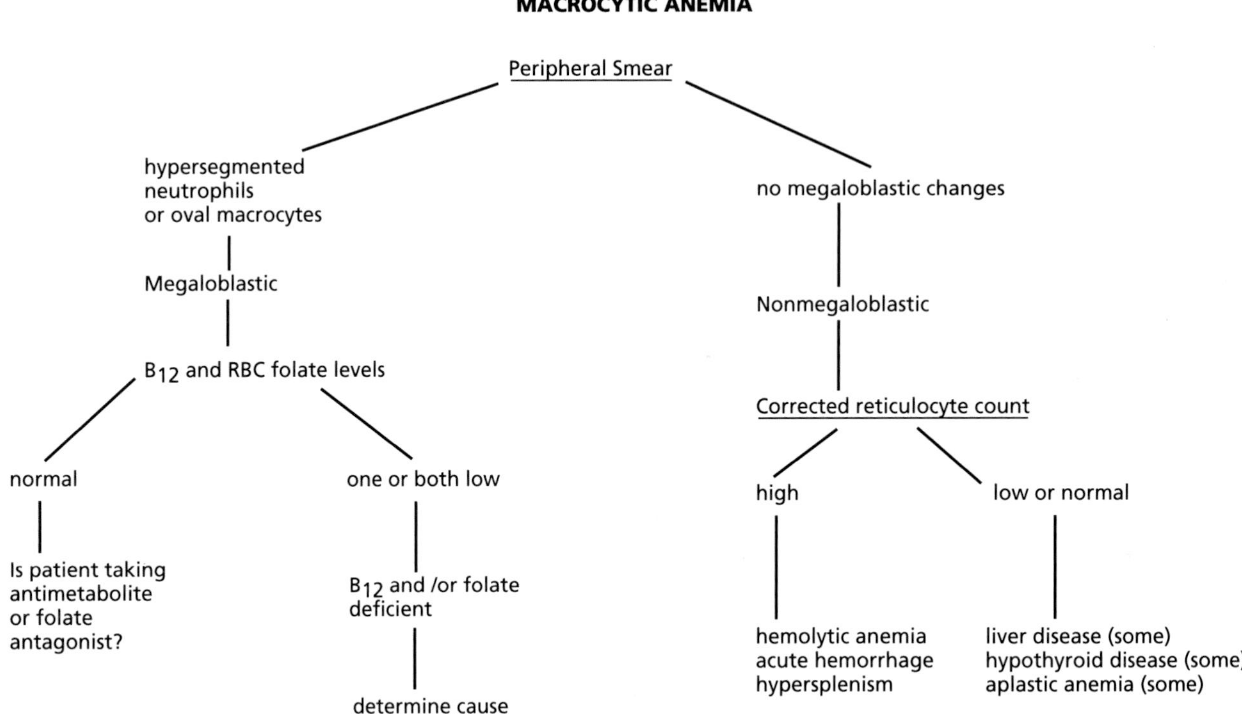

Fig 16.3 Algorithm with differential for macrocytic anemia.

Box 16.2 Causes of B_{12} and Folate Deficiency

B_{12} Deficiency

- Pernicious anemia
- Gastrectomy
- Ileal resection or disease
- Fish tapeworm infestation
- Pregnancy (increased requirement)
- Dietary deficiency (rare; vegan diet)

Folate Deficiency

- Dietary (alcoholic, old age, chronic disease)
- Malabsorption
  - Sprue
  - Drug induced (phenytoin, alcohol, oral contraceptives)
  - Small bowel resection or bypass
- Chronic hemolysis (increased requirement)

algorithm for differential diagnosis is presented in Figure 16.3.

Summary

Anemia is a condition, not a disease; therefore, an underlying cause must be sought. By classifying according to RBC size and morphology, an orderly and cost-effective work-up can be pursued. Iron deficiency anemia is the most common form of all anemias and has a spectrum of presentations. Thalassemia is also common and should be differentiated from iron deficiency because treatment with iron could be detrimental and genetic counseling is indicated. Although other causes of anemia are less common, the primary care physician should be able to diagnose these and treat or refer the patient when necessary.

CHAPTER 17

COAGULATION DISORDERS

Pradip K. Rustagi

Hemostasis is the process by which bleeding is controlled after vascular injury. The mechanisms that constitute hemostasis ensure that blood flow is re-established after thrombus formation and that blood remains fluid in the absence of trauma. Failure of hemostasis manifests as bleeding and leads to ischemia and circulatory collapse. However, dysfunctional hemostasis (thrombus formation within undisturbed blood vessels or persistent vascular occlusion despite control of bleeding) also compromises blood flow and leads to tissue damage. Thus, a dynamic balance between opposing procoagulant and anticoagulant forces helps maintain adequate tissue perfusion. This chapter deals mainly with the recognition and management of disorders of coagulation, which regularly account for bleeding in adult women. A conceptual approach is offered rather than detailed consideration of individual abnormalities. Bleeding due to primary hyperfibrinolysis is rare unless a consequence of thrombolytic therapy and is only briefly mentioned. A short section on hypercoagulability is included. Quantitative platelet disorders and thrombotic microangiopathy are discussed elsewhere.

Interview and Examination of the Bleeding Patient

A review of subjective complaints and objective findings is paramount to the proper management of bleeding. A broad sweep of the history and medical record is necessary to make sense of isolated or scattered signs and symptoms of blood loss, to interpret results of laboratory testing, and to accurately assess the need and urgency to intervene therapeutically. An individual's hemostatic competence is most reliably established by recognizing evidence of successful responses to previous trauma or surgery. Such challenges to vascular integrity provide an overall measure of hemostasis with far more predictive value for the risk of clinically significant bleeding in the future than results of laboratory testing. A laboratory evaluation is indicated to identify the basis for an increased risk of bleeding so that specific treatment may by instituted and response to treatment may be properly monitored.

Symptoms of Bleeding

It must first be established that unintended bleeding has in fact occurred. Such an obvious task should not be dismissed without due consideration: blood loss can be falsely blamed for medical or surgical problems and is occasionally self-induced. Anemia may be a result of intravascular hemolysis, but can be erroneously attributed to bleeding if, for example, care is not taken to distinguish cell-free hemoglobin from intact red blood cells in a patient complaining of bloody urine. Bleeding may be occult or unsuspected. Details with regard to the amount of blood loss and degree of anemia may be volunteered or elicited. Information should be sought with regard to apathy, irritability, easy fatigability, generalized weakness, exertional dyspnea, pica (the irrational ingestion of clay, starch, or ice). Among red blood cell indices, microcytosis, occurs late in the course of iron deficiency (after drop in hemoglobin level, decrease in red cell number, and development of hypochromia) and should be distinguished from the microcytosis of thalassemia. Brisk bleeding can be conveyed by the presence of symptoms attributable to loss of intravascular fluid volume (postural light-headedness, palpitations, confusion) or by information provided at the bedside or in the contemporaneous medical record (the recent development of a measurable transfusion requirement, a rapid 10 mm Hg fall in systolic blood pressure indicating the loss of 10% of intravascular volume, or 1 gm/dL drop in hemoglobin or 3% drop in hematocrit representing the loss of 500 mL of blood). Ancillary supportive evidence of a risk or apparent cause of bleeding (platelet count <20,000/μL, serum chemistries showing azotemia, etc) may also be derived from screening laboratory studies. Unanticipated intra- or postoperative bleeding is most often due simply to the need for additional surgical intervention and is only occasionally a manifestation of a systemic defect of hemostasis that was not suspected preoperatively.

Cardinal symptoms of bleeding such as menometrorrhagia may be subjectively construed as being unworthy of notice if a woman has become so accustomed to them that they are not considered to be unusual. Conversely, minute amounts of bleeding or bruising can provoke unnecessary anxiety. It is important to determine whether the bleeding is appropriate or unexpected in the situation at hand. Almost two thirds of healthy women perceive themselves to suffer from some sort of a bleeding disorder despite the rarity of true systemic coagulation defects in the general population, and it is often necessary to make an assessment of the validity of any individual claim. Familiarity with an individual patient or corroborative information from alternate sources is often necessary.

Causes of Bleeding

An important purpose of the initial evaluation is to determine whether the bleeding can be attributed to a hematologic rather than a structural cause. The absence of unusual postpartum bleeding, worrisome postoperative bleeding, metrorrhagia, or easy bruisability is reliable in excluding the presence of a systemic hemostatic disorder. More than 3 days of heavy menstrual flow or more than an average duration of 7 days for menses should be considered excessive. Although increased bleeding after tooth removal may not reliably identify a patient with a significant defect, it is extremely unusual for someone with a definite coagulation disorder to escape having untoward bleeding after molar extraction. It may be instructive to ask if increased bleeding from minor cuts such as those from shaving with a razor have led to use of an electric shaver. Systemic hemostatic defects are characterized by spontaneous or excessive bleeding from multiple, anatomically distinct sites, either simultaneously or sequentially. The generalized rather than confined location, fast pace or severity (expulsion of clots, rapid accumulation of blood in an operative field, wound, or hematoma, need for hemodynamic support), volume of blood loss (disproportionately severe for the extent of injury), and temporal relationship (delayed rather than immediately following surgery, resumption of bleeding from a previously secure site) should be noted. Repetitive or even solitary bleeding from an apparently restricted site (e.g., the respiratory, gastrointestinal, or urinary tract) is usually caused by a specific tissue defect even if not strictly localized (e.g., angiodysplasia). Nevertheless, anatomically confined bleeding may reflect a generalized propensity to bleed and bring timely attention to an otherwise occult lesion. An unusual but notable situation occurs when a malignant lesion is associated with the development of a cross-reactive autoantibody to a specific coagulation factor with resultant local or distant bleeding and fortuitous identification of the tumor at an early, potentially curative stage.

Information about the onset of a patient's bleeding symptoms contributes greatly to determination of the specific cause. Difficulty with hemostasis since birth or associated with a familial tendency suggests an inherited condition, whereas symptoms that have appeared later in adult life are probably acquired or associated with a systemic illness. One must not construe the history of easy bruisability due to a normally active childhood as a bleeding tendency unless the manifestations are compelling. Persitent bleeding symptoms in first-degree relatives are informative. These defects tend to involve single coagulation proteins with preservation of clinical expression (severity, laboratory features) through several generations. Fresh occurrences continue to maintain the frequency of these defects despite the apparent detrimental effect they have on health. Absence of a family history does not eliminate the possibility of a genetic basis. Isolated factor deficiencies can also be acquired as the result of an antibody or accelerated clearance and do not necessarily indicate congenital deficiency. Despite their congenital origin, bleeding due to vascular defects tends to present in adulthood.

Congenital Causes of Bleeding

The two major types of hemophilia, factor VIII and factor IX deficiency, are sex linked, recessive and occur with a combined incidence of around 1 to 2/10,000 people; this low incidence has been consistent throughout history and across varied geographic and cultural boundaries. Factor IX deficiency accounts for 10% to 15% of hemophilia and, although the clinical presentation of factor IX deficiency is identical to that of factor VIII deficiency, its management is distinct. Because the genes for factor VIII and factor IX are on the X chromosome, defects in those genes are naturally expressed in males. A single defective X-linked gene would be sufficient in women with Turner's syndrome or testicular feminization. When factor VIII or IX levels of less than 25% with normal von Willebrand factor activity are encountered in symptomatic XX women, homozygosity, consanguinity in a family with hemophilia, or fresh mutation or excessive inactivation of the normal gene due to lyonization in an obligate carrier should be considered. An unusually severe bleeding tendency in women also raises the possibility of significant factor VIII deficiency due to absence of von Willebrand factor or presence of von Willebrand factor unable to bind factor VIII (autosomal hemophilia). In contrast, factor XI deficiency is an autosomal recessive condition, expressed equally in both sexes, but quite variable clinically. The incidence of factor XI deficiency can be as high as 30/10,000 in individuals of Ashkenazi Jewish descent but is much less common in other ethnic groups.

Most of the other isolated coagulation factor deficiencies and platelet function defects are inherited as autosomal recessive disorders and are exceedingly rare. Mild congenital platelet storage pool diseases are being recognized more frequently. Although the family history is characteristically negative in these situations, suspicion may be raised by the remote history of bleeding from the umbilical stump or by appearance of a hematoma after mandated vitamin K injection at birth. Pregnant women with factor XIII deficiency are particularly prone to recurrent fetal loss and uterine bleeding.

von Willebrand's disease is a highly prevalent hereditary defect in a coagulation protein that predominantly affects platelet function. Most familial vessel wall structural defects (e.g., hereditary hemorrhagic telangiectasia and collagen vascular or connective tissue disorders) are expressed frequently and equally in both sexes because they are inherited in an autosomal dominant fashion. von Willebrand's disease has an incidence of 15 to 50/10,000, but the diagnosis requires careful interpretation of laboratory studies. In view of the relatively high incidence of von Willebrand's disease, its often subclinical nature, and its frequent presentation at an inopportune moment, it is an important diagnostic consideration in patients with menorrhagia, epistaxis, easy bruisability, worrisome postoperative or postpartum bleeding, or simply iron deficiency anemia without an obvious source of blood loss. Vessel wall defects are generally diagnoses of exclusion, which depend largely on their familial nature or clinical associations.

Acquired Causes of Bleeding

Acquired platelet disorders are far more common than congenital ones. Uremia due to renal insufficiency affects platelet function by inducing metabolic derangements. Hepatic failure, most commonly due to alcoholic liver disease, causes complex hemostatic abnormalities because almost all coagulation proteins (including those that are vitamin K dependent) are produced in the liver, activated coagulation factors and the byproducts of clot formation and dissolution are cleared by the liver, and splenic sequestration of platelets may accompany portal hypertension and produce thrombocytopenia. Chronic liver disease is also generally associated with excessive fibrinolysis due to decreased fibrinogen production, defective clearance of fibrin split products that interfere with fibrin formation and platelet aggregation, and an imbalance in the control of the fibrinolytic process, which favors increased plasminogen activation and reduced plasmin inhibition. Immunologic illnesses are occasionally associated with bleeding due to development of autoantibodies directed against various specific coagulation factors, resulting in decreased activity or accelerated clearance, or against platelets, resulting in thrombocytopenia. Medications or other drugs are the most frequent cause of thrombocytopenia. Bone marrow problems such as myeloproliferative disorders or myelodysplasia may result in abnormal maturation of megakaryocytes leading to reduced numbers of platelets or to defective platelet function. History of radiation or chemical exposure can provide clues to the cause of reduced platelet production.

Particular attention should be paid to generous use of aspirin or other nonsteroidal anti-inflammatory drugs (NSAIDs) because innumerable proprietary formulation contain aspirin and most coagulation disorders are exacerbated by aspirin-related inhibition of platelet function. A partial list of nonprescription medications containing aspirin is provided in Table 17.1. Therapy with oral contraceptives or conjugated estrogens may mask vascular defects because of their poorly understood procogulant properties; also, hormonal variation is responsible for cyclic fluctuation in clinical manifestations of various coagulation disorders, especially von Willebrand's disease. Synthesis and release of von Willebrand factor into the bloodstream are governed by estrogen stimulation.

Table 17.1 Aspirin-Containing Products

This following list is not all inclusive; other drugs or compounds may contain aspirin (acetyl-salicylate), salicylates, or salicylamides. Similar products may also be reformulated to include or exclude substances with platelet-inhibitory properties.

Alka-Seltzer	Gensan
Anacin	Goody's Powder
Arthritis Pain Formula	Lortab ASA
Arthropan	Maxiprin
A.S.A. Enseals	Measurin
Ascriptin	Megaprin
Aspergum	Micrainin
Bayer Children's Cold Tablets	Midol
BC Powder	Mepro-Analgesic
Bufferin	Mobigesic
Buffets	Momentum
Cama	Os-Cal-Gesic
Congespirin	Pabalate
Cope	P-A-C
Cosprin	Pepto-Bismol
CP-2	Persistin
Doan's Pills	S-A-C
Duradyne	St. Joseph's
Easprin	Saleto
Ecotrin	Sine-Off
Efficin	Sloprin
Empirin	Stanback
Equagesic	Supac
Excedrin	Synalgos-DC
Fiorinal	Triaminicin
Fortabs	Trigesic
4-Way	Uracel
Gaysal-S	Ursinus
Gelpirin	Vanquish
Gemnisyn	

A common problem in debilitated patients is deficiency of vitamin K, which is required for the production of several active coagulation factors. One half of the vitamin K needed is supplied by endogenous colonic bacteria; bile salts are required for absorption. Patients undergoing surgery or with an infectious illness are particularly vulnerable to becoming deficient because of dietary restriction or poor oral intake in combination with broad-spectrum antibiotic therapy. The intensity of anticoagulation with warfarin, an antagonist of vitamin K, is highly dependent on the existence of a diet stable in the amount of vitamin K_1-containing foods such as leafy green vegetables and on the contribution of vitamin K_2 by bacteria, as well as the degree of warfarin binding to plasma proteins. A number of concomitant drugs increase bioavailability of warfarin by displacing it from its binding sites and anticoagulation must be carefully monitored whenever a new medication is taken.

Bleeding occurs in as many as one fourth of pregnancies but is usually nonhematologic in origin, albeit potentially serious: threatened abortion; inevitable, incomplete, or complete abortion; placenta abruptio or previa; and ectopic pregnancy. Postpartum bleeding should be evaluated carefully for the contribution of uterine tone, trauma, and coagulopathy to the volume of blood loss, before search for a hemostatic disorder is begun.

Physical Examination

Physical examination can usually be limited and rapidly done to document stigmata of active or past bleeding and confirm the relevance of documented laboratory abnormalities. Extensive detailed inspection and palpation are usually unnecessary to determine whether observed or subjectively worrisome bleeding is truly excessive or due to systemic rather than anatomic causes. A reasonably directed examination can help narrow possibilities by making note of findings indicating chronic hepatic dysfunction (jaundice, spider telangiectasias, ascites, etc) or renal failure (uremic frost, peripheral edema, etc). Joint deformities attributable to inflammation raise concerns about autoimmune illness.

Petechiae are reliable signs of platelet (decreased number or adequate number with poor function) and vessel wall defects. They are reddish, punctate, nonpalpable, cutaneous lesions, usually occurring as a cluster in dependent regions of limbs or distal to an occlusion (e.g., blood pressure cuff related), which reflect disruption of capillary integrity. Petechiae will occur if the platelet count falls below 20,000/μL due to failure of production, unless young (hemostatically more effective) platelets are present, as in idiopathic thrombocytopenic purpura.

Complaints of easy bruisability ("black and blue marks") or subjectively increased bleeding after minor lacerations ("free bleeding") are frequent and often frustrating. This frustration is usually a consequence of previous experience with similar patients in whom no cause of an increased bleeding tendency could be discerned despite exclusion of NSAID use and occult trama. The cosmetic consequence of subcutaneous bleeding is of no minor concern to the suffering individual. Simple easy bruisability or purpura simplex is not associated with a higher risk of operative bleeding, but is a diagnosis of exclusion. Purpura associated with discomfort, at predictable sites, or at sites easily accessible to a patient's hands or mouth, raise the possibility of psychogenic origin. An important feature of purpura is its nonpalpable nature; when palpable, a vasculitic process is suggested (e.g., allergic purpura). Erythematous lesions are distinguished by the ability to blanche with pressure and are due to an entirely unrelated process. Flimsy or paper-thin scar formation following surgery or injury is indicative of poor wound healing, a feature of factor XIII deficiency, fibrinolytic disorders, and connective tissue defects. The characteristic habitus of a patient with Marfan's syndrome (upper-lower body segment ratio of <0.85, arm span 2 cm $>$ height) or evidence of hyperextensibility of the joints in Ehlers-Danlos syndrome support the existence of a connective tissue defect underlying purpura.

It is valuable to try to separate defects of fibrin formation involving coagulation factors (such as hemophilia) from defects of platelets or the blood vessel wall (such as von Willebrand's disease). Important distinguishing features are outlined in Table 17.2. Bloody joint effusions (hemarthroses) are usually painful, associated with restricted range of movement, and lead to severe and debilitating joint deformities. Such episodes of closed cavity bleeding indicate defective fibrin formation, whereas mucosal bleeding events (epistaxis, gum bleeding, menorrhagia) indicate defective platelets or vessels. However, in attributing nosebleeds to a coagulation disorder, it is important to exclude local mucosal defects (septal perforation, dry/friable mucosa, limitation to a single nostril) and hypertension; similarly, gum bleeding is more commonly due to gingivitis. Another historical feature of bleeding, which supports the existence of a platelet or vessel defect, is its immediate (posttraumatic or postoperative) or spontaneous nature. Delayed or prolonged bleeding or bleeding that recurs after initial cessation is characteristic of defective fibrin formation, even when the instigating event is not readily apparent. Soft-tissue bleeding such as intramuscular hematoma is more likely to be seem with hemophilia than with von Willebrand's disease, but can be seen with both types of defects, as are gastrointestinal and urinary tract bleeding. Complex or combined defects of hemostasis will have overlapping symptomatology.

Table 17.2 Mode of Presentation of Bleeding Disorders

	Vascular and Platelet Disorders	Coagulation Disorders
Location	Subcutaneous, mucosal	Deep (soft tissue, occult), closed cavity
Temporal	Spontaneous, immediately after injury	Delayed after injury
Physical	Petechiae, ecchymoses, hematomas	Hemarthroses, hematuria, hematomas

The Coagulation Mechanism

Coagulation refers to discrete events that culminate in the formation of a fibrin clot and involve noncellular components of blood, including ionized calcium. The overall mechanism of hemostatic thrombus formation relies heavily on significant contributions by cellular components of blood and blood vessels and by substances in the extracellular matrix whose activities are difficult to measure. Circulating platelets adhere to subendothelial collagen and von Willebrand factor exposed on vessel injury and initiate formation of a platelet plug held together largely by fibrinogen. This loose platelet plug quickly disintegrates unless stabilized by fibrin. Potent but fleeting enzymes (particularly thrombin) are generated from corresponding inactive circulating proteins with the participation of critical procofactors (such as factor VIII) when previously sequestered or unavailable materials (including tissue factor and platelet factor 3) are brought in contact with blood, induced on the surface of endothelial cells, or expressed on activated monocytes or platelets. Thrombin recruits additional platelets by activating them directly and causing them to aggregate. It enhances its own production by activating factors V and VIII and activates factor XIII. The action of thrombin on fibrinogen yields fibrin which, when stabilized by activated factor XIII, forms an insoluble net with the ability to trap cellular components, congeal blood, and arrest bleeding. Coagulation reactions characteristically involve the sequential conversion of an inactive zymogen to an enzyme that then activates several molecules of another zymogen. Progress toward clot formation depends on the cooperative participation of amenable surfaces and key cofactors, which confine enzymatic amplification to a target area. In our current understanding of the clot-forming process, the extrinsic or tissue factor pathway is considered to be important in initial thrombin generation, with the intrinsic pathway assuming a key role in sustaining thrombin generation until hemostasi is achieved. It is estimated that, in an unfettered system, association of a single molecule of factor VII with tissue factor is responsible for the production of more than 100 million molecules of fibrin monomer.

Formation of the initial platelet plug depends on von Willebrand factor, a multimeric protein with extreme size heterogeneity, which is synthesized and released from endothelial cells into both the vessel lumen and subendothelial matrix. Platelets adhere passively to collagen and to high molecular weight von Willebrand factor localized to subendothelial tissue by means of specific platelet surface membrane receptors. The turbulence in blood flow that results from vascular disruption also alters platelets such that circulating low molecular weight von Willebrand factor can bind to specific receptors on the platelet surface, promoting platelet agglutination and recruiting factor VIII to the platelet surface for activation and thrombin generation. This membrane perturbation activates quiescent platelets so that they produce thromboxane A_2, a potent platelet-aggregating substance that is a product of prostaglandin metabolism in platelets. The platelets express receptors on their surface important for fibrinogen (and later fibrin)-mediated platelet aggregation and present platelet factor 3, a reconfiguration of platelet membrane phospholipid that supports subsequent coagulation reactions and ensures that thrombus formation will occur locally on the developing platelet plug. Thromboxane alters intracellular calcium fluxes by affecting cyclic adenosine monophosphate levels, causing the release from storage granules of substances, including adenosine diphosphate (which activates and recruits nonadherent platelets), ionized calcium, platelet factor 4 (which inhibits heparan and heparin anticoagulant activity), and platelet-derived growth factor (a peptide that stimulates fibroblast and smooth muscle cell proliferation, processes thought to be involved in healing as well as atherosclerosis). Thrombin generated by coagulation is also a potent agonist for platelet degranulation. Each one of these processes can be examined and measured by specialized testing; in contrast to the macroscopic phenomenon of platelet adhesion and aggregation, the impact of each of these molecular platelet events on clinical management is not clear.

Regulation of Coagulation

The reactions that constitute hemostasis are carefully regulated. On injury, the anticoagulant nature of vascular endothelium is disrupted and reflex vasoconstriction occurs. The effects of nitric oxide, the endothelium-derived relaxing factor, and prostacyclin, a platelet inhibitory agent that is the main product of endothelial cell prostaglandin metabolism, decline, leading to vasoconstriction and platelet aggregation. The loss of thrombomodulin, an endothelial membrane cofactor that dramatically alters the specificity of thrombin so that it activates the anticoagulant protein C instead of cleaving fibrinogen, and the removal of heparan sulfate proteoglycan, which normally coats endothelial cells and augments antithrombin III activity, contribute to a localized procoagulant state. The fall in endothelial cell tissue plasminogen activator (tPA) from endothelial cells, release of platelet type 1 plasminogen activator inhibitor (PAI-1), and presence of α_2-proteinase inhibitor in blood outside of the clot protect fibrin from plasmin, allowing fibrin to linger for the necessary period of time. However, tPA released from adjacent endothelial cells binds to freshly formed fibrin, beginning the process that will lead to restoration of blood flow. Plasminogen is activated to plasmin by tPA when the two are bound to the fibrin surface. Plasmin and elastase (released from neutrophils caught in the thrombus) degrade fibrin into fragments termed fibrin split products, permitting re-establishment of the circulation and subsequent healing. Elastase activity is controlled by α_1-proteinase inhibitor. Activated protein C degrades factors Va and VIIIa and inactivates PAI-1. Both unactivated factor V and protein S are nonenzymatic cofactors for the action of activated protein C. Protein S is inactive when bound to C4b-binding protein, a regulatory protein of the classic pathway of complement, which retains its inhibitory activity. Only free protein S participates in regulation of thrombin generation. Thus the temporary, limited procoagulant state created by the exposure of blood to subendothelium stems the loss of blood, but also initiates the process of clot dissolution to restore vascular patency.

Physiology of Coagulation Proteins

Plasma coagulation proteins are normally present in excess and have widely ranging biologic half-lives. These parameters have important implications for prophylaxis and replacement therapy (Table 17.3). Factor VII may need to be replaced every 4 to 6 hours to keep levels above 20% in a bleeding patient, whereas factor XIII may only need to be replaced every 4 weeks to keep levels above 5% to prevent spontaneous bleeding.

Procoagulant factor activity levels generally increase with oral contraceptive therapy and pregnancy until term. Levels of von Willebrand factor and factors VIII and VII typically double; the remainder increase by 15% to 50%. Factor IX is unpredictable during pregnancy and factor V activity does not change significantly. Levels return to baseline 6 weeks after parturition. In contrast, levels of the physiologic anticoagulant proteins remain fairly constant during pregnancy, except for protein S, which decreases by a third due to an acute phase increase in C4b-binding protein, and PAI activity, which increases at least fourfold. PAI-1 level is not affected by oral contraceptive use, but antithrombin III activity decreases.

Although most coagulation proteins are produced by liver cells and then released into the circulation, factor VIII is also produced in extrahepatic sites (possibly reticuloendothelial cells). Therefore, factor VIII activity tends to be preserved in chronic liver disease as compared to factor V activity. Approximately 30% of factor V is associated with platelets. Consequently, a parallel decline in factor VIII and factor V points toward a state of excessive thrombin activity (such as disseminated intravascular coagulation [DIC]) rather than liver failure, factor VIII levels tend to be preserved in chronic liver disease, and liver transplantation can cure hemophilia. The von Willebrand factor subunits and PAI-1 are produced by endothelial cells and bone marrow megakaryocytes, explaining their presence in platelets and extracellular matrix. High molecular weight multimeric forms of von Willebrand factor accumulate in the subendothelial matrix where they participate in platelet adhesion. Lower molecular weight forms of von Willebrand factor and factor VIII circulate as a complex; this association protects factor VIII from rapid clearance and recruits factor VIII to the platelet surface when shear forces in blood enhance binding of von Willebrand factor to platelet glycoprotein Ib or when platelets are activated. The association of von Willebrand factor and factor VIII in blood led to the erroneous designation of von Willebrand factor as "factor VIII-related antigen"; this term should be avoided because von Willebrand factor and factor VIII are products of genes on distinct chromosomes. tPA is produced mainly by endothelial cells. Urokinase, a plasminogen activator that is probably responsible for the fluidity of urine, is secreted by renal epithelial cells. The bacterial product streptokinase

Table 17.3 Coagulation Requirements for Hemostasis

Plasma Coagulation Protein	Minimal Hemostatic Level (% of normal)	Approximate Biologic Half-Life (Days)	Preferred Replacement Source
Contact			
Factor XII	0	–	–
Prekallikrein	0	–	–
High molecular weight kininogen	0	–	–
Procoagulant			
Factor XI	25	2	FFP
Factor VII*	25	0.2	FFP
Factor IX*	25	1	Concentrate
Factor VIII	25	0.5	Concentrate
Factor X*	25	1.5	FFP
Factor V	25	0.5	FFP
Prothrombin*	25	3	FFP
Fibrinogen	(100 mg/dL)	4	Cryoprecipitate
Factor XIII	5	7	Cryoprecipitate
von Willebrand factor	50	0.5	Certain factor VIII concentrates
Anticoagulant			
Antithrombin III	50	2.5	Concentrate
Protein C*	50	0.5	–
Protein S*	50	2.5	–

*Vitamin K dependent.
FFP, fresh frozen plasma.

activates plasminogen to plasmin only when complexed with plasminogen; preexisting antibodies often limit its usefulness. Factor XIII activity is found in liver and extracellular tissues as well as platelets, thereby explaining the beneficial effect of bone marrow transplantation in congenital factor XIII deficiency.

Vitamin K in its reduced form confers calcium ion (and thereby phospholipid)-binding ability to several of the coagulation proteins for whom orientation on platelet or endothelial surfaces is crucial for their function, namely, the procoagulant factors II (prothrombin), VII, IX, and X, and the anticoagulant proteins C and S. Normal internal stores of vitamin K last 1 week, but the minimal dietary requirement of vitamin K is estimated to be only 2 to 3 μg/kg per day. Patients receiving broad-spectrum antibiotic therapy for more than 1 week should receive parenteral supplementation. β-Lactam antibiotics also interfere with synthesis of vitamin K-dependent factors unrelated to their effects on colonic bacteria. Vitamin K-dependent proteins accumulate in their descarboxy forms during warfarin therapy and are converted to active zymogens when vitamin K is given to reverse the anticoagulant effect, promoting a thrombotic tendency. Only 40% of the normal serum ionized calcium concentration is required for hemostasis; hypocalcemic tetany occurs before hemostasis is affected. Serum, formed when blood is allowed to clot in a test tube, is devoid of platelets, von Willebrand factor, fibrinogen, prothrombin, factor XIII, and variable amounts of the other coagulation proteins. Chelation of calcium in blood by citrate affords a method of obtaining plasma that can be conveniently recalcified to assess the adequacy of coagulation proteins involved in fibrin formation. Ethylenediaminetetraacetic acid (EDTA)-treated or heparinized plasma is not suitable for clotting tests.

Laboratory Assessment of Coagulation

Exposure of blood to tissue factor precipitates a series of reactions termed the *extrinsic pathway of coagulation.* Tissue factor is a specific phospholipid-associated protein present in a wide variety of extravascular tissues, but it can also be induced on endothelial cells and macrophages as a consequence of pathologic stimuli, such as hypoxia and endotoxemia. A simplified diagram of the reactions that lead to fibrin formation after the presentation of tissue factor to blood is depicted in Figure 17.1*A*.

In contrast to endothelial and platelet function, fibrin formation is reasonably accessible to clinical laboratory testing. However, coagulation testing introduces significant artifacts into the physiologic mechanism of clot formation and should be ordered only when warranted because test results cannot replate the clinical history in the determination of bleeding risk. In the absence of a history of bleeding or of physical examination findings compatible with bleeding, but with a history of hemostatic stress, a preoperative laboratory evaluation (screening prothrombin time [PT], partial thromboplastin time [PTT], and platelet count) is unnecessary, unless a high-risk procedure is contemplated. In the absence of a record of hemostatic stress, however, the threshold for laboratory evaluation is lower. In the actively bleeding patient without a previously established cause for bleeding, the underlying problem is often acquired and results of laboratory studies are more likely to be helpful than the history. In contrast, an uneventful history provides sufficient assurance that a significant hemostatic defect is not present if a patient has been challenged (such as by accidental trauma) in the past.

Tests with clot formation as an end point are useful clinically despite their lack of specificity. Plasma is recalcified in the presence of an activating substance, and the time taken to form non–cross-linked fibrin polymer is detected electronically. Lipemic and icteric conditions affect clot detection. Clotting times reflect the cumulative activities of the various factors and physiologic inhibitors involved in the activated pathway as compared to normal plasma. Shorter than normal times are not clinically useful. Clotting times are considered abnormal when they are more than 10% beyond the upper limit of the normal range and are generally not prolonged unless there is less than 25% activity of one of the plasma factors involved in the pathway being tested. Because factor levels as low as 25% are often sufficient for casual hemostasis, these tests are valuable in the recognition of factor deficiencies which may contribute to bleeding. These tests and the factors measured are depicted in Figure 17.1*B*. Although activities of 25% may be sufficient for prevention of spontaneous or minor bleeding, 50% to 100% levels are required for major surgery or serious injury; lesser amounts will suffice in given situations.

Prothrombin Time

The prothrombin time (protime or PT) results when thromboplastin (phospholipid-bound tissue factor) and calcium are added to plasma and the time taken to form fibrin (typically 10.0 to 12.5 seconds) is measured. This coagulation time reflects the extrinsic pathway and is particularly sensitive to deficiencies in the activities of the vitamin K-dependent procoagulant factors (especially factor VII), factor V, and clottable fibrinogen. The variability of thromboplastin preparations has led to the use of better standardized reagents such as recombinant human tissue factor for assessment of anticoagulation with warfarin. PTs are also sensitive to hepatic dysfunction, but it is important to note that the intensity of anticoagulation achieved by prolongation of the PT with warfarin therapy is not equivalent to that reflected by prolongation of the PT due to liver failure because deficiencies of different combinations of factors and regulatory proteins are involved.

Activated Partial Thromboplastin Time

The activated partial thromboplastin time (aPTT or simply PTT) results when plasma is preincubated with an activator of factor XII (such as the negatively charged surface provided by ellagic acid) and phospholipid (termed partial thromboplastin) before the addition of calcium. The time taken to form fibrin after addition of calcium (typically 25 to 40 seconds) is most sensitive to the amount of XIIa generated during the preincubation, moderately sensitive to the amount of factors VIII and IX, and variably sensitive to factor XI activity. Because the PTT cannot distinguish

THE COAGULATION MECHANISM IN HEMOSTASIS

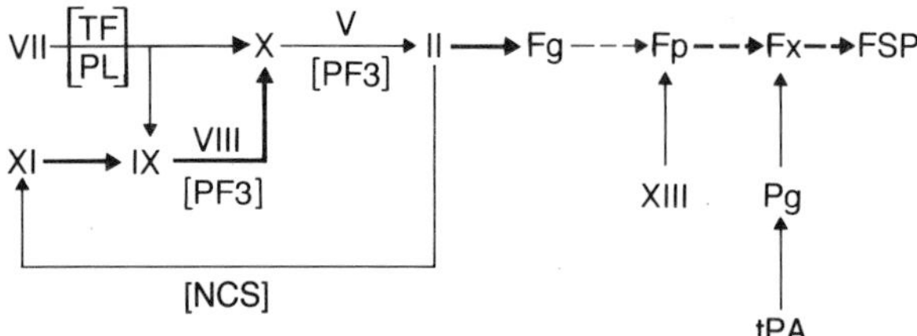

A

THE COAGULATION MECHANISM IN PLASMA TESTING

PT > VII [TF/PL] → X —V/[PL]→ II → Fg → Fp

TCT

PTT > XII —HMWK/[NCS]→ XI → IX —VIII/[PL]

PK

B

Fig 17.1 Comparison of the coagulation mechanism in hemostasis and in plasma testing. In these simplified diagrams, arrows with solid lines indicate sequential activation of zymogens to serine proteinases and arrows with dashed lines indicate product conversions. *A*, During hemostasis, the capture of circulating factor VII or VIIa by tissue factor forms a VII/TF/PL complex, in which factor VII is activated to VIIa, or an enzymatically active VIIa/TF/PL complex. The VIIa/TF/PL complex is capable of activating either factor X or factor IX. A regional excess of TF in the microenvironment of endothelial injury apparently favors the activation of factor X. Xa binds and activates factor V on the activated platelet surface, which provides PF3, creating a Xa/V/PF3 complex, which can activate factor II (prothrombin) to IIa (or thrombin). The loss of its calcium-binding domain releases thrombin from phospholipids on the platelet surface. However, further factor X activation is limited by tissue factor pathway inhibitor (TFPI), an efficient Xa-dependent inhibitor of the VIIa/TF/PL complex, and by the low amount of activated factor V. Thrombin rapidly generated by this extrinsic pathway serves several key functions, including the activation of the nonenzymatic procofactors, factor V and factor VII, which accelerates their cofactor activity, but the small amount is inadequate for hemostasis. Additional thrombin must be generated by a VIIa/TF-independent alternative pathway, which is provided by thrombin-mediated activation of factor XI on an unspecified negatively charged surface. Factor XIa can then activate factor IX on the platelet surface and factor X can be activated by the IXa/VIIIa/PF3 complex. The Xa/Va/PF3 complex activates factor II, generating substantial amounts of thrombin. The importance of alternative pathway of Xa generation is indicated by the severity of bleeding that accompanies hemophilia (the congenital deficiency of factors VIII, IX, or XI). Thrombin sequentially cleaves firbinopeptides A and B form fibrinogen to generate fibrin monomers, which polymerize spontaneously. Fibrin polymer is cross-linked by XIIIa, a transamidase formed on activation of factor XIII by thrombin, stabilizing the fibrin clot. Plasminogen is activated to plasmin on the newly generated fibrin surface by tissue plasminogen activator released from endothelial cells and degrades fibrin into fibrin split products, including D-dimer.

B, Under pathologic circumstances, factor XI can also be activated by XIIa, formed on the exposure of factor XII to certain nonphysiologic surfaces. This reaction requires two additional proteins, the zymogen prekallikrein (or Fletcher factor) and the nonenzymatic cofactor high molecular weight kininogen (or Fitzgerald factor), which is the carrier in plasma for prekallikrein and factor XI. Fibrin polymerization, which occurs following activation of factor XII during in vitro testing, is termed the intrinsic pathway and forms the basis for the PTT. The lack of bleeding due to deficiencies of factor XII, prekallikrein, and high molecular weight kininogen indicates that these factors are not involved in hemostasis; deficiencies of the regulatory proteins involved in the control of XIIa and prekallikrein (C1-esterase inhibitor) and in the control of XIa (α_1-proteinase inhibitor) produce angioneurotic edema or emphysema and cirrhosis, rather than thrombosis. However, the intrinsic pathway appears to be responsible for inflammation and other pathophysiologic events mediated by production of the serine proteinase kallikrein and the oligopeptide bradykinin, which accompany exposure of blood to foreign materials such as vascular grafts and dialyzer or oxygenator membranes.

The excess of tissue factor (as thromboplastin) added to plasma along with ionized calcium during performance of the PT results in preferential activation of factor X and bypasses the need for factors VIII and IX, explaining the observation that the PT is normal in hemophilia. In performance of the PTT, factor XII is first activated by ellagic acid in a 5-minute preincubation, followed by the addition of phospholipid and ionized calcium. In the TCT, thrombin and ionized calcium are added.

Coagulation factors are indicated by their commonly used Roman numeral designations. Fg, fibrinogen; Fp, fibrin polymer; FSP, fibrin split products; Fx, cross-linked fibrin; HMWK, high molecular weight kininogen; NCS, "negatively charged surface"; PF3, platelet factor 3; Pg, plasminogen; PK, prekallikrein; PL, phospholipid; PT, prothrombin time; PTT, activated partial thromboplastin time; TCT, thrombin clotting time; TF, tissue factor; tPA, tissue plasminogen activator.

between abnormalities of factor XII, high molecular weight kininogen, or prekallikrein (three factors that contribute to the amount of activated factor XIIa generated, but are not involved in hemostasis), and hemophilia, it does not correlate with bleeding risk. The PTT is also sensitive to abnormalities of the conversion of fibrinogen to fibrin and is useful in the monitoring of heparin therapy, which inhibits thrombin and activated factor X by enhancement of endogenous antithrombin activity. However, clinically irrelevant effects of heparin (antithrombin III-mediated inhibition of activated factor XII and several other enzymes), which cause prolongation of the PTT, and acute phase increases in factor VIII activity and release of heparin-binding proteins from platelets, which shorten the PTT, explain the lack of consistent correlation between PTTs, bleeding, and the antithrombotic effect of heparin. Prolongation of the PTT by lupus anticoagulants (autoantibodies that appear to interfere with phospholipid-binding proteins) are rarely associated with a bleeding tendency.

Thrombin Clotting Time

The thrombin clotting time measures the formation of fibrin polymer from fibrinogen. Bovine thrombin is added to plasma; calcium is included, but phospholipid is not required. It is normal in plasma containing the lupus anticoagulant. When excess thrombin is used, the thrombin clotting time directly reflects the amount of fibrinogen available to participate in clot formation and is reported as the concentration, in mg/dL, of "clottable" fibrinogen. The thrombin clotting time can be prolonged by a deficiency of fibrinogen, by dysfibrinogenemia, by interference with the action of thrombin (such as by heparin-induced augmentation of antithrombin III activity), or by inhibitors of fibrin monomer polymerization (such as fibrinogen/fibrin degradation products and paraproteins). Paraproteins inhibit polymerization of fibrin in vitro or impair automated optical clot detection and generally do not cause bleeding.

Fibrinogen/Fibrin Degradation Products

Fibrinogen/fibrin degradation products are created by the action of plasmin (as well as elastase released from neutrophils) on fibrinogen or fibrin. They are measured immunologically by the agglutination of latex beads coated with antibody that recognizes fibrin antigenic determinants in serum or plasma. In the standard assay, serum is used rather than plasma to eliminate cross-reactivity with the fibrinogen normally present in plasma. Spurious elevation of fibrin split products may occur if incomplete clotting occurs during the production of serum, such as when there are high amounts of heparin contamination. D-dimer, a specific fibrin split product created when cross-linked fibrin is degraded by plasmin, can be measured in plasma when the assay beads are coated with highly specific monoclonal antibody. The presence of D-dimer in plasma is unique to fibrinolysis, which has occurred after fibrin has been stabilized by factor XIIIa, such as occurs in DIC. Slightly elevated levels of D-dimer (titer of 1:4 or $<2000\,\mu g/mL$) may be due to rheumatoid factor, renal insufficiency, or hepatic failure, but high or increasing levels in the appropriate clinical setting indicate DIC. Increased D-dimer is not seen when fibrinogen is preferentially cleaved before fibrin formation (termed primary or systemic fibrinolysis).

Other Tests

Platelet counts are routinely determined by automated particle counters, but must be confirmed by microscopic examination. Thrombocytopenia may be artifactual, caused by processing of the blood sample (unintentional clot formation, EDTA anticoagulant- or cold-dependent platelet agglutinins) rather than by actual conditions, by the presence of large platelets or megakaryocyte fragments electronically mistaken for red or white blood cells, or not be as low as would be predicted by the severity of findings, due to an excess number of fragmented red blood cells. Only minor information about the function of platelets can be obtained from the count and routine microscopic examination of the blood film.

The skin or template bleeding time is generally not useful for screening purposes and has no predictive value for operative bleeding. It is predominantly a function of initial platelet plug formation and is therefore normal in patients with hemophilia. Although not very dependent on fibrin formation, it is greatly affected by the experience of the performer, anatomic site of testing, and vessel and connective tissue abnormalities. Bleeding times may have some utility in measuring the effect of various therapeutic manipulations in patients with uremia and von Willebrand's disease, in whom bleeding due to platelet dysfunction is a consistent finding.

Clinical Approach

Due to the complexity of coagulation disorders and particularly because of the contribution of hematology and coagulation laboratories and the institutional blood bank to patient management, primary care physicians should seek clinical consultation with a laboratory medicine physician or hematologist early in the medical decision-making process or when routine physical and laboratory assessment is insufficient. The need to have factor assay results for diagnosis or treatment would be an appropriate trigger point for seeking consultation because of the complexity (or idiosyncracies) of these tests and their interpretation.

Patients with coagulation disorders may experience bleeding due to an established or undiscovered hemostatic defect and require timely medical intervention, or alternatively, they may have unimpressive bleeding or a history of bleeding precipitated by stressful circumstances, which requires diagnostic or anticipatory evaluation. Whereas the care of actively bleeding patients raises therapeutic issues, patients at risk for future bleeding present a diagnostic challenge. A third category of patients are those without current or past bleeding who have abnormal screening or special coagulation test results obtained for other (often unnecessary) reasons, but which command attention because hemostatic evaluation may be hindered at a later time. Proper clinical management of coagulation disorders depends on the level of urgency and ascertainment of the specific defect. A basic laboratory evaluation is indispensable because confirmation of bleeding rarely provides enough information to determine specific treatment.

Three scenarios that consider both the evidence of bleeding and the results of initial laboratory test results can account for the diversity of clinical presentations: 1) varying degrees of hemorrhage associated with abnormal routine coagulation screening tests, which suggest a specific cause of bleeding, 2) abnormal routine coagulation tests for no apparent reason, or 3) hemorrhage with normal or unimpressive coagulation test results.

Bleeding with Abnormal Coagulation Test Results

Laboratory evaluation of patients with a prolonged PT or PTT is quite logical. However, clinical interpretation of the results depends on whether an individual is having or has had hemostatic difficulties. A prolonged PTT (to twice normal) with normal PT suggests the diagnosis of classic hemophilia (factor VIII deficiency) in a patient with an appropriate medical or family history, but may be misleading in one without a history of bleeding (Fig 17.2).

The degree of clotting time prolongation is of minor help and the diagnosis should be substantiated by specific factor assays. The PTT is dramatically prolonged by deficiency of factor XII, prekallikrein, and high molecular weight kininogen, but deficiencies of these proteins are not associated with a risk of bleeding nor with protection against thrombosis.

Patients with severe hemophilia have factor activities less than 1% and are prone to significant spontaneous bleeding episodes. Those with moderate hemophilia have factor activities of 1% to 5% and have less severe, but variable symptoms. Patients with mild hemophilia have factor activities of 5% to 25%, which command attention only at times of hemostatic stress. Patients with severe hemophilia require prophylactic treatment, whereas those with mild hemophilia require counseling and avoidance of risky situations. Guidelines for treatment depend on the type of hemophilia and site of bleeding, but need to be individualized. When factor VIII or IX levels of less than 25% with normal von Willebrand factor activity are encountered in symptomatic women with XX genotype, homozygosity, consanguinity in a family with hemophilia, or fresh mutation, or excessive inactivation of the normal gene due to lyonization in an obligate carrier should be considered. Recognition of factor XI deficiency is problematic because of the lack of correlation between levels and clinical bleeding. Replacement of factor XI to "hemostatic levels" may be detrimental if the patient's individual and family history are benign. A prolonged PT with normal PTT suggests isolated factor VII deficiency, a rare congenital condition, but one commonly acquired early in the course of vitamin K deficiency; activities of the other vitamin K-dependent coagulation proteins fall over time. It has not been possible to correlate the degree of

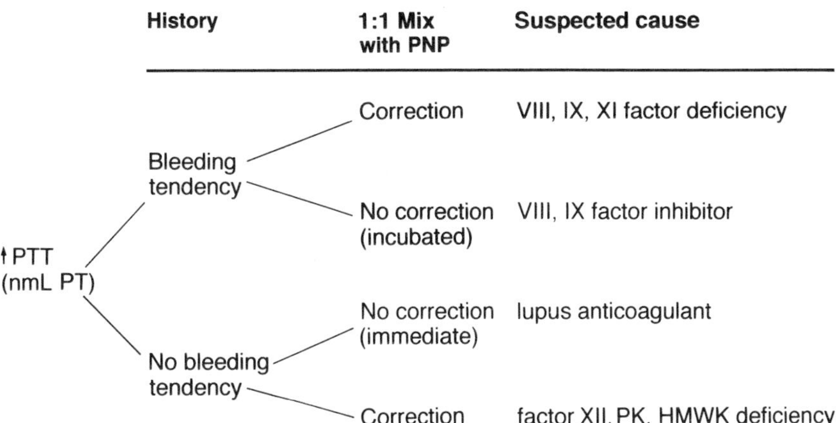

Fig 17.2 Evaluation of a prolonged PTT. Determination of the cause of a prolonged PTT when the PT is normal depends on the existence of a bleeding tendency. Performing the PTT on a mixture of patient plasma with pooled normal plasma (PNP) indicates the presence or absence of a circulating anticoagulant or factor inhibitor. Correction on an immediate mix does not exclude the existence of an inhibitor to factor VIII because it is characteristically time and temperature dependent. Analogous procedures are used to evaluate combined prolongation of the PT and PTT. A prolonged PT with normal PTT indicates decreased factor VII activity. Refer to Fig 17.1*B*.

factor VII deficiency with clinical bleeding symptoms in the past, but this appears to have been resolved by the use of improved thromboplastin preparations in the performance of the PT and the factor VII assay.

It may be reasonable to assume that combined prolongation of both the PT and the PTT is due to deficiencies of individual factors in the common pathway (factor X, factor V, prothrombin, or fibrinogen), but combined deficiencies are more frequently seen in practice and are due to dietary or iatrogenic vitamin K deficiency and chronic liver disease.

Clotting tests performed on a mixture of patient plasma and plasma of known composition provide clinically useful information. Correction of an abnormal clotting time with an equal volume of normal plasma indicates deficiency of one or possibly more procoagulant factors because 30% activity of a single factor is generally adequate for a normal clotting time and complete absence of a factor would be corrected to 50% by mixing with normal plasma. Thus, "correction on a mix" suggests that factor replacement therapy is likely to benefit the patient by improving the test result (or at least would not be contraindicated). A situation in which replacement therapy may not be sufficient to correct the test result would be one in which there was excessive or rapid consumption or utilization of a coagulation factor. Acquired factor X deficiency due to deposition of factor X in tissues occurs in secondary amyloidosis due to pneumonia and is only transiently corrected by fresh frozen plasma transfusion, even though the prolonged PT and PTT correct on mixing with normal plasma. Lack of correction with plasma known to be deficient in a specific factor indicates deficiency of that factor in the patient's plasma; this method of testing provides the basis for quantitative factor assays and suggests specific therapy.

Lack of correction by normal plasma indicates a circulating anticoagulant or inhibitor (specific factor inhibitor, heparin or other agent-inducing antithrombin III activity, or lupus anticoagulant). Specific factor inhibitors (particularly antibodies to factor VIII) characteristically become noticeable with incubation (they are "time and temperature dependent"). There may be initial correction of the PTT on mixing with normal plasma, providing the false assurance that a factor deficiency is present; prolongation on incubation of the mixture indicates the presence of an inhibitor. A Bethesda inhibitor titer represents that dilution of patient plasma that reduces factor VIII activity of normal plasma by 50% when the two are preincubated together for 2 hours at 37°C. Inhibitors to factor VIII are usually found in patients with hemophilia who have had prior replacement therapy. The presence of an inhibitor indicates that in most situations standard replacement therapy is not likely to benefit the patient. More importantly, factor replacement may be detrimental by further augmenting the patients' immune response to the coagulation protein and exacerbating the bleeding tendency. Management of bleeding due to specific factor inhibitors is problematic and strains hospital resources. Occasionally, an inhibitor develops as part of an autoimmune illness or spontaneously. Rarely, a pregnant or postpartum woman will unexpectedly develop antibodies of factor VIII; the inhibitor may not simply be due to an immunologic response to antigens displayed during pregnancy although it generally occurs following birth of the first child. Bleeding can be severe and life-threatening because of location (retropharyngeal hematoma, cerebral hemorrhage), but hemarthroses occur less frequently than they do in patients with congenital hemophilia and factor replacement is less of a problem. Treatment of bleeding is directed at overcoming the inhibitor with high amounts of purified factor VIII, bypassing the inhibitor with porcine factor VIII (if the inhibitor does not cross-react with the porcine protein), or transfusing with activated coagulation factor concentrates ("anti-inhibitor coagulant complex"). A course of IV γ globulin may quickly, but transiently, decrease the inhibitor titer, but immunosuppressive therapy for long-term control is usually not necessary because unlike inhibitors that develop in hemophiliacs, postpartum inhibitors resolve spontaneously in 12 to 18 months and do not recur in subsequent pregnancies.

Acquired deficiency of factor V may be due to an autoantibody induced by viral illness. The prolonged PT and PTT are found to be due to severe factor V deficiency and there is lack of complete correction on a mix. Bleeding symptoms seem to be less severe than predicted, but inhibition of factor V on platelets may also cause platelet dysfunction.

Abnormal Coagulation Test Results Without Bleeding

Valid coagulation testing requires a properly procured blood sample. An inadequate amount of blood, blood improperly drawn from an IV or intra-arterial line, or blood obtained from patients with high hematocrit can lead to erroneous results. Careful repeat testing is necessary to avoid a pointless search for a hemostatic defect. The most important cause of an unsuspected abnormal coagulation test result is the presence of a lupus anticoagulant.

Lupus anticoagulants are circulating inhibitors that prolong phospholipid-dependent coagulation tests (particularly the PTT). Most appear to be autoantibodies directed against plasma prothrombin and specific phospholipids. Many also appear to be directed against serum β_2-glycoprotein I (apolipoprotein H) as well as other phospholipid-binding proteins present in blood such as prothrombin or proteins C and S, and are identifiable immunologically as anticardiolipin antibodies. Lupus anticoagulants can cause clotting tests performed with diluted phospholipid reagents to remain prolonged when mixed with normal plasma and immediately retested and can be neutralized by the addition of a platelet substitute. The term lupus anticoagulant is an unfortunate misnomer because it occurs in only 25% of patients with systemic lupus erythematosus and is rarely associated with a bleeding tendency. Lupus anticoagulants are often recognized in patients on chlorpromazine or other medications and in patients with human immunodeficiency virus (HIV) infection, but they are usually clinically silent. Most patients without an underlying reason to develop the lupus anticoagulant appear to be paradoxically predisposed to thrombosis, clinically manifest as recurrent spontaneous fetal loss, in the third as well as first trimester, transient ischemic attacks, and unusually situated deep venous thrombosis.

Factor assays performed on blood samples containing the lupus anticoagulant will be factitiously low and therefore results should not be interpreted without proper clinical correlation. Bleeding does occur in patients with lupus anticoagulant, but only when there is accompanying thrombocytopenia, platelet dysfunction, or prothrombin deficiency.

Bleeding with Normal Coagulation Test Results

Based on our understanding of hemostasis, it is not surprising that bleeding (whether congenital or acquired) can occur in the setting of a normal PT, PTT, and platelet count (Box 17.1). Possible causes of bleeding include: platelet dysfunction, often drug-related and usually due to aspirin or other NSAIDs, although storage pool disorders, renal failure, or

Box 17.1 Causes of Bleeding with Normal PT, PTT, and Platelet Count

Platelet dysfunction
Mild factor VIII and factor IX deficiency
- von Willebrand's disease

Factor XIII deficiency
Increased fibrinolysis
Vascular or connective tissue defect
- Hereditary hemorrhagic telangiectasia
- Vasculitis
- Collagen vascular disease
- Amyloidosis

Factitious bleeding
- Physical abuse

superimposition on another hemostatic defect should be kept in mind; mild deficiency of factor VIII or factor IX, such as in von Willebrand's disease and in hemophilia carriers with disproportionate inactivation of the X chromosome carrying the normal gene; factor XIII deficiency (rare, but undetected by assays of clotting times, which reflect fibrin formation before cross-linking), increased fibrinolytic activity (primary systemic fibrinolysis due to unregulated plasminogen activation, as in α_2-proteinase inhibitor deficiency and rarely PAI-1 deficiency) or occasionally dysfibrinogenemia; and vascular or connective tissue defects (hereditary hemorrhagic telangiectasia, vasculitis, collagen vascular disease, hypercortisolism, degenerative skin disease, allergic or senile purpura, scurvy, amyloid deposition). Pinch purpura or purpura simplex are not associated with any hemostatic abnormalities. Factitious or self-induced injury and physical abuse should not be discounted without proper attention.

Platelet Dysfunction

Exposure of platelets in blood to as little as one ingested baby aspirin (80 mg) immediately inhibits their function for up to 10 days. Their adhesive capacity is not affected. The aspirin is cleared within a few hours, but the affected platelets continue to circulate and their function as a group only improves as fresh, unexposed platelets are produced. Because the lifespan of platelets is normally 7 to 10 days, about 10% to 15% of the total number of platelets are replaced each day to maintain a steady level until, eventually, only unexposed platelets are circulating. Aspirin irreversibly acetylates and inactivates the enzyme cyclooxygenase in both platelets and endothelial cells, where it interferes with membrane phospholipid mobilization and arachidonic acid metabolism. In platelets, the preferred product of the cyclooxygenase pathway is thromboxane, a potent vasoconstrictive and platelet aggregatory substance. In endothelial cells, the favored product is prostacyclin, a vasodilatory and antiaggregatory substance. Platelets are non-nucleated cells and incapable of new protein synthesis, but endothelial cells can replace inactivated enzyme. Thus the resultant effect of ingested aspirin on circulating platelets is inhibitory. At high doses of aspirin (3 adult tablets or 1000 mg PO per day), this differential effect appears to be lost and the endothelial antiplatelet effect is also suppressed. For elective procedures, it is sensible to wait until the aspirin effect has worn off. For urgent surgery, platelet transfusion can be given; however, bleeding complications are usually not severe in normal individuals and no measures need be taken. To avoid transfusion, desmopressin or antifibrinolytic agents can be administered empirically.

In contrast to aspirin, other NSAIDs such as ibuprofen are reversible inactivators of cyclooxygenase. Their effect on the enzyme dissipates as the drug is cleared. Depending on the rate of clearance (usually a few hours), platelet function normalizes quickly and holding treatment for 1 day is adequate to restore hemostasis to baseline before a surgical procedure.

Acquired platelet storage pool disorders are seen with a variety of conditions. They are partially responsible for bleeding following cardiopulmonary bypass and other procedures in which blood is exposed to foreign surfaces. The activation of platelets depletes the contents of their granules, affecting their hemostatic function. A similar situation appears to occur on binding of β-lactam antibiotics (penicillins and cephalosporins) to platelets.

Uremia is a common cause of platelet dysfunction. Other accompanying abnormalities contribute to bleeding in patients with renal disease: the moderately severe anemia forces platelets away from the vessel wall where they participate in hemostasis and the frequent coexistence of gastrointestinal mucosal angiodysplasia often provides a site for occult blood loss. Bleeding can be ameliorated to some extent by correction of the uremia, but chronic DIC should be excluded. Hemodialysis, conjugated estrogens, desmopressin, and possibly erythropoietin have roles in treatment.

Mild Factor VIII or Factor IX Deficiency

Daughters of men with hemophilia, mothers having more than one son with hemophilia, and mothers having one son with hemophilia and one other relative with hemophilia are obligate heterozygotes. The incidence of spontaneous (postzygotic or germ-line) mutations resulting in the hemophilic defect is as high as 15% for the factor VIII gene and about 8% for the factor IX gene. Mothers and maternal relatives of boys with hemophilia, but without a family history, and sisters of boys with hemophilia are candidates for carrier testing. A worthwhile preliminary evaluation consists of measurement of the ratio of factor VIII activity to the immunologic level of von Willebrand factor. A ratio of less than 0.6 identifies obligate carriers of factor VIII hemophilia in more than 90% of instances. DNA hybridization studies are necessary in the remainder and for reliable identification of factor IX hemophilia carriers. Detection of carriers is important because of the variable risk of bleeding and because of family planning considerations. The variability is due to nonrandom lyonization. Also, it is not unusual for levels of less than 50% to be associated with bleeding during major surgery. Levels should be monitored during pregnancy and for 5 days postpartum and supplemented before delivery if less than 20%. Whereas procoagulant factor levels generally increase with oral contraceptive use and duration of gestation, this is not the case with factor IX. When factor VIII or IX activities of less than 25% with normal von Willebrand factor levels are encountered in symptomatic women, consanguinity in a family with hemophilia or a fresh mutation or excessive inactivation (lyonization) of the normal gene in an obligate carrier should be considered.

von Willebrand's Disease

Because of its prevalence (by far the most common hereditary defect causing hemostatic failure), the diagnosis of von Willebrand's disease should be considered in any patient with mucosal bleeding, particularly posttraumatic or postsurgical, positive family history (usually autosomal dominant), or evidence of iron deficiency. Patients usually present with a history of lifelong increased bruisability, often exacerbated by aspirin. Fluctuations in von Willebrand factor multimer synthesis and release from endothelial cells (increased with stress, oral contraceptive use, etc) cause variability in presentation, course, and test results. Individuals with blood type O typically have 25% lower levels than the rest of the population. Increased levels during pregnancy protect women from obstetric complications until delivery. Diagnosis, especially of the variant forms, requires interpretation of specialized laboratory studies. Classic or type I von Willebrand's disease, in which decreased von Willebrand factor activity in blood is due to defective release from endothelial stores, accounts for over 75% of von Willebrand's disease. von Willebrand factor is responsible for optimal synthesis of factor VIII by unknown mechanism. Factor VIII activity is variably reduced, generally in parallel with von Willebrand factor levels because von Willebrand factor prevents the rapid degradation of factor VIII and maintains its intravascular distribution. Decreased ristocetin cofactor activity is seen in more than 90% of patients, von Willebrand factor antigen is variably decreased in proportion to ristocetin cofactor, and VIII activity is variably reduced. Type II or variant forms have abnormal von Willebrand factor multimeric composition. Bleeding in thyroid disorders may be due to acquired von Willebrand's disease (or von Willebrand syndrome).

The aim of therapy for von Willebrand's disease is to anticipate and be prepared for bleeding problems rather than treat prophylactically. The careful avoidance of antiplatelet agents, especially aspirin, cannot be overstated. IV or intranasal instillation of desmopressin, a nonvasospastic synthetic analogue of antidiuretic hormone, appears to release von Willebrand factor (as well as other substances, such as tPA) from endothelial stores and avoids blood products, but must be used cautiously in variant forms. A therapeutic trial of desmopressin is indicated in all types of von Willebrand's disease. For prolonged support of von Willebrand factor levels after surgery, transfusion therapy is necessary: the most appropriate products are purified factor VIII concentrates, which contain substantial amounts of von Willebrand factor.

Oral contraceptives or conjugated estrogens have a definite role in controlling chronic mucosal bleeding in women with von Willebrand's disease. During pregnancy, von Willebrand factor (ristocetin cofactor) levels should be monitored, especially during the third trimester, when levels may drop. At the time of delivery, levels can be increased to the level needed for hemostasis by von Willebrand factor-containing factor VII concentrate.

Agents for Treatment of Bleeding

Medical therapy is instituted once mechanical and surgically approachable avenues have been addressed. Several products are available for treatment and replacement therapy. In all situations, consideration must first be given to prescribing agents not derived from human blood to alleviate the risk of transmitting viral and other illnesses.

Vitamin K

If the clinical setting permits the luxury of waiting about 12 hours and the pattern of clotting test results confirms deficiency of vitamin K (prolongation of both the PT and the PTT due to reduced activities of vitamin K-dependent factors, but not other factors, such as factor V and factor VIII), 5–10 mg vitamin K should be administered, rather than fresh frozen plasma or a combination of factor concentrates. However, vitamin K is of limited value in improving factor activity in patients with severe parenchymal liver disease and of no value in congenital deficiencies of prothrombin, factor VII, factor IX, or factor X, and of protein C or protein S. A parenteral dose of 5 mg (SQ or IV would be preferable to IM in patients at risk of bleeding) should be sufficient to correct or nearly correct the PT in 6 to 12 hours. Vitamin K_1 (phytonadione, 10 mg) for injection costs about $5 as compared to $200 for preparation and administration of fresh frozen plasma.

Desmopressin

Desmopressin or DDAVP, a nonvasospastic synthetic analogue of antidiuretic hormone (vasopressin), appears to release von Willebrand factor, as well as other stored substances, including tPA, from endothelial cells, and can obviate the need for blood products in a large number of clinical situations, including von Willebrand's disease, mild hemophilia, and platelet storage pool disease. The platelet count should be at least 100,000/μL for desmopressin to be effective. It is given in an IV dose of 0.3 μg/kg over 20 minutes and can be repeated daily. von Willebrand factor levels typically rise two- to threefold and maximum levels are achieved in 30 to 60 minutes and gradually wane over 6 hours. Levels of factor VIII rise threefold and last 24 hours. In responsive patients, desmopressin can be given 1 hour preoperatively and then daily for 2 to 3 days. Repetitive therapy is limited by tachyphylaxis or diminished efficacy due to depletion of stored substances, which require an additional 2 to 3 days to replete. Overtreatment may result in hyponatremia preventable by water restriction. Desmopressin should not be given before delivery. Desmopressin costs about $125. Intranasal instillation of desmopressin (150 μg once in each nostril for adults) has recently become available and holds promise for ambulatory prophylaxis but is expensive ($500 for 24 instillations of 300 μg).

Antifibrinolytic Agents

Antifibrinolytic agents such as ε-aminocaproic acid and tranexamic acid are orally active short-acting lysine analogue inhibitors of fibrinolysis that block the action of plasmin by interfering with the ability of plasminogen or plasmin to bind to fibrin. They are useful for mild bleeding problems in patients with thrombocytopenia due to decreased platelet production, patients with mild to moderate hemophilia, and most patients with von Willebrand's disease. An antifibrinolytic agent should probably accompany desmopressin treatment because of the enhancement of resulting fibrinolytic activity, but this is not universal. The oral dose of ε-aminocaproic acid, 100 mg/kg followed by 25 mg/kg every 3 hours for 5 days, is somewhat cumbersome; the corresponding dose of tranexamic acid, 25 mg/kg every 6 hours, is more reasonable. The cost of 12 gm of ε-aminocaproic acid is about $24; an equivalent 6-gm dose of tranexamic acid costs around $40. Antifibrinolytic agents should be used extremely cautiously in patients with DIC, liver dysfunction, upper urinary tract bleeding, and pregnancy because of the risk of facilitating thrombosis; chronic use is not recommended because of microvascular thrombosis and rhabdomyolysis.

Fresh Frozen Plasma

Purification procedures, which have for all practical purposes eliminated the risk of HIV transmission, appear to allow low level transmission for parvovirus B19 infection and raise the possibility of transmitting as yet unrecognized agents of disease. Thus, fresh frozen plasma contains acceptable amounts of all circulating coagulation proteins (including those with anticoagulant function) except factors V and VIII, which are labile with storage. By definition, each milliliter of fresh frozen plasma contains 1 unit of activity for each clotting factor. An appropriate dose of fresh frozen plasma is 10 mL/kg, which should raise procoagulant factor activity by 20%; each unit of fresh frozen plasma has a volume of about 200 mL. Plasma lacks activated factors that might precipitate thrombus formation and has the ability to immediately reverse factor deficiency. Cryoprecipitate is prepared from fresh frozen plasma; each unit of cryoprecipitate contains about half the fibrinogen available in 1 unit of fresh frozen plasma, but in one twentieth the volume. An appropriate dose of cryoprecipitate is 2 mL/kg; each unit has a volume of about 10 mL. Therapeutically useful amounts of von Willebrand factor (with associated factor VIII) and XIII are also present in cryoprecipitate, but several units have to be infused together.

Factor Concentrates

Safer (because of viral inactivation) and higher purity products such as specific factor concentrates should be used whenever feasible to conserve plasma, reduce adverse effects, and dose patients more effectively. Each unit per kilogram of factor VIII concentrate would be expected to raise factor VIII levels by 2% (because of the intravascular association of factor VIII with von Willebrand factor) and each unit per kilogram of factor IX would be expected to raise factor IX levels by 1% (because of its extravascular distribution). The goals of therapy depend on the clinical indication for replacement and past response. A number of formulations of factor VIII concentrate are available varying from intermediate purity to immunoaffinity-purified or "monoclonally" isolated plasma-derived products and recombinant factor. Recombinant factor VIII is appropriate in previously untreated patients or pregnant women because of safety concerns. Inasmuch as a minimal hemostatic level of 25% is needed for hemostasis during delivery in hemophilia carriers or women with hemophilia, replacement can be accomplished with a single dose of 25 U/kg, which should keep levels above 25% for 24 hours. Each unit of factor VIII activity costs on the order of $1 but prices vary considerably (from as low as $0.20/U for intermediate purity products to as high as $1/U for recombinant products) and are subject to availability and economies of scale. A single 25 U/kg prophylactic dose of factor VIII concentrate in a 60-kg patient with severe deficiency may cost $750. Cryoprecipitate costs $120/U. In patients with inhibitors to factor VIII and factor IX, the Bethesda inhibitor titer can be useful in management. If the reactivity with porcine factor VIII is less than 5 U, porcine factor VIII, 50–100 U/kg, can be given to raise factor VIII activity by 30%. If unsuccessful, factor VIII concentrate at a dose of 150 U/kg followed by 1000 U/h infusion can work. For a titer, greater than 30 U, various maneuvers can be attempted to reduce the intensity of the inhibitor: plasmapheresis with or without staphylococcal protein A extracorporeal immunoadsorption followed by factor VIII infusion may give a better result. Otherwise, anti-inhibitor coagulant complex is given at dose of 75 U/kg every 12 to 24 hours, monitored clinically.

Purification of certain factor VIII concentrates such as Humate-P and Alphanate result in products containing therapeutically useful amounts of von Willebrand factor. These have been accepted as alternatives for therapy when desmopressin and antifibrinolytic agents are not sufficient.

Platelet Transfusion

Platelet transfusion should be reserved for patients whose bleeding is due to a reduced number (<20,000/μL) of normally functioning platelets because of the risk of transmitting blood-borne disease and because of the likelihood that sensitization to platelets will occur with repetitive use. One apheresis unit of platelets or 6 to 8 U of platelet concentrate should raise the platelet count immediately by 60,000/μL in a 60-kg individual and last about 5 days. Less than 20% of the expected increment suggests alloimmunization, whereas a significant fall after 24 hours suggests increased utilization. Transfusion is unlikely to be of significant value in idiopathic thrombocytopenic purpura, when antiplatelet antibody seems to be responsible for platelet destruction, or uremia, when forces extrinsic to circulating platelets are responsible for poor function.

Disseminated Intravascular Coagulation

Acute DIC is a life-threatening thrombotic disorder in which uncontrolled bleeding is often the predominant feature. It may be acute (decompensated) or chronic (compensated). The term DIC is a misnomer because the disorder may not be disseminated or originate intravascularly and may manifest as thrombosis, hemorrhage, or both. It is always secondary to an underlying disease process and is due to unregulated thrombin generation. Twenty-five percent of DIC is due to sepsis, 20% is due to malignancy (usually occurring in the compensated form), 20% is a complication of surgery, 10% is due to liver disease (usually occurring in the compensated form), 5% is due to obstetric complications, and 5% is due to trauma. The source of thromboplastin in obstetric catastrophes is generally extravascular (retained dead fetus, amniotic fluid embolism, saline-induced abortion, hydatidiform mole, retained placenta, etc). Intravascular sources of thromboplastin are found in severe liver injury; endotoxic shock and anoxia are responsible for vascular injury. As a result of excess thrombin activity in the circulation, nonhemostatic fibrin formation occurs systemically and stimulates fibrinolysis. Coagulation factors (especially VIII and V, as well as platelets) are consumed (termed "consumptive coagulopathy"), generalized proteolysis occurs (activation and degradation of many proteins), physiologic anticoagulant proteins (especially antithrombin III) are used, and plasmin action depletes fibrinogen and produces high levels of circulating fibrin split products, including D-dimer. Increased fibrin split products interfere with platelet aggregation (small fragments) and fibrin polymerization (large fragments), thrombocytopenia, platelet dysfunction, defective clot formation, and systemic fibrinolysis lead to increased bleeding (clots may form, but are friable). Microinfarctions can occur in any organ, especially the kidney. DIC develops when the normal capacity to regulate thrombin activity has been overcome. Both arterial and venous thromboses occur, but bleeding is the predominant manifestation.

Laboratory correlates of DIC include thrombocytopenia or decreasing platelet count and increased fibrinogen turnover (inappropriately normal fibrinogen levels of decreasing levels despite replacement), prolonged PTT and PT (insensitive and due mainly to elevated fibrin split products), schistocytes (often, but not universally seen on peripheral blood film), and decreased antithrombin III (reflecting increased utilization, helpful in directing treatment). Thrombotic microangiopathy (thrombotic thrombocytopenic purpura and hemolytic-uremic syndrome) is distinguished from DIC by the lack of an underlying etiology and lack of systemic coagulopathy.

Management of DIC requires first and foremost recognition and appropriate treatment of the primary problem. Maintenance of hemodynamic stability and urine output, replacement of regulatory proteins (especially antithrombin III) with fresh frozen plasma, and replacement of fibrinogen with cryoprecipitate are important therapeutic measures. Antithrombin III concentrate is available for preoperative prophylaxis and during pregnancy in patients who are congenitally deficient in antithrombin III, but its role in acquired deficiencies is still being investigated. Replacement of antithrombin III in acute fatty liver of pregnancy may have some value. Platelet transfusions are rarely indicated and often not helpful. Low-dose heparin (10 U/kg per hour by continuous IV infusion) can be used judiciously to augment antithrombin III activity. Antifibrinolytic agents may exacerbate thrombotic complications because increased fibrinolysis is actually protective in DIC. The aim of therapy is prevention of irreversible organ damage.

Recognition of Prethrombotic Conditions

Its pathogenesis notwithstanding, the predominant clinical manifestation of acute DIC is bleeding; reductions of the regulatory proteins of coagulation occur secondarily. However, primary deficiency of the regulatory proteins involved in hemostasis are known to predispose affected individuals to clinical thrombosis; indeed it is precisely the deficient activity of these proteins in patients and their families with deep venous thrombosis that has identified them a important regulatory proteins. Conditions responsible for congenital prethrombotic states are more often associated with recurrent venous thromboembolic disease such as lower extremity deep venous thrombosis and pulmonary embolism than arterial thromboembolic disease such as stroke, myocardial infarction, and peripheral microvascular occlusion, in which endothelial injury and platelet activation appear to be involved.

Venous Thrombosis

A number of conditions are responsible for a heightened propensity to venous thrombosis. Both acquired and inherited causes are recognized, but the great majority of events are idiopathic. Precipitating factors include advanced age; immobilization due to bed rest, paralysis, operative anesthesia, surgery, or trauma; low flow states such as congestive heart failure; obesity, varicose veins, or previous deep venous thrombosis with consequent anatomic abnormality; and major gynecologic surgery or the postpartum (but not specifically the pregnant) state. Inherited prethrombotic conditions should be considered in young adults with consistent family histories who suffer recurrent venous thromboembolic disease in unusual sites without provocation (Box 17.2). They are inherited in an autosomal dominant fashion and so appear in each generation and to the same extent in both men and women. Dysplasminogenemias are very rare and represent less than 1% of the potential causes. Congenital dysfibrinogenemias occur in 1% to 2%. Eighty percent of patients with dysfibrinogenemia are asymptomatic and only 10% of them are predisposed to thrombosis. Deficiencies of protein S, protein C, and antithrombin III only account for 10% to 20% of familial thrombotic tendencies. Recently, resistance to activated protein C has been found in about 50% of individuals suspected of having a prethrombotic condition; this resistance appears to be due to a polymorphism in the factor V molecule at the site where it is activated by thrombin. Testing during pregnancy is problematic because of gestational effects on levels of these proteins. Furthermore, warfarin reduces the activities of protein S and protein C increases the activity of antithrombin III. The reverse is true with heparin therapy. If necessary, patients can be switched to subcutaneous heparin at prophylactic doses for a couple of weeks before testing. When patients cannot be properly tested, evaluation of asymptomatic relatives often provides useful diagnostic information. Diagnosis before the first thrombotic episode is beneficial: awareness of the symptoms of venous occlusion allows early attention and intervention, which may prevent serious problems and possibly postphlebitic syndrome, a frustrating complication of venous valvular damage from thrombosis. Heparinization is necessary before institution of warfarin in patients with protein C deficiency because of the risk of exacerbating the prethrombotic state and the risk of causing skin necrosis.

Box 17.2 Risk Factors for Venous Thrombosis

Inherited	Acquired
Resistance to activated protein C	Lupus anticoagulant
Protein S deficiency	Myeloproliferative/myelodysplastic syndromes, paroxysmal nocturnal hemoglobinuria
Protein C deficiency	Malignancy, cancer chemotherapy
Antithrombin III deficiency	Nephrotic syndrome
Dysfibrinogenemia	Estrogen therapy for infertility
Plasminogen deficiency	Reduction in postoperative fibrinolytic activity

Acquired causes of recurrent venous thromboembolic disease include the lupus anticoagulant (more correctly the antiphospholipid-binding protein antibody syndrome), myeloproliferative/myelodysplastic disorders (polycythemia vera, essential thrombocythemia, paroxysmal nocturnal hemoglobinuria), nephrotic syndrome (associated with decreased antithrombin III activity and increased C4b-binding protein with resultant decreased protein S activity), disseminated malignancy (manifesting as migratory superficial thrombophlebitis), and cancer chemotherapy (possibly due to decreased synthesis of physiologic anticoagulant proteins).

Arterial Thrombosis

Conditions predisposing to arterial thrombosis are distinctly different from those predisposing to venous thrombosis (Box 17.3). Although the causes are not as well defined, the possibilities of hereditary dyslipoproteinemia (hypercholesterolemia, increased lipoprotein [a]), diabetes mellitus, and heterozygous or homozygous homocysteinemia need to be addressed. Numerous acquired situations contribute to arterial occlusive disease, including atherosclerosis, cigarette smoking, vasculitis, impaired fibrinolysis, and heparin therapy complicated by thrombocytopenia. DIC and lupus anticoagulants are acquired conditions associated with both arterial and venous thrombosis.

Agents for Treatment of Thrombosis

Thrombolytic therapy should be considered early in the course of venous thrombosis because the incidence of postphlebitic syndrome can be reduced by better than one half, but it should not be used indiscriminately. It is relatively contraindicated in pregnancy and is absolutely contraindicated when there is active bleeding or any evidence of a central nervous system event within the previous 2 months. Streptokinase, urokinase, and recombinant tPA are used; despite the relative fibrin specificity of tPA, all fibrinolytic agents result in a systemic "lytic state" with an associated risk of serious hemorrhage. In contrast to venous thrombosis, the first line of therapy for arterial thrombosis is surgical. Within the proper time frame (not more than a week from the event) and in the appropriate setting (absence of contraindications), thrombolytic therapy should also be considered for arterial thrombosis. Even when thrombectomy or thromblytic therapy is successful, anticoagulation is necessary to prevent immediate recurrence.

Heparin

Whereas fibrinolytic agents dissolve existing thrombi, anticoagulant drugs prevent further thrombus formation. Anticoagulant therapy with heparin and warfarin has been found to be highly efficacious. The rapidity and stability of anticoagulation with heparin make it preferable to warfarin in the acute setting. In the treatment of acute deep venous thrombosis, adequate anticoagulation achieved during the first 24 hours is critical in lowering the high risk of recurrence. The pharmacologic effect of heparin depends on its dose, route of administration, availability of antithrombin III, presence of heparin-neutralizing proteins in blood, and the degree of activation of coagulation. Close monitoring is necessary and is usually best accomplished by frequent PTT testing. An IV bolus dose of 80 U/kg is given. A continuous infusion dose of 20 U/kg per hour is begun and should prolong the PTT to 1.5 to 2.5 times control, given normal baseline values. Heparin resistance may be due to preexisting or acquired antithrombin III deficiency and require correction. Five days of heparin infusion are followed by warfarin or similar oral anticoagulant medication. The elimination half-life of heparin is dose dependent; half of a 200 U/kg IV bolus is cleared in 1.5 hours.

Bleeding due to heparin is best dealt with by adjusting the dose or discontinuing treatment; neutralization with protamine is rarely necessary. Platelet counts should be monitored in patients receiving heparin; a greater than 30% drop in count will occur in 5% of patients; in 10% of those, the fall will be associated with antibodies that stimulate platelets, release platelet factor 4 (forming heparin-platelet factor 4 complexes), interfere with endothelial anticoagulant function, and precipitate arterial thrombosis. In heparin-associated thrombocytopenia, the platelet count characteristically begins to fall 5 to 8 days after institution of heparin. Heparin must be discontinued and alternative anticoagulation (such as with fibrinolytic agents, rheologically active substances, nonheparin heparinoid drugs, accelerated dosing with warfarin, etc) instituted. Long-term heparin therapy is associated with osteoporosis and should be used judiciously in women; bone densitometry is recommended after 6 months. Low molecular weight heparin has recently become available and has several attractive features: reduced bleeding complications for the same level of anticoagulation, reduced need for laboratory monitoring when adjusted-dose heparin regimens are indicated, potential for ambulatory therapy, and more convenient dosing. Conventional porcine heparin (10,000 U) costs about $2. Some preliminary evidence suggests low molecular weight heparin, like standard unfractionated heparin, is safe for use in pregnancy.

Box 17.3 Risk Factors for Arterial Thrombosis

Inherited	Acquired
Homocysteinemia	Atherosclerosis
Dyslipoproteinemias	Arteritis, thromboangiitis obliterans
Diabetes mellitus	Lupus anticoagulant

Warfarin

Warfarin inhibits the dithiol-dependent reductases involved in regeneration of reduced vitamin K. Interference with the γ-carboxylation of glutamic acid residues in the vitamin K-dependent proteins results in decrease of the activities of factor VII, protein C, factor IX, factor X, prothrombin, and protein S in the order of their biologic half-lives. Although the PT is sensitive to changes in factor VII activity, the therapeutic effect of warfarin is a function of reduction in factor X and prothrombin activity; thus oral dose adjustments should be made more frequently than every other day. Standardization of testing of the intensity of anticoagulation achieved by warfarin therapy among different laboratories has been accomplished by expressing the prolongation of the PT as an international normalized ratio (INR). Therapeutic INR ranges are defined for various clinical indications (anticoagulation for venous as well as arterial thromboembolic disease), but apply only to patients on stable doses of warfarin. Warfarin therapy is rarely complicated by skin necrosis, attributable to initiation of anticoagulation with high doses of warfarin without heparin coverage, or protein C or S deficiency. Bleeding due to over-anticoagulation with warfarin may be serious or life-threatening and manifest as intramural bleeding causing intestinal obstruction or retroperitoneal bleeding causing impairment of urinary flow. Because of the delay in normalization of the activities of long-lived vitamin K-dependent factors with vitamin K administration, treatment with fresh frozen plasma is preferable despite the risk of transmitting viral infection and the potential to overextend intravascular volume. In situations requiring normalization of the PT, but in which the indication for anticoagulation remains active (such as intercurrent surgery), fresh frozen plasma is also preferred over vitamin K, particularly because the proteins induced by vitamin K antagonism would have accumulated during warfarin therapy and would become active with vitamin K administration, creating a prothrombotic situation.

Lifelong ambulatory prophylaxis against thrombosis is indicated for prethrombotic states when the cause has been documented and once there has been at least one episode of venous thrombosis. An INR goal of 2.0 to 3.0 is recommended for most instances. An INR of 2.5 to 3.5 is recommended for patients with lupus anticoagulants or mechanical prosthetic heart valves. In asymptomatic individuals with a laboratory abnormality, chronic oral anticoagulation is not indicated because of the lack of certainty that thrombosis will occur and because of the risks of therapy. However, even asymptomatic individuals should receive prophylaxis in high-risk situations such as postoperatively, during the immediate postpartum period, or when being treated with estrogen-containing oral contraceptives. The low doses of conjugated estrogens used for alleviation of postmenopausal symptoms do not appear to increase thrombotic risk.

Special Considerations

Warfarin is contraindicated during pregnancy, especially from 6 to 12 weeks, because of embryonapathy. Women on oral anticoagulation should protect against becoming pregnant. During pregnancy, SQ heparin prophylaxis can be safely administered. For patients with two previous thrombotic episodes regardless of cause or prethrombotic conditions with at least one previous thrombosis, the dose of heparin should be adjusted to increase PTT to 1.5 to 2.5 times normal 4 hours after a dose and administered every 8 hours. Improved monitoring of anticoagulation is possible using anti-Xa activity (a laboratory method to accurately measure heparin concentration) with therapeutic goal of 0.2 to 0.4 U/mL. Patients who have had a single episode of thrombosis without an established prethrombotic state need low-dose heparin or 5000 U SQ every 8 to 12 hours. Patients with asymptomatic prethrombotic states can receive this regimen during the immediate postpartum period. If there is a history of one episode of deep venous thrombosis with some sort of provocation, anticoagulation is not necessary and noninvasive monitoring during pregnancy is recommended, such as by serial venous Doppler imaging or impedance plethysmography. Warfarin can be restarted postpartum; vitamin K supplements can be administered to breast-feeding infants. Warfarin costs $0.50 for 5 mg.

The management of patients with lupus anticoagulants is controversial although the guidelines outlined for other prethrombotic states can be followed. Successful pregnancies have resulted in patients with recurrent fetal loss due to the lupus anticoagulant with low-dose aspirin (80 mg/day) and moderate prednisone (40 mg/day). Aspirin is safe during the second and third trimesters, and probably safe during the first. Adjusted-dose SQ heparin can also be effective and should be continued for 3 to 4 days immediately postpartum.

Aspirin is used for prophylaxis of arterial thrombotic disease and is of limited usefulness for venous thromboembolism. In patients who experience recurrence of thrombosis despite adequate warfarin anticoagulation, the addition of aspirin can be considered, but its use must be balanced with the risk of gastrointestinal bleeding. Ticlopidine can be considered for aspirin failures. Dextran-40 is a plasma expander given IV with anticoagulant and antiplatelet properties, which has some value when heparin treatment is not feasible.

SUGGESTED READINGS

Colman RW, Hirsh J, Marder VJ, Salzman T, eds. Hemostasis and thrombosis basic principles and clinical practice. 3rd ed. Philadelphia: JB Lippincott, 1994.

Furie B, Limentani SA, Rosenfield CG. A practical guide to the evaluation and treatment of hemophilia. Blood 1994;84:3–9.

Greengard JS, Eichinger, Griffin JH, Bauer KA. Brief report: variability of thrombosis among homozygous siblings with resistance to activated protein C due to an Arg-Gln mutation in the gene for factor V. N Engl J Med 1994;331:1559–1562.

Hathaway WE, Goodnight SH Jr. Disorders of hemostasis and thrombosis. A clinical guide. New York: McGraw-Hill, 1993.

Hoffman R, Benz EJ Jr, Shattil SJ, et al., eds. Hematology, Basic principles and practice. 2nd ed. New York: Churchill Livingstone, 1995.

Rossi EC, Simon TL, Moss GS. Principles of transfusion medicine. Baltimore: Williams & Wilkins, 1991.

Roubey RAS. Autoantibodies to phospholipid-binding plasma proteins: a new view of lupus anticoagulants and other "antiphospholipid" autoantibodies. Blood 1994;84:2854–2867.

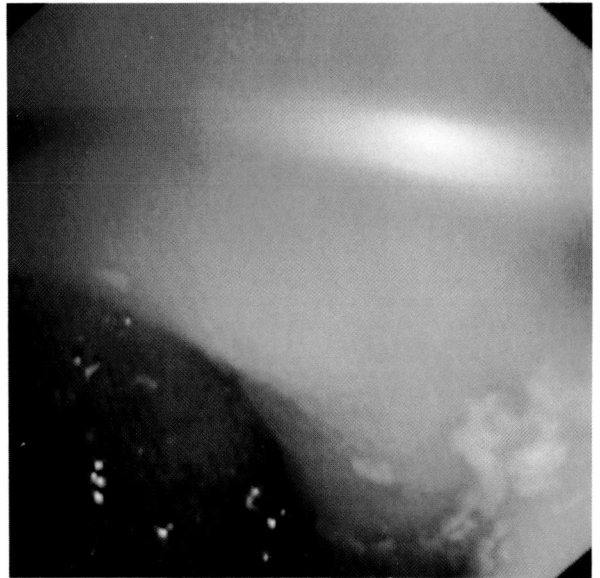

Plate 1: Normal colonoscopy (see page 178).

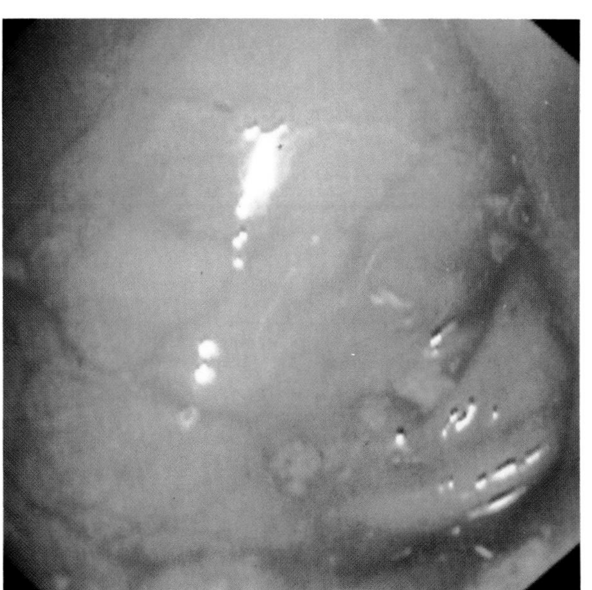

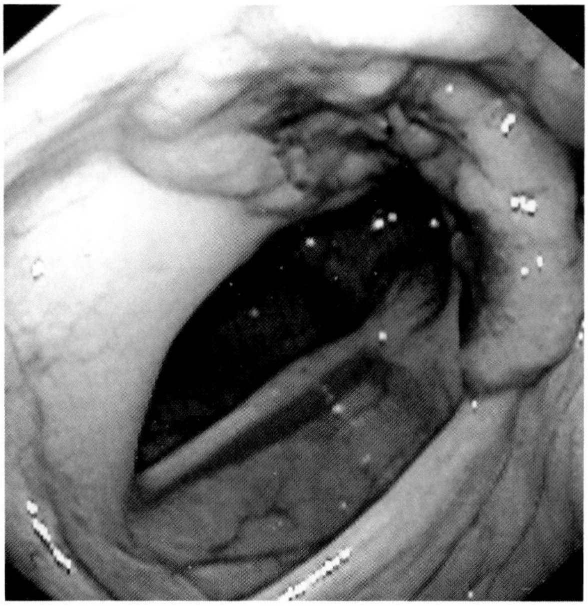

Plate 2: Colonoscopy demonstrating cancer (see page 179).

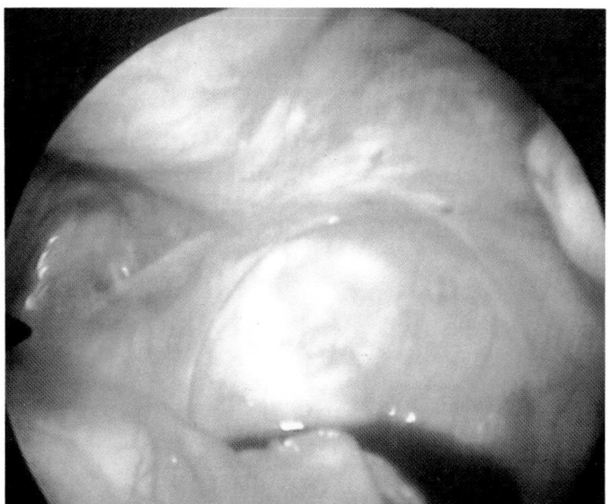

Plate 3: Implants of endometriosis on the uterosacral ligament (see page 180).

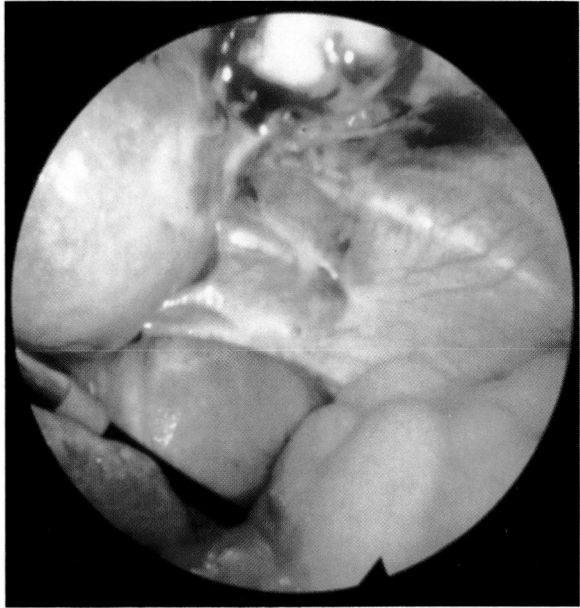

Plate 4: Fixation of bowel to posterior aspect of uterus with endometriosis (see page 180).

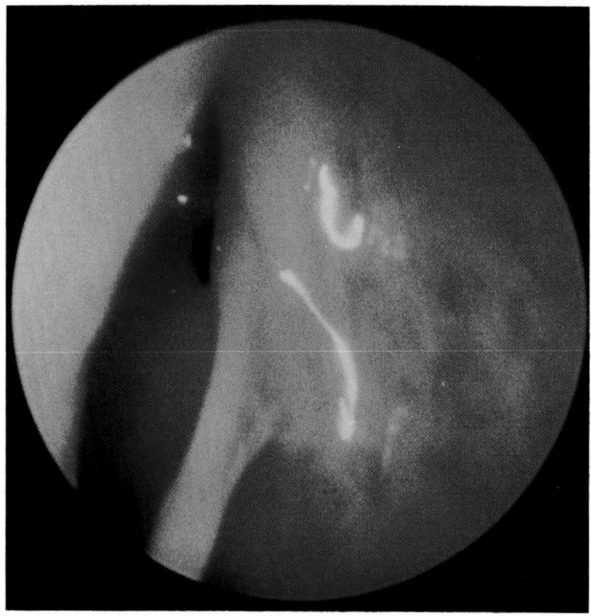

Plate 5: Purulent drainage from maxillary sinus ostium (see page 367).

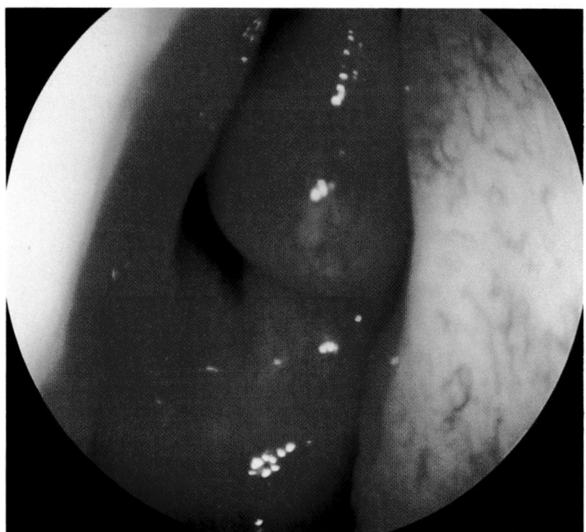

Plate 6: Right nasal cavity with polyps in right middle meatus (see page 367).

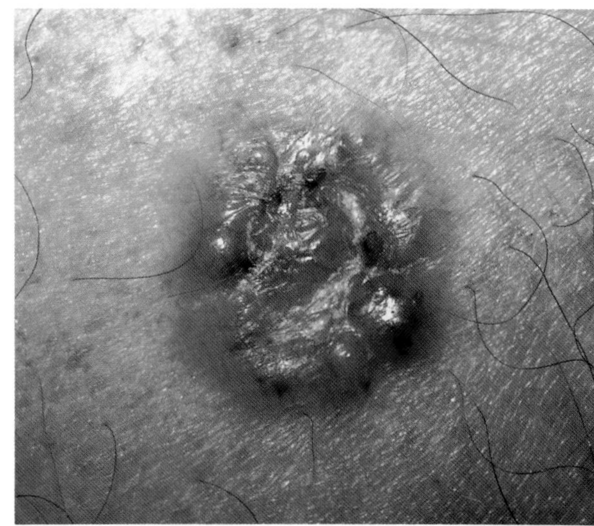

Plate 7: Classic basal cell carcinoma. Note the rolled edges (see page 494).

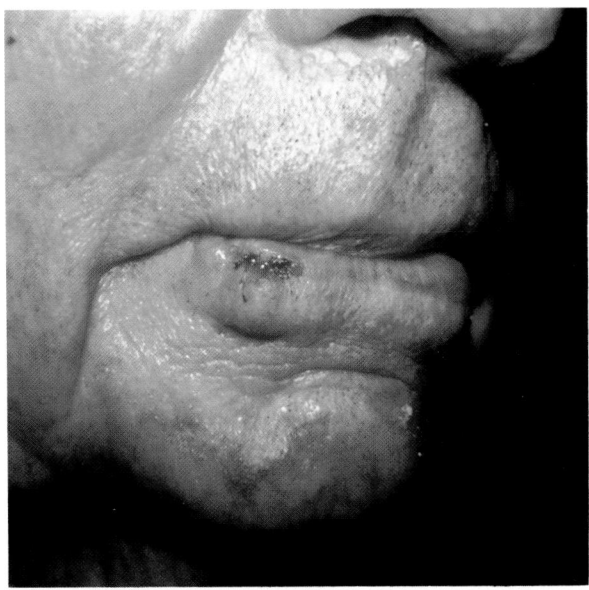

Plate 8: Squamous cell carcinoma of the lower lip. The area of induration around the ulcer is a typical, presenting finding (see page 495).

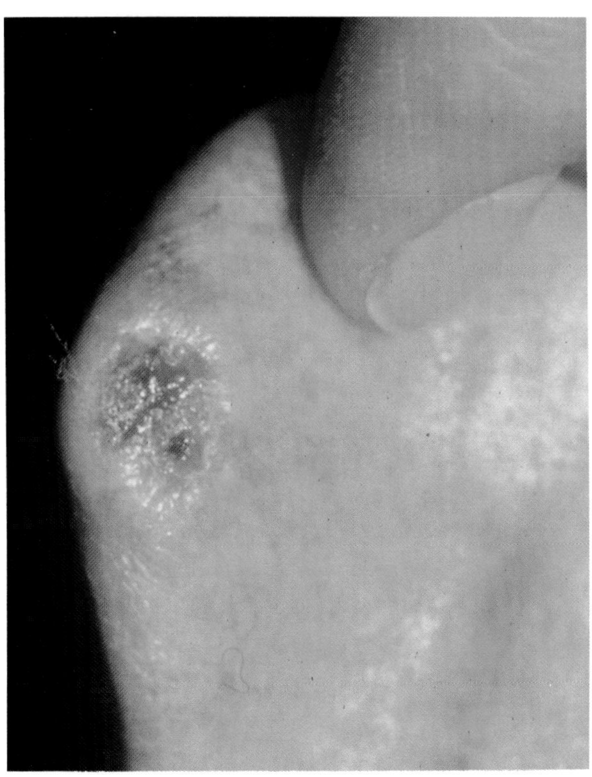

Plate 9: Squamous cell carcinoma of the posterior aspect of the pinna is often overlooked by the patient (see page 495).

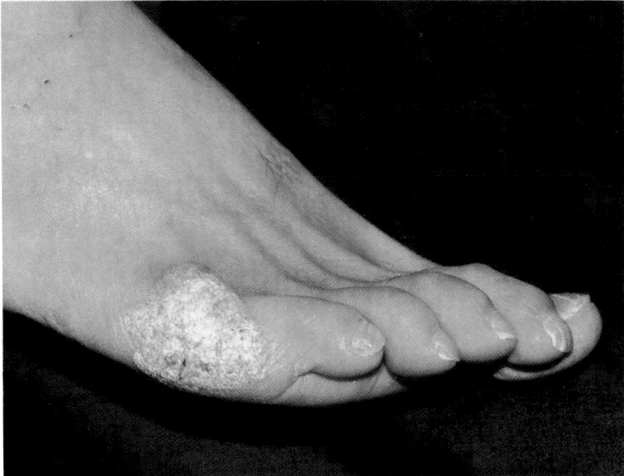

Plate 10: Squamous cell carcinoma of the foot is often mistaken for a verruca or callus (see page 495).

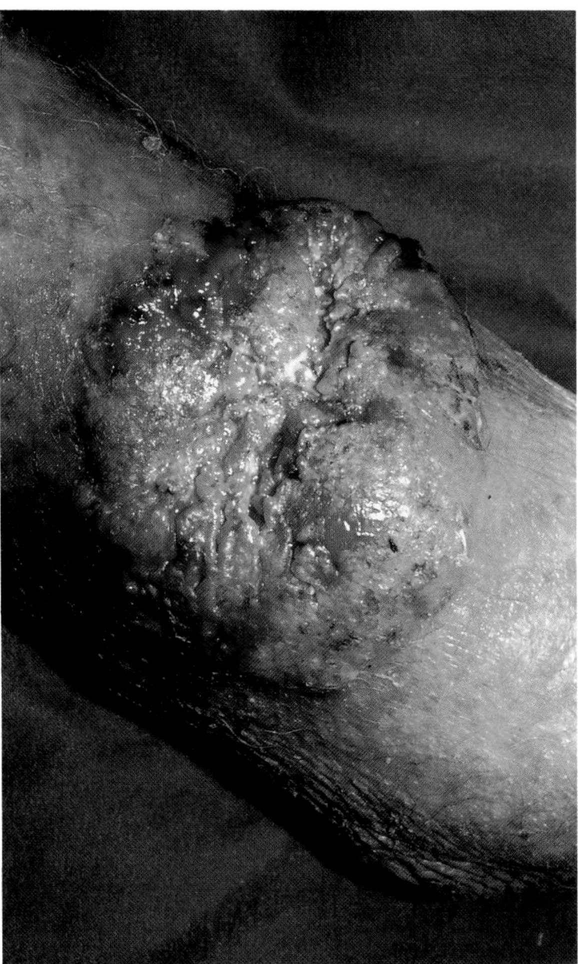

Plate 11: Large squamous cell carcinoma with typical, denuded or ulcerated surface (see page 495).

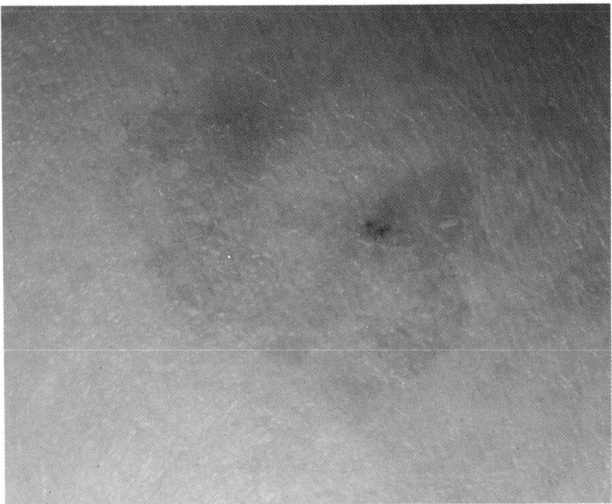

Plate 12: Bowen's disease or squamous cell carcinoma, in situ (see page 496).

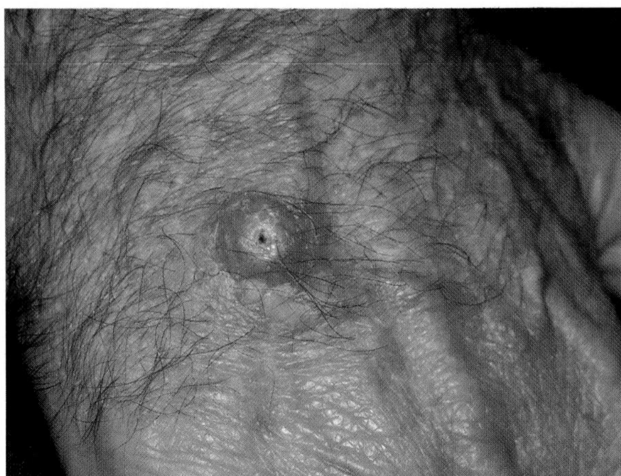

Plate 13: Keratoacanthoma. Note the typical "volcano" appearance with a central, keratinous core (see page 496).

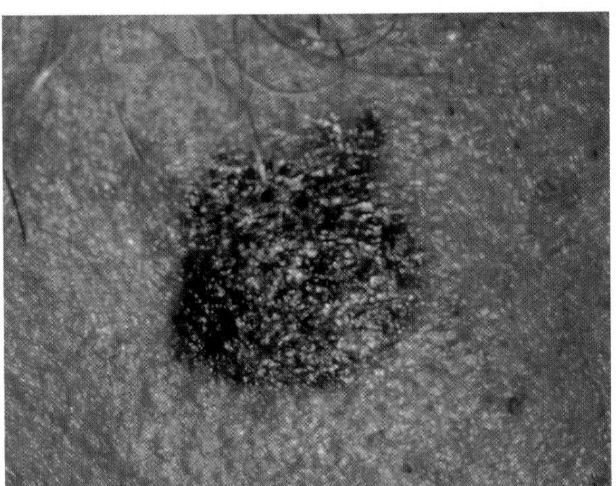

Plate 14: Cutaneous malignant melanoma. Note the ABCDs of diagnosis (see page 497).

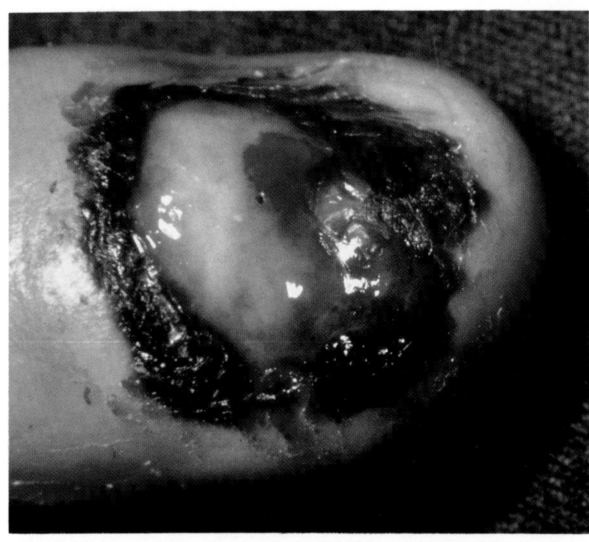

Plate 15: Acral-lentiginous melanoma with proximal nail fold involvement (Hutchinson's sign) (see page 497).

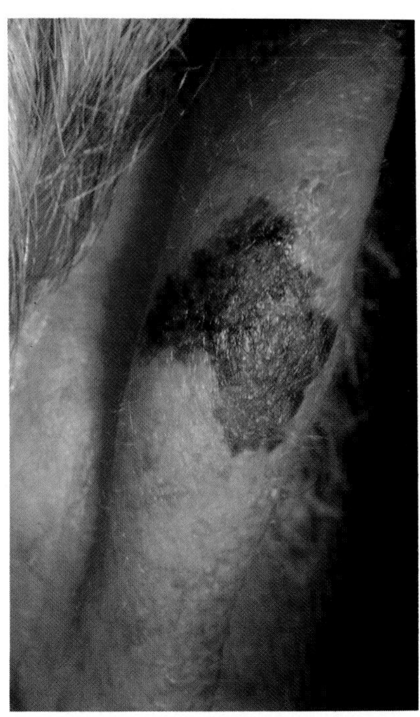

Plate 16: Lentigo malignant melanoma almost always occurs on sun-exposed skin of elderly patients. (see page 497).

SECTION SIX

ENDOCRINE DISORDERS

CHAPTER 18

THYROID DISEASE

Elizabeth J.v.B. Stahl,
Elizabeth Delionback Ennis,
Robert A. Kreisberg

The thyroid is the first endocrine gland to appear in fetal development. By 10 weeks of gestation, it is able to trap and organify iodine. Thyroxine (T_4) and thyroid-stimulating hormone (TSH) are detectable in the blood soon after, and they increase in concentration during the second trimester (1). Maternal TSH does not cross the placenta and the transfer of thyroxine is inefficient, emphasizing the importance of fetal thyroid hormonogenesis.

The thyroid is not only the first to develop but is the largest human endocrine gland, weighing approximately 20 gm in the adult. The gland consists of two lobes connected by an isthmus, often described as the shape of a butterfly.

Embryology

Thyroid tissue is derived from endoderm at the base of the tongue. It may remain attached to this region in adult life if the embryonic thyroglossal duct persists. Portions of the duct may survive as the pyramidal lobe of the thyroid, which extends upward from the isthmus, or as thyroglossal duct cysts. Because of the growth of structures in the neck, the thyroid may occasionally be displaced to a level below the larynx. Some or all of the thyroid may remain embedded in the base of the tongue as lingual thyroid. Most patients with a lingual thyroid are hypothyroid.

Anatomy

The isthmus of the thyroid overlies the second or third tracheal ring. It is attached to the anterior and lateral aspects of the trachea by loose connective tissue. The upper border of the isthmus is usually just below the cricoid cartilage, providing a landmark for the location of the gland. The carotid arteries and the sternocleidomastoid muscles are lateral to the gland. The recurrent laryngeal nerves lie in grooves between the lateral lobes of the gland and the trachea. Two pairs of parathyroid glands are situated on or beneath the posterior surface of the thyroid lobes.

Two main vessels, the superior thyroid artery, from the external carotid artery, and the inferior thyroid artery, from the subclavian artery, supply the gland. Blood flow to the thyroid has been estimated at 4 to 6 mL/min per gram (compare to the kidney at 3 mL/min per gram). In hyperthyroidism, blood flow may increase to 1 L/min and is responsible for the bruit heard over the gland. Microscopically, the gland is composed of closely spaced sacs, called follicles, which have a rich capillary network. The interior of each follicle is filled with colloid, a clear proteinaceous material, which is the major part of the total thyroid mass. Colloid contains a unique protein, thyroglobulin, within which T_4 and tri-iodothyronine (T_3) are synthesized and stored. The wall of the follicle is lined with a single layer of cuboidal cells.

The thyroid also contains other cells, known as parafollicular or C cells, which are the source of calcitonin, a calcium-lowering hormone. C cells become hyperplastic early in the course of medullary carcinoma of the thyroid and give rise to this tumor in its familial and sporadic forms.

Physiology

The thyroid secretes sufficient amounts of thyroid hormone to meet the demands of peripheral tissues. The active hormones are L-thyroxine (T_4) and 3,5,3'-tri-iodo-L-thyronine (T_3).

Thyroid hormone synthesis and secretion involve four sequential steps: 1) Active inward transport of iodide (trapping) from plasma into the thyroid follicle. This occurs at a rate greater than the passive diffusion of iodide out of the gland, thereby maintaining a concentration gradient for iodide. The average iodine intake in the United States is approximately 1000 μg daily. 2) Oxidation of iodide for iodination of tyrosyl residues in thyroglobulin. Iodide oxidation occurs via the action of iodide peroxidase and produces two hormonally inactive precursors, mono-iodotyrosine (MIT) and di-iodotyrosine (DIT); 3) Coupling of MIT and DIT, also mediated by iodide peroxidase, to form a variety of iodothyronines, including T_4 and T_3, the active hormones. 4) Release of T_4 and T_3 into the bloodstream. T_3 accounts for about 80% to 85% of the biologic effect of thyroid hormone secretion. T_3 is derived by direct secretion from the thyroid gland and by peripheral conversion of T_4 to T_3 by enzymatic removal of 5′-iodine from the outer ring of thyroxine. Peripheral conversion is responsible for about 80% of the daily T_3 production rate, whereas direct secretion accounts for about 20%.

The four steps in the synthesis and release of thyroid hormones may be inhibited by a variety of chemicals and drugs, known as goitrogens, because by inhibiting hormone synthesis they reduce circulating hormone levels that stimulate TSH secretion, leading to goiter formation. Perchlorate and thiocyanate inhibit iodide transport and reduce the amount of substrate available to form hormone. The antithyroid medications, methimazole and propylthiouracil (PTU), inhibit the oxidation of iodide, decrease the amounts of DIT and MIT, and block coupling of MIT and DIT to form active hormone. When iodine is given in large doses, it acutely blocks organic binding and coupling reactions, an action known as the Wolff-Chaikoff effect. The fetal thyroid is quite sensitive to the effect of iodide; therefore, pregnant women should not be given iodine in large doses because of the danger of producing goitrous hypothyroidism in the fetus. Lithium has several effects on thyroid metabolism, including inhibition of hormone release. Dexamethasone in large doses also inhibits thyroid hormone release by inhibiting TSH secretion.

Both T_4 and T_3 are almost entirely bound to plasma proteins. Normally, only about 0.03% of T_4 and 0.3% of T_3 are free. As a consequence, the proportion of free T_3 is about 10 times greater than that of T_4. Only free hormone or hormone loosely bound to protein is available to tissues; therefore, an individual's metabolic state correlates best with the concentration of free hormone, rather than total hormone concentration.

Approximately 30% of T_4 is converted to T_3 ($0.3 \times 100\,\mu g/day = 30\,\mu g/day$), whereas 40% is converted to reverse T_3 (rT_3), a biologically inert metabolite. When patients with hypothyroidism are treated with synthetic T_4 in doses sufficient to maintain normal blood levels of T_4, the T_3 concentration will be maintained at a normal level as well because of peripheral conversion of T_4 to T_3. Consequently, it is unnecessary to use preparations for replacement that contain T_3.

Thyroid hormones influence the growth and function of all tissues, energy use, substrate turnover, and the rates of metabolism of vitamins, other hormones and importantly, drugs.

Thyroid Hormone Regulation

The thyroid gland is primarily regulated by TSH, a glycoprotein secreted by thyrotropes in the anterior pituitary. It regulates thyroid growth, enhances synthesis of thyroglobulin, and stimulates all steps in the synthesis and secretion of thyroid hormones. TSH binds to specific cell surface receptors located on the follicular cell and activates the enzyme, adenylate cyclase. Cyclic 3′,5′-adenosine monophosphate (cAMP) is responsible for mediating almost all of the actions of TSH.

Secretion of TSH by the thyrotropin-producing cells of the anterior pituitary is regulated by the hypothalamus and by the level of circulating thyroid hormone. Thyrotropin-releasing hormone (TRH), a product of the hypothalamus, stimulates the synthesis and secretion of TSH, and subsequently the synthesis of T_4 and T_3, while the circulating levels of T_4 and T_3 influence TSH secretion by the process of negative feedback at the level of the thyrotrope. TSH secretion is affected in a negative feedback manner by thyroid hormones; the feedback inhibition threshold is set by TRH. Thyroid hormones do not influence TRH secretion but reduce the number of TRH receptors on the surface of the thyrotrope, decreasing the cell's responsiveness to TRH. Circulating T_3 and T_3 derived from T_4 conversion to T_3 within the thyrotrope regulates TSH secretion.

Physical Examination of the Thyroid Gland

The thyroid gland may be examined from the front or back of the patient. The thyroid gland is located by first finding the thyroid cartilage, and then proceeding one to two fingerbreadths inferiorly. Once the isthmus is located, the lobes are easily identified by moving laterally. Using both hands is helpful; one hand may be placed on the border of the sternocleidomastoid muscle, gently pushing it laterally and posteriorly, to more accurately assess the thyroid tissue. The patient should be asked to turn her head first to one side, and then the other, as the thyroid gland is palpated; when the patient turns her head, the ipsilateral muscle is relaxed, and the thyroid may be more easily palpated on that side. It is helpful to have the patient drink from a cup of water during the examination, swallowing several times, which allows the gland to be observed as well as palpated. The normal gland weighs 20 to 30 gm and is often not palpable if not enlarged. The lobes of the thyroid gland are often asymmetric. Palpation behind the sternum is useful for finding substernal extension of the thyroid. The overall size, consistency (multinodular goiters are often described as "lumpy or bumpy" while the gland in Graves' disease is usually firm, smooth, and warm to the touch), presence of nodules, and lymphadenopathy should be noted. Nodules should be characterized by size, consistency (soft, firm, rock hard), and the presence of lymphadenopathy. When the gland is enlarged, measurement of the size of each lobe may be helpful for future comparisons after treatment of the underlying disease. Vascular bruits over thyroid may be heard in thyrotoxic patients and a thrill may also be detected with careful palpation. Because thyroid nodules and goiter are quite common among women, the thyroid gland should be examined yearly.

Laboratory Tests

An extensive number of tests are available to assess thyroid function. The levels of free and total T_4 and T_3 can be measured, thyroid-binding globulin (TBG) levels can be assessed indirectly with the T_3 resin uptake (T_3RU) or quantitated by radioimmunoassay (RIA), and thyroid gland activity can be quantified by measuring radioactive iodine uptake (RAIU), using ^{131}I or ^{123}I. The adequacy of circulating thyroid hormone levels is determined by the measurement of TSH. Thyroid anatomy is defined with thyroid scans using radioiodine or technetium or with thyroid ultrasound. Measurement of antithyroid antibody levels and levels of human thyroid-stimulating immunoglobulin (TSI) may be helpful in patients with autoimmune thyroid disease. A description of each type of test follows.

Hormone Concentration and Binding

The free T_4 is currently the best test for assessment of thyroid hormone levels because it is a measure of the free (unbound) hormone. The normal range varies with the assay. The normal value is higher in newborns and children. The free T_4 is superior to the measurement of total T_4 because it is not affected by changes in binding proteins, but like the total T_4 it may be reduced by severe nonthyroidal illness. Free T_4 levels are useful in making a diagnosis of hyper- or hypothyroidism, as well as for following therapy in these diseases.

The total T_4 immunoassay measures the total serum concentration of T_4, both bound and free. Its major shortcoming is that it is affected by alterations in binding proteins; therefore, it has been largely supplanted by the free T_4.

The T_3 radioimmunoassay (T_3RIA) is a useful test when hyperthyroidism due to T_3 thyrotoxicosis is suspected; however, this disorder is uncommon. In this setting, the T_4 concentration will be normal, and hyperthyroidism may be missed in the absence of a T_3 measurement. Because reduced levels of T_3 occur with acute and chronic medical illness, it is not a useful test for the diagnosis of hypothyroidism. The free T_3 concentration can be helpful in rare situations but is not a routine test.

The T_3RU is an indirect test of serum TBG and when used with a T_4 measurement allows calculation of the free T_4 index. It has been replaced by the free T_4; however, if a free T_4 measurement is not available, it is useful. The free T_4 index requires measurement of the T_4 and T_3RU. The T_3RU assay involves adding labeled T_3 to a sample of the patient's serum. It is then allowed to compete and equilibrate with the patient's T_4 for binding to TBG in the sample. This mixture is then added to a resin that will bind the T_3 that is not bound by TBG. The resin is then assayed for its uptake of the labeled T_3. A high RU indicates that the patient's serum either contains a high amount of thyroid hormone and has saturated TBG or that a decreased level of TBG is present. Conversely, when the T_3 resin uptake is decreased, there are either increased levels of TBG (as is seen with estrogen therapy) or understaturation of TBG (as seen in hypothyroidism). Many factors alter thyroid-binding proteins (1) (Box 18.1) and confound the use of the T_3RU.

Regulation of Thyroid Function

Measurement of the serum TSH is useful in the diagnosis of both hyper- and hypothyroidism. The immunoassays for TSH have become increasingly more sensitive, with first-generation assays able to detect TSH levels down to 1 mIU/L, second-generation assays to 0.1 mIU/L, and the third-generation assay (currently used) down to 0.03 mIU/L. TSH is used to distinguish primary from secondary hypothyroidism because it will be elevated in primary and decreased or normal in secondary hypothyroidism. TSH is suppressed to undetectable levels in most cases of hyperthyroidism, but it is normal to slightly increased in the rare situation when hyperthyroidism is of pituitary origin. TSH may also be suppressed to low or undetectable levels in patients with a toxic multinodular goiter or toxic nodule, or in a patient taking excessive thyroid hormone replacement.

TSH level may be normal, low, or high in patients with severe nonthyroidal illness, depending on when it is measured during the illness. It may also be suppressed by certain commonly used drugs, including dopamine, high-dose glucocorticoids, and diphenylhydantoin.

Box 18.1 Factors Associated with Altered Thyroid-Binding Protein Concentration

Increased TBG	Decreased TBG
Pregnancy	Androgenic and anabolic steroids
Oral estrogens	Chronic liver disease (cirrhosis)
Newborn state	Severe systemic illness
Acute viral hepatitis	Active acromegaly
Tamoxifen	Nephrotic syndrome
Biliary cirrhosis	Genetic
Genetic	

TBG, thyroid-binding globulin

Source: Adapted from Ingbar S. Diseases of the thyroid. In: Braunwald E, Isselbacher KJ, Petersdorf RG, et al., eds. Harrison's principles of internal medicine. 11th ed. New York: McGraw-Hill, 1987:1732–1752.

Direct Tests of Thyroid Gland Function

The thyroid RAIU is the most common of these tests. ^{131}I has most commonly been used in the past, but ^{123}I is preferable because it delivers a lower radiation dose. The small dose of radioiodine administered to the patient mixes with the endogenous iodide pool and is used to assess iodine uptake by the thyroid. The RAIU is usually measured at 24 hours after the patient has received the isotope. In Graves' disease maximum iodine uptake may be reached earlier; consequently, 4 or 6 hour uptakes are often done in these patients. The RAIU usually correlates with the functional state of the thyroid. However, trapping of iodide and synthesis and release of T_4 may be dissociated leading to situations in which the uptake is misleading. At usual levels of iodine intake (in the United States, up to 1000 μg/day), the normal range for the 6-hour uptake is 5% to 15% and for the 24-hour uptake is 10% to 30% of the given dose. This test is not useful for evaluation of hypothyroidism because of the lower normal values; values above the normal range are useful in the diagnosis of hypethyroidism.

The idoine uptake is most useful when hyperthyroidism is associated with a low uptake, such as thyroiditis (postpartum or subacute), thyrotoxicosis factitia, or iodine-induced hyperthyroidism (2) (Box 18.2).

Thyroid Imaging—Scans and Ultrasound

A thyroid scan allows localization of sites of accumulation of radioiodine (^{123}I) or sodium pertechnetate (^{99m}Tc). It is useful for defining areas of increased (hot) or decreased (cold) function within the thyroid and for detecting retrosternal thyroid tissue, ectopic tissue, abnormal location of thyroid tissue (retrosternal, thy-

Box 18.2 Causes of Elevated and Reduced Radioactive Iodine Uptake

Elevated	Low
Graves' disease	Antithyroid medications
Iodine deficiency	Administration of iodine (drugs, contrast dye)
Toxic nodular goiter	Subacute thyroiditis
Pregnancy	Thyroid hormone administration
Early Hashimoto's thyroiditis	Thyroid gland damage
Recovery from subacute thyroiditis	Hypopituitarism with decreased thyroid-stimulating hormone
Recovery from thyroid hormone	Ectopic functioning thyroid tissue
Suppression	

Source: Adapted from Fitzgerald PA. Endocrine disorders. In: Tierney LM Jr, McPhee SJ, Papadakis MA, eds. Current medical diagnosis and treatment. 33rd ed. East Norwalk, CT: Appleton & Lange, 1994:912–976.

roglossal duct cysts, lingual thyroid tissue), and, under certain circumstances, functioning metastases of thyroid carcinoma. These radioisotopes are contraindicated in pregnant or lactating women.

The usual dose of ^{123}I is 200 μCi PO. It is trapped by functioning thyroid tissue, organified, and retained. The scan is generally done within 4 to 24 hours after giving the ^{123}I. If a patient has had radioiodide contrast studies (as used in computed tomographic procedures), at least 4 weeks should intervene before proceeding to a thyroid scan. The previously administered iodide will expand the body iodide pool and reduce the uptake of the radioisotope.

Pertechnetate is given by IV injection. It is trapped by the thyroid but not organified. Imaging must be done early, before the isotope leaks out of the gland, and is usually begun 10 to 20 minutes after the injection. The dose given ranges between 1 and 10 mCi. Compared to ^{123}I, ^{99m}Tc is readily available in nuclear medicine departments, delivers a lower radiation dose to the thyroid (but a higher dose to the rest of the body), and is less expensive. ^{123}I is thought, by some, to give a better quality thyroid scan. As in the case of radioiodine, ^{99m}Tc is inhibited by excess iodine and drugs that inhibit the iodide-trapping mechanism of the thyroid. The commonly used antithyroid drugs, PTU and methimazole, do not impair iodide trapping; therefore information may be obtained about the thyroid gland during treatment with these medications.

Thyroid ultrasound is a commonly performed test. However, it should be reserved for selected and relatively few patients and should not be routinely ordered for the evaluation of a thyroid nodule. Ultrasound is the most definitive technique for demonstrating the cystic or solid nature of a thyroid nodule. It is also often used to follow the size of a thyroid nodule in response to therapy. It is most useful in patients in whom there is uncertainty about the origin of a neck mass and in guiding needle biopsies of nodules that are not easily palpable. Thyroid ultrasound may also be the imaging procedure of choice in evaluating thyroid nodules in pregnant women in whom clinical uncertainty exists and who cannot have isotopic scanning done. Approximately 20% of the adult population has thyroid nodules on ultrasound, most of which are clinically undetectable. The significance of finding a small thyroid nodule by ultrasound in an asymptomatic patient is unclear and there are no protocols for evaluation that can be justified on a cost–benefit basis. Consequently, an ultrasound examination should not be ordered unless the patient has a palpable nodule and cannot undergo fine needle aspiration biopsy.

Miscellaneous Tests

Thyroid Antibodies

Antibodies against several constituents of the thyroid (thyroglobulin and microsomal) are most commonly seen in Hashimoto's thyroiditis, but they are also found in patients with Graves' disease. Antithyroid antibodies occur in 5% to 10% of the normal population, with increasing incidence with age. In Graves' disease, the serum also contains antibodies against the TSH receptor. These inhibit both the binding of TSH to its receptor (TSH-binding inhibitory immunoglobulins or TBII) and stimulate the production of cAMP within the thyroid (thyroid-stimulating immunoglobulin, or TSI). Both of these anti-TSH antibodies have the ability to cross the placenta and produce transient hyperthyroidism (TSI) or hypothyroidism (TBII) in the newborn.

Thyroglobulin

Thyroglobulin is used as an index of endogenous thyroid activity and is present in all normal persons. It is useful in the diagnosis of thyrotoxicosis factitia where thyroid hormone levels are high but thryoglobulin is absent, indicating an exogenous source of thyroid hormone. It can also be used as a tumor marker to follow the course of differentiated thyroid cancer, provided that all functioning thyroid tissue has been surgically removed or ablated. Thyroglobulin levels cannot be used for the diagnosis of differentiated thyroid cancer. Thyroglobulin will be absent unless there is residual metastatic thyroid tissue. Serial (annual) thyroglobulin measurements may be useful for follow-up of a patient with treated differentiated thyroid cancer, both in assessing the adequacy of therapy, as well as monitoring for recurrence of disease.

Fine Needle Aspiraton of the Thyroid

This test is done in the initial evaluation of a thyroid mass. The usefulness of the test is only as good as the physician performing the aspiration and the pathologist reading the cytology. A patient is probably best served by referral to an endocrinologist for this procedure.

Hyperthyroidism

Thyrotoxicosis is a common clinical problem that is due to an excess of circulating thyroid hormone; it is caused by a variety of disorders (1) (Box 18.3). It is important to differentiate among these disorders to optimize therapy and management. The more common causes of hyperthyroidism are discussed below.

Graves' Disease

This is an autoimmune disorder with diffuse toxic goiter, ophthalmopathy, and dermopathy. This triad may appear together or separately, and each component often runs an independent course. Graves' disease is a fairly common disorder that may occur at any age but is most common in the third and fourth decades. It accounts for approximately 70% of all patients with hyperthyroidism and is more common in women than men, in a ratio approaching 7:1 in the United States. There is a familial predisposition to Graves' disease, with certain HLA haplotypes occurring more frequently in patients with the disease.

Pathogenesis

Patients with Graves' disease have a serum IgG antibody directed against the TSH receptor of the thyroid gland, known as thyroid-stimulating immunoglobulin (TSI). After binding to the receptor, this antibody acts as a TSH agonist, stimulating thyroid hormone production as well as glandular growth. In most cases, both hyperactivity and hyperplasia occur; however, patients with Graves' disease particularly the elderly, may not have a goiter.

Clinical Features and Physical Findings

The clinical presentation of the thyrotoxic patient is variable (3) (Box 18.4). Patients with thyrotoxicosis commonly present with nervousness, heat intolerance, inability to sleep, tremor, excessive sweating, frequent bowel movements, and weight loss. Features specific to Graves' disease include a diffuse hyperfunctioning goiter, ophthalmopathy, and dermopathy. The goiter may be asymmetric. A bruit may be present over the gland, reflecting increased thyroid vascularity and suggesting that the patient is thyrotoxic. Ophthalmopathy may take a number of forms, including stare, lid lag, and lid retraction, as well as proptosis, chemosis, conjunctivitis, and periorbital swelling. The dermopathy of Graves' disease involves the pretibial and foot areas and is termed pretibial myxedema. The affected area is well demarcated, raised and thickened, with a peau d'orange appearance. It may be pruritic and hyperpigmented.

More prolonged disease is associated with features of a chronic catabolic illness, including muscle wasting and a proximal myopathy. A severe cardiomyopathy with congestive heart failure may occur, especially in the older patient. Cardiac arrhythmias, especially atrial fibrillation, are a common presenting feature in the elderly thyrotoxic patient.

Diagnosis

A typical case of Graves' disease is easily diagnosed based on the history and physical findings. Laboratory

Box 18.3 Causes of Thyrotoxicosis

Illness Associated with Thyroid Hyperfunction; Increased RAIU	Illness Not Associated with Thyroid Hyperfunction; Decreased RAIU
Graves' disease	Subacute thyroiditis
Excess TSH production	Silent thyroiditis
Trophoblastic tissue (due to abnormal thyroid stimulator)	Transient thyrotoxicosis
Hyperfunctioning adenoma	Thyrotoxicosis factitia
Toxic multinodular goiter	Ectopic thyroid tissue

RAIU, radioactive iodine uptake; TSH, thyroid-stimulating hormone
Source: Adapted from Ingbar S. Diseases of the thyroid. In: Braunwald E, Isselbacher KJ, Petersdorf RG, et al., eds. Harrison's principles of internal medicine. 11th ed. New York: McGraw-Hill, 1987:1732–1752.

Box 18.4 Clinical Features of Thyrotoxicosis

Symptoms	Signs
Nervousness	Thyroid enlargement
Heat intolerance	Lid lag
Palpitations	Warm skin
Tremulousness	Tremor
Muscle weakness	Onycholysis
Emotional lability	Tachycardia, atrial fibrillation
Hyperdefecation	Proptosis, ophthalmoplegia*
	Pretibial myxedema*

* Graves' disease only
Source: Adapted from Andreoli TE, Carpenter CCH, Plum F, Smith LH Jr, eds. Cecil essentials of internal medicine. Philadelphia: WB Saunders, 1986:452–456.

studies are confirmatory and reveal an elevated free T_4 and suppressed TSH. If Graves' disease is suspected but the T_4 is normal, a T_3RIA should be ordered, because T_3 thyrotoxicosis is present in some patients. Further testing at the time of diagnosis is unnecessary unless treatment with radioiodine is planned and then an iodine uptake is required.

In some patients, especially the elderly, the clinical picture may be one of masked or apathetic hyperthyroidism. In the absence of ophthalmopathy and goiter, the diagnosis may be overlooked. In such patients, cardiovascular abnormalities predominate, and patients may present with unexplained heart failure or atrial fibrillation. Laboratory confirmation is required to make the correct diagnosis.

Therapy

The treatment of Graves' disease takes three forms: medication, radioactive iodine, or surgery. Most patients will require medical management at the outset; some will require ablative therapy with RAI or surgery after the signs and symptoms of hyperthyroidism have been controlled.

β-Blocking agents should be used in all hyperthyroid patients (unless contraindicated) to modify the severity of their symptoms. Their principal mechanism of action is to antagonize β receptor-mediated effects of catecholamines (4). The usual drug is propranolol, in a dose of 40–80 mg every 6 hours. The dose should be titrated until hyperadrenergic symptoms are controlled. Large doses may be required because thyrotoxic patients can rapidly metabolize β blockers. The long-acting form of propranolol can also be used, but dose titration is always necessary. The target heart rate with β-blocker therapy is 60 to 70 beats/min ideally, but rates under 90 to 100 beats/min are acceptable provided that the patient is not undergoing surgery. Other β-blocker drugs are also effective. Potential adverse reactions to these drugs include bronchospasm, decreased cardiac output, hypotension, bradycardia, and masking of the symptoms of hypoglycemia. Their use is relatively contraindicated in patients with asthma, congestive heart failure, and heart block. They play a significant role as adjunctive therapy with thionamides, radioactive iodine, and surgery.

The thionamides PTU and methimazole (Tapazole) inhibit the synthesis of thyroid hormone by blocking the peroxidase enzyme within the thyroid gland. They can restore a euthyroid state within 4 to 8 weeks of treatment provided that the correct dose is used. Tapazole is approximately 10 times more potent than PTU. Because of different half-lives, the initial dose of PTU is 100–200 mg every 6 to 8 hours, and for methimazole 10–20 mg every 8 to 12 hours. Recent literature suggests that methimazole is effective given as a once daily dose of 20–40 mg (5,6). Each patient should have a complete blood count and a set of liver function tests before therapy is begun with either of these medications. Side effects of the medications are similar and can be grouped into minor (rash, arthralgias, fever) and major (agranulocytosis, liver dysfunction, vasculitis, and lupus-like syndromes) (7). The toxicity rate is similar with both agents; about 5% for minor reactions and 0.5% for agranulocytosis. When given in small doses, however, methimazole is associated with less risk of agranulocytosis than PTU (7). Minor side effects are generally dose related and can be controlled with a decrease in dose. The rash that may occur is not dose related and generally resolves despite continuation of therapy. Agranulocytosis is idiosyncratic and not predictable based on complete blood counts; therefore there is no value to obtaining these routinely. Patients should be advised to watch for fever or sore throat and to report such symptoms immediately. The majority of patients recover from agranulocytosis once the medication is stopped. If a minor side effect develops, the patient may be switched to the other drug, but there is a fairly high degree of cross-reactivity between the two. Patients should also be cautioned regarding weight gain; the thyrotoxic state allows patients to lose or maintain their weight despite the consumption of a large amount of calories. Once the hypermetabolism of thyrotoxicosis is controlled with antithyroid medications, patients are susceptible to weight gain if their eating habits do not change.

If medication is chosen for long-term therapy, it is continued for at least 6 to 12 months. Medical therapy is the treatment of choice for children and teenagers. Patients should be seen every 4 to 6 weeks for clinical and laboratory evaluation. As the thyrotoxic state comes under control, the antithyroid medication dosage may be reduced. Recently it has been suggested that addition of a T_4 supplement to antithyroid medication after the patient becomes euthyroid increases the likelihood of remission (8). Careful follow-up is required to avoid either hypothyroidism or recurrent hyperthyroidism.

Radioactive iodine (^{131}I) offers a relatively easy and effective way to treat thyrotoxicosis. The dose given is designed to render the patient euthyroid, but immediate and delayed hypothyroidism occur commonly, thus requiring lifetime follow-up because 50% to 70% will require thyroid hormone replacement therapy. This, however, is preferable to recurrence of hyperthyroid symptoms. If patients are followed closely, there is little likelihood that they will become severely hypothyroid before thyroid hormone supplementation is begun. Therapy with ^{131}I is the treatment of choice for the thyrotoxic adult and is best supervised by an endocrinologist. Complications are rare and may include thyroiditis, with pain and swelling in the area of the thyroid gland. It can be managed with nonsteroidal anti-inflammatory drugs (NSAIDs).

Surgical treatment of thyrotoxicosis is an option for the young patient in whom antithyroid drug therapy is unsuccessful, in any patient who refuses ^{131}I, and in the patient with a very large thyroid gland in whom therapy with ^{131}I is unlikely to be successful. Generally, a subtotal thyroidectomy is done. In the hands of an experienced surgeon, this procedure is relatively safe, and complications are few. If complications occur they include recurrent laryngeal nerve damage and hypoparathyroidism. Hypothyroidism occurs frequently with surgery (approximately one half the frequency as with ^{131}I), and should not be considered a complication because it is easier to treat hypothyroidism than recurrent thyrotoxicosis.

Toxic Multinodular Goiter

Thyrotoxicosis associated with toxic multinodular goiter develops over a number of years and occurs in patients with a previous multinodular goiter, when the number of follicles with autonomous iodide metabolism become sufficiently large that overall hormone production exceeds individual needs. This is a slow process that requires years. It mostly affects older women with a long history of multinodular goiter. Subclinical hyperthyroidism (suppressed TSH secretion with normal free T_4 and T_3 levels) often precedes overt hyperthyroidism (9).

The symptoms of thyrotoxicosis in the elderly patient are often difficult to detect and are frequently superimposed on other underlying diseases. Patients who present with unexplained tachycardia, atrial fibrillation, weight loss, and psychiatric disorders should be examined closely for the presence of multinodular goiter, with attention to the results of thyroid function tests to determine if thyrotoxicosis is present.

Radioiodine or surgery may be used for treatment of toxic multinodular goiter. In a younger patient in good general health, with a large gland, surgery is often the best option. Radioiodine therapy may be the treatment of choice in the elderly patient with multiple medical problems. Euthyroidism should be established with medical management before either surgery or radioiodine therapy to avoid aggravation of the thyrotoxicosis.

Autonomously Functioning Thyroid Nodules

Autonomously functioning thyroid nodules (AFTNs) are nodules that function independently of the pituitary–thyroid negative-feedback control mechanism (10). The autonomous secretion of thyroid hormone eventually suppresses TSH secretion, resulting in atrophy of surrounding extranodular thyroid tissue. These may be solitary nodules in otherwise normal thyroid glands or may appear as single or multiple nodules in preexisting multinodular goiters. These nodules are, by definition, hyperfunctioning; however, depending on the mass of hyperfunctioning thyroid tissue, the patient may be either euthyroid or hyperthyroid. In a series of 361 patients with AFTNs, 76% were euthyroid, 19% were thyrotoxic, and 5% were borderline thyrotoxic (11).

The diagnosis of AFTN has changed in recent years. As fine needle aspiration of the thyroid has become the first step in the diagnosis of a thyroid nodule, fewer AFTNs are being picked up on scan. Suppressed TSH concentrations are the first indication that an asymptomatic patient has autonomous thyroid function.

In a patient with an AFTN and thyrotoxicosis, ablation of the nodule is indicated. An asymptomatic patient with an AFTN may be observed closely until symptoms appear, especially if the patient is young and healthy (12). In the older patient, or in any patient with a nodule greater than 3 cm in diameter in whom the risk of developing thyrotoxicosis is greater, ablation of the nodule may be indicated. Two options are available—surgery or ^{131}I therapy. Surgery is the procedure of choice for the younger patient. ^{131}I therapy may be as effective as surgery, but because the nodules are relatively radioresistant, larger doses are required and hypothyroidism may be more likely. As with all patients, careful follow-up is required.

TSH-Induced Hyperthyroidism

Hyperthyroidism is rarely TSH dependent. However, this diagnosis must be considered in the patient with thyrotoxicosis who has a normal or elevated TSH level. This combination suggests a TSH-secreting pituitary adenoma. The patient often presents with clinical features (headaches, visual disturbances) that are consistent with a pituitary tumor, goiter, and thyrotoxicosis. The associated features of Graves' disease, such as ophthalmopathy and dermopathy, are not present. Patients may have partial hypopituitarism, particularly loss of gonadal function because of encroachment of the tumor on normal pituitary tissue. The tumor may also cosecrete other hormones, such as growth hormone, follicle-stimulating hormone, and prolactin. This occurs in up to one third of patients. Laboratory investigation reveals elevated free thyroid hormone levels and TSH levels within the normal or elevated range, rather than suppressed as they are in Graves' disease, toxic multinodular goiter, and hyperfunctioning thyroid nodules.

Pituitary surgery is the only rational therapy for these patients; however, ablation of the thyroid may be necessary if the tumor is unresectable. Patients may be treated with antithyroid medications and β blockers in preparation for surgery. Somatostatin may be useful to control pituitary tumor growth if the lesion cannot be completely resected.

Thyrotoxicosis Factitia

The term thyrotoxicosis factitia is used to describe thyrotoxicosis produced by ingesting exogenous thyroid hormone. Thyroid hormone has been used in the past for many diseases other than hypothyroidism. Obesity and menstrual irregularities were common reasons to begin patients on thyroid hormone. Because patients treated in this way did not improve, the dose was gradually increased to the point of producing hyperthyroidism. Many patients are still taking thyroid hormone for inappropriate reasons.

Another common cause of thyrotoxicosis factitia is the secretive use of thyroid hormone by patients with underlying psychiatric disorders. This is often difficult to establish because the patient will not usually admit to using the medication. Occasionally ingestion is inadvertent (several epidemics of hyperthyroidism have been reported due to ingestion of hamburger meat contaminated with thyroid tissue).

The clinical manifestations are identical to those of hyperthyroidism of thyroid origin, except that there is no thyroid enlargement, ophthalmopathy, or dermopathy. The laboratory reveals elevated free T_4 and T_3RIA levels, with decreased TSH and thyroglobulin values. Thyroid uptake of ^{131}I or ^{99m}Tc is low.

If a history of ingestion is obtained from the patient, diagnosis is not difficult. The thyroid hormone should be stopped, with repeat clinical and laboratory evaluation 1 month later. If the use of thyroid hormone is surreptitious, however, diagnosis of the underlying cause of thyrotoxicosis may be more challenging. A low serum thyroglobulin level may be valuable in helping to confirm clinical suspicion of thyroid hormone (ab)use. Treatment involves confrontation of the patient with an explanation of the deleterious effects of inappropriate thyroid hormone use.

Hypothyroidism

Hypothyroidism is the most common functional disorder of the thyroid. It may result from a variety of diseases that lead to inadequate synthesis of thyroid hormone (10) (Box 18.5). The most common of these conditions are discussed below. It is most often due to decreased thyroid hormone production from the thyroid gland; this is known as primary hypothyroidism. Less often, it occurs because of a decrease in TSH, due to either pituitary disease or a deficiency of TRH from the hypothalamus. In this situation, the hypothyroidism is central or secondary (or tertiary, when the deficiency is of TRH). Thyroid hormone deficiency may affect any or all body functions. The degree of severity ranges from mild, unrecognized states to life-threatening myxedema. Hypothyroidism dating from birth is known as cretinism. The term myxedema refers to severe hypothyroidism in which there is accumulation of mucopolysaccharides in the skin and other tissues.

The clinical features of hypothyroidism are independent of the cause (10) (Box 18.6). Hypothyroidism affects all ages and both sexes and may be obvious or subclinical. Subclinical hypothyroidism is defined by normal levels of free T_4, T_4, and T_3, in the face of an elevated TSH. Several factors influence the features of hypothyroidism in the individual patient. These include the age of the patient, the presence of other medical problems, and the rate at which the hypothyroidism develops. In infants, hypothyroidism may result in irreversible mental and physical retardation unless treatment is initiated quickly on diagnosis. In children and adults, the effects are usually reversible with treatment.

Autoimmune Thyroiditis

Autoimmune thyroid dysfunction occurs commonly and has been described in up to 4.5% of the population (13). Autoimmune thyroiditis was first described in 1912 by Hashimoto, thus is widely known as Hashimoto's thyroiditis. Patients with this type of thyroiditis have elevated levels of antithyroid antibodies in their serum; the disease process results in thyroid cell damage and often, but not inevitably, hypothyroidism. Goiter formation occurs in most patients due to widespread lymphocytic infiltration of the thyroid, subsequent hypothyroidism, and TSH stimulation of the failing gland.

Patients with Hashimoto's thyroiditis have an increased incidence of other autoimmune diseases, including insulin-dependent diabetes mellitus, autoimmune adrenal disease with adrenal insufficiency, hypoparathyroidism, autoimmune oophoritis, and hypophysitis (14). Nonendocrine autoimmune diseases associated with autoimmune thyroid disease include pernicious anemia, vitiligo, myasthenia gravis,

Box 18.5 Common Causes of Hypothyroidism

Primary Hypothyroidism	Central Hypothyroidism	Transient Hypothyroidism
Autoimmune thyroiditis	Pituitary disease	Silent thyroiditis
Radiation	Hypothalamic disease	Subacute thyroiditis
Surgical removal		Postpartum thyroiditis
Infiltrative diseases		
Iodine deficiency or excess		
Antithyroid drugs		
Inherited enzymatic defects		

Source: Adapted from Braverman LE, Utiger RD. Introduction to hypothyroidism. In: Braverman LE, Utiger RD, eds. Werner and Ingbar's the thyroid: a fundamental and clinical text. 6th ed. Philadelphia: JB Lippincott, 1991:919–920.

Box 18.6 Signs and Symptoms of Hypothyroidism

Symptoms	Signs
Fatigue	Slow movements
Lethargy	Bradycardia
Mental impairment	Dry skin
Depression	Hoarseness
Cold intolerance	Nonpitting edema (myxedema)
Hoarseness	Delayed relaxation phase of reflexes
Dry skin	Diffuse or nodular goiter
Weight gain	Visual field, cranial nerve abnormalities*
Menorrhagia	
Constipation	
Headache, visual disturbance*	

* Central hypothyroidism due to pituitary tumor
Source: Adapted from Braverman LE, Utiger RD. Introduction to hypothroidism. In: Braverman LE, Utiger RD, eds. Werner and Ingbar's the thyroid: a fundamental and clinical text. 6th ed. Philadelphia: JB Lippincott, 1991:919–920.

Sjögren's syndrome, chronic active hepatitis, thrombocytopenic purpura, and alopecia (15).

Most patients with Hashimoto's thyroiditis have an enlarged thyroid gland. The goiter is nontender and rubbery or firm, but not hard. Early in the disease, the only abnormality may be an elevated TSH with normal free T_4 concentration. Thyroid autoantibodies will be present in the serum. Later, especially when a patient has symptoms of hypothyroidism, the free T_4 level will be decreased with an elevated TSH. A thyroid scan usually reveals decreased radionuclide uptake, but it may have an irregular pattern, described as "salt and pepper."

The frequency of lymphoma of the thyroid, a rare disorder, is increased in patients with Hashimoto's thyroiditis.

Treatment involves T_4 replacement, whether hypothyroidism is subclinical or clinical. Treatment is generally lifelong because hypothyroidism recurs if the dose is discontinued. The treatment of the patient with a goiter who is euthyroid is not quite as clear. T_4 replacement may cause regression in the size of the goiter, but this is variable. For most patients, T_4 supplementation should be considered (15) with careful attention to avoidance of a suppressed TSH. Surgical therapy should be considered only in certain situations—enlargement of the goiter despite T_4 supplementation, or thyroid enlargement sufficient to cause local symptoms of dysphagia, stridor, or dyspnea.

Postoperative Hypothyroidism

The frequency of hypothyroidism after subtotal thyroidectomy for Graves' disease is estimated, in the first year, at 10% to 60% (16), with late-onset hypothyroidism developing at a rate of 1% to 3% a year. The risk of hypothyroidism after partial thyroidectomy for toxic or nontoxic multinodular goiter is low.

Hypothyroidism After Radioiodine Therapy

Hypothyroidism after ^{131}I therapy for Graves' disease is common, occurring in as many as 50% of patients in the first year after therapy when a relatively high dose (≥10 mCi, or ≥150 μCi/gm tissue) is given. About 70% of patients are hypothyroid 10 years after therapy. If lower doses are given (40–70 μCi/gm tissue), there is a decreased incidence of hypothyroidism at 1 year (12%), but an increased risk of recurrent hyperthyroidism (33%). Patients who have received ^{131}I therapy should be followed closely with thyroid function tests (free T_4 and TSH), to determine if and when thyroid hormone supplementation is appropriate.

Drug-Induced Hypothyroidism

Primary hypothyroidism is a known side effect of numerous commonly used drugs. Iodide in quantities 50- to 1000-fold greater than the recommmended dietary allowance can cause hypothyroidism or goiter. This may occur in the patient who must take amiodarone or in people who consume large amounts of seaweed. Amiodarone contains a large amount of iodide. It has numerous effects on thyroid hormone production, metabolism, and action and may cause either thyrotoxicosis or hypothyroidism. The hypothyroidism associated with amiodarone use is most likely due to inhibition of thyroid hormone synthesis and secretion. These patients require cautious thyroid hormone replacement, a process best supervised by an endocrinologist or by a physician familiar with amiodarone-induced hypothyroidism.

Lithium may cause subclinical or overt hypothyroidism. In a study of patients treated with lithium for an average of 5 years, 15% developed symptomatic hypothyroidism requiring thyroid hormone supplementation. Lithium blocks thyroid hormone release. These patients should be monitored for changes in thyroid function and symptoms of hypothyroidism.

The anticonvulsant drugs, carbamazepine and phenytoin, enhance hepatic degradation of thyroid hormones and decrease serum free T_4 levels. Curiously, the TSH concentration is not elevated, indicating a second effect at the level of the pituitary. Clinically significant hypothyroidism is rare. However, in the patient with preexisting treated hypothyroidism who must take one of these drugs, the dose of thyroid hormone should be increased by about 50% to maintain the euthyroid state.

Central Hypothyroidism

This condition is caused by a deficiency of TSH or hypothalamic TRH. The etiology is most frequently a pituitary adenoma, which may be either functional or nonfunctional. Varying degrees of hypopituitarism may result from compression of the normal pituitary by the adenoma. Hypopituitarism may also result from hemorrhage within an adenoma. Craniopharyngioma is a frequent cause of central hypothyroidism in the younger age group. Meningiomas and gliomas are rare causes of central hypothyroidism (17).

Postpartum pituitary necrosis (Sheehan's syndrome) is a relatively common cause of adult panhypopituitarism. Pituitary insufficiency does not occur unless most of the anterior pituitary is affected.

The clinical presentation of the patient with central hypothyroidism varies widely, depending on the severity of thyroid failure, other associated hormonal deficiencies, the age of the patient, and the nature of the underlying lesion. The features of hypothyroidism resulting from TSH deficiency are similar to those of primary hypothyroidism, but may be less pronounced. The condition should be suspected in the patient with signs and symptoms of hypothyroidism in association with other hormonal deficiencies and clinical evidence of a pituitary mass lesion. The diagnosis is based on the finding of low or inappropriately normal TSH in the face of low serum thyroid hormone levels. The patient should be evaluated for other hormonal deficiencies as well as have an imaging study performed of the pituitary region.

Treatment is directed toward the underlying disorder, including surgery, if appropriate. Hypofunction of other endocrine glands should be addressed, as well as restoration and maintenance of a euthyroid state in the patient. Patients with central hypothyroidism should have thyroid hormone supplementation just as a patient with primary hypothyroidism, unless there is coexisting corticotropin deficiency. In this case, glucocorticoid replacement should be initiated before or with T_4 therapy. The administration of thyroid hormone may precipitate an adrenal crisis in a patient with occult or subtle adrenal insufficiency. Patients should be followed clinically and free T_4 levels should be used to adjust the dose. The TSH level is not a helpful measurement because it is low or inappropriately normal, by definition.

Thyroid Hormone Replacement

Thyroid hormone replacement is widely prescribed; more than 15 million prescriptions are filled yearly.

Synthetic and natural thyroid hormone preparations are available. The synthetic preparations are levothyroxine (T_4), liothyronine (T_3), and liotrix (T_4/T_3, 4:1 ratio by weight). Natural preparations, prepared from beef and pork thyroid tissue, include desiccated thyroid (Armour, others), which is a mixture of T_4 and T_3 standardized by iodine content, and thyroglobulin (Proloid), which contains T_4 and T_3 in an approximate ratio of 2.5:1. Natural products are available in oral forms only.

Although combination therapy ($T_4 + T_3$) was recommended in the past, knowledge that T_4 is converted in the body to T_3 makes it necessary to provide only T_4 under most circumstances. Synthetic T_4 is available in oral and injectable forms. Liothyronine (T_3) (Cytomel), available in IV and oral forms, should be used only in the preparation of thyroid cancer patients for scanning or specific testing and in the therapy of myxedema coma. Otherwise, the use of T_3 is strongly discouraged.

Levothyroxine is efficiently absorbed from the small intestine (80% of administered dose). It is highly protein bound (>99%), with most binding by TBG, thyroid-binding prealbumin, and albumin. Several medical conditions and medications may alter the absorption/metabolism of thyroid hormone (18) (Box 18.7). These conditions should be considered in each patient receiving thyroid hormone therapy.

The half-life of T_4 is 6 to 7 days, which makes it well suited for single daily dosing. It also indicates that patients be monitored at 28- to 30-day intervals for dose assessment since a new steady state is achieved after four half-lives. We recommend that thyroid status be evaluated 4 weeks after a change in dose.

The goal of routine therapy in patients with hypothyroidism is to normalize the TSH level. Iatrogenic thyrotoxicosis, overt or subclinical (manifested only by a suppressed TSH), should be avoided, because it may be associated with reduced bone mineral density and osteoporosis, and perhaps potential cardiovascular morbidity.

The average dose of T_4 required for normalization of TSH in the hypothyroid adult is 112 μg/day. Most patients require 75–150 μg/day for replacement (1.63 ± 0.42 μg/kg per day) (19). In elderly patients or patients with known or suspected coronary artery disease, we suggest starting at lower doses (25–50 μg/day) with frequent clinical and laboratory assessment. The replacement dose of T_4 in the elderly is about 1.1 μg/kg per day, lower than in young or middle-aged

Box 18.7 Altered Levothyroxine Requirements/Metabolism

Increased Levothyroxine Requirements

Pregnancy
Malabsorption
  Diabetic diarrhea
  Mucosal disease
  Postjejunoileal bypass/small bowel resection

? Estrogen therapy in hypothyroid patients on thyroxine replacement

Altered Metabolism/Bioavailability

Decreased absorption

- Sucralfate
- Ferrous sulfate
- Cholestyramine
- Aluminum hydroxide

Increased metabolism

- Carbamazepine
- Rifampin

Decreased T_4 conversion to T_3

- Propranolol
- Amiodarone

Decreased Requirements

Advancing age

Source: Adapted from Mandel S, Brent G, Larsen PR. Levothyroxine therapy in patients with thyroid disease. Ann Intern Med 1993;119:492–502.

adults. New or worsening angina should prompt cessation of the drug with reinstitution of a previously tolerated dose 1 week later. Appropriate cardiac evaluation should commence immediately. In patients with thyroid cancer a T_4 dose of 2.69 ± 0.48 μg/kg per day is required to suppress TSH to values observed in hyperthyroidism (19). Although the suppression of TSH to undetectable levels has not been fully assessed, the benefits of diminished cancer recurrence are believed to outweigh the risks (18).

Thyroid Nodules and Goiter

Solitary Thyroid Nodule

A solitary thyroid nodule is a common reason for referral of a patient to an endocrinologist. A single palpable nodule in an otherwise normal gland, is four to five times more common in women than men. They are commonly asymptomatic and found on routine examination. However, patients may present with sudden pain and enlargement of the thyroid due to hemorrhage into a previously unnoticed nodule. Rarely, a patient will present with compressive symptoms, hoarseness or dysphagia.

The majority (about 95%) of single thyroid nodules are benign. It is important to determine whether a nodule is benign or malignant to reduce unnecessary neck exploration and thyroidectomy. The widespread use of fine needle aspiration and biopsy has greatly changed the evaluation of thyroid nodules. In published surgical reports, an estimated 42% to 77% of nodules are benign colloid nodules, 15% to 40% are adenomas, and 8% to 17% are cancer (20).

Initial evaluation of the patient with a solitary thyroid nodule should include risk factor assessment (21) (Box 18.8), a history and physical examination, and directed laboratory studies. A family history of thyroid nodules or malignancy, previous head or neck irradiation, age, rapidity of growth, and accompanying symptoms of compression/invasion such as hoarseness or dysphagia are important. Particular attention must be paid to the size, consistency, and mobility of the nodule. Laboratory evaluation should include a TSH and a free T_4. In some patients a T_3RIA may be necessary if the TSH is suppressed and the free T_4 is normal. This evaluation should identify those patients with unsuspected hyperthyroidism. A diagnosis of hyperthyroidism in a patient with a thyroid nodule does not, however, complete the evaluation.

All patients with solitary thyroid nodules should have a fine needle aspiration biopsy. The flow diagram (Fig 18.1) provides a reasonable method of evaluation. Patients may be informed that the biopsy (with a 23- or 25-gauge needle) is an office procedure of 10 to 15 minutes duration. Three to six samples are required to have satisfactory diagnostic material. Local anesthesia with 1% lidocaine may be used but is often unnecessary. The specimen is promptly prepared by the cytologist. Patients tolerate the procedure well with little if any residual ecchymosis or discomfort. Diagnosis is commonly available within 24 hours. At that time definitive recommendations can be made. The procedure has greatly reduced the need for ultrasound and radionuclide scanning of thyroid nodules. In special situations these studies may be helpful, but due to cost considerations and lack of sensitivity and specificity we do not routinely recommend these studies.

Box 18.8 Risk Factors for Thyroid Carcinoma

Age
- <20 or >60 yr

Male sex
Radiation
- Low-dose head or neck
  - Tonsils
  - Tinea capitis
  - Acne
  - Hemangioma
- Mantle—e.g., Hodgkin's lymphoma
- Atomic bomb survivors

Family history of thyroid cancer—e.g., multiple endocrine neoplasia, type II
Iodine deficiency
Cold nodule
Hard consistency
Fixation
Adjacent lymphadenopathy
Hoarseness
Dysphagia
Rapid growth
History of Graves' disease

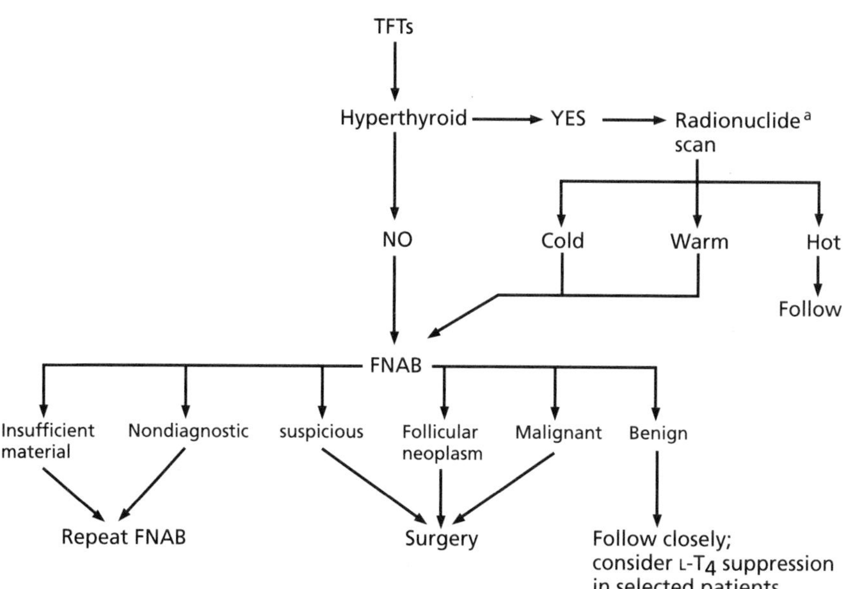

Fig 18.1 Evaluation of the thyroid module. Endocrine consultation for all patients with thyroid nodules is recommended. [a] Scanning is contraindicated in pregnancy. FNAB, fine needle aspiration biopsy

Fine needle aspiration biopsy can also be used for evaluation of a solitary thyroid nodule during pregnancy (22). Radioisotope evaluation and therapy are contraindicated during pregnancy. Thyroid cancer is probably not adversely affected by pregnancy (23).

Approximately 10,000 to 12,000 cases of thyroid cancer are diagnosed each year. The definitive therapy for thyroid cancer is surgery. A surgeon who is experienced in thyroid surgery is most important because the complications of hypoparathyroidism and vocal cord paralysis are substantially reduced in experienced hands.

Papillary variants and follicular cancer benefit from adjunctive postoperative radioactive iodine. Therapy for anaplastic carcinoma is disappointing, with 5-year survival rates less than 4% (24). Medullary carcinoma of the thyroid (MCT) is clearly a surgical disease. Neither radiation, to control local metastatic MCT, nor chemotherapy, to treat advanced disease, is effective. Five-year survival rates for MCT patients approach 78% to 82%, substantially lower than rates for papillary or follicular lesions. When MCT recurs, the best approach is re-exploration with meticulous dissection and removal of local disease.

Thyroid lymphoma and rare metastatic disease to the thyroid are treated with regimens that are most appropriate for the specific tumor type.

All patients with differentiated thyroid cancer benefit from suppressive doses of L-T_4. For patients with no known residual disease, and no residual thyroid tissue, due to near total thyroidectomy and adjunctive RAI ablation, maintenance of the TSH level at about 0.3 mIU/L is suggested. For patients with metastatic or incompletely resected cancer or those who have refused RAI ablation, suppression of TSH levels to undetectable levels is advised (25). In either case, appropriate care includes periodic total body scanning and thyroglobulin measurements. These studies should be performed 6 weeks after withdrawal of thyroid hormone.

Benign thyroid nodules should be followed carefully. Growth of a nodule, hoarseness, compressive symptoms, fixation, or any combination should prompt immediate repeat evaluation and referral. Controversy exists over the use of L-T_4 for the suppression of benign solid thyroid nodules. Therapy is directed to prevent further growth of the nodule or to induce regression. The data on the efficacy of this approach are conflicting (25). It may be acceptable in certain patients (<60 years) to administer L-T_4 in a dose sufficient to reduce the TSH to 0.05 to 0.1 mIU/L (about 100–150 μg/day). In some patients (>60 years), doses sufficient to reduce TSH to 0.1 to 0.3 mIU/L are suggested (18). Therapy should be continued for 1 year with clinical evaluation every 3 months. If the nodule increases in size, fine needle aspiration biopsy should be performed. If it remains stable or decreases in size, therapy is continued.

Three-dimensional ultrasound sizing of the nodule before and at the conclusion of the trial should dictate the continuance of L-T_4 therapy. We do not recommend continued L-T_4 therapy in patients without an objective response.

Levothyroxine is beneficial in the postsurgical patient with radiation-induced benign thyroid nodules, where recurrence occurs in 36% of untreated versus 8.4% of treated patients (25). The incidence of recurrent malignant disease in these patients is not altered by L-T_4 therapy.

Multinodular Goiter

Multinodular goiter is diagnosed by careful palpation of the thyroid gland, by ultrasound, or by radionuclide scanning. In the past a multinodular gland was thought to indicate a benign process, but recent data indicate that the risk of malignancy in a dominant nodule in such a gland is similar to that in a solitary nodule. Fine needle aspiration biopsy is indicated for all dominant nodules in multinodular goiter (26). If malignant disease is found, surgery is recommended. If the cytology is benign, expectant observation with attempts at nodule suppression are suggested. Functional activity of the multinodular goiter should be assessed before biopsy. The growth pattern of any of the nodules and their chances of becoming autonomous depend on size. Nodules larger than 3 cm in size have the greatest chance of achieving autonomy, producing hyperthyroidism in about 20% of patients (25). Thyroid hormone use in patients with multinodular goiter may produce hyperthyroidism because hormone production by the gland is fixed and autonomous.

Sporadic Goiter

Simple goiter is less common in North America than in other parts of the world due to abundant dietary sources of iodine. Because TSH is a growth factor for sporadic goiter, its suppression may cause regression of goiter in 50% of euthyroid patients (27).

We recommend a trial of T_4 in patients who are able to tolerate therapy, but exclude all patients with baseline low TSH levels of 1.0 mIU/L or less. Assessment of thyroid function with thyroid function tests, and thyroid ultrasound with three-dimensional measurements are performed before therapy. Patients are re-evaluated at 3-month intervals. If therapy has been successful it is continued for 1 year with subsequent evaluation at that time. Goals of therapy include reduction of the goiter without producing hyperthyroidism. Ideally TSH levels should be maintained in the low normal range, 0.5 to 1.0 mIU/mL. If successful, therapy should be continued indefinitely with yearly thyroid function tests and examination.

Some elderly patients, particularly those with coronary artery disease, will be unsuitable candidates for L-T_4 suppression. These patients are best followed expectantly. Thyroid function tests should be performed to exclude subclinical hyperthyroidism or hypothyroidism. Surgical removal of the gland may be necessary for selected patients.

Thyroiditis

Autoimmune thyroiditis (Hashimoto's thyroiditis) has been discussed previously in the section on hypothyroidism. This section will concentrate on the other major forms of thyroiditis, including subacute, silent, and postpartum thyroiditis.

Subacute Thyroiditis

Subacute thyroiditis is also known as granulomatous, giant cell, or de Quervain's thyroiditis. The female-male ratio is about 3 to 6:1; it occurs most commonly between the second and fifth decades and is recognized most often during the summer months (28). It often follows an upper respiratory infection. The histologic findings are pathognomonic in this disorder and are characterized by granulomatous giant cell inflammation. The clinical presentation is that of pain in the region of the thyroid, which may radiate to the ear or jaw. Patients often complain of systemic symptoms, including malaise, myalgias, feverishness, and anorexia. The gland is often enlarged and exquisitely tender to palpation, with one lobe more severely affected than the other. The overlying skin may be warm and erythematous. Occasionally, the focus of involvement migrates from one part of the gland to another. Approximately half the patients affected by subacute thyroiditis will have thyrotoxicosis, which generally resolves in 4 to 10 weeks (28). As the acute phase of the disease progresses, thyroid hormone stores are depleted, and the patient returns to a euthyroid state. In more severe cases, transient hypothyroidism occurs and usually lasts 1 to 2 months. As the gland recovers, thyroid follicles are regenerated, and normal thyroid function is restored. The disease usually resolves in a few months, but may remit and recur, with hypothyroidism the end result. Permanent hypothyroidism is rare.

Laboratory findings early in the course of disease include elevated serum free T_4 and T_3 levels, with a decrease in the TSH. As hormone stores are depleted, T_4 and T_3 levels decrease to normal. In the subset of patients who progress to transient hypothyroidism, the hormone levels fall to subnormal before returning again to normal. Because of damage to the follicular cells, the thyroid ^{131}I uptake is reduced and radioisotope scans (either iodine or technetium) reveal little or no uptake in the gland or in the affected area.

Diagnosis is based on history and the physical examination, with confirmatory laboratory tests including an increased erythrocyte sedimentation rate, elevated free T_4 and T_3RIA levels, and decreased thyroid ^{131}I uptake. Fine needle aspiration provides the correct diagnosis in at least 90% of patients but is seldom required (28).

Salicylates and other NSAIDs have been used successfully to reduce inflammation and to relieve pain and tenderness. If the patient is thyrotoxic, β-adrenergic blockade may be used to control symptoms. Antithyroid drugs have no role in this disease. Glucocorticoids should be avoided unless absolutely necessary. In contrast to salicylates and NSAIDs, a recurrence of signs and symptoms often accompanies tapering and discontinuation of steroids.

Silent Thyroiditis

Silent thyroiditis is the term used to describe lymphocytic thyroiditis with transient thyrotoxicosis. Postpartum thyroiditis is often described as silent thyroiditis, but because of the wide spectrum of clinical presentation of the postpartum patient, this entity is described separately.

Silent or painless thyroiditis has been identified with increasing frequency. It was initially described as a painless form of subacute thyroiditis, but biopsy has shown it to be a separate disease, with lymphocytic infiltration of the thyroid gland that is similar to but less extensive than that found in chronic autoimmune thyroiditis or follicle disruption.

This disorder accounts for 2% or 3% of all cases of thyrotoxicosis (28). The male-female ratio is approximately 2:1, a clearly different gender ratio than that reported for most other types of thyroid disease. Most patients are between 20 and 50 years of age. No specific initiating event in this illness has been identified.

The onset and severity of silent thyroiditis is variable. Thyrotoxicosis is usually mild, with the usual symptoms and signs of thyrotoxicosis. Exophthalmos and dermopathy do not occur. The thyroid gland is enlarged in only about half the patients, is usually symmetric, and when enlarged is rarely greater than two to three times normal size. Thyroid pain and tenderness are rare. Most patients present in the thyrotoxic phase of this illness, which generally lasts for about 3 months. They then enter a hypothyroid phase, which may last approximately 3 months, but may persist indefinitely. Finally, patients recover and euthyroidism is restored.

Laboratory findings vary, depending on the phase of the disease present at the time of diagnosis. Initially, when the thyroid gland is inflamed and the follicles are damaged, there is leakage of thyroid hormones into the bloodstream, resulting in elevated T_4 and T_3 levels and a decreased TSH. If a ^{131}I uptake is done, it will be decreased because of the suppressed TSH and the inability of the damaged gland to take up iodine. As the thyrotoxic phase resolves, serum T_4 and T_3 levels decrease into the normal range, and then further, as the hypothyroid phase is entered.

Patients with silent thyroiditis are generally treated supportively. Thyrotoxicosis, if symptoms warrant, may be treated with a β blocker. Antithyroid medications are not useful because increased thyroid hormone synthesis is not the cause of the thyrotoxicosis. When patients enter the hypothyroid phase, they benefit from thyroid hormone supplementation, which may then be slowly withdrawn. If the hypothyroidism lasts for greater than 6 months, it is probably permanent, and there is no need for further attempts at withdrawal. Patients should be counseled about the transient nature of their illness, and that they will likely recover in 8 to 12 weeks. About 10% will have recurrent episodes. Permanent hypothyroidism occurs in less than 5% of patients (28).

Postpartum Thyroiditis

Postpartum thyroid dysfunction is an autoimmune disease occurring in as many as 5% to 10% of postpartum women during the first year after delivery. It is a form of chronic autoimmune thyroiditis, and lymphocytic infiltration of the gland has been observed. The presence of antimicrosomal antibodies before or during pregnancy increases the risk of developing this disorder. It may manifest itself as transient hypothyroidism, transient thyrotoxicosis, or thyrotoxicosis followed by hypothyroidism (29). It typically consists of a transient thyrotoxic phase occurring at 1 to 3 months postpartum, followed at 3 to 6 months by a hypothyroid phase. The severity of the thyroid dysfunction varies. Symptoms are often mild, with fatigue as the most common complaint; however, patients often have typical findings of hyper- or hypothyroidism, depending on the stage of their illness at diagnosis. Physical examination reveals a nontender goiter. If the TSH and free T_4 measurements are consistent with thyrotoxicosis, and the patient is not nursing, a ^{131}I uptake is done. If uptake is low, the diagnosis of thyroiditis is confirmed. A low free T_4 with an elevated TSH confirms that the patient is in the hypothyroid phase of the disease. If thyroid autoantibodies are measured, they are often positive.

Thyrotoxic patients may benefit from therapy with a β-blocking medication. Patients with hypothyroidism should be treated with thyroid hormone supplementation. Close follow-up of these patients is necessary because their thyroid status may change, requiring adjustments in therapy. Approximately 20% of patients will develop permanent hypothyroidism (30). Patients with postpartum thyroiditis, who recover normal thyroid function, are at risk for the disorder with subsequent pregnancies.

Thyroid Economy and Therapy in Pregnancy

Thyroid Economy

Pregnancy has a profound effect on thyroid homeostasis. Increased levels of thyroid binding proteins, increased urinary loss of iodide, and circulating thyroid stimulators such as β-human chorionic gonadotropin (βHCG) contribute to altered thyroid economy.

Estrogen increases the sialylation of TBG and prolongs its half-life in the serum (31,32). TBG levels increase 2.5-fold during pregnancy, reaching their peak about the 21st week of pregnancy (23). These changes increase the protein-bound levels of circulating thyroid hormones.

During the first trimester, free T_4 and free T_3 levels increase, returning to normal by the 20th week of gestation. The peak levels coincide with peak βHCG production, thus implicating βHCG as being a weak thyroid stimulator. During this interval βHCG and TSH levels are inversely related. Elevated βHCG levels with elevated free T_4 and free T_3 levels are also seen in hyperemesis gravidarum.

The second and third trimesters of pregnancy are marked by a progressive but very mild decrease in free T_4 and free T_3 levels from those seen in early pregnancy. Most patients maintain elevated TSH levels within the normal range, whereas some have reported elevated TSH levels, thus suggesting a decline in thyroid hormone production (23).

Goiter

Goiter in pregnant women is multifactorial with early stimulation by βHCG and potentiation by relative iodide deficiency. Iodine intake in iodine-sufficient areas, such as North America, precludes the development of goiter during pregnancy. Consequently, an enlarging thyroid gland in a pregnant woman in the United States requires immediate thyroid evaluation. TSH, free T_4, and thyroid antibody studies should be performed. At the first prenatal visit, patients with signs or symptoms of thyroid dysfunction and those with a previous history of hyper- or hypothyroidism should have thyroid function studies. Pituitary disease is a rare cause of hypothyroidism in pregnancy because pituitary pathology most commonly affects gonadotropins before TSH, thus precluding pregnancy.

Hypothyroidism

Hypothyroidism increases fetal wastage, with a twofold increase in miscarriage. Euthyroid women with increased antithyroid antibody levels are, curiously, at increased risk of miscarriage. Women who are able to maintain their pregnancies are predisposed to abruptio placentae and pre-eclampsia (23). Maternal hypothyroidism has an adverse effect on the development of the fetus; mental retardation and motor abnormalities occur with increased frequency in the offspring of severely hypothyroid women (23).

Hormone replacement with T_4 should begin immediately in a patient with hypothyroidism. Initial therapy should begin at the anticipated full daily dosage of L-T_4 (1.63 μg/kg per day). Thyroid function studies should be repeated at 4-week intervals and the adequacy of the dose monitored with TSH measurements.

The mean dose increment required during pregnancy in previously hypothyroid women on replacement is approximately 50%, the majority of which occurs during the first trimester. The increase is independent of the cause of hypothyroidism and persists throughout pregnancy. After delivery the dosage should be reduced to that before pregnancy (32).

Thyrotoxicosis

Thyrotoxicosis, excluding that caused by molar pregnancy or choriocarcinoma, occurs in 0.2% of all pregnancies (23). The causes of hyperthyroidism in pregnancy are similar to those in an age-matched population, with Graves' disease being the most common (see Box 18.3).

Many of the normal features of pregnancy can be clinically indistinguishable from hyperthyroidism. The mild tachycardia, peripheral vasodilatation, heat intolerance, hyperphagia, and increased cardiac output often seen in thyrotoxicosis are part of a normal pregnancy. The severity of symptoms, presence of goiter, eye findings suggestive of Graves' disease, or history of previous remitted hyperthyroidism should prompt evaluation.

The diagnosis of hyperthyroidism is made on the basis of the clinical symptoms and confirmed by a suppressed TSH and elevated free T_4 levels. Laboratory methods should be used that will not be influenced by TBG. If surreptitious ingestion of exogenous thyroid hormone is suspected, a thyroglobulin level (reflecting endogenous production of thyroid hormone) will be helpful. Any scanning or uptake procedures using radionuclides are contraindicated.

Therapy of the hyperthyroidism of Graves' disease in pregnant women must be modified. The intensity of Graves' disease changes during the pregnancy, being most active in the first trimester and gradually lessening in the second and third trimesters due to increased levels of TBG and suppression of the immunologic disease process that causes Graves' disease (23). The goal of antithyroid therapy in pregnancy is to make the mother euthyroid with the lowest possible dose of PTU, thereby preserving fetal thyroid function.

The placenta allows transfer of both antithyroid drugs available in the United States (methimazole and PTU). Fetal availability of methimazole in human beings is approximately four times greater than PTU (23). PTU causes less neonatal goiter and hypothyroidism by virtue of its decreased placental transfer and is the preferred antithyroid drug. Methimazole may be associated with aplasia cutis in the fetus (33,34) although this is largely unsubstantiated.

Propylthiouracil, in doses of 100–150 mg every 8 hours, should be initiated when the diagnosis is made. Higher doses may be required in some patients. The goal of therapy is to maintain the free T_4 level in the high-normal or slightly elevated range. A response to the therapy, indicated by decreasing free T_4 levels, should occur in 1 to 2 weeks (23). As pregnancy progresses, medication requirements decrease. Pregnant women should not be allowed to become hypothyroid. Antithyroid regimens that combine high doses of antithyroid drugs with thyroid hormone supplementation are undesirable during pregnancy because the antithyroid drug crosses the placenta more readily than T_4, leading to neonatal goiter.

The β blocker, propranolol, commonly used in the therapy of the autonomic hyperactivity of thyrotoxicosis, may cause fetal growth retardation, delayed spontaneous respiration, neonatal hypoglycemia, and bradycardia in some newborns. The studies to date have been conflicting. At any rate, minimizing drug exposure for the fetus seems the most prudent course. Consequently we recommend use of β blockers in pregnancy only under emergent conditions where maternal or fetal health may be acutely threatened (23,35). Iodide has no role in the management of hyperthyroidism during pregnancy except for thyroid storm. Surgical therapy for thyrotoxicosis in pregnancy may be necessary at times due to intolerable side effects of antithyroid drugs. It can be safely performed during the second trimester but is not routinely recommended.

Although it has been traditional to advise against breast-feeding for mothers taking PTU, its concentration in breast milk is too low to influence newborn thyroid function. The lowest possible dose of drug should be used to guarantee a euthyroid infant, and infant thyroid function should be monitored.

Neonatal complications of maternal therapy of thyrotoxicosis include both hypothyroidism and hyperthyroidism. Nonetheless, about 1% of infants exposed to antithyroid drugs in utero develop significant transient neonatal hypothyroidism (35). Neonatal hyperthyroidism may occur secondary to placental transfer of the TSI responsible for thyroid stimulation in Graves' disease. Consequently, the concentration of TSI should be assessed in patients with Graves' disease as well as in patients with previously treated Graves' disease, particularly those who were cured with surgery or RAI and who are on replacement doses of L-T_4.

Compulsive care of the pregnant woman with thyroid dysfunction and anticipation of potential complications is essential. A multidisciplinary effort involving the obstetrician, neonatologist, and endocrinologist is recommended.

Thyroid Emergencies

Thyroid storm and myxedema coma are uncommon thyroid emergencies with high mortality rates ($\geqslant$20%).

Thyroid Storm

Thyroid storm may occur in any patient with thyrotoxicosis, but it is usually due to worsening of Graves' disease. It is characterized by fever (out of proportion to other findings), delirium, and cardiovascular instability in a patient with thyrotoxicosis. The cardiac abnormalities include atrial arrhythmias and congestive heart failure.

The diagnosis of thyroid storm is strictly clinical. It has been associated with or precipitated by many conditions: surgery, acute medical illness, infection, iodine administration (radiocontrast dyes, iodine-containing foods/medications), trauma, uncontrolled diabetes mellitus, child delivery, and general anesthesia (36).

The mechanism of storm is not well defined and thyroid laboratory indices are not helpful. Increased sensitivity of peripheral tissues to circulating catecholamines is a well recognized phenomenon in patients with thyrotoxicosis. This is due to increased numbers of tissue catecholamine receptors. The combination of increased catecholamines and high levels of thyroid hormones sets the stage for this disorder. However, absolute levels of T_4 and T_3 do not differ in patients with storm from those with severe hyperthyroidism. It is very likely that stress or illness decreases the binding of T_4 and T_3 to TBG increasing the free hormone levels without substantially changing total levels.

The patient suspected of having thyroid storm should be thoroughly evaluated to identify precipitating factors. The history should specifically address a previous history of thyroid disease, thyroid surgery, medication/health food usage, a family history of endocrine disease, and recent symptomatology. The possibility of pregnancy should be considered. Manifestations of thyroid storm are variable and include agitation or restlessness progressing to coma, nausea, emesis, diarrhea/hyperdefecation, and liver dysfunction. Virtually any organ system can be affected by the severe hypermetabolism associated with thyroid storm.

The physical examination in thyroid storm is dominated by fever. The vasodilated skin is moist unless the patient is hypotensive. Peripheral manifestations of autonomic hyperactivity such as tremor and lid lag are seen. Tachycardia with a wide pulse pressure and cardiac arrhythmias may be present. The size, texture, and symmetry of the thyroid, as well as the presence of a bruit, are helpful in establishing the diagnosis. Baseline chemistries including a hemogram, liver function tests, coagulation parameters, and cardiac enzymes should be obtained. An ultrasensitive TSH, T_3RIA, and free T_4 should be ordered, but these results will be delayed and cannot be used for decision-making. Cultures of blood, urine, and cerebrospinal fluid (CSF) should be obtained when indicated.

There are two basic principles in the management of thyroid storm. Supportive care should be initiated immediately and continued throughout the illness. This may include but not be limited to mechanical ventilation, cardiac monitoring, pulmonary artery catheterization, arterial pressure monitoring, nutritional support, anticoagulation when appropriate, as well as other indicated procedures. Cardiac problems should be managed as in the nonthyrotoxic patient. Anticoagulation for atrial fibrillation is indicated because systemic embolization occurs in 10% to 40% of these patients, particularly those with atrial dilatation (37).

The therapy of thyroid storm involves prevention of synthesis of thyroid hormone by the gland, prevention of release of previously formed or stored thyroid hormone, and reduction of peripheral T_4 to T_3 conversion. Antithyroid drug therapy is the only way of preventing further synthesis of thyroid hormone. However, release of previously synthesized hormone will not be influenced with this therapy. Release can be blocked by administration of an antithyroid drug followed by high doses of sodium iodide. Traditionally PTU has been the preferred drug for use during thyroid storm because it also blocks T_4 to T_3 conversion. Whether this is clinically important remains unclear. Decreased T_4 to T_3 conversion is theoretically advantageous because T_3 is the biologically active form of thyroid hormone. PTU may be administered PO or per rectum by retention enema. A dose of 1000–1400 mg/day in divided doses every 4 to 6 hours is recommended. Therapy with PTU should precede the administration of iodine to prevent further hormone synthesis.

Blocking the release of previously formed and stored thyroid hormone is a critical element in management. Lugol's solution, sodium iodide, or radiocontrast dyes (Oragrafin and Telepaque) may be used. Their use in the management of thyroid storm in the pregnant woman should be restricted to minimize effects on the fetal thyroid (35). Several alternatives exist: Lugol's solution given as 20 drops PO every 8 hours, saturated solution of KI 8 drops PO every 6 hours, or Oragrafin or Telepaque as 1 gm PO daily may be used. Alternatively NaI may be administered at a rate of 1–2 gm/24 hours by IV infusion.

β-Blocking drugs, such as propranolol, are clearly beneficial. An additional benefit may be a reduction in T_4 to T_3 conversion. The dose required to maintain the heart rate between 80 and 90 beats/min varies greatly between patients. IV doses of 1–2 mg every 5 to 10 minutes may be used if necessary. The usual oral dose is 40–120 mg PO every 6 hours. We recommend initial IV administration with close monitoring and dosage alteration based on patient response. Calcium channel blockers such as verapamil and diltiazem have been used with success. They and other β blockers such as metoprolol and labetalol may be used but do not have the advantage of blocking T_4 to T_3 conversion. Although propranolol carries some risk to the fetus, we believe that the short-term benefits outweigh the risks in the pregnant woman with thyroid storm.

Adjunctive therapy includes the administration of glucocorticoids for the relative "adrenal insufficiency" that has been postulated to occur in thyroid storm. Additionally, steroids also block the conversion of T_4 to T_3 and act in a synergistic manner when given with PTU. Dexamethasone 2 mg IV every 6 hours or hydrocortisone 100 mg IV every 8 hours is recommended initially, with rapid tapering thereafter.

Nonaspirin-containing products are recommended for the management of fever. Aspirin is avoided because it displaces T_4 and T_3 from their binding protein, TBG, when used in large doses thus elevating the free fraction of these hormones.

In patients refractory to conventional management, peritoneal dialysis or plasmapheresis is a rapid means by which thyroid hormone levels can be reduced. Bile acid-binding resins will also block the enteroenteric reabsorption of T_4. Although lithium and amiodarone may be helpful in selected patients, their routine use is not suggested.

Following recovery from thyroid storm, conventional therapy for thyrotoxicosis should be continued. Definitive therapy, after delivery, should be considered for patients with a history of thyroid storm.

Myxedema Coma

Myxedema coma represents the other end of the spectrum of decompensated thyroid disease. It is a result of long-standing, severe, untreated hypothyroidism. This condition most commonly affects elderly patients, particularly women in the winter months. Classically, features of severe hypothyroidism are present. The diagnosis is usually obvious with the proviso that "to make the diagnosis you have to think of it." Despite vigorous early therapy, mortality rates may be as high as 60% (38).

Although most patients with myxedema coma have a history of previous hypothyroidism, radioactive iodine therapy, or surgery, a rare patient may present with newly diagnosed primary hypothyroidism (38). Some patients with myxedema coma (<10%) will have pituitary or hypothalamic disease as a cause of their hypothyroidism. Precipitating factors are listed in Box 18.9.

The clinical presentation of the patient in myxedema coma is dominated by hypothermia, found in 75% of patients (may be severe, <80°F, 26.6°C), and an altered sensorium progressing to coma. Other neuropsychiatric manifestations include amnesia,

Box 18.9 Myxedema Coma Precipitating Factors

Drugs

- Anesthetics
- Sedatives
- Narcotics
- Tranquilizers
- Lithium
- Amiodarone

Infection
Cerebrovascular accident
Congestive heart failure
Trauma
Gastrointestinal bleeding
Hypothermia
Noncompliance with L-T_4 therapy

Source: Adapted from Wartofsky L. Myxedema coma. In: Braverman LE, Utiger RD, eds. Werner and Ingbar's the thyroid: a fundamental and clinical text. 6th ed. Philadelphia: JB Lippincott, 1991:1084–1091.

cerebellar signs, depression, hallucinations, and disorientation. Paranoia, otherwise known as "myxedema madness" may be seen. Generalized edema is present and may be severe. Facial characteristics include sparse coarse hair, lateral eyebrow loss, periorbital edema, and macroglossia.

Respiratory drive is depressed leading to hypercapnia and respiratory acidosis; when severe, it may cause coma (38). Pleural effusions and myxedematous infiltration of the upper airways may complicate the presentation. The cardiac manifestations are bradycardia, reduced stroke volume, and reduced cardiac output. Severe congestive heart failure may be seen, but is rarely due to hypothyroidism alone. An enlarged cardiac silhouette is common, due generally to pericardial effusion. The effusion typically accumulates slowly over time and is rarely hemodynamically significant. Any effusion, however, should be evaluated by echocardiogram with further study as indicated. Gut motility is severely affected. Paralytic ileus and gastric atony may require surgical intervention (38).

Total body water is increased in myxedema. Extracellular volume is augmented while intravascular volume is reduced, predisposing to hypotension. Decreased glomerular filtration rate results in deficient water excretion, causing hyponatremia (38). This hyponatremia may contribute to the central nervous system (CNS) alterations seen in myxedema coma.

Laboratory evaluation of the patient should include routine chemistries, hematologic studies, arterial blood gas determination, and cultures and CSF analysis, if indicated. TSH, free T_4, and T_3RIA levels should be obtained. A Cortrosyn stimulation test should be performed to rule out the presence of concomitant primary adrenal insufficiency (Schmidt's syndrome) or secondary adrenal insufficiency. The TSH level should be elevated if due to primary hypothyroidism but will be low or normal in secondary hypothyroidism. Free T_4 and T_3RIA levels should be low. Rarely, critically ill patients may not have an elevated TSH of the expected magnitude because life-threatening illness and certain medications (dopamine, corticosteroids, dilantin) inhibit its release. Other laboratory abnormalities in myxedema coma include hypercholesterolemia, anemia, hypercapnia, hyponatremia, and increased lactic dehydrogenase and creatine kinase levels. Lumbar puncture reveals increased opening pressure with an increased CSF protein (38). The electrocardiogram may show evidence of pericardial effusion with low voltage, and ST-T wave changes.

Therapy

Therapy should begin when the diagnosis is suspected clinically. Intensive care including ventilatory support may be required for the first 48 to 72 hours. Hypothermia should resolve as thyroid hormone levels are replenished. Blankets or increased room temperature may be helpful. External warming should be undertaken cautiously because it may result in vasodilatation with subsequent hypotension and vascular collapse. Pulmonary artery pressure monitoring should be considered for these patients.

For patients with mild hyponatremia ($sNa^+ >$ 125 mEq/L and no hypotension), mild fluid restriction and thyroid hormone supplementation may be all that is required for correction. In the severely hyponatremic or the hypotensive patient, therapy with normal saline (NS) or D_5NS is indicated. Therapy should be monitored closely with hemodynamic parameters and electrolyte determinations. Vasopressors should be used, if indicated.

The possibility of concomitant adrenal insufficiency (Schmidt's syndrome—first-degree adrenal insufficiency and first-degree hypothyroidism) should always be considered. Patients should be given glucocorticoids until the results of the Cortrosyn stimulation test are available. We prefer dexamethasone initially (2 mg IV) because it does not interfere with cortisol measurements during the Cortrosyn stimulation test. After testing, hydrocortisone is administered by continuous infusion at a dose of 200–300 mg over 24 hours. Glucocorticoids may be discontinued after adrenal insufficiency has been ruled out.

The empiric use of antibiotic therapy has been recommended in these patients because they often do not have fever with infection. Because infection is a common precipitating factor for myxedema coma in elderly patients, empiric antibiotics after indicated culture material has been obtained are appropriate. Review of culture data and clinical correlation should dictate further therapy.

Myxedematous patients metabolize all medications slowly, which predisposes to excessive CNS depression with sedative-hypnotics and analgesic agents. Care must be taken to avoid drug toxicities.

The most controversial aspect of management concerns the dosage and preparations of thyroid hormone to be used. Because of the infrequency of this disorder, randomized trials are not possible; consequently, optimal therapy remains undefined. The extrathyroidal pool of thyroid hormone is estimated to be 300 to 600 μg in the 70-kg individual. The circulating thyroid pool is replenished with a single IV dose of 300–500 μg L-T_4 with subsequent daily doses of 0.075–0.100 mg. Because the conversion of T_4 to T_3 is decreased in critically ill patients and because T_3 is the active form of thyroid hormone, it has been suggested that T_3 also be rapidly restored to normal. An IV preparation of T_3 has become available for treatment of these patients. The recommended dose is 10 μg every 12 hours, to be used in addition to L-T_4 in the acute therapy of myxedema coma. The IV route of administration of thyroid hormone is preferred in all myxedema coma patients. When the patient is improved, L-T_4 should be given orally at a dose of 1.6 μg/kg per day. In the elderly patient/cardiac patient, the administration of T_3 should be avoided and the maintenance L-T_4 dose should also be reduced.

Although most thyroid disorders are easily managed by the primary physician with endocrine consultation, endocrine emergencies are best managed by a multidisciplinary team. Endocrine consultation is required for patients suspected of having endocrine emergencies.

REFERENCES

1. Ingbar S. Diseases of the thyroid. In: Braunwald E, Isselbacher KJ, Petersdorf RG, et al. eds. Harrison's principles of internal medicine. 11th ed. New York: McGraw-Hill, 1987:1732–1752.
2. Fitzgerald PA. Endocrine disorders. In: Tierney LM Jr, McPhee SJ, Papadakis MA, eds. Current medical diagnosis and treatment. 33rd ed. East Norwalk, CT: Appleton & Lange 1994:912–976.
3. Andreoli TE, Carpenter CCJ, Plum F, Smith LH Jr, eds. Cecil essentials of medicine. Philadelphia: WB Saunders, 1986:452–456.
4. Geffner DL, Hershman JM. β-adrenergic blockade for the treatment of hyperthyroidism. Am J Med 1992;93:61–68.
5. Bouma DJ, Kammer H. Single daily dose methimazole treatment of hyperthyroidism. West J Med 1980;132:13–15.
6. Roti E, Gardini E, Minelli R, et al. Methimazole and serum thyroid hormone concentrations in hyperthyroid patients: effects of single and multiple daily doses. Ann Intern Med 1989;111:181–182.
7. Cooper DS. Which anti-thyroid drug? Am J Med 1986;80:1165–1168.
8. Hashizume K, Ichikawa K, Sakurai A, et al. Administration of thyroxine in treated Graves' disease. Effects on the level of antibodies to thyroid-stimulating hormone receptors and on the risk of recurrence of hyperthyroidism. New Engl J Med 1991;324:947–953.
9. Belfiore A, Sava L, Runello F, et al. Solitary autonomously functioning thyroid nodules and iodine deficiency. J Clin Endocrinol Metab 1983;56:283–287.
10. Braverman LE, Utiger RD. Introduction to hypothyroidism. In: Braverman LE, Utiger RD, eds. Werner and Ingbar's the thyroid: a fundamental and clinical text. 6th ed. Philadelphia: JB Lippincott, 1991:919–920.
11. Hamburger JI. Should all autonomously functioning thyroid nodules be ablated to prevent the subsequent development of thyrotoxicosis? In: Hamburger JI,

Miller JM, eds. Controversies in clinical thyroidology. New York: Springer-Verlag, 1981:69–104.

12. Burman KD, Earll JM, Johnson MC, Wartofsky L. Clinical observations on the solitary autonomous thyroid nodule. Arch Intern Med 1974;134:915–919.

13. Hawkins BR, Cheah PS, Dawkins RL, et al. Diagnostic significance of thyroid microsomal antibodies in randomly selected population. Lancet 1980;2:1057–1059.

14. Volpe R. Immunology of human thyroid disease. In: Volpe R, ed. Autoimmune diseases of the endocrine system. Boca Raton; FL: CRC Press, 1990:73–239.

15. Volpe R. Autoimmune thyroiditis. In: Braverman LE, Utiger RD, eds. Werner and Ingbar's the thyroid: a fundamental and clinical text. 6th ed. Philadelphia: JB Lippincott, 1991:921–933.

16. Toft AD, Irvine WJ, Sinclair I, et al. Thyroid function after surgical treatment of thyrotoxicosis. A report of 100 cases treated with propranolol before operation. New Engl J Med 1978;298:643–647.

17. Pinchera A, Martino E, Faglia G. Central hypothyroidism. In: Braverman LE, Utiger RD, eds. Werner and Ingbar's the thyroid: a fundamental and clinical text. 6th ed. Philadelphia: JB Lippincott, 1991:968–984.

18. Mandel S, Brent G, Larsen PR. Levothyroxine therapy in patients with thyroid disease. Ann Intern Med 1993;119:492–502.

19. Fish LH, Schwartz HL, Cavanaugh J, et al. Replacement dose, metabolism and bioavailability of levothyroxine in the treatment of hypothyroidism. New Engl J Med 1991;316:764–770.

20. Mazzaferri EL. Management of a solitary thyroid nodule. N Engl J Med 1993;328:553–559.

21. Ridgway EC. Clinical evaluation of solitary thyroid nodules. In: Braverman LE, Utiger RD, eds. Werner and Ingbar's the thyroid: a fundamental and clinical text. 6th ed. Philadelphia: JB Lippincott, 1991:1197–1203.

22. Hamburger JI, Kaplan MM, Husain M. Diagnosis of thyroid nodules by needle biopsy. In: Braverman LE, Utiger RD, eds. Werner and Ingbar's the thyroid: a fundamental and clinical text. 6th ed. Philadelphia: JB Lippincott, 1991:544–549.

23. Emerson CH. Thyroid disease during and after pregnancy. In: Braverman LE, Utiger RD, eds. Werner and Ingbar's the thyroid: a fundamental and clinical text. 6th ed. Philadelphia: JB Lippincott, 1991:1263–1279.

24. Robbins J, Merino MJ, Boice JD, et al. Thyroid cancer: a lethal endocrine neoplasm. Ann Intern Med 1991;115:133–147.

25. Ridgway EC. Clinician's evaluation of solitary thyroid nodule. J Clin Endocrinol Metab 1992;74:231–235.

26. Belfiore A, LaRosa GL, LaPorta GA, et al. Cancer risk in patients with cold thyroid nodules: relevance of iodine intake, sex, age, and multinodularity. Am J Med 1992;93:363–369.

27. Studer H, Gerber H. Clinical manifestations and management of nontoxic diffuse and nodular goiter. In: Braverman LE, Utiger RD, eds. Werner and Ingbar's the thyroid: a fundamental and clinical text. 6th ed. Philadelphia: JB Lippincott, 1991:1114–1118.

28. Nikolai TF. Silent thyroiditis and subacute thyroiditis. In: Braverman LE, Utiger RD, eds. Werner and Ingbar's the thyroid: a fundamental and clinical text. 6th ed. Philadelphia: JB Lippincott, 1991:710-727.

29. Jansson R, Bernander S, Karlsson A, et al. Autoimmune thyroid dysfunction in the postpartum period. J Clin Endocrinol Metab 1984;58:681–687.

30. Othman S, Phillips DIW, Parkes AB, et al. A long-term follow-up of postpartum thyroiditis. Clin Endocrinol 1990;32:559–564.

31. Robbins J. Thyroid hormone transport proteins and the physiology of hormone binding. In: Braverman LE, Utiger RD, eds. Werner and Ingbar's the thyroid: a fundamental and clinical text. 6th ed. Philadelphia: JB Lippincott, 1991:111–143.

32. Mandel SJ, Larsen PR, Seely EW, Brent GA. Increased need for thyroxine during pregnancy in women with primary hypothyroidism. N Engl J Med 1990;323:91–96.

33. Milham S Jr. Scalp defects in infants of mothers treated for hyperthyroidism with methimazole or carbimazole during pregnancy. Teratology 1985;32:321. Letter.

34. Milham S, Elledge W. Maternal methimazole and congenital defects in children. Teratology 1972;5:125–126.

35. Becks GP, Burrow GN. Thyroid disease and pregnancy. Greenspan FS, ed. In: Medical clinics of North America. Philadelphia: WB Saunders, 1991;75:121–150.

36. Wartofsky L. Thyrotoxic storm. In: Braverman LE, Utiger RD, eds. Werner and Ingbar's the thyroid: a fundamental and clinical text. 6th ed. Philadelphia: JB Lippincott, 1991:871–879.

37. Ladenson PW. Recognition and management of cardiovascular disease related to thyroid dysfunction. Am J Med 1990;88:638–641.

38. Wartofsky L. Myxedema coma. In: Braverman LE, Utiger RD, eds. Werner and Ingbar's the thyroid: a fundamental and clinical text. 6th ed. Philadelphia: JB Lippincott, 1991:1084–1091.

CHAPTER 19

DIABETES MELLITUS

Christine Heckemeyer

Diabetes Mellitus

Presentation

The classic symptoms of diabetes mellitus include polydipsia, polyuria, and weight loss in the face of increased food intake. If the patient has type I (insulin-dependent) diabetes mellitus, such symptoms may progress to nausea, vomiting, and nonspecific abdominal pain. She will complain of generalized fatigue and orthostatic dizziness (caused by dehydration). Family and friends may note some difficulty with concentration and sleepiness. Frank coma is less common.

The woman with type II diabetes mellitus is often asymptomatic at the time of diagnosis. She may complain of increased thirst, polyuria and nocturia, and increased appetite. Depending on her food intake, she may experience weight loss or weight gain. Generalized chronic fatigue is a common complaint, accompanied by dyspnea on exertion. She may give a history of large babies or complications during pregnancies. She may have recurrent yeast infections or other skin problems such as boils or cellulitis. Generalized pruritus is frequent. Paresthesia may interfere with sleep. Blurred vision may be present. She may experience leg cramps with or without evidence of peripheral vascular disease. Occasionally, the individual with type II diabetes mellitus presents with an unexplained neuropathy (i.e., diplopia or foot drop).

Differential Diagnosis

Polydipsia and polyuria are seen in diseases that affect the renal concentrating mechanism. These would include central and nephrogenic diabetes insipidus, hypercalcemia, hypokalemia, renal sodium wasting, drugs or toxins (such as lithium, diuretics, ethanol, amphotericin, and propoxyphene), and tubulointerstitial disease (such as sickle cell anemia, multiple myeloma, amyloidosis, analgesic nephropathy, post-obstructive nephropathy, and chronic pyelonephritis). High solute loads from contrast dyes, mannitol, or high-protein tube feedings may cause diuresis. The loss of renal concentration associated with chronic renal failure may cause polyuria. Primary polydipsia associated with sarcoidosis or psychiatric disease may wash out the intramedullary gradient, causing decreased urinary concentration.

Few problems cause weight loss accompanied by *increased* appetite and food intake. Malabsorption associated with sprue, chronic pancreatitis, or other bowel diseases may cause a decreased ability to use food. This is usually, but not always, accompanied by complaints of increased stool frequency or frank diarrhea. Increased caloric needs may accompany hypermetabolic states such as thyrotoxicosis or pheochromocytoma.

As any practitioner can attest, chronic fatigue may have many etiologies. Frequent causes in the adult include anemia, chronic infections, heart failure, subclinical renal disease, lung disease, malignancy, arthritis, and poor nutrition. Fatigue may be a prominent feature of endocrine disorders such as hyperthyroidism, hypothroidism, adrenal insufficiency, Cushing's syndrome, and panhypopituitarism. Often patients suffering from depression complain of fatigue, which is present on awakening and which may improve as the day progresses. Prescription and over-the-counter medications may cause sedation and complaints of fatigue.

Nausea, vomiting, and dehydration occur frequently with pyelonephritis, nephrolithiasis, salpingitis, gastroenteritis, and hepatitis. Ketoacidosis may mimic acute abdominal problems such as cholecystitis, intestinal obstruction, or appendicitis. Pancreatitis may be difficult to differentiate from ketoacidosis because elevated serum amylase levels occur with both. High urinary ketone levels may accompany peptic ulcer disease with gastric outlet obstruction although serum ketone levels should be low. Ingestion of methanol, ethylene glycol, or salicylate may cause an accompanying increased anion gap. The hyperventilation associated with salicylate ingestion may resemble Kussmaul's respirations. However, serum ketone levels should be low.

Inferior myocardial infarction often presents with severe nausea and vomiting. Congestive heart failure with associated hepatic congestion may induce nausea. A mildly elevated anion gap may be present because of associated lactic acidosis.

Patients with endocrine disorders such as adrenal insufficiency hypothyroidism and thyrotoxicosis with storm may present with nausea and vomiting.

The neuropathies associated with diabetes mellitus are legion, involving the motor, sensory, and autonomic nervous systems. If the average blood sugar elevation is mild, the patient may have no other symptoms to suggest the diagnosis of diabetes mellitus. Fasting blood sugars may be normal. An oral glucose tolerance test may be necessary to make the diagnosis in this setting.

Focal entrapment neuropathies such as carpal tunnel syndrome occur with overuse, pregnancy, hypothyroidism, acromegaly, trauma, amyloidosis, rheumatoid arthritis, and localized granulomatous disease. Ulnar and radial entrapment syndromes and tarsal tunnel syndrome may also be present.

Exposure to toxins such as heavy metals, hydrocarbons, organophosphorus compounds, and alcohol; infections such as infectious mononucleosis, hepatitis, leprosy, or syphilis; vitamin B_{12} deficiency; hypothyroidism; amyloidosis; uremia; sarcoidosis; porphyria; vasculitis; and malignancy may cause stocking-glove peripheral neuropathies.

Mononeuropathies may result from pressure, trauma, vasculitides occurring with polyarteritis nodosa or rheumatoid arthritis, malignancy with local neural invasion, herpes zoster, leprosy, and sarcoidosis.

Although cranial nerve palsies caused by diabetes mellitus usually happen in the setting of long-standing disease, they may be the initial presentation of glucose abnormalities. Third cranial nerve palsies caused by diabetes mellitus tend to spare the pupil. Palsies caused by intracranial masses or aneurysms do not. Sixth nerve palsies caused by diabetes mellitus are indistinguishable from those caused by vascular disease, intracranial masses, or viral disease. Herpes zoster infection, central nervous system (CNS) lesions, trauma, otitis media, and Guillain-Barré syndrome may cause Bell's palsy.

Peripheral vascular disease may accompany severe atherosclerotic disease of any etiology. In a young person with a heavy smoking history, Buerger's disease may be present. Drugs that cause vasospasm, such as ergot compounds and β blockers may be responsible. Raynaud's disease may occur in isolation or in association with connective tissue disorders or other immune disorders, environmental exposures, or oral contraceptive use. Cardiac arrhythmias, coagulopathies, and vasculitis may cause acute arterial lesions.

Physical Findings

Diabetic ketoacidosis typically presents with orthostatic hypotension, tachycardia, Kussmaul's respirations with a fruity odor, nausea, vomiting, and poorly localized abdominal tenderness. The patient has dry mucous membranes and peripheral vasoconstriction. She is somnolent but usually arousable. She may note decreased visual acuity.

Patients with poorly controlled diabetes often appear mildly dehydrated without pulse or blood pressure tilt. They may have evidence of *Candida* infections, especially involving the vaginal and intriginous areas. Folliculitis and furuncles may be present.

With associated peripheral neuropathy or vascular insufficiency, the skin on the extremities becomes dry and cracked. Absent hair growth on the legs may indicate the level of vascular insufficiency. There may be atrophy in the skin and in the subcutaneous fat from small vessel disease. This skin is more susceptible to injury from relatively minor trauma. Sweating may be absent below the level of nerve damage. Pressure ulcers, cellulitis, or infected areas around foreign bodies may be present. In addition, gangrene of the distal digits may occur. Peripheral pulses may be decreased or absent. However, with thickened arterial walls, palpable pulses may accompany significant evidence of peripheral vascular compromise. Appropriate maneuvers may elicit dependent rubor and elevation pallor. She may have had an amputation.

If her hands are in water and harsh detergents, periungual infections may be a problem. Ingrown and thickened toenails may be hard to trim and prone to onychomycosis.

Granuloma annulare may appear several years before the onset of diabetes mellitus. Necrobiosis lipoidica diabeticorum may disfigure the anterior shins with yellow or red telangiectatic plaques that tend to ulcerate. They heal very slowly and often incompletely. Eruptive xanthomas on the flexor surfaces may indicate an accompanying lipid abnormality. Patients taking oral hypoglycemic agents may have sunburn or eczema in the sun exposed areas.

Musculoskeletal abnormalities are also frequent in long-standing diabetes mellitus. Thickening of the subcutaneous connective tissues may lead to flexion deformities of the small joints in the hands and decreased ability to oppose the palmar surfaces. Loss of pain sensation and proprioception may induce Charcot changes in the ankle, knee, and smaller joints of the foot. Loss of interosseus muscle strength may lead to hammer toe deformities and loss of grip strength. Ligamentous swelling makes the person with diabetes more prone to carpal and tarsal tunnel syndromes, as well as ulnar compression. Marked muscle wasting and weakness may accompany mononeuropathies.

Decreased ventricular compliance may produce an audible gallop on auscultation. Congestive heart failure may develop secondary to volume overload from accompanying nephropathy. Reversible left ventricular failure of abrupt onset, with diffuse bilateral crackles and gallops, may be the only manifestation of otherwise silent myocardial ischemia.

Cataracts may obscure visualization of the retina. Ophthalmoscopic examination may reveal a glaucomatous disc or changes of diabetic retinopathy.

Neurologic examination frequently reveals loss of light touch, pain, position, and vibratory sensation in a stocking-glove distribution. This gradually progresses to involve the distal ends of truncal sensory nerves. Dysesethesias involving truncal nerves may resemble angina or an acute abdomen requiring surgical intervention. Diabetic radiculopathy may simulate a herniated disc. Deep tendon reflexes may be absent. Isolated cranial nerve palsies, peripheral mononeuropathies, and mononeuropathy multiplex may occur.

One of the first manifestations of autonomic neuropathy may be loss of respiratory variation in the pulse or an otherwise unexplained resting tachycardia. Orthostatic hypotension may be most prominent on arising in the morning or after a meal. There may be no change in heart rate to compensate for the marked postural blood pressure change.

Laboratory and Other Work-Up

Diagnostic criteria for diabetes mellitus, impaired glucose tolerance, and gestational diabetes are included in Table 19.1.

In addition to blood glucose values and glycosylated hemoglobin levels, obtain a fasting lipid profile including high-density lipoprotein cholesterol, low-density lipoprotein cholesterol, and triglycerides. Screen renal function with a complete urinalysis and serum creatinine and blood urea nitrogen (BUN) determinations. Because of an increased frequency of hypothyroidism in patients with type I diabetes mellitus, thyroid function tests (T_4 or thyroid-stimulating hormone) are recommended. In adults who may be at increased risk for silent cardiovascular disease, an electrocardiogram is also advisable. In the patient with type I diabetes mellitus, electrolytes may show a decreased serum bicarbonate and an increased anion gap. It is important to realize that normal or near-normal blood glucose levels do *not* exclude diabetic ketoacidosis. Urine ketones are usually high, but may be confusing in patients with severe dehydration and renal shutdown. Serum ketone levels are helpful in this situation. In patients with ketoacidosis, serum potassium, phosphate, and magnesium levels should also be determined so that appropriate repletion may be made. (See section on complications and management).

Basic Pathophysiology

Selective cell-mediated immune attack on the β cells within the pancreas causes most type I (insulin-dependent) diabetes mellitus. In rare genetic disorders such as Wolfram's syndrome β cell loss occurs in the absence of immune attack. Circulating islet cell antibodies and anti-insulin antibodies may serve as markers for increased risk of developing insulin-dependent

Table 19.1 Diagnostic Criteria for Diabetes Mellitus, Impaired Glucose Tolerance, and Gestational Diabetes

NONPREGNANT ADULTS

Criteria for Diabetes Mellitus: Diagnosis of diabetes mellitus in nonpregnant adults should be restricted to those who have *one* of the following:

- A random plasma glucose level of ⩾200 mg/dL *plus* classic signs and symptoms of diabetes mellitus including polydipsia, polyuria, polyphagia, and weight loss
- A fasting plasma glucose level of ⩾140 mg/dL on at least two occasions
- A fasting plasma glucose level of <140 mg/dL *plus* sustained elevated plasma glucose levels during at least two oral glucose tolerance tests. The 2-hr sample and at least one other between 0 and 2 hr after the 75-gm glucose dose should be ⩾200 mg/dL. Oral glucose tolerance testing is not necessary if the patient has a fasting plasma glucose level of ⩾140 mg/dL.

Criteria for Impaired Glucose Tolerance: Diagnosis of impaired glucose tolerance in nonpregnant adults should be restricted to those who have *all* of the following:

- A fasting plasma glucose of <140 mg/dL
- A 2-hr oral glucose tolerance test plasma glucose level of 140–200 mg/dL
- An intervening oral glucose tolerance test plasma glucose value of ⩾200 mg/dL

PREGNANT WOMEN

Criteria for Gestational Diabetes: Following an oral glucose load of 100 gm, the diagnosis of gestational diabetes may be made if two plasma glucose values equal or exceed the following:

Fasting	105 mg/dL
1 hr	190 mg/dL
2 hr	165 mg/dL
3 hr	145 mg/dL

Reprinted by permission of *The Physician's Guide to Type II Diabetes (NIDDM): Diagnosis and Treatment.* Copyright © 1984 by the American Diabetes Association, Inc.

diabetes mellitus (IDDM). Their role in the disease process is still unclear. Antibodies against islet cells and insulin may be present for many years before frank diabetes mellitus develops. Indeed, some individuals with the antibodies never develop diabetes mellitus.

Individual genetic susceptibility appears to control the rate of islet destruction. HLA DR3 or DR4 are present in 90% of individuals with IDDM. However, genetic studies indicate that some sort of environmental factor, as yet not fully identified, must be present to initiate the autoimmune process. Destruction of 80% to 90% of the islet cell mass causes fasting hyperglycemia. Depending on the rate of loss of residual islet cell function, the individual may not initially manifest ketoacidosis, and thus be mistakenly diagnosed as having type II diabetes mellitus. As the islet cell loss continues, the correct diagnosis and necessity of insulin therapy becomes evident.

Ketoacidosis is due to absolute insulin deficiency. Lack of insulin induces a catabolic state. Elevated counterregulatory hormones compound the problem by increasing glycogenolysis, gluconeogenesis, and lipolysis. Glucagon induces ketone body formation. Elevations in catecholamine, cortisol, and growth hormone levels antagonize the effects of any residual endogenous insulin. Hyperglycemia and osmotic diuresis ensue, associated with electrolyte losses. Poor oral intake secondary to nausea and vomiting compound the dehydration and electrolyte abnormalities.

A "honeymoon phase" requiring little or no exogenous insulin therapy may be noted after correction of the initial episode of ketoacidosis. Correction of glucotoxicity and electrolyte abnormalities allows resumption of insulin secretion by residual islet cells. As islet cells continue to be destroyed, insulin dependence recurs, usually within several months to 1 year.

Insulin resistance and abnormal endogenous insulin secretion cause type II diabetes mellitus. In the liver and peripheral tissues, decreased insulin binding to cell membrane receptors in combination with decreased intracellular response to insulin cause tissue resistance. Initially, decreased insulin sensitivity is accompanied by a compensatory increase in insulin secretion. Hyperinsulinemia causes "down regulation" of peripheral insulin receptors, requiring further increases in basal insulin secretion to maintain normal fasting blood sugars. As the disease progresses, the pancreatic β cells are unable to maintain the increased insulin production. Insulin levels decrease and are no longer sufficient to suppress hepatic glucose production in the fasting state. Fasting hyperglycemia ensues.

Medications and Their Pharmacology

By definition, type I diabetes mellitus requires insulin therapy to prevent ketoacidosis. Oral agents have no place in the treatment of type I diabetes mellitus. Individuals with type II diabetes mellitus may also require insulin therapy to obtain adequate control of elevated blood sugars. Insulin preparations vary according to their time of action and species of origin. In the U.S. market, Regular, NPH and Lente insulins of animal origins are being replaced by biosynthetic human preparations (Table 19.2).

The Diabetes Complications and Control Trial (DCCT) has proved that tight glycemic control slows the onset of neuropathic, renal, and retinal complications from type I diabetes mellitus, albeit at the price of more frequent hypoglycemic episodes and some weight gain. The trial used either a multidose insulin injection regimen or a SQ insulin infusion pump. The multidose injection regimen tries to replicate physiologic insulin secretion. Long-acting or intermediate insulin preparations provide basal insulin requirements. Preprandial Regular insulin imitates endogenous meal boluses in the normal individual (see Table 19.2). Both multidose injection and an insulin pump require a patient who is willing to do self-monitoring of blood glucose before each meal and at bedtime, and who can adjust premeal boluses according to a variable insulin dose schedule developed to maintain euglycemia. Some individuals may need to monitor blood glucose response to exercise and prevent nocturnal hypoglycemia with 3 AM blood glucose determinations.

Conventional insulin therapy consists of one or two injections of mixed intermediate and short-acting insulin, usually before breakfast and supper. It is appropriate for patients who are unable or unwilling to comply with the requirements of a multidose regimen and in individuals with increased risk of complications from hypoglycemia, such as those with cardiovascular or cerebrovascular disease, or those with severe autonomic neuropathy and hypoglycemia unawareness. The individual amounts of each insulin are adjusted according to preprandial blood glucose patterns, with adjustments for exercise.

Erratic blood sugar levels may make it difficult to determine the correct insulin dosage. One of the most common causes for erratic sugars is a problem in communication between the health practitioner and the patient. Ask her how she is actually taking her insulin,

Table 19.2 Pharmacology of Insulin

Type of Insulin	Species of Insulin	Onset of Action (HR)	Peak of Action (HR)	Usual Duration (HR)	Maximum Duration (HR)
Regular	Human	0.5–1	2–3	3–6	4–6
NPH	Human	2–4	4–10	10–16	14–18
Lente	Human	3–4	4–12	12–18	16–20
Ultralente	Animal	8–14	minimum	24–36	24–36
	Human	6–10	?	18–20	20–30

and do not rely on medical records for the dosage. Other causes of erratic blood sugar values include malingering, factitious disease, concomitant drug use (prescription, over-the-counter, and recreational), alcohol, improper self-injection technique, and intercurrent illness. Counterregulatory hormone insufficiency and gastrointestinal motility disturbances are more common in patients with neuropathy. Anti-insulin antibodies are an uncommon cause in the absence of evidence of other autoimmune disorders or a previous history of marked insulin resistance.

The initial therapy of choice for uncomplicated type II diabetes mellitus is dietary (Table 19.3). Even individuals who present with marked hyperosmolarity may be controlled with diet alone, or combined with oral hypoglycemic agents, once their metabolic abnormalities have been rectified.

In patients who are markedly symptomatic, or who are already at their ideal body weight, simultaneous initiation of oral hypoglycemic or insulin therapy may be appropriate. The choice of the oral hypoglycemic agent depends on the age of the patient, her hepatic and renal function, her eating schedule, and other medications she may be taking. Chlorpropamide is not recommended in individuals over the age of 65, in those with variable food intake, or in those taking diuretics. Patients with poor renal function are especially prone to complications from chlorpropamide, but may have problems with the other agents that have renal metabolism or urinary excretion of active metabolites (Table 19.4). A rule of thumb would be to avoid such agents in patients with serum creatinine levels greater than 2 mg/dL.

A serious side effect of sulfonylurea therapy is hypoglycemia. This appears to be more frequent with long-acting agents. Underlying renal or liver disease and older age appear to increase the risk of this problem. Alcohol use may increase the risk. Concomitant prescription or over-the-counter medication use may also increase the incidence of hypoglycemia, especially with first-generation agents that are highly protein bound. Use of a short-acting agent without active metabolites may decrease the risk.

Other infrequent side effects seen with sulfonylurea therapy include nausea, skin rashes, photosensitivity, and headache. Hyponatremia may occur with chlorpropamide therapy, especially with concomitant diuretic use. Rare hematologic reactions such as thrombocytopenia, hemolytic anemia, and agranulocytosis have been reported. Occasionally, cholestatic jaundice may occur.

Insulin therapy should be given during pregnancy and during times of stress such as surgery, infection, or myocardial infection. Individuals who do not respond to an oral hypoglycemic agent may be tried on a second agent, but usually require initiation of insulin therapy. Such "primary failures" are especially common in patients with near-normal body weight. Another group of patients respond initially to an oral hypoglycemic agent, but then lose responsiveness (probably because of decreased endogenous insulin production). With such "secondary failure" it is wise to rule out dietary noncompliance, subclinical infections, interference from other medications, and electrolyte disturbances (particularly hypokalemia).

Table 19.3 Diet

- 55–60% carbohydrate
- 15–20% protein (0.8 mg/kg per day)
- <30% fat
- <300 mg/day cholesterol
- Dietary prescriptions:

1. Age 0–12 yr	1000 cal for 1st yr, then 100 cal/yr over age 1.
2. Age 12–15 yr	1500–2000 cal + 100 cal/yr > age 12 for females 2000–2500 cal + 100 cal/yr > age 12 for males
3. Age 15–20 yr	13–15 cal/lb IBW for females 15–18 cal/lb IBW for males
4. Adults	10–12 cal/lb IBW for sedentary 12–14 cal/lb IBW for moderate activity 14–16 cal/lb IBW for active
5. Pregnancy	12–16 cal/lb IBW
6. Lactation	15–17 cal/lb IBW

- Sorbitol, fructose—calorically equivalent to table sugar.
- Limit ethanol to 2 oz twice a week.
- Nonnutritive sweeteners may be used within established safe limits.

IBW, idealbody weight.
Source: Based on American Diabetes Association. National recommendations principles for individuals with diabetes mellitus. *Diabetes Care* 1987;10:126–132.

Table 19.4 Pharmacology of Oral Hypoglycemic Agents

Agent	Duration of Action (HR)	Dosage in mg	Site of Metabolism	Notes
tolbutamide (Orinase)	6–12	500–3000	Liver	
tolazamide (Tolinase)	12–24	100–750	Liver/renal excretion	Active metabolite
chlorpropamide (Diabinese)	24–72	100–500	Liver/renal excretion	Active metabolite
acetohexamide (Dymelor)	12–24	100–1500	Liver/renal excretion	Active metabolite
glyburide (Micronase, Glynasen, DiaBeta)	16–24	1.25–20.0	Liver/bile and renal excretion	
glipizide (Glucotrol)	12–18	2.5–40.0	Liver	

Another oral agent may be tried, but usually insulin is required for adequate control of blood glucose levels.

Combination therapy with insulin and oral hypoglycemics has been advocated as a means of decreasing the total amount of insulin necesssary to obtain adequate glucose control. The reduction in insulin requirements is relatively small, and combination therapy may increase the cost by as much as 50% over insulin alone.

Indications for Referral

A dietitian may instruct patients in the diabetic diet and any adjustments necessary because of lipid or renal disorders. A diabetic educator can be invaluable in teaching proper self-care, insulin self-injection, home blood glucose monitoring, and sick day management.

Given the findings of the DCCT trial, individuals with type I diabetes mellitus should be referred to a diabetologist if the primary care provider is unable to supply the support necessary for intensive insulin therapy.

Young women of childbearing age need a frank discussion of the need for excellent blood glucose control before initiation of pregnancy. Birth control needs should be addressed, either by the primary care physician or by referral to a gynecologist.

Individuals with type I diabetes mellitus require annual ophthalmologic evaluation for possible retinopathy, beginning 5 years after the onset of their disease. Individuals with type II diabetes may have had subclinical disease for some time and should see an ophthalmologist soon after diagnosis, with annual follow-up visits. Immediate referral should be made if proliferative retinopathy involves more than 25% of the optic disk or with neovascular disease and preretinal or vitreous hemorrhage. Hard exudates within the macula (suggesting macular edema) also require immediate referral. In addition, women beginning or planning to begin a pregnancy should be evaluated by an ophthalmologist for proliferative retinopathy. Obviously, any patient experiencing decreased vision should be referred.

Once an individual has developed overt proteinuria (>500 mg/24 hr) or elevated serum creatinine levels, management should be coordinated with a nephrologist. Urinary retention from neurogenic bladder may lead to worsening renal function and should be managed with the help of urologic consultants, if conservative therapy such as use of the Credé maneuver are unsuccessful.

Orthopedic intervention may prevent loss of function from carpal tunnel syndrome and ulnar entrapment. Physical therapy is helpful in minimizing loss of muscle mass with mononeuropathies involving the lower extremities.

Podiatrists can be helpful in management of callouses, bunions, plantar ulcerations, and toenail infections. Vascular surgical intervention may be necessary if peripheral vascular disease contributes to poor wound healing or claudication and rest pain are present. Orthopedic consultation is indicated if osteomyelitis or Charcot joint changes from peripheral neuropathy are present.

Diagnostic Testing for Complications

The major acute complications of diabetes mellitus are diabetic ketoacidosis, hyperosmolar nonketotic coma, and hypoglycemia. All can be diagnosed by obtaining serum electrolyte and serum ketone levels in the appropriate clinical setting. Management is outlined in the next section.

Annual urinalyses to screen for proteinuria are the usual means of diagnosing nephropathy. (Newer tests for microalbuminuria may pick up problems at an earlier stage. Ongoing studies are assessing the value of intervention at this earlier stage.) Urine cultures should be done to diagnose and treat any infection that may be contributing to the problem. A 24-hour urine collection for creatinine, creatinine clearance, and protein can be helpful in assessing the severity of the problem. A renal ultrasound to evaluate kidney size and rule out obstructive lesions is also indicated. In individuals with accompanying hypertension that is difficult to control, a renal scan may diagnose unilateral renal vascular stenosis.

Foot and leg pain may be due to vascular disease, neuropathy, or a combination of the two. A complete physical examination should include special attention to auscultation for femoral bruits, palpation of pedal pulses, and evaluation of hair growth on the feet and legs, along with evaluation of vibratory sensation over the lower extremities. Foot ulcers should be x-rayed to rule out an occult foreign body or underlying osteomyelitis. Peripheral vascular disease may be noninvasively assessed with Doppler studies. If proximal (and potentially surgically correctable) disease is present, an arteriogram may be indicated. Nerve conduction velocity studies may be helpful in discriminating between distal symmetric polyneuropathy and lumbosacral radiculopathies or entrapment syndromes, which may benefit from orthopedic or neurosurgical intervention.

Gastroparesis may be manifested by early satiety, anorexia, abdominal distention, nausea, and vomiting (especially several hours after eating). Impaired gastric emptying may cause widely fluctuating blood sugar values because nutrients are being absorbed from the intestine at irregular intervals—if at all. An upper gastrointestinal series should be done to rule out other gastric diseases such as gastric or duodenal ulcer. However, a normal upper gastrointestinal series does not rule out gastroparesis because it evaluates the emptying of liquids, but not solid foods from the stomach. A radionuclide gastric emptying study is more specific for the diagnosis of gastroparesis.

Chronic diarrhea should be evaluated with the same modalities as in a nondiabetic individual. In particular, steatorrhea might indicate accompanying pancreatic insufficiency, bacterial overgrowth, or celiac sprue—all amenable to appropriate treatment.

Treatment for Complications

Ketoacidosis

Presenting symptoms of diabetic ketoacidosis include polyuria, polydipsia, nausea, vomiting, nonspecific abdominal pain, and decreased mental status. Patients have tachycardia, orthostatic hypotension, hyperventilation, evidence of dehydration, and weight loss. In the majority of individuals a precipitating cause is noted. These include infection, trauma, stroke, and myocardial infarction. More frequently insulin has been omitted because of inability to eat. Frequent episodes of ketoacidosis may indicate poor compliance. Counseling to improve psychological adjustment to the illness may be required.

Serum calcium, phosphate, and magnesium levels, as well as arterial blood gases, should be checked on admission. Electrolytes should be checked every 2 to 4 hours to ensure adequate replacement and appropriate administration of IV fluids. Urine ketones should be monitored although they may lag behind serum ketones in clearance. Complete blood count, urinalysis, and chest x-ray should be obtained to evaluate a possible source of infection. An electrocardiogram will give a quick estimation of serum potassium levels and may show an ischemic event that precipitated the ketoacidosis.

Volume repletion, insulin, and correction of electrolyte abnormalities are the cornerstones of therapy for diabetic ketoacidosis. Isotonic saline is used until adequate blood pressure and urine output are established. This usually requires 1 to 2 liters over the first 2 hours of treatment. (Hypernatremia or underlying cardiac or renal disease obviously may alter the choice and rate of administration hydration fluid.) Thereafter, 0.5% saline may be used. When the blood glucose level drops to 300 mg/dL, dextrose is added to enable continued administration of insulin until the ketoacidosis is broken and serum bicarbonate is normalized. The blood glucose level should be maintained around 250 mg/dL during the first 12 to 24 hours to avoid cerebral edema. Strict intake and output is mandatory to ensure adequate volume repletion in the face of continuing osmotic diuresis.

Preferably, regular insulin should be administered IV if adequate nursing supervision is available to monitor the infusion rate. An intensive care setting or specialized diabetic unit is recommended. Dehydration and variable perfusion of the subcutaneous tissues make SQ insulin administration less reliable in this situation. A bolus dose of 0.1 U/kg is given initially, followed by infusion of 0.1 U/kg per hour. The blood glucose level should be closely monitored. If it does not drop by 75 to 100 mg/dL per hour, the patient has some insulin resistance, and the infusion rate should be increased. When blood glucose levels drop below 300 mg/dL, the insulin infusion rate should be decreased by 50%. IV insulin should be continued until ketoacidosis has cleared and SQ insulin administration has been resumed.

Diabetic ketoacidosis causes marked potassium depletion. Acidosis usually causes initial laboratory determinations to be normal or increased. Unless potassium levels are above 6 mEq/L or the patient is anuric, potassium chloride should be added to the initial IV fluids. Ten to 30 mEq/hr is usually adequate. Potassium chloride may be alternated with potassium phosphate to prevent hyperchloremia and treat accompanying phosphate deficiencies. This is especially important if the phosphate value is less than 1 or if there is evidence of rhabdomyolysis. Repletion should be cautious because administration of more than 90 mEq potassium phosphate over a 24-hour period may induce hypocalcemia.

If the patient has low initial potassium values, it might be preferable to administer IV fluids and potassium supplementation alone, holding initiation of insulin therapy until the serum values have normalized. Otherwise, insulin-induced sequestration of potassium in the cells may worsen the hypokalemia. In these patients, higher infusion rates (40 to 80 mEq/hr) may require central venous lines and electrocardiographic monitoring.

Caveats of care:

- The need for IV insulin is based on continuing acidosis, not on blood glucose levels.
- Frequent observation of cardiovascular status is necessary to avoid congestive heart failure.
- Nausea and vomiting may require placement of nasogastric suction to prevent aspiration. Intubation may be necessary to protect the airway in comatose patients.
- Children are susceptible to cerebral edema if blood glucose levels are lowered too quickly.

Hyperosmolar Hyperglycemic Coma

Presenting symptoms of hyperosmolar hyperglycemic coma include depressed sensorium and evidence of severe dehydration. New-onset seizures or focal neurologic deficits may resolve with therapy of the hyperosmolar state. Blood pressure may be low, and underlying chronic renal disease may be present. The individual is usually over 50 years of age and may not have been previously diagnosed with diabetes mellitus. Often she is debilitated or has decreased access to fluid intake. Patients being treated with IV hyperalimentation, dialysis, phenytoin, glucocorticoids, β blockers, and diuretics are susceptible to hyperosmolar hyperglycemic coma. It may be precipitated by any severe stress, including myocardial infarction, surgery, trauma, sepsis, stroke, gastrointestinal hemorrhage, and pancreatitis.

Plasma glucose levels are usually above 600 mg/dL. Acidosis may be present although serum ketone levels are usually low to moderate. Lactate levels may be elevated. Severe dehydration may be associated with elevated BUN and creatinine levels. Total body potassium levels are usually depleted although initial serum potassium values may be low or elevated.

Therapy is initiated with isotonic saline until blood pressure is acceptable, then changed to 1/2 normal saline. Replace half the volume deficit over the first 24 hours, then decrease the rate of hydration to replace the remainder over the next 24 to 36 hours. Because the individual may have underlying renal or cardiac disease, central venous pressure monitoring can be helpful. Potassium repletion should be held until adequate urinary output is established, unless the patient is frankly hypokalemic on presentation. Administration should be less aggressive than in diabetic ketoacidosis, with frequent monitoring of serum sodium and potassium levels. Dropping the serum sodium level too quickly, especially to hypotonic levels, has been associated with central pontine myelinosis in some individuals.

Normal signs of infection such as fever, leukocytosis, and infiltrates on chest x-rays may be masked in the hyperosmolar state. In very ill individuals, it may be advisable to obtain appropriate cultures and initiate broad-spectrum antibiotic coverage until the clinical picture clarifies with treatment. Acute respiratory distress syndrome may present as tachypnea in the absence of acidosis.

Prophylactic SQ heparin may be advisable. Thromboembolic complications may occur several days after the hyperosmolar state has been corrected. In severely dehydrated individuals, acute tubular necrosis may complicate treatment and require a nephrology consultation.

Hypoglycemia

The symptoms of hypoglycemia are autonomic and neuroglycopenic. Autonomic symptoms include hunger, sweating, nervousness, tachycardia, and palpitations. In individuals with autonomic neuropathy or with tightly controlled blood glucose levels, autonomic symptoms may be minimal, with the exception of sweating. As the blood sugar level drops, neuroglycopenic symptoms including headache, decreased concentration or frank confusion, slowed or slurred speech, and weakness may be more prominent. Severe hypoglycemia may cause marked mental status changes, coma, and seizures. Nocturnal hypoglycemic symptoms may include night sweats and nightmares, as well as headaches on awakening.

Hypoglycemia may be caused by errors in insulin administration or erratic insulin absorption. Dietary changes including late or skipped meals and snacks, or decreased intake due to gastroenteritis, depression, or desire to lose weight may induce low blood glucose levels. Exercise without appropriate adjustments in insulin dosage or carbohydrate intake may be responsible. Alcohol and recreational drug use may be responsible. In addition, new prescription and over-the-counter medications may change insulin requirements. Renal impairment may decrease insulin and oral hypoglycemic drug metabolism. Rarely, concomitant adrenal or thyroid insufficiency may have developed in an individual with type I diabetes. Finally, hypoglycemia may be the presenting indication of pregnancy in a previously well controlled diabetic woman.

Mild and moderate hypoglycemic episodes usually respond to ingestion of 15 to 20 gm of carbohydrate, such as 1/2 can of carbonated beverage, 6 Lifesavers, or 4 teaspoons or packets of sugar. If there will be a significant delay until mealtime, ingestion of some form of protein is appropriate. Family members and coworkers should know how to treat a reaction because the patient's ability to recognize a reaction may be impaired. An unconscious patient may respond to parenteral glucagon, supplemented by carbohydrate ingestion, when consciousness is restored. With severe hypoglycemia and impaired consciousness, the risk of aspiration requires IV glucose administration by trained personnel. Hypoglycemic agents with long half-lives may require hospitalization and parenteral glucose administration for several days.

Definitive therapy requires recognition of the cause and adjustment of medications or patient education.

Natural History

Life expectancy for individuals with diabetes has improved markedly since the introduction of insulin therapy in 1921. However, individuals with poor glucose control and complications such as nephropathy or atherosclerotic cardiovascular disease still have a higher mortality than the general population.

Abnormalities in the retinal vessels begin to develop in a few individuals within 4 to 5 years of the onset of the disease, and incidence increases thereafter. Retinopathy develops in 90% of the population within 15 years of onset of type I diabetes mellitus. Prepubertal individuals appear to be protected until they enter puberty. Proliferative retinopathy begins to occur in poorly controlled individuals within 8 to 10 years of the onset of their diabetes. Good metabolic control delays the onset of proliferative vessel disease although it has not been proven to prevent eventual problems.

Nephropathy also develops after a lag period of 5 years and increases during the next 15 years. Individuals with a family history of renal disease or hypertension appear to be more susceptible to this complication. Poor glycemic control also increases the risk. Mortality is increased in these individuals, with 50% being dead within 10 years of the onset of proteinuria, often from concomitant atherosclerotic disease.

Atherosclerotic cardiovascular disease is markedly increased in the population with type I diabetes mellitus. The Framingham study showed a cumulative mortality of 33% by age 55. Women lose the protective effect of estrogen present before menopause.

The time course for presentation of complications may differ in the patient with type II diabetes mellitus. Because of the long period of glucose intolerance that may precede diagnosis, these individuals may manifest retinopathy, proteinuria, neuropathy, and atherosclerotic disease at the time of diagnosis. Atherosclerotic disease incidence is increased over that of the general population. In addition, patients with type II diabetes are more likely to suffer complications and death from myocardial infarctions than nondiabetic individuals.

Hypoglycemia

Presentation

Hypoglycemia presents as symptoms of autonomic activation and decreased mentation. Autonomic symptoms include sweating, nervousness, tremor, palpitations, headache, and hunger or nausea. These often occur after a rapid decrease in blood glucose levels.

Central neuroglycopenia produces decreased coordination, irritability, visual changes (including blurring and transient color blindness), decreased concentration or frank confusion, memory loss, and slurred speech. Severe hypoglycemia may result in coma, localized neurologic deficits or seizures. Neuroglycopenic symptoms usually occur with hypoglycemia of more gradual onset, or after autonomic symptoms are ignored.

"Whipple's triad" requires that the symptoms suggest hypoglycemia, that hypoglycemia be biochemically documented at the time of the symptoms, and that the symptoms resolve with food ingestion.

Differential Diagnosis

The possible etiologies for hypoglycemia differ, depending on whether it is present in the fasting or postprandial state. Diseases that cause fasting hypoglycemia may also cause postprandial symptoms, especially more than 4 to 5 hours after eating.

In individuals with previous gastric surgery, postprandial hypoglycemia may occur. Hypoglycemia usually occurs within 2 hours after eating. "Reactive" hypoglycemia occurs in individuals with impaired glucose tolerance. In contrast to alimentary hypoglycemia, the blood sugar level tends to drop in the third to fourth hour after the meal. "Reactive" hypoglycemia may rarely present in individuals with normal insulin secretory dynamics.

Congenital abnormalities of metabolism such as hereditary fructose intolerance, galactosemia, and leucine sensitivity usually present in childhood.

When hepatic, renal, or cardiac problems cause fasting hypoglycemia, the disease is usually so far advanced that the cause is evident. The same is true of severe inanition and severe sepsis.

The history should include all prescription, over-the-counter, and recreational drugs. Drugs such as pentamidine, disopyramide, acetominophen, and salicylates may be responsible. Occasionally a patient may have received an oral hypoglycemic agent due to dispensing error. Alcohol may induce hypoglycemia by blocking gluconeogenesis in an individual with depleted glycogen stores. This usually occurs in someone who has been drinking without eating for several days. However, it has happened with alcohol ingestion after an overnight fast.

Surreptitious use of insulin or oral hypoglycemic agents may be difficult to document. Obtain a social history regarding medical background or access to medications through family members with diabetes mellitus.

Deficiencies in counterregulatory hormones such as growth hormone, glucagon, and epinephrine cause hypoglycemia more commonly in children than adults. However, exclude adrenal insufficency.

Rarely, large tumors may cause severe fasting

hypoglycemia suggestive of insulinoma, but with low serum insulin levels. These tumors include mesenchymal tumors such as spindle cell tumors, sarcomas, and hemangiopericytomas, hepatomas, adrenal cell carcinomas, and carcinoids. Rarely epithelial tumors of the gastrointestinal and genitourinary tract are responsible. These tumors are usually quite large and often found in the retroperitoneal area.

Inappropriate elevations in fasting insulin levels may be caused by insulinomas or nesidioblastosis. A rare autoimmune disorder of insulin antibody production has also been described.

Physical Findings

The physical examination is often normal. During an episode, an individual may manifest tachycardia, diaphoresis, and decreased visual acuity. Slurred speech, decreased mentation, and inappropriate behavior may be present. Examination may reveal dermal hyperpigmentation, stigmata of liver or cardiac disease, or bruising from insulin self-injection. Careful examination of the abdomen may rarely reveal a mass.

Laboratory and Other Work-Up

Initial evaluation requires documentation of "Whipple's triad." In normal women, fasting blood glucose levels may fall below 30 mg/dL, so it is important to document symptoms at the time of the sample and resolution of the symptoms with food ingestion.

Evaluate patients with postprandial hypoglycemia with a 5-hour mixed meal tolerance test. If they have a history of previous gastric surgery, radiologic studies of gastrointestinal motility may be helpful. A glucose determination after an overnight fast should also be done to rule out fasting hypoglycemia.

Fasting hypoglycemia requires plasma samples for insulin, C-peptide, cortisol, and ethanol levels. If the above tests are negative, the problem usually requires a hospital admission for observation during a 72-hour fast. Monitor glucose levels every 4 hours. Determine plasma insulin, C-peptide, cortisol, and growth hormone levels at the time of symptomatic hypoglycemia. If hypoglycemia has not occurred after 72 hours, an hour of exercise may induce a symptomatic drop in the blood glucose level. With endogenous hyperinsulinemia, plasma insulin levels are 6 μU/mL or greater and C-peptide levels are above 0.2 nmol at the time of hypoglycemia. Assay an extra sample of plasma for sulfonylureas, which may duplicate the biochemical findings of insulinoma. Markedly elevated plasma insulin levels may indicate either surreptitious insulin use or insulin antibodies. C-peptide levels are suppressed with exogenous insulin administration.

Radiologic evaluation with abdominal computed tomography (CT) scanning may be helpful once there is biochemical evidence of insulinoma. At the Mayo Clinic, ultrasound studies are used. It is important to recognize that insulinomas are usually small and may be missed with both studies.

Because insulinomas are associated with multiple endocrine neoplasia, type I syndrome, one should screen for parathyroid and pituitary disease. Hypercalcemia and hypophosphatemia require measurement of intact parathyroid hormone levels. Serum prolactin levels should be determined. Hypersecretion of other pancreatic hormones, most commonly gastrin, may also be present. An elevated level of human chorionic gonadotropin (HCG) may indicate a malignant tumor.

Basic Pathophysiology

A mismatch between ambient insulin and circulating glucose causes hypoglycemia. With alimentary reactive hypoglycemia, the rapid absorption of ingested carbohydrate within the first hour after eating causes a marked rise in glucose levels. This signals the pancreas to secrete large amounts of insulin. Unfortunately, the glucose absorption from the gut ceases before insulin secretion can be adequately adjusted, and hypoglycemia occurs.

Insulin secretion in normal persons consists of a brief initial spike of insulin, followed by a more prolonged second phase. In individuals with glucose intolerance or a family history of diabetes mellitus, reactive hypoglycemia develops within the third to fourth hour after eating. The initial insulin spike is lost. The delayed and increased second phase of insulin secretion overshoots absorption of carbohydrate from the gut.

Rarely, individuals with normal insulin secretion dynamics develop reactive hypoglycemia. Possibly counterregulatory hormone deficiencies are responsible for their symptoms although this has not yet been proven.

Fasting hypoglycemia associated with severe hepatic disease, severe cachexia, alcohol ingestion, or congenital enzyme defects is caused by a breakdown in gluconeogenesis. Because cortisol facilitates gluconeogenesis, this may also be the mechanism of hypoglycemia in adrenal and pituitary insufficiency. The liver is unable to manufacture enough glucose to meet body needs because of inadequate hepatocyte function or lack of precursors. Decreased insulin catabolism may also play a part in severe hepatic or renal disease.

Drugs such as sulfonylureas and pentamidine may increase insulin secretion. Others, such as β blockers, decrease counterregulatory hormone response to insulin-induced drops in blood glucose levels. Individuals with underlying renal or hepatic disease or congestive heart failure are particularly prone to drug-induced hypoglycemia. Poor nutritional status also may be a predisposing factor.

Large extrapancreatic tumors may cause hypoglycemia by increasing their glucose uptake beyond the body's ability to compensate. Elevated levels of insulin-like growth factor have been found in some cases and may suppress gluconeogenesis by binding to insulin receptors.

Rare cases of autoimmune antibody production may cause hypoglycemia. In this situation, the antibody interacts with the insulin receptor, mimicking insulin action.

Insulinomas and nesidioblastosis fail to adequately suppress insulin secretion in the face of hypoglycemia. Although insulin levels may be within the "normal" range of the assay, they should be suppressed below 5 μU/mL when the blood glucose level is low.

Medications and Their Pharmacology

Dietary adjustment is the treatment of choice for reactive hypoglycemia. Counsel individuals abusing sulfonylureas or insulin to desist. Patients with poor renal or hepatic function may benefit from discontinuing oral sulfonylureas and initiating insulin therapy. Hypoglycemia induced by sulfonylureas with long half-lives, (glyburide, chlorpropamide) requires hospitalization, IV glucose infusion, and frequent carbohydrate feedings, with frequent monitoring of blood glucose levels.

Surgery is the primary therapy for insulinoma and nesidioblastosis. With malignant metastatic disease, streptozocin and 5-fluorouracil have been used with some success. The nephrotoxicity of streptozocin may limit therapy. Doxorubicin has been added in some studies. Excessive insulin secretion may be treated with diazoxide (400–600 mg/day). Gastrointestinal disturbances and fluid retention may be dose limiting. Starting with lower doses and titrating upward may help the patient tolerate these side effects.

Somatostatin analogues may provide palliation of hyperinsulinemia. SQ injections of 50 μg twice a day are gradually increased to control of symptoms. Steatorrhea, glucose intolerance, and cholelithiasis are the main side effects of this therapy.

Indications for Referral

Dietetic counseling is the mainstay of therapy for reactive hypoglycemia. Psychiatric consultation may be helpful when surreptitious insulin or sulfonylurea use has been documented.

Refer patients with biochemical evidence of insulinoma to a surgeon and center with experience in dealing with these tumors. Because radiologic studies may be unrewarding in tumor localization, the experience of the surgeon may be crucial in finding and removing the tumor intraoperatively.

Likewise, an experienced oncologist working in association with an endocrinologist is most important in treating patients with metastatic insulinoma.

Diagnostic Testing for Complications

Islet cell tumors usually metastasize first to the regional lymph nodes, then to the liver. Elevated liver enzymes, accompanied by an elevated HCG level and defects on abdominal CT scanning may indicate metastatic disease.

Treatment for Complication

Hypoglycemia associated with metastatic insulinoma may be particularly difficult to treat. Simultaneous administration of several of the agents listed above may be necessary. L-Asparaginase may also be helpful in this situation. Hepatic artery embolization has also been tried.

Natural History

The prognosis of hypoglycemia depends on the cause. Most cases of reactive hypoglycemia are amenable to dietary therapy. Morbidity is limited to the episodic symptoms, and long-term survival is not an issue.

Individuals with fasting hypoglycemia tend to have more severe problems. Severe hypoglycemia of long duration may cause permanent damage to the CNS, with focal neurologic deficits or organic brain syndrome. If the hypoglycemia is not discovered, patients may die from the acute episode. If the cause of the hypoglycemia is determined and adequately treated, however, their life expectancy should be normal. Patients with metastatic insulinomas have a limited life expectancy, less than 2 years. Present chemotherapy is palliative but may extend life expectancy for a few months.

SUGGESTED READINGS

Davis MD. Diabetic retinopathy: a clinical overview. Diabetes Care 1992;12:1844–1874.

Diabetes Control and Complications Trial Research Group. The effect of intensive treatment of diabetes on the development and progression of long-term complications in insulin-dependent diabetes mellitus. N Engl J Med 1993;329:977–986.

Krolewski AS, Kosinki EJ, Warram JH, et al. Magnitude and determinants of coronary artery disease in juvenile-onset insulin-dependent diabetes mellitus. Am J Cardiol 1987;59:750–755.

Lebovitz HE, ed. Therapy for diabetes mellitus and related disorders. Alexandria, VA: American Diabetes Association, 1991.

Lebowitz MR, Blumenthal SA. The molar ratio of insulin to C-peptide. An aid to the diagnosis of hypoglycemia due to surreptitious (or inadvertent) insulin administration. Arch Intern Med 1993;a53(5):650–655.

Levine SN, Sanson TH. Treatment of hyperglycaemic hyperosmolar non-ketotic syndrome. Drugs 1989;38: 462–472.

Seltzer HS. Drug-induced hypoglycemia. Endocrinol Metab Clin North Am 1989;163–183.

Service JF. Hypoglycemias. J Endocrinol Metab 1993;269–272.

Stone PH, Muller JE, Hartwell T, et al. The effect of diabetes mellitus on prognosis and serial left ventricular function after acute myocardial infarction: contribution of both coronary disease and diastolic left ventricular dysfunction to the adverse prognosis. J Am Coll Cardiol 1989;14:49–57.

CHAPTER 20

OBESITY

Donald D. Hensrud,
Roland L. Weinsier

Presentation

An active medical practice almost certainly includes many obese patients. Despite the more than $30 billion that is spent on diet and diet aids each year in the United States (1), encounters with the obese patient are unlikely to decrease in the future because the prevalence of obesity is increasing. For many women, contact with their obstetrician or gynecologist is their main source of primary care. Thus, the initial treatment of obesity should be an essential part of the armamentarium of all primary care physicians and is likely to assume more importance in the future as increased emphasis is placed on health promotion and disease prevention.

In the United States approximately one fourth of adults, or 34 million Americans, are overweight (2). The prevalence of obesity is slightly greater in women compared with men, in blacks and Hispanics compared with whites, and in lower socioeconomic groups. Among women, the prevalence of overweight is approximately 15% greater in Hispanics and 20% greater in blacks compared with whites. The variability of weight change is greater in women than men, and women are at twice the risk of a major weight gain compared with men. It is somewhat disconcerting that preliminary data from the third National Health and Nutrition Examination Survey (NHANES III) have confirmed that the prevalence of obesity is continuing to increase among all groups.

It is not hard to identify the severely obese patient. But, what constitutes obesity, or overweight? By definition obesity is an excess of body fat. Body composition and total fat can be estimated, usually in research settings, by various methods including underwater weighing, dual-energy x-ray absorptiometry, bioelectrical impedance analysis, and total body potassium. Because it is not practical to measure body fat directly in clinical practice, surrogate measures of body fat are commonly used, such as body weight or body mass index (BMI). BMI is defined as wt/ht^2 where wt is weight in kilograms and ht is height in meters. The advantage of BMI is that it normalizes weight for height. One definition of overweight in women is a BMI of 27.3 kg/m^2 or greater, which corresponds to the 85th percentile of BMI distribution among women in the NHANES II study. A BMI of 32.3 kg/m^2 or greater is defined as severe overweight (95th percentile) and greater than 39.4 kg/m^2 is classified as morbid obesity.

The degree of obesity can also be estimated by comparing actual body weight with desirable body weight derived from standard weight/height tables (Table 20.1) (3). However, it is important to realize the limitations of these tables (4). Desirable weight in weight/height tables is based on survival data from insurance policy holders. This is a selected group and may not be representative of the general population. The tables do not take into consideration body composition. Moreover, although some attempt is made in the 1983 Metropolitan Life weight/height tables to estimate frame size, it is a rough approximation. For these reasons, an individual with a large amount of lean tissue, such as a muscular body builder, may be falsely classified as obese. In addition to body composition, age is not considered. Finally, the data from which weight/height tables are derived are susceptible to confounding and may falsely indicate that lower weights are less healthy. For example, smokers tend to weigh less and have a higher mortality rate than nonsmokers. Terminal

Table 20.1 Weight/Height Table for Adult Women

HEIGHT (NO SHOES)		REFERENCE WEIGHT	
Feet/Inches	Centimeters	Pounds	Kilograms
4′10″	147	101	46
4′11″	150	104	47
5′0″	152	107	49
5′1″	155	110	50
5′2″	157	113	51
5′3″	160	116	53
5′4″	162	120	54
5′5″	165	123	56
5′6″	167	128	58
5′7″	170	132	60
5′8″	172	136	62
5′9″	175	140	63
5′10″	178	144	65
5′11″	180	148	67
6′0″	183	152	69

Source: Data adapted from Metropolitan Life Insurance Company. Build and Blood Pressure Study, 1959.

wasting diseases at the end of life may produce a similar effect.

There is some controversy about what constitutes the healthiest weight. The 1983 Metropolitan Life weight/height tables were criticized because of an increase in desirable weight at all heights compared to the 1959 tables. This may be secondary to secular trends in weight and may not reflect health status. Many experts prefer the 1959 tables for this reason. Recently, data from the Harvard Alumni Health Study showed that after accounting for smoking and illness-related weight loss, the lowest mortality in men was found in those 20% below the U.S. average (5).

After taking into consideration the limitations discussed above, weight/height tables are still useful in clinical practice. They are the easiest and simplest reference standard to use and intuitively make sense. Moreover, body weight is a readily obtainable clinical parameter, can be easily followed over time, and is a relatively useful measure of health risk. A weight greater than 20% above desirable is considered obese and approximately corresponds to a BMI of 25 kg/m^2 in women. Another definition of morbid obesity is greater than 100% of desirable weight.

In recent years increasing attention has been given to body fat distribution as a better indicator of health risk. Individuals with large amounts of visceral or intra-abdominal fat (also known as central obesity, upper body obesity, android pattern, or "apple" distribution) are at increased risk of morbidity and mortality compared to subjects with a distribution of body fat predominantly in the hips, thighs, and buttocks (peripheral obesity, lower body obesity, gynoid pattern, or "pear" distribution). In research settings visceral fat can be accurately measured by magnetic resonance imaging or computed tomography scanning. Other methods used to describe body fat distribution include combinations of skin-fold thickness measurements at the thigh, abdomen, triceps, or subscapular regions and circumferences such as the waist or hip. One of the most commonly used measures is the ratio of the waist circumference to the hip circumference or waist-to-hip ratio (WHR). The validity of these anthropometric measurements can vary, however. A subject with a large waist circumference could potentially have either a large amount of visceral fat and a small amount of subcutaneous fat, or the reverse situation. These two individuals would, in all likelihood, have different health risk profiles. Another problem with anthropometric measurements of body fat distribution is that standardization is not uniform, probably because no one measure has been shown to be clearly superior. The waist circumference has been measured at the minimal diameter, lower rib margin, and umbilicus, and the hip circumference has been measured at the maximum diameter, greater trochanters, and iliac crests. It has been suggested that increased health risks are associated with a WHR of greater than 1.0 in men and 0.85 in women. However, this should not be interpreted as a threshold effect; rather, the risk is probably continuous.

Differential Diagnosis

Less than 1% of obesity is due to endocrine and metabolic diseases, including hypothyroidism, hypopituitarism, Cushing's syndrome, ovarian failure, polycystic ovary syndrome, insulinoma, hypothalamic lesions, and rare genetic conditions such as Frohlich's syndrome, Laurence-Moon-Biedl syndrome, and Prader-Willi syndrome. Usually, secondary causes of obesity do not result in severe degrees of overweight.

These patients should be referred to the appropriate subspecialist and nutrition specialist for management.

Pathogenesis

Etiology

The etiology of obesity is presumed to be a chronic imbalance of energy ingested and energy expended. Adoption and twin studies have shown there is a genetic component to body weight (6,7). Moreover, a familial dependence of the resting metabolic rate (RMR) has been demonstrated in Pima Indians (8). However, it is not known by what mechanism(s) genetic factors contribute to variation in body weight. Environmental factors ultimately determine an individual's weight.

The determinants of total daily energy expenditure include the RMR, the thermic effect of food (TEF), and the thermic effect of exercise (TEE). The RMR is an approximation of the basal metabolic rate and differs from it only by steady-state conditions before measurement. It is the amount of energy expended in maintaining bodily functions and is generally the largest component of daily energy expenditure, accounting for approximately 60% to 75%. It includes energy expended by the brain, liver, heart, and kidneys, which together comprise about 70% of the RMR. In clinical practice, the RMR can be measured by indirect calorimetry. The TEF, or diet-induced thermogenesis, is the energy required to digest, assimilate, and metabolize nutrients and comprises approximately 10% of total energy expenditure. Physical activity is the most variable component of daily energy expenditure and usually contributes about 15% to 20%, but this can be greater in cases of increased physical activity.

The major determinant of the RMR is the amount of fat-free mass (FFM) (9). FFM is much more metabolically active compared to fat, which has a very low metabolic rate. There is no evidence the obese have a lower RMR or total energy expenditure compared to lean subjects. In fact, the obese, in general, have a greater RMR than the lean because approximately 25% to 40% of excess body weight is FFM. When corrected for FFM, however, there is no significant difference in RMR between the obese and the lean. Women, on average, weigh less than men, have a proportionately lower FFM, and higher percentage of body fat. Therefore, they have a lower absolute RMR, and need to consume fewer calories to maintain or reduce weight. A lower TEF in obese compared to normal-weight subjects has been demonstrated in some studies (10), and this appears to be a contributor to obesity rather than a consequence (11). However, the differences observed between normal-weight and obese subjects are relatively small.

Decreased levels of physical activity have been found in obese compared to lean subjects. Many of the studies in this area of research have been cross-sectional, so it is difficult to determine whether the decreased activity was a cause or a consequence of obesity. In a small number of studies, decreased spontaneous physical activity, or "fidgeting," has been observed in obese subjects, which may contribute to decreased overall physical activity (12).

Eating to satiety is a normal desire and probably achieved by most members of a population as long as food is available. Despite this, there are marked differences among populations in the prevalence of obesity. It follows that because most people eat to satiety, these differences in obesity may result from factors other than the amount or volume of food ingested, for example, the fat content of the diet. Traditional societies that consume a diet low in fat have a low prevalence of obesity. However, increased physical activity in these populations is a potential confounding factor.

Contrary to wide belief, it has been difficult to demonstrate that the obese eat more than the lean, after correcting for FFM. It is not clear to what extent underreporting of energy intake by obese subjects has affected the results of these studies, but it probably operates to some extent. In some studies obese subjects have been shown to underestimate their caloric intake by up to 47% (13). This may not be a totally conscious act as even volunteers trained to record their dietary intake underestimate intake by about 18% (14). Despite the lack of a clear relationship between obesity and total energy intake, there is more evidence that the obese consume a greater percentage of energy as fat (15,16).

Other data support the notion that diet composition may influence weight gain. Animal studies have shown that mice fed ad lib will gain weight in proportion to the fat content of the diet (17). Early human studies showed that it was much easier to gain weight when excess energy was provided as fat compared to a mixed diet of carbohydrate and fat (18). Increased fat intake does not increase fat oxidation, in contrast to carbohydrate and protein, which will increase their rates of oxidation in response to increased dietary intake (19). In short-term metabolic studies, it has been estimated that the metabolic "cost" of converting dietary carbohydrate to body fat is approximately 23% (20). That is, 23% of energy is lost as heat in this conversion. Converting dietary fat to body fat it is a much more efficient 3%. Very large amounts of carbohydrate have to be ingested before net lipogenesis occurs; de novo lipogenesis from carbohydrate is negligible under normal circumstances (21). Therefore, energy balance appears to be equivalent to fat balance (19), and is affected little by carbohydrate and protein intake under usual conditions. Although the effect of fat on energy balance may be largely due to its inherent high caloric density, the previous studies suggest that diet composition may influence energy balance separate from energy intake.

There are other reasons why dietary fat may contribute to obesity. As mentioned, fat has a very high energy density. On the other hand, complex carbohydrates, such as fruits, vegetables, and starches, have a low energy density. Because of this, eating to satiety and consuming equivalent amounts of high-fat or high-complex carbohydrate foods will result in considerably less energy ingested from the high-carbohydrate foods (22). This may partially explain the previously mentioned differences in the prevalence of obesity among populations that consume different amounts of fat.

There are also differential effects of fat and carbohydrate on appetite. After ingestion, excess fat is stored as adipose tissue. The ability of the body to store fat is impressive. An obese female weighing 200 lb and of average body composition may have approximately 80 lb of fat equivalent to 280,000 stored kcal. Once stored, fat has little effect on appetite—obese people still get hungry. Carbohydrate is stored as glycogen which, unlike fat stores, may contribute to decreased energy intake through feedback inhibition on appetite (23). Because the ability of the body to increase glycogen stores is extremely limited (maximum of approximately 1 kg) compared to fat stores, carbohydrate has a greater potential effect on appetite than fat. Other evidence indicates that carbohydrate can affect appetite, much greater than fat, both during and after meals (24).

Certain life events seem to be associated with weight gain including pregnancy, quitting smoking, and stressful periods in life. Pregnancy may be associated with a sustained weight gain of 3 to 5 lb, and women who gain more weight during pregnancy are less likely to return to a normal postpartum weight. Smoking is associated with lower body weight through several potential mechanisms. Quitting smoking is associated with a mean increase in weight of from 4 to 8 lb in women, although more than 10% of women may gain more than 25 lb (25). Adhering to some of the same principles used in the treatment of weight loss, which will be discussed later, may help prevent this gain in weight. Due to the marked adverse effects of smoking on health, which exceed the small mean gain in weight, fear of gaining weight should not be used as an excuse for not quitting smoking.

Small reductions in energy expenditure have been postulated to result from abnormalities in energy metabolism and predispose to obesity. A recent study examined this issue by using mathematical models to predict the theoretical effect of a persistent reduction in energy expenditure on long-term weight gain, assuming no adaptation in energy intake (26). This analysis found the magnitude of weight gain due to chronic small reductions in energy expenditure would be only about 3 to 15 kg, an amount which does not explain severe degrees of obesity. Therefore, it is unlikely that abnormalities in energy expenditure explain the etiology of this highly prevalent disease. By contrast, there is interesting circumstantial evidence that reduced exercise and excessive fat intake play a central role in determining weight status.

Health Complications

Obesity is associated with an increased risk of diabetes mellitus, hypertension, certain cancers, lipid abnormalities and coronary heart disease, degenerative arthritis, gallstones and other gallbladder problems, respiratory problems, and an increase in overall mortality as the degree of obesity increases. Many obese individuals are healthy and do not have any associated comorbidities. However, the risk for many of these complications increases with the degree and duration of obesity. Because overweight is a strong risk factor for developing these conditions, maintaining normal body weight through healthy dietary and other lifestyle habits has a huge potential impact on the primary prevention of premature morbidity and mortality.

Obesity is associated with increased fasting insulin levels, decreased insulin sensitivity in peripheral tissues, and increased risk of diabetes. Approximately 90% of diabetes mellitus is adult onset (type II) and the vast majority of individuals with type II diabetes are obese. Because of the known genetic component in type II diabetes, it is possible that obesity unmasks a diabetic tendency in susceptible individuals.

It is not clearly established if obesity itself is responsible for the increase in low-density lipoprotein (LDL) and total cholesterol observed in obese persons in some studies, or if dietary factors associated with obesity are responsible. It is well accepted, however, that obesity is associated with higher triglycerides and lower levels of high-density lipoprotein (HDL) cholesterol. This lipoprotein pattern is associated with small, dense LDL cholesterol, which is particularly atherogenic. In some studies obesity has been shown to be an independent risk factor for coronary heart disease (27). The lack of association in other reports may have been due to unrecognized bias (28). Because of its association with risk factors for coronary heart disease, including hypertension, diabetes, and dyslipidemia, obesity contributes to coronary heart disease mainly through other mechanisms. Although it may also be an independent risk factor, the relative risk is probably less compared to other established risk factors.

Obesity is associated with hypertension although the mechanism(s) are not entirely clear. Recently, the fifth report of the Joint National Committee on Detection, Evaluation, and Treatment of High Blood Pressure concluded that health risks increase above a blood pressure of 120/80, and optimal blood pressure is below this level (29). There are a great number of people with hypertension or with blood pressures between 120 and 140 systolic and 80 and 90 diastolic, many of whom are also obese. Therefore, increased weight has a large potential effect on blood pressure and its associated health risks.

Cholelithiasis is associated with obesity, especially in women. There is also a 15- to 25-fold greater incidence of cholelithiasis during periods of rapid weight loss, such as results from using very low calorie diets (VLCDs) (30). Many of these gallstones are symptomatic and require surgical intervention. Obesity is associated with hepatic steatosis, which is sometimes expressed as mild elevations of liver function tests.

Osteoarthritis of weight-bearing joints appears to be more prevalent in the obese. There may also be an increased prevalence of osteoarthritis in non–weight-bearing joints such as the hands, indicating factors other than weight are involved. In severe cases, joint arthroplasties may be required. Obese individuals in this situation are in a difficult bind because weight loss is desirable before surgery to prolong the life of the artificial joint. For many patients, this can be difficult to achieve, as will be discussed later. Uric acid levels appear to correlate with body weight, as does the prevalence of gout.

The risk of cancers of the endometrium, breast, and perhaps ovary and gallbladder is increased in obese women. For endometrial and breast cancers the risk appears highest in women with predominantly central distribution of body fat.

Respiratory disturbances in obesity include obesity–hypoventilation syndrome and sleep apnea. In obesity–hypoventilation syndrome increased weight can lead to decreased compliance of the chest wall, decreased functional residual capacity, and underventilation of parts of the lungs. Sleep apnea due to obesity can be obstructive or central. Respiratory disturbances can lead to cor pulmonale in severe cases.

Studies have shown increased visceral fat to be associated with many of these conditions, including hypertension, hypertriglyceridemia, low HDL cholesterol, small dense LDL cholesterol, insulin resistance, hyperinsulinemia, and glucose intolerance. These associations are independent of the overall degree of obesity. Collectively, this group of conditions has been referred to as a "metabolic syndrome" or syndrome X. Prospective studies have reported abdominal obesity to be associated with increased mortality from stroke and coronary heart disease. At least seven prospective studies have demonstrated an association between increased abdominal fat and overall mortality. A recent study in 42,000 women reported a dose–response relationship between the WHR and total mortality within all quintiles of BMI (31). In fact, as also demonstrated in a previous Swedish study (32), those at highest risk of mortality were those with a high WHR and a *low* BMI, that is, relatively thin individuals who carry most of their excess adiposity in the abdominal region.

Different mechanisms have been postulated for these relationships. Visceral obesity is associated with endocrine abnormalities of several hypothalamoperipheral axes including increased corticosteroids, decreased growth hormone, and altered sex steroid hormones. Mesenteric and omental fat cells are metabolically more active than peripheral adipoctyes. They have high basal and catecholamine-stimulated lipolytic activities. These fat cells are unique in that they empty their fatty acids directly into the portal circulation, exposing the liver to high concentrations of free fatty acids. Increased concentrations of free fatty acids inhibit the uptake of insulin by the liver, which may lead to peripheral hyperinsulinemia and eventually other components of the metabolic syndrome. Increased free fatty acid flux to the liver may also increase triglyceride production and very low-density lipoprotein secretion.

Lifestyle factors, including smoking, lack of physical activity, and alcohol intake, especially beer, have been associated with increasing abdominal obesity. It has been proposed that genetic susceptibility combined with an unhealthy lifestyle and positive energy balance may predispose an individual to the endocrine abnormalities and visceral obesity, ultimately leading to expression of the metabolic syndrome described above.

Pregnancy in obese women is associated with increased risk of gestational diabetes mellitus, hypertension, toxemia of pregnancy, and cesarean section. However, pregnancy is not the appropriate time to attempt weight loss. The incidence of maternal and fetal complications increases with either very small or very large amounts of weight gain in both lean and obese women. For women of normal weight (BMI 19.8 to 26.0 kg/m^2) before pregnancy, recommended weight gain during pregnancy should be from 11.5 to 16.0 kg. For obese women (BMI $>$ 29.0 kg/m^2) total weight gain during pregnancy should still be at least 6.8 kg (33).

Social and Psychological Consequences

A subject that is not frequently discussed is the discrimination and adverse social consequences to which obese individuals are subjected (34). Overweight persons are often described physically and psychologically using negative terms, even by physicians. Young obese people make less money and are less likely to be married than their non-overweight counterparts (35). Despite this prejudice, obese persons, in general, do not appear to have greater psychological disturbance than normal-weight persons. Among overweight and normal-weight individuals, however, dieting may contribute to the development of eating disorders. When working with obese patients, increased awareness of and sensitivity to the stigmas associated with being overweight is necessary.

Work-Up

History

A weight history should be obtained from obese patients (Box 20.1). A history of obesity in family members may indicate a genetic tendency toward increased weight but does not prove it because family members are also exposed to similar environmental factors. Medications should be recorded because certain medications can predispose to weight gain, such as coriticosteroids and tricyclic antidepressants. Use of laxatives or diuretics for weight loss should be inquired about. Associated medical conditions should be noted, particularly comorbidities associated with obesity and musculoskeletal or other problems that may inhibit physical activity. Patients with significant life stresses or history of a psychiatric disorder often find it difficult to make the necessary lifestyle changes to lose weight and may benefit from therapy to address these problems before focusing on weight management. Any other barriers to successful weight loss and maintenance should be determined. The preceding information can be used to address potential problems that may inhibit weight loss.

Physical Examination

A complete physical examination should be performed, and particular attention should be given to the physical signs in Box 20.2 that may indicate an underlying endocrine abnormality or associated comorbidity. Height and weight can be used to calculate the BMI. Anthropometric measurements can be recorded if desired, but are probably beyond the scope of practice of most primary care physicians. Body fat distribution can be grossly assessed by visual inspection or measured at the waist and hip circumferences to determine the WHR.

Box 20.1 Pertinent Information in the Medical History of the Obese Patient

Factors predisposing to or associated with obesity

Weight during childhood and at high school graduation (to help determine age of onset)
Life events associated with weight gain (pregnancy, quitting smoking, other stressful periods such as a job change or change in marital status)
Family history of obesity
Medications
Diet history (breakfast, lunch, dinner, snacks, fluids [soda, alcohol], favorite foods, foods which are avoided)
Activity and exercise patterns
Current life stresses
Symptoms of endocrine abnormalities
- Hypothyroidism: cold intolerance, lethargy, constipation, menstrual abnormalities, paresthesia of the hands or feet
- Cushing's syndrome: hypertension, glucose intolerance, menstrual abnormalities, weakness, back pain (compression fractures), easy bruisability
- Polycystic ovary syndrome: menstrual abnormalities, infertility

Associated comorbidities

Hypertension
Diabetes mellitus or impaired glucose tolerance
Hyperlipidemia
Cancer (especially endometrium and breast)
Respiratory disease (sleep apnea or obesity–hypoventilation syndrome)
Osteoarthritis
Hepatobiliary disease (gallstones or hepatomegaly)

Previous treatments and outcome

Supervised programs
Self-imposed methods of weight loss (caloric restriction, liquid protein supplements)
Surgical procedures
Weight cycling pattern, including peak adult weight

Factors warranting precaution or that may preclude weight reduction

Age < 20 or > 65
History of anorexia nervosa or bulimia
Psychiatric disorders
Pregnancy or lactation

Box 20.2 Physical Examination of the Obese Patient

Vital signs: Height, weight, pulse, blood pressure, waist-to-hip ratio. Blood pressure should be taken using a cuff appropriate for arm size. Bradycardia is seen in hypothyroidism.

Skin: Purple striae, hirsutism, ecchymoses, thin skin, and "moon" facies with plethora suggest Cushing's syndrome. Hirsutism is also seen in polycystic ovary syndrome. Dry, coarse, and cool skin, along with thin, dry hair are seen in hypothyroidism. Tendon, eruptive, or tuberous xanthomas, or xanthelasma suggest hyperlipidemia.

Fat distribution: Truncal distribution with fat accumulation in the supraclavicular and dorsocervical ("buffalo hump") areas suggest Cushing's syndrome.

Thyroid gland: Enlargement may be seen in hypothyroidism.

Edema: Periorbital edema may be seen in myxedema of hypothyroidism. In addition, enlargement of the tongue, wrists, and ankles may occur.

Neurologic examination: A delayed relaxation phase of deep tendon reflexes is suggestive of hypothyroidism.

Laboratory Studies

Fasting blood glucose, thyroid function tests, and serum lipid levels should be performed on patients if they have not recently been done. Measurement of resting energy expenditure is probably best reserved for selected patients, such as those who are unable to lose weight but presumed to be compliant with therapy. Patients with symptoms compatible with sleep apnea should be referred for a formal sleep evaluation and possibly to an otolaryngologist to determine if upper airway obstruction is present. If gallstones are suspected, ultrasonography can be performed. In patients with suspected Cushing's syndrome, a 24-hour urine collection for free cortisol followed by a low-dose dexamethasone suppression test may be helpful. For patients with signs, symptoms, or laboratory studies consistent with a secondary cause for obesity, referral to the appropriate subspecialist should be considered.

Treatment and Results

General Comments

The fact that there are so many different treatments available, including many untested and unproven therapies touted in the lay press, attests to the difficulty of realizing the goals of weight loss and long-term weight loss maintenance. Long-term results from any weight loss program are disappointing to say the least. One year after losing weight approximately one third to two thirds of weight is regained, and 5 years later, almost all of the lost weight is regained (1). Successful long-term weight maintenance involves much more than "going on a diet," which implies eventual discontinuation. Changes in lifestyle behaviors conducive to obesity and consistency over time in continuing indefinitely behaviors that promote weight maintenance are necessary to realize sustained weight loss. The poor long-term results demonstrated across studies to date underscore the difficulty in accomplishing this feat.

At any one time, as many as 40% of women are trying to lose weight (1). The reasons for seeking weight loss and individual perceptions of the need to lose weight for health reasons vary among people. Many who are trying to lose weight are trying to lose "the last 10 pounds" and have relatively few reasons other than cosmetic to do so. In this situation, the potential for doing physical and psychological harm through extreme "dieting" or unhealthy approaches to weight loss can be greater than the minimally increased health risks associated with the slight increase in weight. On the other hand, many obese patients who would benefit from weight loss for health reasons are either not attempting it or are unable to do so. Other obese subjects have few health complications but are at increased risk for developing them. It is important to determine the motives and goals of those patients desiring weight loss, to place health risks in perspective, and communicate an estimate of risk to all obese patients regardless if they are seeking weight loss or not.

Many patients will want to lose weight and see results immediately, which is one reason why VLCDs and surgical approaches seem attractive. However, rapid weight loss is usually followed by rapid weight gain, if the lifestyle behaviors that influenced the development of obesity in the first place are not changed. Gradual but sustained weight loss is more likely to result in long-term weight loss maintenance, which should also result in sustained improvement in associated comorbidities. Patients should be aware that a reasonable and realistic goal is loss of from 1 to 3 lb/week. Faster weight loss than this will be mostly fluid and may also result in increased loss of FFM. An important concept is to encourage the patient to focus on "patterns, not pounds." By making changes in behavior patterns to ones that promote long-term weight management, the pounds will take care of themselves. Weighing every day should not be encouraged because any short-term weight changes are probably a reflection of changes in fluid status or measurement error. Weighing once per week is adequate to document trends in weight over time.

Risks of Weight Loss

Losing weight is not risk free. Improperly designed diets increase the risk of nutritional deficiencies. Patients losing weight rapidly may experience physical symptoms such as nausea, fatigue, weakness, hair loss, and hypotension. The degree of weight loss is proportional to the incidence of symptomatic cholelithiasis. Refeeding after weight loss is associated with edema (and corresponding weight gain), electrolyte disturbances, cholecystitis, and cardiac arrhythmias. Dieting can also lead to emotional and psychological disturbances. Restrictive dieting may promote a feeling of restraint and lead to binge eating behavior (36).

Benefits of Weight Loss on Comorbid Conditions

Weight loss results in marked improvement in many of the comorbidities associated with obesity. Weight reduction improves insulin sensitivity, decreases insulin concentrations, and improves glucose control in type II diabetic patients. The degree of blood pressure lowering is related to the amount of weight loss, although modest amounts of weight loss can result in some improvement. Sleep disturbances can improve markedly with weight loss. Many, but not all, studies show an improvement in the lipid profile after weight loss. In many studies, it has been difficult to separate the effects of weight loss and energy restriction. In tightly controlled studies, weight loss, distinct from energy restriction, resulted in lower triglyceride and LDL cholesterol concentrations, insulin levels, and blood pressure (37,38). Some reports have suggested that temporary weight loss may lead to sustained improvement in these parameters. However, a recent well controlled long-term study found that the improvement in the comorbidities associated with obesity were related to the magnitude and persistence of weight loss maintenance (39). Previously, it was mentioned that physical inactivity, smoking, and alcohol intake were associated with increased abdominal obesity. It follows that improvements in these areas could lead to decreased central distribution of weight although further studies are needed to support this contention.

Guidelines for Weight Control Programs

The weight loss industry is largely unregulated. Unfounded claims of rapid weight loss and guaranteed success are common. As previously discussed, the health risks associated with obesity and the need to lose weight vary among individuals, and there are potential risks associated with weight loss. For these reasons, it is important to use guidelines for weight control programs.

Expert panels have recommended that a weight loss program should consist of three main components: dietary change, exercise, and behavioral modification (40,41). The nutritional program should have a sound scientific rationale, be safe and nutritionally adequate, and practical enough to allow long-term compliance. Exercise should be safe, promote increased energy expenditure and fat loss while minimizing loss of FFM, and become a permanent part of an individual's lifestyle. Behavioral treatment should focus on methods of acquiring new behaviors that will promote weight loss and maintenance and address psychological and social problems that patients encounter as a result of weight loss. Health care professionals working in the areas of diet, exercise, and behavioral modification should possess training and experience in these areas.

In general, the level of medical care in a weight control program should be proportional to the patient's health risk and level of treatment. Subjects should be screened for individuals for whom weight loss is not appropriate (see Box 20.1). Patients with a history of an eating disorder or other psychiatric condition, pregnant or lactating women, or the very young or old should be excluded from treatment. Medical supervision should be available for patients with comorbid conditions or other health risks that may complicate treatment.

Diet Treatment

Very Low Calorie Diets

VLCDs provide 800 kcal/day or less. Early use of VLCDs resulted in serious health complications, including death. Subsequent modification of these diets has shown them to be generally safe under medical supervision. Restricting energy under 800 kcal/day does not seem to result in increased weight loss and is not recommended. Energy restriction causes a lowering of the RMR in proportion to the degree of restriction, which is, in essence, an adaptive response to starvation. This decrease in RMR may be one factor responsible for the lack of increased amounts of weight loss with severe degrees of energy restriction less than 800 kcal/day.

Patients on VLCDs have shown large amounts of weight loss initially, up to 20 kg in 12 to 16 weeks (42). Of the weight that is lost, however, a greater proportion is composed of FFM compared to less calorically restricted diets. Early results of VLCDs showed rapid regain after stopping the program, often to levels above pretreatment weight. In recent years, in an attempt to improve long-term results, VLCDs have been used initially followed by a moderate calorie-restricted diet and behavior modification. Limited data have shown this to be slightly more effective, but long-term results remain no better than with behavioral modification alone.

Low-Calorie Diets

An underrecognized dietary principle that has important implications for weight loss is the energy density of the food consumed. In pure form fat contains 9 kcal/gm, protein 4 kcal/gm, and carbohydrate 4 kcal/gm. Whole foods, on the other hand, vary widely in their energy density. For example, vegetables contain only an average of about 10 kcal/oz compared with fats at 175 kcal/oz. One cup of roasted peanuts contains 875 kcal, which is approximately the same amount of calories as *24* cups of popcorn. One and a third sticks of butter contain the same amount of calories as 10 to 15 medium apples, 10 to 11 *heads* of lettuce, or *35* cups of green beans. Because satiety is determined primarily by the volume of food consumed, foods with a high energy density will lead to an increased rate of energy intake and an overall increase in calories ingested compared to foods with a low energy density. Therefore, to maximally promote weight loss, foods that are low in energy density and high in bulk such as vegetables, fresh fruits, and whole-grain starches should be emphasized at the expense of high-fat foods. By doing this, the rate of energy intake is slowed, and satiety is reached at a lower total intake of calories. Moreover, consuming a diet high in carbohydrate and low in fat may prevent the decrease in RMR observed in energy-restricted diets (43).

The EatRight program at the University of Alabama at Birmingham has reported success in treating obesity using this principle. This program uses an exchange list approach whereby foods are grouped, in order of increasing energy density, into vegetables, fruits, starches, meat and dairy, and fats (44). The intake of foods from the meat and dairy, and especially fat groups, is limited. However, starches are encouraged, and unlimited amounts of fruits and vegetables are allowed. Simple sugars, alcohol, soda, candies, and processed foods are allowed only in very limited quantities; the emphasis is on unprocessed starches, fruits, and vegetables.

Studies have shown this program has a sound scientific rationale (22), is safe, nutritionally adequate (45), palatable, and appropriate for long-term weight control (46). Another advantage is that by allowing unlimited access to certain foods, feelings of restraint may be minimized, unlike many restrictive diets. The restrained eater phenomena has been proposed as leading to less compliance and binge eating behavior. A retrospective study of 213 consecutive subjects enrolled in this program reported the mean weight loss was 6.3 kg (47). After 2 years of follow-up (74% follow-up rate), mean weight loss had increased to 8.0 kg and more than 50% of subjects had maintained their original amount of weight loss or more. There was no significant trend for greater weight rebound with increasing length of follow-up. Because this was a review of consecutive patients and not a selected study group, the results are even more impressive.

Behavioral Modification

Behavioral modification consists of the analysis of factors leading to or following behaviors conducive to obesity (overeating or lack of physical activity) and the subsequent modification of these factors. The various treatment components of behavioral modification programs include self-monitoring (recording of behaviors), stimulus control (restricting environmental factors), contingency management (rewarding appropriate behaviors), changing behavior parameters directly, and cognitive behavior modification (48). An important example of self-monitoring is keeping dietary records, which has been associated with greater success at weight loss. Behavioral modification programs combined with moderate caloric restriction have shown more modest degrees of weight loss compared to VLCDs. In recent studies, the average length of treatment is 18 weeks and mean weight loss is 10 kg. Long-term results are somewhat better than VLCDs, yet still modest. One year after completing a behavioral modification program, two thirds of the weight loss is maintained. However, 5 years after treatment, most of the weight that was lost is regained.

Exercise and Physical Activity

Increasing energy expenditure by increasing physical activity is an essential part of any weight loss program. Exercise can increase the amount of weight loss compared to diet alone. It may also help to minimize the loss of FFM during weight loss, especially during rapid weight loss. Of particular relevance is that exercise is one of the most important factors related to long-term weight loss maintenance (49). Other benefits of exercise include improvements in cardiovascular conditioning, glucose tolerance, mood and sense of well-being, and serum lipids (increased HDL cholesterol and decreased triglycerides). The energy expended during exercise results from the activity itself and the replacement of energy stores in the few hours following activity. Most studies show that there is no sustained effect on RMR, other than indirectly by increasing FFM.

Physical activity recommendations should be tailored to the patient, taking into consideration the patient's lifestyle. There are basically two ways to increase physical activity: through formal exercise and through daily activities. The advantage of increased energy expenditure throughout the day's normal activities is that no special effort is needed to schedule exercise, which may save time. The advantage of formal exercise is greater energy expenditure per unit of time. However, intensity should be balanced with duration. Preferably, the type of exercise chosen should be enjoyable, or it is less likely to be maintained over time. Finally, exercise should become a part of the patient's lifestyle and be continued indefinitely, similar to diet and other behavioral changes, all of which should focus on long-term goals.

Surgery

Surgery has been used to treat obesity by creating anatomic changes in the gastrointestinal tract that lead to malabsorption or decreased energy intake. Earlier procedures, including the jejunoileal bypass, were plagued by complications. In recent years, the most commonly used procedures are the vertical banded gastroplasty and the Roux-en-Y gastric bypass. Some centers are also using the biliopancreatic diversion in selected cases of severe obesity. The amount of weight loss and the risk of nutrient deficiencies is greatest in the biliopancreatic diversion, followed by the gastric bypass and the vertical banded gastroplasty. This is partly related to the degree of malabsorption.

Patients should be carefully selected for surgical procedures. In general, they should fulfill the following criteria: 1) severe obesity (BMI $> 40\,kg/m^2$ or 100% above desirable body weight) or less severe with significant complications; 2) refractory to conservative treatment with diet, exercise, and behavioral modification; and 3) medical complications that are likely to improve with weight loss. In addition, it is imperative the patient be well informed about the procedure, the potential short- and long-term complications, expected results, and long-term treatment and follow-up recommendations following the procedure. Prospective patients should be evaluated by an experienced team with expertise from surgical, medical, nutritional, and psychological disciplines. The operation should be performed by a surgeon with considerable experience with the procedure.

Short-term complications of gastric reduction procedures include perioperative morbidity and mortality. Although reported mortality is low, postoperative complications may be as high as 10% and include wound infections and dehiscence, stomal stenosis, and staple-line leaks, in addition to deep venous thrombosis and other problems related to surgery. Long-term complications include nutritional deficiencies of vitamin B_{12}, folate, and iron, dumping syndrome (gastrointestinal distress, diarrhea, and other symptoms), persistent vomiting, cholecystitis, and pouch and esophageal dilatation.

Many of the patients who undergo surgical procedures for obesity are women of childbearing age. Of particular concern is the risk of fetal damage due to nutrient deficiencies in pregnancy after obesity surgery. This risk should be discussed with all premenopausal women considering such surgery and an effective method of birth control ensured. Pregnancy should be discouraged until weight has stabilized and nutritional status is adequate. Patients considering pregnancy should understand the importance of the increased nutritional requirements and adequate weight gain during pregnancy. Women who become pregnant after a surgical procedure for obesity should be followed closely and nutritional status monitored. The National Institutes of Health Consensus Development Panel has published a statement and recommendations on the use of gastrointestinal surgery for severe obesity (50).

Drugs

Pharmacologic agents have been used for many years to treat obesity. Earlier agents have largely been abandoned because of side effects. Noradrenergic and serotonergic agents, both of which act by suppressing appetite, are two main classes of drugs used to promote weight loss. Examples of noradrenergic agents include benzphetamine (Didrex), phendimetrazine (Plegine and others), diethylpropion (Tenuate), mazindol (Sanorex), phentermine (Fastin and others), and phenylpropanolamine (Dexatrim). Serotonergic drugs include fenfluramine (Pondimin), and fluoxetine (Prozac), which is currently licensed as an antidepressant. Overall, significantly greater amounts of weight loss have been demonstrated in studies using these agents compared with placebo (51). However, the amount is modest (usually < 5 kg) and weight regain is the rule after cessation of treatment. In addition, long-term benefits have not been adequately documented. Newer agents that are currently being studied include thermogenic adrenergic agonists, drugs which promote fat malabsorption by inhibiting lipase, and agents that stimulate lipid oxidation. At the present time pharmacologic agents cannot be recommended for general use and should be used only by persons experienced in their use. There is no role for using thyroid hormone, diuretics, laxatives, or similar therapeutic agents to promote weight loss.

Criteria for Success

The results of treatment for obesity are traditionally judged by the amount of weight lost. Weight loss is obviously an important criterion and may reflect improvement in other parameters. However, weight alone should not be the only criterion used to measure success (52). For example, if a patient is exercising vigorously, body composition may change by increasing FFM and losing fat mass. Because lean tissue is more dense than fat tissue, body weight may not change as much as expected. Other measures of success that can be used include changes in anthropometrics (inches lost), maintenance of weight loss, and improvements in comorbid conditions such as hypertension, dyslipidemia, and diabetes mellitus.

Summary

Obese patients should be encouraged to make changes in lifestyle behaviors to lose weight and reduce the risk of future morbidity and mortality. Weight loss should be particularly encouraged in patients with central distribution of body fat or any of the comorbidities associated with obesity. Lifestyle changes should include increased daily physical activity and exercise, decreased dietary fat, and increased consumption of fresh fruits, vegetables, and whole grain starches. These habits should be continued indefinitely to maintain weight loss and enhance health status. Although results to date suggest that most people will regain their weight loss over time, sustained changes from behaviors conducive to obesity to those that promote weight loss and maintenance offer the best chance at success. Fad diets and overly restrictive diets should be discouraged. Consultation with a registered dietitian for specific dietary instructions is helpful and necessary for most patients. Medically supervised weight loss programs can be considered for any obese patient, especially those refractory to initial therapy or with comorbid conditions.

REFERENCES

1. NIH Technology Assessment Conference on Methods for Voluntary Weight Loss and Control. Ann Intern Med 1992;116:942–949.

2. Kuczmarski RJ. Prevalence of overweight and weight gain in the United States. Am J Clin Nutr 1992;55:495S–502S.

3. Metropolitan Life Insurance Company. New weight standards for men and women. Stat Bull Metropol Life Insur Co 1959;40:1–4.

4. Knapp TR. A methodological critique of the "ideal weight" concept. JAMA 1983;250:506–510.

5. Lee I, Manson JE, Hennekens CH, Paffenbarger RS. Body weight and mortality: a 27-year follow-up of middle-aged men. JAMA 1993;270:2823–2828.

6. Stunkard AJ, Sorensen TIA, Hanis C, et al. An adoption study of human obesity. N Engl J Med 1986;314:193–198.

7. Stunkard AJ, Harris JR, Pedersen NL, McClearn GE. The body-mass index of twins who have been reared apart. N Engl J Med 1990;322:1483–1487.

8. Bogardus C, Lillioja S, Ravussin E, et al. Familial dependence of the resting metabolic rate. N Engl J Med 1986;315:96–100.

9. Ravussin E, Bogardus C. Relationship of genetics, age, and physical fitness to daily energy expenditure and fuel utilization. Am J Clin Nutr 1989;49(suppl):968–975.

10. D'Alessio DA, Kavle EC, Mozzoli MA, et al. Thermic effect of food in lean and obese men. J Clin Invest 1988;81:1781–1789.

11. Nelson KM, Weinsier RL, James LD, et al. Effect

of weight reduction on resting energy expenditure, substrate utilization, and the thermic effect of food in moderately obese women. Am J Clin Nutr 1992;55:924–933.

12. Ravussin E, Lillioja S, Anderson TE, Christin L, Bogardus C. Determinants of 24-hour energy expenditure in man: methods and results using a respiratory chamber. J Clin Invest 1986;78:1568–1578.

13. Lichtman SW, Pisarska K, Berman ER, et al. Discrepancy between self-reported and actual caloric intake and exercise in obese subjects. N Engl J Med 1992;327:1893–1898.

14. Mertz W, Tsui JC, Judd JT, et al. What are people really eating? The relation between energy intake derived from estimated diet records and intake determined to maintain body weight. Am J Clin Nutr 1991;54:291–295.

15. Romieu I, Willett WC, Stampfer MJ, et al. Energy intake and other determinants of relative weight. Am J Clin Nutr 1988;47:406–412.

16. Miller WC, Lindeman AK, Wallace J, Niederpruem M. Diet composition, energy intake, and exercise in relation to body fat in men and women. Am J Clin Nutr 1990;52:426–430.

17. Salmon DMW, Flatt JP. Effect of dietary fat content on the incidence of obesity among ad libitum fed mice. Int J Obesity 1985;9:443–449.

18. Sims EAH, Danforth E, Horton ES, et al. Endocrine and metabolic effects of experimental obesity in man. Recent Prog Horm Res 1973;29:457–496.

19. Swinburn B, Ravussin E. Energy balance or fat balance? Am J Clin Nutr 1993;57(suppl):766S–771S.

20. Flatt JP. The biochemistry of energy expenditure. In: Bray GA, ed. Recent advances in obesity research. Vol. 2. London: Newman, 1978:211–228.

21. Acheson KJ, Schutz Y, Bessard T, et al. Glycogen storage capacity and de novo lipogenesis during massive carbohydrate overfeeding in man. Am J Clin Nutr 1988;48:240–247.

22. Duncan KH, Bacon JA, Weinsier RL. The effects of high and low energy density diets on satiety, energy intake, and eating time of obese and nonobese subjects. Am J Clin Nutr 1983;37:763–767.

23. Flatt JP. Importance of nutrient balance in body weight regulation. Diabetes Metab Rev 1988;6:571–581.

24. Blundell JE, Green S, Burley V. Carbohydrates and human appetite. Am J Clin Nutr 1994;59(suppl): 728S–734S.

25. Williamson DF, Madans J, Anda RF, et al. Smoking cessation and severity of weight gain in a national cohort. N Engl J Med 1991;324:739–745.

26. Weinsier RL, Bracco D, Schutz Y. Predicted effects of small decreases in energy expenditure on weight gain in adult women. Int J Obesity 1993;17:693–700.

27. Pi-Sunyer FX. Medical hazards of obesity. Ann Intern Med 1993;119(7 pt 2):655–660.

28. Manson JE, Stampfer MJ, Hennekens CH, Willett WC. Body weight and longevity. A reassessment. JAMA 1987;257:353–358.

29. Joint National Committee on Detection, Evaluation, and Treatment of High Blood Pressure, Fifth report of the Joint National Committee on Detection, Evaluation, and Treatment of High Blood Pressure. Arch Intern Med 1993;153:154–183.

30. Weinsier RL, Ullman DO. Gallstone formation and weight loss: a review. Obesity Research 1993;1:51–56.

31. Folsom AR, Kaye SA, Sellers TA, et al. Body fat distribution and 5-year risk of death in older women. JAMA 1993;269:483–487.

32. Larsson B, Svardsudd K, Welin L, et al. Abdominal adipose tissue distribution, obesity, and risk of cardiovascular disease and death: 13 year follow up of participants in the study of men born in 1913. Br Med J 1984;288:1401–1404.

33. Institute of Medicine, Food and Nutrition Board, Committee on Nutritional Status During Pregnancy and Lactation. Nutrition during pregnancy, part 1, weight gain. Washington, DC: National Academy Press, 1990.

34. Wadden TA, Stunkard AJ. Social and psychological consequences of obesity. Ann Intern Med 1985;103:(6 pt 2):1062–1067.

35. Gortmaker SL, Must A, Perrin JM, et al. Social and economic consequences of overweight in adolescence and young adulthood. N Engl J Med 1993;329:1008–1012.

36. Polivy J, Herman CP. Dieting and binging: a causal analysis. Am Psychol 1985;40:193–201.

37. Weinsier RL, James LD, Darnell BE, et al. Obesity-related hypertension: evaluation of the separate effects of energy restriction and weight reduction on hemodynamic and neuroendocrine status. Am J Med 1991;90:460–448.

38. Weinsier RL, James LD, Darnell BE, et al. Lipid and insulin concentrations in obese postmenopausal women: separate effects of energy restriction and weight loss. Am J Clin Nutr 1992;56:44–49.

39. Hensrud DD, Weinsier RL, Darnell BE, Hunter GR. Relationship of comorbidities of obesity to weight loss and four-year weight maintenance/rebound. Obesity Research (in press).

40. Weinsier RL, Wadden TA, Ritenbaugh C, et al. Recommended therapeutic guidelines for professional weight control programs. Am J Clin Nutr 1984;40:865–872.

41. Council on Scientific Affairs, American Medical Association. Treatment of obesity in adults. JAMA 1988;260;2547–2551.

42. Wadden TA. Treatment of obesity by moderate and severe caloric restriction. Ann Intern Med 1993;119(7 pt 2):688–693.

43. Hammer RL, Barrier CA, Roundy ES, et al. Calorie-restricted low-fat diet and exercise in obese women. Am J Clin Nutr 1989;49:77–85.

44. Weinsier RL, Johnston M, Doleys D. Time-calorie displacement: approach to weight control. Philadelphia: George F. Stickley, 1983.

45. Weinsier RL, Bacon JA, Birch R. Time-calorie displacement diet for weight control: a prospective evaluation of its adequacy for maintaining normal nutritional status. Int J Obesity 1983;7:539–548.

46. Weinsier RL, Johnston MH, Doleys DM, Bacon JA. Dietary management of obesity: evaluation of the time-energy displacement diet in terms of its efficacy and nutritional adequacy for long-term weight control. Br J Nutr 1982;47:367–379.

47. Fitzwater SL, Weinsier RL, Wooldridge NH, et al. Evaluation of long-term weight changes after a multidisciplinary weight control program. J Am Diet Assoc 1991;91:421–426, 429.

48. Foreyt JP, Goodrick GK. Evidence for success of behavior modification in weight loss and control. Ann Intern Med 1993;119(7 pt 2):698–701.

49. Safer DJ. Diet, behavior modification, and exercise: a review of obesity treatments from a long-term perspective. South Med J 1991;84:1470–1474.

50. Consensus Development Conference Panel. Gastrointestinal surgery for severe obesity: Consensus Development Conference statement. Ann Intern Med 1991;115:956–961.

51. Bray GA. Use and abuse of appetite-suppressant drugs in the treatment of obesity. Ann Intern Med 1993;119(7 pt 2):707–713.

52. Atkinson RL. Proposed standards for judging the success of the treatment of obesity. Ann Intern Med 1993;119(7 pt 2):677–680.

CHAPTER 21

HYPERPROLACTINEMIA

Richard E. Blackwell,
Karen R. Hammond

Hyperprolactinemia is one of the most common endocrine disorders that presents to the primary care physician. Its presentation was described by Chiari and Frommel in 1885 and 1882, respectively. Chiari described two cases of peripheral atrophy of the uterus associated with persistent lactation after pregnancy. Subsequently, Argonz and Delcastillo described the clinical nature of persistent lactation occurring independent of pregnancy, yet associated with the hyposecretion of estrogen. Forbes and Albright described a syndrome of galactorrhea, amenorrhea, and associated low urinary follicle-stimulating hormone (FSH) levels. This was described in 1954 and was found to be associated with pituitary tumors 25% of the time.

Although galactorrhea has been most commonly associated with hyperprolactinemia, it is now known that menstrual dysfunction is a more common presentation. Menstrual dysfunction has been shown to occur approximately 5 years before the onset of galactorrhea in many patients, and any patient presenting with any variant in ovulation (i.e., luteal phase defect, oligo-ovulation, anovulation, or amenorrhea) should be evaluated for hyperprolactinemia. Further, hyperprolactinemia will frequently occur in the pediatric adolescent age group and may present with failure of pubescence, primary amenorrhea, or galactorrhea before the onset of menstruation. These conditions may be associated with headache, which can occur in the presence of either a microadenoma (< 1 cm) or a macroadenoma (>1 cm).

Natural History of Hyperprolactinemia and the Biology of Prolactin Secretion

Prolactin is an ancient molecule that influences many functions in vertebrate organisms. These extend from luteal support and maintenance of lactation and regulation of free fatty acid metabolism in mammals to salt water metabolism in amphibians and the regulation of sexual behavior in bony fish. In 1970, human prolactin was purified and shown to be different from growth hormone. Specific sensitive radioimmunoassays were developed that allowed the measurement of prolactin in vitro and in vivo in the early 1970s. Concomitantly, subsequent studies showed prolactin to be a single polypeptide containing approximately 198 amino acid residues with a molecular weight of 22,000. The structure is folded into a globular form with the folds being connected by three disulfide bonds. There is enormous similarity between the structure of human placental lactogen, human growth hormone, and human prolactin (1). In addition, the gene for human prolactin was cloned in the early 1980s, and it is believed that this gene was derived from a common somatomammotropic precursor. The gene for prolactin is positioned on chromosome 6 and located near the human leukocyte antigen (2). The prolactin molecule exists in at least five forms: little prolactin (molecular weight 22,000) is monomeric and has the highest biologic activity. Big prolactin with a 50,000 molecular weight is a mixture of both diametric and triameric forms; big prolactin has a molecular weight of 100,000 with little biologic activity. Iso-B prolactin has been isolated by isofocusing and is thought to have an effect on reproductive function, and glycosylated prolactin has a molecular weight of approximately 25,000. All of these forms reside in the human lactotrope, which is located in the anterior pituitary. The lactotrope is thought to arise from a common stem cell that gives rise to both somatotropes and lactotropes. The lactotrope is primarily found in the lateral aspect of the pituitary gland and makes up at least 20% of the cell population. The cellular concentration of prolactin varies considerably, reflecting the fact that this is a dynamic hormone, which is released by a variety of agents. Prolactin has been thought to show some variation throughout the menstrual cycle, being highest before ovulation and in the middle of the luteal phase. This is reflected in the studies of Neill, using the reverse hemolytic plaque assay where several populations of cells are described—ones that show little biologic activity and secrete a small amount of prolactin, the others that secrete large amounts of prolactin. Further, it has been suggested that some lactotropes are less responsive to the inhibitory influence of dopamine than others and in fact pituitary tumors have been described that are devoid of dopamine receptors.

At one time prolactin was thought to be unique among the pituitary hormones in that its release was regulated by inhibitory influences from the hypothalamus. This concept was developed following the observation that prolactin secretion persists when the pituitary gland is transplanted in vivo, to sites removed from the base of the brain such as the pneumoderma pouch, the kidney capsule, or maintained in vitro in organ or cell culture. The prolactin-inhibiting factor was at one time thought to be a polypeptide; however, despite numerous attempts no such factor has been isolated. Prolactin seems to be regulated by a host of chemicals that are both stimulatory and inhibitory in nature. Although dopamine appears to be the principle inhibitor of prolactin secretion, γ-aminobutyric acid (GABA) may play a role. When L-dopa is administered to test subjects, it crosses the blood–brain barrier and decreases prolactin secretion within about 2.5 hours. A rebound response occurs that is greater in women than in men. In the stalk-transsected monkey, the inhibitory effect of dopamine on the plasma prolactin level varies as a function of the estrogen concentration. Further, in the estrogen-treated stalk-transsected monkey the infusion of dopamine (0.1 mg/kg per minute) in pulses ranging from 2.5 to 7.5 minutes produces a dose–response inhibition of prolactin secretion. It has been demonstrated in vitro in the rodent that infusion of dopamine into animals pretreated with the inhibitor of dopamine synthesis, α-methylparatyrasine, accounts for 70% of prolactin-inhibiting activity. The remaining 30% appears to arise from factors produced in the neurohypophysis (3). These studies have been confirmed in the monkey model but not in the human being. However, infusion of 0.02–8 mg/kg per minute has been carried out in the human being for 3 to 4 hours. A dose-related suppression of prolactin occurs, and although dopamine is thought not to cross the blood–brain barrier, the median eminence and adenohypophysis lie outside this hypothetical barrier. Further, it is noted that dopamine isolated from stalk portal blood is approximately 0.8 ng/mL which is eightfold greater than found in the peripheral plasma of the rhesus monkey. GABA is secreted into the portal system and receptors for GABA have been isolated on human lactotropes. GABA is in fact a more potent inhibitor of prolactin secretion than is dopamine; however, these two agents seem to produce different effects on the lactotrope. For instance, dopamine induces the storage of newly synthesized prolactin, which is rapidly released after withdrawal of the inhibitor, whereas dopamine does not.

Although inhibition appears to be the primary mechanism by which prolactin is regulated, great interest has been shown in prolactin-stimulating factors. In the early 1970s it was shown that the thyrotropin-releasing howmone (TRH) would acutely release prolactin in vivo and in vitro (4). Recently, vasoactive intestinal peptide (VIP) and angiotensin-II have been shown to stimulate both the synthesis and the release of prolactin. The injection of hormones such as TRH cause the release of thyroid-stimulating hormone (TSH). This response is regulated by circulating triiodothyronine (T_3) and thyroxine (T_4). This accounts for the fact that prolactin secretion can occur independent of TSH, for instance, following suckling.

The VIP porcine duodenal duct polypeptide is found throughout the central nervous system (CNS). It has been measured in hypothalamic blood samples, and infusion of VIP into the stalk-resected monkeys at 20 μg/kg induces an acute rise in prolactin secretion (5). Further, it appears that the hormone may be produced in the pituitary gland and serves as an autocrine regulator of prolactin secretion. Likewise, angiotensin-II has been shown to stimulate prolactin release in vivo and in vitro and angiotensin-II receptors are found on the lactotrope. Likewise, its injection brings about the rapid release of prolactin and it appears to be the most potent releasor of this hormone with activity far greater than TRH. Other neurotransmitters and modulators have been shown to modify secretion including serotonin, which causes an acute rise in prolactin secretion; the opioids, which inhibit dopamine turnover; histamine, a hypothalamic neurotransmitter that stimulates prolactin release by acting on the H_1 receptor; neurotensin, a tridecapeptide; and substance P, an undecapeptide, both stimulate prolactin secretion. Their physiologic role is as yet unclear.

Prolactin regulation is complex. Retrograde flow has been demonstrated in the hypothalamic portal system and prolactin has been shown to affect its own secretion via a short feedback loop (6). It has been demonstrated for instance that interventricular injection of prolactin results in increased dopamine turnover in the median eminence. A high rate of turnover has been demonstrated both during lactation and pregnancy and this is decreased by hypophysectomy or treatment with dopamine. In fact, autoradiographs of prolactin-secreting tumors have been associated with reduced pituitary prolactin content. Further, intrahypophyseal mechanisms appear to be involved in the regulation of prolactin secretion. VIP has been demonstrated to be synthesized in the lactotrope from radiolabeled amino acids and has been shown to stimulate prolactin secretion. A number of other reports suggest that gonadotropes may exert regulatory influence on prolactin secretion. In vivo and in vitro studies have shown that synthetic gonadotropin-releasing hormone (GnRH) will release prolactin in the rat using a superfusion model and in vitro in a human pituitary monolayer system (7). Incubation of GnRH with lactotropes separated from large gonadotropes fails to increase prolactin secretion, whereas coaggregation of these two cell types restores the stimulatory effect of GnRH on prolactin. Further, coincubation of a potent GnRH antagonist with GnRH inhibits the release of prolactin, whereas coincubation of this antagonist with synthetic TRH fails to alter prolactin release. Likewise, the incubation of the α chain of luteinizing hormone (LH) has been shown to stimulate the differentiation of rat fetal lactotropes. Further, incubation of β-LH or FSH with human pituitary cells in vitro fails to stimulate prolactin secretion, whereas coincubation of antiserum LH and FSH inhibits the GnRH-mediated release of prolactin (8). Likewise, the GnRH-associated peptide, a peptide component of the precursor of GnRH, has been reported to inhibit prolactin secretion in the rat.

These complex interrelationships perhaps give some insight into the natural history of hyperprolactinemia. Many common neurotransmitters and neuromodulators are involved in prolactin regulation. Many of these, such as dopamine and opioids, interface with the regulators of the menstrual cycle. A number of these factors and their metabolic pathways are influenced by such things body weight, stress, and size. A number of reports in the literature suggest that dysfunction of dopamine metabolism may be part of the natural history of the development of hyperprolactinemia and prolactinomas. These come from studies that show abnormal responses to dopamine-altering drugs after resection of prolactinomas. Support for this notion is also found in the clinical observation that following resection of microadenomas 50% of patients persist in having hyperprolactinemia and 70% of patients have hyperprolactinemia following resection of macroadenomas despite infrequent recurrence of tumors. Therefore, one of the causative agents of hyperprolactinemia may be a dysfunction in dopamine metabolism. A second possible cause of hyperprolactinemia may be the evolution of lactotropes that either have suppressed or absent dopamine receptors. Pituitary tumors have been studied histologically that fail to bind dopamine or its agonists. Those tumors, while rare, are unresponsive to drugs such as bromocriptine.

A third possible cause of hyperprolactinemia stems from the relationship of gonadotropes and other trophic cell types to lactotropes. It is becoming evident that many factors are involved in the paracrine regulation of lactotropes including the various chains of gonadotropins and possibly growth factors. Regardless of the mechanisms involved in the generation of hyperprolactinemia and prolactinomas, it seems to be a rather benign process. Expectant management of pituitary prolactinomas over 8 to 10 years results in a modest 10% growth, yet a 30% resolution of lesions (9). When the majority of hyperprolactinemic patients and those with prolactinomas are treated with dopamine agonists such as bromocriptine, suppression of prolactin occurs and either stabilization or diminution of tumor size is found in the majority of patients. Thus, the hyperprolactinemic states including those associated with prolactinomas behave as an endocrinopathy.

Evaluation of Hyperprolactinemia

The patient who presents with galactorrhea, menstrual dysfunction, or disorders of pubertal development should undergo evaluation of the serum prolactin levels. Prolactin secretion is physiologically stimulated by stress, breast examination, and food intake and follows a sleep-entrained pattern (10). In the past it has been recommended that prolactin be measured an hour away from meals, preferably in the late morning or early afternoon. Recently these beliefs have been challenged in that prospective controlled studies evaluating the effect of amino acid intake such as tryptophan, tyrosine, and arginine in normal cycling reproductive age women failed to show significant elevation of prolactin within an hour's follow-up (Fig 21.1). Likewise, breast examination carried out in a similar group of women failed to result in the acute release of prolactin (Fig 21.2). Although breast examination or suckling will result in an elevated prolactin level in women who are pregnant or in postpartum women and the infusion of pharmacologic doses of arginine or other amino acids may elevate prolactin levels in men, it appears that these events taken in the context of daily practice do not markedly influence our accurate measurement of prolactin.

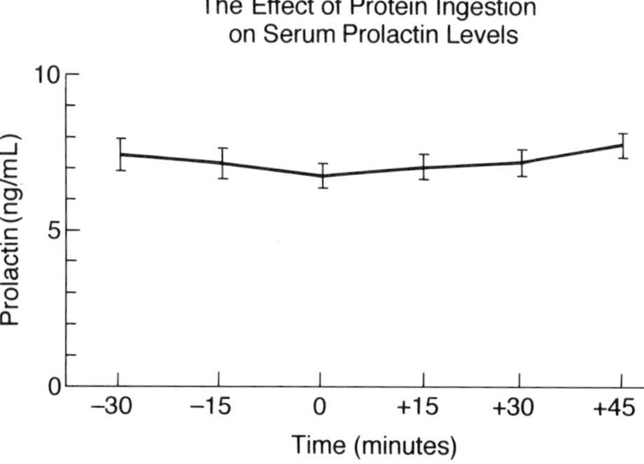

Fig 21.1 Change in serum prolactin level after oral ingestion of a food supplement rich in arginine, tryptophan, and tyrosine. (n=11)

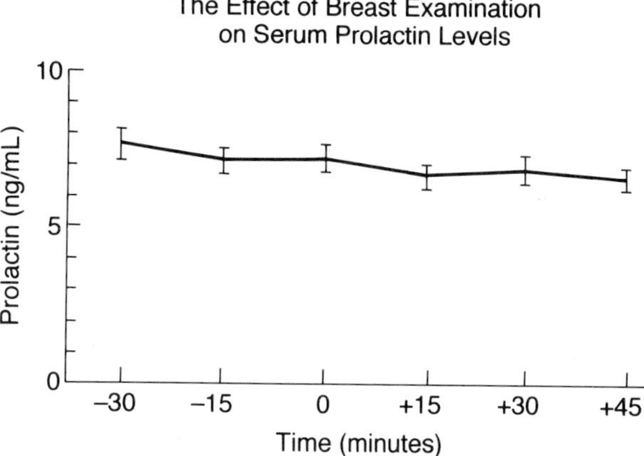

Fig 21.2 Change in serum prolactin level after breast examination. (n=11)

Likewise, physicians have felt it necessary to measure multiple samples of the hormone at different time intervals. This is partially based on the observation that there is great heterogeneity in prolactin assays and the accuracy of its measurement as exemplified by the tabulation of College of American Pathologists standards. In 1985, data suggested that multiple assays carried out in nearly 400 measurements resulted in a mean value of 95 with a range extending from 5 to 135. Considering that most contemporary prolactin assays were developed from monoclonal antibodies and the measurement is carried out on a single serum sample, although analyzed by an automated system, room for error exists. Further, the probability of obtaining a normal level after measurement of an elevated level of prolactin is unclear. Until these issues are resolved by prospective analyses, it is recommended that two elevated prolactin levels be obtained on separate occasions. It is further suggested that in view of the fact that compensated hypothyroidism will occasionally be found in the patient with hyperprolactinemia, that a high sensitivity TSH level be determined simultaneously with a second sample.

In years past, great emphasis was placed on the evaluation of dynamic response of various pituitary hormones to releasing factors and other trophic stimuli. Although numerous reports appeared in the literature suggesting changes in patient populations, these studies are inapplicable to individual situations and have been abandoned. Their use appears to be in the postoperative evaluation of pituitary function following transsphenoidal hypophysectomy.

Likewise, visual field examination using a variety of different systems including Goldman-Bowl perimetry was used for the evaluation of the patient with hyperprolactinemia. It seems clear that patients with large suprasellar macroadenomas have superior bitemporal hemianopsia demonstrated on field examination 68% of the time (Fig 21.3). However, lesions under 1 cm and those that do not have suprasellar extension, cannot, by definition, produce visual field alterations. Therefore, it is recommended that no visual field examination be carried out unless the patient has a suprasellar macroadenoma demonstrated by radiography. Should field defects be detected in the patient with a suprasellar macroadenoma, compensated hypothyroidism should be excluded because these individuals will present with evidence of suprasellar tumor and visual defect secondary to thyrotrope hypertrophy (11). The appropriate treatment of this situation is suppression with Synthroid, not neurosurgery or radiation therapy.

The choice of radiographic technology used to evaluate patients with prolactinomas and hyperprolactinemia is controversial. Both modern computed tomography (CT) scan and magnetic resonance imaging (MRI) are acceptable for differentiating between

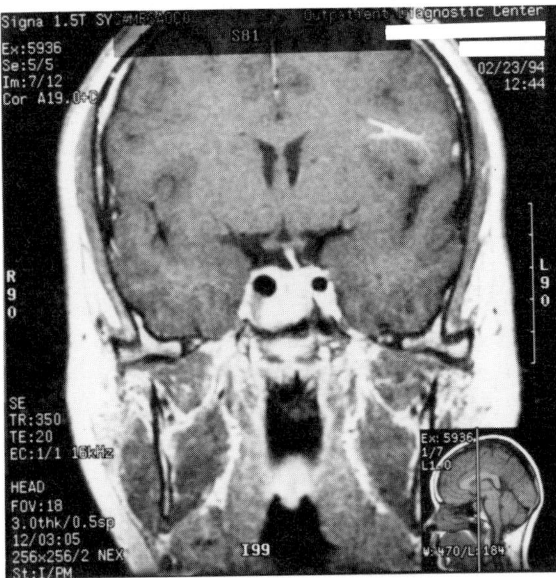

Fig 21.3 MRI of patient with suprasellar macroadenoma and visual field change.

the states of pituitary hyperplasia, microadenoma, and macroadenoma. Because hyperplasia and microadenomas are handled identically, the real issue centers around the ability to differentiate between tumors greater than or less than 1 cm. Either the 9800 CT scan or conventional MRI will scan in 2-mm increments. Therefore, although MRI perhaps gives better resolution of soft tissue, either is acceptable for the evaluation of hyperprolactinemia when one considers the cost difference. Though the incidence of pituitary tumors seems to correlate with serum prolactin levels to some degree, different investigators would choose to scan at different levels. At a prolactin level of 50 ng/mL approximately 25% of individuals will have a microtumor, at a level of 100 ng/mL 50% of individuals will be found to have a tumor, and virtually all patients with levels greater than 200 ng/mL will be found to have a tumor (12). Therefore, many clinicians will institute radiographic surveillance when the prolactin level reaches 100 ng/mL, others at 50 ng/mL, and those of us with a strong interest in hyperprolactinemia will scan all patients with prolactin levels greater than our laboratory normals. Although there seems to be some correlation between prolactin level and incidence of tumors, many women with large endocrine inactive tumors will have slight elevations in prolactin.

A large number of techniques have been used to assess the presence of a prolactinoma by radiography. Posteroanterior and lateral skull films with or without cone-down view can at times detect the largest adenomas, assuming that sellar erosion occurs. These are infrequently used but they may have a rebirth with the advent of managed health care. Sellar tomography has an unacceptably high false-positive and false-negative result rate and has been abandoned. Pituitary arteriography with magnification subtraction technique was used for a brief period; however, patients occasionally developed unwanted central nervous system side effects as a result of this. CT scanning has been the mainstay for the evaluation of pituitary tumors for a number of years (13). New generation machines will produce images in 2-mm sections, which is adequate for evaluation of both microadenomas and macroadenomas. The technique is cost effective; however, patients are exposed to radiation. MRI, the latest of the radiographic techniques, gives excellent visualization of the sella and surrounding areas and requires no radiation exposure; however, it has the disadvantage of being considerably more expensive than CT scanning (Fig 21.4). Payment for MRI scans are often denied by insurance carriers and this should be considered when ordering this test. In the past, radiographic imaging of the pituitary gland was carried out much more frequently in patients who developed adenomas. However, over the last 20 years it has become clear that these lesions grow much slower than originally thought and that scanning requirements can be considerably relaxed. For instance, patients with microadenomas, if untreated, show virtually no change in an 8-year follow-up with a 30% resolution of tumors. Even patients with macroadenomas, particularly those on medical therapy, will fail to show enlargement of lesions and many times the lesions shrink dramatically or are undetectable by the best radiographic technology. Therefore, either CT scanning or MRI is appropriate for making the diagnosis of a pituitary tumor; however, the choice of technique or long-term follow-up may be dictated by whether one is dealing with a small or large tumor.

Treatment of Hyperprolactinemia

The treatment of hyperprolactinemic syndromes depends on several factors: 1) whether a pituitary tumor is present or not and whether this lesion is greater or less than 10 mm, 2) whether fertility is desired by the individual, and 3) whether symptoms are present such as headache or visual field disturbances that require therapy (Box 21.1). Patients with functional hyperprolactinemia (i.e., individuals having no detectable pituitary tumor by either CT scan or MRI) may be followed expectantly if they have regular menstruation, treated with cyclic progestogen if they are euestrogenic, maintained on oral contraceptive agents or cyclic estrogen/progestogen if they are hypoestrogenic, or treated with dopamine agonists such as bromocriptine or pergolide mesylate, which render them euprolactinemic and usually cyclic. Individuals with microadenomas can be treated neurosurgically with transsphenoidal hypophysectomy or with dopamine agonists as can patients who have macroadenomas. In addition, the patient with a macroadenoma or invasive adenoma can be treated with primary or adjunctive radiation therapy.

Perhaps the oldest therapy for the treatment of pituitary tumors is neurosurgical resection of the lesion. Originally, the resections were carried out by craniotomy; however, modern neurosurgeons perform the vast majority of these resections trans-

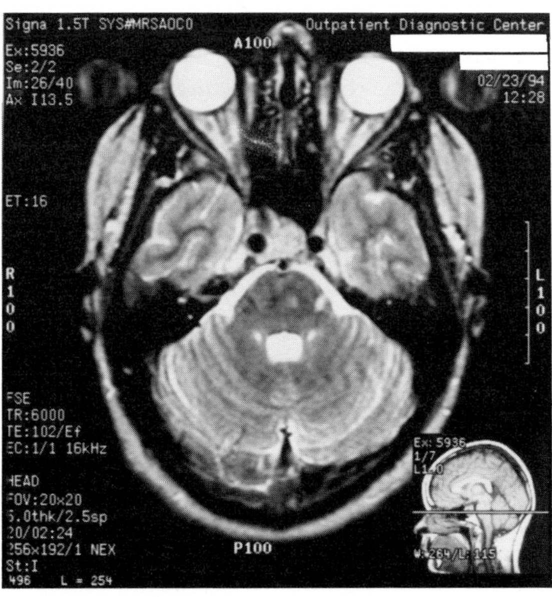

Fig 21.4 MRI of patient with macroadenoma.

Box 21.1 Treatment of Hyperprolactinemia

Hyperplasia

- Observe
- Birth control pill
- Cyclic estrogen and progesterone
- Dopamine agonist
  1. Bromocriptine 1.25–15.00 mg PO four times daily
  2. Pergolide mesylate 50–100 mg every day
  3. CV205-502 80–120 mg every day

Microadenoma

- Same
- Surgery

Macroadenoma

- Dopamine agonist
- Surgery
- Radiation therapy

sphenoidally, working in conjunction with the otolaryngologist. The resectability of lesions depends on size and location and the success of surgery seems to correlate with size of lesion and prolactin level. The general literature suggests that transsphenoidal resection of microadenomas is highly successful from the viewpoint of tumor eradication; however, patients remain hyperprolactinemic approximately 50% of the time (14,15). The failure rate increases markedly when dealing with macroadenomas and large reviews have suggested a 70% failure to resolve either the tumor or hyperprolactinemia (16). Although it has been suggested that prolactinomas arise from single cells, at least eight reports in the literature suggest that patients have abnormal dopamenergic CNS function following resection of such lesions, suggestive of at least a partial neurotransmitter dysfunction in the development of hyperprolactinemia and perhaps adenomas. Therefore, in many centers, the primary neurosurgical approach has been abandoned for the treatment of these lesions with substitution of long-term medical therapy.

It was noted during the Middle Ages that women who ate bread made from rye flour contaminated with the fungus *Claviceps purpura* developed gangrenous ergotism and failure to lactate. A disease called Saint Anthony's fire resulted from the ingestion of ergot alkaloid (ergopeptines). Subsequently, these compounds were extracted for obstetric and other use; however, it was the development of the dopamine agonist bromocriptine (Parlodel) in the mid 1970s that revolutionized the care of the patient with hyperprolactinemia. This compound inhibits prolactin secretion and synthesis in vivo and in vitro, normalizes prolactin levels in the vast majority of patients afflicted with hyperprolactinemia, and at times has caused astounding shrinkage of even the largest prolactinomas (17). Bromocriptine is administered orally in doses ranging from 1.25 mg up to 160 mg in the patient with Parkinson's disease. However, the majority of patients with hyperprolactinemia will respond effectively to doses of 2.5–15 mg/day. Unfortunately, the ingestion of bromocriptine is not without side effects with the vast majority of patients developing gastrointestinal complaints such as nausea. Some patients are hypersensitive to the drug and intractable vomiting develops. Likewise, nasal stuffiness, dysphoria, and lethargy are common side effects and at extremely high doses, psychosis and fatal tachyarrhythmias have been reported. To maximize the effectiveness of bromocriptine therapy and minimize its side effects, it has been demonstrated that this drug is highly effective in suppressing prolactin when taken at bedtime and nausea can be limited by its vaginal administration (18). It is suggested that the drug be begun at 1.25 mg at bedtime and increased until it suppresses prolactin levels over the next 4 weeks.

For patients who are unable to tolerate bromocriptine ingestion or who fail to respond to it, the only alternative is pergolide mesylate (Permax). This drug is a nonergoline dopamine agonist, is three times more potent than bromocriptine, and is taken once a day. Its active dose range is 50–100 μg. It is highly effective in suppressing hyperprolactinemia in patients with and without pituitary tumors (19). The drug is currently approved by the Food and Drug Administration (FDA) for the treatment of Parkinson's disease and is used for the treatment of hyperprolactinemia in Europe and Canada.

The newest agent used to treat hyperprolactinemia is CV205-502. This drug is effective in suppressing hyperprolactinemia in the 60–80 μg dose range and has a 30% better side effect profile than does bromocriptine (20). Like bromocriptine or pergolide mesylate, however, patients still can experience dysphoria, lethargy, nasal stuffiness, and at times nausea. It is unclear when this drug will be approved by the FDA; however, clinical trials are completed.

Finally, radiation therapy is highly effective in the treatment of all types of prolactinomas. The course of therapy is generally divided into four or five fractions over 5 weeks with a dose range falling between 3500 and 5500 rads at the 95% isodose line. A number of radiation sources have been used to treat prolactinomas including radiocobalt teletherapy and 4-MeV line accelerator. Complications from radiation therapy include epilation, optic nerve and chiasm injury, brain necrosis, and sarcoma formation. Likewise, there is loss of trophic hormone secretion and patients can develop both hypoadrenalism and hypothyroidism. In addition to the conventional radiotherapy, proton radiosurgery using open or stereotactic technique is available. Bragg-Peak proton hypophysectomy appears to have the lowest mortality rate and the highest prospect for cure for the treatment of prolactinomas. For instance, Kjellberg and Kliman treated 44 patients with proton therapy with no recurrences. In a series of 678 patients, 5 recurrences or 0.7% were found (21).

Long-Term Management of Hyperprolactinemia

Since human prolactin was separated from growth hormone in 1972 and radioimmunoassays were developed for clinical use, the first generation of patients is now being followed for long periods of time. In addition, some of this cohort of women have entered menopause and must make decisions about estrogen replacement therapy. The primary issue that must be dealt with in the hyperprolactinemic patient without evidence of a prolactinoma appears to be the loss of bone mineral content in the face of both hyperprolactinemia and hypoestrogenism. The rate of bone loss appears to exceed that found in other hypoestrogenic states and this bone loss has been shown to be reversible following bromocriptine therapy (22,23). Therefore, it seems preferable in this group of patients to either treat them with a dopamine agonist or some form of estrogen replacement therapy. In general, this tends to be a life-long process although following pregnancy prolactin levels tend to fall for as yet unexplained reasons, and at times patients will become euprolactinemic following delivery. The same management scheme appears to be applicable to the patient with a microadenoma and neither pregnancy nor estrogen replacement therapy appears to be contraindicated in this group (24). In the past it was felt that because the pituitary hypertrophy occurred during pregnancy and occasionally a tumor was found to expand during this period of time estrogen therapy was contraindicated. In addition, estrogen has a biphasic effect on prolactin secretion as does progesterone. In vitro studies in rabbits and sheep have suggested that sex steroids may stimulate prolactin secretion. However, several prospective trials have demonstrated that birth control pills have only a slight positive effect on prolactin secretion and do not cause the expansion of prolactinomas. The use of estrogen replacement therapy and the achievement of pregnancy in the patient with a macroadenoma appears to be less clear. No prospective trials have dealt with these issues and only antidotal experience is available from a limited number of clinicians worldwide. Two schools of thought exist with regard to the treatment of macroadenomas during pregnancy—expectant management and continuous bromocriptine. The author's limited experience over the last 17 years with approximately half a dozen pregnant patients with macroadenomas have shown no expansion or complication during pregnancy using expectant management (Figs 21.5 and 21.6). Likewise, a limited number of patients with macroadenomas have been treated with estrogen replacement therapy and no increased prolactin secre-

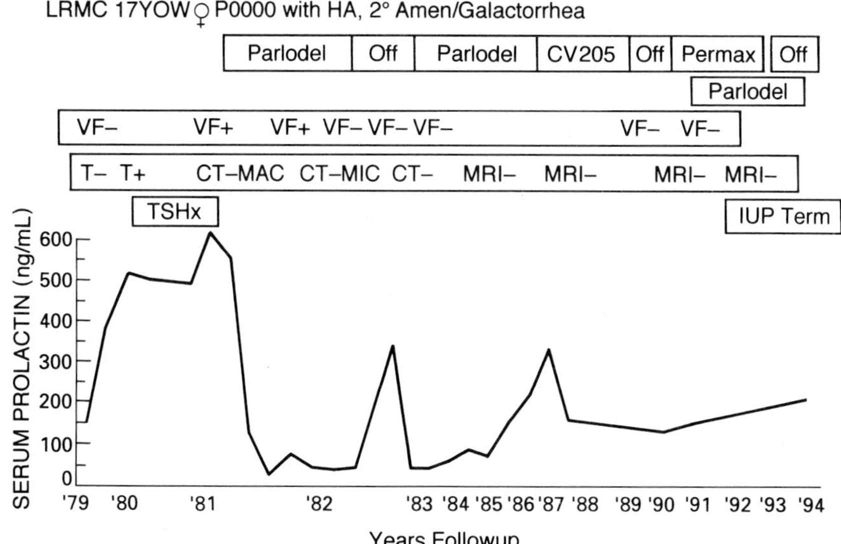

Fig 21.5 Fifteen-year follow-up of a patient with a macroadenoma.

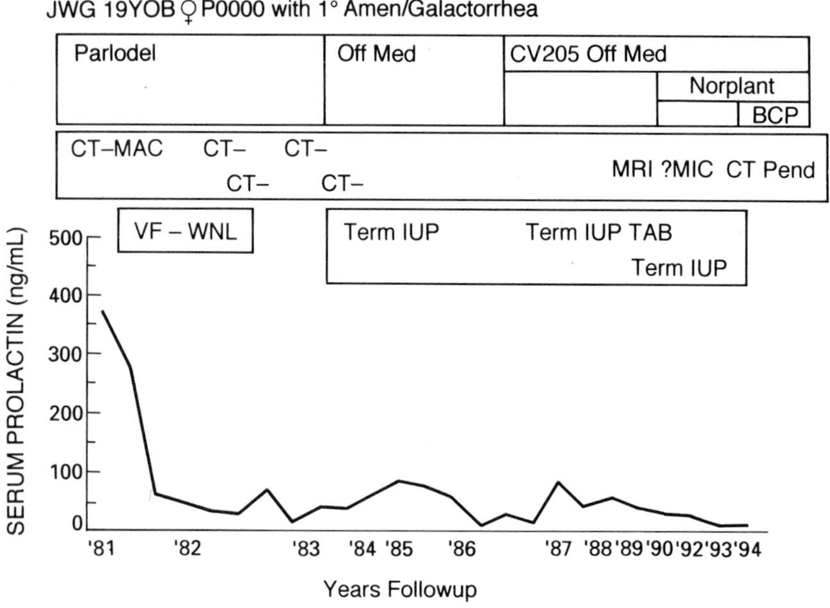

Fig 21.6 Thirteen-year follow-up of a patient with a macroadenoma.

tion or tumor expansion has been noted, although all of these patients are maintained on simultaneous bromocriptine therapy. Patients with microadenomas are being treated with estrogen replacement therapy during menopause and as yet none of these patients followed at our institution have had an increase in prolactin secretion or expansion of tumor. No case series has been reported on the effect of estrogen replacement therapy in the patient with a macroadenoma either with or without dopamine agonist therapy.

The recommendation for follow-up of patients with functional hyperprolactinemia includes yearly general physical examination and prolactin level determination. For the patient with a microadenoma, the same follow-up protocol can be used with CT or MRI scans being performed every 10 years. The patient with a macroadenoma should be seen twice a year and prolactins measured, should be maintained on continuous bromocriptine therapy with radiographic images being performed at every widening interval, generally in the neighborhood of every 5 years. Any abrupt rise in prolactin or change in CNS symptoms should be investigated with measurement of prolactin, evaluation of the pituitary with radiographic imaging, and perhaps visual field examination. Patients with hyperprolactinemia and microadenomas should be managed by the obstetrician/gynecologist either with or without reproductive endocrine consult. Patients with macroadenomas should, in general, be followed in conjunction with a reproductive endocrinologist and neurosurgeon.

REFERENCES

1. Suh HK, Frantz AG. Size heterogeneity of human prolactin in plasma and pituitary extracts. J Clin Endocrinol Metab 1974;39:928–935.

2. Owerbach D, Rutter WJ, Cooke NE, et al. The prolactin gene is located on chromosome 6 in humans. Science 1981;212:815–916.

3. Neill JD, Luque EH, Mulchahey JJ, Nagy G. Regulation of prolactin secretion. In: Blackwell RE, Chang RJ, eds. Prolactin-related disorders. New York: Macmillan Healthcare Information, 1987;5–14.

4. Vale W, Blackwell RE, Grant G, Guillemin R. TRF and thyroid hormones on prolactin secretin by rat pituitary cells in vitro. Endocrinology 1973;93:26–33.

5. Marsushita N, Kato Y, Shimatsu A, et al. Effects of VIP, TRH, GABA and dopamine on prolactin release from superfused rat anterior pituitary cells. Life Sci 1983;32:1263–1269.

6. Bergland R, Page R. Can the pituitary secrete directly to the brain? (Affirmative anatomical evidence). Endocrinology 1978;102:1325–1338.

7. Blackwell RE, Rodgers-Neame NT, Bradley EL, Asch RH. Regulation of human prolactin secretion in gonadotropin releasing hormone in vitro. Fertil Steril 1986;56:26–31.

8. Blackwell RE, Garrison PN. Inhibition of prolactin secretion by antiserum to the alpha- and beta-subunits of gonadotropin. Am J Obstet Gynecol 1987;156:863–868.

9. Weiss MH, Teal J, Gott P, et al. Natural history of microprolactinomas: six-year follow-up. Neurosurgery 1983;12:180–183.

10. Blackwell RE. In: Wallach EE, Kempers RD, eds. Modern trends in infertility and conception control. Vol. 4. Diagnosis and management of prolactinomas. Chicago: Year Book Medical Publishers, 1988:197–208.

11. Yamamoto K, Saito K, Takai T, et al. Visual field defects and pituitary enlargement in primary hypothyroidism. J Clin Endocrinol Metab 1983;67:283–287.

12. Blackwell RE, Boots LR, Goldenberg RL, et al. Assessment of pituitary function in patients with serum prolactin levels greater than 100 ng/mL. Fertil Steril 1970;32:177–182.

13. Newton DR, Witz S, Norman D, Newton TH. Economic impact of CT scanning on the evaluation of pituitary adenomas. Am J Radiol 1983;140:576.

14. Domonigue JN, Richmond IL, Wilson CB. Results of surgery in 114 patients with prolactin-secreting pituitary adenomas. Am J Obstet Gynecol 1980;137: 102–108.

15. Faria MA, Tindall GT. Transsphenoidal microsurgery for prolactin-secreting pituitary adenomas: results in 100 women with the amenorrhea-galactorrhea syndrome. J Neurosurg 1982;56:33–43.

16. Serri O, Rasio E, Beauregard H, Hardy J, Somma M. Recurrence of hyperprolactinemia after selective transsphenoidal adenomectomy in women with prolactinoma. N Engl J Med 1983;309:280–283.

17. Molitch M, Elton R, Blackwell RE, et al., and the Bromocriptine Study Group. Bromocriptine as primary therapy for prolactin secreting macroadenomas: results of a prospective, multicenter study. J Clin Endocrinol Metab 1985;60(4):698–705.

18. Katz E, Weiss BE, Schran HF, et al. Increased levels of bromocriptine following vaginal as compared to oral administration. Fertil Steril 1991;55:882–884.

19. Blackwell RE, Bradley EL Jr, Kline LB, et al. Comparison of dopamine agonists in the treatment of hyperprolactinemic syndromes: a multicenter study. Fertil Steril 1983;39:744–748.

20. Vance ML, Cragun JR, Reimnitz C, et al. CV205-502 treatment of hyperprolactinemia. J Clin Endocrinol Metab 1989;68:336–339.

21. Kjellberg R, Kliman B. Proton radiosurgery for functioning pituitary adenomas. In: Tindall GT, Collins WF, eds. Clinical management of pituitary disorders. New York: Raven Press, 1979:315–334.

22. Klibanski A, Greenspan SL. Increase in bone mass after treatment of hyperprolactinemic amenorrhea. N Engl J Med 1986;315:542–546.

23. Klibanski A, Neer RM, Beitins IZ, et al. Decreased bone density in hyperprolactinemic amenorrhea. N Engl J Med 1986;303:1511–1514.

24. Divers WA, Yen SSC. Prolactin-producing microadenomas in pregnancy. Obstet Gynecol 1983;61:425–429.

CHAPTER 22

HIRSUTISM

Richard E. Blackwell

Next to menstrual dysfunction, hirsutism is probably the most common endocrine complaint that presents to the primary care physician. Many patients who present with the complaint of hirsutism, in fact, have a strong hereditary overtone to their problem. For instance, patients of North European, American Indian, or Oriental background can be expected to have little body hair, whereas individuals from the Balkan region and the Mediterranean areas will have increased amounts of hair growth. It is therefore best to quantify hair growth with a Ferriman-Gallwey score, which evaluates hair distribution on the lip, chin, chest, abdomen, arms, inner thigh, back, and buttocks (Fig 22.1) (1). In addition, it is useful to ask the patient to compare her body hair growth to other female members of her family and to pay particular attention to central axis hair growth when staging hirsutism (Fig 22.2). Further, the age of the patient should be considered because older women who have increased luteinizing hormone (LH) drive to the thecal cells will produce increased androgens.

The patient who does not have a genetic propensity toward hirsutism will either produce excess androgens from the ovary or adrenal gland or metabolize those androgens more efficiently in the periphery (2–4). Therefore, the diagnosis and treatment of hirsutism concentrates on the secretion and metabolism of androstenedione, dehydroepiandrosterone (DHEA), dehydroepiandrosterone sulfate (DHEAS), testosterone, and dehydrotestosterone. The ovary directly secretes testosterone and androstenedione plus DHEA. The adrenal gland secretes testosterone only in conditions of pathology but does secrete androstenedione in amounts equal to that produced by the ovary. The adrenal also secretes DHEAS, the sulfated form of DHEA, in quantities larger than any other systemic androgen. Likewise, both ovary and adrenal glands secrete δ-5-androstenediol; however, a greater amount is produced by the adrenal and 11-β-hydroxyandrostenedione has been demonstrated to be a specific marker for adrenal androgen production.

Although testosterone and DHEAS are frequently measured by the clinician as an index of androgen secretion, DHEAS, androstenedione, and DHEA are relatively weak androgens. The more potent androgen, testosterone, which is converted to a more potent androgen dehydrotestosterone, 3-α-androstenediol and its metabolite 3-α-androstenediol glucuronide, are perhaps better markers of androgen metabolism (5). Further, dehydrotestosterone is tightly bound to sex hormone-binding globulin and is not very useful as a peripheral marker. Further, there is no back conversion of 3-α-androstenediol glucuronide to dehydrotestosterone. Likewise, the glucuronide conversion product of androstenedione is also a good marker of peripheral 5-α-reductase activity.

Not only is the production of the various androgens from the adrenal and the ovary important in the expression of hirsutism, primary transport proteins of androgen sex hormone-binding globulin will have a marked effect on its metabolic clearance (6). A variety of pathologies such as exogenous androgen to estrogen, acromegaly, thyroid dysfunction, liver disease, and obesity can effect the production of sex hormone-binding globulin.

Physiology of Hair Growth

Villus hair, under the influence of androgen, changes to a terminal hair pattern. Hair development passes

HIRSUTISM SCORING STANDARDS
from Hatch et al., Am J Obstet Gynecol
140: 815, 1981
adapted from Ferriman and Gallwey

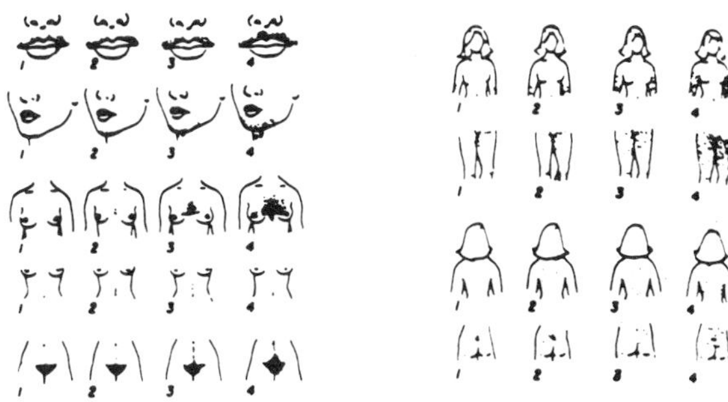

A score of 8 or more indicates Hirsutism

Patients Name ______________________

Medical # ______________________

Total Score ______________________

Date ______________________

Fig. 22.1 Hirsutism scoring sheet used by University of Alabama at Birmingham. It is based on the Ferriman-Gallway system. *(Courtesy of Dr. Ricardo Azziz.)*

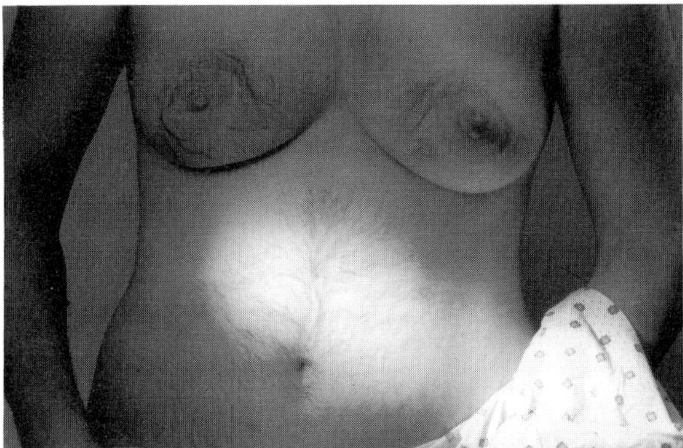

Fig. 22.2 Patient with severe hirsutism.

through several phases; pilogen, catagen, and anagen. Androgens are necessary for the recruitment of terminal hair development, they prolong the time a hair spends in anagen, and they regulate the 5-α-reductase activity, which ultimately modulates androgen signals (7). On the scalp as an example, hair may persist in anagen for 3 years, whereas on the face, this is reduced to 4 months. Androgen on the other hand might average 3 months for both facial and scalp hair.

Causes of Hirsutism

A limited number of conditions result in androgen excess: exogenous drug ingestion, idiopathic, polycystic ovary syndrome, ovarian hyperthecosis, androgen-producing ovarian tumors, congenital adrenal hyperplasia, androgen-producing adrenal tumors, and Cushing's syndrome. Drug-induced androgen excess is quite rare in modern practice and limited almost exclusively to compounds that contain testosterone. These might include testosterone injections, mixtures of estrogen and testosterone, and danocrine. It should be noted that the compound danazol (Danocrine) is actually a very weak androgen; however, it results in a suppression of the sex hormone-binding globulin, therefore, causing a threefold rise in free testosterone (8). Hirsutism is one of its known side effects; therefore, this drug is limited to a 6-month therapeutic trial. However, with the advent of the gonadotropin-releasing hormone (GnRH) analogues such as leuprolide acetate (Lupron) and histrelin acetate (Synarel) for the treatment of endometriosis, danazol is rarely used for therapy of this disorder. Other medications related to testosterone such as 19-nonsteroids and synthetic progestogens (norethindrone and levonorgesterel) can result in hirsutism.

Idiopathic Hirsutism

Idiopathic hirsutism is a common disorder associated with increased androgen expression. This occurs in the face of normal menstrual cycles and normal levels of both testosterone and DHEAS in women. At times women with this disorder may have a slight increase in free testosterone suggesting an alteration in sex hormone-binding globulin production; however, it may also be due to increased 5-α-reductase activity within the hair cell. This is supported by the fundings of an increased 5-α-reductase activity in the skin of patients with idiopathic hirsutism and an increase in 3-α-diol-G metabolism (9).

Polycystic Ovary Syndrome

The polycystic ovary syndrome was derived from the original descriptions of Stein and Leventhal, which discussed obese, slightly hirsute women with menstrual irregularities (Fig 22.3) (10). A more contemporary term for this family of disorders might be hyperandrogenic chronic anovulation. Patients with this disorder can present with hirsutism, obesity, oily skin, acne, primary or secondary infertility, or any combination of the above. Total testosterone levels are usually in the upper limit of normal, free testosterone is frequently slightly elevated, and sex hormone-binding globulin is decreased. Follicle-stimulating hormone (FSH) may be slightly decreased and there may be an altered LH/FSH ratio of greater than 2. Twenty percent of the time prolactin will be elevated and 50% of the time DHEAS will likewise be elevated (11). Hirsutism is a feature of approximately 70% of these women; this diagnosis must be considered in the evaluation of hirsutism, particularly in the younger woman.

Ovarian Hyperthecosis

Ovarian hyperthecosis is often confused with hyperandrogenic chronic anovulatory syndromes. At times these patients may present with temporal balding, clitoral enlargement, and other signs of virilism. Serum testosterone levels are usually markedly elevated in these patients and DHEAS is normal. FSH levels are usually within normal range and LH/FSH ratio is appropriate. This relentless production of androgens is thought to occur through stimulation of the thecal cells (12).

Androgen-Producing Tumors of the Ovary

Virtually any tumor of the ovary has the capacity to produce either androgens or estrogens. These tumors include the Sertoli-Leydig cell-type hilar tumors, adrenal rest tumors, and granulosa cell tumors. Also, any space-occupying lesion in the ovary may affect ovarian stromal production of androgens including the Brenner's tumor, Krukenberg's tumor, and any type of cystadenoma or cystadenocarcinoma. In general, androgen-secreting ovarian tumors will present with the rapid onset of hirsutism and virilism and a marked elevation in testosterone levels. DHEAS levels are usually normal or mildly elevated. The finding of a testosterone level two to three times baseline in association with the rapid onset of virilism is highly suggestive of the presence of a malignancy (13).

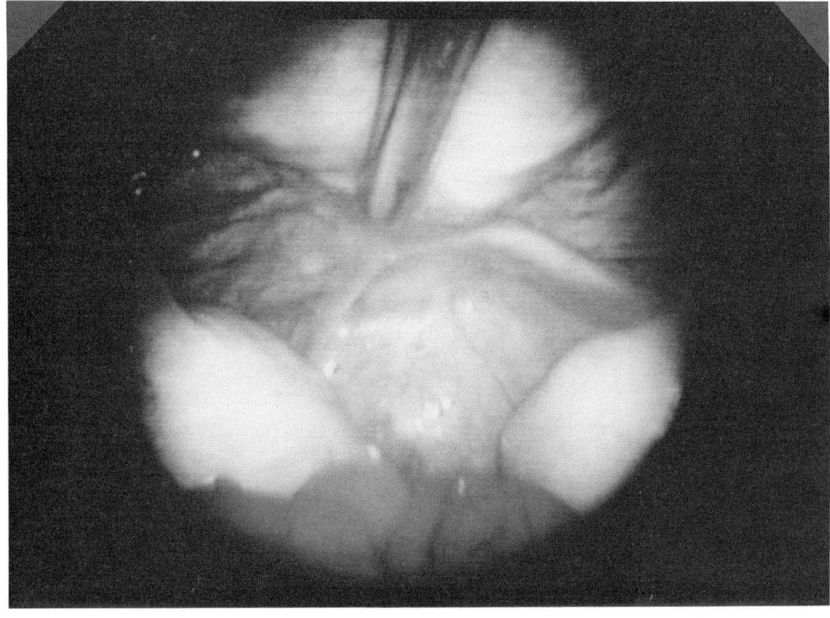

Fig 22.3 Laparoscopy showing polycystic (kissing) ovaries.

Endocrine Active Adrenal Tumors

Adenomas are perhaps the most common type of adrenal androgen-secreting tumor (14). However, both testosterone and nonproducing testosterone carcinomas have rarely been described. Adrenal adenomas can produce DHEA, DHEAS, and androstenedione; however, DHEAS levels are usually markedly elevated with levels ranging between 7 and 37 μg/mL with an average of 17 μg/mL (15). Most of these lesions are unilateral, are greater than 1 cm in size, and can be diagnosed with computed tomography (CT) scanning or magnetic resonance imaging (MRI). These tumors frequently produce hirsutism in association with other signs of virilism.

Congenital Adrenal Hyperplasia

Congenital adrenal hyperplasia of the late-onset type frequently will mimic polycystic ovary syndrome (16). The disorder is caused by a partial deficiency in 21-hydroxylase enzyme activity and its prevalence is concentrated in certain ethnic groups such as Hispanics and Ashkenazi Jews. Not all patients with 21-hydroxylase deficiency will present with hirsutism and cryptic forms may be present. Because there is a failure to metabolize 17-hydroxyprogesterone, the basal level usually will be elevated. A level greater than 8 ng/mL is diagnostic of the disorder; however, adrenocorticotropic hormone (ACTH) stimulation may have to be done to confirm the diagnosis (Fig 22.4) (17). The patient with adrenal hyperplasia may present with an elevated DHEAS level as well, accompanied by hirsutism and amenorrhea. However, enzyme defects of the adrenal gland that may present with hirsutism include an 11-hydroxylase deficiency, which is associated with hypertension, and an elevated level of 11-dioxycortisol following ACTH stimulation and 3-β-OL dehydrogenase-isomerize deficiency.

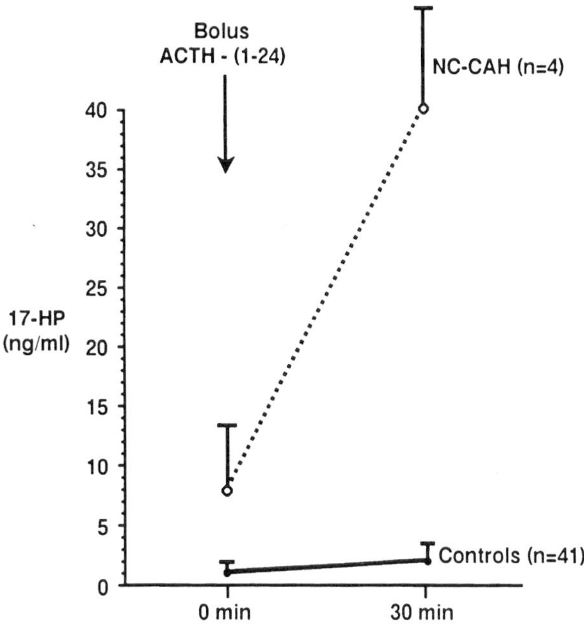

Fig 22.4 Change in serum 17-hydroxyprogesterone level following ACTH administration in patient with congenital adrenal hyperplasia as control. (*Courtesy of Dr. Ricardo Azziz.*)

Therapy of Hirsutism

A number of agents are available for the treatment of hirsutism. The therapy is generally dictated by the source of excess androgen or its point of metabolism and whether these patients present with other signs of androgen excess such as oily skin, acne, or menstrual dysfunction. It should also be noted that therapy does not necessarily have to be directed at the specific offending androgen as long as the overall androgen load to the body is decreased or the expression of the androgen is modified. The primary agents used to treat androgen excess include a variety or oral contraceptive agents, continuous progestogens, GnRH analogues, spironolactone, ketoconazole, cimetidine, flutamide, and dexamethasone (Box 22.1).

Oral Contraceptives

The birth control pill is in general composed of a mixture of estrogen and a mutated 19-nortestosterone or progestogen. These agents affect hirsutism by two mechanisms: 1) by decreasing central nervous system pituitary output of LH and FSH, which results in a diminution of folliculogenesis and decreased stimulation of thecal androgen production, and 2) by stimulating the liver to increase production of the sex hormone-binding globulin, which removes free testosterone from the circulation and alters metabolic clearance rate. Both of these mechanisms result in a decreased availability of bioactive free testosterone to

Box 22.1 Treatment of Hirsutism

Birth Control Pill

- Monophasic pill
- Low androgen properties, i.e., Demulen 1+35

Progestogens

- Medroxyprogesterone acetate 20–30 mg daily
- Norethindrone acetate 10–15 mg daily

Peripheral Androgen Blockers

■ Cimetidine	Unacceptable side effects
■ Flutamide	500 mg daily
■ Spironolactone	100–200 mg daily

Corticosteroids

■ Dexamethasone	0.5–0.7 mg daily
■ Prednisone	2.5–5.0 mg daily

Inidazoles

■ Ketoaconazole	400–1000 mg daily

GnRH Analogues

- Leuprolide acetate 3.75 mg IM 9 mo

interact with the hair cell and be converted to dehydrotestosterone. In the past it was thought to be preferable to choose an oral contraceptive agent that contained a compound such as norethindrone as opposed to norgestrol. These compounds have different androgenic potential, either directly or through metabolites. However, with the advent of new generation birth control pills and the decrease in the amount of both estrogens and progestogen-like compounds in these preparations, there seems to be no specific advantage in choosing one pill over another. The compounds that contain ethynodiol diacetate (Demulen) are the least androgenic and somewhat estrogenic. Other compounds that contain ethinyl estradiol and norethindrone (Ortho-Novum 1+35) are only mildly androgenic and are recommended for therapy. It should be emphasized that a monophasic pill is probably preferable over a triphasic preparation in the treatment of this form of pathology although there is no difference in terms of efficacy as far as contraception is concerned (18).

Continuous Progestogen Therapy

Progestogens can likewise be used for the treatment of hirsutism and many other disorders in gynecology that require cycle disruption. The two most common progestogens are medroxyprogesterone acetate in the dose range of 20–30 mg/day or norethindrone acetate in the dose range of 10–15 mg/day. As opposed to GnRH analogue therapy, which results in the demineralization of bone, therapy with either medroxyprogesterone acetate or norethindrone acetate does not result in bone destabilization. Although there are no progestogen receptors in bone, both of these compounds occupy the cortisol receptor and block the demineralizing effect of this compound. As opposed to oral contraceptive agents, these women will be hypoestrogenic and have signs of estrogen withdrawal such as hot flushes, dysphoria, perhaps lethargy, and mood changes. The availability of depot medroxyprogesterone acetate as an oral contraceptive agent also raises the possibility of using this compound for the suppression of hirsutism. Doses required to suppress androgen production are different from those that produce anovulation. It should also be noted that doses as low as 25 mg produce persistent anovulation for up to 9 months; therefore, this medication is not recommended in individuals who might be contemplating pregnancy in the near future. Also, bleeding problems are frequently encountered with progestogen therapy and the oral preparations have the advantage of being able to control this problem by discontinuing therapy for a short period of time. Unfortunately, the depot form persists in down regulating estrogen receptors in the endometrium for an extended period of time and the control of bleeding is made more difficult by its presence.

The antiandrogen cyproterone acetate is currently used for the treatment of hirsutism in Europe (19). Like progestogens, it inhibits LH secretion resulting in a decrease in ovarian androgen production. It is generally administered in doses of 50 mg/day and may be administered with concomitant doses of ethinyl estradiol. The protocol that has been recommended involves 50–150 mg cyproterone acetate administered on days 5 to 15 with 50 μg ethinyl estradiol being added days 5 to 26. It has been described as the reversed sequential regimen required for menstrual control.

GnRH Analogues

Analogues of GnRH are available clinically in the agonist form (Lupron and Synarel) and in the antagonist form (Nal-Glu) (antide). The antagonist, while having the initial appeal of the rapid onset and cessation of action, has not been brought to the clinical market due to problems with histamine release and lack of solubility. The agonist, on the other hand, will produce down regulation of pituitary LH and FSH production following an initial flair and render women profoundly hypogonadotropic (20). Both estrogen and androgen levels fall dramatically; however, these drugs are not approved for the treatment of hirsutism, only endometriosis or fibroids with a limited therapeutic life of 6 months. GnRH analogue therapy produces demineralization of bone plus vasomotor symptoms and other side effects. Therefore, the concept of add-back either using birth control pill or sequential estrogen/progestogen therapy may ultimately increase the utility of these compounds. Currently, therapy with a GnRH analogue is recommended only for the most severe cases of hirsutism and this therapy may be, in fact, a prelude to endoscopic oophorectomy as a last approach to treating disabling hirsutism and mild virilism.

Imidazole

Ketoconazole, an imidazole derivative, interferes with cytochrome P450-linked steroidogenesis (21). Its primary point of action is on the enzyme 17–20 desmolase and it affects both adrenal and ovarian production. In addition, ketoconazole will inhibit cholesterol side-chain cleavage. The drug has been used in a dose range of 400–1000 mg/day. However, the side effects of this drug has limited long-term use. These include hepatotoxicity with some 10% of patients developing transient dysfunction, 1% of patients with true hepatotoxicity, plus pruritus and gastrointestinal complaints.

Corticosteroids

Adrenal androgen suppression is less commonly used than agents that are directed at suppressing ovarian production or peripheral conversion. The most common therapies involve dexamethasone administered at night in a dose range of 0.50–0.75 mg every day to every other day or prednisone 2.5–5.0 mg at bedtime. These agents effectively suppress adrenal androgen production and are the treatment of choice in patients with adrenal hyperplasia (22,23). These agents produce profound suppression of adrenal androgens, and at a dose of 0.5 mg the recovery of the adrenal from dexamethasone suppression is less than 8 hours. At times corticosteroids can be used every other day at bedtime in combination with either spironolactone or oral contraceptive agents. With any corticosteroid therapy program, problems can be encountered calcium metabolism, vascular fragility, thinning of the skin, and susceptibility to stress or infection.

Peripheral Androgen Blockers

Therapy directed at the disruption of peripheral androgen conversion is one of the most effective treatments of hirsutism. Peripheral blockers bind to the androgen receptor and inhibit 5-α-reductase activity. Two of the compounds mentioned previously, cyproterone acetate and spironolactone, are used as peripheral blockers; however, only spironolactone is available on the U.S. market. It is generally administered in a dose range of 50–200 mg daily and many times it is used in conjunction with oral contraceptive suppression (24). At this dose range the side effects of spironolactone therapy such as hypotension and hyperkalemia are virtually never seen. In fact, in the older patient with hypertension, this is often of benefit. Two other drugs merit discussion as peripheral androgen blockers. Cimetidine is an H_2-receptor antagonist that has some effect at inhibiting the androgen receptor; however, its side effects are generally unacceptable. Further, it induces hyperprolactinemia, which may interfere with fertility. Flutamide has been shown to be as effective as spironolactone in the inhibition of hirsutism at a dose range of 500 mg (25). Like spironolactone, it can be used in conjunction with oral contraceptive therapy.

One of the difficulties in choosing the appropriate therapy for hirsutism is concomitant menstrual dysfunction. In general, drugs such as spironolactone may make this problem worse; therefore, peripheral androgen blockers frequently need to be used in conjunction with either oral contraceptive agents or cycle progestogen. The latter compounds are not considered as contraceptive agents and alternate means must be used with this form of therapy. In patients with dysfunctional uterine bleeding and associated hyperandrogeninemia, the oral contraceptive agent with or without spironolactone is probably the best choice of therapy.

Long-Term Follow-Up

The patient who presents with hirsutism generally expects that therapy will result in a resolution of unwanted hair. It should be emphasized to these individuals that the best response that can be seen will be a *reduction* in the rate of hair growth and a decrease in hair coarseness. Unwanted hair must be removed or camouflaged. For hair on the lip or face, peroxide will often mask its presence. Occasionally hair can be removed by plucking or waxing, but this often traumatizes the hair follicle and will stimulate growth. Shaving has also been used in conjunction with these agents. Ultrasonics can be used for removing hair below the skin; however, this does not destroy the pilosebaceous unit. Only electrolysis will result in the destruction of this entity. This technique must be used sparingly, particularly on the face, to prevent scarring. In general, for the long-term containment of hair growth a combination of these medical and nonmedical therapies should be applied. Patients should be counseled to expect not to see a significant clinical response until 3 to 6 months of therapy as this will allow hairs in various stages of growth to complete their cycles. Finally, all women should probably be counseled as they become older that hair growth may present as a cosmetic problem. As ovarian follicle production wanes, androgen production will increase under the presence of ever-increasing gonadotropin levels. Perhaps estrogen replacement therapy combined with a progestogen or long-term use of oral contraceptive agents through the perimenopausal period will help to control this cosmetic problem as well as furnish the other benefits associated with this mode of therapy.

REFERENCES

1. Hatch R, Rosenfield RL, Kim MH, Tredway D. Hirsutism scoring standards. Am J Obstet Gynecol 1981;140:815–830.
2. Bardin CW, Lipsett MB. Testosterone and androstenedione blood production rates in normal women and women with idiopathic hirsutism or polycystic ovaries. J Clin Invest 1967;46:891–902.
3. Lobo RA, Paul WL, Goebelsmann U. Dehydroepiandrosterone sulfate as an indicator of adrenal androgen function. Obstet Gynecol 1981;57:69–73.
4. Serafini P, Lobo RA. Increased 5α-reductase activity in idiopathic hirsutism. Fertil Steril 1985;43:74–78.
5. Morimoto I, Edmiston A, Hawks D, Horton R. Studies on the origin of androstenediol and androstenediol glucuronide in young and elderly men. J Clin Endocrinol Metab 1981;52:772–778.
6. Cumming DC, Wall SR. Non-sex hormone binding globulin-bound testosterone as a marker for hyperandrogenism. J Clin Endocrinol Metab 1985;61:873–876.
7. Mowszowicz I, Melanitou E, Doukani A, et al. Androgen binding capacity and 5α-reductase activity in pubic skin fibroblasts from hirsute patients. J Clin Endocrinol Metab 1983;56:1209–1213.
8. Buttram VC Jr, Reiter RC, Ward S. Treatment of endometriosis with danazol; report of a six-year prospective study. Fertil Steril 1985;43:353–360.
9. Paulson RJ, Serafini PC, Catalino JA, Lobo RA. Measurement of 3α-, 17β-androstenediol glucuronide in serum and urine and the correlation with skin 5α-reductase activity. Fertil Steril 1986;46:222–226.
10. Yen SSC. The polycystic ovary syndrome. Clin Endocrinol 1980;12:177–207.
11. Lobo RA, Kletzky OA, Kaptein EM, Goebelsman U. Prolactin modulation of dehydroepiandrosterone sulfate secretion. Am J Obstet Gynecol 1980;138:632–636.
12. Judd HL, Scully RE, Herbst AL, et al. Familial hyperthecosis: comparison of endocrinologic and histologic findings with polycystic ovarian disease. Am J Obstet Gynecol 1973;117:976–982.
13. Schwartz U, Moltz L, Brotherton J, Hammerstein J. The diagnostic value of plasma free testosterone in nontumorous and tumorous hyperandrogenism. Fertil Steril 1983;40:66–72.
14. Yuen BH, Moon YS, Mincey EK, Li D. Adrenal and sex steroid hormone production by a virilizing adrenal adenoma and its diagnosis with computerized tomography. Am J Obstet Gynecol 1983;145:164–169.
15. Gabrilove JL, Seman AT, Sabet R, et al. Virilizing adrenal adenoma with studies on the steroid content of the adrenal venous effluent and a review of the literature. Endocrine Rev 1981;2:462–470.
16. Azziz R, Zacur HA. 21-Hydroxylase deficiency in female androgenism: screening and diagnosis. J Clin Endocrinol Metab 1989;69:577–584.
17. Azziz R, Bradley E Jr, Huth J, et al. Acute adrenocorticotropin-(1-24-(ACTH) adrenal stimulation in

eumenorrheic women: reproducibility and effect of ACTH dose, subject weight and sampling time. J Clin Endocrinol Metab 1990;70:1273–1279.

18. Wild RA, Umstot ES, Anderson RN, Givens JR. Adrenal function in hirsutism. II. Effect of anoral contraceptive. J Clin Endocrinol Metab 1982;54:676–681.

19. Kuttenn F, Rigaud C, Wright F, Mauvais-Jarvis P. Treatment of hirsutism by oral cyproterone acetate and percutaneous oestradiol. J Clin Endocrinol Metab 1980;51:1107–1111.

20. Chang RJ, Laufer LR, Meldrum DR, et al. Steroid secretion in polycystic after ovarian disease after ovarian suppression by a long-acting gonadotropin-releasing hormone agonist. J Clin Endocrinol Metab 1983;56:897–903.

21. Sonino N. The use of ketoconazole as an inhibitor of steroid production. N Engl J Med 1987;317:812–818.

22. Rittsmaster RS, Loriaux DL, Cutler GB Jr. Sensitivity of cortisol and adrenal androgens to dexamethasone suppression in hirsute women. J Clin Endocrinol Metab 1985;61:462–466.

23. Sarris S, Swyer GIM, Ward RHT, et al. The treatment of mild adrenal hyperplasia and associated infertility with prednisone. Br J Obstet Gynaecol 1978;85: 251–253.

24. Lobo RA, Shoupe D, Serafini P, et al. The effects of two doses of spironolactone on serum androgens and anagen hair in hirsute women. Fertil Steril 1985;43: 200–205.

25. Cusan L, Dupont A, Gomez JL, et al. Comparison of flutaminde and spironolactone in the treatment of hirsutism: a randomized controlled trial. Fertil Steril 1994;61:281–287.

SECTION SEVEN

INFECTIOUS DISEASES

CHAPTER 23

ANOGENITAL HUMAN PAPILLOMAVIRUS INFECTIONS

Michael Saccente,
Peter G. Pappas

Papillomaviruses are human and animal pathogens that preferentially infect stratified squamous epithelial cells and stimulate cellular proliferation, causing warts and other tumors including invasive cancers. They are grouped with the polyomaviruses to form the papovavirus family. Papillomaviruses are small, nonenveloped viruses that have an icosahedral capsid and a circular, double-stranded DNA genome. The genomic organization of all known papillomaviruses is remarkably similar. Within a given species of host, new types are defined by DNA sequence homology, with new types sharing less than 50% homology with any known type. There are at least 70 different types of human papillomaviruses (HPVs) (Table 23.1). HPVs having specific tropism for anogenital and oral mucosa can be sexually transmitted and are the focus of this chapter.

Anogenital HPV infection is quite common, probably affecting 20% of young and middle-aged people in the United States at any given time. Its prevalence exceeds that of genital herpes simplex infection, making it the most common viral sexually transmitted disease (STD). The clinical manifestations produced by HPVs vary depending on the infecting type and the immune status of the host. Types 6 and 11 are the most common types to cause genital warts (condylomata); types 16, 18, and 31 induce cervical dysplasia and are consistently found in cervical cancer tissue. The mechanism underlying the association between HPV infection and malignant tumors is currently the focus of intensive investigation. That HPVs have been causally linked to anogenital cancers may have important implications with regard to prevention of HPV transmission, screening of sexually active women for evidence of infection, and the manner of follow-up care of women known to be infected with HPV.

Epidemiology

Incidence and Prevalence

The epidemiology of HPV disease has not been completely characterized. The common occurrence of asymptomatic infection and the lack of a sensitive, widely available diagnostic test that can be used to screen large numbers of patients pose obstacles to obtaining accurate incidence and prevalence data. The epidemiology of symptomatic HPV infection is difficult to define because in the United States it is not a reportable disease and contact tracing is usually not performed. Despite these pitfalls, the available data do provide information regarding trends in incidence and prevalence in certain populations of women.

Reports from both the United States and the United Kingdom indicate that the incidence of genital warts has increased significantly over the past 40 years. Investigators in Rochester, Minnesota found that the age-adjusted incidence of condylomata was 106/100,000 population in the mid to late 1970s, an eightfold greater rate than that found in the early 1950s. The highest incidence (617/100,000) was in women between the ages of 20 and 24 years. Although the incidence of clinically inapparent infection is unknown, using koilocytic atypia on Pap smear as an indicator of HPV infection, investigators in Finland in the mid 1980s showed that one half of sexually active women would experience at least one cervical HPV infection within 10 years and that the estimated lifetime risk in this same population was almost 80%.

The determination of HPV prevalence data is highly dependent on the sensitivity of the detection technique. Koutsky and colleagues estimated a prevalence of 20% in men and women in the United States

Table 23.1 Selected Human Papillomavirus Types and Associated Diseases

Type	Associated Diseases
6, 11	Benign anogenital and oral warts, laryngeal papillomas, Buschke-Loewenstein tumors, CIN I–II
16, 18, 31, 35, 33, 52, 58	CIN II–III, anogenital squamous cell cancers some adenocarcinomas
18, 39, 45	Adenocarcinoma of the cervix, some anogenital squamous cell cancers

CIN, cervical intraepithelial neoplasia

between the ages of 15 and 49 in 1987, with 1% of people in this age range having condylomata, 2% having subclinical infection apparent by colposcopy or hand lens magnification, 7% having HPV detectable by nucleic acid probe technology, and another 10% having latent HPV undiagnosed by any of these techniques. Using the polymerase chain reaction (PCR), Bauer and coworkers found the prevalence of HPV infection to be 46% among a group of female college students presenting to a clinic for routine gynecologic examinations. The prevalence of grossly visible genital warts in these 467 women was only 1%.

HPV Transmission and Risk Factors for Disease Expression

It is assumed that sexual contact is the most common mode of transmission of HPV although studies of HPV transmission are limited by available technology. The risk of acquiring HPV increases with increasing numbers of sexual partners. In 1954, the first study to strongly suggest that HPV is sexually transmitted examined an outbreak of condylomata among wives of servicemen who had recently returned from the Korean War. The incubation period in this cohort of women was 4 to 6 weeks, but later studies found the average incubation time to be approximately 3 months.

Abrasions in the epithelium and coexistent genital ulcer disease appear to enhance transmission of HPV by allowing the virus to gain access to deeper layers of the epithelium. Daling and coworkers showed that cigarette smoking and long-term oral contraceptive use, in addition to large numbers of sexual partners, independently increase the risk of developing condylomata.

Anal warts are strongly associated with anal intercourse, but autoinoculation may occur. Infection of the oral mucosa by genital HPV types occurs in individuals who have oral to genital contact with an infected partner. Vertical transmission, especially of types 6 and 11, can result in recurrent respiratory papillomatosis in infants and young children. Thirty to 50% of children with this disorder are offspring of women with genital warts.

Natural History of Uncomplicated HPV Infections

The natural history of condylomata is variable, ranging from spontaneous regression to relentless progression of locally aggressive growths that are recalcitrant to therapy. The rate of spontaneous regression has not been clearly defined, but most warts will resolve over months to many years. In placebo-controlled treatment studies, spontaneous clearing has occurred in 20% to 30% of untreated patients over 3 months.

Cellular immunity appears to be the primary host defense against HPV, and suppression of cell-mediated immunity affects the natural history of HPV-related disease. The main clinical evidence of this is that condylomata are more common, more extensive, more resistant to therapy, and less likely to show spontaneous regression in solid organ transplant recipients and in those infected with the human immumodeficiency virus (HIV). HPV can persist in tissues after resolution of condylomata and may reactivate at a later time, commonly during periods of immunosuppression. In addition, during pregnancy, existing warts tend to increase in size, and subclinical HPV infection may become apparent. Warts usually regress in the postpartum period.

The effect of HPV on the natural history of cervical dysplasia is discussed below.

Pathogenesis and Pathology

Infection begins when the virus gains access to the basal cells of cutaneous or mucosal stratified squamous epithelium, with varying tropism for cutaneous or mucosal cells depending on HPV type. Abrasions and moisture on the surface of the epithelium facilitate access to the deeper basal cells. Interactions between viral gene products and host cellular machinery cause hyperproliferation of the infected epithelial cells. As the basal cells differentiate and mature, viral gene expression changes, with the eventual production of structural proteins and the release of infectious virions.

Histology and Cytology

The characteristic pathologic finding in HPV-infected tissues is the *koilocyte*, an enlarged cell containing a pyknotic nucleus surrounded by a clear halo (Fig 23.1). The presence of koilocytes in histopathologic specimens is diagnostic of papillomavirus infection. Other histologic features of condylomata include deepended rete ridges, acanthosis, parakeratosis, and hyperkeratosis. Examination of regressing warts reveals infiltration with mononuclear cells including T lymphocytes.

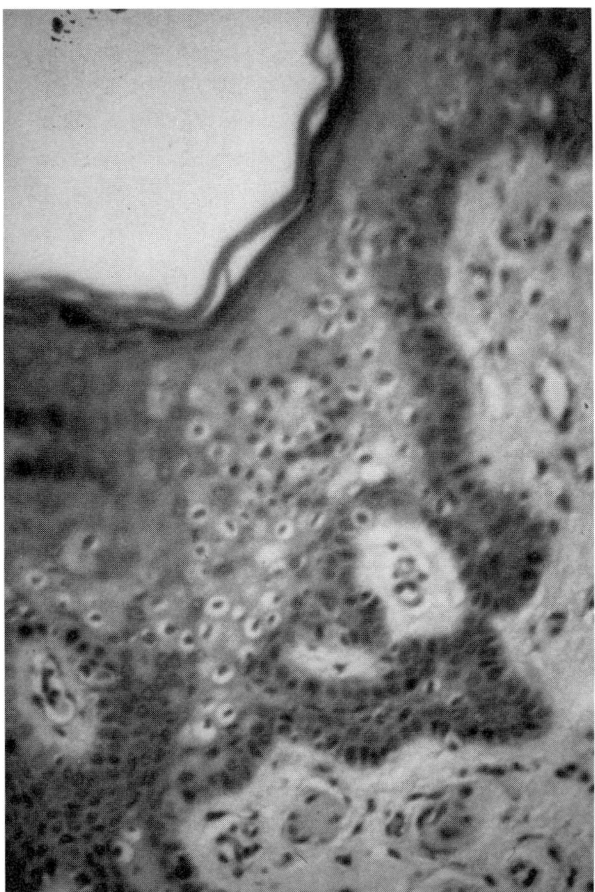

Fig 23.1 Photomicrograph of a condyloma. Note the numerous koilocytes, each of which contains a small, shrunken nucleus with a surrounding clear halo. This cell type is pathognomonic of HPV infection.

Cytologic examination of exfoliated endocervical cells is used to screen for cervical dysplasia (Pap screening). Because of the strong association between HPV and cervical dysplasia, a Pap smear showing dysplastic cells implies HPV infection. If HPV is present, cytology may also reveal pathognomonic koilocytic atypia.

The severity of dysplasia can only be determined by histologic examination of tissue obtained by biopsy. Dysplasia is graded according to the fraction of normal squamous epithelium that has been replaced by undifferentiated cells that resemble malignant cells but which have not breached the basement membrane (Fig 23.2). Such cells occupy the lower one third and lower two thirds of the epithelium in cervical intraepithelial neoplasia (CIN) I (mild dysplasia) and CIN II (moderate dysplasia), respectively. If undifferentiated cells are present in the full thickness of the epithelium, then CIN III (severe dysplasia) is the descriptive term used. Usually, CIN III cannot be distinguished from carcinoma in situ (CIS). In the Bethesda classification scheme, low-grade squamous intraepithelial lesion (SIL) corresponds to CIN I, mild dysplasia and koilocytosis, and high-grade SIL encompasses CIN II, CIN III, moderate and severe dysplasia, and CIS. These premalignant lesions develop on a continuum that may ultimately lead to invasive cervical cancer. Analogous terminology is used to describe intraepithelial and invasive neoplasias of the vulva and vagina.

HPV and Oncogenesis

According to the World Health Organization, cancer of the cervix is second only to breast cancer as the most frequent malignancy in women worldwide. It is expected that over 400,000 women worldwide will be diagnosed with invasive cervical cancer each year. With the use of effective screening programs, the incidence and mortality are decreasing, but such programs are lacking in many developing countries. It is generally accepted that infection with high-risk HPV types is etiologically linked to anogenital cancers, especially involving the cervix. The oncogenic process most likely involves multiple steps occurring over 15 to 30 years.

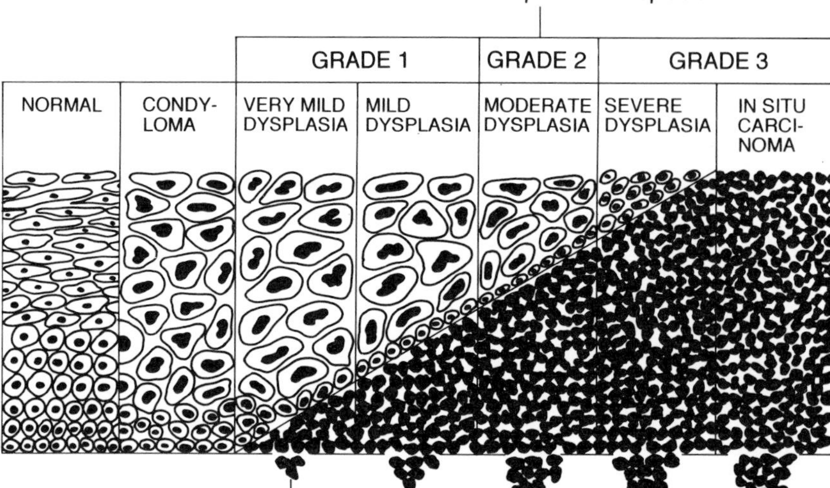

Fig 23.2 This illustration depicts the progression from normal cervical epithelium to carcinoma in situ. Grading is based on the fraction of epithelium replaced by undifferentiated cells. In the Bethesda classification, low-grade SIL encompasses koilocytosis and CIN I; CIN II, CIN III and CIS are grouped together as high-grade SIL (see text). CIN, cervical intraepithelial neoplasia; CIS, carcinoma in situ; SIL, squamous intraepithelial lesion

Sexual behavior influences the risk of developing cervical cancer. The disease is practically nonexistent in virginal women. In contrast, early age at first coitus and increasing numbers of lifetime sexual partners are risk factors for its development. Some studies have shown that the total number of a husband's sexual partners increases his wife's risk of cervical cancer, and women married to men whose previous wives had cervical cancer are at increased risk of developing cervical dysplasia. Smoking, oral contraceptive use, and lower socioeconomic class are associated with higher risk of cancer as well. It has long been suspected that an infectious agent might be involved in the pathogenesis of cervical neoplasia, and over the past 20 years the focus has shifted from herpes simplex virus type II to HPV.

Cervical cancer develops on a continuum from CIN I to CIN III and CIS culminating in invasive disease. The presence of HPV affects this progression. A recent prospective study showed that among women with initially negative cytologic screening, the cumulative incidence of CIN II and III was much greater in subjects who had positive tests for HPV DNA, especially types 16 and 18. All cases of moderate and severe dysplasia were detected within 2 years. Earlier investigators found that detectable HPV 16 DNA is associated with an increased risk of progression from CIN I to CIN III. Koilocytic cytologic atypia has been related to a higher risk of developing CIS. Spontaneous regression of CIN I may occur but is less likely in the presence of HPV 16.

There is compelling evidence that infection with specific oncogenic types of HPV (primarily types 16, 18, 31, and 35) is etiologically linked to invasive anogenital cancers of the vulva, vagina, and anus, in addition to the cervix. DNA from the high-risk HPV types 16 and 18 is found in 90% of anogenital cancers and is also present in moderately and severely dysplastic lesions. Additionally, DNA from these HPV types can be detected in metastases and cell lines derived from cervical cancer tissue. HPV 16 is the most common type associated with squamous cell carcinoma of the cervix, whereas HPV 18 is strongly associated with adenocarcinomas and less so with squamous cell cancers. The molecular basis of the apparent causal association between high-risk HPV types and anogenital cancers is being elucidated.

Because not all women infected with high-risk HPVs develop cancer, other factors are probably involved. A study in 1986 found that smokers had a relative risk of 1.5 compared to nonsmokers with current, heavy, and long-term smokers having the greatest risk. Cervical mucus from smokers is more likely to be mutagenic than that from nonsmokers, and smoking has been shown to induce a local immunologic defect. Data on the effect of oral contraceptive use are conflicting, but long-term use is probably an independent risk factor for cervical cancer. Deficiencies of folate, vitamin C, and vitamin A have also been implicated as contributing factors.

Although the peak age of incidence for genital HPV infection is in the early twenties, that of cervical cancer is approximately 35 years in low incidence populations and 50 years in high incidence groups. This lag time may partly be explained by the cumulative effect of cofactors over time. The age at acquisition of cervical HPV infection appears to be important. The cervical transformation zone (the area where the stratified squamous epithelium of the vagina and ectocervix changes to the glandular epithelium of the endocervix and body of the uterus) migrates up into the endocervical canal as a women ages. The transformation zone, which is a naturally occurring area of metaplasia, is the histologic site where cancer of the cervix usually begins. In the late teens and early twenties, the transformation zone is more easily exposed to HPV, and infection of this area occurring at this time in life may predispose to the later development cervical cancer. The absence of corresponding transformation zones on the vulva and in the vagina may partly explain why cancer at these sites is much less common than cervical cancer.

Clinical Manifestations

The clinical manifestations of genital HPV infection are variable and can depend on the type of HPV involved, the site or sites affected, and the immune status of the host. Disease may be clinically apparent or subclinical. Condylomata acuminata are soft, fleshy, vascular exophytic warts that have multiple papillary surface projections (Fig 23.3). These are the

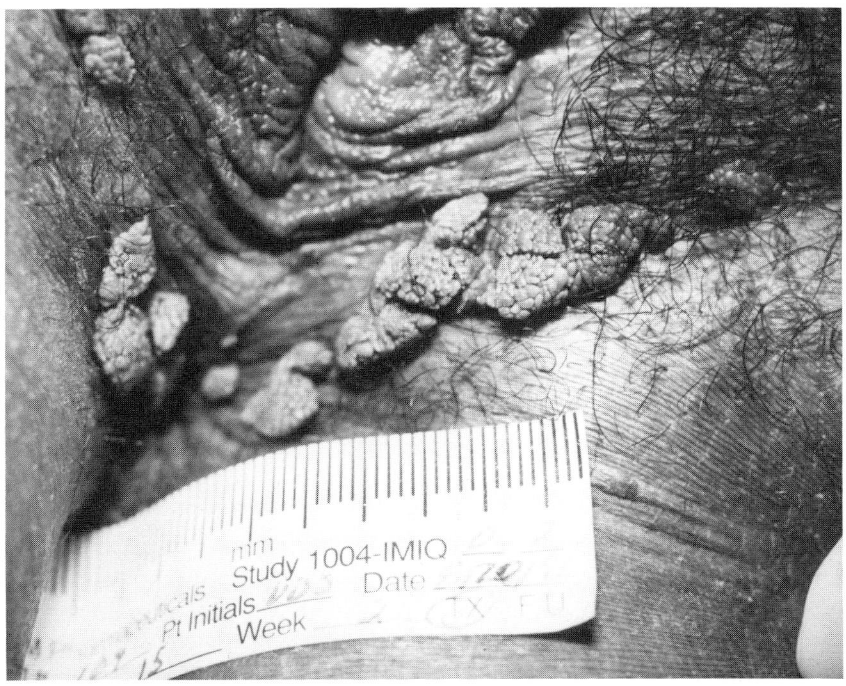

Fig 23.3 Extensive external condylomata acuminata. These fleshy, exophytic growths are covered with small, papillary surface projections. Some of the lesions are pedunculated; others are sessile.

most commonly recognized overt manifestation of genital HPV infection. Mucosal condylomata are not keratinized, and therefore may not have the rough, thickened surface characteristic of cutaneous warts. Aside from the obvious cosmetic effect, symptoms are usually minimal. A Buschke-Loewenstein tumor is a locally aggressive giant condyloma that does not metastasize. Nonexophytic papular warts are smooth and flat and tend to occur in drier areas such as the vulvar skin and inner thighs.

Subclinical disease includes those manifestations of infection that are not visible without magnification by colposcopy, hand lens or light microscopy (i.e., cytologic or histologic examination). Tiny, finger-like mucosal projections or "microwarts" are sometimes visible to the unaided eye, but are more effectively seen with a hand lens or colposcope. Detection of abnormalities by colposcopy is enhanced by application of 3% to 5% acetic acid, which causes whitening of infected areas. Although characteristic of HPV, acetowhitening is not a specific finding. Noncondylomatous, acetowhite lesions are sometimes referred to as flat condylomata. HPV infection can cause cytologic and histologic abnormalities in the absence of warts and acetowhite lesions. These microscopic manifestations are described above.

Latent infection is another variety of subclinical disease and describes the presence of HPV in histologically normal tissue. In this situation, a sensitive DNA detection technique is necessary for diagnosis. These techniques are described below.

Vulvar and Vaginal Disease

Moist areas prone to coital friction are most susceptible to HPV infection. Condylomata acuminata most commonly occur in the posterior introitus and on the adjacent labia minora (Fig 23.4). The warts can quickly spread to other sites on the vulvar skin and vestibule. Infection of the vulvar skin may also cause flat, smooth papules, a condition known as Bowenoid papulosis. Small papillary projections on the mucosa of the vulva (microwarts) can cause dyspareunia, pruritus, and burning discomfort.

Vaginal warts are usually asymptomatic and may easily be missed on examination. When present, they are usually multifocal. Symptoms can include vaginal discharge, postcoital bleeding, and pruritus. In pregnant women, large vaginal warts may complicate delivery by obstructing the birth canal.

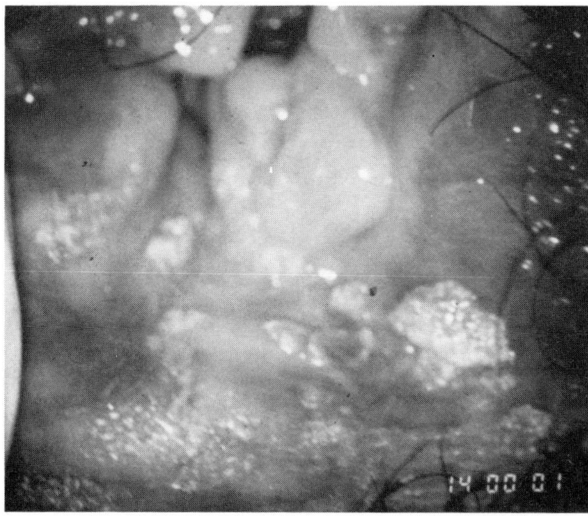

Fig 23.4 Condylomata in the area of the posterior introitus.

Cervical Disease

Even though the cervix is a common site for HPV infection, cervical disease is more likely to be subclinical, with cervical condylomata being relatively rare. Abnormalities occur in the transformation zone and consist either of leukoplakia (areas that are white before the application of acetic acid) or areas that turn white only after acetic acid is applied. The lesions are slightly raised and have a roughened appearance. Various vascular atypias are also manifestations of cervical HPV infection. The sharpness of the demarcation between normal and abnormal tissue, the vascular pattern, and the color tone of the lesion are correlated with the likelihood of biopsy-confirmed intraepithelial neoplasia.

Cervical warts may be multifocal and can become confluent (Fig 23.5). Extension into the endocervical canal may occur. Although an exophytic wart is virtually always caused by a low-risk HPV type (6 or 11) and has little malignant potential, coexistent CIN is present in at least 20% of patients with condylomatous cervical lesions. All patients with cervical condylomata should have colposcopy with biopsy of suspicious lesions to rule out CIN.

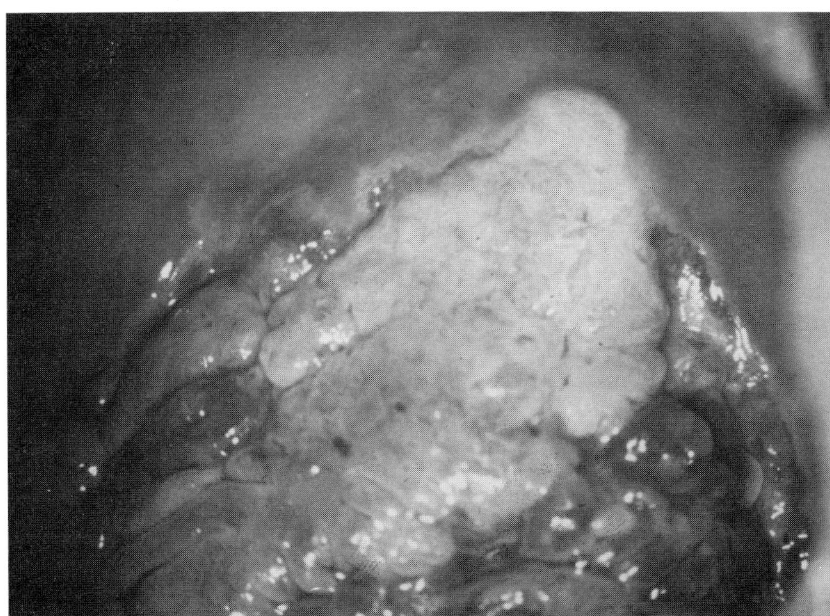

Fig 23.5 This close-up view of the cervix demonstrates confluence of multiple condylomata with an overlying area of leukoplakia.

Anal Disease

In approximately 20% of women with vulvar warts, lesions will spread posteriorly to involve the anal area. Condylomata in the perianal region tend to be large and multifocal, commonly causing pain and bleeding on defecation. Ten percent of patients will have intra-anal or distal rectal lesions.

Other Sites of Disease

Genital HPVs can infect the urethral and bladder epithelia, causing condylomata at these sites. Exophytic warts of the oral mucosa and the adult form of respiratory papillomatosis may occur in patients who have acquired HPV through oral to genital contact with an infected partner.

Differential Diagnosis

Genital warts must be differentiated from other infections that can cause similar-appearing lesions, normal anatomic variants, and malignant neoplasms. Condylomata lata of secondary syphilis occur on the moist mucosa of the anogenital area, but these lesions are more rounded and smoother than condylomata acuminata. Darkfield microscopy will usually reveal motile spirochetes. Other lesions of secondary syphilis such as a rash or diffuse lymphadenopathy may be present, and serologic tests for syphilis will be strongly positive. The dome-shaped papules of molluscum contagiosum have a characteristic central dimple, and although they tend to appear in the genital region and on the skin of the inner thighs (as well as other skin sites), these lesions do not involve mucosal surfaces. Histopathology is the only means by which benign tumors can be definitively differentiated from those which are malignant. Genital warts that are atypical in appearance or refractory to conventional therapy should be biopsied to confirm the diagnosis and rule out malignanacy.

Evaluation of the Patient with Genital Warts

History and Physical Examination

A detailed sexual history is an essential part of the evaluation of all patients with STDs. While remaining sensitive to the personal nature of sexual activities, physicians must not allow fear of embarrassing the patient interfere with taking a thorough history. Women should be asked about previous history of genital warts and the treatment they received. The diagnosis of concomitant HIV infection should be considered in all women with genital warts especially if the lesions are particularly extensive or resistant to therapy.

Women with clinically evident condylomata should be thoroughly examined for signs of HPV infection at other anogenital sites. Although low-risk HPV types (primarily 6 and 11) most commonly cause exophytic warts, their presence serves as a marker for possible coexistent HPV infection elsewhere in the lower genital tract. Evaluation should include colposcopy with application of 3% to 5% acetic acid to identify flat cervical and vaginal condylomata and a routine Pap smear. All suspicious lesions should be biopsied. Patients with perianal warts require anoscopy to look for distal rectal warts.

Laboratory Evaluation

Cytologic examination of exfoliated cells from the cervical transformation zone (Pap smear) can be an effective technique to screen for cervical dysplasia. When used appropriately, Pap screening has contributed to the decrease in incidence of invasive cervical cancer in some populations. The rate of false-negative Pap smears varies widely, and some properly screened women will present with severe dysplasia or invasive cancer as their initially detected lesion, implying that lower grade lesions were missed earlier. If the Pap smear meets criteria for dysplasia, histologic examination of colposcopically directed biopsy tissue is necessary to grade the dysplasia and rule out invasive disease. Dysplasia on cytology or histopathology is an insensitive indicator of HPV infection.

No cell culture of serologic test is currently available to diagnose HPV infection. However, several techniques have been used for detection and typing of HPV DNA in clinical specimens. DNA hybridization is the basis for the dot blot, Southern blot, filter in situ hybridization, and in situ hybridization detection tests. A full description of these methods is beyond the scope of this chapter. ViraPap and ViraType are commercially available kits that are based on dot blotting. Dot blotting and filter in situ hybridization are inexpensive, easy to perform, and quick, but quality varies among laboratories. Southern blotting is highly specific and sensitive but is time consuming and expensive. In situ hybridization involves examination of intact tissue sections, thereby making it possible to look at HPV infection in the context of preserved histology. Both Southern blotting and in situ hybridization are used primarily in research settings.

Polymerase chain reaction technology has been applied to the detection of HPV infection, and studies comparing PCR with dot blotting and Southern blotting have shown PCR to be more sensitive for the detection of HPV DNA. The sensitivity of PCR is so great that false-positive results are a potential problem. At the current time PCR is a research tool.

It is not yet clear how to use HPV detection techniques in clinical practice. There are no data to indicate that screening women for the presence of HPV will alter outcome compared to Pap screening aimed at detecting dysplasia. HPV typing may help to determine prognosis and influence management in certain situations, but no available data support its routine use.

Treatment of Condylomata

The goal of therapy is to eliminate signs and symptoms; eradication of HPV is not currently possible. Several modalities are available for the treatment of anogenital warts, and others are being studied in clinical trials (Table 23.2). Recurrences, which are most commonly due to reactivation of latent virus, are not adequately prevented by any currently used therapy. Clinical efficacy is measured by the elimination of visible lesions and rate of recurrence. In general, warts that are new and small are more likely to respond to therapy than those that are larger or have been present for months or years. Because the spontaneous regression of warts is common, treatment efficacy data should always be viewed in comparison to a placebo group.

Destruction of lesions by direct application of cytotoxic or caustic agents and surgical removal are the mainstays of therapy. Immunomodulation with interferons has also been studied in the treatment of genital warts. The Centers for Disease Control and Prevention has recently published guidelines for the treatment of HPV infection.

Table 23.2 Treatment of Condylomata

Therapy	Comments
Topical	
Podophyllin	Systemic absorption, contraindicated in pregnancy
Podophyllotoxin	No reported systemic toxicity, approved for self-application, more expensive than podophyllin, contraindicated in pregnancy
Trichloroacetic acid	Depth of tissue destruction difficult to control
5-Fluorouracil	Severe local reactions
Ablative	
Cryotherapy	Inexpensive, moderately painful
Electrocautery	Contraindicated in patients with implanted electrical devices
Surgical excision	Moderate to severe postoperative pain
CO_2 laser	Expensive, risk of perforation, severe postoperative pain, prolonged healing time
Immunotherapy	
Systemic interferon	Expensive, many patients develop significant systemic toxicity
Intralesional interferon	Expensive, painful, and difficult to administer, not free of toxicity

Topical Therapy

Direct application of podophyllin resin is a widely used treatment for anogenital warts. Podophyllin is derived from the May apple plant *Podophyllum peltatum* and *Podophyllum emodi.* It contains cytotoxic lignins that cause tissue necrosis by binding to microtubules and interfering with cell division. A 10% to 25% solution in tincture of benzoin is applied to the wart and washed off within 4 to 8 hours. Treatment may be repeated weekly up to six times, but if the warts persist, another therapy should be tried because the lesions will probably not respond to further podophyllin, and excessive use is potentially carcinogenic. Warts in moist areas are more likely to clear than those in drier areas that are more heavily keratinized. Because systemic absorption and toxicity can occur, not more than 0.5 mL of a 20% solution should be applied in any given session, and the area treated should not exceed 10 cm^2. Local side effects include burning pain, irritation, swelling, and erosions. Initial response rates range from 30% to 80% with recurrence rates of at least 30%. Internal use of podophyllin is discouraged because of the greater potential for systemic absorption. Podophyllin is contraindicated in pregnancy because of possible teratogenicity.

Podofilox is a 0.5% solution of podophyllotoxin, one of the active components in podophyllin resin. In contrast to podophyllin, podofilox is approved for self-application by the patient, does not need to be removed once applied, and is more stable. One disadvantage of self-application is that it can only be used on warts that the patient can easily see and reach. It is applied twice daily for 3 days followed by 4 days of no therapy, with this cycle being repeated up to four times. As with podophyllin, heavily keratinized warts are less apt to respond. Although no systemic adverse effects have been reported, the manufacturer recommends that no more than 0.5 mL be applied daily. Podofilox has local side effects and clinical efficacy similar to those of podophyllin and is also contraindicated in pregnancy.

Trichloroacetic acid (TCA) applied as an 80% to 90% solution causes chemical destruction of tissues and can be used weekly for up to 6 weeks for the treatment of genital warts. Most patients experience moderate pain, and TCA is caustic to surrounding skin or mucosa so care must be taken to apply it only to the wart. Depth of tissue destruction is difficult to control, and scarring may result if the underlying dermis is affected. Few efficacy data are available for TCA, but it is probably comparable to podophyllin.

Ablative Therapy

Cryotherapy can be achieved with liquid nitrogen or a specialized cryoprobe that uses nitrous oxide. Pain is moderate, and treatment of more than one or two small warts requires local anesthesia. There is no scarring if performed correctly. Quoted clearance and recurrence rates are from 60% to 90% and 20% to 40%, respectively.

Electrodesiccation and electrocautery are other forms of ablative therapy. Treatment of extensive disease is performed under general anesthesia. In one trial the clearance and recurrence rates with electrodesiccation were 94% and 22%, respectively. These procedures are contraindicated in patients with implanted electrical devices (e.g., cardiac pacemakers) and should not be attempted on lesions near the anal verge. Carbon dioxide laser therapy and general surgery should be reserved for treatment of extensive disease that has been unresponsive to other modalities. Both procedures may require general anesthesia, and postoperative pain may be severe. The rate of complications with either procedure depends on the skill and experience of the operator and include perforation and scarring.

Topical 5-fluorouracil is a cytotoxic agent that has not been sufficiently evaluated in clinical trials to recommend its use. It can cause significant local irritation, sometimes resulting in vaginal discharge and vulvitis.

Immunotherapy

Interferons have antiviral and immunomodulatory activity and have been evaluated in clinical trials for the treatment of condylomata. Unlike the other therapies described above, interferons given systemically could have an effect on latent HPV. However, two placebo-controlled trials of systemic interferon-α showed no benefit of treatment over placebo. A study comparing interferon-α with placebo following debulking with laser also failed to show any benefit. More recent data reveal that interferon-α, -β and -γ provide no advantage over placebo when combined with cryotherapy, with all study groups having about a 65% resolution rate. A substantial proportion of patients given systemic therapy develop significant side effects including fever, chills, headache, fatigue, and cytopenias.

An alternative to systemic interferons is local administration. Data on topically applied interferons are conflicting, but two placebo-controlled trials showed no benefit compared to placebo. Intralesional injection has been shown to be more effective than placebo in controlled trials (36% versus 17% clearance in one study using interferon-α_2b). However, intralesional injection of interferon is painful, cumbersome to perform, and not completely free of systemic toxicity.

Treatment of Warts at Other Sites

Exophytic condylomata of the cervix are rare, but when present are often accompanied by cervical dysplasia. Management in this situation is centered on the detection and treatment of coexistent dysplasia and is not affected by the presence or absence of HPV. There is no recommended therapy for non-condylomatous HPV infection of the cervix without dysplasia.

Vaginal condylomata should be treated with liquid nitrogen, TCA, or podophyllin. In using the latter agent, the treated area must be dry before the speculum is removed. Concern about increased systemic absorption through the vaginal mucosa has led to the recommendation that the area treated should be less than 2 cm^2. The nitrous oxide cryoprobe should not be used to treat vaginal warts because of the risk of perforation. Anal warts are treated with liquid nitrogen, TCA, or surgical removal.

Prevention

General guidelines for the prevention of transmission of STDs are applicable to HPV. Health care providers need to inform patients that sexual activity can result in infection of partners. This may be true whether or not overt clinical manifestations are present at the time of the activity because of the infectious potential of latent virus. The use of condoms should reduce the risk of transmission. Although it is reasonable to advise patients not to delay seeking medical attention when lesions appear and to be compliant with therapy and follow-up, there is no evidence to suggest that therapeutic interventions decrease transmissibility.

Because there is no effective therapy for incubating HPV, treatment of case contacts solely on the basis of exposure is not applicable to this disease. Clinically evident lesions can be treated as outlined above. Women exposed to HPV who do not have clinically apparent lesions do not require any intervention other than routine yearly Pap smears to screen for dysplasia.

Vertical transmission of HPV may lead to recurrent respiratory papillomatosis in infants and children. Although it is assumed that most transmission occurs during exposure to infected secretions during the birthing process, cases occurring in children delivered by cesarean section suggest that in utero transmission is possible. Thus, the presence of genital warts is not, by itself, an indication for cesarean section.

The World Health Organization has outlined strategies for vaccine development. Many questions remain unanswered. It is unknown whether antibody is protective, or to which antigens the antibodies should be directed. Vaccination with a live attenuated virus could be dangerous because of the oncogenic potential of HPV. Because genital HPVs are mucosotropic, it is probable that circulating antibody is not protective and that stimulation of mucosal IgA production will be an important feature of a successful vaccine.

Conclusion

As the epidemiology of anogenital HPV infection has become more clearly defined, it is apparent that this disorder is exceedingly common in sexually experienced women. Consequences of HPV infection include condylomata and under certain conditions, anogenital malignancies, the most notable of which is invasive cervical cancer. The treatment of genital warts is suboptimal, and novel therapies are being evaluated in clinical trials. As our understanding of the epidemiology and pathogenesis of HPV infection increases, more effective strategies can be implemented for early detection, treatment, and prevention of this potentially serious infectious disease. Over the next several years, physicians will have to determine how to best use the growing body of basic science knowledge and molecular technology in the management of their female patients with HPV disease.

SUGGESTED READINGS

Epidemiology

Daling JR, Sherman KJ, Weiss NS. Risk factors for condyloma acuminatum in women. Sex Transm Dis 1986;13:16–18.

Koutsky LA, Galloway DA, Holmes KK. Epidemiology of genital human papillomavirus infection. Epidemiol Rev 1988;10:122–163.

Syrjänen K, Hakama M, Saarikoski S, et al. Prevalence, incidence and estimated life-time risk of cervical human papillomavirus infections in a nonselected Finnish female population. Sex Transm Dis 1990;17:15–19.

HPV and Cancer

Paavonen J, Koutsky LA, Kiviat N. Cervical neoplasia and other STD-related genital and anal neoplasias. In: Holmes KK, Mårdh PA, Sparling PF, Wiesner PJ, eds. Sexually transmitted diseases. 2nd ed. New York: McGraw-Hill, 1990:561–592.

Clinical Manifestations

Campion MJ. Clinical manifestations and natural history of genital human papillomavirus infection. Obstet Gynecol Clin N Am 1987;14:363–388.

Diagnostic Tests

Lörincz AT. Human papillomavirus detection tests. In: Holmes KK, Mårdh PA, Sparling PF, Wiesner PJ, eds. Sexually transmitted diseases. 2nd ed. New York: McGraw-Hill, 1990:953–960.

Treatment

Centers for Disease Control and Prevention. Human papillomavirus infection. In: 1993 Sexually transmitted diseases treatment guidelines. MMWR 1993;42 (RR-14):83–88.

Kraus SJ, Stone KM. Management of genital infection caused by human papillomavirus. Rev Infect Dis 1990;12(suppl 6):S620–S632.

CHAPTER 24

VIRAL HEPATITIS AND ITS IMITATORS

Dirk J. van Leeuwen,
Andree Dadrat

Viral hepatitis refers to hepatic inflammation caused by viruses that primarily target the liver. At least five such viruses have now been identified and named: hepatitis A (HAV), B (HBV); C (HCV), D (HDV), and E (HEV) virus. The viruses have distinctive characteristics, which are summarized in Table 24.1. No doubt, further letters of the alphabet will follow, as additional viruses are identified. Other viral illnesses affecting the liver are usually childhood ailments or occur in the immunocompromised host and include measles, rubella, mumps, herpes, cytomegalovirus (CMV), and Epstein-Barr virus. These viruses may occasionally cause severe and even fatal liver injury in both children and adults. In addition, there are exotic viruses that will not be discussed in this chapter. However, conditions that may clinically imitate viral hepatitis will briefly be discussed.

Although infectious causes of jaundice have been recognized for a long time, major break-throughs have come in the last three decades. The first of many discoveries was the detection of HBV by Blumberg and colleagues in 1965 ("Australia antigen"), which was identified as the cause of previously so-called serum hepatitis. This was followed by the identification of the HAV in 1973 by Feinstone and coworkers as the cause of so-called infectious hepatitis. The HDV ("delta agent"), a small RNA virus that needs HBV for its replication, was described in 1978 by Rizetto and associates and finally the HCV in 1989 by Houghton and colleagues. In 1983, Balayan transmitted a water-borne form of hepatitis to monkeys that was later shown to be HEV. It has now become clear that a majority of cases of hepatitis previously called non-A, non-B hepatitis are caused by HCV (parenterally transmitted non-A, non-B hepatitis) and hepatitis E (enterically transmitted non-A, non-B hepatitis). The identification of the viruses has been accompanied by the rapid development of diagnostic tests and both passive and active immunization, which have already greatly contributed to reducing the transmission of viral disease. Antiviral therapy has been developed and liver transplantation is possible for certain patients with viral hepatitis who develop liver failure. (For historical reviews, see Suggested Readings, General Reviews.) Women are as likely to be affected by viral hepatitis and viral illnesses as men although certain differences are notable. They may transmit the virus to their newborns, and they will suffer a high mortality if they contract hepatitis E during pregnancy. A large number of women are occupationally exposed to these diseases, especially in the health care professions and the sex trade. Recent data also suggest that spouses of patients with HCV viremia and chronic liver disease have a somewhat increased risk of acquiring HCV, proportional to the duration of marriage.

This chapter reviews the current knowledge on hepatitis with particular emphasis on the diagnosis and management of these diseases by the nonspecialist and most importantly, the efforts at prevention and possible eradication of this disease with its large global impact on public health care.

Epidemiology

All hepatitis viruses may cause *acute* hepatitis of variable severity, but only HBV, HCV, and HDV are important causes of *chronic* liver disease. Worldwide chronic viral hepatitis B is the most frequent cause of cirrhosis with an estimated 400 million people, or 5% of the world population, being HBV carriers. Up to 50% of these may develop cirrhosis or hepatocellular

Table 24.1 Characteristics of Hepatitis Viruses

Virus	Abbreviation	Genome	Family	Transmission	Chronicity	Risk of Hepatocellular Carcinoma
Hepatitis A	HAV	RNA	Picornavirus	Water	No	No
Hepatitis B	HBV	DNA	Hepadnavirus	Blood	Yes	Yes
Hepatitis C	HCV	RNA	Flavivirus	Blood	Yes	Yes
Hepatitis D	HDV	RNA	Satellite	Blood	Yes	Yes
Hepatitis E	HEV	RNA	Calcivirus	Water	No	No

carcinoma (HCC) as a consequence. The worldwide distribution of HCV, and its contribution to the number of HCC cases is currently being studied, but it is already evident that HCV is another major cause of chronic liver disease and HCC.

In the United States, an estimated 1 million people are affected by chronic hepatitis B and 2 to 3 million by hepatitis C. Most of these patients are asymptomatic and estimates suggest that up to 90% of chronic viral hepatitis patients are detected by elevated liver tests incidentally noted on routine screening or when trying to donate blood. In the United States, chronic viral hepatitis is the second most frequent cause of cirrhosis after alcohol abuse. The Centers for Disease Control and Prevention (CDC) has established it to be the second most common reported disease after gonorrhea, despite the fact that only about 50% of the cases of viral hepatitis are recognized.

Hepatitis A and Hepatitis E (Waterborne Hepatitis)

Hepatitis A is a waterborne disease that is spread by fecal–oral transmission. The annual incidence of hepatitis A infection in the United States is placed somewhere between 30,000 and 50,000 cases. HAV is typically found in association with poor hygiene and sanitation, and consequently more prevalent in developing countries, where the majority of the population will have developed hepatitis A antibodies in the first decade of life. Hepatitis A in children is usually a minor disease, if recognized at all. However, in the developed world, which has much higher levels of hygiene, the prevalence of antibodies to HAV increases only gradually with advancing age, to reach approximately 50% at age 30 and almost 60% to 80% at age 60. In developed countries, hepatitis A epidemics also occur and these seem to be on a 10-year cycle that is presumably related to population susceptibility. HAV epidemics also occur in the developed world in areas of natural disasters with breakdown of normal sanitation and, to a smaller extent, in institutionalized populations (day-care centers, residences for mentally handicapped). Hepatitis A is found at an increased rate among the homosexual population.

Hepatitis E is the second waterborne hepatitis virus and was first recognized as a cause of epidemics in the Far East and on the Indian subcontinent. It is very rare in the United States, but the disease needs to be considered in people who have visited endemic areas. The disease seems to affect mainly young adults of both genders and has a devastating effect on pregnant women with mortality figures as high as 15% to 40%.

Hepatitis B, C, and D (Bloodborne Hepatitis)

Hepatitis B, C, and D are diseases that are spread via blood and body fluids. Approximately 300,000 new hepatitis B infections and 200,000 cases of hepatitis C are estimated to occur among 260 million Americans each year.

Risk factors for HBV infection are related to its hematogenous and body fluid spread, which is in many ways similar to the spread of the HCV. A major difference is that HCV is much less (1000-fold) contagious than HBV. However, if HCV is contracted, up to 80% of cases become chronic. Risk factors for developing these illnesses include blood or blood product transfusions, intravenous (IV) drug use, tattoos, and homosexuality. Health care workers, especially nurses, dental technicians, and IV teams, are at high risk. HBV in endemic areas accounts for a high prevalence of vertically transmitted disease from mother to child around birth and a high horizontal transmission rate in the first few years of life with intimate contacts with numerous carriers. This leads to the high incidence of chronic hepatitis and its complications (cirrhosis, HCC). The ability to clear the virus appears to be related to the age at which the infection is contracted: the younger the age of infection, the less likely the patient is able to clear the virus. Newborn infants therefore may become carriers in up to 98% of cases, whereas healthy adults may eradicate the virus in over 95% of patients infected. The clearance rate of the virus is somewhat higher in female patients compared to male patients, indicating that genetic or hormonal aspects of immune competence play a role. It is important to realize that in 20% to 40% of the cases of hepatitis B and C, *no* specific risk factors can be identified. Previously it was believed that we easily could determine which mothers were at risk of transmitting the HBV to their children on history of endemic background, IV drug abuse, and other factors. However, it now appears that up to 8% of children were missed using these criteria. This recognition is one of the reasons why universal vaccination of newborns is now recommended.

Hepatitis D virus occurs in conjunction with hepatitis B, either as a coinfection or superinfection. HDV is endemic in countries bordering the Mediterranean, particularly Italy and the Middle East. A second area of high prevalence is in the Amazon basin in South America where it affects primarily children and results in a high mortality. In nonendemic areas HDV is most commonly found in IV drug abusers. The combined pathology due to HBV and HDV tends to be worse compared to HBV alone.

Pathogenesis

Some simplified concepts are helpful to understand the pathology of viral hepatitis. Both direct cytotoxic and immune-mediated mechanisms of injury are proposed and probably both are relevant, even if one mechanism prevails. The HAV is thought to act through a *direct cytopathic* effect on the hepatocytes, leading to hepatocellular death. The clearance of the virus and death of cells is sometimes accompanied by a transient deepening of jaundice. In hepatitis E, probably similar mechanisms are responsible for liver damage; therefore, the clinical picture is also similar.

The pathology caused by HBV is the result of cytotoxic T cell-mediated processes. Cytotoxic T cells recognize as their target the viral antigen (predominantly HBcAg) bound to HLA-1 at the hepatocyte surface and as a consequence eliminate the hepatocyte. Therapy with interferon is believed to work by a combination of inhibiting viral replication and enhancing the immune response to eliminate the virus and the disease. One of the postulated modes of action of interferon is the enhancement of HLA-1 expression on the hepatocyte with subsequent enhancement of T cell recognition and elimination. Persistence (chronicity) of the disease is caused by an insufficient immune response.

The HDV is an RNA virus that needs HBsAg for its replication. If the patient is already a carrier, superinfection with HDV can take a dramatic course because "the factory is ready for immediate replication." HBV and HDV coinfection tend to run a less severe course because HBsAg production is required before significant HDV replication can occur.

The pathology caused by hepatitis C virus is less well understood. There is increasing evidence that the HCV genotype plays a role in the pathology. Factors (alcohol and iron) in addition to the virus itself are crucial as well. The virus probably acts as a cytopathic agent. Recent data suggest that cellular immunity also plays a part in the pathology.

Clinical Aspects of Viral Hepatitis

Viral hepatitis, both acute and chronic, can present as a spectrum from subclinical to fulminant disease (Fig 24.1). Clinically, all types of viral hepatitis may have a similar presentation. The history may be more revealing than physical examination.

Acute viral hepatitis can be *icteric* or *nonicteric*. If symptoms develop at all, they usually start with a prodrome lasting from 3 to 5 days to 3 or more weeks and consisting of headaches, malaise, flulike symptoms, arthalgias, low-grade fevers, and frequently loss of taste for food and cigarettes. Some patients develop nausea, vomiting, and right upper quadrant pain, occasionally even diarrhea.

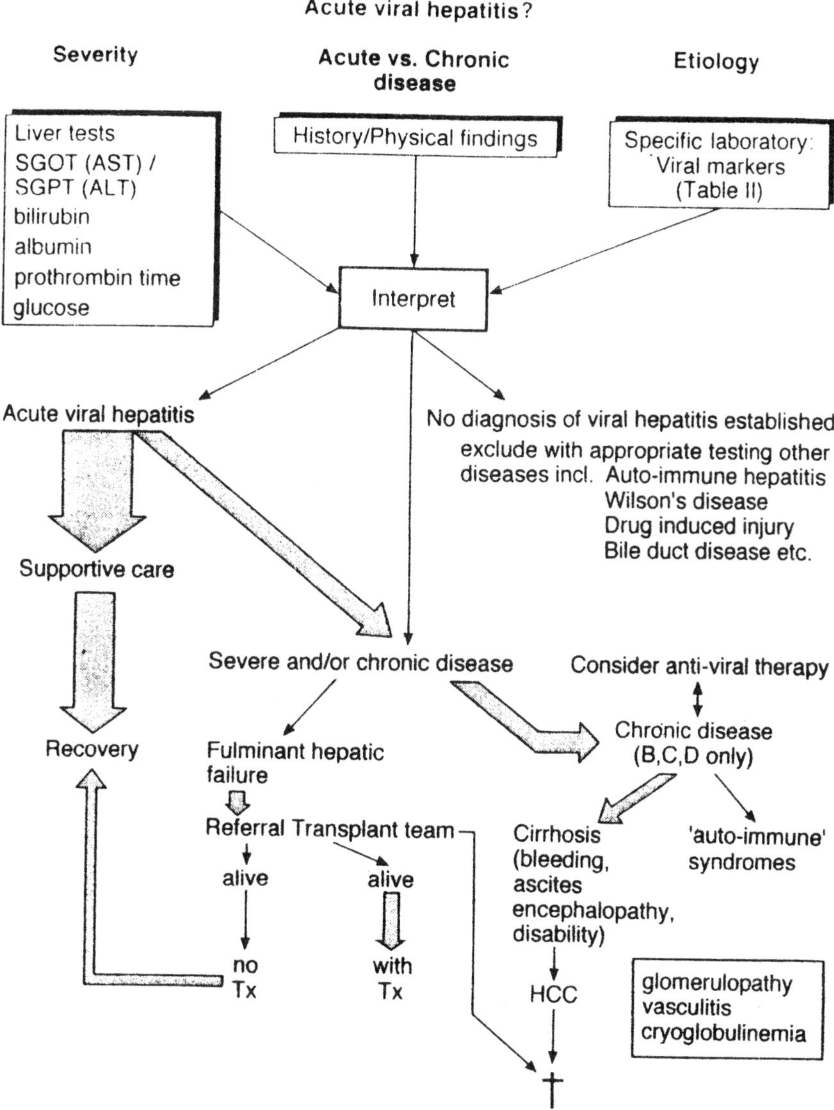

Fig 24.1 Algorithm for diagnostics and management of acute viral hepatitis.
HCC, hepatocellular carcinoma; SGOT, serum glutamic-oxaloacetic transaminase (AST, aspartate transaminase) ; SGPT, serum glutamate pyruvate transaminase (ALT, alanine transaminase)

The physical findings are also nonspecific. The patient may develop lymphadenopathy, mild splenomegaly, and mild hepatomegaly with some tenderness in the right upper quadrant due to the stretch of Glisson's capsule. In addition, jaundice accompanied by occasional pruritus as well as excoriated skin lesions from scratching can be found in patients with icteric hepatitis. Unlike viral hepatitis, certain symptoms are helpful in differentiating some causes of jaundice not related to hepatitis. For example, obstructive jaundice due to gallstone disease is suggested by biliary colic, whereas malignant jaundice often presents with few or no other symptoms.

Extrahepatic manifestations, although rare, may be induced by chronic viral hepatitis. These include skin manifestations (rashes, vasculitis), joint symptoms, kidney disease (nephrotic syndrome, glomerulonephritis), polyarteritis, and mixed cryoglobulinemia.

Work-up of the Patient with Presumed Viral Hepatitis

A physician faced with a potential case of viral hepatitis has to establish a specific *etiologic* diagnosis, obtain an impression about the *severity* of the disease, establish if the condition is *acute* or *chronic*, and determine why the disease has become symptomatic (see Fig 24.1). An increasing number of tests are available (Table 24.2) to aid in diagnosis. However, not all tests are appropriate in all patients. Which tests should be ordered in case of suspicion of acute viral hepatitis?

Table 24.2 Viral Markers and Their Interpretation

Virus	Tests	Interpretation	Comments
HAV	anti-HAV IgM	Acute hepatitis	Can remain positive for >1 yr
	anti-HAV IgG	Past hepatitis, immunity	Life-long!
HBV	HBsAg	Acute *or* chronic disease	
	anti-HBc IgM	Acute infection (high titer) Chronic infection (low titer)	
	anti-HBc IgG	Any past or recent HBV contact	Can be only serum indicator of past infection
	HBe	Active viral replication	Is becoming obsolete. Has played major role in diagnosing replication
	anti-HBe	Low or absent replicative state	Typically present in long-standing HBV carriers
	anti-HBs	Immunity	Immunity, after vaccination
	HBV-DNA	Active viral replication	Expensive; may replace HBeAg if price declines
HCV	anti-HCV	Past *or* current infection	Not a neutralizing antibody
	RIBA	Test for various viral components	Expensive, limited indications
	HCV-RNA	Active viral replication	Expensive, limited indications (treatment)
HDV	anti-HDV IgM	Acute or chronic infection	Consider HDV only if HBsAg positive
	anti-HDV IgG	Chronic infection (high titer and IgM positive) Past infection (low titer and IgM negative)	
	HDV-RNA	Replication of delta	
HEV	anti-HEV IgM	Acute hepatitis	Not commercially available in United States
	anti-HEV IgG	Past hepatitis	CDC may test in selected cases
	HEV-RNA	Viral replication	

Most laboratories have an "acute hepatitis panel," that includes anti-HAV (IgM) to diagnose acute hepatitis A, HBsAg and anti-HBc (IgM) as indicators of acute HBV hepatitis; and, increasingly, anti-HCV (IgG) testing.

As can be seen from Table 24.2, hepatitis A tends to be straightforward. Anti-IgM reflects acute disease, but may remain positive for up to a year, whereas IgG antibodies indicate immunity and a past HAV infection.

For HBV, a great number of markers are available, which reflect the various viral components and related antibodies to the virus. The interpretation of a positive HBsAg is subject of much confusion and depends to a great extent on the clinical circumstances: if accompanied by clinical and biochemical tests of acute hepatitis, the latter diagnosis is likely. Further support may be obtained from a positive anti-HBc (IgM). If the patient has stigmata of chronic liver disease on examination (palmar erythema, spider naevi, gynecomastia, wasting, etc.), but the clinical picture of acute hepatitis, other causes of hepatitis need to be considered, including other viral infections (A, C, D), alcohol, and hepatoxic drugs. If physical signs and laboratory findings suggest chronic liver disease (low platelets, prolonged prothrombin time, low albumin, etc.), chronic hepatitis B infection that has progressed to cirrhosis, should be considered. If abdominal pain, wasting, or general deterioration occurs, HCC and intra-abdominal infection need to be excluded.

Traditionally, HBeAg positivity has been used as a marker for active viral replication. However, HBV-DNA testing has now become widely available and this test is the best indicator of active viral replication and should probably replace HBeAg testing. HBV-DNA testing is expensive and, therefore, not routinely used in the diagnosis of hepatitis B. HBV-DNA levels are particularly valuable to monitor the effect of antiviral therapy.

Testing for HCV only became available in 1989. The sensitivity and specificity of testing has rapidly increased. A patient who is anti-HCV positive with the newest second-generation enzyme-linked radioimmunoassay tests has a high likelihood of having a hepatitis C infection. However, it may take 6 months before the anti-HCV becomes positive. In rare difficult cases, reversed immuno-blotting assay (RIBA testing) can be used to increase the specificity somewhat. HCV-RNA testing is still a costly tool, but it is increasingly used in clinical protocols. The significance of anti-HCV is that it indicates past or ongoing HCV infection. Anti-HCV is *not* a neutralizing antibody. The presence of HCV-RNA indicates viral replication. This test guides treatment with interferon therapy.

Hepatitis D testing should be done in HBsAg positive patients, particularly in patients from an endemic area or IV drug abusers with unexpected severe hepatitis B.

Hepatitis E testing is not yet commercially available in the United States, but the CDC does it, if indicated. In many other countries commercial testing can be done. In many parts of the world it is rarely indicated due to the prevalence of the disease.

Course of the Disease

In addition to the clinical findings and course of the disease, the use of certain tests can be helpful (see Fig 24.1). Elevated transaminases, SGPT/SGOT, for example, indicate hepatocellular necrosis. Although they are imprecise with respect to prognosis, they certainly reflect the extent of damage. Severe viral hepatitis may be accompanied by transaminase values as high as 10,000 IU. A rapid increase to very high levels followed by a rapid decrease within a few days may reflect acute (transient) ischemia. An indicator of poor prognosis is the combination of rapidly declining transaminases in a deteriorating patient with rising prothrombin time. This usually denotes nearly complete hepatocellular necrosis with no further liberation of aminotransferases. Hypoglycemia, a low factor V, and impaired renal function may be other indicators of severe disease.

Hepatic synthetic function is reflected in the albumin level and prothrombin time. The bilirubin is an indicator of hepatic excretory function. In the chronic setting, a drop in albumin may presage further decompensation and a low platelet count is often the reflection of splenomegaly and portal hypertension. A rise in bilirubin value in a cirrhotic patient may indicate irreversible deterioration of liver function. None of these tests are in fact true function tests.

Anicteric Viral Hepatitis

An estimated 20% to 50% of all cases of viral hepatitis are believed to run an anicteric course. Anicteric cases of acute hepatitis are generally milder but more frequently (HBV, HCV) evolve into chronic disease. Although there is currently no good explanation for this phenomenon, it has been suggested that in HBV infection severe jaundice reflects an aggressive immune attack with a higher likelihood of HBV clearance.

Differential Diagnosis of Viral Hepatitis

The diagnosis of viral hepatitis is based on clincial suspicion, substantiated by the appropriate laboratory investigations. The clinician must be aware of conditions that mimic viral hepatitis. The patient who presents with the clinical picture of acute hepatitis, but whose test results do not confirm acute viral hepatitis, may require consultation with a specialist. There are several considerations in this situation.

First, viral hepatitis may be present, but testing is still negative. It may take months before antibodies become detectable against hepatitis C; or the HBsAg has just become negative but anti-HBs is not yet detectable ("window phase").

Second, other viruses may be responsible for abnormal liver test results. Infectious mononucleosis is sometimes forgotten outside childhood although occasionally children may infect their parents or grandparents. Severe CMV hepatitis is not uncommon in the immunocompromised host and particularly human immunodeficiency virus (HIV)-infected and transplant patients. Herpes virus sometimes should be considered and the presence of herpetic lesions may help in making this diagnosis. However, disseminated herpes infection in adults is rare and when it occurs, skin lesions may be absent.

Another possibility is bacterial infection, which, however, only rarely mimics viral hepatitis. Pronounced cholestatic disease may be seen in the setting of septicemia (particularly due to gram-negative organisms) and total parenteral nutrition. Leptospirosis is characterized by high bilirubin, kidney failure that is not a hepatorenal syndrome and conjunctivitis: a history of water and rats remains crucial in making this diagnosis.

Hepatotoxic drugs are a frequent cause of hepatitis and a detailed drug history should be obtained. This should include questions about over-the-counter medications (nonsteroidals, acetaminophen), herbal teas, and other alternative medicines.

Autoimmune hepatitis can be a diagnostic challenge. In many liver diseases, autoimmune markers may be present but are not specific for autoimmune hepatitis. Autoimmune hepatitis can present at any age with a variety of symptoms and frequently has a fluctuating course. This sometimes causes a diagnostic delay with missed opportunities for medical treatment and potentially a fatal outcome unless transplantation is used. A hepatitis patient in whom no satisfactory explanation is found for an apparent acute viral hepatitis requires specific testing including autoimmune markers, protein electrophoresis, and a liver biopsy. Wilson's disease may occasionally present with acute hepatitis. Kayser-Fleischer rings, impaired clotting, hemolysis, and a low ceruloplasmin level should help in making the diagnosis.

Reason for admission to a hospital are the development of complications such as dehydration, hypoglycemia, coagulopathy, infections, and mental status changes, or fulminant hepatitis.

Fulminant hepatitis is defined as major impairment of liver function and development of hepatic encephalopathy within 2 months of developing hepatitis in a patient without preexisting liver disease. Early recognition of this syndrome is important to initiate appropriate treatment.

Role of Liver Biopsy

In case of typical acute viral hepatitis, a liver biopsy does not provide further diagnostic information and is therefore not indicated. In cases of acute disease mimicking viral hepatitis where the etiology is unclear, a liver biopsy may prove helpful. In chronic disease, there are a number of indications for liver biopsy including the assessment of cirrhosis, disease activity, and defining etiology in some patients. Biopsy guided by ultrasound or computed tomography (CT) scanning will help to diagnose malignancy in case of focal liver lesions.

Role of Imaging Techniques

Ultrasonography and CT scanning of the abdomen are helpful in assessing liver disease. Aspects that can be assessed include the liver size, architectural changes, spleen size, and the presence of vascular abnormalities and collaterals. Bile duct obstruction can be recognized and gallstones or tumors may be seen. Scintigraphy is no longer a first choice for imaging technique.

Viral Hepatitis in Pregnancy

Up to 1% of pregnancies are complicated by viral hepatitis. For the obstetrician, the differential diagnosis of jaundice in pregnancy includes disorders of variable severity, such as intrahepatic cholestasis of pregnancy, acute fatty liver of pregnancy, pre-eclampsia/eclampsia, and infectious etiologies. The management of jaundice is determined by the underlying etiology.

In the United States, viral hepatitis is the most common cause of jaundice during pregnancy and the clinical presentation and outcome are no different between pregnant and nonpregnant patients. Reports from certain countries with less well developed medical care suggest a higher infant and mother mortality and morbidity, which may be in part related to referral bias. As mentioned, hepatitis E has a high mortality in areas where HEV is endemic (India, Middle East, and Africa). It is unclear whether the high mortality of HEV infection in pregnancy is an inherent function of the virus or mainly related to the poor prenatal care and nutritional status of the woman. Viral hepatitis does not appear to adversely affect pregnancy, and there is generally no clear reason to terminate the pregnancy solely due to the fact that the patient has viral hepatitis. In contrast, acute fatty liver of pregnancy and toxemia may be an indication for termination of pregnancy. A pregnancy complicated by toxemia or a delivery with resulting shock from blood loss may cause significantly elevated liver function test results, mimicking fulminant hepatitis. The vertical transmission of hepatitis A virus is not a clinical problem. In the rare circumstance where acute hepatitis A occurs during the last few weeks of pregnancy, passive immune prophylaxis of the neonate with a single shot of immunoglobulins shortly after delivery is the only therapy required.

The CDC recommends that all pregnant women be tested for hepatitis B. This is directed particularly at women who are carriers of HBV and the risk transmitting the disease during birth, when the baby is at direct contact with the mother's blood. Transplacental transmission probably does not occur. Cesarean section is not a means of protecting or reducing the incidence of vertical transmission. The possibility of transmitting hepatitis via breast milk is controversial. However, in the developed world with its ready availability of safe infant formula that can be kept in optimal condition, the potential risk of breast-feeding probably outweighs its benefit in HBV-positive mothers. Fortunately, the newborn can be protected from developing the disease with the help of active/passive immune prophylaxis (Table 24.3). This consists of HBV vaccination. The first dose is given within 24 hours of birth, combined with 0.5 mL of hepatitis B immunoglobulin (HBIG) within 48 hours of birth, and the second at 1 month with a booster dose at 6 months. HBIG adds somewhat to the highly protective effect of active vaccination. The CDC now recommends universal vaccination against HBV for all newborns as part of the general vaccination program for children.

Vertical transmission of HCV is believed to be rare. It seems to be enhanced by conditions of immune compromise such as HIV positivity of the mother. When vertical transmission does occur, the risk

Table 24.3 Guide to Postexposure Immunoprophylaxis for Hepatitis B Virus

Type of Exposure	Immunoprophylaxis
Perinatal	Vaccination + HBIG 0.5 mL
Sexual	
Acute infection	Vaccination + HBIG 0.06 mL/kg
Chronic carrier	Vaccination
Household contacts	
Acute case	
Incidental contact	None unless exposure known
Known exposure	Vaccination ± HBIG 0.02 mL/kg
Infant (<12 mo) (acute hepatitis in primary caregiver	Vaccination + HBIG 0.5 mL
Chronic case	Screening and vaccination
Inadvertent occupational exposure (percutaneous /permucosal)	Vaccination ± HBIG 0.06 mL/kg

HBIG, hepatitis B immunoglobulin

correlates with the level of HCV-RNA in the mother. The presence of anti-HCV in the newborn does not necessarily indicate infection and infection may be present in the absence of anti-HCV. HCV-RNA testing is helpful in this setting. No specific protective measure for newborns to HCV-positive mothers exists. Although some authorities recommend immune serum globulin injection, there is as yet no sound basis for this recommendation.

HDV infection in newborns is extremely rare. Hepatitis B vaccination will protect because HDV cannot replicate in the absence of HBsAg. Prevention of HBV is prevention of HDV as well.

Despite its high maternal morbidity, no cases of vertical transmission of HEV have been documented.

Maternal chronic persistent hepatitis (minor parenchymal disease) causes no significant increase in fetal or maternal mortality or morbidity. In women with chronic active hepatitis, pregnancy is less common because secondary amenorrhea is common and may occasionally be the first presentation of liver disease. Pregnancy does occur without noticeable effect on the underlying disease. In case of cirrhosis, maternal morbidity and mortality increase sharply and these patients are subject to all the complications of end-stage liver disease including ascites and development of spontaneous bacterial peritonitis, portal hypertension, esophageal varices and bleeding, hepatic encephalopathy, and hepatorenal syndrome. Almost all patients with end-stage liver disease have amenorrhea or are infertile. The management of viral hepatitis during pregnancy is supportive only, with the exception of requiring close maternal and fetal monitoring for the development of complications.

Treatment and Prevention

Acute Hepatitis

The Patient

The majority of patients with acute hepatitis will recover without chronic sequelae. The mainstay of treatment has remained supportive care, avoidance of additional hepatic toxins, and consideration of liver transplantation in the deteriorating fulminant cases. The latter will occur in fewer than 1% of the cases.

The majority of patients with viral hepatitis can be managed as outpatients but should be followed closely enough to recognize any deterioration. Reasons for admission include alteration in mental status, inability to maintain hydration or nutrition due to persistent nausea and vomiting, or significant biochemical deterioration with rapidly rising prothrombin time, transaminases, and bilirubin, or falling albumin. Acute hepatitis may contribute to malabsorption, and this, in addition to the anorexia frequently found in hepatitis patients, may lead to significant weight loss. Adequate calorie intake should be encouraged, and no dietary restrictions should be imposed.

The Environment

New cases of viral hepatitis should be reported to the public health department. This is in the interest of the patient, the environment, and the public. The public health team will bring in specific expertise and often arrange screening and vaccination for close contacts of the affected patient. The household contacts of a newly diagnosed patient should receive appropriate active (A and B) and passive (A) immunization as soon as possible. This may not always prevent the outbreak of disease, but will mitigate the severity.

Acute viral hepatitis requires adequate hygiene. If possible, a separate bathroom and separation of toilet equipment should be available. A patient with clinically overt hepatitis A is usually no longer highly contagious. Studies have shown that viral presence in feces rapidly diminishes, when jaundice presents; however, more recent data would suggest that the virus may circulate somewhat longer in the serum (up to a week after the onset of jaundice) than previously believed.

Medical personnel have always been at increased risk to contract the virus from patients than vice versa. The current protection of health care personnel, increased levels of hygiene and specific precautions (gloves, screening of blood products, needle-stick policies), and the implementation of vaccination programs have greatly contributed to the reduced incidence of hepatitis in the medical community. A former policy of specifically labeling risky patients has been abandoned: "The most dangerous specimen is the unidentified dangerous specimen."

Chronic Viral Hepatitis

In cases of hepatitis B, C, and D, the identification of a carrier would require protection of the intimate partner and household contacts. This is possible with vaccination for HBV, which prevents HDV as well, but unfortunately no vaccine against HCV is as yet available. The psychosocial impact of the HBV carrier state is too often greatly underestimated by physicians as to fears regarding risks of sexual intercourse, kissing grandchildren, or casual contacts in the community. Patient education is important and it should be emphasized that all those close to HBV patients should be vaccinated. The disease will not be transmitted by shaking hands or the incidental kiss, but contact with blood or body fluids via open wounds is a potential means of transmission and therefore more risky. As mentioned, hepatitis B is probably at least 1000 times more contagious compared to HCV infection. Therefore, unprotected intercourse should be avoided by the nonimmune partner of an HBV carrier, unless already immune or vaccinated. Most physicians will be much less restrictive in case of hepatitis C because of the much lower transmission rate.

Immune Prophylaxis (see Table 24.3)

Passive Immunization

Immunoglobulins are used for *passive* immune prophylaxis. This is usually recommended for protection over a limited period as well as postexposure protection. Administration of immunoglobulins is now safe because they are tested for and guaranteed to be HIV negative and HBsAg negative. Both γ globulin and HBIG are felt to be safe for use as hepatitis prophylaxis in pregnant and lactating women.

Hepatitis A

Conventional immunoglobulins (γ globulins) are a stabilized protein solution containing antibodies to HAV in excess of 1 in 1000. Unfortunately, with a half-life of approximately 3 weeks following administration, the protection afforded by these immunoglobulins is relatively short lived.

Hepatitis B

The second immunoglobulin is HBIG, which has a high titer of antibody to HBsAg (>1:100,000). HBIG is used to prevent HBV recurrence after liver transplantation. The unacceptable high cost for repeated doses is a major setback for extensive use.

Active Immunization

The second form of immune prophylaxis is *active* immunization with a vaccine that provides long-term if not lifelong immunity.

Hepatitis A

A vaccine has become available in many countries outside the United States. Approval from the Food and Drug Administration (FDA) has been obtained. Of interest is the fact that one injection already may provide years of immunity. There is no doubt that in the near future a liberal vaccination policy will be recommended.

Hepatitis B

A number of recombinant DNA vaccines have become available with a high protective efficacy. Two are FDA approved and available in the United States and provide immunity in 90% to 95% of patients vaccinated. The usual protocol involves the first two injections 4 weeks apart, with a booster dose at approximately 6 months after the first inoculation. The protective antibody is anti-HBs, which will be present in sufficiently high titers (>20 IU) in over 90% of people following the third inoculation. The longevity of the response is not known due to the relatively short period of use of the vaccine. The low risk of vaccination in contrast to the potentially deleterious effect of viral hepatitis and chronic hepatitis with its complications have led the CDC to recommend universal vaccinations against hepatitis B of all newborn infants and gradually the population at large. This policy was developed to protect children and young adults (sex, IV drugs) from a potentially devastating disease. It is increasingly believed, that even if antibody titers drop, boosters after 5 to 10 years are not indicated due to the quick memory response of the immune system. For those who do not develop antibodies, a second course of vaccine can be attempted with double dose vaccine at monthly intervals. A group of nonresponders, including immunocompromised patients, will remain.

Needle Stick Injury: In persons accidentally exposed to HBV by a needle stick, a combination of active and passive immune prophylaxis with HBIG and vaccine is now standard of care (see Table 24.3). Similarly, neonates born to HBV-positive mothers should receive two doses of HBIG 4 weeks apart and starting within 24 to 48 hours after birth in addition to the recombinant vaccine. The need to vaccinate the sexual partner was already discussed. An exception can be made for individuals who have documented anti-HBs in their blood.

Hepatitis C

Although there are currently no vaccines available yet, aggressive research is ongoing and hopefully vaccines will become available in the near future.

Therapy for Chronic Viral Hepatitis

General Aspects

Antiviral therapy aims to eliminate the virus and infectivity, to reduce symptoms, to halt inflammation and progression toward cirrhosis, and prevent the development of HCC.

Although no effective antiviral therapy can be recommended for the acute infection as yet, chronic hepatitis B, C, and possibly D show a response to therapy with interferon alfa-2b in selected patients. Other agents are currently under investigation.

Interferon therapy is associated with a number of side effects. In practice, the therapy is tolerated by most patients, particularly at lower dosages. General malaise, flulike symptoms and arthralgias are commonly experienced side effects. Less common side effects include drop in white blood cell and platelet counts, which rarely causes bleeding or infectious problems, and depression. Depression can be severe; a history of significant depression in the past is a relative contraindication, and ongoing depression is an absolute contraindication to therapy. Interferon therapy should be supervised by physicians experienced with its use. There are pitfalls including insidious development of hypothroidism following interferon therapy. This can be easily missed or occasionally be interpreted as worsening liver disease.

Patients need to be screened to assess their suitability for therapy and calculate the likelihood of a response. A liver biopsy is part of this assessment to document the severity of the disease and the histologic activity and to exclude other pathology.

Hepatitis B: Several factors can be used as positive and negative predictors of response to interferon in clearance of HBV (Table 24.4). HBV-infected patients (HBsAg positive, HBeAg positive and preferably documented HBV-DNA positive) should have documented elevation of transaminases for 6 months and lack evidence of decompensated liver disease (jaundice, ascites, end-stage cirrhosis with varices or hepatic encephalopathy). With the currently recommended regimens (daily 5 million IU or three times weekly 10 million IU for 4 to 6 months), 30% to 40% of patients will respond (loss of HBeAg and normalization of transaminases) of which up to 10% will relapse with time. The effect of interferon needs to be followed after stopping therapy because markers may disappear 6 to 12 months later. Spontaneous seroconversion may occur as well, on average in 10% of the chronic carriers.

Hepatitis C: Patients with HCV considered for interferon therapy should show no sign of decompensated liver disease, have their transaminases monitored for a period of about 6 months due to the inherent fluctua-

Table 24.4 Predictors of Response to Interferon Therapy

HEPATITIS B	
Positive Predictors	Negative Predictors
Heterosexual	Homosexual
Female	Male
White	Asian
HIV negative	HIV positive
Anti-HDV negative	Anti-HDV positive
HBV-DNA low	Low ALT
HBV DNA high	
High ALT	Histology with little inflammation
Histology with active inflammation	
HEPATITIS C (POSITIVE PREDICTORS, LIMITED DATA AS YET)	
Chronic persistent hepatitis on liver biopsy	
Absence of cirrhosis	
Low serum ferritin	
Genotype 2	
Low serum HCV-RNA level	

ALT, alanine aminotransferase; HIV, human immunodeficiency virus

tion of levels, and have a liver biopsy before therapy is started. The current recommendation is interferon-α 3 million IU three times weekly for 6 months. The expected response rate is about 50% of patients treated, but, unfortunately, about half of the initial responders will relapse in time. This results in a long-term response rate of only 20%.

Predictors of response are less well identified, but certain viral subtypes and low levels of HCV-RNA at the start of therapy may increase the likelihood of response. Excess liver iron may contribute to a diminished response. A variety of dosages and time schedules are under investigation, and longer treatment (up to 12 months) may increase the long-term response rate. If the patient shows no sign of response to the above regimens by 6 (or even 3) months, further interferon is unlikely to have any beneficial effect.

Hepatitis D: HDV responds best to 9 million IU interferon every other day. On this schedule about two thirds of patients have shown improvement or normalization of aspartate transaminase, but one half of these patients relapsed. Although the histology improved, it did not result in a sustained loss of HDV-RNA.

Treatment of Complications of Chronic Liver Disease

Although general malaise, fatigue, and wasting are often accompanying features of chronic liver disease, the three major complications of chronic liver disease are *bleeding varices*, *ascites*, and *portosystemic encephalopathy*.

Bleeding varices are usually treated with sclerotherapy or banding. Shunt surgery is indicated in a limited number of patients. β-Blocking agents (propranolol) and nitrates play a role in the prevention of bleeding. Ascites is treated with salt restriction, diuretics (spironolactone and furosemide), and large volume paracentesis. Transjugular intrahepatic shunts are increasingly used in the treatment of refractory bleeding and ascites. The treatment of portosystemic encephalopathy includes lactulose (with the goal of two to three soft bowel motions daily), avoidance of benzodiazepines, and protein restriction if medical therapy is unsuccessful.

Liver Transplantation

Liver transplantation has become a viable treatment option for both acute fulminant hepatitis and end-stage chronic liver disease. Whereas HAV, HCV, and HDV infected patients tend to do well, HBV infection is associated with a high clinical and histologic recurrence rate in the new liver and an accelerated course of disease. Many centers will deny HBV-infected patients transplantation or will select HBV-DNA-negative patients and protect them with HBIG indefinitely.

Patients need a thorough pretransplant evaluation. This evaluation includes the assessment of suitability with respect to medical, psychosocial, and economic factors.

Fulminant Hepatic Failure

The mortality of fulminant hepatitis previously was 60% to 90%. This has dramatically changed with the increase of acute liver transplantation. Acute liver transplantation for fulminant hepatic failure is associated with a 1-year survival rate of 60% to 90%. Therefore, any suitable candidate with this syndrome should be referred to a transplant center for optimal treatment. These patients are threatened by rapid deterioration and can develop a number of problems such as coagulopathy, volume and electrolyte disturbances, hypoglycemia, infections, and others. Mental status changes (hepatic coma) may develop and be worsened by any of the aforementioned conditions. Early involvement of a transplant team is essential and the timing of transplantation is critical.

Chronic Liver Disease

As soon as the patient deteriorates or medical treatment starts to fail, suitable candidates should be evaluated by a liver transplant team. A patient whose only complication is bleeding varices usually can be managed with sclerotherapy or other measures to control bleeding. A patient who starts to miss work, has increasingly disabling symptoms, or has refractory ascites and signs of encephalopathy, requires evaluation for liver transplantation. These patients are in certain countries (United States) prone to lose their job and health insurance first, before transplantation is considered. This can greatly add to the constraints for the patient and transplant team. The patient with very advanced disease who is referred late may survive transplantation but with increased morbidity and expense.

Summary

Viral hepatitis can be a severe disease with a variety of presentations, but recovery is the rule in the majority of patients. An increasing number of causes have been identified over the last three decades. The possibilities for prevention at many different levels are rapidly increasing and should lead to a further reduction and possible elimination of viral hepatitis.

Improved socioeconomic circumstances have dramatically reduced exposure to HAV in the developed world. This has created a shift toward an elderly population contracting the disease with increased morbidity and mortality. Vaccination should solve this problem.

Although in many areas preventive measures have helped to reduce the problem of HBV and HCV, millions of carriers worldwide will suffer the consequences of end-stage liver disease and its complications, including HCC, which is a major cause of death in many areas of the world. The need for treatment of these complications will remain a problem for many years to come. In view of the organ shortage and problems of recurrence of disease, alternatives to liver transplantation are desperately needed.

Although progress has been made in the medical treatment of chronic viral hepatitis, success rates do not exceed 30% to 40%. Major efforts are ongoing to find new and better antiviral agents to prevent progression of disease.

Molecular biology will further unravel the relationship between disease expression and the many variables in the genome of viruses. A number of mutants have already been recognized and the further study will add to our understanding.

Acknowledgements

The authors are grateful to Drs. A. S. F. Lok, M. Fleenor, and W. G. Blackard for their most helpful comments.

SUGGESTED READINGS

General Reviews

Craske J. Hepatitis C and non-A, non-B hepatitis revisited: hepatitis E, F, and G. J Infect 1992;25:243–250.

Johnson PJ. Hepatitis viruses, cirrhosis, and liver cancer. J Surg Oncol 1993;(suppl 3):28–33.

Krugman S. Viral hepatitis: A,B,C,D, and E-infection. Pediatr Rev 1992;13:203–212.

Purcell RH. The discovery of the hepatitis viruses. Gastroenterology 1993;104:955–963.

Hepatitis A

Koff RS. Clinical manifestations and diagnosis of hepatitis A infection. Vaccine 1992;10(suppl 1):S15–S17.

Yotsuyanagi H, Shiro I, Kazuhiko K, et al. Duration of viremia in human hepatitis A viral infection as determined by polymerase chain reaction. J Med Virol 1993;40:35–38.

Hepatitis B

de Franchis R, Meucci G, Vecchi M, et al. The natural history of asymptomatic hepatitis B surface antigen carriers. Ann Intern Med 1993;118:191–194.

Maruyama T, McLachlan A, Lino S, et al. The serology of chronic hepatitis B infection revisited. J Clin Invest 1993;91:2586–2595.

Uchida T. Genetic variations of the hepatitis B virus and their clincial relevance. Microbiol Immunol 1993;37:425–439.

Hepatitis C

Choo Q-L, Kuo G, Weiner AJ, et al. Isolation of a cDNA clone derived from blood-borne non-A, non-B viral hepatitis genome. Science 1989;244:359–362.

Kao JH, Chen PJ, Yang PM, et al. Intrafamilial transmission of hepatitis C virus: the important role of infection between spouses. J Infect Dis 1992;166:900–903.

Merican I, Sherlock S, McIntyre N, Dusheiko GM. Clinical, biochemical and histological features in 102 patients with chronic hepatitis C infection. Q J Med 1993;86:119–125.

Seef LB, Buskell-Bales Z, Wright EC, et al. Long-term mortality after transfusion-associated nonA, nonB hepatitis. N Engl J Med 1992;327:1906–1911.

Hepatitis D

Hadziyannis SJ, Taylor JM, Bonino F. Hepatitis delta virus: molecular biology, pathogenesis and clinical aspects. New York: Wiley-Liss, 1993.

Rizetto M. The delta agent. Hepatology 1983;3:729.

Hepatitis E

Favorov MO, Fields HA, Purdy MA, et al. Serologic identification of hepatitis E virus infections in epidemic and endemic settings. J Med Virol 1992;36:246–250.

Krawczynski K. Hepatitis E. Hepatology 1993;17:932–941.

Treatment

Davis GL, Balart LA, Schiff ER, et al. Treatment of chronic hepatitis C with recombinant interferon alfa. A multicenter randomized controlled trial. N Engl J Med 1989;321:1501–1506.

Davis GL. Prediction of response to interferon treatment of chronic hepatitis C. J Hepatol 1994;21:1–3.

Di Bisceglie A. Interferon therapy for chronic viral hepatitis. N Engl J Med 1994;330:137–138. Editorial.

Farci P, Mandas A, Coiana A, et al. Treatment of chronic hepatitis D with interferon alfa-2A. N Engl J Med 1994;330:88–94.

Perillo RP. Antiviral therapy of chronic hepatitis B past, present and future. J Hepatol 1993;17(suppl 3): S56–S63.

Prevention and Vaccination

Akahane Y, Kolima M, Sugai, et al. Hepatitis C virus infection in spouses of patients with type C chronic liver disease. Ann Intern Med 1994;120:748–752.

Beasley RP, Hwang LY, Lee GC, et al. Prevention of perinatally transmitted hepatitis B infection with hepatitis B immune globuline and hepatitis B vaccine. Lancet 1983;2:1099.

Bloom BS, Hillman AL, Fendrick AM, Schwartz JS. A reappraisal of hepatitis B virus vaccination strategies using cost-effectiveness analysis. Ann Intern Med 1993;118:298–306.

Centers for Disease Control. Hepatitis surveillance report no. 53, 1990:23. (Case fatality rate of viral hepatitis related to age is discussed).

Centers for Disease Control. Protection against viral hepatitis. Recommendations of the Immunization Practices Advisory Committee (ACIP). MMWR 1990;39:5–22.

Delage G, Remy-Prince S. Montplaisir S. Combined active-passive immunization against the hepatitis B virus: five-year follow-up of children born to hepatitits B surface antigen-positive mothers. Pediatr Infect Dis J 1993;12:126–130.

Gluck R, Mischler R, Brantschen S, et al. Hepatitis A vaccines: past, present and future. Gastroenterology 1993;105:943–946.

Green MS, Tsur S, Slepon R. Sociodemographic factors and the declining prevalence of antihepatitis A antibodies in young adults in Israel: implications for the new hepatitis A vaccin. Int Epidemiol 1992;21:136–141.

Hou MC, Wu JC, Juo BIT, et al. The heterosexual transmission as the most common route of hepatitis B infection among adults in Taiwan: the importance of extending vaccination to susceptible adults. J Infect Dis 1993;167:938.

Koff RS. The low efficiency of maternal-neonatal transmission of hepatitis C virus: how certain are we? Ann Intern Med 1992;117:967–969. Editorial.

Lai C, Wong BC, Yeoh E, et al. Five-year follow-up of a prospective randomized trial of hepatitis B recombinant DNA yeast vaccine vs. plasma-derived vaccine in children: immunogenicity and anmnestic responses. Hepatology 1993;18:763–767.

Lau Y, Tam AYC, Ng KW et al. Response of preterm infants to hepatitis B vaccine. J Pediatr 1992;121:962–965.

Lee WM. Pregnancy in patients with chronic liver disease. Gastroenterol Clin North Am 1992;21:889–903.

Margolis HS. Prevention of acute and chronic liver disease through immunization: hepatitis B and beyond. J Infect Dis 1993;168:9–14.

Misra L, Seeff LB. Viral hepatitis, A through E complicating pregnancy. Gastroenterol Clins North Am 1992;21:873–887.

Ohta H, Sousuke T, Sasaki N, et al. Transmission of hepatitis C virus from mother to infant N Engl J Med 1994;330:744–750.

Reinus JF, Leikin EL, Alter HJ, et al. Failure to detect vertical transmission of hepatitis C virus. Ann Intern Med 1992;117:881–886.

Schiff ER. Hepatitis C among health care providers: risk factors and possible prophylaxis. Hepatology 1992;16:1300–1301. Editorial.

Shapiro CN, Coleman PJ, McQuillan GM, et al. Epidemiology of hepatitis A: seroepidemiology and risk groups in the USA. Vaccine 1992;10(suppl 1):S59–S62.

Silverman N, Jenkin BK, Wu C, et al. Hepatitis C virus in pregnancy; sero prevalence and risk factors for infection. Am J Obstet Gynecol 1993;169:583–587.

Steffen R. Risk of hepatitis A in travellers. Vaccine 1993;10(suppl 1):S59–S62.

Liver Transplantation

Devictor D, Desplanques L, Debray D, et al. Emergency liver transplantation for fulminant liver failure in infants and children. Hepatology 1992;16:1156–1162.

Fagiuoli S, Shah G, Wright HI, van Thiel DH. Types, causes, and therapies of hepatitis occurring in liver transplant recipients. Dig Dis Sci 1993;38:449–456.

Lake JR. Changing indications for liver transplantation. Gastroenterol Clin 1993;22:213–229.

Samuel D, Muller R, Alexander G, et al. Liver Transplantation in European patents with the hepatitis B surface antigen. N Engl J Med 1993;329:1842–1847.

Wright TL. Liver transplantation for chronic hepatitis C viral infection. Gastroenterol Clin 1993;22:231–242.

CHAPTER 25

THE APPROACH TO THE PATIENT AT RISK FOR SEXUALLY TRANSMITTED DISEASES

David M. Ennis

Over 15% of the population of the United States between ages 18 and 50 report having one or more sexually transmitted disease (STD) in their lifetime and this figure likely underestimates the true cumulative prevalence of these common infections two to threefold. In addition to the classic bacterial STDs such as gonorrhea and syphilis, the spectrum of common STD pathogens now includes over 20 microorganisms, of which chronic, incurable viral infections such as herpes and human papillomavirus infections are most common. Unrecognized or improperly treated, STDs may result in severe or lifelong morbidity such as chronic pelvic pain, infertility, ectopic pregnancy, and cancer. STDs can also lead to severe or life-threatening complications in pregnant patients and their neonates. The true cost of STD-related morbidity is not immediately apparent to patients and their health care providers because the rates of STD acquisition in women and STD-related morbidity are greatest in the young, in whom the sequelae of infection may not be manifest for many years after initial infection. In recent years, it has become apparent that a significant majority of women with STDs may have mild or absent symptoms, thereby increasing the likelihood that infections will go undiagnosed, worsening the chance of sequelae. Thus, it is essential that physicians be aware of the often subtle manifestations of STDs, as well as the basic management and counseling of patients with STDs (Table 25.1). Further complicating the picture is the understanding that many common sexual practices and the types of birth control used may alter both the risk of infection and the symptoms of patients with an STD.

Epidemiology

The epidemiology of STDs in American women is nearly as diverse as the numbers of pathogens. Relatively few STDs are reportable to the U.S. Public Health Service (gonorrhea, syphilis, chancroid, and human immunodeficiency virus [HIV] and even figures for these diseases probably underestimate true infection rates. Epidemiologic studies of other STDs (chlamydia, herpes, and trichomonas) provide only partial data on the characteristics of infected persons. Factors such as age, race, geography, sexual behavior, community disease prevalence, and health care opportunities all influence STD incidence and distribution. Thus, understanding of the epidemiologic features of different STDs may help clinicians assess their patients' STD risks and guide clinical evaluation. Although overall the prevalence of traditional bacterial STDs has been decreasing, rates of STD acquisition are highest in younger age groups, possibly because of relatively greater rates of sex partner turnover. For example, in 1991 gonorrhea rates among 10- to 14-year-old girls and 10- to 19-year-old boys were up to 51% higher than in 1981, whereas over the same period overall gonorrhea rates declined 42%. Likewise, although no national data are available, most studies of *Chlamydia trachomatis* indicate that the highest rates of infection are among the youngest patients. Similarly, the rate of primary and secondary syphilis for girls 10 to 19 years old between 1981 and 1991 showed increases in excess of 100% (1).

Rates of STDs among inner city, minority populations tend to be disproportionately high. In 1992, gon-

Table 25.1 Sexually Transmitted Pathogens

Bacteria	Viruses	Protozoans	Ectoparasites
Neisseria gonorrhoeae	Herpes simplex	*Trichomonas vaginalis*	*Sarcoptes scabeie*
Chlamydia trachomatis	Cytomegalovirus		*Phthirus pubis*
Treponema pallidum	Human papillomavirus		
Haemophilus ducreyi	Hepatitis B and C		
Calymmatobacterium granulomatis	Human immunodeficiency virus 1 and 2		
	Human T-cell leukemia virus 1 and 2		
	Molluscum contagiosum		

orrhea rates among blacks were 39 times greater than for non-Hispanic whites, despite an overall decline. Similarly, syphilis rates that year were 60-fold higher in blacks than in non-Hispanic whites, again despite an overall decrease in disease prevalence (2).

Finally, disease rates are higher in some regions of the country than in others. The southeastern United States reports some of the nation's highest rates of gonorrhea and syphilis. In 1992, of the 10 states with the nation's highest gonorrhea prevalence, 8 were located in the South, as were 92% of the counties with the highest syphilis rates (2).

The reasons for the disparities noted between races and regions of the country are unknown, but they may be related to variables such as education level, income, and access to health care. Reporting bias may also contribute to the apparent differences of STDs between races, because most reporting is done by health departments, which mainly serve minorities and poorer members of society. Disease rates among whites may be falsely low due to nonreporting by private physicians although this alone cannot account for the huge differences in STD rates. Disease prevalence in Native Americans is likewise probably underestimated (3).

Risk for STD Acquisition

As mentioned above, STDs are far more common than suspected by the population at large or, in many cases, by their health care providers. All sexually active individuals are at risk for STDs, if not on the basis of their own behavior, then potentially because of the past or present behaviors of their sex partners. In the United States, the average age of onset of sexual activity for young women is 16 years and rates of partner change are greatest in the years following onset of sexual activity. Thus, STD acquisition is less often the result of having multiple contemporaneous sexual partners than a consequence of change in sexual partners. In general, rates of partner exchange are greater in younger patients, making STD incidence greater in younger patients.

Certain behaviors other than partner choice may also modify risk for STD acquisition. These include alcohol ingestion, tobacco use, and drug use. The association of increased risk for STD with tobacco and other drugs in some instances is less of a biologically active risk factor than a risk marker, indicative of an individual's overall willingness to take part in activities that place her at risk for STD acquisition despite knowledge that it might occur. In either instance, changes in decision-making due to the direct effect of alcohol or drugs on risk assessment (i.e., intoxication) may increase risk of STD acquisition. Finally, in some cases, addiction to drugs such as cocaine may lead individuals to participate in behaviors such as exchange of sex for drugs or money to buy drugs despite knowledge that such behaviors increase risk of STDs.

Contraceptive Methods and STDs

A patient's choice of contraception may also modify STD risk. Great progress has been made over the past few decades in the development of safe and effective birth control methods. These diverse methods vary greatly in their abilities to prevent pregnancy and to modify risk for STD or STD complications. Optimally, recommendations regarding contraceptive choice should incorporate a potential contraceptive measure's impact on risk for STD, as well as birth control efficacy.

Barrier and Spermicidal Contraceptives

Barrier contraceptives constitute a diverse group of contraceptive methods that includes the male and female condoms, the diaphragm, the cervical cap and film, and the contraceptive sponge. Spermicidal products are often used in conjunction with barrier contraceptives either as lubricants (for condoms) or to increase the contraceptive efficacy of female barrier methods. In addition, some women may choose to use spermicidal preparations (foams, gels, or wafers) without barrier methods. For STD prevention, the physical barrier provided by contraceptives such as condoms reduces STD risk; spermicidal products reduce STD risk through the microbicidal effect of the detergents that are the active ingredients of these agents.

In North America, the male condom has been widely promoted for prevention of HIV and STD acquisition, often without stressing its potential as a method of birth control. This practice has inadvertently stigmatized condoms for potential users, and in some instances may actually make individuals less likely to use them. Theoretically, the condom should provide absolute protection against pregnancy and infection. In vitro studies show that latex condoms are impervious to all bacterial and viral pathogens (4). The larger pores of natural—as opposed to latex—condoms may allow the passage of viral particles and are not suitable for disease prevention. In actual practice, whether due to breakage or misuse, condoms are less than 100% effective, for both pregnancy and STD prevention. Pregnancy rates in condom users range from 2.1% to 36.8%, tending to be lower in experienced users (5). Likewise, condoms appear to be partially protective against gonorrhea, chlamydia, and human papillomavirus, genital ulcer disease, and viral STDs, such as HIV (6,7). The efficacy of the male condom may be improved by the concomitant use of a spermicide (5,8). Recently, a female condom has been approved and though it appears impermeable to STD pathogens, its efficacy for STD prevention has not been proven. The utility of other barrier methods to prevent STDs has not been well studied, but failure rates in preventing pregnancy ranges from 0.3% to 55.7% (5). Each is likely to offer the user some, but not complete, protection from STD acquisition.

The most commonly used spermicidal preparation is nonoxynol-9. Its antimicrobial activity appears to be due to its detergent effect on cell membranes (4). Laboratory studies of nonoxynol-9 show that it has activity against *Neisseria gonorrhoeae*, *Trichomonas vaginalis*, *Treponema pallidum*, herpes simplex virus, and HIV. Its effects on *C. trachomatis*, candida, and human papillomavirus are controversial. Clinical studies have shown that nonoxynol-9 reduces risk for gonorrhea, chlamydia, and trichomoniasis. Nonoxynol-9 may cause a dose-related toxic effect on vaginal epithelium. However, for most potential users, the benefits in terms of STD prevention are likely to outweigh the risks.

Hormonal Contraceptives

Although hormonal contraceptives are widely used and are highly effective in preventing pregnancy, their impact on STD risk is uncertain. Increased numbers of cervical infections with *C. trachomatis* and *N. gonorrhoeae* have been reported in users of oral contraceptives (4,9). Paradoxically, hormonal contraceptives reduce the risk of development of pelvic inflammatory disease (PID) in infected women, possibly by the effect of progestins on cervical mucus.

Intrauterine Devices

After years of scientific and legal debate, the safety of intrauterine devices (IUDs) is being re-evaluated. Recent studies indicate that IUDs are safe and effective methods of birth control, if used in an appropriate patient. Except for the first 3 weeks after insertion, there is no significant increase in risk of PID. Early IUDs such as the Dalkon Shield and Lippes Loop were associated with increased risk of PID in women who acquired STDs. However, more recently developed IUDs are not associated with significantly increased risk for PID. Thus, the IUD remains a good contraceptive measure for many women.

Douching

Douching is practiced by approximately 67 million American women each year. It has been associated with PID and ectopic pregnancy. Whether this practice is a risk marker for disease or acts as an independent risk factor by overcoming the host's defenses and spreading infection is unknown (4).

The Sexual History

A complete sexual history is an essential component of the evaluation of any patient. It not only provides clues to a patient's illness, but allows the clinician to identify risk factors for counseling and intervention. Unfortunately, numerous studies have shown that many physicians perform this task poorly (10,11). Reasons for this include the lack of familiarity with STDs, the belief that their patients are not at risk for infection, and the fear that questioning patients about sensitive topics will be offensive. Actually, studies suggest that clinicians who take detailed sexual and STD histories from patients are considered by the patients to be better prepared to care for them. Given the frequency with which STDs occur and their potential to cause lifelong complications, it is incumbent on physicians to take an adequate sexual history from every patient, regardless of age, seen for the first time.

How physicians address questions related to sexual behavior and STDs affects not only the patient's reactions to the questions but the reliability of the answers. Patients should be questioned in a confident, nonaccusatory, nonjudgmental manner. They should be assured that any answers will be completely confidential. The components of an adequate sexual history, including pertinent historical features and physical symptoms, are outlined in Table 25.2.

The Physical Examination and Specimen Collection

In general, each patient at risk for STDs should be evaluated in the same standardized fashion. In this way, coexistent STDs that may be present but unrelated to the patient's presenting complaints are unlikely to be overlooked. The examination of the female patient will be familiar to most practitioners. However, a few special points of the examination should be emphasized, especially for patients with a suspected STD.

Each patient should undergo a visual examination of the oropharynx. Although relatively rare, the presence of findings such as ulcers, mucous patches (a sign of secondary syphilis), or oral hairy leukoplakia (associated with HIV infection) may provide the first clue to diagnosis. Women who have performed fellatio, particularly those currently infected with or exposed to

Table 25.2 Components of the Sexual History

Historical Features	Symptoms

New partner in the last 30 days	Vaginal discharge
	  Difference from usual discharge
	  Color, quantity, quality, and duration

Number of partners in the past 6 mo	Vaginal pruritus Internal versus external
Number of lifetime partners	Abnormal bleeding Pelvic pain (acute versus chronic)
Known prior STDs Does partner have symptoms?	Dysuria Fever
Sites of sexual exposure—oral, anal, vaginal	Lesions Changes in appearance, pain, prior episodes

Contraceptive practices
  Current and past
  Type and frequency of use
	Warts

Drug and alcohol use	
Menstrual history	

gonorrhea, should have pharyngeal cultures for gonorrhea. Because chlamydial pharyngitis is rare, cultures are not usually indicated.

Lymphadenopathy is a manifestation of several STDs. Thus, lymph node palpation should be part of routine evaluation. If enlarged, the location, size, firmness, tenderness, and mobility of the nodes should be carefully noted. Blood tests or other procedures should be performed as determined by the clinical situation.

Dermatologic examination is also important because STDs such as secondary syphilis, disseminated gonococcal infection, and HIV often have cutaneous manifestations that may not be mentioned by patients. It is beyond the scope of this chapter to describe each lesion in detail. However, close examination of the skin, including the palms and soles, may provide clues to an underlying disease.

During the pelvic examination, the patient should be closely inspected for evidence of ulcers or vesicles. The color, amount, consistency, and odor of any vaginal discharge should be noted. The cervix should be examined for purulent or mucopurulent drainage, edema at the zone of ectopy, or easily induced bleeding.

Due to the fastidious nature of many STD pathogens, proper collection and processing of specimens is essential. In general, unless they represent previously diagnosed recurrent disease, vesicular lesions and ulcerative genital lesions should be cultured for herpes. Specimens should be sent for darkfield microscopy, if available. In endemic areas, culture for *Haemophilus ducreyi*, the agent of chancroid, should be considered. Specimens of vaginal discharge for wet prep and KOH examination should be obtained from the vaginal wall and not from pooled vaginal secretions. Cervical specimens should be obtained for testing for gonorrhea and chlamydia, especially for women at risk, because signs of infection are often absent. Specimens to be tested by commercially available antigen detection or DNA probe tests should be obtained using the special collection devices provided by manufacturers. In settings where culture is used for diagnosis, the swab type used may influence the sensitivity of chlamydia (but not usually gonorrhea) culture. Dacron-tipped swabs are considered to be the best for chlamydia culture, but cotton-tipped aluminum or steel swabs are also acceptable. Swabs tipped with calcium alginate (Calgiswabs) or those with shafts made from wood or plastic are the least acceptable (12). Furthermore, because *C. trachomatis* is isolated only from intact epithelial cells and not leukocytes, swabs for chlamydia testing should be obtained last, when most of the cervical debris has been cleared.

Clinical Syndromes

Vaginal Discharge

Although vaginal discharge is a common symptom, its numerous etiologies such as vaginal disease, cervicitis, and neoplasm make it a highly nonspecific complaint. Other symptoms frequently associated with vaginal discharge—abnormal vaginal bleeding and dyspareunia—are no more specific. Thus, even with careful questioning, the clinician can seldom make a diagnosis from history alone and must rely on the physical examination and laboratory testing.

Vaginal Diseases

Exact figures for the number of cases of vaginal diseases are lacking. However, they rank as some of the most common complaints seen in the physician's office. In 1992, the Centers for Disease Control and Prevention (CDC) estimated that trichomonas accounted for approximately 250,000 office visits. Other vaginal complaints were associated with another 3,500,000 visits (2).

The most common causes of vaginal diseases are bacterial vaginosis (BV), vulvovaginal candidiasis (VVC), and trichomonas. Although the proportion caused by each will vary with the population studied, BV appears to be most common, accounting for 30% to 35% of cases. VVC is associated with 20% to 25% of cases of vaginal diseases; trichomonas causes only 10%. More than one cause can be found in about 20% of patients (13). Noninfectious causes that may mimic these vaginal diseases include chemical irritation from soaps, contraceptives, deodorants, topical medications, as well as foreign bodies and collagen vascular diseases such as Behçet's syndrome (13,14). Of the three major causes of vaginal diseases, only trichomonas is a sexually transmitted pathogen. BV is not considered to be an STD by most experts. Only trichomonas and BV will be discussed here (Table 25.3).

Table 25.3 Signs and Symptoms of Vaginal Diseases

	Bacterial Vaginosis	Vulvovaginal Candidiasis	Trichomonas Vaginalis
Symptoms			
	Malodorous discharge	Vulvar pruritus Abnormal discharge Tenderness Dyspareunia Dysuria	Abnormal discharge Vaginal pruritus Dyspareunia Dysuria
Signs			
	Moderate-profuse often frothy adherent, homogeneous white or gray discharge	Minimal-moderate discharge, often "curdlike"	Profuse, often frothy discharge
	Vulvar, labial, vaginal Inflammation absent	Vulvar and labial erythema and swelling	Vulvar and vaginal erythema
		Vaginal erythema	"Strawberry cervix" rare

Trichomonas Vaginalis (TV)

Trichomonas vaginalis is not only the most common sexually transmitted parasitic infection, but may also be the most common STD in the world. Rates of trichomoniasis in the United States vary according to the clinical setting. Various studies report rates of 5% in family planning clinics, 0.9% to 39.6% in STD clinics, and 50% to 75% in prostitutes. Risk factors for trichomonal infection include multiple sex partners, race, prior STDs, coexistent infection with gonorrhea, and type of birth control (nonuse of hormonal or barrier contraceptives) (15).

Trichomonas vaginalis is a flagellated, motile, anaerobic parasite that adheres only to squamous epithelium, such as that found in the vagina and in associated glands. The risk of transmission from an infected man to a woman is 85%, with an incubation period of 3 to 28 days. Transmission by fomites is extremely rare. As with other causes of vaginal diseases, the signs and symptoms of TV are neither sensitive nor specific. Up to 50% of patients with culture-proven trichomonal infection may be asymptomatic. Among symptomatic patients, a malodorous vaginal discharge is seen in 50% to 70%. The classic green, frothy discharge is noted in fewer than half the patients (15). A gray discharge, resembling that of BV, is noted with an equal frequency (16). Other symtoms of TV are vulvovaginal irritation, vaginal erythema, dyspareunia, dysuria, and, rarely, lower abdominal pain. Of note, the "strawberry cervix" associated with TV is seen in only 2% of patients (15).

Diagnosis: The diagnosis of TV is primarily based on examination of the wet prep. The pH is usually above 4.5 and is frequently greater than 5.0. Motile trichomonads are seen in 60% to 80% of wet mount samples. A positive "whiff test" on addition of KOH is noted in 50%. Culture is about 95% sensitive with the combination of culture and wet prep being considered 100% sensitive. Newly developed monoclonal antibodies may be superior to wet prep alone (15).

Bacterial Vaginosis

Bacterial vaginosis is not considered an STD by most experts. Technically, BV is not an inflammatory process, because generally few leukocytes are noted in the discharge. Neither is there significant vaginal erythema or irritation. BV appears to be caused by an absolute or qualitative reduction in the number of the vaginal lactobacilli, which constitute more than 90% of the normal vaginal flora. The lactobacilli suppress other vaginal flora by maintaining a low pH and by the production of antibacterial factors. The loss of these protective bacteria allows the overgrowth of anaerobic gram-negative organisms and genital mycoplasmas.

The prevalence of BV depends on the population

sampled. The prevalence in private physician's offices is 16%, whereas STD clinics report rates of 33% to 64%. In obstetric and family planning clinics, rates are 10% to 26% and 23% to 29%, respectively. Purported risk factors include the number of sex partners and IUD use (17).

A malodorous vaginal discharge is the hallmark of BV and is the most frequent complaint among women seeking attention for this disorder. Physical examination reveals a homogeneous, thin, often profuse, white or gray discharge, which is adherent to the vaginal walls.

Diagnosis: No definitive tests exist for the diagnosis of BV. Consequently, the diagnosis is based on Amsel's criteria. A diagnosis of BV requires that at least three of the four following criteria be present: a typical vaginal discharge, vaginal fluid pH above 4.5, the presence of at least 20% clue cells, and a positive "whiff test" on the addition of KOH. The sample should contain few or no white blood cells. The sensitivity of these criteria is considered to be very high, though there has been no "gold standard" against which to judge them. Other diagnostic tests include Gram stain of the vaginal sample and gas-liquid chromatography, which has been primarily used for research. Although not often performed, the Gram stain revealing abundant gram-negative bacteria and relatively few lactobacilli may be more sensitive than other techniques. The presence of clue cells on Pap smears is of unknown significance.

Complications: BV has been increasingly linked with severe complications. It has been associated with PID, preterm birth, premature rupture of the membranes, chorioamnionitis, lower gestational age at birth, and postpartum and postcaesarean endometritis. In the neonate, BV may also cause scalp abscesses and umbilical wound infection (18).

Cervicitis

The symptoms of cervicitis are essentially the same as those described for the vaginal disease. However, the majority of women with cervicitis are asymptomatic and may have no physical signs of disease, emphasizing the need for a thorough physical and laboratory evaluation. *C. trachomatis* and *N. gonorrhoeae* are the most common causes. Other etiologies include herpes and chemical irritants.

Chlamydia Trachomatis

Chlamydia trachomatis is an obligate intracellular parasite consisting of several biovars. Types D through K are responsible for urethral, cervical, and pelvic infections, whereas types A, B, and C cause neonatal disease and types L1, L2, and L3 cause lymphogranuloma venereum. The life cycle of the organism is complex. The infectious particle, the elementary body, is metabolically inert and is able to withstand most extracellular conditions. The elementary body attaches to the host cell membrane and is internalized into a phagosome. Within 8 to 12 hours of entry, the elementary bodies transform into metabolically active reticulate bodies and begin to reproduce. Twenty-four to 36 hours later, the reticulate bodies begin to reorganize into elementary bodies, which are later released from the cell to continue the cycle of infection (19). Only the reticulate bodies are affected by antibiotic therapy.

Neisseria Gonorrhoeae

Neisseria gonorrhoeae are fastidious gram-negative diplococci. The gonococcus is particularly well adapted for the human genital tract infection because it adheres preferentially to the epithelial lining the urethra and cervix. The risk of transmission of gonorrhea from an infected man to a woman is 60% to 90%. The risk of infection from an infected woman to a man is 20% to 40% (20). Extragenital gonorrhea is not uncommon. Rectal infection is found in 35% to 50% of women with cervical gonorrhea, usually resulting from exposure of infected vaginal secretions. The rectum is rarely the sole site of infection and is usually asymptomatic. Pharyngeal infection, which is usually asymptomatic occurs in 10% to 20% of women; few have any symptoms. As with cervical infection, women are at greatest risk for pharyngeal infection because fellatio more efficiently transmits infection than does cunnilingus. Despite the fact that pharyngeal gonorrhea has been linked to an increased risk of disseminated gonococcal infection, almost all cases resolve without treatment (25).

Diagnosis of Cervicitis

The diagnosis of cervicitis (Table 25.4) can be elusive because most women will have few or no signs of infection. This is especially true for chlamydia due to the difficulty in diagnosing infection without culture or other special diagnostic tests. Consequently, numerous investigators have attempted to develop criteria

Table 25.4 Etiologic Agents of Cervicitis and Their Preferred Diagnostic Test and Therapies

Etiology	Preferred Diagnostic Tests	Therapy of Choice
Neisseria gonorrhoeae	Gram stain of cervical smear culture	Third-generation cephalosporin Quinolone
Chlamydia trachomatis	Direct fluorescent antibody Enzyme Immunoassay Nucleic acid hybridization (DNA probe) Nucleic acid amplification (polymerase chain reaction)	Doxycycline Azithromycin Ofloxacin Erythromycin

for predicting chlamydial cervical infection and women at risk for infection based on demographic data and clinical observations. In many models, various risk factors are combined with specific symptoms and signs, such as cervical friability or suspicious vaginal discharge (22,23). Others support the diagnosis of chlamydia based on the Gram stain of cervical mucus revealing varying numbers of polymorphonuclear cells (10 to 30) in the absence of evidence of gonorrhea (24–27). However, the reliability and reproducibility of these criteria are debatable because they are based on data derived from differing populations, using different diagnostic tests. Thus, many experts believe that chlamydial cervicitis should be strongly suspected in any patient at risk for infection based on historical or demographic data and in whom cervical friability is noted during the physical examination.

No such criteria exist for the diagnosis of endocervical gonorrhea. Like chlamydia, the diagnosis by Gram stain of the cervical smear is difficult. Although the sensitivity of a urethral smear in a man infected with gonorrhea is > 95%, the sensitivity of a cervical smear is only about 50% (21).

Consequently, clinicians must rely on other diagnostic methods. For both organisms, the most commonly used and thoroughly evaluated method is culture. Proper collection and processing of specimens are essential because the ability to isolate an organism may be adversely affected if these seemingly trivial details are ignored. Assuming that proper care has been taken in obtaining a specimen, the sensitivity of a culture for gonorrhea varies by site. Cervical cultures are the most sensitive, 80% to 90%, whereas anal and pharyngeal cultures are 40% to 60% and 50% to 70% sensitive, respectively (20,21). Nonculture tests for gonorrhea include a genetic probe, which is very sensitive and rapid, but does not allow for antimicrobial resistance testing. Newer tests using polymerase chain reaction (PCR) technology are being developed.

Culture for *C. trachomatis* has been considered the "gold standard." However, the sensitivity of chlamydial culture can be adversely influenced by numerous factors, including the type of swab, transport media, and cell culture technique. Furthermore, there appears to be laboratory variability in technique and sensitivity. In experienced laboratories sensitivity may be as high as 90%, although it is much lower in most facilities. Although culture has the advantage of allowing determination of serovars and antimicrobial sensitivities, this technique has several important disadvantages, including the special training required and the delay in reporting results (28). Consequently, noncultured techniques (described below) may be more appropriate in most settings.

Given the time and uncertainties of culture techniques for chlamydia, nonculture methods have been developed. The direct fluorescent antibody technique uses a dried specimen treated with a monoclonal antibody that binds to chlamydial antigens. This test has the advantage of not having stringent transportation requirements and of being relatively fast. Disadvantages include subjective interpretation of results and cross-reactivity with other bacteria (29). The reported sensitivity is 68% to 100%, with a specificity of 98% (12,30).

The enzyme immunoassay (EIA) uses an antibody labeled with an enzyme that binds to a component of the chlamydial cell membrane. The intensity of the colored product is read by a spectrophotometer. This product also has the advantages of being easy to transport and providing results in 3 to 4 hours. Disadvantages of the EIA are a "gray zone" in differentiating definitely positive and negative readings (29) and cross-reactivity with other bacteria, which requires an additional step for confirmation (28). The sensitivity of EIA is about 88%, with a specificity of 99% (29,30).

The DNA probe test for chlamydia involves the binding of a chemiluminescent DNA probe that is complementary to a specific sequence of chlamydial ribosomal RNA. These products are then adsorbed to magnetic particles, which are detected in a luminometer. This test, like the EIA, requires special training and may cross-react with other chlamydial species (21). The sensitivity of the test in women is 80% to 95% and the specificity greater than 98% (31).

The newest addition to the diagnostic armamentarium is PCR. This test uses DNA primers that bind to specific DNA sequences in the sample being tested. Through a series of cycles, these DNA fragments are lengthened and multiplied until several million identical copies are produced. The products then undergo an enzyme-linked immunosorbent reaction, resulting in a color change, which is then read by a spectrophotometer. As with other nonculture tests, PCR has the advantage of ease of transport and providing results quickly. The disadvantages of this test are its cost, the training required to perform the process optimally, and the risk of false-positive results. The sensitivity of PCR in diagnosing chlamydia in cervical specimens is 89% to 100%, with a specificity of greater than 96% (31,32). Of note, there is no cross-reactivity with other chlamydial species.

The proper use of these tests for the diagnosis of chlamydia is essential to avoid unnecessary expense, overdiagnosis, and undertreatment. Culture has generally been the most widely used method for diagnosing chlamydial infection. However, its lack of widespread availability and the technical problems mentioned above have made nonculture techniques more desirable. The validity of these tests depends greatly on the prevalence of chlamydial infection in a clinic population. In a high incidence population ($\geq$5%), the chance that a positive test represents true infection is very high. In a low prevalence population (<5%), the chance of a false-positive result increases dramatically. This places such a patient at significant risk for unnecessary treatment, in addition to causing psychological and social problems. If a nonculture test is positive for chlamydia in a woman in a low prevalence population, a second test should be performed to ensure the accuracy of the first. Although culture is the preferable method, another type of nonculture test may be used. Alternatively, a second specimen may be taken and subjected to the same test. A positive test in a patient from a high prevalence group or in whom the likelihood of infection is great does not usually require confirmation (28).

Complications of Cervicitis

Pelvic Inflammatory Disease: Although the majority of women with the diseases described here suffer no serious consequences, a few will develop severe, even life-threatening complications. One of the most common complications is PID, which affects 15% to 20% of women of reproductive age in the United States (33). PID is responsible for hundreds of thousands of hospitalizations and surgical procedures each year, costing the country over $4 billion in 1990 (16,34). Over half the cases of PID are caused by *N. gonorrhoeae*, *C. trachomatis*, or both. Other organisms implicated in PID are *Escherichia coli*, *Ureaplasma urealyticum*, *Mycoplasma hominis*, anaerobic streptococci, and gram-negative anaerobes associated with BV. Risk factors for PID include young age, race, low socioeconomic status, multiple sex partners, and type of contraception used. Barrier and hormonal contraceptive methods appear to decrease the risk of PID (16,33,34).

Diagnosis of PID: The diagnosis of PID is controversial. Most clinicians rely on clinical criteria (Table 25.5). However, the sensitivity of these criteria, as confirmed by laparoscopy, is only 80% (35). Laparoscopy is considered to be the "gold standard." This procedure may detect asymptomatic PID, as well as other causes for pelvic pain such as appendicitis. However, its utility is limited by its cost and the need for special training. Endometrial biopsy has been proposed as alternative to laparoscopy. This procedure, though having a sensitivity as high as 90% compared to lapar-

Table 25.5 Criteria for the Clinical Diagnosis of Pelvic Inflammatory Disease

Each much be present
1. History of lower abdominal pain with tenderness noted on examination (rebound tenderness not required)
2. Cervical motion tenderness
3. Unilateral or bilateral adnexal tenderness
One must be present
1. Temperature ⩾38°C (⩾100.4°F)
2. White blood cell count ⩾10,500/µl
3. Presence of an inflammatory mass on physical or sonographic examination
4. Culdocentesis revealing leukocytes and bacteria
5. Erythrocyte sedimentation rate >15 mm/hr
6. Evidence of cervical infection with gonorrhea or chlamydia on examination, Gram stain, culture, or nonculture test

oscopy, is compromised by possible sampling error and by the delay in reporting results (16).

This condition is associated with severe complications. The risk of tubal factor infertility is increased 11% by one episode of PID, with higher risk for each subsequent episode. The risk of ectopic pregnancy is likewise increased. Chronic pelvic pain occurs in up to 18% of women with PID.

Disseminated Gonococcal Infection: Disseminated gonococcal infection (DGI) is an uncommon complication of PID, occurring in fewer than 3% of patients (21). It usually occurs 7 to 30 days after menstruation or during the third trimester of pregnancy (16,21). The course of disease is divided into two stages. The first is the bacteremic phase, characterized by fever, chills, and skin lesions. The classic skin lesions are tender, necrotic pustules on erythematous bases. They usually number less than 30 and are located on the extremities. The second phase is the arthritis phase, manifested by swollen, tender joints containing a purulent exudate. The knees, wrists, ankles, and metacarpophalangeal joints are most commonly involved. The diagnosis is difficult because blood cultures are positive in fewer than half of the patients. Synovial fluid cultures are variably positive. Consequently, the diagnosis should be suspected in any patient at risk for gonorrhea presenting with typical symptoms and signs. In such a patient, a rapid response to appropriate antimicrobial therapy supports the diagnosis (21).

Genital Ulcer Disease

Genital ulcer disease (GUD) is responsible for 5% to 10% of patient visits to STD clinics. The most common causes of this syndrome in the United States are herpes, syphilis, and chancroid, with herpes causing the vast majority of cases. Common nonvenereal causes of GUD are cancer, trauma, drug eruptions, and skin infections. In the developing world, lymphogranuloma venereum and granuloma inguinale are frequently seen but are rarely encountered in the United States. Given the broad differential diagnosis and the similar appearance of the lesions, the diagnosis can be extremely difficult in the absence of laboratory data. Studies have shown that even experienced clinicians make the correct diagnosis in only 60% to 80% of cases of GUD. No diagnosis is made in up to 30% of patients, despite thorough physical and laboratory evaluations (36). GUD has been the object of intense study for years because of the potential health risks to pregnant women and their babies. Understanding and control of these diseases has become more urgent due to the strong correlation between GUD and the acquisition of HIV infection. Clinical characteristics and diagnostic tests for the common causes of GUD are listed in Table 25.6.

The History and Physical Examination

In addition to the standard sexual history outlined earlier, additional information should be sought from the patient presenting with a genital ulcer. Questions about prior history of similar lesions, changes in the lesion's appearance, and tenderness may assist in making a diagnosis. Sexual contact with a person from an area with endemic lymphogranuloma venerum, granuloma inguinale, or chancroid should be investigated because these infections often require special testing.

The physical examination should include close inspection of the ulcer, noting tenderness, induration, the presence of an exudate, and undermining of the edges. The presence of adenopathy should also be noted, particularly tenderness or fluctuence.

Table 25.6 Clinical and Diagnostic Characterics of Genital Ulcer Disease

Disease	Herpes	Syphilis	Chancroid
Etiologic Agent	Herpes simplex virus	*Treponema pallidum*	*Haemophilus ducreyi*
Appearance of Lesion	Tender, nonindurated vesicles progressing to pustules. Often coalesce in primary episode.	Macule progressing to an ulcerating papule. Ulcer is sharply demarcated with an indurated, nontender, clean base	Tender papule progressing to a tender, ragged, nonindurated ulcer with a purulent base. Often nontender in women.
Number of Lesions	Multiple	Usually single; multiple in up to 40% of cases.	Multiple
Adenopathy	Common in primary episode. Usually tender and bilateral. Uncommon in recurrence	Usually bilateral, nontender, and small.	Usually unilateral. Tender, sometimes fluctuent and draining.
Systemic symptoms	Common in primary episode.	None	Sometimes mild symptoms.
Diagnosis (see text)	Culture Tzank prep or Pap smear Serology for antibody	Darkfield microscopy Serologies RPR VDRL FTA-ABS MHA-TP No culture routinely available.	Gram stain not useful Culture of ulcer and/or lymph node.
Preferred Therapy	Acyclovir	Penicillin	Azithromycin Ceftriaxone Erythromycin

FTA-ABS, fluorescent treponemal antibody absorption test; MHA-TP, microhemagglutination-*Treponema pallidum*; RPR, rapid plasma reagin; VDRL, Venereal Disease Research Laboratory

Herpes Simplex Virus

Herpes is the most common cause of genital ulcer disease in the United States. An estimated 500,000 new cases of herpes are diagnosed each year (16). Serologic studies show that up to 20% of the population of the United States has antibodies for herpes simplex virus type 2 (HSV-2) (37), which is responsible for the vast majority of genital infections. Many of the risk factors associated with herpes infection resemble those described for other STDs—low socioeconomic status and education levels and Hispanic or black race. In addition, antibodies for HSV-2 become more prevalent as age increases, suggesting that the cumulative number of sex partners is important in acquiring infection. Herpes is also more common in homosexual men and in patients infected with HIV (38).

Studies using new serologic techniques have shown that symptomatic infection represents only a small proportion of those actually infected with the virus. Of women with antibodies to HSV-2, the vast majority have no history of prior of lesions (38). Antibodies to HSV-2 have been found in 32% of pregnant women with no prior history of herpes (39). This knowledge has become particularly important because other studies have shown that a significant number of women shed HSV asymptomatically. As many as 1% of infected women shed virus asymptomatically each day. Although the amount of virus shed may be small, the risk of infection to a seronegative male partner is about 4%. Overall, about 10% of seronegative individuals exposed to a partner with HSV-2 acquire herpes each year (40).

Diagnosis of Herpes

Viral culture remains the "gold standard" for the diagnosis of herpes, especially during the primary episode before antibodies are formed. Culture will be positive in 90% of vesicular primary lesions, dropping to 30% with crusted lesions. Culture of recurrent lesions is positive in about 40% of cases. Papincalaou and Tzank preparations, EIA, and direct fluorescent antibody, are less sensitive than culture (40). Commercial serum antibody tests are able to detect prior infection with herpes, but are unable to discern reliably HSV-1 from HSV-2. More specific antibody tests have been developed but are available for research purposes only (38).

Syphilis

Though less common than herpes, syphilis remains one of the major causes of GUD in the United States and in the rest of the world. The epidemiology and risk factors for syphilis were described earlier. The lesion of primary syphilis is the chancre, which develops about 21 days after exposure. In women, chancres are most commonly found on the vulva—especially on the fourchette—and on the cervix. The chancre persists for 3 to 6 weeks if not treated. Exposure to a person with primary syphilis carries a risk of infection of 18% to 51% (41,42).

Diagnosis of Syphilis

As with herpes, the diagnosis of syphilis depends on the clinician's clinical suspicion, aided by laboratory testing. A specimen should be taken for darkfield examination, if available. This technique is particularly useful in early syphilis, when serologies may be negative. No satisfactory culture method for *T. pallidum* has been developed. Thus, if the microscopic evaluation is negative or unavailable, the clinician must rely on serologic tests. The most commonly used screening tests are the nontreponemal tests, the rapid plasma reagin (RPR) and the Venereal Disease Research Laboratory (VDRL). These tests take advantage of serum antibodies that cross-react with certain nontreponemal antigens. Unfortunately, these tests may not become reactive until 2 weeks after the appearance of the chancre, missing up to 41% of cases of primary disease (43). The specificity of the nontreponemal tests is compromised by positive reactions in patients with a variety of conditions, including other spirochetal diseases, HIV, tuberculosis, pregnancy, and advanced age. Consequently, positive reactions should be confirmed with a specific treponemal test, either the fluorescent treponemal antibody absorption test or microhemagglutination-*T. pallidum*. These tests, which detect antibodies by direct exposure to treponemal antigens, are generally more sensitive and specific than the RPR and VDRL. However, due to expense and labor, they are generally used to confirm the less-specific nontreponemal tests.

Chancroid

Although not a common cause of GUD in this country, chancroid—caused by *H. ducreyi*—is endemic in the United States. In 1992, 2000 cases were reported (2). Risk factors for infection include crack cocaine and alcohol use and prostitute exposure (44). Transmission appears to occur only in the presence of an ulcer. In women, ulcers may be subclinical (45). The diagnosis of chancroid requires a careful history and physical examination, with confirmation by culture. Gram stain of purulent material is unreliable. Special media are necessary to maximize the yield from culture. However, the sensitivity of culture for *H. ducreyi* remains only 60% to 80% (46).

Lymphogranuloma Venereum

Lymphogranuloma venereum, caused by *C. trachomatis* types L1, L2, and L3, is sporadically seen in the United States. Most cases are acquired by persons visiting endemic areas. The disease is characterized by the appearance of a papule or asymptomatic ulcer, followed by the onset of acute adenitis and fever. Serologic tests may confirm a diagnosis. Consultation with an expert is strongly suggested.

Granuloma Inguinale

Granuloma inguinale (Donovanosis), caused by *Calymmatobacterium granulomatis*, is also rarely seen in this country. The first manifestations of the disease are small, subcutaneous nodules that eventually erode, enlarge, and form areas of heaped-up, red granulation tissue. The diagnosis is confirmed by microscopic examination of a crushed specimen revealing Donovan bodies. In cases of suspected granuloma inguinale, expert advice should be sought.

Screening for STDs

Universal screening for STDs would probably be effective in preventing long-term complications and in reducing the spread of infection. However, given the limitations of available diagnostic tools, such an effort would be prohibitively expensive and lead to considerable overdiagnosis and overtreatment. Consequently, numerous investigators have attempted to devise clinical and physical criteria to identify groups at high risk for STDs and who may thus benefit from screening. Unfortunately, no criteria have been shown to be sufficiently sensitive or specific. However, the following criteria are reasonable guidelines for the screening of asymptomatic women. Universal screening for gonorrhea and chlamydia should be performed on all women in areas of high prevalence. In populations with lower disease prevalence, screening should be strongly considered in patients with a new sex partner or those with multiple partners (two or more) in the last year. Cervical friability on physical examination should also prompt appropriate testing. Syphilis testing should be provided for women in high-risk groups. HIV testing should be offered to all patients, especially those with GUD. The frequency at which screening should be performed is unknown, but every 3 to 6 months seems reasonable in groups at high risk of recurrent infection. All pregnant women should be screened at intake, with subsequent testing—especially during the third trimester—if the patient continues to engage in risky behavior. Women with STDs or visiting an STD clinic should have a Pap smear every 12 months.

Conclusion

Despite major advances in the understanding of the epidemiology, pathogenesis, and treatment of STDs, they continue to be major health problems. The cost to the country of managing these diseases and their complications is staggering. Furthermore, they afflict the youngest portion of society, who have the greatest risk of developing permanent complications. These facts, in combination with increasing numbers of heterosexual, noninjection drug users becoming infected with HIV, make the development of more effective screening and prevention programs a top research priority for the 1990s.

Acknowledgment

The author wishes to thank Dr. EW Hook III for his guidance and invaluable assistance in preparing this manuscript.

REFERENCES

1. Centers for Disease Control and Prevention. Surveillance for gonorrhea and primary and secondary syphillis among adolescents, United States—1981–1991. MMWR 1991;42(SS-3):1–11.

2. Centers for Disease Control and Prevention. Sexually transmitted disease surveillance 1992. U.S. Department of Health and Human Services, Public Health Service, 1993:5–21.

3. Toomey KE, Moran JS, Beckett GA. Epidemiological considerations of sexually transmitted diseases in underserved populations. Infect Dis Clin 1993;7:739–752.

4. McGregor JA, Hamill HA. Contraception and sexually transmitted diseases: interactions and opportunities. Am J Obstet Gynecol 1993;168:2033–2041.

5. Stratton P, Alexander NJ. Prevention of sexually transmitted infections: physical and chemical barriers. Infect Dis Clin 1993;7:841–859.

6. Barbone F, Austin H, Louv WC, Alexander WJ. A follow-up study of methods of contraception, sexual activity, and rates of trichomoniasis, candidiasis, and bacterial vaginosis. Am J Obstet Gynecol 1990;163:510–514.

7. Judson FN, Bodin GF, Levin MJ, Ritmeijer CAM. In vitro evaluations of condoms with and without nonoxynol 9 as physical and chemical barriers against *Chlamydia trachomatis*, herpes simplex virus 2, and human immunodeficiency virus. Sex Trans Dis 1989;16:51–56.

8. Austin H, Louv WC, Alexander WJ. A case-controlled study of spermicides and gonorrhea. JAMA 1984;251:2822–2824.

9. Louv WC, Austin, Perlman J, Alexander WJ. Oral contraceptives and the risk of chlamydial and gonococcal infections. Am J Obstet Gynecol 1989;160:396–402.

10. Lewis CE. Sexual practices: are physicians

addressing the issues?. J Gen Intern Med 1990;5-(Suppl):S78–S81.

11. Bowman MA, Russell NK, Bockeloo BO, et al. The effect of educational preparation on physician performance with a sexually transmitted disease-simulated patient. Arch Intern Med 1992;152:1823–1828.

12. Tarylor-Robinson D. Laboratory methods for chlamydial infections. J Infect 1992;25(suppl):61–67.

13. Sobel JD. Vaginal infections in adult women. Med Clin North Am 1990;74:1573–1602.

14. Sharp HC. Vulvovaginal conditions mimicking vaginitis. Clin Obstet Gynecol 1993;36:129–136.

15. Heine P, McGregor JA. *Trichomonas vaginalis*: a reemerging pathogen. Clin Obstet Gynecol 1993;36:137–144.

16. Sweet RL, Gibbs RS. Infections of the female genital tract. 2nd ed. Baltimore: Williams & Wilkins, 1990:218.

17. Thomason JL, Gelbert SSM, Scaglione NJ. Bacterial vaginosis: current review with indications for asymptomatic therapy. Am J Obstet Gynecol 1991;165:1210–1217.

18. Spiegal CA. Bacterial vaginosis. Clin Microbiol Rev 1991;4:485–502.

19. Pearlman MD, McNeely SG. A review of the microbiology, immunology, and clinical implications of *Chlamydia trachomatis* infections. Obstet Gynecol Surv 1992;47:448–461.

20. Judson FN. Gonorrhea. Med Clin 1990;74:1353–1366.

21. Hook III EW, Handsfield HH. Gonococcal infections in the adult. In: Holmes KK, Mårdh PA, Sparling PF, et al., eds. Sexually transmitted diseases. 2nd ed. New York: McGraw-Hill, 1990:149–165.

22. Weinstock HS, Bolan GA, Kohn R, et al. *Chlamydia trachomatis* infection in women: a need for universal screening in high prevalence populations? Am J Epidemiol 1992;135:41–47.

23. Ramstedt K, Forssman L, Giesecke J, Granath F. Risk Factors for *Chlamydia trachomatis* in 6810 young women attending family planning clinics. Int J STD AIDS 1992;3:117–122.

24. Sellors JW, Pickard L, Gafni A, et al. Effectiveness and efficiency of selective vs universal screening for chlamydial infection in young sexually active women. Arch Intern Med 1992;152:1837–1844.

25. Holmes KK. Lower genital tract infections in women: cystitis, urethritis, vulvovaginitis, and cervicitis. In: Holmes KK, Mårdh PA, Sparling PF, et al., eds. Sexually transmitted diseases. 2nd ed. New York: McGraw-Hill, 1990:527–545.

26. Winter L, Goldy AS, Baer C. Prevalence of epidemiologic correlates of *Chlamydia trachomatis* in rural and urban populations. Sex Trans Dis 1990;17:30–36.

27. Katz BP, Caine VA, Jones RB. Diagnosis of mucopurulent cervicitis among women at risk for *Chlamydia trachomatis* infection. Sex Trans Dis 1989;16:103–106.

28. Centers for Disease Control and Prevention. Recommendations for the prevention and management of *Chlamydia trachomatis* infections, 1993. U.S. Department of Health and Human Services, 1993.

29. Ridgway GL, Taylor-Robinson D. Current problems in microbiology: chlamydial infections: which laboratory test?. J Clin Pathol 1991;44:1–5.

30. Schubiner HH, Lebar W, Jemal C. Hershman B. Comparison of three new nonculture tests in the diagnosis of chlamydia genital infections. J Adolesc Health Care 1990;11:505–509.

31. Chapin-Robertson K. Use of molecular diagnostics in sexually transmitted diseases: critical assessment. Diagn Microbiol Infect Dis 1993;16:173–184.

32. Wu CH, Mey-Fann L, Sui-chu Y, et al. Comparison of polymerase chain reaction, monoclonal antibody based immunoassay, and cell culture for detecton of *Chlamydia trachomatis* in genital specimens. Sex Trans Dis 1992;19:193–197.

33. National Institutes of Health. Pelvic inflammatory disease: research directions in the 1990's. Sex Trans Dis 1991;18:46–64.

34. McCormack WM. Pelvic inflammatory disease. N Engl J Med 1994;330:115–119.

35. Waerström L, Mårdh PA. Acute pelvic inflammatory disease (PID). In: Holmes KK, Mårdh PA, Sparling PF, et al., eds. Sexually transmitted diseases. 2nd ed. New York: McGraw-Hill, 1990:593–613.

36. Hook EW III. Approach to sexually transmitted diseases and genital tract infections. In: Kelly WN, ed. Textbook of internal medicine. 2nd ed. Philadelphia: JB Lippincott, 1992:1602–1609.

37. Prober CG, Corey L, Zane AB, et al. The management of pregnancies complicated by genital infections with herpes simplex virus. Clin Infect Dis 1992;15:1031–1038.

38. Mertz GJ. Epidemiology of genital herpes infections. Infect Dis Clin 1993;7:825–839.

39. Frenkel LM, Garraty EM, Shen JP, et al. Clinical reactivation of herpes simplex virus type 2 infection in seropositive pregnant women with no history of genital herpes. Ann Intern Med 1993;118:414–418.

40. Mertz GJ. Genital herpes simplex virus infections. Med Clin 1990;74:1433–1454.

41. Schrijvers D, Jose R, Trebucq A, et al. Transmission of syphilis between sexual partners in Gabon. Genitourin Med 1989;65:84–85.

42. Schober PC, Gabriel G, Feton WF, Thin RN. How infectious is syphilis? Br J Vener Dis 1983;59:217–219.

43. Hutchinson CM, Hook EW III. Syphilis in adults. Med Clin 1990;74:1389–1416.

44. Dicarlo RP, Martin DH. Risk factors for genital ulcer disease. 33rd ICAAC, New Orleans, October 17–20, 1993. Abstract.

45. Ronald AR, Albritton W. Chancroid and *Haemophilus ducreyi*. In: Holmes KK, Mårdh PA, Sparling PF, et al., eds. Sexually transmitted diseases. 2nd ed. New York: McGraw-Hill, 1990:263–271.

46. Jessamine PG, Ronald AR. Chancroid and the role of genital ulcer disease in the spread of human retroviruses. Med Clin 1990;74:1417–1431.

SECTION EIGHT

OTOLARYNGOLOGY

CHAPTER 26

NASAL AND SINUS DISEASE

C. Elliott Morgan

Rhinology is a diverse and expanding subspecialty in the field of otolaryngology. The causes of rhinitis cover many etiologies, expanding into many disciplines of medicine. This chapter is meant to be a concise, accessible overview for the practicing primary care physician. It is hoped that the material presented here will be beneficial in both treatment of diseases of the nose as well as in providing vital information when consultation with a otolaryngologist is warranted.

Nasal Anatomy

External Nose

The external nose is pyramidal in shape and is formed primarily by the nasal bones superiorly, which are wedge shaped and articulate with the frontal bone, and the frontal processes of the maxilla laterally and the upper lateral cartilages inferiorly. Upper lateral cartilages form a portion of the nasal valve and prevent collapse of the nasal vestibule on inspiration. The lower lateral cartilages form the lower one third of the nose and provide structural stability to the vestibule laterally and inferiorly.

Septum

The nasal septum is the bony and cartilaginous partition that divides the nasal passages into right and left sides. The bony part consists of the perpendicular plane of the ethmoid bone, the vomer, the bony crest of the maxilla, and the palatine bone. This bone is articulated anteriorly with the quadrilateral cartilage with a small contribution from the upper and lower lateral cartilages. Inferiorly, the septal cartilage sits in the groove of the maxillary crest and anteriorly it abuts the medial crura of the lower lateral alar cartilages. The cartilaginous septum is important in the development of the mid-third of the face and damage to this area in birth through infancy can cause dramatic alterations to the growth of this area.

Lateral Nasal Wall

The lateral nasal wall is occupied by the nasal turbinates, which create turbulence in the inspired air, thus absorbing heat and moisture and filtering particles of dust and bacteria from the air. This makes the air more pleasant to breathe. There are usually three turbinates on each lateral nasal wall: the inferior turbinate, middle turbinate, and superior turbinate. Occasionally, there is a supreme turbinate.

Blood Supply to the Nasal Cavity

The lateral nasal wall in the septum receives blood from the external and internal carotid systems. The anterior and posterior ethmoid arteries contribute to the blood supply superiorly and branches of the internal maxillary artery supply the posterior and inferior portions of the nasal cavity.

Nerve Supply

Sensation to the nasal septum is supplied by the maxillary division of the trigeminal nerve. Postganglionic sympathetic fibers to the blood vessels accompany the sensory fibers. Postganglionic parasympathetic secretomotor fibers pass to the glands. Olfactory fibers innervate the olfactory epithelium in the upper part of the septum.

Infective Rhinitis

Viral Rhinitis

Viral rhinitis is most commonly manifested as the

common cold. Many viruses have been associated with upper respiratory tract infections and more than 100 types of rhinoviruses have been identified. It is estimated that most adults suffer from two to three viral upper respiratory tract infections a year.

Predisposing factors that may cause viral rhinitis include climate changes, especially in the winter months when the temperature is colder, and environmental changes such has humidity and chilling. People with immunodeficiencies or decreased levels of immunoglobulins in their nasal secretions are more susceptible to the infections. Nutrition, fatigue, and stress have all been cited as factors that can lead to viral rhinitis. Close contact and exposure to airborne droplets of virus from coughing or sneezing also contribute significantly to the progression and development of viral infections in the nose.

Acute inflammation caused by the virus initially causes edema with increased secretions from the glands within the nasal cavity and desquamation of the surface epithelium within the nasal cavity with regeneration over several days following the initial infection.

Clinical features of viral rhinitis and viral upper respiratory tract infection include muscle aches, headaches, and loss of appetite. The nose feels congested and swollen with frequent episodes of sneezing. The catarrhal phase follows a few hours after viral exposure with profuse rhinorrhea, anosmia, and increased hyperemia of the mucous membranes of the nose. The phase of active mucoid discharge then follows with resolution of the symptoms over the next few days if the infection is not complicated by secondary bacterial infection.

Other areas of the upper aerodigestive tract may be affected with resulting pharyngitis, otitis media, tonsillitis, possibly bronchitis, and there may be lymphadenitis associated with the infection as well.

Treatment of viral rhinitis involves avoidance of contact with infected persons and symptomatic treatment including topical and oral decongestants. Antibiotics are reserved for secondary bacterial infections.

Influenza also is responsible for viral upper respiratory tract infections. These have a more serious nature with more necrosis of the nasal epithelium, which further facilitates secondary bacterial infections with more significant morbidity and mortality in susceptible populations. The attempted use of vaccines for influenza has been somewhat successful but is generally limited due to the potential for viral mutation.

The nasal manifestations of human immunodeficiency virus (HIV) infection can and do occur at any stage of the disease. After initial exposure to the virus, the patient may have a short-lived acute upper respiratory tract infection that may mimic a common cold. In chronic HIV infection, a rhinitis similar to sarcoid and granulomatous nasal diseases may be seen with the associated symptoms of nasal congestion and signs of nasal crusting, bleeding, and bacterial infections. In fully developed acquired immunodeficiency syndrome (AIDS), Kaposi's sarcoma may be noted on the mucous membranes but is rarely found within the nasal cavity.

Bacterial Infections

The normal bacterial flora of the nose includes species of corynebacteria, staphylococci, and α-hemolytic streptococci. Between 20% and 50% of adults are chronic carriers of *Staphylococcus aureus* in the nasal vestibule and this may play a role in the epidemiology of hospital-acquired infections and postoperative wound infections.

Specific bacterial infections such as furunculosis can occur in the nasal vestibule. The usual offending agent is *S. aureus* that invades a pilosebaceous follicle to produce an infection around the follicle with induration, which will spontaneously rupture and discharge purulent contents after 3 to 4 days. These infections are usually caused by digital manipulation of the nasal vestibule or trauma to the face or puncture or compression of acneiform lesions. Treatment for nasal vestibulitis includes local cleansing and systemic antibiotics, which should have coverage for *Staphylococcus* both coagulase-negative and coagulase-positive strains.

The potential complications from nasal vestibulitis can be extremely serious due to retrograde flow of the organisms through the veins of the face. The angular vein and superior ophthalmic veins are valveless, which allow flow of organisms, both antegrade and retrograde, and have the potential for the complication of cavernous sinus involvement with these infections.

Infections caused by diphtheria are rare today due

to widespread immunization programs. However, these cases do occur and may be overlooked. Diphtheria can occur in an acute form with neurologic complications or a more chronic form that may resolve over several months. The pseudomembrane that occurs over the mucosa consists of neutrophils, necrotic epithelium, and a diphtheria bacilli, and when removed, causes bleeding. Treatment is with parenteral penicillin with antitoxin being reserved for acute cases.

Rhinoscleroma

Rhinoscleroma is endemic in southeastern Europe, northern Africa, Central America, northern South America, Pakistan, and Indonesia. However, sporadic cases may occur anywhere, including the United States. The causative organism is *Klebsiella rhinoscleromatis*.

The disease occurs in three phases: rhinitic, infiltrative, and nodular, finally resulting in adhesions and nasal stenosis and atresia. The tumor-like masses of the nodular phase are characterized by the presence of Mikulicz's cells, which are large cells with clear cytoplasm containing the bacilli. Plasma cells containing intracytoplasmic gobules of secretory product are numerous and stained deeply red on hematoxylin-eosin stain.

Treatment of rhinoscleroma is by large doses of streptomycin or tetracycline over a 4- to 6-week period and until two consecutive nasal biopsies are negative for the bacteria. Reconstructive nasal surgery may be required to correct cosmetic changes in the lobule of the nose and to relieve nasal obstruction due to stenosis and scarring.

Tuberculosis

Primary tuberculosis is rare in the United States. However, with the increasing population of immunosuppressed people, it has become a more common infection in the past 5 years. Nasal involvement is almost always secondary to pulmonary involvement. Early symptoms include mucopurulent discharge from the nose, pain, partial nasal obstruction, and intermittent epistaxis. Examination may reveal an ulcerated, isolated tender nodule in the anterior part of the nasal septum, sometimes associated with septal perforation. The lesions may also occur on the anterior ends of the inferior turbinates.

The usual organism is *Mycobacterium tuberculosis*. Histologic examination of the tissue reveals tubercles with central caseation necrosis. On acid-fast staining, the organism will be found in epithelioid cells or free within the tubercle. Treatment includes isoniazid (INH) and usually one of the following drugs: rifampin, streptomycin, ethambutal or para-amino salicylic acid. Negative culture is the guide to control of the disease and the discontinuation of therapy.

Lupus vulgaris is a tuberculous infection of the skin. It is found most commonly in young adult women in northern climates. The clinical picture is similar to that described for tuberculosis of the nasal cavity with the exception that the nasal vestibule, external nose, and adjacent face may be involved with more resultant scarring from the infection. Classic "apple jelly" nodules are found at the myocutaneous junction of the vestibule. Treatment is the same as for tuberculosis.

Syphilis

Infection of the nose with *Treponema pallidum* can occur at any age. It is generally uncommon today. Three phases of the infection can affect the nose: primary, secondary, and tertiary. This infection can also present in its congenital form. Involvement of the nose in congenital syphilis begins usually in the third or fourth week of life with purulent rhinorrhea (snuffles) that is associated with fissures and erosion of the tissue around the anterior nares. Granuloma formation may cause destruction of the growth centers in the cartilage with the resulting saddling of the nasal dorsum.

Primary syphilis can occur on the external nose or the vestibule 3 to 4 weeks after contact. This is an ulcerated, painless lesion that will disappear within 6 to 10 weeks. This lesion may also be associated with cervical adenopathy. Smears of the lesion at this time examined under darkfield illumination may reveal the *Treponema* organism, although serology may be negative in the early stages. Treatment at this stage is with systemic penicillin.

Secondary syphilis may appear 6 to 10 weeks after the initial exposure to the *Treponema* organism. Patients may have mucopurulent rhinitis with crusting and fissuring around the anterior nares. Normal mucous patches seen in the oral mucosa are not usually apparent in the nose. A serologic diagnosis can be made during this phase.

The tertiary syphilis is characterized by gumma formation, which invades the mucous membrane, periosteum, and bone, and especially involving the septum, producing tenderness over the bridge of the nose, septal perforations, and nasal collapse. Serology is positive in 90% of these cases. Treatment is with systemic high-dose penicillin for up to 3 months.

Fungal Rhinitis

Aspergillus is a frequent fungal organism affecting the sinuses; however, it infrequently will affect the nasal cavity as well. Signs and symptoms include nasal obstruction with mucosal edema, mucopurulent nasal discharge, and extensive crusting within the nose. Smears of the nasal exudate and crusting lesions may reveal the fungal organisms. In general, the lesions are treated by local excision, by local nasal cleaning, and with topical antifungal agents; occasionally systemic amphotericin or ketoconazole is given for significant invasive infection.

Mucormycosis is another fungal infection of worldwide distribution. It usually affects patients with underlying debilitative diseases and severe immunodepression. Approximately 70% of the affected patients have diabetes mellitus. The organism may exist in seven different forms. It invades along vascular channels and prefers the internal elastic lamina of arterial structures. Arterial occlusion results in ischemic infarction of involved structures, which may include the entire mid-face, the orbit, and eye, resulting in blindness and ophthalmoplegia. Intracranial extension is also common with this fungus, which may produce brain abscess, stroke with associated hemiplegia, severe infections, and death. Diagnosis is made by fungal stain and culture of the organism. Fungal stains will show irregularly branched nonseptate hyphae. Treatment is radical debridement and drainage of the affected areas with debridement of devitalized tissue. IV amphotericin B in high doses over a prolonged period of time, at least a month, may be required to eradicate the organism. Management of the underlying debilitating disease also improves prognosis.

Rhinosporidium is another fungal organism that is endemic to the areas of India and Sri Lanka. Innoculation may occur from inhaling dust-borne organisms. A characteristic clinical finding is a bleeding polyp within the nose. This lesion is usually painless and friable and usually originates from the nasal septum. It may fill the entire the nasal cavity or nasopharynx. The patient will complain of intermittent epistaxis, nasal obstruction, and foul-smelling nasal discharge. Diagnosis of this fungal infection is best made by histologic section because culture is usually not revealing. Surgical excision is the primary treatment with amphotericin B reserved for recurrent cases.

Blastomycosis and histoplasmosis infections may also cause abscesses in the nose. This is rare but may occur especially in endemic areas.

Candidiasis has been reported in the nose; however, it is normally a harmless parasitic infection. In severely debilitated patients, particularly AIDS patients, candidiasis can affect the nasal mucosa with erosion of the mucosa, purulent drainage, and destruction of the septal cartilage. Treatment is surgical debridement with systemic administration of amphotericin B.

Allergic Rhinitis

Allergic rhinitis can be defined as congestion of the nasal mucous membrane accompanied by rhinorrhea and sneezing. The two factors that are required for its development are an immunologic sensitivity to an allergen and a recurrent or continuous exposure to it. About 17% of the U.S. population suffers from allergic disease. Allergic rhinitis is triggered by a variety of allergens and can be classified into four different types of reactions. Types I through III include the immediate and late reactions that are humoral in nature. Type IV is a delayed reaction and is mediated by cellular mechanisms.

Allergic rhinitis is a distinct clinical entity and can be distinguished from other forms of rhinitis by the following characteristics: early onset (age 1 to 20 years), strong familial tendency, propensity to be associated with other allergic disorders, elevated serum IgE levels, increased specific IgE antibodies that can be demonstrated by skin testing or in vitro procedures (radioallergosorbent test [RAST]), and increased lower airway reactivity.

Histologic findings in patients with allergic rhinitis consist of mucosal edema within infiltration of eosinophils, lymphocytes, and plasma cells. These cells are attracted to the site of mass cell degranulation with the release of chemical mediators including histamine, a slow-reacting substance of anaphylaxis, eosinophil chemotactic factor of anaphylaxis, platelet-activating factor, and arachidonic acid metabolites.

The main clinical features of allergic rhinitis are sneezing, watery rhinorrhea, and nasal congestion. Itching of the eyes, nose, and throat is associated typically with seasonal rather than perennial rhinitis. The histamine release resulting in the edema and obstruction of the nasal passages indirectly produces the sneezing and watery rhinorrhea.

Other symptoms include venous congestion under the eyes (allergic shiners), conjunctivities, chronic mouth breathing due to nasal obstruction, nocturnal tooth grinding, and complaints of a dry, irritated, frequently sore throat with repeated throat clearing. Laboratory testing to confirm allergic rhinitis includes nasal cytology, skin testing, and in vitro testing. Nasal smears are obtained by wiping the nasal cavity with a cotton-tipped applicator, transferring the secretions to a slide, and staining with Wright-Giemsa stain. An increase in eosinophils, goblet cells, and mast cells is highly associated with allergic rhinitis and provides indication as to whether skin testing or in vitro testing should be pursued to identity specific allergens. Skin testing using available dilutions of the allergens can confirm reactions to specific allergens based on the skin response after injection. Disadvantages of skin testing include variations due to antihistamine ingestion and steroid ingestion. Skin testing may be variable in response to certain food allergens and is dangerous in patients taking β blockers. If an anaphylactic reaction were to occur, epinephrine would be ineffective to reverse the reaction. In vitro testing involves the measurement of IgE levels in the blood stream. RAST measures the level of allergen-specific IgE in the blood. The technique uses a paper disc with antigen bound to the surface. The allergen-specific IgE that may be present in the serum binds to the antigen on the disc. After excess IgE is washed away, radiolabeled anti-IgE is added, which binds to the patient's IgE bound to the antigen on the disc and the amount of radioactivity is counted to determine allergen sensitivity. The advantages of RAST include the elimination of variability of the skin test. It eliminates the effects of antihistamines, can be done with one blood test, and may be more specific than skin testing. It is also safe for patients taking β blockers. The disadvantages of RAST are that it is relatively expensive, requires specialized laboratory equipment and technician training, and may be less sensitive than skin testing.

Treatment of Allergic Rhinitis

Treatment of allergic rhinitis involves three phases: environmental control, pharmacotherapy, and immunotherapy.

Environment

Environmental control involves decreasing the amount of allergen the patient is exposed to by attempting to control the patient's environment. Patients are advised to avoid living in damp places, avoid moisture accumulation indoors around air conditioners and pipes, and avoid storing magazines, papers, or clothing in the house, especially in the bedroom. Dust precautions to eliminate the dust mite antigen include use of synthetic carpets, frequent vacuuming, regular filter changes of the air conditioners, and the use of plastic sheets, covers, and pillow covers on mattresses. Avoiding cats or dogs if the patient is allergic to animal dander also aids in reducing symptoms.

Pharmacotherapy

Pharmacotherapy of allergy can be divided into three classes of medications: antihistamines, decongestants (systemic and topical) and steroids (systemic and topical).

Antihistamines: The H_1-receptor antagonists are useful in the management of allergic rhinitis. Their onset is usually rapid and reduces sneezing, pruritus, and rhinorrhea, but they do not relieve congestion. Activation of H_1 receptors causes smooth muscle contraction, increases vascular permeability, and increases the production of mucus. Activation also induces sensory nerves to generate pruritus and reflexes such as sneezing. Traditional antihistamine drugs used in the treatment of allergic rhinitis are lipophilic and cross the blood–brain barrier and, therefore, produce sedation. The newer H_1 antihistamines, such as terfenadine, astemizole and loratadine, are less lipophilic, which reduces their ability to cross the blood–brain barrier and reduces their sedative and cholinergic actions. Antihistamines are effective for the treatment of sneezing and watery rhinorrhea. They work better in seasonal and episodic allergic rhinitis than they do in perennial rhinitis in which congestion is a greater problem. With the introduction of the newer nonsedating antihistamines, the traditional antihistamines have been reduced to a lesser role in management of allergic rhinitis due not only to their sedative side effects, but also due to associated dizziness, blurred vision, and alterations in motor function with their ingestion.

Many antihistamines produce cholinergic effects ranging from dryness of the eyes, urinary retention, tachycardia, and constipation. In children and elderly persons, extremely high doses may also cause central cholinergic blockade manifested by irritability. Antihistamines can have a quinidine-like effect on cardiac muscle and prolong the QT interval and occasionally can lead to torsade de pointes.

Decongestants: These drugs are used orally and topically and are primarily directed against nasal obstruction. These medications are α-adrenergic agonists that cause vasoconstriction and reduce the blood supply to the nasal mucosa, thus decreasing the volume of blood in the tissue and the amount of mucosal edema. These medications are often combined with antihistamines. Topical administration produces a more rapid onset of action and is generally more efficacious than systemic administration. However, prolonged topical administration will lead to rhinitis medicamentosa. This term refers to the progressive shortening of the duration of efficacy of the topical decongestants with repeated use and to rebound rhinitis after treatment is discontinued. Topical decongestants should be used to manage allergic rhinitis only for the following purposes: to facilitate diagnostic evaluation of the upper airway, to permit introduction of topical steroids, and to facilitate sleep during severe rhinitic exacerbations.

Pseudoephedrine hydrochloride and phenylpropanolamine hydrochloride are the prototypes of the systemic decongestants. These medications also will cause constriction of other vascular beds and this accounts for their many side effects.

The most frequently reported adverse reactions to decongestant medication are insomnia and irritability. Agitation, tachycardia, palpitations, nausea, and vomiting may also occur. The medications are contraindicated in children with behavioral disorders; in elderly men with potential prostate problems; in patients with coexisting hypertension, angina, diabetes mellitus, and glaucoma; and in patients who are taking monoamine oxidate inhibitors or tricyclic antidepressants.

Cromolyn has been effective in the treatment of allergic rhinitis. Cromolyn sodium functions as a mast cell stabilizer and is best used before the onset of seasonal allergic rhinitis and as prophylaxis before exposures to inhalant allergens. The medication is delivered intranasally as a 4% spray through a metered-dose inhaler containing 5 mg of drug per actuation. The medication is poorly absorbed and has as a few side effects of any antiallergic medication. When the medication is effective, its potency is similar to that of antihistamines and less than that of topical steroids.

Steroids: Glucocorticoids are the most potent medications available to treat allergic rhinitis. Cortisol is the apparent molecule from which synthetic and natural anti-inflammatory steroids are derived. These agents act by regulating gene expression, which accounts for their delay in onset of action.

Treatment with prednisone has little effect on the immediate response to nasal provocation with antigen but it markedly diminishes the late phase hyperresponsiveness to antigen.

The development of topical steroids has dramatically reduced the need for systemic steroid treatment. In contrast to systemic steroids, topical steroids also affect the early allergic response. They not only inhibit the influx of eosinophils but also inhibit the influx of neutrophils as well.

The preparations available include flunisolide, beclomethasone, and dexamethasone. In adults, the recommended starting dose is 2 sprays per nostril twice a day. The patient should be re-evaluated in 1 to 2 weeks to look for signs of local irritation from the medication. The maintenance dose can be adjusted according to clinical response. Clinical studies have shown that flunisolide seems to depress mucociliary function more so than the beclomethasone preparations.

The principal side effect of intranasal steroids is local irritation and about 10% of patients will experience this. Rarely, with long-term use, has bloody nasal discharge and septal perforation occurred. Overgrowth of candidiasis has occurred with prolonged use of topical inhalation steroids as well. The systemic side effects, however, are minimal and, with proper dosing, these medications can be used for a prolonged period of time with good benefit and without any adverse long-term effect.

Vasomotor Rhinitis

Hyperactive parasympathetic stimulation of nasal mucosa is the pathologic basis of vasomotor rhinitis. This produces symptoms of vasodilation, edema, and hypersecretion of mucus. Patients will complain of nasal stuffiness, profuse rhinorrhea, occasional sneezing episodes, and facial pressure with headache. These symptoms can be aggravated by certain irritants, including cigarette smoke, air pollutants, aerosols, certain perfumes, and noxious odors. Also, extreme temperature changes and changes in the humidity as well as stress and anxiety can worsen the symptoms.

Diagnosis is one of exclusion of other types of rhinitis, including infective rhinitis, sinusitis, and allergic rhinitis. The diagnosis is usually made primarily by history to rule out pregnancy, hypothyroidism, or medications that can contribute to nasal congestion and alterations of the nasal physiology.

Systemic decongestants can be prescribed to treat the congestion, but the side effects are not well tolerated at times and tachyphylaxis also occurs as the medication develops. Antihistamines may decrease nasal secretions from their anticholinergic effects and intranasal steroids can reduce inflammatory-mediator release.

Ipratropium bromide has been used with some success in the treatment of vasomotor rhinitis. The drug antagonizes acetylcholine transmission from the synapse in parasympathetic nerves reducing submucosal gland secretion. The drug is primarily effective in reducing the symptoms of watery rhinorrhea. The medication is applied as an inhalant into the nasal cavities using 80 μg every 6 hours.

For patients who fail medical therapy and have particularly troublesome symptoms, surgical therapy may be necessary. The procedures that have been used involve reduction of the size of the inferior turbinates. Various techniques have been used to do this and range from unipolar, bipolar submucosal cauterization to actual submucous resection of the turbinates. Complications from this will include prolonged nasal crusting and atrophic rhinitis. Turbinoplasty or turbinectomy has had varying results on vasomotor rhinitis. Cryosurgery on the inferior turbinates has also been used with varying degrees of success.

Recently, laser turbinectomy has been performed for swollen inferior turbinates. However, there is significant postoperative crusting during the 4- to 8-week healing period and again the results have been variable with this technique.

Rhinitis During Pregnancy

During pregnancy increased estrogen levels appear to inhibit acetylcholinesterase, thereby promoting the cholinergic effects within the nasal cavity. This will cause increased mucous gland activity, changes in the mucosa, and increased vascularization of the nasal turbinate mucosa. These factors may be coupled with an already preexisting allergic rhinitis, bacterial rhinosinusitis, or vasomotor rhinitis, which can further aggravate the symptoms.

In diagnosing and treating rhinitis during pregnancy, the safety of the fetus must be of prime concern. RAST can be done instead of skin testing to avoid the dangers of anaphylaxis. Nasal cytology may be performed to assess for neutrophils or eosinophils, which may aid in ruling out allergic or bacterial sinusitis. Ultrasound may be performed to rule out fluid collections in the frontal or maxillary sinuses. Treatment of pregnancy-induced rhinitis should first be with nonpharmacologic approaches, such as avoiding things that may trigger the rhinitis (noxious fumes, temperature changes, or humidity changes). Systemic steroids and antihistamines are contraindicated but judicious use of topical steroid preparations may help in this situation and the condition will resolve after delivery.

Rhinitis Medicamentosa

Nasal obstruction can be caused by chronic use of topical or oral decongestants and produce persistent nasal obstruction. The nasal decongestant may be used to treat an underlying disorder such as septal deviation, allergic rhinitis, or nasal polyposis.

Rhinitis medicamentosa is attributed to rebound vasodilatation after prolonged vasoconstriction with topical agents. Continued use of the drug will diminish vasoconstriction and increase vasodilitation. Management of rhinitis medicamentosa involves discontinuation of the offending medication and treatment with topical steroid nasal spray and, in certain extreme cases, a short-term course of oral prednisone for 7 to 10 days.

Nasal Polyposis

The pathogenesis of nasal polyps is poorly understood. Polyps seem to arise in areas where the secretions and particulate matter from the paranasal sinuses are deposited. Three factors are thought to be important in polyp pathogenesis: chronic mucosal inflammation, abnormal vasomotor response, and mechanical problems related to increased interstitial edema. Major basic protein from eosinophils may also damage the basement membrane in allowing prolapse of the lamina propria. Histamine release secondary to certain antigens may cause increased vascular permeability followed by tissue edema and ultimately polyp formation.

Nasal polyps are usually bilateral and if they are not they should be regarded with suspicion for neoplasia. The earliest signs of nasal polyposis include nasal obstruction, loss of senses of smell and taste, and persistent nasal discharge. Expansion and erosion of bone can result in complications including visual changes and proptosis of the eye. Cranial neuropathies have been caused by extreme expansion of the polyps with compression and inflammation around cranial nerves II through VI.

There is no cure for nasal polyposis and the recurrence rate after treatment is high. Medical and surgical treatment are often complimentary. Causative factors should try to be identified and eliminated. Medical treatment includes certain elimination diets, aspirin avoidance, desensitization for antigens, antihistamines, and systemic and topical steroids. Surgical treatment of the nasal polyps is indicated if there is inadequate response to medical therapy with persistent severe nasal obstruction or impendng or actual complication of rhinosinusitis secondary to the polyposis.

Nasal Trauma

Nasal fractures rank third in incidence behind fractures of the clavicle and the wrist. Many fractures of the nasal bones go unrecognized and untreated at the time of initial injury. Symptoms of nasal fracture include nasal deformity, swelling, pain, tenderness, mobility of the nasal bones, nasal obstruction, and epistaxis.

The nose must be inspected internally and externally to rule out deformity and septal hematoma. Lacerations and mucosal tears should be repaired as early as possible. Plain radiographs may give some indication of the extent of the fracture. However, at times, these may be confusing with suture lines, vascular markings, and prior fractures obscuring the findings of the present injury.

Other common associated injuries such as dental fractures, lacrimal system involvement, or cerebrospinal fluid fistula should also be sought and treated as early as possible.

Delayed treatment of nasal fractures generally involves a rhinoplasty, septorhinoplasty or, in certain cases of severe nasal trauma, an open rhinoplasty approach. Splints are usually applied to stabilize the septum and an external nasal splint is usually applied for 7 to 10 days.

The Nose and Systemic Disease

Sarcoidosis

Sarcoidosis is a systemic condition of unknown etiology characterized by noncaseating epithelioid granulomas. It primarily affects the lower respiratory tract but can involve the upper respiratory tract including the nose. The disease is found throughout the world. There is usually a higher incidence in the rural southeastern United States and Scandinavia. Black people are affected more commonly and it is more common in the female population. The patient usually experiences nasal obstruction, some mucopurulent blood-stained discharge, and nasal crusting. Physical examination reveals small yellow crusts covering the septum and crusting of the lateral nasal wall. There may be spontaneous septal perforations and this can produce saddling of the nasal dorsum.

Laboratory studies usually include erythrocyte sedimentation rate and serum calcium, both of which are sometimes elevated. The Kveim test is usually positive in 90% of the patients and the majority of the patients will have an elevated angiotensin-converting enzyme level. Sinus radiographs and computed tomography

(CT) scans will usually show mucosal thickening and occasionally cystic lesions of the nasal bones. Differential diagnosis involves other diseases that cause the formation of granulomas including tuberculosis, atypical microbacteria, leprosy, Wegner's granulomatosis, and AIDS.

Treatment of the nasal symptoms is usually with nasal douches and beclomethasone nasal spray. The majority of patients may also require oral corticosteroids to control their other pulmonary symptoms.

Autoimmune Tissue Diseases

A number of autoimmune connective tissue disorders can also affect the nose and sinuses. These are usually diagnosed by a combination of the clinical history and histology.

Systemic lupus erythematosus may manifest as reddish patches over the nasal dorsum, which extend to the cheeks in a classic butterfly rash. There may also be nasal crusting as well as intranasal lesions.

Takayasu's disease is an obliterative arteritis that can affect the nasal septum, producing septal perforation and saddling.

Relapsing polychondritis usually affects aural cartilage but nasal chondritis may occur in up to 60% of the cases with erythema and swelling of the nasal dorsum, which eventually leads to collapse of the nasal dorsum.

Wegner's Granulomatosis

This is a systemic disease that initially may present in the nose before pulmonary and renal manifestations develop. A limited form of this disease affects just the nose and lungs. The histologic diagnosis may be difficult at times because this usually is a nonspecific chronic inflammation with areas of necrosis and Langhan's and foreign body giant cells. The vasculitis usually affects small vessels, producing certain circumscribed lesions in the lungs, which heal by fibrosis and focal necrotizing glomerulonephritis.

The symptoms are usually insidious and progress to nasal obstruction, discharge, and gradual collapse of the nasal dorsum. Systemic symptoms may occur with cough, hemoptysis, hematuria, and malaise. Sometimes the condition may be more aggressive and may be rapidly fatal. The disease usually responds dramatically to high-dose corticosteroids and immunosuppressive agents such as azathioprine.

The erythrocyte sedimentation rate is usually raised and can be used as a monitor of therapeutic response. Sinus radiographs show nonspecific inflammatory change.

Leukemia

Acute and chronic leukemic infiltrates can present in the nose. These can be confirmed histologically and hematologically.

During the course of multiple myeloma, patients may present with an extramedullary plasma cytoma that can develop intranasally. Biopsy is used for confirmation of diagnosis and these lesions are usually treated with radiation therapy.

Sinuses and Sinus Disease

Sinusitis can be defined as inflammation of the mucosal linings of the sinuses. This can be caused from various etiologies. The most common, however, is viral from the common cold. Sinusitis is one of the most common illnesses in the United States, and it affects more than 31 million people yearly. Sinusitis usually presents in either the acute form or in the chronic form with long-standing patient complaints. This section reviews the anatomy and physiology of the paranasal sinuses and discusses the diagnosis, imaging, and treatment of sinusitis.

Anatomy of Paranasal Sinuses

There are eight paranasal sinuses, four on each side of the nose. These consist of the frontal, ethmoid, maxillary, and sphenoid sinuses. The sinuses are lined with a mucous membrane that protects against viral and bacterial invasion. The sinus secretions contain antibacterial enzymes and immunoglobulins to provide a natural defense against infection. Under normal conditions, these sinuses are filled with air and the mucus within the sinuses is sterile. Each sinus communicates with the nasal cavity through an ostium.

The ethmoid sinuses appear during the third or fourth fetal month as evaginations of the lateral nasal wall in the region of the middle meatus. At birth, there are usually three or four ethmoid air cells present on each side. They usually reach an adult size by the time a child is 12 years old.

Maxillary sinuses will appear on radiographs at about age 4 months, and growth of these sinuses is not complete until about 14 or 15 years of age. The maxillary sinus is the largest of the paranasal sinuses, and the floor of this sinus is closely related to the roots of the maxillary teeth.

The frontal sinus begins development in the fourth month of gestation. It can usually be demonstrated radiographically about the second year of life and continues to grow until it reaches full size around age 17 or 18. Five to 10% of the population has failure of development of one of the frontal sinuses. The posterior table of the frontal sinus separates the sinus from the anterior cranial fossa.

The sphenoid sinuses originate in the third month of fetal life. They become pneumatized around age 9 to 10 and achieve their final size around age 12 to 15 years. The sphenoid sinus lateral wall lies adjacent to the optic nerve and the carotid artery, and the hypophysis lies immediately above the posterior wall.

Acute Sinusitis

Pathophysiology

Three factors must be present to maintain the normal physiology of the paranasal sinuses: patency of the sinus ostia, functional cilia, and normal quality of the nasal secretions.

The cilia require the fluid medium to function properly. Therefore, when the nasal secretions are altered, the ciliary function is impaired and the normal sinus physiology is altered.

The most significant factor leading to sinusitis is mucosal edema in and around the sinus ostium. The obstruction of the ostium will cause decreased oxygen tensions in the involved sinus. This further disturbs the ciliary function and then alters the mucous blanket as well. As secretions are altered, they become retained in the sinus as a result of the obstruction of the ostium. Negative intrasinal pressure is created and nasal breathing is decreased as a result of factors causing mucosal edema. This produces further hypoxia, and along with sneezing, sniffling, or nasal blowing, bacteria may enter the sinus ostium. The change in viscosity of nasal secretions occurs and this provides an ideal culture medium for bacteria. Epithelium that lines the nose and paranasal sinuses is pseudostratified columnar ciliated epithelium. The mucociliary transport is important in maintaining normal sinus and nasal physiology and factors that impair this transport are critical to the initiation of a sinus infection.

Local Factors Causing Sinusitis

Trauma that may alter the anatomy of the sinus outflow tracts may predispose to sinusitis. Any mechanical obstruction including septal deviation, turbinate hypertrophy, or choanal atresia may interfere with drainage of the nose and drainage of the paranasal sinuses. Inspiration of cold or dry air can also cause alterations in the function of the cilia and lead to sinus infection. Edema around the sinus ostium, from upper respiratory tract infection, can cause reduced mucous clearance of the sinus and ultimately a bacterial infection. Barotrauma related to air travel or diving can also produce edema of the sinus ostium and allow bacteria to multiply within the sinus, thus producing an infection. Nasal polyps, foreign bodies, or nasal packing can all alter the ventilation of the sinuses and produce sinusitis. Certain syndromes that alter the ciliary motility or the development of normal cilia may lead to sinusitis due to poor mucociliary clearance.

Systemic Factors Causing Sinusitis

Patients with debilitating diseases such as diabetes and certain blood dyscrasias may be more predisposed to developing sinusitis. Long-term steroid therapy, chemotherapy, and periods of malnutrition also predispose certain patients to persistent or recurring sinus infections. Sinusitis may also be a manifestation of IgG deficiency. Patients with AIDS should be examined for signs and symptoms of sinusitis because it has been reported that at least 85% of AIDS patients have some symptoms or signs of sinusitis. In fact, sinusitis may be one of the first manifestations of AIDS in the HIV-positive patient.

Classification of Sinusitis

Sinusitis can be classed into three categories: acute sinusitis, which is any infection lasting from 1 day up to 4 weeks; subacute sinusitis, which lasts from 4 weeks to 3 months where the disease process is still reversible; and chronic sinusitis in which the sinusitis persists longer than 3 months.

Classification of sinusitis enables the physician to determine which patients will respond to medical management alone and which will require surgical intervention to resolve the disease.

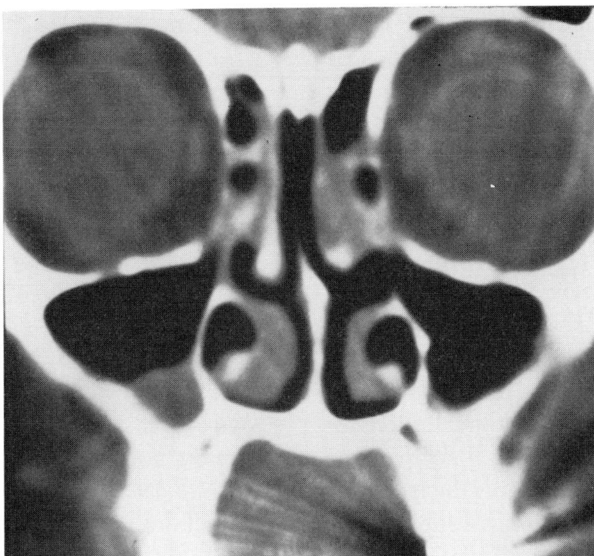

Fig 26.1 Chronic bilateral ethmoid and maxillary sinusitis.

Symptoms of Acute Sinusitis

Symptoms of sinusitis usually relate to the location of the sinus involved and the duration of the disease. Pain over the involved sinus is a common complaint along with headache, either directly over the sinus or referred headache pain. The patient may also complain of nasal obstruction and discolored nasal discharge. In children, the primary symptoms may only be halitosis or persistent nasal discharge. Associated symptoms may include fever, malaise, and lethargy.

Pain associated with ethmoid sinusitis is usually located in the medial portion of the nose and the retro-orbital area. Sphenoid sinusitis may present as a vertex or bitemporal headache. Frontal sinusitis usually defers pain to the forehead area, whereas maxillary sinusitis can cause pain over the cheek area or in the maxillary posterior teeth on the affected side.

The majority of cases of acute bacterial sinusitis usually follow an upper respiratory tract infection. However, localized maxillary sinusitis can be from a dental etiology and trauma of varying sorts may precipitate sinusitis by causing bleeding into the sinuses with secondary bacterial infection.

Physical Examination

Examination of the nasal passages and the sinus ostia has been made easier with the advent of rigid nasal endoscopy. This allows the physician to determine the sinus or sinuses involved and the presence of any local associated factors important in the etiology of the sinus infection.

In performing the nasal examination, special features of the nasal anatomy are examined such as deviated nasal septum and large middle turbinates. Also, pathologic changes such as polyps or obstructing masses in the middle meatus are easily observed. Mucopurulent discharge is also easily visualized through endoscopic methods and the source of the purulent mucus is usually easily determined (Plates 5 and 6).

Computed tomography imaging of the paranasal sinuses has become the "gold standard" to fully evaluate the sinuses and any disease process that may be present. The CT scan affords an excellent view of the sinus ostia as well as the sinus outflow tracts and of the sinus cavities themselves (Figs 26.1 and 26.2). These images are usually done in the axial and coronal views.

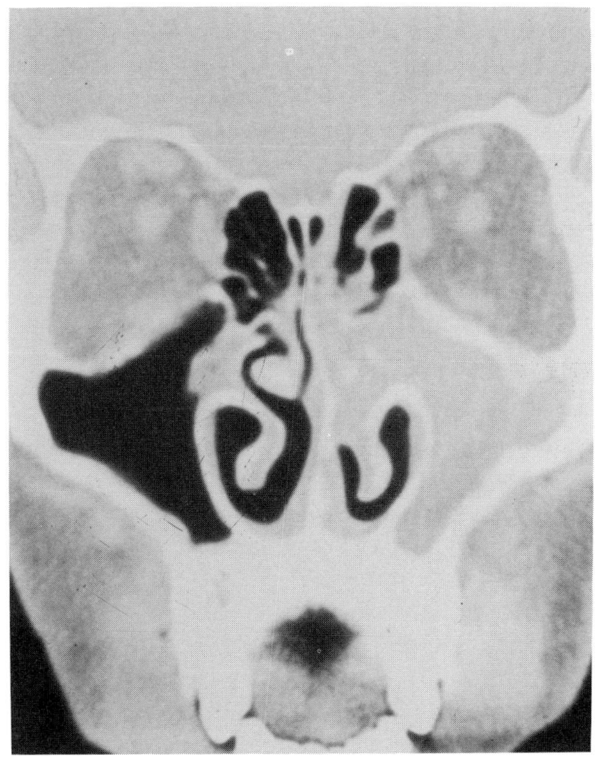

Three- to 5-mm cuts provide better detail of the nasal and sinus anatomy. Plain films are only useful to assess whether or not a fluid accumulation is present in the maxillary sinus. A screening CT scan of the paranasal sinuses is just as cost efficient as a three-view plain sinus series and gives the physician a great deal more information.

Bacteriology of Acute Sinusitis

Not all episodes of acute sinusitis are bacterial in origin. Many episodes of sinusitis will follow a viral upper respiratory tract infection and this alters the mucociliary function and facilitates invasion of the sinuses by the bacteria that are present.

If bacterial infection is present, the most common organisms are *Streptococcus pneumoniae* and *Haemophilus influenzae*, which account for approximately 50% of maxillary sinus infections. There are other organisms that are responsible for acute sinusitis as well including the hemolytic streptococcus A, B and C, and *S. aureus*. In children with acute sinusitis, the common organisms are *Streptococcus pneumoniae*, *Branhamella catarrhalis*, *H. influenzae*, *Streptococcus pyogenes* groups A and C, and streptococcus of the α-hemolytic type.

Cultures obtained from the nasal cavity correlate poorly with the organisms present in the sinus cavities. Therefore, to get an accurate culture of the organisms, the maxillary sinus cavity may have to be aspirated and lavaged in certain situations to retrieve culture material so that the antibiotic therapy can be directed toward the appropriate organisms.

Management of Acute Sinusitis

Management of acute sinusitis can be divided into two categories, medical management and surgical management. Antibiotics are the mainstay of medical management in acute sinusitis. A broad-spectrum penicillin is a good choice for initial therapy for gram-positive and gram-negative bacillae and gram-negative cocci. Amoxicillin has been used to cover for *H. influenzae*. However, in recent years, there have been emergent strains of β-lactimase-positive and amoxicillin-resistant *H. influenzae* and *B. catarrhalis*. In these cases, cefaclor, trimethoprim sulfate, amoxicillin and potassium clavulanate, or cefuroxime axetil may be used successfully to treat these resistant organisms.

The antibiotic therapy should be continued for at least 10 days and possibly up to 2 weeks. If there is poor distribution of antibiotics to the involved sinuses, prolonged treatment with high-dose antibiotic therapy is usually necessary to achieve adequate tissue levels. Topical and systemic decongestants may be used in conjuction with the antibiotics to decrease mucosal edema and improve the ventilation of the paranasal sinuses and the drainage of the purulent secretions from the affected sinuses.

Antihistamines should be avoided in acute sinusitis unless the patient has a proven allergic history that may be the underlying predisposing factor as the cause for the sinusitis. Mucolytics are also helpful in mobilizing thick secretions and saline nasal irrigations also improve sinus ventilation and drainage.

Surgical management is reserved for patients with acute sinusitis who do not respond to aggressive medical therapy. In the acute sinusitis setting, the surgical management is usually aspiration and drainage of one of the affected sinuses with irrigation of the sinus with saline. This is both diagnostic and therapeutic because the secretions can then be cultured to give an accurate picture of the bacteriology and this also lowers the bacterial count in the affected sinus.

Complications of Acute Sinusitis

Complications of acute sinusitis can be divided into two categories, extracranial and intracranial. The rate of significant complications is low and usually related to the area of the involved sinus.

Orbital and periorbital complications can occur from infections in the ethmoid and frontal sinuses that may produce signs from diplopia to blindness if left untreated. In acute ethmoid disease in children, the eyes are frequently affected and an abscess, either subperiosteal or orbital, may develop and may require drainage.

Osteomyelitis may involve the frontal bones of the maxilla but this is a very rare complication of acute sinusitis.

Intracranial complications include epidural and subdural abscesses, meningitis, brain abscess, and cavernous sinus thrombosis. These patients must be aggressively treated with IV antibiotics along with appropriate surgical intervention to drain any collections of pus that may have accumulated.

Chronic Sinusitis

Pathophysiology

Chronic sinusitis results from acute sinusitis that has been ineffectively treated or not treated at all. When the patient reaches this stage, the mucosal changes that have developed are usually irreversible. The mucosal edema has developed to such an extent that the sinus outflow tracts are totally obstructed and fail to open with aggressive medical management. The sinus cavities become severely hypopsic and there is marked reduction in ciliary function with retained thick secretions in the sinus cavities.

Symptoms

The symptoms of chronic sinusitis usually include persistent postnasal drainage, which is usually thick and may or may not be discolored, and chronic nasal obstruction; pain is usually not present. The patient is usually not febrile and usually does not complain of headache.

Physical Examination

The diagnosis of chronic irreversible sinusitis is made using nasal endoscopy and CT imaging of the paranasal sinuses. Nasal endoscopy will allow the clinician to visualize the significant edema in the sinus outflow tracts. Polypoid masses may be present that are obstructing the sinus outflow tracts and the nature of the secretions can also be evaluated as well as the origin of secretions that can implicate the sinus that is involved. CT scanning of the paranasal sinuses becomes invaluable in diagnosing chronic sinusitis because these symptoms are subtle and have been persisting for a longer period of time. Both axial and coronal views are obtained on the scan, allowing the clinician to evaluate the anatomy and abnormalities of the sinus outflow tracts and extent of the sinus involvement.

Bacteriology of Chronic Sinusitis

The organisms in chronic sinusitis differ significantly from the organisms found in acute sinusitis. Most of the common organisms include *H. influenzae*, *S. aureus*, and streptococci.

Management of Chronic Sinusitis

The management of chronic sinusitis is primarily surgical although extended medical management may be of some benefit in selected cases.

Antibiotic coverage in chronic sinusitis should include coverage for anaerobic bacteria. The antibiotics that have been most effective in treating chronic sinusitis include amoxicillin with clavulanic acid, cefuroxime axetil, clindamycin, and metronidazole.

Topical or oral steroid medication may be indicated in adjunctive treatment of chronic sinusitis. Topical steroid preparations reduce mucosal edema and improve the ventilation and oxygenation of the sinus cavities. However, sometimes topical therapy alone is not sufficient and a short course of oral steroids tapering over 7 to 10 days may be necessary to reduce the massive mucosal edema that has developed over a period of time. Topical and systemic decongestants are also useful in reducing mucosal edema and in mobilizing secretions. Antihistamines should be avoided unless there is a proven etiology of allergy as the causative factor for the chronic sinusitis.

Even with aggressive medical management, there is a large population of patients who fail to improve and surgical intervention becomes necessary. With the advent of the rigid sinus endoscopes, endoscopic sinus surgery has become an efficient means to treat chronic sinusitis surgically with minimal patient morbidity. The philosophy behind the endoscopic technique is to remove only the obstructing, inflamed mucosa leaving the majority of the mucosal surfaces untouched. After the sinuses are opened by this procedure and normal ventilation and drainage can occur, the remainder of the sinus mucosa will return to normal over a period of time, usually 6 weeks to 2 months. This procedure can be performed in the outpatient setting either under local or general anesthesia and is done entirely intranasally. Most patients are usually fully recovered within 7 days and only require postoperative cleaning visits to remove the crusts that develop within the sinus cavities. The actual description of the surgical technique is beyond the scope of this chapter.

Fungal Sinusitis

Invasive fungal sinusitis usually presents in patients who are immunosuppressed either from chemotherapy, chronic steroid therapy, or HIV infection. These sinus infections can take a rapidly destructive fulminant course manifested by angioinvasion with extension of the infective process into the orbit and brain. Fungal sinusitis may also occur in patients who are atopic or have asthma with associated nasal polyps. The infection is extra mucosal and does not involve tissue invasion. There is also a true allergic response to the fungal elements present in the sinus passages. Documentation of the allergy can be done with allergic testing to the appropriate fungi. The treatment of extramucosal noninvasive forms of fungal sinusitis is the removal of the fungus and accompanying mucus with restoration of mucocilliary drainage and sinus ventilation. Antifungal agents have not been advocated in this patient population because invasion does not occur in this condition. However, current studies are still ongoing to determine whether or not this patient population would benefit from a short term of antifungal therapy along with systemic and topical corticosteroids.

Conclusion

The treatment of infections and diseases of the nose and paranasal sinuses can become a challenge in certain situations. The acute infections can usually be managed by the primary care physician. However, if diagnostic dilemmas occur or inability to adequately examine the area in question is a problem, then referral to an otolaryngologist is warranted. The otolaryngologist can perform a systematic examination of the nasal cavity and paranasal sinuses using endoscopic techniques and provide the proper treatment plan based on the history and physical findings. Patients with chronic sinusitis refractory to medical management should be referred promptly to the otolaryngologist so that a thorough endoscopic examination along with CT scanning of the paranasal sinuses can be performed and an accurate diagnosis can be rendered and proper therapy instituted.

SUGGESTED READINGS

Bailey BJ, ed. Otolaryngology—head and neck surgery. Philadelphia: JB Lippincott, 1993:269–301.

Blitzer A, Lawsen, Friedman Surgery of the paranasal sinuses. Philadelphia: WB Saunders, 1985.

Cummings CW, ed. Otolaryngology—Head and neck surgery. St. Louis: CV Mosby, 1986:651–672.

DeShazo RD, Smith DL. Primer on allergic and immunologic disease. JAMA 1992;268:2807–2829.

Lee KJ. Essential otolaryngology. 5th ed. New York: Medical Examination Publishing, 1991.

Maran AGD, Lund VJ. Clinical rhinology. New York: Thieme Medical Publishers, 1990.

Stammberger H, Hawke M. Essentials of endoscopic sinus surgery. St. Louis: CV Mosby, 1993.

SECTION NINE

NEUROLOGY

CHAPTER 27

CHRONIC FATIGUE

William Fulcher

In the early seventeenth century, Rene Descartes developed a philosophy of mind–body dualism that was to form the foundation for much of twentieth century medical research, teaching, and the understanding of disease processes. Unfortunately, many clinician–philosophers feel that this concept has reached its limits of usefulness as an explanation of many common primary care complaints. For example, this "mind set" has led to the often bitter debate regarding whether the etiology of chronic fatigue is an infection or a mental illness (1). The primary care understanding of chronic fatigue threatens to further undermine the Cartesian separation of mind and body because most recent research suggests that these patients suffer from a combination of physical, mental, and sociocultural conditions. Considering the frequency of patients presenting with this complaint and its potential costs to society, it is imperative, therefore, that the primary care physician understand the multifactorial nature of chronic fatigue.

Fatigue is one of the most common subjective experiences that persons experience at times especially after vigorous exercise, hard work, inadequate sleep, or an acute illness. When fatigue becomes persistent or chronic and coexists with or transforms into "lassitude," patients frequently consult their physicians for an explanation or diagnosis of the problem. Because of the highly subjective nature of fatigue and its potential to herald a wide variety of serious illnesses, physicians have been duly concerned about diagnosing these patients but generally unable to find a universally successful approach to evaluation and management. The evaluation and management of chronic fatigue, therefore, tests the skills of the best primary care doctor in every area of diagnosis and treatment. Furthermore, it has seriously questioned the adequacy of a purely biomedical approach to diagnosis and treatment of patients with this common presenting complaint.

Background

Fatigue is listed as the seventh most common presenting complaint to primary care doctors (2). Between 15% and 20% of men and women in the United States describe themselves as being tired "all the time" (3). This translates into almost 11 million patient visits a year in the United States for fatigue. Up to 25% of a primary care physician's patients may state that fatigue was the major reason for coming to the doctor on that visit (4,5). In other developed countries as well, 25% to 30% of adult patients, surveyed over various lengths of time, state that they have experienced significant chronic fatigue (6,7). Clearly all primary care physicians must be prepared to encounter and manage patients with primary complaints of fatigue.

Many syndromes of chronic fatigue have existed for decades and the multiplicity of names for them reveal the medical profession's heretofore inability to categorize patients into a unifying etiology or diagnosis: neurasthenia, nervous exhaustion, DaCosta syndrome, Royal Free disease, chronic brucellosis, chronic Epstein-Barr virus (EBV) or mononucleosis, benign myalgic encephalomyelitis, and chronic candidiasis (8,9). A common unifying concept put forward by our social scientists to explain the emergence and subsequent decline in popularity (though not in prevalence) of the chronic fatigue syndromes has been described in relating to sociocultural issues and their effect on an individual's perceptions and definitions of the illness and the illness behavior than on variations in infectious disease agents (10). For example, during times of severe sociocultural strife or in situations when individuals are expected to endure extreme physical or psychological stress without recognition of their suffering, tolerance, or effort, epidemics of chronic fatigue have emerged. As sociocultural expectations then lessen and, concomitantly, the chronic fatigue condition is given legitimacy by the medical community, the frequency of these complaints lessens. Theoretically, the increasing expectations by our modern industrial society on the middle class (especially women), to "do it all and do it now" may explain some of the epidemiology of patients suffering from the current chronic fatigue syndrome (women more frequently than men, high achievers, high income and high education) (11). Furthermore, in 1987, the Centers for Disease Control and Prevention (CDC) "legitimized" a subset of the population with chronic fatigue into a syndrome to better define a group in which to conduct research concerning its etiology and treatment (12). The usefulness of this classification has been criticized recently and has not led to any real advances in understanding or treatment of this small subset of patients or those with chronic fatigue in general (13). Consequently, what follows is a general approach to the patient with chronic fatigue that should be useful to all patient subgroups. This is based on recent literature evaluating chronic fatigue patients in both referral and general practice populations.

Classification and Presentation

It is useful to consider the patient's presentation and description of fatigue in the history when considering appropriate evaluation and management. *Fatigue* usually refers to an individual's inability to do physical work or the failure to sustain required muscular activity. *Lassitude*, on the other hand, refers to a purposelessness, lack of energy, ennui, depletion of enthusiasm, and inordinately easy exhaustion with daily activities. *Weakness* is usually reported by the patient as a specific, localized loss of strength in a part of the body's neuromuscular system. Although many patients with chronic fatigue complain of some weakness, it is usually *not* their *primary* complaint. Additionally, because weakness usually denotes a specific neuromuscular disease state (i.e, myopathy, deconditioning, myasthenia gravis, multiple sclerosis) it will not be discussed here.

Fatigue can be further divided into acute, chronic, and multifactorial (14). Each classification has some overlap. The general distinctions are useful in determining the need for further evaluation. *Acute fatigue* usually accompanies the other symptoms of an obvious acute illness (infection, hemorrhage, metabolic disorders). Generally it is of less than 2 weeks' duration and patients rarely complain of acute fatigue as their primary reason for visiting the doctor. Acute fatigue may become chronic (>30 days) in patients predisposed to chronic fatigue (i.e., history of depression, chronic dysphoria, or somatization disorder) or after illnesses with significant convalescent periods: influenza, major surgery, adverse drug reactions.

Multifactorial fatigue refers to patients with multiple ongoing illnesses or conditions or lifestyle and psychological predispositions to fatigue. The sedentary, smoking executive suffering with allergic rhinitis who takes diphenhydramine for an antihistamine would be a good example of a patient who may have or may develop multifactorial fatigue. This is a much underreported form of fatigue in primary care because physicians recognize many of these predisposing diseases and appropriately address each one separately.

Chronic fatigue is defined as significant daily fatigue of greater than 30 days' duration. It *is* usually the patients *primary* or only complaint and it often has no easily recognized onset or recognized change in the patients health or routine. A subgroup of patients with chronic fatigue have been further categorized by the CDC as having a chronic fatigue syndrome (CFS), many of whom *do* report a sudden onset of their symptoms with a viral type illness (5,9,15). By definition, patients with CFS must have significant fatigue that reduces their individual daily activity below 50% of normal, be of 6 months' duration or greater, and not be due to another organic disease. Initially, these patients were required to be free of depression to qualify for CFS. The high prevalence of concomitant depression in these patients, however, and the overlap of symptoms of CFS with the neuropsychiatric criteria for depression (especially atypical depression) has made this distinction controversial and, at least, confusing. Currently, patients may be diagnosed with CFS even with a diagnosis of depression especially if they have the "signs" of CFS (13). In summary, the initial history should allow the primary care physician to determine the type of fatigue the patient is suffering from but may only touch on the many possibilities in the differential.

The complaint of fatigue has been described as having more than just informational meaning, however. Because it is a subjective experience for patients, it often reflects their current psychological, social, and psychiatric milieu. These unrevealed experiences or meanings, usually hidden initially from the physician, have been called the *transactional meanings* (14). They reflect the patient's unspoken fears and expectations, pleas for explanation and understanding, concern about "What is wrong with me?" and "How am I going to cope?" After patients have visited many prior physicians, they may also mean "Can you or anyone help me?" If primary care physicians are unwilling or unable to acknowledge these meanings, they will be ineffective in the thorough evaluation of each patient's unique problem. However, if physicians are lured into the trap of promising to find a cure for these patients, they will be set up for failure when the tests return normal or patients fail to respond to treatment. This may lead to frustration by the physicians and eventual rejection of the patients. Physicians caring for fatigued patients, must, therefore enter into an honest relationship with these patients that is sensitive to their needs and their suffering, with courage to just "be there," be reliable, and be competent for the duration of the relationship.

Obese, sedentary, smoking persons as well as those with high-stress lifestyles report significantly more fatigue than controls (16,17). Chronic fatigue patients are usually young (25 to 60 years), white, highly educated, and high achievers. Women outnumber men 2:1 in reporting significant chronic fatigue. These characteristics have led to the inaccurate and pejorative label "Yuppie flu," which may represent more these patients' willingness and ability to seek and receive medical care than their susceptibility to this condition. Chronic fatigue patients have higher levels of perceived exertion than controls at similar workloads. They have lower levels of physical activity than controls, but the studies are conflicting as to whether they are actually deconditioned. Chronic fatigue sufferers also score higher on rating scales of depression and anxiety than controls (18). In fact, studies of depression in chronic fatigue patients have shown significantly higher rates of depression than in controls even when the complaint of fatigue is eliminated from the diagnostic criteria for depression (19).

Differential Diagnosis

Fatigue, in the absence of fever, has the broadest differential in all of medicine. This, combined with the fact that some of the illnesses in the differential can be serious and life-threatening, places an enormous, perceived burden on the physician to make a timely and correct diagnosis. This is further heightened by the suffering patient's urgency to remedy the fatigue condition. There is no other area where the primary care physician must have more courage to deal with uncertainty than in the management of chronic fatigue.

The causes of acute fatigue are usually recognizable from the history and physical and any indicated laboratory or x-ray studies. The causes of chronic fatigue are not always readily apparent on the initial evaluation and may cover all the major categories of disease from neoplasm to metabolic problems (Box 27.1). It should be reassuring to the primary care provider that the clinical reviews of chronically fatigued patients in primary care practices find few serious organic illnesses in patients with no other symptoms than fatigue. Furthermore, the physician should be able to discover some underlying, treatable illness in at least 70% to 75% of patients with a thorough history and physical (20,21). Subsequent laboratory or x-ray testing should be focused on other specific symptoms or signs. A "shotgun" approach to laboratory testing for all patients with chronic fatigue is not indicated and is not cost effective (5).

Although a small number of chronic fatigue patients will have no identifiable cause for their illness after a thorough history, physical, and laboratory examination, the single largest group of illnesses discovered will be psychiatric diagnoses (18,22). The three most common psychiatric illnesses detected in chronic fatigue patients are depression, anxiety disorders (panic disorder, general anxiety disorder), and

Box 27.1 Differential Diagnosis of Chronic Fatigue

1. Psychiatric illness (depression, generalized anxiety disorder, panic disorder, somatization)
2. Chronic infection (systemic lupus erythematosus, tuberculosis) brucellosis, parasite infestation
3. Chronic anemia
4. Nutritional abnormalities (malnutrition, obesity, acute and chronic dieting)
5. Exogenous toxins (alcohol, nicotine, carbon monoxide, heavy metals, pesticides)
6. Endogenous toxins (uremia, liver failure)
7. Endocrine disorders (diabetes mellitus, pituitary/adrenal/thyroid)
8. Malignancy (infrequent)
9. Medicatons (sedatives, tranquilizers, antihistamines, corticosteroids, digitalis, most analgesics, tetracycline)
10. Physiologic fatigue (inadequate inefficient rest or sleep, sedentary life-style, decreased cardiopulmonary reserve, pregnancy, advancing age)
11. Atopic disease (allergic rhinitis)
12. Multifactorial (combination of several possible etiologies, very common in primary care)
13. Unknown (chronic fatigue syndrome)

somatization disorder (12). Consequently, primary care physicians who evaluate and test patients with chronic fatigue must be skilled in recognizing these disorders. They must also be prepared for the resistance most patients will exhibit to being labeled with a psychiatric illness for what they perceive as a medical problem (23). The primary care physician often becomes the initial counselor and psychiatrist for many patients with CFS. To successfully manage patients with chronic fatigue, the primary care physician must initiate the evaluation and treatment of any concurrent psychiatric illness at the beginning of the standard biomedical evaluation. If the primary care physician does not find an obvious psychiatric condition initially, he or she should be vigilant in future surveillance because 1) there is a high incidence of depression developing in chronic illnesses like chronic fatigue and 2) many chronic fatigue patients present with atypical depression, which is more difficult to recognize. Primary care physicians have been notoriously inaccurate in detecting atypical depression because they perceive (incorrectly) that patients cannot be depressed unless they report a depressed mood (24). This is often absent in fatigue patients who have difficulty reporting their symptoms as depression. Furthermore, fatigued, depressed men quite often reveal their depression as anger, dissatisfaction with a career or marriage, or loss of interest in hobbies and other daily routines.

Finally, the managing physician should remember that many patients may have multifactorial fatigue with several conditions contributing to their problem. Just like the "straw that broke the camel's back," a minor condition can trigger a major fatigue. The physician will often have to relieve the suffering patient's burden of more than "one straw" to get the patient back on his or her feet.

In 1987, the CDC defined CFS (12). The specific criteria are shown in Table 27.1. The major criteria have been mentioned earlier and the minor criteria must include 8 of the 11 symptoms listed or 6 of the 11 symptoms and 2 of the 3 signs listed. Fortunately, for primary care doctors, suggested additions or revisions to this description have been made by Schluederberg and colleagues in 1992 (Table 27.2). CFS has accounted for 5% or less of the fatigued patients seen in primary care practices (15,22).

Pathogenesis

The etiology of chronic fatigue (CFS in particular) has undergone considerable speculation as our sophistication in medical testing has increased. Entities as varied as EBV (25–27), herpes virus-6 (28), coxsackie B, and chronic brucellosis have been investigated and rejected as causative agents of CFS. The search continues because numerous immunologic abnormalities have been identified in chronic fatigue sufferers (29,30). Although most all CFS patients have some measurable immunologic abnormality, they are of

Table 27.1 CDC Criteria for Chronic Fatigue Syndrome

Case must satisfy both major criteria plus either 8 symptoms or 6 symptoms and 2 physical criteria.

Major Criteria

1. New onset of fatigue lasting 6 mo reducing activity to <50% normal
2. Other conditions causing fatigue must be ruled out

Minor Criteria

1. Low-grade fever (37.5°–38.6°C; 99.5°–102.4°F) orally or chills
2. Sore throat
3. Painful cervical or axillary lymph nodes
4. Generalized muscle weakness
5. Muscle pain
6. Postexertional fatigue lasting 24 hr
7. Headache
8. Migratory arthralgias
9. Neuropsychological complaints (photophobia, transient scotomata, forgetfulness, irritability, confusion, difficulty thinking, decreased concentration, depressed mood)
10. Sleep disturbances
11. Acute onset of symptoms over a few hours to a few days

Physical signs: documented by a physician at least twice 1 mo apart

1. Low-grade fever: 37.6°–38.6°C (100°–102°F) orally or 37.8°–38.8°C (100°–102°F) rectally
2. Nonexudative pharyngitis
3. Palpable cervical or axillary nodes up to 2 cm in diameter

Source: Adapted from Holmes G, Kaplan J, Grantz N, et al. Chronic fatigue syndrome: a working case definition. Ann Intern Med 1988;108:387–389.

such wide variety among patients that none have been found to have significant sensitivity or specificity to aid in diagnosis or treatment. Research suggests that higher levels of perceived stress result in decreased

Table 27.2 National Institute of Allergy and Infectious Disease/National Institute of Mental Health's Modifications of CDC Criteria for CFS

A. Exclusions
- I. Psychiatric disorders
  - a. Psychoses
    1. Psychotic depression
    2. Bipolar depression
    3. Schizophrenia
  - b. Substance abuse
- II. Postinfections fatigue (must include a, b, and c)
  - a. Established etiology determined
  - b. Etiologic agent is known to regularly produce chronic active infection
  - c. Clinical picture compatible with chronic active infection
    1. Chronic hepatitis B or C with active liver disease
    2. Infections with human immunodeficiency virus
    3. Lyme disease inadequately treated
    4. Tuberculosis

B. Inclusions (in patients who meet the CDC criteria)
- I. Fibromyalgia
- II. Postinfections fatigue
  - a. Lyme disease with adequate treatment
  - b. Brucellosis after appropriate treatment
  - c. Acute infections mononucleosis with significant debilitating, convalescent fatigue
  - d. Acute cytomegalovirus infection
  - e. Acute toxoplasmosis (adequately treated)
- III. Nonpsychotic depression
- IV. Somatiform disorders
- V. Generalized anxiety/panic disorder

Source: Adapted from Schluederberg A, Strauss SE, Peterson P, et al. Chronic fatigue syndrome research: definition and medical outcome assessment. Ann Intern Med 1992;117:325–331.

immunocompetence and, theoretically, enhanced vulnerability to the disease, but CFS patients do not develop opportunistic infections or other symptoms of classic immune system deficiencies (31). Furthermore, premorbid personality traits and individual characteristics on Minnesota Multiphasic Personality Inventory tests correlate with altered natural killer T-cell activity (a frequent finding in patients with CFS) (32). Currently, the immunologic abnormalities are considered a nonspecific marker of increased immune system activity though of unknown significance or cause (33).

Atopic disease(s) has a strong correlation with CFS. Up to two thirds of patients classified with CFS have premorbid allergies to food or other airborne (household) allergens. These collective observations have led to the speculation that a unifying hypothesis for the illness involves a hyperresponsive immune system (manifested by atopy) that responds to (interferon and interleukin) release, which in turn leads to CFS symptoms. Anxiety and depression may magnify the deranged immune response or perpetuate a prolonged vicious cycle consisting of aberrant immune function, inappropriate cytokinin release, CFS symptoms, depression, and continued aberrant immune function (34).

A promising area of research for the cause of all chronic fatigue is currently in the realm of central nervous system neurotransmitters and their role in the control of perceptions of fatigue (35). Strauss and others have documented altered functioning of the hypothalamic-pituitary-adrenal axis in patients with CFS (36,37). Other research in this area has improved our understanding and therapy of depression, anxiety, and pain and may one day provide new insights into chronic fatigue. In summary, it seems to be clear that stress whether physical, mental, or sociocultural can alter an individual's immune system sufficiently such that many ordinary infections and illnesses result in chronic fatigue. The question remains how to remedy this once it happens.

Work-Up

Undeniably, the most cost effective diagnostic procedure for chronic fatigue patients is the extended history. During a busy clinic, one cannot often take the time for a complete history and physical on the fatigued patient's initial presentation. Furthermore, some have recommended that the extended history should not be done on the first visit because 1) some of the fatigue problems will be self-limiting or have straightforward treatment, 2) the patient should have time to prepare for the long history and think about any psychosocial contributors to the condition, and 3) it allows the physician to stage and pace the biomedical evaluation, decrease frustration in trying to squeeze a long examination into a busy day and increase doctor–patient rapport (38). This delay will also allow the physician to assemble any old records for review. What then is important to do in the brief examination on initial presentation? Solberg recommends six items the physician should accomplish with the brief examination (Box 27.2) (38). This initial brief examination should take no longer than 10 to 15 minutes. At this point the physician can determine whether he or she is willing or able to conduct the thorough history and physical the patient needs for management. If not, this is an appropriate place for a referral to a family physician or general interest with experience in managing chronic fatigue.

Referrals should be made to a physicians sensitive to psychiatric and psychosocial issues and well versed

Box 27.2 Initial Brief Encounter with the Fatigued patient

1. Establish the true complaint
2. Determine the patient's and family's expectations
3. Rule out serious medical or psychiatric illness
4. Diagnose and treat simple problems
5. Complete the necessary examination and tests to accomplish steps 3 and 4
6. Negotiate a plan of evaluation with the patient

If no serious illness found, reassure patient and schedule an unhurried extended history and physical or refer to other primary care family physician with experience managing chronic fatigue

Source: Adapted from Solberg L. Lassitude: a primary care evaluation. JAMA 1984;25:3272–3276.

in the evaluation and management of chronic fatigue. If the primary care physician does complete the initial extended history and physical and then later needs a consultant to evaluate specific problems, he or she should heed the same advice regarding the selection of consultants. Patients are easily upset or influenced by the promise of a quick cure or one more diagnostic test only to be let down and rejected as incurable by the physician with less than a comprehensive focus.

When the patient returns for the extended history, the physician should attempt to allow the patient to "tell the story" with as few interruptions as possible. The physician should carefully review social history, family and work history, and sexual history and take a thorough oral intake history (type of diet, prescription or over-the-counter medication, drug, alcohol, cigarette use). Up to 50% of the diagnoses of chronic fatigue may be readily apparent through the extended history alone. Many times physicians will find themselves saying "no wonder you are tired!" Reflecting this back to the patient in terms of reality therapy and support (I'm impressed you could go on so long) can be powerful "therapy" in a trusting physician–patient relationship.

The physical examination should focus also on areas of the body that are many times overlooked such as the skin, lymph nodes, ear-nose-throat area, pelvis and rectum, and other areas suggested by the history. A careful heart examination may reveal the click of mitral prolapse (up to 30% of these patients complain of significant fatigue) (39). Another 20% to 30% of the diagnoses in chronic fatigue may be detected or determined by the physical examination.

Screening laboratory data have been of little use in the diagnosis and evaluation of chronic fatigue patients (33,40). Most experts recommend basic laboratory studies including a complete blood count, chemistry profile, and thyroid screen. Others also recommend a urinalysis and erythrocyte sedimentation rate. More specific or costly tests have not been shown to be cost effective in the initial evaluation of chronic fatigue. The specific use of chest x-ray, electrocardiogram, Holter monitor, and the like should depend on the specific symptoms reported by the patient. Immunologic studies, including titers for EBV antibody, have not been shown to be useful in general practice and should not be routinely ordered. The physician should perhaps consider obtaining a second opinion from a trusted colleague rather than spending money on tests with unproven benefit.

During the initial extended and follow-up examinations, the physician must be on the look out for depression. With a 15% lifetime risk of death from suicide, major depression is one of the most common, curable, life-threatening illnesses in primary care (41). The symptoms of depression can be remembered with the mnemonic SIG E: CAPS to represent a "script" for energy capsules: *S*leep disturbance, decreased *I*nterest in usual activities, *G*uilt or low self-esteem, lack of *E*nergy, altered *C*oncentration, altered *A*ppetite, *P*sychomotor agitation or retardation, *S*uicide ideation or potential. The "colon" in the mnemonic is to remind the physician of the somatic complaints that patients use as depressive equivalents: abdominal symptoms, fatigue, chronic pain, or headaches. If a patient has five of these symptoms plus a depressed mood or lack of interest in usual activities for greater than 2 weeks, which is not due to normal grieving, the diagnosis of depression should be made. Depression may be the primary cause of chronic fatigue or secondary to it. In fact, depression is so common in patients with chronic illnesses, especially those with pain or fatigue, that one should ask why it is not present in a particular patient if the symptoms are not readily obvious. Detectable depression should be treated whether it is primary or secondary to chronic illness or fatigue because it is equally disabling and life-threatening in either case.

Patients who seem to have numerous other body symptoms or distressing symptoms of tension and anxiety may have a somatization disorder or anxiety disorder. Most of the anxiety disorders respond well to the newer antianxiety medications and some tricyclic antidepressants. Primary care doctors not familiar with these therapies may desire to refer patients to a family or general interest physician or psychiatrist with such experience.

Patients with somatization disorders can be difficult for any physician to manage. They often present with many symptoms at each office visit and cause the physician to feel frustration because, despite best efforts, most do not improve with traditional therapy. Patients with somatization disorders generally express their psychological states or stress through bodily symptoms and should be given frequent, albeit brief, appointments to express these concerns. Physicians should firmly insist on evaluating only one or two symptoms per visit. This should be done during the first 5 minutes of the visit and the rest of the encounter used to allow the patient to express his or her current feelings or situation. Physicians should also state that they will not always prescribe medicine for the symptoms, especially the ones they feel are not serious but will keep a close watch on the patient for the development of serious illness. This will greatly reduce polypharmacy and possible medication side affects. Often the number of complaints will subside and these patients will improve until their next life crisis comes along.

The primary care physician should work up suspected CFS in the same manner as any chronically fatigued patient. If the physician finds an elevated temperature (>37.9°C or 100.4°F), significant weight loss, or a particular emphasis on any one symptom such as abdominal pain, he or she should consider the diagnosis of CFS suspect. Patients with CFS often keep extensive dairies of their symptoms. The major dilemma facing the primary care doctor is the need to sift through these symptoms and exclude the many diagnoses that can cause fatigue. A thorough history and physical and simple screening laboratory tests mentioned above should assist in making 90% to 95% of diagnoses for fatigued patients in primary care settings.

Box 27.3 Management for all Chronically Fatigued Patients

1. Treat any obvious diseases including psychiatric illness
2. Stress prevention to avoid conditions with convalescent fatigue
3. Stress adequate, efficient rest/sleep
4. Recommend daily moderate exercise, walking
5. Recommend well balanced, low fat diet
6. Avoid unnecessary medications, over-the-counter or illicit drugs
7. Discontinue tobacco and alcohol
8. Encourage greater patient involvement in treatment
9. Avoid discouraging "harmless" home remedies or nontoxic vitamins
10. Recommend psychological counseling to improve coping skills
11. Schedule brief regular follow-up visits to detect developing illnesses

Above all, "express concern but be optimistic"

Treatment

The treatment for all types of chronic fatigue is multifaceted (Box 27.3). Because the cause of the CFS is not known, there is no *specific* treatment for it. In all fatigued patients the physician should obviously treat any detected diseases *including* mood disorders, somatization, and anxiety disorders. Patients should be encouraged to get adequate rest, daily moderate exercise, and good nutrition. They must be cigarette, alcohol, and drug free, if possible. If medications are necessary, the physician should use those with a minimum of side effects, especially fatigue. Patients need to be given permission to rearrange their work and life priorities to accomplish the above and to remain as involved with their premorbid activities as their fatigue will permit.

Concomitant cognitive behavioral therapy (CBT) has been shown to hasten the resolution of fatigue in many patients (42). Very simply, CBT assists patients in moving from an "all-or-nothing" lifestyle orientation to a more functional style of coping with fatigue with day-to-day activity. This allows the patient to move the locus of control internally and often results in more rapid improvement in daily functioning.

Physicians would also do well to arrange monthly visits for the first 6 months to monitor the patient for developing depression or other illness. This also builds trust and rapport. Physicians should avoid discouraging alternative therapies (nontoxic vitamin doses, massage, meditation) unless these are obviously harmful. The physician should show concern but be optimistic and hopeful. The physician who acknowledges small gains or improvements made by the patient is more likely to see improvements. Finally, patients may be referred to the chronic fatigue support group listed below although the usefulness and accuracy of the lay literature has been questioned.

Chronic Fatigue and Immune Dysfunction Syndrome Association
c/o CFIDS Chronicle
P.O. Box 220398
Charlotte, NC 28222-0398

Specific CFS Treatment

Many specific modalities have been tried for resolution of the CFS. Acyclovir (43), liver extract–folic acid–cyanocobalamin (44), and IV immunoglobulin are the most recent. In a placebo-controlled trial of high-dose IgC (2 gm/kg per month) for 3 months (45), many patients experienced transient improvement but 43% experienced serious toxicity. Lower-dose IgC (1 gm/kg per month) for 6 months showed no significant benefit to patients (46). However, both studies and the studies of acyclovir and other therapies have demonstrated a significant placebo affect in controls. IV IgC is currently *not* recommended for the CFS nor routine chronic fatigue patients (47). Finally, Ampligen (a mismatched, double-stranded RNA) has been suggested to provide some relief of CFS symptoms (48). Further research with this agent is expected. The primary care physician may also, however, benefit from a significant placebo affect by "prescribing himself" in a skillful way: reliable trusting relationship that skillfully treats the significant, treatable illnesses or symptoms and encourages the patient to do the best he or she can with those that cannot be treated.

Summary

The long-term management of patients with chronic fatigue can be viewed as a glass either half empty or half full. There is no specific therapy other than treating obvious diseases (depression, etc.) for chronic fatigue or CFS. On the other hand, there is no evidence to date that chronic fatigue sufferers progress to more serious illness or cancer any more often than the general public (5,49). Up to 25% to 50% of patients will improve in 1 year and the majority will experience relief of fatigue and return to normal functioning over several years (21). For the few who experience chronic, long-term fatigue, it is a disease of "morbidity not mortality" (8). Their primary care physicians will do well to remember the French medical adage "to cure sometimes, relieve often, and comfort always."

REFERENCES

1. Beard G. Neurastemia or nervous exhaustion. Boston Medical and Surgical Journal 1869;3:217–220.

2. National Ambulatory Medical Care Survey; 1975. Summary U.S. Department of Health and Human Services. Publication (phs) 78–1784, 1978.

3. Chen MK. The epidemiology of self perceived fatigue among adults. Prev Med 1986;15:74–81.

4. Kroenke K, et al. Chronic fatigue in primary care. JAMA 1988;260:929–934.

5. Kroenke K. Chronic fatigue: frequency, causes, evaluation and management. Compr Ther 1989;15:3–7.

6. Lloyd AR, Hickie I, et al. Prevalence of chronic fatigue syndrome in an Australian population. Med J Aust 1990;153:522–528.

7. Cox B, Blaxter M, et al. The health and lifestyles survey. London: Health Promotion Research Trust, 1987.

8. Shafran S. The chronic fatigue syndrome. Am J Med 1991;98:730–739.

9. Strauss SE. The history of chronic fatigue syndrome. Rev Infect Dis 1991;13(suppl)1:S2–S7.

10. Ware NC, Kleinman A. Culture and somatic experience: the social course of illness and neurasthenia and chronic fatigue syndrome. Psychosom Med 1992;54:546–560.

11. Abbey SE, Garfinkle PE. Neurasthenia and chronic fatigue syndrome: the role of culture in the making of a diagnosis. Am J Psychiatry 1991;148:1638–1646.

12. Holmes G, Kaplan J, Grantz N, et al. Chronic fatigue syndrome: a working case definition. Ann Intern Med 1988;108:387–389.

13. Schluederberg A, Strauss SE, Peterson P, et al. Chronic fatigue syndrome research: definition and medical outcome assessment. Ann Intern Med 1992;117:325–331.

14. Rockwell D, Burr B. The tired patient. J Fam Pract 1974;1:62–65.

15. Manu P, Lane TJ, Matthews DA. The frequency of chronic fatigue syndrome patients with symptoms of persistent fatigue. Ann Intern Med 1988;109:554–556.

16. Blakely A, Howard R, Sosich R, et al. Psychiatric symptoms personality and ways of coping in chronic fatigue. Psychol Med 1991;21:347–362.

17. Keller R, Sheffield BF. The one week prevalence of symptoms in neurotic patients and normals. Am J Psych 1973;130:102–105.

18. Manu P, Matthews DA, Lane TJ. The mental health of patients with a chief complaint of chronic fatigue—a prospective evaluation and follow-up. Arch Intern Med 1988;148:2213–2217.

19. Wessely S, Powell R. Fatigue syndromes: a comparison of chronic post viral fatigue with neuromuscular and affective disorders. J Neurol Neurosurg Psychiatry 1989;52:940–948.

20. Elnicki D, Shockcor W, Brick J. Evaluating the complaint fatigue in primary care: diagnoses and outcomes. Am J Med 1992;93:303–306.

21. Matthews DA, Manu P, Lane TJ. Evaluation and management of patients with chronic fatigue. Am J Med Sci 1991;302:269–277.

22. Turgeon S. Chronic fatigue syndrome: review of the literature. Can Fam Physician 1989;35:2061–2065.

23. Matthews DA, Manu P, Lane TJ. Diagnostic beliefs among patients with chronic fatigue. Clin Res 1989;37;820A. Abstract.

24. Davis TC, Nathan RG, Cash MV. Diagnosing depression in primary care. South Med J 1986;79: 1273–1279.

25. Bell D. Chronic fatigue syndrome. Postgrad Med 1992;91:245–252.

26. Jones JF, Ray CG, et al. Evidence for active Epstein Barr virus infection in patients with persistent unexplained illnesses: elevated anti-early antigen antibodies. Ann Intern Med 1985;102:107.

27. Horwitz CA, et al. Long term follow-up of patients for Epstein Barr virus after recovery from infectious mononucleosis. J Infec Dis 1985;151: 1150–1153.

28. Buchwald D, Cheney P, et al. A chronic illness characterized by fatigue, neurological and immunological disorders and active human herpes virus type 6 infection. Ann Intern Med 1992;116:103–113.

29. Morague A, Toby M, et al. Increased (2′–5′) oligoadenylate activity in patients with prolonged illness associated with serological evidence of persistent Epstein Barr virus infection. Lancet 1982;1:744.

30. Landay AL, Jessop C, Lennette ET, Levy JA. Chronic fatigue syndrome: clinical condition associated with immune activation. Lancet 1991;338:707–712.

31. Rosenhan DL, Serigman ME. Abnormal psychology. 2nd ed. New York: Norton, 1988.

32. Hersel JS, Locke SE, Krauss LJ, Williams MJ. Natural killer cell activity and MMPI scores of a cohort of college students. Am J Psy 1986;143:1382–1386.

33. Buchwald D, Komaroff AL. Review of laboratory findings for patients with chronic fatigue syndrome. Rev Infect Dis 1991;13(suppl)1:S12–S18.

34. Klonoff DC. Chronic fatigue syndrome. Clin Infect Dis 1992;15:812–823.

35. McDaniel J. Psycho-immunology: implications for future research. South Med J 1992;85:388–396.

36. Ur E, White PD, Grossman A. Hypothesis: cytokines may be activated to cause depressive illness and chronic fatigue syndrome. Eur Arch Psychiatry Clin Neurosci 1992;241:217–222.

37. Devietrack MA, Dale JK, Strauss SE. Evidence for impaired activation of the hypothalamic-pituitary-adrenal axis in patients with chronic fatigue syndrome. J Clin Endocrinol Metab 1991;73:1224–1234.

38. Solberg L. Lassitude: a primary care evaluation. JAMA 1984;25:3272–3276.

39. Gonzales ER. The non neurotic approach to mitral valve prolapse. JAMA 1981;246:2113–2114, 2119–2120.

40. Lane TJ, Matthews DA, Manu P. The low yield of physical examination and laboratory investigations of patients with chronic fatigue. Am J Med Sci 1989;299:313–318.

41. Guze SB, Robins E. Suicide and primary affective disorders. Br J Psychiatry 1970;117:437–480.

42. Lloyd A, Hickie I, Brockman A, et al. Immunologic and psychologic therapy for patients with chronic fatigue syndrome: a double blind placebo controlled trial. Am J Med 1993;94:197–203.

43. Strauss SE, Dale JK, Toby M, et al. Acyclovir treatment of chronic fatigue syndrome. N Engl J Med 1988;319:1692–1698.

44. Kaslow JE, Rucker L, Onishi R. Liver abstract-folic acid-cyanocobalamin versus placebo for chronic fatigue syndrome. Arch Inter Med 1989;149:2501–2503.

45. Peterson PK, Sheppard J, Macres M, et al. A controlled trial of intravenous immunoglobulin G in chronic fatigue syndrome. Am J Med 1990;1989:554–560.

46. Lloyd A, Hickie I, Wakefield D, et al. A double blind placebo controlled trial of intravenous immunoglobulin in patients with chronic fatigue syndrome Am J Med 1990;1989:561–568.

47. Strauss SE. Intravenous immunoglobulin treatment for the chronic fatigue syndrome. Am J Med 1990;1989:551–553.

48. Strayer D, Gillespie D, Peterson P, et al. Treatment of CFIDS with poly (I): poly ($C_{12}U$). In: Program supplements to the 31st Literscience Conference on Antimicrobial Agents and Chemotherapy. Washington, DC: American Society for Microbiology, 1991.

49. Valdini AF, Steinhardt S, Valcenti J, Jaffe A. One year follow-up of fatigued patients. J Fam Pract 1988;26:33–88.

CHAPTER 28

HEADACHES

Bradley K. Evans

Headaches are common: about half of all women, on at least one occasion, will consult a physician for evaluation and treatment of headache. More than 1% of visits to primary care physicians are for a headache problem (1). Headaches are responsible for 30 million days of work lost each year in the United States and lost productivity is estimated at $12 billion (2). Although the economic aspects can be estimated, headaches adversely affect the quality and enjoyment of life in ways that are not easily measured.

This chapter reviews the clinical evaluation of the patient with headaches and the practical aspects of the common chronic headache syndromes—migraines, tension headaches, and mixed headaches. These three syndromes account for over 95% of diagnoses in headache specialty clinics. About 30% of women, at some point, are diagnosed as having migraine and about 40% with tension headaches. For more information regarding headache problems, consult good textbooks on headache (3–5).

In general, it can be said that each person's headache problem is unique and that, in the same individual, headaches change. For instance, a person can have migraine without aura, then migraine with aura, then aura without headache. Despite this variability, the International Headache Society has published an exhaustively comprehensive and detailed classification of headaches (6). This system will be important for clinical studies of headaches.

The History

Evaluating a patient with chronic headaches usually requires an office visit dedicated to this problem. Not only does the symptom of headache need proper evaluation, but, in the treatment of headache, there is a placebo effect (7), which depends mainly on physician factors: the more thorough the physician seems to be, the more a physician explains to the patient, and the more confidence the patient has in the physician, the greater the placebo effect.

A good first question is to ask the patient whether she is "headachy." Her answer gives the clinican an idea as to whether she has chronic headaches, a sudden and severe headache, or a new and different type of headache. "Sudden, severe headache" and "new, different headaches" may be symptoms of a more serious cause of headaches.

In characterizing the headaches, the clinician needs the answers to 10 key questions (Box 28.1). The answers to these questions describe the headaches and give important clues to diagnosis (8). Head pain brought on by drinking hot or cold liquids suggests dental disease; a headache that comes on with sitting and resolves with lying down is characteristic of a post-lumbar puncture headache; and jaw pain brought on by chewing suggests temporal arteritis. It is also important to find out how many other physicians the patient has seen for headaches, what medicines and dosages have been tried, how often does she miss work, and how many times has she been to the emergency room. Patients with chronic headaches commonly overuse analgesics and are depressed and under stress. These should be asked about specifically. For instance, the history may reveal that there is a major illness in a close relative, that she is a single mother, working 40 hours a week and attending college full-time, that she is unwillingly taking care of four grandchildren, that she is married to an alcoholic and abusive husband, or that she has been hospitalized several times for depression.

Box 28.1 Ten Key Questions

How long have you had these headaches?

How often do you have headaches?

What brings on a headache?

Is there a warning before a headache begins?

Where is the headache located?

During a headache, what happens to your appetite and vision?

What else happens during a headache?

During a headache, given your druthers, what do you do?

How long does a headache last?

What have you found that relieves a headache?

Physical Examination and Testing

The physical examination of the patient with headaches is usually normal (8). It is nevertheless important to measure blood pressure, do a fundoscopic examination, and examine the neck. Although population studies show that high blood pressure and headaches do not correlate unless the diastolic blood pressure is above 130 mm Hg (9), the identification and treatment of hypertension often leads to improvement in headaches. On fundoscopy, physicians are primarily looking for papilledema and hypertensive changes in retinal arteries. Neck pain and tenderness are common in patients with chronic headaches, and vice versa, chronic headaches are common in patients with neck pain. Kerr proposed that this association was a form of referred pain, due to a convergence of sensory input (10): primary sensory afferents from the forehead synapse in the high cervical cord, near the synapses of primary sensory afferents from the neck. Often, patients with chronic headaches will be found to have exquisitely tender areas in the shoulders and neck, known as "trigger points," located along the hairline, near the mastoids, in the posterior neck and trapezii, at the periphery of the scapulae, and over the bicipital grooves. Patients with trigger points have limitation of all neck movements (*Note*: Do not test neck movements if there is a history of trauma or if an unstable cervical spine is suspected.) In contrast, patients with meningitis have extensor rigidity of the neck, limitation of neck flexion, and little or no limitation of neck rotation. Patients with meningitis may have fever, altered mental status, and other meningeal signs, such as Kernig's and Brudzinski's signs.

In the evaluation of headache patients, laboratory tests—blood, cerebrospinal fluid (CSF), and cranial imaging—are often normal (8). Blood tests that may be considered include a complete blood count (anemia can cause headaches), a biochemical profile, and thyroid tests. In a patient who is over 50 years old and who has a new or different headache, an erythrocyte sedimentation rate (ESR) may be ordered. In headache patients, cranial imaging is often performed although its exact clinical indications are unknown (11,12). In patients with an acute, severe headache, when acute subarachnoid hemorrhage is suspected, noncontrast cranial computed tomography (CT) scanning should be done (11,12). In a patient with chronic headaches, when the clinician feels cranial imaging is needed, either cranial CT scanning or cranial magnetic resonance imaging (MRI) can be done. Cranial CT scanning is cheaper and quicker. Because cranial MRI produces better images of the base of the brain and posterior fossa (11,12), it is the test of choice when the clinician suspects a lesion in these areas. MRI can be done without and with

Table 28.1 Subarachnoid Bleed or Traumatic Tap? General Guidelines

Finding	Subarachnoid Bleeding	Traumatic Tap
CSF clots	No	Sometimes
Decrease in red blood cell count from first to last tube	No	Yes
CSF has xanthochromia	Yes	Usually no
Repeat tap at higher level is still bloody	Yes	No

CSF, cerebrospinal fluid

gadolinium contrast. Gadolinium contrast administration is safer than the iodine contrast required for CT scanning.

In patients with an acute, severe headache and a normal noncontrast cranial CT scan, a lumbar puncture may be indicated to examine the CSF for subarachnoid hemorrhage. It can be difficult to differentiate subarachnoid bleeding from a traumatic tap (13). Table 28.1 lists characteristic differentiating features. When in doubt, consult a specialist.

Benign Head Pain Syndromes

Migraine

Pain

The term "migraine" is derived from Galen's "hemicrania," headache on one side of the head. Unilateral, pulsating headache that alternates sides from attack to attack is characteristic of migraine. However, many patients with migraine have bilateral head and neck pain, and unilateral headache can be seen in other headache syndromes. Many migraine patients have pain over the sinuses, perhaps because the sinuses are highly vascular, richly innervated, and sensitive to the vascular changes seen in migraine. In these patients, migraine can mimic sinus disease. A few patients have pain in the anterior neck, associated with carotid tenderness (15). This can mimic carotid artery dissection. Patients may complain, not of head pain, but of paresthesia—tingling, burning, or creeping and crawling. "Icepick-like," sharp, jabbing pains in the orbits and temples can occur in migraine patients as well (14). Some patients with migraine do not have head pains at all (migraine equivalent).

A person with migraines may have a few headaches in her life or daily headaches. Sometimes migraines will "cluster," meaning that the patient has periods of frequent headaches separated by headache-free intervals. In women, migraines may cluster during the menses, associated with declining estrogen levels (16). "Clustering" does not mean the patient has "cluster headaches," which is a specific headache syndrome. Features differentiating cluster and migraine headaches are listed in Table 28.2. Acute cluster headaches are treated with intranasal 4% lidocaine, 100% oxygen at 8 to 10 L/min by tight-fitting mask, or dihydroergotamine SQ or IM. Because an acute cluster headache lasts 30 to 45 minutes, the goal of acute treatment is to administer medication so that high blood levels are achieved quickly. For prevention of cluster headaches, lithium verapamil, ergotamine, dihydroergotamine, prednisone, or methysergide can be used.

Onset and Causes

The onset of migraines is before the age of 40 in 90% of patients. Migraines also begin after head trauma and cranial surgery. Constant, uncomfortable, or painful paresthesia near the site of trauma or near the surgical scar are characteristic of posttraumatic headaches. Migraines tend to improve with time: 15 to 20 years after first diagnosis, 30% of patients no longer have headaches and headaches are markedly improved in another 50% (17). The reasons for improvement are not known.

Many patients with migraines will notice specific *trigger factors*. The most common are stress and depression. For instance, students have more headaches at the time of final examinations. Some patients notice the opposite—the sudden release of stress

Table 28.2 Some Features Differentiating Migraine and Cluster Headaches

	Migraine	Cluster
Prevalence?	Common	<1% as common as migraine
Sex?	Females, 3:1	Males, 10:1
Unilateral headache?	Yes, alternates	Yes, does not alternate
Frequency?	At most, 1–2/day	Many attacks/day
More common at night?	No	Yes
Nausea and vomiting?	Often	No
During a headache, ...	I lie down	I pace
Duration of headache?	>2 hr	30 min to 2 hr
Family history?	67% positive	No

triggers a headache. These people have their headaches after examinations are over, on weekends, or on vacations. Changing eating and sleeping patterns may trigger headaches: patients may be unable to follow a diet, do shift work, or sleep late on weekends. Specific foods, in some patients, can trigger a headache. The most commonly incriminated foods are chocolate, ethanol-containing beverages (especially red wine), foods with monosodium glutamate as a preservative, cheeses, and citrus fruits. Sometimes, changes in the weather, febrile illnesses, exercise, head trauma (18), sexual intercourse (19,20), caffeine withdrawal, strong smells, bright lights, and loud noises trigger migraines. Certain medicines can also worsen migraines. These include vasodilators commonly prescribed for hypertension (hydralazine, minoxidil, and prazosin) and nitrates prescribed for coronary artery disease. One old-time headache remedy, acetanilide, produced methemoglobinemia and headaches in susceptible patients. The neuropharmacologists Brody and Axelrod discovered that acetanilide's major active metabolite, acetaminophen, was an effective analgesic and did not produce methemoglobinemia. Their discovery led to the common use of acetaminophen for headaches.

Migraine headaches sometimes are related to estrogen and progesterone levels. About 60% of women have worsening of headaches at the time of their menses; this is thought to be related to declining estrogen levels (16). During pregnancy, perhaps because of sustained high estrogen levels, migraine headaches usually abate. High-estrogen oral contraceptive pills worsen migraines, but only about 5% of women will have worsening, or first appearance, of migraine while taking low-estrogen oral contraceptives. About 30% to 40% of these patients will have fewer headaches if they stop taking oral contraceptives (3). Some women have improvement of migraines after beginning low-estrogen oral contraceptives. Menopause and bilateral oophorectomy have no effect on migraines. Postmenopausal replacement therapy also has no clear effect on migraines. Headache improvement has been reported to occur in some patients if the estrogen dose is increased, if it is decreased, if a synthetic estrogen is substituted for an organic, equine-derived, conjugated estrogen preparation, or if this preparation is substituted for a synthetic estrogen preparation.

Headache Phase

By the recent International Headache Society criteria, most migraines are either "migraine without aura" (the old "common migraine") and "migraine with aura" (the old "classic migraine"). Migraine without aura is much more common than migraine with aura. "Aura" typically refers to symptoms heralding a migraine, which begins about 25 minutes after the aura starts. However, an aura may occur at the time the headache begins, after the headache, or even unrelated temporally to the headache. Typical aura symptoms are white or colored scintillations, paracentral scotomata (blind spots), fortification spectra (a scotoma surrounded by bright jagged edges, like a fort), homonymous hemianopia, reading difficulty, unilateral paresthesia or numbness, unilateral weakness, and speech difficulty. The visual symptoms are due to occipital lobe dysfunction. In some patients, visual symptoms progressively enlarge or "march." In 1941, Karl Lashley, a Harvard neuropsychologist, measured the progression of his own visual aura. He estimated that the dysfunction spread across his visual cortex at the rate of about 3 mm/min (21). This is approximately the same rate as the "spreading depression of Leao," a progressive, but reversible, shutdown of cortical function produced in experimental animals after many different types of cortical stimulation (22). Spreading depression is accompanied by electrolyte changes in the extracellular spaces in the brain, and a negative DC voltage shift. This hypothesis of aura pathogenesis is known as the "spreading depression" hypothesis, Alternatively, the aura may be due to vasospasm. This is known as the vascular hypothesis, first proposed by Wolff (23). Cerebral blood flow studies, designed to differentiate between the two hypotheses, are contradictory (24,25).

During the headache phase of a migraine, patients commonly lose their appetite. Many complain of nausea and some vomit. Gastrointestinal absorption of food and medicines is delayed and incomplete. Patients often notice that bright lights, sounds, and smells bother them; these are popularly known as photophobia, phonophobia, and osmophobia. Patients with a migraine tend to seek a dark, quiet room, lie down, and try to sleep. They notice that sitting up, standing up, coughing, and sneezing make the headache worse. Patients generally look pale and sick. Many are orthostatic during a migraine and some black out. Thinking slows and speech can be slurred. Patients may notice other phenemona, such as facial flushing, swelling, temporal tenderness, and Horner's syndrome.

Although migraine without aura and migraine with aura are the most common migraine syndromes, there are other varieties of migraine. These are summarized in Table 28.3.

There is an increased risk of stroke in patients who have migraine with aura. The relative risk has been estimated at 2.6-fold (26). At one referral center, 25% of all strokes in patients less than 50 years old were attributed to migraine, and 0.4% of patients diagnosed with migraine also had a migraine-associated stroke (27). Advancing age, hypertension, diabetes mellitus, oral contraceptive use, cigarette smoking, and the lupus anticoagulant–anticardiolipin antibody syndrome are additional risk factors for stroke. A "crescendo" headache—a progressively worsening migraine headache problem—is often seen in the month before a cerebral infarction occurs (28,29). Migraine-associated strokes are characteristically occipital lobe infarctions with a homonymous hemianopia (27), but strokes can occur in any arterial distribution (28). A migraine patient with a stroke needs thorough investigation before attributing the stroke to migraine (30). This evaluation commonly includes cerebral angiography although patients with migraine-associated stroke may have an increased risk of ischemic stroke as a complication of this procedure (30).

Table 28.3 Other Varieties of Migraine

Hemiplegic migraine	Often autosomal dominant; strokelike hemiplegia with migraine, usually resolving in 24 hr
Basilar artery migraine	Occipital headaches accompanied by various combinations of visual disturbance, diplopia, vertigo, ataxia, dysarthria, tinnitus, bilateral dysesthiae, mental confusion, and loss of consciousness
Ophthalmoplegic migraine onset <10 yr old	Third cranial nerve palsy with migraine; usually males;
Retinal migraine	Monocular blindness, thought to be due to retinal artery spasm, in association with migraine
Migraine equivalent	Migraine aura without headache
Abdominal migraine	Attacks of vomiting in a child, thought to be a migraine equivalent
Benign paroxysmal vertigo	Episodic vertigo in a child, possible migraine equivalent

The increased risk of ischemic stroke in patients who have migraine with aura supports Wolff's vascular hypothesis: the aura is a consequence of cerebral arterial vasospasm and the head pain is due to vasodilation in scalp and meningeal arteries. This hypothesis also helps explain the pulsating nature of the pain, the vasodilator-induced exacerbations of migraine, the increased amplitude of pulsations in the superficial temporal artery associated with headache, the relief of headache by compression of this artery, and the relief of headache and diminution of arterial pulsations after successful ergotamine treatment (31). However, the amplitude of temporal artery pulsation does not correlate well with headache intensity (32) and the exacerbation of migraine headache by coughing, sneezing, and straining suggests there is an intracranial component of the headache.

Total plasma serotonin level falls at the onset of migraine (33). Many antimigraine treatments interact with serotonin receptors: for instance, sumatriptan, a new antimigraine agent, is a serotonin $5HT_{1D}$-receptor agonist. These facts suggest that abnormal serotonin neurotransmission may play a role in the genesis of a migraine attack. More recent theories of migraine pathophysiology attempt to unify the serotonin/neuronal hypothesis and the vascular hypothesis. Moskowitz has proposed that local "axon-reflexes" of trigeminal nerve fibers innervating cranial blood vessels is responsible for vasodilation during migraine headaches (34). Lance has hypothesized that migraine headaches involve positive feedback between serotonergic fibers from the brain stem to cranial blood vessels and trigeminal nerve sensory fibers from blood vessels to the brain stem (4).

Tension Headaches

In tension headaches, pain is worse in the occiput, neck, and shoulders. A common complaint is that it is hard to enter freeways while driving because the neck rotation required exacerbates the pain. More than half of patients complain of inability to sleep well. In addition to occipital, neck, and shoulder pain, some patients have forehead pain, perhaps on a referred-pain basis. Unilateral headache, poor appetite, nausea, vomiting, and sensitivity to light, sound, and smells are uncommon unless the patient has migraines too. Many patients have both tension and migraine headaches. Sometimes it seems that each type of headache makes the other worse. Tension headaches usually last days and may be continuous ("I always keep a headache"). Headaches are worse with prolonged driving, stress, and depression, and after trauma, such as a whiplash injury. Smoking seems to worsen these headaches, not because of anything in cigarettes, cigars, or pipe tobacco, but because of the chronic coughing these patients have.

The examination usually shows trigger points—discrete tender areas—in the occiput, near the mastoids, in the posterior neck, and in the shoulders. Tension headaches may be part of the chronic pain syndrome known as tension myalgia, fibromyalgia, or fibromyositis. Despite the fact that nearly all these patients have neck pain, only rarely is a patient with tension headaches found to have a cervical disease, such as a herniated disc or rheumatoid arthritis (35).

The pathogenesis of tension headaches is not known. They were thought to be caused by muscle spasms because trigger points lie over ligaments and because measures designed to relax muscles improve the headaches. However, electromyographic studies have not confirmed excessive muscle fiber activity.

Analgesic Rebound Headaches

Daily use of some medications can lead to "rebound" headaches when the medicines are stopped. Commonly incriminated drugs include caffeine, nicotine, ergot derivatives, sympathomimetic agents, opiates, and barbiturates. Many patients with chronic daily headaches overuse these medicines and add to their headache problems. The pathophysiology of rebound headaches may involve drug withdrawal effects or reflex vasodilation. Simple treatment—advising patients to discontinue these medicines and prescribing amitriptyline 10 mg each evening and naproxen 500 mg daily—is surprisingly effective (36). Some patients may need inpatient drug withdrawal and 48 hours of IV prochlorperazine and dihydroergotamine 0.2–1.0 mg every 8 hours (see below) (3).

Chronic Paroxysmal Hemicrania

This is a rare type of headache. The male-female ratio is 1:5. The headache consists of 5- to 45-minute episodes of sharp. stabbing hemicranial pains. Patients can have a dozen or more attacks each day. The headache responds well to indomethacin 25–50 mg three times daily.

Postlumbar Puncture Headache

About 10% of people will have a headache after a lumbar puncture. It begins within 4 days of the procedure and is often accompanied by photophobia. The headache is provoked by sitting or standing and relieved by lying down. It lasts about 7 days, remitting spontaneously. Reynolds has reported that relief of this headache by gradual abdominal compression is a physical examination finding diagnostic of postlumbar puncture headache (37). In addition to the classic postlumbar puncture headache, patients may also have migraine and tension headaches, brought on by the stress of having the procedure. There have been a few reported cases of subdural hematoma following diagnostic lumbar puncture (37). The pathophysiology of postlumbar puncture headaches probably involves low CSF pressure and stretching of pain-sensitive structures at the base of the brain. Occasionally patients will have a transient sixth cranial nerve palsy, presumably due to traction on this nerve. To prevent this headache, Fishman recommends using a small gauge needle, inserting it with the bevel parallel to the dural fibers, and having the patient rest in bed for 15 to 30 minutes after the spinal tap (13). These preventive measures are only partially effective. Simple treatments—bed rest, caffeine, and analgesics—are often not effective. Time improves all patients. A "blood patch"—the epidural injection of 10 to 20 mL of the patient's venous blood in the epidural space near the location of the previous spinal tap—is successful 80% to 90% of the time (13,37).

Trigeminal Neuralgia (Tic Douloureux)

This is a unilateral, sharp, lancinating pain syndrome, located in the second or third division of the trigeminal nerve. Patients, usually elderly, can have dozens of episodes of pain each day although the pain relents at night. The pains can be spontaneous but more commonly are set off by stimulation of trigger zones, certain areas of the face or mouth. In fear of setting off pain, patients may be unable to eat, brush the teeth, wash, or talk. Although the condition itself is benign, the pain of trigeminal neuralgia is severe enough that patients may become suicidal. Sometimes meningiomas adjacent to the trigeminal nerve may cause trigeminal neuralgia, but more commonly, the cause is a tortuous blood vessel impinging on the trigeminal nerve as it enters the pons. Treatment options are medicines, such as baclofen or carbamazepine, or surgery, either ablation procedures of the gasserian ganglion or posterior fossa operations designed to relieve pressure on the trigeminal nerve from the aberrant blood vessel.

Differential Diagnosis

Temporal Arteritis or Giant Cell Arteritis

Patients with temporal arteritis are always more than 50 years old. Consider temporal arteritis in any woman in this age group who has a new or different type of headache. The history gives clues to the correct diagnosis. She may complain she "feels ill," with fever, generalized soreness and stiffness, and anemia. Some patients complain of jaw or tongue claudication. Others complain of temporal soreness, associated with sharp, jabbing pains. In 90% of patients with temporal arteritis, the ESR is greater than 50 mm/hr. Often, it is above 100 mm/hr. Although some patients with temporal arteritis have a normal ESR, this test is important in the evaluation of patients suspected of having temporal arteritis. An ESR determination needs to be done within 2 hours of the blood being drawn, otherwise the results can be falsely low. The ESR can also be falsely low in patients with abnormally shaped red blood cells (e.g., sickled cells).

The main serious complication of temporal arteritis is sudden, permanent blindness in one or both eyes, from ischemic optic neuropathy. Preventing this requires treating the patient with high-dose glucocorticoids for a prolonged time. Although treatment can begin when the diagnosis is suspected, definitive diagnosis by temporal artery biopsy is required. Patients should be referred to a large medical center where the surgeon (typically an ophthalmologist or vascular surgeon) and pathologist have experience diagnosing temporal arteritis. Treatment should be monitored by an experienced clinician—usually an ophthalmologist, neurologist, or rheumatologist.

Subarachnoid Hemorrhage

Subarachnoid hemorrhage causes a sudden, severe headache. Common descriptions are "like a sledgehammer," and "the worst of my life." There is accompanying neck stiffness, nausea, vomiting, and mental confusion. This headache may be triggered by physical exertion such as sexual intercourse. The physical examination shows neck stiffness and, sometimes, preretinal hemorrhages in the eyegrounds. In 80% of patients, noncontrast cranial CT scanning shows subarachnoid blood. For the other 20%, the scan is unremarkable. For these patients, diagnosis requires lumbar puncture (see above and Table 28.1).

Meningitis

Classic symptoms of meningitis are headache, fever, and altered mental status. Raskin reports that patients with meningitis characteristically have a headache with prominent retro-orbital pain (3). This is not pathognomonic of meningitis—it is also seen with migraine and optic neuritis—but, in the setting of new-onset headaches, should suggest the possibility of meningitis. Diagnosis of meningitis requires lumbar puncture.

Pseudotumor Cerebri (Benign Intracranial Hypertension)

Affected patients are often obese women. Sometimes this syndrome is a reaction to taking tetracycline, nitrofurantoin, nalidixic acid, or excessive vitamin A, chlordecone exposure, or to withdrawal of glucocorticoid medication. Patients with pseudotumor cerebri have headache, transient visual obscurations, and pulsatile tinnitus. There is nothing that distinguishes the headaches of pseudotumor cerebri. Transient visual obscurations are brief, bilateral white-outs of vision, lasting seconds. These may occur dozens of times daily. In comparison, amaurosis fugax lasts minutes. Examination shows papilledema. About 25% of patients have a sixth cranial nerve palsy. Cranial imaging often shows slitlike ventricles. At lumbar puncture, the opening pressure is greater than 250 mm H_2O, often above 500 mm H_2O, and the CSF protein is low. The pathogenesis of this syndrome is not known. Probably it is due either to increased pressure in the cerebral venous system or to increased outflow resistance at the arachnoid villi. Treatment is acetazolamide 1 gm daily, repeated lumbar punctures, and a weight-loss diet. Treatment which produces resolution of symptoms and returns opening pressure to normal, is continued for about a year or two, after which the syndrome of pseudotumor cerebri usually spontaneously remits.

Pseudotumor cerebri is not a "benign" headache syndrome. There is a risk of permanent visual loss. Because of this risk, referral to an ophthalmologist for periodic visual fields is indicated. Progressive visual field defects and failure of symptoms to improve with treatment may indicate that visual loss is imminent and that surgical therapies (optic nerve fenestration, subtemporal decompression, or lumbar-peritoneal shunt) should be considered.

Carotid Dissection

Dissection of carotid arteries may occur spontaneously or may occur in association with trauma, Marfan's syndrome, or fibromuscular dysplasia. Affected patients may be young or old. They usually complain of a new or different headache, with prominent anterior neck pain. Many patients have symptoms of transient ischemic attacks or stroke. On examination, about 67% have an ipsilateral Horner's syndrome. The combination of anterior neck pain, ipsilateral Horner's syndrome, and focal cerebral symptoms is not specific for carotid dissection, but can also be seen in migraine. Diagnosis requires carotid imaging: carotid ultrasound, magnetic resonance angiography, or carotid angiography. The classic finding on angiography is the "string sign," gradual tapering of the vessel lumen, sometimes leading to an occlusion. Carotid dissections often heal spontaneously. Heparin therapy may be beneficial (38).

Brain Tumors, Including Colloid Cyst of the Third Ventricle

Brain tumor headaches are generally described as dull, rather than throbbing. Coughing, sneezing, straining, and changes in position often worsen the headaches of brain tumors, and brain tumor headaches are worse first thing in the morning. However, these symptoms are not specific: for each of these symptoms, the diagnosis of migraine is still more likely than brain tumor. It is a general rule that the location of the head pain early on (before there are complications such as increased intracranial pressure) indicates the location of the tumor. Also, more rapidly growing tumors tend to cause more headaches than slowly growing tumors do. Tumors in the posterior fossa may present with headaches alone or headaches with papilledema, whereas tumors elsewhere often have other neurologic symptoms and signs. Diagnosis of brain tumor is made by cranial imaging.

Colloid cysts of the third ventricle are benign tumors at the foramen of Monro, the opening of the lateral ventricles into the third ventricle. Because of its characteristic location, this tumor can produce sudden obstruction of CSF flow, and cause sudden death in young patients. Patients present with new, worsening headaches associated with alteration in consciousness. Noncontrast cranial CT scanning shows a small, round, hyperdense tumor in a characteristic location, and makes the diagnosis. Treatment is surgery.

Subdural Hematoma

Patients with subdural hematoma present with headaches, altered mental status, and hemiparesis. All these symptoms fluctuate, a clue to the diagnosis of subdural hematoma. There may be a history of head trauma or falls, but elderly patients, patients with seizures, and alcoholics may not have a history of head trauma, either because the head trauma was mild or the patient does not remember the trauma. Patients with clotting disorders—patients who take coumadin, who are uremic, or who are alcoholic—are at increased risk of subdural hematoma. Diagnosis is generally made by cranial CT scanning.

Acute Narrow-Angle Glaucoma

Patients have the sudden onset of blurred vision and eye pain, which can mimic migraine headache. However, the headache is new or different, the eye is red and swollen, and the pupil is fixed. Anticholinergic medication may precipitate this syndrome. Diagnosis is obvious once the disease is considered. This is an ophthalmologic emergency.

Treatment of Migraine and Tension Headaches (39)

No medicine will cure headaches forever. No treatment is guaranteed effective. The goals of treatment are to decrease the frequency and severity of headaches so that they do not interfere with the patient's life, and to provide her some control over her headaches. In general, the treatment of migraine and tension headaches must be individualized. This requires the active participation of your patient: she must note the efficacy and side effects of therapy so that the therapeutic regimen can be altered accordingly. The treatment options that will be discussed are only general guidelines. The physician must be flexible and fit the treatment to the patient, who is looking for a simple routine relatively free of side effects.

Studies of placebo treatment of headache show that 20% to 40% of patients respond. Interestingly, response does not seem to be dependent on patient factors (you cannot predict which patient will have a placebo response), but is dependent on physician factors, such as thoroughness of examination, completeness of explanations, perceived empathy, and time spent with the patient.

The first step in treatment of any recurrent headache problem is the obvious: review precipitating factors with the patient and find ways to avoid them. The patient should be advised to cut down on consumption of coffee and alcohol, sleep regular hours, eat at regular times, avoid—if possible—extremely stressful situations, and, if necessary, take treatment for depression. Women being sexually harassed at work or abused at home may present to the physician complaining of headaches. Headache remedies may not be effective in these situations until her job changes or she gets a divorce.

Acute Headaches, Outpatient Treatment

These types of treatment (Table 28.4) are designed to relieve an occasional headache. For many of these remedies, when they are taken more than twice a week chronically, there is a danger of analgesic rebound headaches (see above).

Analgesics

For an acute headache, simple analgesics are usually the best first-line treatment (40). This includes aspirin, acetaminophen, and nonsteroidal anti-inflammatory drugs (NSAIDs). Aspirin and NSAIDs inhibit prostaglandin synthetase, thereby reducing inflammation (including sterile inflammation that may occur in

Table 28.4 Medicines for an Acute Headache

Medicine	Typical Dose (mg)	Side Effects
Analgesics		
Acetaminophen	1000	
Aspirin	1000	Dyspepsia, gastrointestinal bleeding
Ibuprofen	800	Dyspepsia, gastrointestinal bleeding
Antiemetics		
Metoclopramide	10–20	Acute dystonic reaction
Promethazine	25	Acute dystonic reaction
Ergot alkaloids		
Ergotamine	1–2	Nausea, vomiting, vasoconstriction
Dihydroergotamine	0.5–1.0	Same as ergotamine, but less severe
Serotonin receptor agonist		
Sumatriptan	6	Chest tightness, flushing
Opiates		
Codeine	60–120	Constipation, addiction
Meperidine	50–200	Constipation, addiction

migraine), altering neurotransmitter release, and decreasing pain transmission on both a peripheral and central basis. Acetaminophen's analgesic action may be due to inhibition of a central nervous system prostaglandin synthetase, relieving pain on a central basis (41). For a typical migraine, patients take 1000 mg acetaminophen, 1000 mg aspirin, or 600–800 mg ibuprofen. Many patients prefer enteric-coated aspirin. Some physicians prescribe effervescent formulations of aspirin and acetaminophen, which are absorbed more quickly and more effectively (40). Some physicians prescribe the antiemetics metoclopramide (10–20 mg) or promethazine (25 mg) to be taken in conjunction with simple analgesics (40). These antiemetics both speed the effect of the analgesics and relieve the nausea and vomiting of migraine. Suppositories of analgesics and of antiemetics are available if needed. The maximum aspirin dose is 6 gm/day; the maximum acetaminophen dose is 4 gm/day. Many combination-type medicines contain aspirin or acetaminophen; patients may inadvertantly take more than the maximum dose. Aspirin and NSAIDs should be avoided in patients with aspirin hypersensitivity, a syndrome of nasal polyps, asthma, and allergy to aspirin and aspirin-like drugs. Aspirin and NSAIDs taken in the last trimester of pregnancy are associated with delayed and prolonged labor, increased blood loss, increased incidence of stillbirths, and patent ductus arteriosus in the newborn. Acetaminophen is generally considered safe in pregnancy. Metoclopramide is in pregnancy category B; promethazine is category C.

When simple analgesics are inefective or contraindicated, there are still a variety of medicines that can be considered (see Table 28.4). Each has advantages and disadvantages.

Ergot Alkaloids

Ergot preparations are often used to abort a migraine. Ergot alkaloids are agonists at serotonin $5HT_1$-receptors; this may or may not be the mechanism by which they improve an acute migraine. Ergotamine is typically prescribed at a dose of 2 mg for each headache. It is commonly given orally (these formulations often have caffeine too) or sublingually. A suppository preparation is available as well. Because ergot alkaloids can cause nausea and vomiting, an antiemetic is often prescribed with them. If a patient takes more than 6 mg ergotamine in a day, there is a risk of ischemia of the extremities. Although many patients take both ergot alkaloids and propranolol without problems, there have been anecdotal reports that, with the combination, there is an increased risk of gangrene (42). There is definitely an increased risk of gangrene with the concomitant use of erythromycin and ergot alkaloids (43). Because of their vasospastic effects, ergots should not be given to patients with coronary artery or peripheral vascular disease. If patients use them more than three times a week, physical dependence and rebound headaches can result. Ergotamine, and other ergot alkaloid derivatives, are contraindicated in pregnancy.

Dihydroergotamine (DHE), among the ergot alkaloids, has the least arterial vasospastic effects. DHE can be given SQ, IM, or IV (an intranasal DHE spray, which has proven safe and effective in clinical trials, may soon be available in the United States). Drug levels of DHE are highest after IV administration, next highest after IM, and least after SQ. The half-life of DHE is about 20 hours. A typical dose of DHE is 0.5–1.0 mg. Nausea and vomiting can occur, especially with IV administration. For patients receiving IV DHE, it is best to premedicate with an IV antiemetic (10 mg metoclopramide or 10 mg prochlorperazine (44). IM DHE can be given with or without antiemetics (45). If antiemetics are given, it is useful to remember that DHE is miscible with promethazine, so they can be given together in the same injection. DHE is contraindicated in pregnancy and in patients with coronary artery or peripheral vascular disease. Because of a risk of vasospasm and gangrene, the manufacturer recommends that no more than 6 mg DHE be given each week. Some physicians prescribe up to 9 mg in a 3-day period, provided the patient is hospitalized, so that vasospastic effects can be closely monitored. DHE and sumatriptan should not be given together; wait 6 hours after the last dose of sumatriptan before administering DHE. DHE and any vasospastic agent (cocaine, epinephrine, phenylephrine, isometheptene, other ergot alkaloids, and nicotine patches) should not be given concurrently. DHE and erythromycin also should not be given together because of an increased risk of vasoconstriction.

Serotonin Receptor Agonist

Sumatriptan is a new medication for aborting a

migraine headache. It acts as an agonist at serotonin $5HT_{1D}$-receptors. Sumatriptan does not cross the blood-brain barrier. In the United States, it is available only by SQ injection (although it may soon be available in an oral formulation [46], which may largely replace SQ injections). The SQ dose is 6 mg, which the patient can inject herself. Although SQ sumatriptan is highly effective in aborting an acute migraine (72% to 90% response rate [47,48]), it is expensive—about $35/6 mg injection, and $14 for each 100-mg sumatriptan tablet (49)—and its duration of action is only about 2 hours. In contrast to the ergot alkaloids, which can cause nausea and vomiting, sumatriptan tends to relieve nausea and vomiting. If the first injection does not relieve a headache, another dose will also be ineffective (50). In about 40% of patients with initial relief the headache returns. In this situation, another SQ injection—a "rescue" dose—is highly effective. No more than two SQ doses should be given in 24 hours. Side effects of sumatriptan include tingling and flushing and chest tightness in 33%. Sumatriptan is contraindicated in patients with angina or uncontrolled hypertension. It should not be given within 24 hours of an ergot derivative (ergotamine or DHE). Sumatriptan is in pregnancy category C.

Opiates

Oral opiates can also be considered for these patients if simple analgesics fail or are contraindicated. As long as the total dose of opiates is less then 20 pills each month, the risk of addiction is small. Constipation is the major side effect of opiates. Codeine 60–120 mg can be effective in aborting headaches, without inducing drowsiness or sedation. However, about 20% of the population is unable to metabolize codeine to its active metabolite. For them, codeine will be ineffective. Oral meperidine, propoxyphene, hydrocodone, and oxycodone are also effective for acute headaches. A newer agent is intranasal butorphanol for an acute migraine (51,52). Dosage is 1 mg (1 spray in one nostril) with the headache, and the patient may repeat it once if necessary. One bottle provides 15 sprays. No more than two bottles should be prescribed each month. Intranasal butorphanol's disadvantage is a high frequency of sedation. Opiates, in general, are in pregnancy category C. However, codeine and meperidine have been used frequently in pregnant women and are generally considered safe by experienced clinicians (3,16). These medicines are generally prescribed if acetaminophen is not effective. Meperidine is used at a dose of 50–200 mg per headache.

Combination Drugs

A number of combination medications are available for the treatment of migraines. Two commonly prescribed ones are the combination of isometheptene, acetaminophen, and dichloralphenazone; and aspirin, caffeine, butalbital, and codeine. Combination medicines may contain sympathomimetic vasoconstrictor agents (such as isometheptene), muscle relaxants, barbiturates, aspirin, acetaminophen, and opiates. Combination medicines are less effective in treating severe migraine and can cause rebound headaches.

Treatment of Acute Headache in the Office or Emergency Room

When a patient presents to the emergency room or physician's office because of an acute headache, evaluation and treatment often proceed simultaneously. The main serious causes of headache to be considered in this situation are subarachnoid hemorrhage, acute meningitis, and temporal arteritis. The clinical characteristics of these conditions and the diagnostic tests needed were discussed above.

For an acute, severe headache unresponsive to self-administered medications, the drugs of choice are DHE given IM or IV, or sumatriptan SQ (Table 28.5). Intranasal DHE (when it becomes available) or intranasal butorphanol may also be considered. IV or IM narcotics, traditionally used to treat headaches in the emergency room, are not the drugs of choice because they are sedating, addictive, and less effective for an acute headache than DHE and sumatriptan. The NSAID ketorolac can be given IM and is effective in

Table 28.5 Parenteral Medicines for an Acute Headache

Medicine	Route	Dose
Dihydroergotamine	IM/IV	0.5–1.0 mg
Sumatriptan	SQ	6 mg
Ketorolac	IM	30–60 mg
Meperidine	IM/IV	50–100 mg
Prochlorperazine	IM/IV	10 mg
Metoclopramide	IM/IV	10 mg
Promethazine	IM/IV	25 mg

treating acute headaches. Parenteral antiemetics are often given with DHE, narcotics, and ketorolac.

Chronic Headaches

In general, patients are ready to consider taking daily antimigraine preventive medicines when they have more than two headaches a month.

Patients with very frequent—daily or nearly daily—headaches often have tension headaches or mixed tension—migraine headaches. Improving these headaches may not be easy. For tension headaches, conservative measures should be tried first. This includes regular massage of the trigger points, daily exercise (typically walking), wet heat treatments (long, hot baths and showers), relaxation exercises (53), losing weight, and stopping smoking. In refractory cases, referral to a physical therapist for evaluation and treatment may be helpful. A tricyclic antidepressant, such as amitriptyline 10 mg nightly, helps patients sleep. Regularly prescribed NSAIDs may improve pain. Muscle relaxants—benzodiazepines, cyclobenzaprine, and others—are not very effective and should only be used for short periods (<2 weeks) because of the risks of addiction and rebound headaches.

Four categories of drugs are effective in preventing migraine headaches and have few major side effects (Table 28.6).

The first category is β blockers. Propranolol and nadolol seem to be the most effective in preventing migraines. Usual doses of propranolol are 60–320 mg daily. For the patient, the long-acting form is more convenient and just as effective. About 67% of patients respond to propranolol. Contraindications to β blockers include congestive heart failure, asthma, and insulin-dependent diabetes mellitus. β Blockers sometimes worsen depression. Although many migraine patients become orthostatic during a headache and one might expect that β blockers would worsen orthostatic hypotension, this has not been a prominent side effect, in my experience. The mechanism by which these medicines prevent migraine is not known. Propranolol is in pregnancy category C.

The calcium channel blockers verapamil and diltiazem prevent migraine headaches. Both can worsen heart failure and cardiac conduction defects. Verapamil causes constipation. Both are available in long-acting preparations. Typical doses are 180–360 mg daily for diltiazem and 240 mg daily for verapamil. The mechanism of migraine prevention is not known, but they are effective in preventing migraines in about 67% of patients. Diltiazem is in pregnancy category C.

Some tricyclic antidepressants prevent migraines effectively in 67% of patients. These medicines are also effective in treating tension headaches. Amitriptyline, nortriptyline, and desipramine seem to work best. Although these medicines prevent serotonin reuptake, it seems that their effectiveness correlates best with their ability to block serotonin $5HT_2$-receptors. Typical doses of amitriptyline are 10–150 mg nightly. Amitriptyline is associated with the most side effects: dry mouth, orthostatic hypotension, increased appetite, weight gain, drowsiness, mental confusion, blurred vision, and urinary retention. Although

Table 28.6 Preventive Medicines for Migraines

Medicine	Typical Dose	Side Effects
β blockers		
Propranolol	60–320 mg/day	Fatigue, depression
Nadolol	40–240 mg/day	Fatigue, depression
Calcium channel blockers		
Verapamil	240 mg/day	Constipation
Diltiazem	180–360 mg/day	
Tricyclic antidepressants		
Amitriptyline	10–150 mg/day	Dry mouth, weight gain, drowsiness, mental clouding
Nortriptyline	10–100 mg/day	Mild drowsiness
Desipramine	25–200 mg/day	Mild drowsiness
Analgesics		
Naproxen	550 mg twice a day	Dyspepsia, gastrointestinal bleeding
Aspirin	650 mg twice a day	Dyspepsia, gastrointestinal bleeding

amitriptyline is in pregnancy category C ("risk cannot be ruled out"), it is regarded as the preventive medication of choice during pregnancy: amitriptyline has "a long record of safe use during pregnancy" (16).

Nonsteroidal anti-inflammatory drugs, taken regularly, can prevent migraines. The best studied are naproxen 550 mg taken twice daily and aspirin 650 mg twice daily.

If none of the above measures are ineffective, other medicines can be tried. Cyproheptadine 12–24 mg daily is sometimes effective but is associated with dyspepsia and drowsiness. It is in pregnancy category B. Methysergide 2–8 mg daily is effective in preventing migraines in about 67% of patients. It is contraindicated in pregnancy and can cause retroperitoneal fibrosis. To prevent the fibrotic complications, methysergide should be used at the lowest possible dose and patients should interrupt treatment for 1 month of every 4 months. Methysergide also causes muscle aching. It should not be used in patients with thrombophlebitis, arterial vaso-occlusive disease, severe hypertension, and pregnancy. Valproic acid 800–1000 mg daily is reportedly effective in some patients. Because of its association with neural tube defects, it should not be prescribed to pregnant women for headaches (category D). Valproic acid can cause gastrointestinal upset, particularly at the start of therapy. This can be avoided by using divalproex sodium instead of valproic acid, beginning at low doses, and increasing slowly. Valproic acid can also cause weight gain, tremors, thrombocytopenia, pancreatitis, hair loss, hepatic dysfunction, and hyperammonemia.

Monoamine oxidase (MAO) inhibitors, such as phenelzine, are sometimes recommended as migraine prophylaxis. However, there is a severe, sometimes fatal drug interaction between MAO inhibitors and meperidine, between MAO inhibitors and dextromethorphan, and between MAO inhibitors and serotonin selective reuptake inhibitors such as fluoxetine and sertraline. Taking any of these combinations can cause delirium, coma, fever, convulsions, and death. Avoid MAO inhibitors in the treatment of migraine.

REFERENCES

1. Rivo ML, Saultz JW, Wartman SA, DeWitt TG. Defining the generalist physician's training. JAMA 1994;271:1499–1504.

2. Rapoport AM. Update on severe headache with a focus on migraine. Neurology 1994;44(suppl 3):S5.

3. Raskin NH. Headache. 2nd ed. New York: Churchill Livingstone, 1988.

4. Lance JW. Mechanism and management of headache. 5th ed. Boston: Butterworth-Heinemann, 1993.

5. Sacks O. Migraine: revised and expanded. Berkeley: University of California Press, 1992.

6. Headache Classification Committee of the International Headache Society. Classification and diagnostic criteria for headache disorders, cranial neuralgias and facial pain. Cephalalgia 1988;8(suppl 7):19–28.

7. Turner JA, Deyo RA, Loeser JD, et al. The importance of placebo effects in pain treatment and research. JAMA 1994;271:1609–1614.

8. Kunkel RS. Evaluating the headache patient: history and workup. Headache 1979;19:122–126.

9. Al Badran RH, Weir RJ, McGuiness JB. Hypertension and headache. Scott Med J 1970;15:48–51.

10. Kerr FWL. Structural relation of the trigeminal spinal tract to upper cerviceal roots and the solitary nucleus in the cat. Exp Neurol 1961;4:134–148.

11. Kent DL, Haynor DR, Longstreth WT Jr, Larson EB. The clinical efficacy of magnetic resonance imaging in neuroimaging. Ann Intern Med 1994;120:856–871.

12. American College of Physicians. Position paper: magnetic resonance imaging of the brain and spine: a revised statement. Ann Intern Med 1994;120:872–875.

13. Fishman RA. Cerebrospinal fluid in diseases of the nervous system. 2nd ed. Philadelphia: WB Saunders, 1992:157–188.

14. Raskin NH, Schwartz RK. Icepick-like pain. Neurology 1980;30:203–205.

15. Raskin NH, Prusiner S. Carotidynia. Neurology 1977;27:43–46.

16. Donaldson JO. Neurology of pregnancy. 2nd ed. Philadelphia: WB Saunders, 1989:217–228.

17. Whitty CWM, Hockaday JM. Migraine: a follow-up study of 92 patients. Br Med J 1968;1:735–736.

18. Matthews WB. Footballer's migraine. Br Med J 1972;2:326–327.

19. Paulson GW, Klawans HL. Benign orgasmic cephalgia. Headache 1974;13:181–187.

20. Lance JW. Headaches related to sexual activity. J Neurol Neurosurg Psychiatry 1976;39:1226–1230.

21. Lashley KS. Patterns of cerebral integration indicated by the scotomas of migraine. Arch Neurol Psychiatry 1941;46:331–339.

22. Leao AAP. Spreading depression of activity in the cerebral cortex. J Neurophysiol 1944;7:359–390.

23. Wolff HG. Headache and other head pain. New York: Oxford University Press, 1963:227–386.

24. Lauritzen M, Olsen TS, Lassen NA, Paulson OB. Changes in regional cerebral blood flow during the course of classic migraine attacks. Ann Neurol 1983;13:633–641.

25. Olsen TS, Friberg, L, Lassen NA. Ischemia may be the primary cause of the neurological deficits in classic migraine. Arch Neurol 1987;44:156–161.

26. Henrich JB, Horwitz RI. A controlled study of ischemic stroke risk in migraine patients. J Clin Epidemiol 1989;42:773–780.

27. Broderick JP, Swanson JW. Migraine-related strokes: clinical profile and prognosis in 20 patients. Arch Neurol 1987;44:868–871.

28. Bogousslavsky J, Regli F, Van Melle G, et al. Migraine stroke. Neurology 1988;38:223–227.

29. Gardner, JH, Hornstein S, van den Noort S. The clinical characteristics of headache during impending cerebral infarction in women taking oral contraceptives. Headache 1968;8:108–111.

30. Rothrock JF, Walicke P, Swenson MR, et al. Migrainous stroke. Arch Neurol 1988;45:63–67.

31. Editorial. Vasodilatation and migraine. Lancet 1990;335:822–823.

32. Brazil P, Friedman AP. Craniovascular studies in headache: a report and analysis of pulse volume tracings. Neurology 1956;6:96–102.

33. Lance JW, Anthony M, Hinterberger H. The control of cranial arteries by humoral mechanisms and its relation to the migraine syndrome. Headache 1967;7:93–102.

34. Sakas DE, Moskowitz MA, Wei EP, et al. Trigeminovascular fibers increase blood flow in cortical gray matter by axon reflex-like mechanisms during acute severe hypertension or seizures. Proc Natl Sci USA 1989;86:1401–1405.

35. Edmeads J. The cervical spine and headache. Neurology 1988;38:1874–1878.

36. Hering R, Steiner TJ. Abrupt outpatient withdrawal of medication in analgesic abusing migraineurs. Lancet 1991;337:1442–1443.

37. Reynolds F. Dural puncture and headache. Br Med J 1993;306:874–875.

38. Caplan LR. Stroke: a clinical approach. 2nd ed. Boston: Butterworth-Heinemann, 1993:299–304.

39. Welch KMA. Drug therapy of migraine. N Engl J Med 1993;329:1476–1483.

40. Wilkinson M. The treatment of acute migraine attacks. Headache 1976;15:291–292.

41. Vane J. Towards a better aspirin. Nature 1994;367:215–216.

42. Baumrucker JF. Drug interaction—propranolol and cafergot. N Engl J Med 1973;288:916.

43. Leroy F, Asseman P, Pruvost P, et al. Dihydroergotamine-erythromycin-induced ergotism. Ann Intern Med 1988;109:249.

44. Jones J, Sklar D, Dougherty J, White W. Randomized double-blind trial of intravenous prochlorperazine for the treatment of acute headache. JAMA 1989;261:1174–1176.

45. Saadah HA. Abortive headache therapy with intramuscular dihydroergotamine. Headache 1992;32:18–20.

46. Goadsby PJ, Zagami AS, Donnan GA, et al. Oral sumatriptan in acute migraine. Lancet 1991;338:782–783.

47. The Subcutaneous Sumatriptan International Study Group. Treatment of migraine attacks with sumatriptan. N Engl J Med 1991;325:316–321.

48. Cady RK, Dexter J, Sargent JD, et al. Efficacy of subcutaneous sumatriptan in repeated episodes of migraine. Neurology 1993;43:1363–1368.

49. The Medical Letter. Sumatriptan for migraine. Med Lett 1992;34:91–93.

50. Cady RK, Wendt JK, Kirchner JR, et al. Treatment of acute migraine with subcutaneous sumatriptan. JAMA 1991;265:2831–2835.

51. Baumel B. Migraine: a pharmacologic review with newer options and delivery modalities. Neurology 1994;44(suppl 3):S13–S17.

52. Markley HG. Chronic headache: Appropriate use of opiate analgesics. Neurology 1994;44(suppl 3):S18–S24.

53. Turner JA, Chapman CR. Psychological interventions for chronic pain: a critical review. I. Relaxation training and biofeedback. Pain 1982;12:1–21.

SECTION TEN

RHEUMATOLOGY

CHAPTER 29

OSTEOPOROSIS

Jiri Dubovsky

Definition and Etiology of Osteoporosis

Osteopenia, Osteoporosis, and Fractures

Osteoporosis is a systemic skeletal disease characterized by low bone mass and microarchitectural deterioration of bone tissue with consequent increase in bone fragility and risk of fractures. The concept of osteoporosis has changed in recent years primarily because of the technology that allows measurement of bone density (mass) with great accuracy by noninvasive procedures. There has been a controversy whether the presence of insufficiency fracture(s) is a necessary criterion for the diagnosis of osteoporosis.

Definitions recommended recently by the expert panel of the World Health Organization are as follows. A decrease of bone mass of mild to moderate degree (between 1.0 and 2.5 SD below race- and gender-matched peak mean value—T score) is called *osteopenia.* Severe loss (T score is <2.5 SD) is *osteoporosis*, irrespective whether fractures are or are not present. Consequently, a prefracture stage of osteoporosis is acknowledged. Nonetheless, fractures and their complications are the principal clinical manifestations of osteoporosis. Osteoporotic fractures represent a major public health problem. In the United States osteoporosis predisposes yearly to 500,000 vertebral fractures and 250,000 hip fractures. The importance of osteoporotic fractures is increasing with the current increase in the age of the population.

Types of Osteoporosis

Classification of osteoporosis helps to some degree in assessment and management. Unfortunately, the several types overlap substantially. *Primary osteoporosis* is not associated with typical medical disorders known to produce bone loss. It includes idiopathic and involutional (i.e., postmenopausal and senile types).

Secondary osteoporosis includes a long list of disorders known to be associated with bone mass loss. The most common types are listed in Table 29.1. The complete list of secondary osteoporosis is important for diagnosis of rare cases of bone loss in a specialized clinic; the present selection shows the most important items for differential diagnostic approach in everyday practice. The overlap of osteoporosis types (i.e., involutional with secondary) is caused by the fact that causes of secondary osteoporosis appear also on the lists of factors in involutional osteoporosis such as physiologic primary hypogonadism of menopause and variable degree of calcium malabsorption in late involutional osteoporosis (Box 29.1). The difference between causes (of secondary osteoporosis) and factors (in involutional osteoporosis) is based on intensity and duration, which is more limited in factors than in causes.

The following text discusses only involutional osteoporosis in women and mentions the other types only as differential diagnosis issues. Primary idiopathic osteoporosis in women presents as either preadolescent or adult types. Both are rare and diagnosis follows from exclusion of all common causes of primary and secondary osteoporosis, obviously a task for a speciality clinic.

Involutional osteoporosis in women has a different pathogenesis and presentation in the early (<10 years) and late (>10 years) postmenopausal age. The early and late types have been labeled as type I and type II, respectively. Type III is a subtype of type II. The differences are listed in Table 29.2.

Table 29.1 Common Types of Secondary Osteoporosis

1. Endocrine disorders
   Glucocorticoid excess, endogenous, iatrogenic
   Hypogonadism in premenopausal female, endogenous, iatrogenic
   Thyroid hormone excess, endogenous, iatrogenic
   Parathyroid hormone excess, primary and secondary

2. Hematologic disorders
   Myeloma
   Chronic anemic states with bone marrow hyperplasia

3. Chronic systemic diseases
   Intestinal malabsorption, postgastrectomy state
   Severe liver disease
   Chronic renal failure
   Chronic inflammatory diseases including rheumatoid arthritis

4. Drugs and substances
   Anticonvulsants
   Immunosuppressants
   Alcohol
   Hormonal manipulations (overlaps with 1, e.g., antagonists of gonadotropin-releasing factor)

5. Deficiency states
   Vitamin D
   Calcium, phosphate

6. Disuse
   Protracted immobilization

7. Inborn errors
   Late presenting osteogenesis imperfecta
   Subtle disorders of collagen presenting as idiopathic or primary osteoporosis

This terminology will be used in this text for brevity.

Pathogenesis of Low Bone Mass—The Bone Bank

Cross-sectional and longitudinal studies of bone mineral content by accurate noninvasive procedures allow us to construct a lifetime profile of bone mass starting with initial growth, additional mineral gain after completion of growth (bone consolidation), peak bone mass, and subsequent age-related bone loss, accentuated for 3 to 6 years after menopause (Fig 29.1). The rate of loss in the spine is low before menopause, less than 1%/yr. In the first 3 years after menopause the loss totals an average 10% with substantial individual variation (slow and fast losers). About 6 years after menopause the rate is again 1%/yr or less. Cancellous bone, such as in the vertebral bodies and trochanters of proximal femur, has much higher surface per volume than cortical bone; it shows higher remodeling activity and bone loss, which appears early and is easily recognized by density measurement. During her lifetime a women loses an average 50% of bone from spine (predominantly cancellous) and 30% of cortical bone in appendicular skeleton.

Box 29.1 Factors in Involutional Osteoporosis in Women

White and Oriental race
Family history of involutional osteoporosis
Thin and small habitus
Postmenopausal age
Premature menopause
Amenorrhea in athletes
Cigarette smoking
Alcohol abuse
Sedentary life-style
*Low dietary calcium
*Vitamin D deficiency in the elderly
Falls in the elderly
*Current or previous corticoid medication
*Antiepileptic medication
*Thyroid replacement or suppression

*Overlap with secondary osteoporosis

The bone mass at a given time in adulthood depends on the initial peak value and on the rate of subsequent bone loss. The ideal course of bone mass profile (see Fig 29.1) may be disrupted by the effect of factors that, for a limited duration, accelerate the bone loss (e.g., secondary or type II osteoporosis).

When the absolute bone mass decreases to a level that substantially increases the incidence of insufficiency fractures (so-called *fracture threshold*), the woman suffers osteoporosis. In advanced age many apparently healthy women reach this degree of bone

Table 29.2 Types of Involutional Osteoporosis (Riggs and Melton)

Type	I	II	III
Etiology	Menopause	Aging	—
Age at presentation	50–70 yr	>70 yr	>70 yr
Bone loss	Rapid	Slow	Slow
Fracture type	Vertebral (crush)	Vertebral (multiple wedging)	
	Distal radius	Proximal femur	
Parathyroid function	Decreased*	Increased[a] statistically	Increased[a] measurably
Calcium absorption	Low (low 1,25-D)	Low (low 1,25-D, mucosal defect)	
Calcitriol (1,25-D)	Low (low PTH)	Low (production defect)	

* Parathyroid hormone (PTH) decreased because estrogen deficiency increases sensitivity to PTH
[a] Secondary hyperparathyroidism

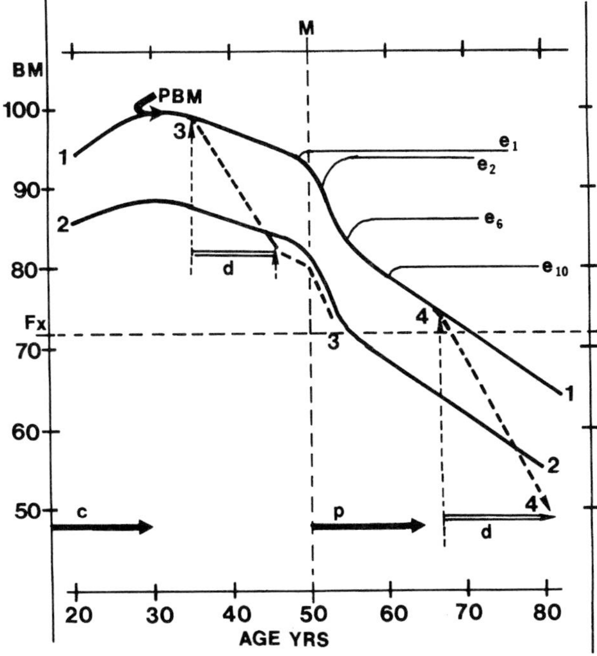

Fig 29.1 Lifetime profile of bone mass in women. BM, bone mass in percent of peak value (PBM). Curve 1–1, profile in an average woman showing bone gain after termination of growth (c, bone consolidation) and accelerated bone loss after menopause (M). Clinical presentation of postmenopausal osteoporosis extends into the seventh decade (p) though accelerated bone loss ceases after 4 to 5 years. Curve 2–2, profile in a woman with low peak mass (hereditary, environmental). Curve 3–3, accelerated bone loss due to transient factor (d), such as pharmacologic corticoid medication in premenopausal age. Curve 4–4, accelerated bone loss starting in postmenopausal age due to disorder (d) that persists, such as untreated calcium malabsorption in type II osteoporosis. Lines e1, e2, e6, and e10, effect of estrogen replacement at different times (in years) after onset of menopausal estrogen deficiency. The bone mass gain depends on the turnover of bone (reflected by the rate of bone loss) at the time of initiation of replacement. Fx, fracture threshold.

loss. The fracture threshold line is a favorite feature of bone density reports but provides only a rather incomplete description of patient's bone status because 1) as a function of bone mass fracture risk is a continuum, and consequently fractures may occur also in patients with bone mass above the threshold; 2) age increases risk of fracture independently of bone mass by a factor of two for each decade; and 3) previous fractures multiply the risk but are not considered in the threshold value.

Bone Remodeling—The Key to Understanding of Adult Bone

Understanding of the most important aspects of adult bone physiology—the bone remodeling process—is essential for understanding the pathogenesis of bone loss and the mechanisms of effects of agents used to prevent and treat osteoporosis. Many preventive and therapeutic decisions are based on this knowledge.

In the adult skeleton practically all bone activity is derived from bone remodeling. Bone remodeling is a focal and time-limited sequence of bone resorption that removes a definite volume of bone, followed by bone formation that replaces the volume of bone removed (Fig 29.2). Duration of resorption in adult women is about 1 month, whereas formation takes 3 to 4 months. The biologic function of bone remodeling is the removal of old bone damaged by material fatigue and microcracks and replace it with new, functionally more efficient bone. The main stimuli for the generation of this focal process are signals of

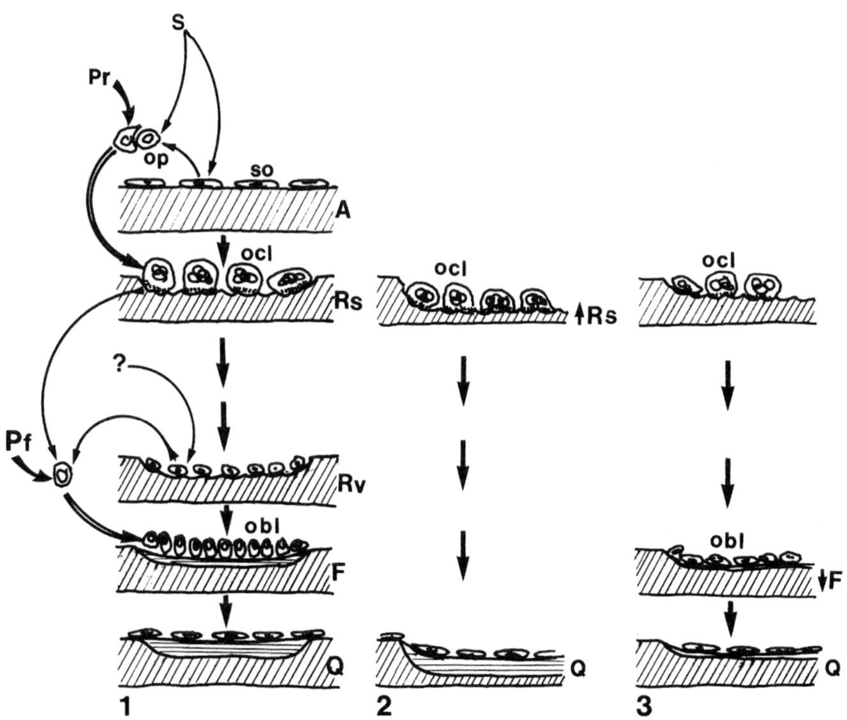

Fig 29.2 Remodeling cycle, remodeling balance. Panel 1, Activation (A). Initial stimulus (S) interacts with surface osteocytes (so) and osteoblast precursors (op), which in turn interact with osteoclast precursors (Pr) to stimulate differentiation and activity of osteoclasts (ocl), and initiate bone resorption (Rs). Rv, reversal. Osteoclasts are replaced by mononuclear cells of uncertain origin (?) and function. Humoral factors released from resorbed bone matrix and from resorbing cells interact with osteoblast precursors (Pf) to differentiate osteoblasts (obl) and initiate bone formation (F). New bone replaces removed bone completely and bone surface becomes quiescent (Q). Panel 2, Negative remodeling balance due to excessive osteoclastic activity (increased depth of resorption cavity) results in bone loss despite adequate osteoblast function. Important mechanism in early postmenopausal bone loss. Panel 3, Negative remodeling balance due to low osteoblastic activity. Important factor in type II and glucocorticoid osteoporosis.

bone damage possibily mediated by local autocrine and paracrine factors such as cytokines and prostaglandins.

Systemic factors such as hormones increase the generation of remodeling foci (bone remodeling units), possibly by triggering the remodeling process at lower threshold or independently of local damage signals, or suppressing the remodeling by opposite action. Parathyroid hormone, thyroid hormones, and growth hormone stimulate the generation of remodeling units, whereas corticoids, gonadal hormones, and practically all current agents used in treatment of osteoporosis have an inhibitory effect.

Changes of bone remodeling explain, among others, the irreversibility of bone loss and the fact that most current osteotropic drugs increase bone mass without stimulating bone formation (Figs 29.2 through 29.4). The most important implications are as follows. 1) A part of bone volume is always missing—at the sites of bone resorption as resorption cavities and at the sites of bone formation as osteoid and incompletely filled resorption cavities. This missing bone—called *bone remodeling space*—increases bone porosity and thins the trabeculae. Increased remodeling space is the pathogenetic basis of high turnover osteoporosis, a potentially reversible bone disease. 2) Under ideal circumstances, such as in young adults, the amount of bone removed is equal to the amount of bone replaced—the remodeling is in zero balance. However, in adults past the fourth decade of age the remodeling balance is negative; there is a small deficit in bone after each remodeling cycle. This is the cause of age-related bone loss. Because of negative remodeling balance, an increase of the number remodeling units produces accelerated bone loss in pathologic states. 3) Bone formation follows bone resorption and can occur only on preexisting bone surfaces. Complete removal of trabecular and cortical endosteal structures is an important cause of irreversibility of osteoporosis. 4) The phenomenon of transient states of bone remodeling reflects the definite duration and sequence of the processes of resorption and formation. Sudden application of a stimulus of bone remodeling, for example, overdose with L-thyroxine or oophorectomy, will produce a histologic and biochemical image of prevalent bone resorption and accelerated bone loss that will be followed only after several months by increased formation. Conversely, application of a factor or agent that inhibits bone resorption, such as estrogen in an estrogen-deficient woman, or calcitonin or bisphosphonate, will produce an image of prevalent bone formation and bone mass gain for up to 2

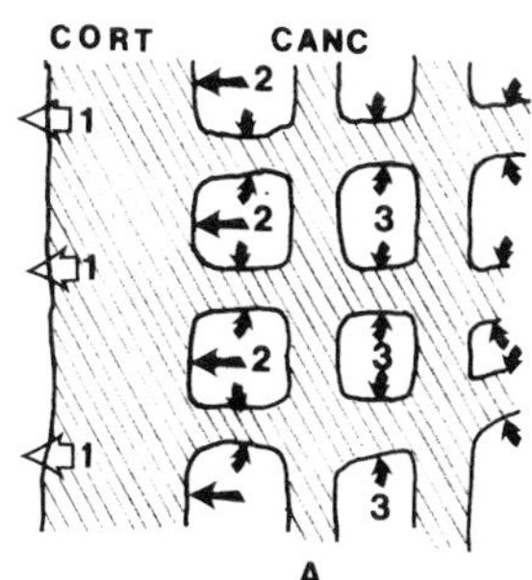

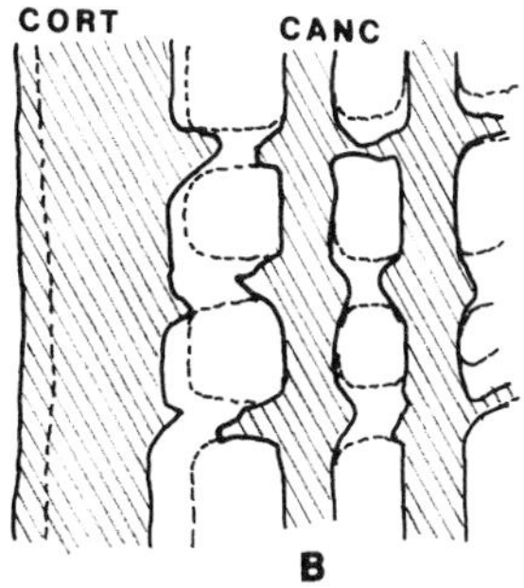

Fig 29.3 Structural changes. Bone expansion, cortical thinning, disconnnectivity. *A*, Cortical bone (CORT) and adjacent cancellous bone (CANC). Weight-bearing stress acts in the vertical direction. In cancellous bone loss the horizontal non-weight-bearing structures (trabeculae, plates) are resorbed (3) preferentially. Also the inner (endosteal) surface of cortex is resorbed (2) at higher rate, which expands the cancellous bone cavity. Periosteal bone tends to increase (1) but the cortical expansion is small and the balance of process (2) and (1) results in cortical thinning despite some bone expansion. *B*, The main result of process (3) is the loss of horizontal supportive structures, which results in buckling and fractures of weight-bearing structures—disconnectivity of cancellous bone increases fragility disproportionally to bone loss.

In addition, the complete loss of trabecular structures results in interruption of remodeling cycles because of loss of available surfaces for bone formation phase of remodeling—an important cause of irreversibility of osteoporosis. Endosteal bone loss is irreversible because of the same reason, in addition to the effect of prevailing negative remodeling balance on that surface.

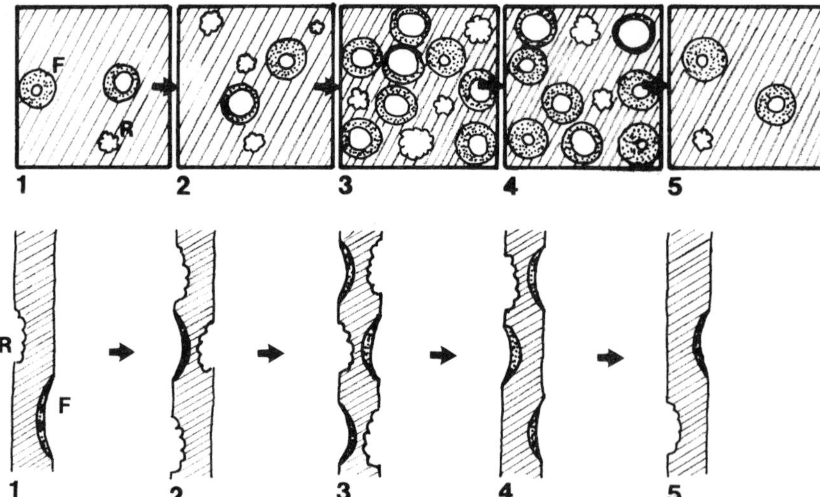

Fig 29.4 Bone turnover, remodeling space, transient states in remodeling. Upper panels, cortical bone, lower panels trabeculae of cancellous bone. Remodeling units present as holes in cortical bone and as surface defects on trabeculae. Resorption (R) marked as scalloped outlines, formation (F) as double surfaces with osteoid seams (*dotted areas*). Time sequence from left to right. Segments 1→2: bone turnover (activation frequency) increased four times. For the duration of resorption phase of remodeling, resorption activity predominates over formation, bone mass is lost. Segment 3: after 3 to 4 months, formation in balance with formation, bone mass decreased to minimum, in high turnover and steady state. Segments 3→4: stimulus that caused high turnover removed, activation frequency returned to baseline. Bone resorption decreased but bone formation units persist until formation in all remodeling units completed (3 to 4 months), formation predominates over resorption. If a researcher started to treat high turnover state (segment 3) with an antiresorptive agent he seemingly stimulated bone formation—the agent produced histologic and biochemical picture of increased formation over resorption. Segment 5: Bone activity and mass returned to baseline state in segment 1: high turnover osteoporosis present in segment 3 was reversible.

Remodeling space is the sum of bone deficit in the cavities of resorption and formation units. It represents a potential bone because the cavities will be filled with new bone when remodeling cycle is completed. Still it reduces bone mass, e.g., as measured by bone densitometry and increases the risk of fractures. It is potentially reversible if the cause of increased bone turnover is removed or—less specifically—the activity of osteoclasts inhibited.

years to be followed by a state of equally decreased resorption and formation (see Fig 29.4).

Bone Turnover

The level of resorptive and formative activity in the bone—the *bone turnover*—is determined primarily by the number of remodeling sites. In bone diseases high bone turnover usually signals the risk of rapid bone loss because of remodeling imbalance described above, which may be further aggravated by a specific effect of the disease itself, such as bone formation inhibition in corticoid excess, tobacco and alcohol abuse, and nutritional deficiencies. Low bone turnover, on the other hand, usually signals the absence of rapid bone loss but may result in a decline of bone quality because of accumulation of old bone with microcracks and decreased elasticity. This is a factor in the increased fragility of bone with advancing age and with glucocorticoid excess. Assessment of bone turnover is an important step in evaluation of osteoporosis and provides crucial information pertinent to use of antiresorptive agents.

Qualitative Changes Resulting in Fragility

Numerous studies document that decreased bone mass increases the risk of insufficiency fracture. The risk of fracture is a statistical concept that indicates that part of the population with a given decreased bone mass does not have insufficiency fractures. However even with this limitation it appears that bone mass as measured with current technology predicts up to 70% of fracture risk in the adult population. In the very old, bone quality and exogenous factors such as frequency and mechanics of falls play increasingly greater roles compared with bone mass.

Trabecular disconnectivity is one of qualitative changes that increases bone fragility. The process of thinning of trabeculae in cancellous bone such as vertebrae affects primarily the horizontal structures (see Fig 29.3) and may result in complete loss of trabeculae. The consequence is buckling and loss of strength of vertical weight-bearing trabeculae. In addition, the loss of structures, bone surfaces on which bone formation may start, causes abortive remodeling and limits the effectiveness of therapeutic agents that increase bone formation.

Material fatigue is the second qualitative change. Bone remodeling serves bone renewal. If bone remodeling fails to keep pace with generation of microcracks, the structural damage will accumulate without bone mass loss. Ultimately the structure fails and bone breaks. This is probably an important factor in increased fragility of bone with advancing age. This mechanism of qualitative bone damage generates a potential risk in excessive use of antiresorptive agents in osteoporosis (primarily bisphosphonates). Fortunately, thus far, no adverse effects of that nature have been observed.

Etiology of Postmenopausal (Type I) Osteoporosis

Decrease in estrogen level at the time of menopause increases bone turnover and accentuates the negative bone remodeling balance. The resorption phase of remodeling produces deeper resorption cavities, which are refilled with relatively smaller amounts of new bone. In addition, the deep resorption removes some trabecular structures completely and also removes the endosteal surfaces of bone cortices from within. Both mechanisms remove surfaces on which the formation phase of remodeling would proceed and thus interrupt the remodeling cycle. Substantial bone loss occurs, primarily of the cancellous bone, in the first 3 to 5 years after menopause. The rate and degree of bone loss varies substantially: about 26% of women lose bone at a yearly rate of 3% to 7.5%, but about 45% of women lose bone at a much slower rate (0% to 1%). Measurement of markers of bone turnover helps to identify the fast losers.

The mechanism of estrogen action is mediated by receptors on osteoblasts. In the absence of estrogen osteoblasts signal to osteoclast precursors and differentiated osteoclasts to enhance differentiation and activity. The details of signaling at this level are unknown.

Because of increased turnover in the early postmenopausal period, the bone will be more vulnerable to incidental pathogenic factors such as seen with concurrent thyroid, parathyroid, and corticoid hormone excess. The same holds true for nutritional deficiencies including calcium deficiency. The fact that bone mass loss due to estrogen deficiency cannot be prevented by high calcium intake cannot be interpreted as indicating that early postmenopausal women cannot become calcium deficient. Replacement of estrogen reverses the bone loss and actually increases the bone mass temporarily because of completion of ongoing remodeling sites—reduction of remodeling space. In addition, estrogen therapy may stabilize the bone mass so that even the slow, age-related bone loss disappears. Because of the mechanism of bone loss nonspecific antiresorptive agents such as calcitonin and bisphosphonates (preferably new-generation compounds) may be effective as alternative therapy if estrogens are contraindicated. Discontinuation of estrogen replacement results in accelerated bone loss similar to that after oophorectomy. There are no controlled studies but from what we know about the protective estrogen action the loss after estrogen discontinuation will be the greatest in early postmenopausal years and less pronounced at older age.

Other Hypoestrogenic States

The postmenopausal state is the most common but not the only hypoestrogenic state. In the premenopausal age bone mass loss (and amenorrhea) has been demonstrated with extreme physical activity in top athletes, ballet dancers, and anorexia nervosa, all associated with estrogen deficiency. Other endocrine disorders such as hyperprolactinemia, hypopituitarism, premature ovarian failure, ovarian agenesis, and women treated with gonadotropin-releasing hormone antagonists deserve similar attention.

Etiologic Factors in Type II Involutional Osteoporosis

The structual bone failure in older age is apparently a multifactorial disease in which both the cancellous and cortical bone are affected. Previous low peak bone mass and severe postmenopausal loss may set the stage. Additional factors increase the age-related bone loss.

Calcium deficiency due to low dietary intake is often present and documented in national studies. It is aggravated by inadequate conservation of calcium by renal tubular reabsorption, which constitutes the obligatory renal calcium loss related to high salt and protein intake. *Calcium malabsorption* has been documented in many elderly women. Decreased response of the intestine to calcitriol (1,25-dihydroxyvitamin D), the principal regulatory factor of calcium absorption, was documented in some patients and a decreased production of calcitriol from calcidiol (25-hydroxyvitamin D) in others. In addition, this population may be subject to *vitamin D deprivation* because of insufficient dietary sources of vitamin D, indoors confinement, decreased production of vitamin D in the skin (lower levels of precursors), and probably higher requirements.

Vitamin K deficiency has been described in this population and may aggravate the calcium balance by the mechanism of insufficient production of renal proteins involved in calcium reabsorption.

Vitamin D and calcium disturbances result in *secondary hyperparathyroidism,* which represents the ultimate cause of accelerated bone loss. An extreme degree of this condition with persistent presence of measurable elevation of serum parathyroid hormone is designated type III osteoporosis. In addition, histology demonstrates a *declining function of osteoblasts* reflected by diminished amount of bone deposited at the end of remodeling cycle. Age-related accumulation of old bone due to ineffective remodeling decreases the quality of bone.

Osteoporotic fractures of the elderly show much less dependence on bone mass, apparently because of substantial reduction of bone mass in most subjects in that population and because of an increasing role of substantial qualitative deterioration of bone and increasing frequency of falls. Falls to the side rather than forward or backward are especially important. Increased incidence of falls is related to sensorimotor deterioration, lack of coordination, visual impairment, and associated diseases of the musculoskeletal, cardiovascular, and nervous systems. Polypharmacy plays a definite role.

Clinical Presentation

Insufficiency Fractures

In general the gradual bone loss is asymptomatic until structural failure manifests itself as an *insufficiency (osteoporotic) fracture* also called a fragility fracture. The term indicates a fracture that occurs with inappropriate, minimal, or apparently no force. These terms are relative to expected bone strength and consequently somewhat vague. Any bone may fracture in osteoporosis, but typical are wrist, vertebral, and proximal femur (hip) fractures in typical order of appearance in women. Whereas wrist and hip fractures are most likely associated with falls, vertebral compression fractures happen most likely without an obvious impact injury. In her lifetime, a 50-year-old white woman has a 16% risk of wrist fracture, 32% of vertebral fracture, and 15% of hip fracture.

Vertebral Compression Deformity

Vertebral compression fracture is a hallmark of postmenopausal osteoporosis. Unlike other fractures it leaves permanent deformity even after healing, that is, after disappearance of callus, biochemical evidence of bone turnover, and focal accumulation of radionuclide on bone scan. Typically vertebrae from T4 down are involved with maximum at the peak of thoracic kyphosis (T7–T8) and at the thoraolumbar transition (T12–L1). On lateral radiograms of the spine the vertebral body shows wedging from decreased anterior height, or central compression from decreased central height, or crush (vertebra plana) deformity with decreased anterior and posterior height (Fig 29.5). The prevalence of vertebral deformities increases with age after menopause, from about 5/100 in the sixth decade to close to 30/100 in the eighth decade.

Not all vertebral deformities are diagnostic of osteoporotic fractures. Some are sequelae of old injuries, forgotten or unrecognized as fractures at the time of accident, others are due to juvenile kyphosis (Scheuermann), and still others reflect benign or ma-

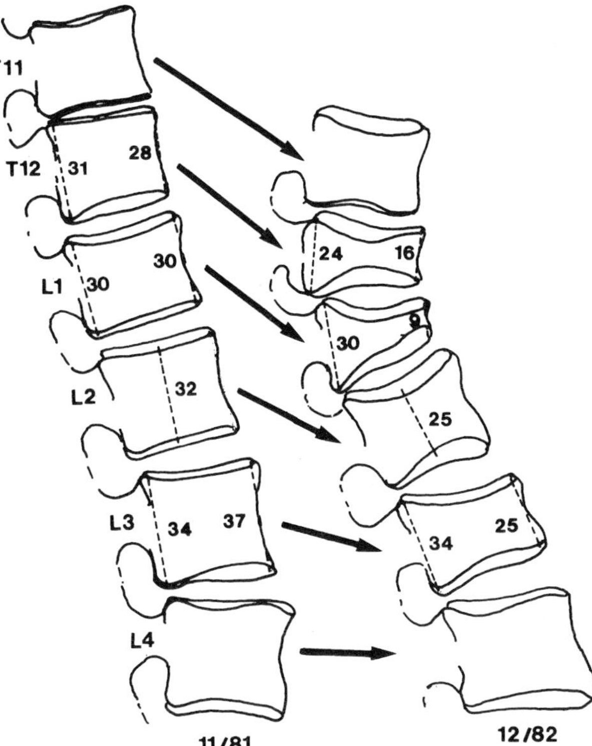

Fig 29.5 Vertebral deformities. Tracings of lateral radiograms of lower thoracic and lumbar spine of a 60-year-old white woman with postmenopausal osteoporosis accelerated by surreptitious alcohol abuse. Radiograms obtained in November 1981 and December 1982 show rapid development of vertebral compression deformities: in T12 crush fracture with substantial decrease of both posterior and anterior vertebral height; in L1 and L3 wedging deformity with decreased anterior height; in L2 central compression with decreased central height. Measurements (in mm) are of posterior, central, and anterior heights of vertebral bodies in vertebrae of interest. Sites of measurement marked with interrupted vertical lines. Both films were obtained with standard radiographic techniques. The shortening of spine (stature) and development of low thoracic kyphosis reflect actual changes in the patient.

lignant local disease. It is probable that a number of thoracic wedging deformities result from adjustment of vertebral shape to habitual slumped posture. Such wedging is typically of mild to moderate degree, fairly uniform in several vertebrae, and associated with thoracic hyperkyphosis without measurable osteopenia.

Quantitation of vertebral deformity has developed from plain inspection of radiograms through measurement of vertebral heights, widths, and wedging angles into digitizing of images and computerized processing of data including comparision with normative data automatically. Some recent instruments originally designed for bone density measurement have the capability of concurrent assessment of compression deformities in lateral vertebral images.

Thoracic vertebral wedging results in accentuation of thoracic kyphosis, which, in turn forces cervical and lumbar hyperlordosis. Shortening of thoracic and lumbar spine results in loss of body height, protrusion of abdomen, and contact between lower ribs and pelvic rim (Fig 29.6).

Hip Fractures

Cervical and transtrochanteric fractures of the proximal femur in osteoporosis do not differ from other fractures on radiography. Their incidence in white women increases with age rather rapidly from about 1/100 patient-years at age 50 to 16 at age 75 to 80 to 33 at age over 80. Risk of fracture increases with decreased bone density by a factor 2.6 for each 10% to 15% of decrease of bone mass. In addition, the length of femoral neck is directly proportional to fracture risk. Unlike vertebral fractures hip fractures are typically associated with trauma (falls) in a majority (90%) of cases. Hip fractures are trypical for older women and cause substantial morbidity and increased mortality. Five to 20% of fracture victims do not survive the first year after fracture and over 50% become incapacitated and dependent.

Pain in Osteoporosis

The typical acute compression fracture is a clinically distinct event with sudden onset of pain of great intensity localized at the level of fracture that lasts several weeks and gradually improves. Involvement of lower thoracic segments may produce abdominal symptomatology of adynamic ileus. Spasm of paravertebral muscles aggravates the misery. The acute pain is followed by much less intense discomfort often localized at the lower spine level, most likely reflecting strain from the changes of spinal configuration. Epidemiologic studies indicate that many vertebral compressions, possibly over 50%, are asymptomatic. The

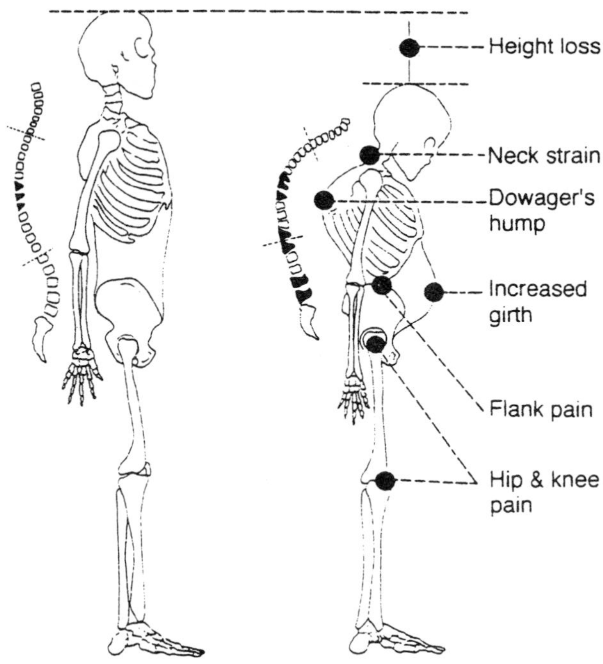

Fig 29.6 Secondary events in spinal osteoporosis with compressions. A number of symptoms in patients with vertebral compressions are not from bone pain at the site of fracture.

reason is not clear. In many patients the pain may be relatively mild and misinterpreted as strain, disc disease, or spondylosis. Radiography may not be performed or may be misleading because of delayed development of overt deformity.

Chronic pain in osteoporotic vertebral deformities is mostly due to changed spinal anatomy. Low back and neck pain is due to compensatory hyperlordosis; abdominal pain is due to contact of lower ribs with pelvic rim and hip pain is from abnormal pelvic tilt. Secondary osteoarthrosis of vertebral joints is another source. All these types of pain are frequently sources of anxiety in patients who worry about new fractures and progression of osteoporosis. Even though osteoporosis is called the silent thief it is probable that severely decreased bone mass without overt fractures (prefracture stage of osteoporosis) may hurt, most likely because of subclinical fractures, quite often demostrable as focal lesions on bone scintigrams. In addition to spine (from T4 down), the pelvis and lower extremities may be affected by this type of pain.

Diagnosis of Osteoporosis (Fig 29.7)

Bone Mass Measurement

From the definition of osteoporosis it follows that assessment of bone mass is part of the diagnostic process. Bone densitometry measures bone mineral content with great precision and at sites subject to osteoporotic fractures—spine, proximal femur, and distal forearm. Inspection of radiograms cannot provide information of comparable sensitivity, accuracy, and precision. A number of longitudinal studies confirm the common sense notion that decreased bone mass increases the risk of insufficiency fractures. A decrease of 10% to 15% below age-matched normal mean value (−1 SD, Z score) increases the risk of fracture by a factor of 2 to 2.5.

Dual Energy Absorptiometry

This noninvasive procedure of bone mineral content measurement developed from single- and dual-pho-

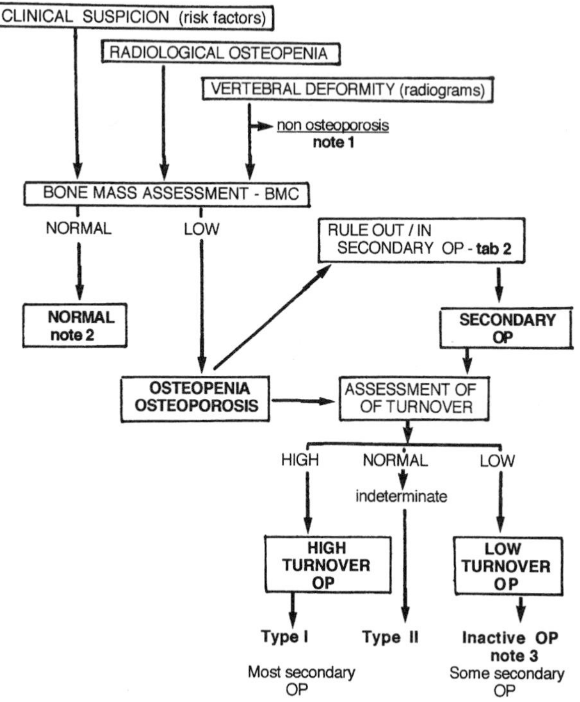

Fig 29.7 Diagnosis and assessment of osteoporosis (OP).

ton absorptiometry into the current procedure, the dual energy x-ray absorptiometry (DEXA, DXA). DXA uses x-rays of two definite energies that are absorbed to different degrees in the soft tissues and in the bone. Computation eliminates the contribution of soft tissues and net absorption of the radiation in the bone is converted into units of mass of bone mineral. The dose of radiation is small. Typical sites of measurement are L1–L4 vertebrae, proximal femur, and forearm bones. Because osteoporosis is a systemic disease, in many cases measurement at one site is sufficient. The lumbar spine is the traditional site, most commonly used and most accurate, but the proximal femur is probably more relevant and informative. Results of measurement are reported as bone mineral content and bone mineral density, the latter is derived from the former by correcting for the size of projected bone image and thus for bone size. The report also contains a comparision with normative data and some assessment of fracture risk (due to decreased bone mass), such as the fracture threshold.

Quatitative Computed Tomography

This procedure uses multipurpose computed tomography (CT) scanners with additional software and calibration accessories. The advantage of the procedure is its capability to measure bone density separately in the cancellous and cortical bone of the vertebral body and minimal interference of extravertebral calcified structures such as osteophytes and aortic calcifications. Disadvantages are its limitation to spine measurement, lower accuracy, high radiation dose (an order higher than DXA), and cost.

Ultrasound in Bone Assessment

Ultrasound techniques for measurement of bone quantity, and possibly quality, differ from ultrasound used in medical imaging in their lower frequency (100 to 300 kHz versus 1000+ kHz) and mode of application. Accessible bone (calcaneus, patella) is placed between sending and receiving transducers. The instrument measures changes of ultrasound velocity and attenuation in the bone. Changes in sound velocity and attenuation are thought to reflect—in addition to bone density—bone elasticity and architecture, respectively. Commercially produced instruments are available. The advantages of procedure are the absence of ionizing radiation, low cost, and assessment of bone quality. Large scale evaluations and validations of the technique are not available.

Interpretation and Indications of Bone Densitometry

A patient's measurements are compared with reference values for healthy young subjects of the same sex (peak bone mass) and with an age-matched population. The difference is expressed as percent of expected value or, statistically more correctly, in units a standard deviation from the peak value (T score) and from age-matched value (Z score). For the purpose of orientation the values of standard deviation are close to 10%. Even though black women show 3% to 5% higher bone mass, this correction is rarely applied and has to be considered in the interpretation.

A single value of bone density, for example, in an early postmenopausal woman, cannot distinguish between a subject with a low peak bone mass at age 30 to 35 years, from a subject with previous normal peak bone mass and subsequent bone loss, or a combination of both. Neither can a low value indicate whether the patient is losing bone at the time of evaluation or whether the loss occurred in a time-limited event (disease, treatment) years ago and the condition is stable and inactive at the present. Absolute value of bone density is, however, always an index of fracture risk and thus represents important information pertinent to management.

In 1989, the American Society for Bone and Mineral Research with the National Osteoporosis Foundation published a report on clinical indications for bone mass measurement primarily because of problems with reimbursement for the test. In that report the principal indications are 1) estrogen deficiency, premenopausal and postmenopausal, 2) abnormal radiologic findings on the vertebrae, that is, vertebral deformity (compression) and the radiologist's impression of low bone density, 3) mild primary hyperparathyroidism to help the decision about neck exploration, and 4) treatment with glucocorticoids to weigh risks versus benefits of pharmacologic corticoids. Additional potential indications originally mentioned but not recommended were universal screening for osteoporosis prophylaxis and repeated measurements to assess the efficacy of therapy and identify "fast losers" of bone for more aggressive therapy.

Follow-up bone mass measurements are now more frequently recommended in management of osteoporosis. Their usefulness depends on the precision of the instrument in relation to expected changes of bone mass. Precision error has decreased substantially with the current instruments (e.g., for vertebral measurements from 3% for dual photon to <1% for DEXA). This has improved our ability to detect changes between two measurements from 8.3% to 2.7% of bone mass. Obviously only the higher precision instruments can detect changes expected in clinical practice, such as age-associated ("normal") loss at about 1%, accelerated at 2% to 3%, and rapid postmenopausal at 5% to 6%. The clinician using follow-up data of densitometry for decision-making should be aware of the precision factor and should inquire about the precision of the procedure, especially because the precision may vary substantially among laboratories depending on their quality control.

Bone Turnover Assessment

The sum of bone resorption and formation activities of all remodeling units in the skeleton reflects the bone turnover, and in systemic bone disease such as osteoporosis, the activity of bone disease. Histologic studies indicate that in randomly selected osteoporotic women the turnover may be low, normal, or high. More carefully selected populations show more consistent changes, such as increased bone turnover in early postmenopausal years, or in involutional osteoporosis with secondary hyperparathyroidsm due to calcium or vitamin D disturbances.

Because of remodeling imbalance we can presume that high bone turnover signals rapid bone loss at the time of observation. Long-term observations showed that in normal postmenopausal women indices of bone turnover predict the rate of bone loss for years ahead.

Assessment of bone turnover helps in selecting immediate measures, specifically how aggressively to use antiresorptive agents (e.g., estrogens in postmenopausal women) and in secondary osteoporosis how aggressively to treat the underlying cause.

Biochemical Indices of Bone Turnover

Routine "sequential multiple analysis" is a part of initial evaluation along with blood count and urinalysis. Among those data the level of (total) serum alkaline phosphatase provides some information on bone turnover; however, because of the presence of other than bone fractions of alkaline phosphatase the test has a low sensitivity. An array of more specific tests has been described and validated against histomorphometric data.

Bone formation is reflected by bone specific serum alkaline phosphatase, which is produced by osteoblasts. Serum osteocalcin, another bone-specific protein produced by osteoblasts and split products of processing of procollagen I (C and N extension peptides) in the process of bone matrix synthesis are more specific but less readily available and more expensive markers. Bone resorption is reflected by urinary excretion of collagen split products, hydroxyproline peptides, and with more specificity by remnants of cross-links of mature collagen, the pyridinolines. Fasting calciuria may reflect the same, if interference of a number of physiologic and pathologic factors is considered. It is important to consider also the presence of a substantial local bone lesion such as extensive comminutive fracture or bone surgery, which will affect biochemical markers in the same manner as systemic bone disease.

Because of the variable sensitivity of individual tests it is impossible to make a quantitative judgment as to the prevalence of either resorption or formation in osteoporosis. The use of biochemical markers of bone turnover will depend mostly on the clinical setting and therefore on the clinician's decision. It will not be necessary in early postmenopausal women with negative history of diseases and taking no medication potentially affecting the bone; it may be mandatory if there is a history of rapid sequence of fractures or apparent failure of usual therapy, such as an effective dose of estrogen.

Substantial information on calcium and phosphate, calcium-regulating hormones, and bone turnover can be obtained on an outpatient basis as follows. A 2-hour second void urine specimen is collected after an overnight fast along with a blood specimen drawn in the middle of urine collection period. Blood and urine are submitted for calcium, phosphorus, and creatinine and for additional tests as indicated, for example, serum osteocalcin, parathyroid hormone, and 25-hydroxyvitamin D, urine for total hydroxyproline or pyridinolines. Data on urine are expressed per mg (mmol) of urinary creatinine to avoid inaccuracy of short-time urine collection and to normalize for lean body mass. The phosphorus indices, tubular reabsorption and theoretical renal threshold of phosphate, are computed from serum and urine data.

Technetium Bisphosphonate Scintigram

The bone scan is primarily used to detect the multifocal image of metastatic bone disease in the differential diagnosis of osteoporosis, but it is also useful for detection of subclinical fractures as a source of pain and differentiation of new from old compression deformities. The procedure can be modified to a quantitative method and uptake of the radionuclide can be measured as an index of bone turnover, that is, bone formation. An experienced radiologist may provide similar information semiquantitatively from a diffusely increased uptake of the nuclide, especially in the metaphyseal regions of bones on a technically satisfactory scintigram.

Bone Biopsy and Histomorphometry

Bone histomorphometry has been the principal source of knowledge on bone physiology and pathogenesis of osteoporosis. It is rarely used in clinical diagnosis of osteoporosis because it is invasive, time consuming, and expensive. The patient has to be prepared by two doses of tetracycline about 10 days apart, and after the second dose the bone is obtained from the anterior superior ilium with a large-bore trocar. The specimen is processed in undecalcified state in a polyacrylic resin. A number of data are measured pertinent to bone resorption and formation, typically by computerized image analysis.

Differential Diagnosis of Secondary Osteoporosis

History and physical examination often raise suspicion and lead to referral to a specialized clinic for appropriate diagnostic procedures to identify the underlying disorder in secondary osteoporosis, such as documentation of excessive production of corticoids (urinary free cortisol-creatinine ratio in a 24-hour specimen), parathyroid hormone (serum calcium and pararthyroid hormone by a double antibody procedure), or thyroid hormones (serum free thyroxine and thyroid-stimulating hormone).

It appears that 20% to 30% of women of postmenopausal age presenting for evaluation of osteoporosis have an important pathogenetic factor besides estrogen deficiency. Only minor degrees of biochemical abnormalities may be present when such factors are present in involutional osteoporosis and may require substantial testing (e.g., for primary renal hypercalciuria, hypercorticism—surreptitious from self-administration or endogenous presenting without cushingoid features, iatrogenic T_3 overdose from thyroid extract, endogenous T_3 toxicosis in multinodular goiter, denied alcohol abuse, phosphate depletion from aluminum hydroxide antacid abuse, etc.).

The presence of such contributing factors in involutional osteoporosis may be discovered if routine management of osteoporosis fails to result in satisfactory clinical response. The clinician should follow patients after institution of therapy and if in doubt should order follow-up bone densitometry and biochemical markers of bone turnover to rule out continuous bone loss and persistence of high bone turnover because current therapeutic approaches invariably contain an antiresorptive agent, which is expected to decrease bone turnover.

In older women, calcium status is an issue because of the possibility of calcium malabsorption and vitamin D disturbances. Therefore type II osteoporosis overlaps with secondary osteoporosis (see Table 29.1). Serum levels of calcium are mostly normal and nondiagnostic because of calcium homeostasis mechanisms that are the cause of bone loss in such clinical setting. There is no easy way to assess the efficacy of calcium absorption outside of research protocols. Demonstration of a low fasting and 24-hour urinary calcium-creatinine ratio is the best available approach if a problem is suspected. Response of calciuria to calcium and vitamin D (or calcitriol) administration further clarifies this issue. Because vitamin D depletion may be present and calcium malabsorption results in secondary hyperparathyroidism, look for low levels of serum 25-hydroxyvitamin D, increased parathyroid hormone, and evidence of increased bone turnover by biochemical markers.

Such detailed biochemical testing is not warranted in most patients with type II osteoporosis. Careful follow-up will reveal therapeutic failure and indicate the need for detailed studies, most likely in a speciality clinic.

Management of Osteoporosis

Management aims at pain relief, termination of bone loss, and restoration of bone mass. Assessment of severity and activity of bone disease on presentation is necessary for a decision about how aggressively to use antiresorptive agents to stop bone loss. Search for evidence of substantial participation of factors known to produce bone loss (secondary osteoporosis) leads to measures that remove the causes (e.g., exogenous thyrotoxicosis, unrecognized hyperparathyroidism, unindicated doses of glucocorticoids) or to additional measures against noxious factors that cannot be removed (e.g., immunosuppression in transplant patients or antiepileptics in seizure patients). After initial measures take effect long-term management is implemented. Unfortunately current means are ineffective to restore bone mass in involutional osteoporosis.

Pain Management

Bed rest usually need not to be ordered because the patient is bedridden with pain. Duration of rest is 7 to 10 days. Mild narcotics (e.g., propoxyphene or codeine) and diazepam for muscle spasm are given. Many patients are overwhelmed with pain, especially if they experienced a series of recurrent compressions. Active counseling about the transient nature of pain in compressions is often effective in relieving anxiety and depression. Narcotics should not be used indefinitely. Spinal bracing helps when the patient resumes upright activity. When the acute stage resolves with bed rest, the patient is allowed upright activity starting with the minimum necessary for independence at home and increasing gradually. For exacerbation of pain the patient is advised to recline flat for 15 to 20 minutes. Sitting down does not decrease the weight-bearing stress on the spine and therefore does not relieve pain. Concurrent measures taken to stop bone loss most likely do not affect the initial pain. It is honest to tell the patient that improvement of pain she experiences at that time is the natural course of events rather than an effect of an osteotropic agent, with the possible exception of calcitonin.

Calcium Supplementation and Vitamin D

Numerous studies indicate that postmenopausal women on estrogen replacement require 1000 mg of elemental calcium daily and those without replacement 1500 mg. These are guideline values recommended to cover the broad population and presume a vitamin-repleted state. In healthy subjects the individual variation of calcium requirement is substantial. It results in part from obligatory urinary calcium loss, which increases with intake of salt (sodium excretion) and protein (excretion of acid load, primarily sulfate from sulfur containing amino acids).

Providing calcium from dietary sources and supplements will prevent calcium depletion also in early postmenopausal women. The fact that estrogen-dependent early rapid postmenopausal bone loss cannot be prevented with calcium should not result in denial of adequate calcium intake. Recent studies on the involutional osteoporosis of the elderly indicate that routine administration of 800 U vitamin D daily along with calcium supplements prevents progression of osteoporosis and protects against fractures. Serum level of 25-hydroxyvitamin D is used to assess vitamin D repletion in a subject. Even though the normal range is 12 to 55 mg/mL, the target value in this population is in the upper range of normal (30 to 35 ng/mL). A smaller proportion of elderly women will not respond to supplemental vitamin D with increased levels of 1,25-dihydroxyvitamin D and improved calcium absorption. Again the only practical way to find out is to measure urinary calcium. If persistent malabsorption is proven, the patient should receive calcitriol (1,25-dihydroxycholecalciferol) 0.25-0.50 μg PO daily.

The most common source of supplemental calcium is calcium carbonate, including oyster shell calcium. Tablets are labeled by the content of elemental calcium, except possibly USP calcium carbonate tablets 650 mg (equals 250 mg elemental calcium). Bioavailabilty may be a problem in some generic formulations. Carbonate should be used with meals to ensure absorption in gastric anacidity. Other calcium compounds such as citrate and malate are water soluble and more effectively absorbed even if taken on empty stomach. One brand of calcium phosphate is available for limited but important use in patients with concurrent need for calcium and phosphate supplementation, such as in corticoid osteoporosis. Many over-the-counter preparations of vitamin D (vitamin D_2, ergocalciferol), 400 U dose are available, some mixed with calcium carbonate. Calcitriol is available as a prescription (Rocaltrol) in 0.25 and 0.5 μg strength. It is rather expensive for continuous use.

Physical Activity and Exercise

There is no doubt that disuse from immobilization and a weightless state result in bone loss that may occur at a rate of 3% to 4% a month and the bone density difference between habitually active and sedentary women may be 6% to 7%. Controlled exercise programs usually result in a modest gain of 2% to 3% at best; they cannot counteract the effects of estrogen deficiency and disappear if activity ceases. Consequently increased physical activity to the extent applicable to osteoporotic patient population has rather limited effect on bone mass. Other effects of physical activity and exercise are probably more important. Resistance exercise improves muscle strength, flexibility, and coordination. Back muscle exercises as described from the Mayo Clinic prevent deterioration of postural deformities in spinal compressions, and simple walking in the elderly maintains coordination to prevent falls.

Antiresorptive Agents

All agents used to inhibit rapid bone loss by inhibiting the function of osteoclasts decrease the generation of new remodeling units at the same time. Their mechanism of action on the process of remodeling is the same whether they are administered as replacement for physiologic estrogens or nonspecific inhibitors such as bisphosphonates. Antiresorptive agents produce a transient remodeling state characterized by relative predominance of formation over resorption activity and by temporary gain of bone mass due to filling of remodeling spaces. The changes are transient and limited in quantity of bone gain. They disappear in 1 to 2 years depending on the duration of the remodeling cycle, despite continuation of therapy. The bone mass gain is higher in a high turnover bone state than in a low turnover state when it may not be demonstrable at all. This, of course, again reflects the effect of bone remodeling space. Prolonged, much slower, bone gain (>2 years) has been observed with some antiresorptive agents. It may have to do with a decrease of remodeling (less effect of remodeling imbalance), or improvement of remodeling imbalance due to restriction of the resorption depth without affecting the formation that follows, or due to accumulation of old, highly mineralized bone (Fig 29.8). The temporary gain in bone mass has been frequently misinterpreted as stimulation of bone formation.

Estrogens

Estrogens are indicated for prevention and treatment of osteoporosis in early menopause and at that time they are considered hormonal replacement therapy. Their effect on bone remodeling, bone mass, and prevention of insufficiency fractures has been well documented and constitutes the principal indication for their use. Because of the time limitation of the rapid bone loss to 3 to 6 years after menopause, in the recent past the use of estrogen replacement was thought to be limited to 5 to 6 years. Subsequent studies demonstrated estrogen effectiveness also in type II osteoporosis. Moreover, discontinuation of estrogen resulted in rapid bone loss similar to that after menopause or oophorectomy. It is a matter or semantics whether the use of estrogens a long time after menopause is called hormonal replacement or antiresorptive therapy with a suitable physiologic agent (see Fig 29.1).

Oral forms of estrogens, such as conjugated equine estrogens (Premarin, mixture of several equine estrogens, effective component is estrone sulfate), other estrone conjugates (e.g., sulfate, piperazine sulfate [Ogen]), or micronized estradiol (Estrace) are all converted in the intestine and liver into estrone, which is in biochemical equilibrium with estradiol, the active hormone. The high levels of estrogens reaching the liver after oral administration induce biochemical changes, some beneficial (changes in lipoproteins, especially increase of high-density lipoproteins), some possibly adverse, such as angiotensinogen.

The effective doses have been established in clinical studies using bone mass as a criterion. For conjugated equine estrogens the dose is 0.625 mg, for micronized estradiol 0.5–1.0 mg, and for some estrone conjugates (Ogen) possibly 1.25 mg.

From parenteral preparations, the transdermal system of estradiol (Estraderm) has been evaluated and found effective in a 0.05-mg dose. There is not enough information on long acting-injectable estradiol esters (valerate, cypionate).

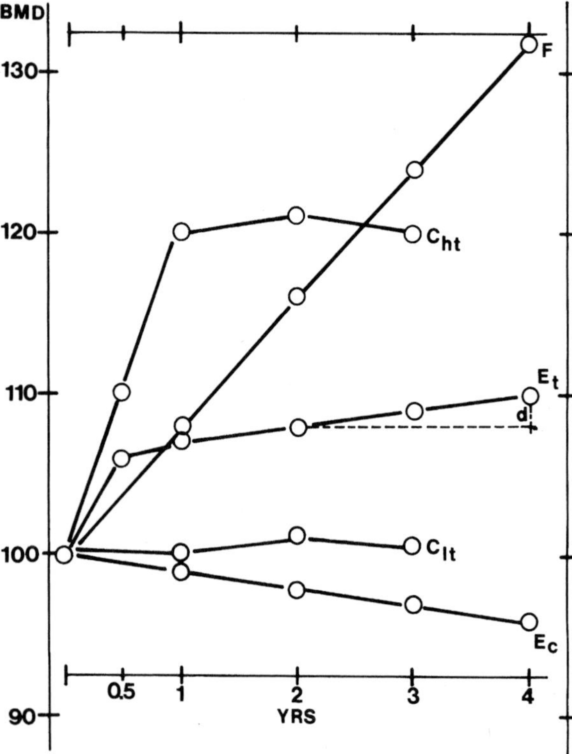

Fig 29.8 Response of bone density to therapy of osteoporosis. The graph is a schematized composite of work of several research groups. Vertebral bone mineral density (BMD) is expressed as percent of initial value (100%) and is plotted against duration of treatment (years, yrs) with active agent. Line E_c is data on typical control group, showing loss of BMD at about 1% a year. Curve C_{ht} shows the marked effect of salmon calcitonin injections in patients with high bone turnover (by biochemical markers), whereas the same treatment in patients with low turnover had no effect (C_{lt}). E_t shows effect of intermittent oral etidronate in osteoporotic patients with unknown turnover status, probably a mix of high, normal, and low turnover. As with other antiresorptive agents (e.g., C_{ht}) the rate of bone gain slows down after 12 to 24 months (depending on the average duration of remodeling cycle in the group of patients). With bisphosphonates there may be a continuous slow gain after 2 years (d) probably reflecting a decreased depth of osteoclastic resorption with normal thickness of newly formed bone—a positive remodeling balance. Curve F shows an almost linear and continuous increase after fluoride, the only agent that stimulates bone formation.

With an effective dose the clinician can expect a satisfactory response. The question of nonresponders to estrogens has not been resolved; estimates are that the range between 0% to 5% of patients are nonresponders. Part of the problem is uncertainty about serum levels of estrogens in replacement therapy. Follicle-stimulating hormone level is not a suitable marker of effective estrogen levels because normalization to premenopausal levels is not expected in estrogen replacement. In cases when impaired intestinal absorption (or noncompliance) is suspected serum levels of estradiol can be considered. Experts agree that levels above 40 pg/mL (in laboratories with early follicular reference 40 to 60) are effective. Serum levels of estrone are very high with oral preparations and substantially vary with time from administration. Assay of estrone does not provide useful information. Because the effect of estrogens on biochemical markers of bone resorption is quite profound and reproducible, biochemical studies may be indicated 2 to 3 months after initiation of treatment. With bone densitometry it takes at least 1 year or more (depending on instrument precision) of treatment to show changes in the rate of bone loss.

An estrogen agonist/antagonist, tamoxifene, shows a substantial estrogenic activity on bone (and endometrium) in women while conveniently lacking an effect on the mammary gland. It decreases bone turnover by biochemical and histologic criteria and bone loss by densitometry. It exerts a protective effect on bone if used in patients with breast cancer who cannot take estrogens. An analogue of tamoxifene, raloxifene, shows similar activity on bone without affecting either the breast or endometrium. Study of this group of drugs reflects a search for an ideal substance with partial estrogenic activity.

Progestins

Progestins are used along with estrogens in women who did not have hysterectomy to prevent endometrial hyperplasia and increased risk of endometrial cancer. Several dosage patterns have been recommended primarily to decrease the chance of monthly vaginal bleed in postmenopausal women. The efficacy of *all* regimens depends on the estrogen dose.

In general, high doses of progestins slow down cortical bone loss. There are two types of progestins: 1) derivatives of 21 carbon steroid 17-hydroxyprogesterone, such as medroxyprogesterone acetate (Provera and other brands) and 2) derivatives of 19-nortestosterone such as norethindrone acetate (Norlutate). The former type is commonly used in combination with estrogen and appears to have a small additive effect if estrogen is used in low dose. The latter has possibly mild anabolic action—stimulates bone formation. If confirmed this beneficial effect probably reflects the chemical relationship to androgens, which is expressed also in the adverse effect on high-density lipoproteins. Norethindrone was used successfully in postmenopausal women with primary hyperparathyroidism to reduce calcemia and biochemical markers of bone turnover.

Anabolic androgens, such as nandrolone decanoate (Decadurabolin injections), and stanozolol (Winstrol tablets), are also primarily antiresorptive agents, but probably also stimulate bone formation. This group of agents produced the expected increase of bone density and unlike estrogens also an increase of muscle mass. The increase of muscle mass created artifacts resulting in overestimation of bone density by techniques used at that time. Virilizing effects and potentially adverse effects on cholesterol fractions make this group of hormones unacceptable to most women irrespective of age.

Calcitonin

Calcitonin in one of the calcium regulation hormones of low potency in physiologic concentrations. In pharmacologic doses it inhibits osteoclasts by direct interaction with osteoclastic receptors. Synthetic salmon calcitonin is most commonly used because of high potency. Besides its antiresorptive activity it appears to have a direct analgesic effect, the mechanism of which is unknown. Injectable and intranasal forms are available. The doses vary between 50 and 100 U/day; the dosage varies from continuous to a variety of intermittent schedules used to avoid a decline of activity of the hormone, due to blocking antibodies or down regulation of receptors, or both. Concomitant calcium supplements are necessary to avoid hypocalcemia and secondary hyperparathyroidism, which counteracts the effects of calcitonin.

There is disagreement whether intranasal calcitonin is effective in prevention of bone loss in early osteoporosis. The cost of therapy is substantial, especially if intended for continous application. A typical indication for limited treatment is a patient with acute pain and evidence of high turnover bone disease who probably benefits most from parenteral application of calcitonin. Duration of treatment depends on the response (pain, biochemical markers) and availability of a feasible alternative antiresorptive agent. If estrogens are contraindicated calcitonin itself becomes an alternative.

Bisphosphonates

Bisphosphonates are analogues of pyrophosphate. Unlike pryrophosphate they are resistant to the effect of pyrophosphatase and show a portracted action. Similarly to pyrophosphate they bind to the surface of crystals of bone mineral, but the mechanism of their action is not clear and probably varies in different derivatives. Their therapeutic effect results from inhibition of differentiation and activity of osteoclasts. In high doses bisphosphonates inhibit osteoblasts and bone mineralization.

For many years the first-generation derivative, etidronate, was the only available bisphosphonate in this country. It has the disadvantage of inhibiting bone mineralization, which in high or protracted dosage may result in a fracturing bone disease, a type of osteomalacia. However, in moderate intermittent dosage (400 mg daily for 2 weeks every 3 months) etidronate proved to be safe and resulted in an increase of bone mineral in patients with osteoporosis. The incidence of fractures was reduced in severe osteoporosis. Histology showed a decrease of bone turnover as expected, and probably a positive remodeling balance due to a relative decrease of resorption depth compared with the thickness of newly formed bone. There was no evidence of osteomalacia. If estrogens are contraindicated the drug appears to be an alternative in doses described above. It is not approved for use in osteoporosis.

A number of additional derivatives are presently in clinical trials for use in osteoporosis—tiludronate, alendronate, and risedronate in this country and many others abroad, such as pamidronate (approved in this country for IV treatment of hypercalcemia of malignancy and Paget's disease) and dimethyl derivative of pamidronate. All of these derivatives are much safer than etidronate because inhibition of osteoblasts occurs with doses high above therapeutic and more likely after IV administration.

Calcitriol, 1,25-dihydroxyvitamin D

Calcitriol was mentioned above in connection with calcium malabsorption in elderly women. Calcitriol is one of the calcium-regulating hormones of high potency. Whereas its effect to stimulate intestinal calcium (and phosphate absorption is the most obvious there are multiple additional effects in which calcitriol acts on cell differentiation in bone and many nonosseous tissues. In that capacity calcitriol has been shown to stimulate differentiation and function of both osteoblasts and (via osteoblasts) osteoclasts. Based on these actions calcifrol was tried in treatment of osteoporosis. The hormone worked as an antiresorptive agent because of increased intestinal calcium absorption and suppressed parathyroid hormone. Some authors present circumstantial evidence of increased bone formation.

The preparation (Rocaltrol) is rather expensive and hardly a first choice agent to treat osteoporosis. Probably the only indication beyond doubt is malabsorption of calcium refractory to plain vitamin D or evidence of calcium deficiency with absolute intolerance of dietary sources and usual doses of supplemental calcium.

Fluoride

Fluoride is the prototype of formation-stimulating agent. In chronic exposure such as in cryolite industry or in regions with high fluoride content in drinking water it produces bone disease characterized by excessive bone formation and secondary hyperparathyroidism. In pharmacologic doses used in osteoporosis (30–80 mg NaF) three effects are noted: 1) incorporation of fluoride into the crystals of bone mineral changing hydroxyapatite in part into fluoroapatite, which is resistant to osteoclastic dissolution; 2) mitogenic effect on osteoblast precursors, apparently direct and mediated by enhanced response of receptors for growth factors: an increased amount of active osteoblasts results; and 3) mineralization defect possibly due to interference with the initial mineral deposition in the osteoid. This adverse effect is complicated by secondary hyperparathyroidism if the increased demand for calcium is not met by calcium supplements (1000–1500 mg daily). Disorganized woven bone is produced with inferior structural quality.

In fairly narrow therapeutic range the effect of fluoride results in continuous increase of bone density of cancellous bone (5% to 10% a year) with no evidence of diminshed effect with time. In the spine the vertebral density may return from an osteoporotic range to normal value within 3 to 5 years (see Fig 29.8). The effect on cortical bone is slightly negative with gradual mass loss. The critically important proximal femur appears to gain mass, most likely because of the presence of cancellous bone in the trochanteric region. A patient taking fluoride may suffer from frequent painful insufficiency (incomplete) fractures in the weight-bearing skeleton of the pelvis and lower extremities. These fractures heal well and rapidly with temporary discontinuation of fluoride.

Despite bone mass increase, the incidence of vertebral fractures does not decrease after fluoride doses in the higher therapeutic range (75 mg daily). Consequently the newly formed bone appears mechanically inferior. Less well documented studies with lower doses (50 mg) did not show decreased bone quality, and the frequency of fractures decreased with increased vertebral mass.

Fluoride is not approved for human use except for small-dose tablets for dental caries prevention. It remains an experimental drug with a possible future if proper formulation, fluoride monitoring, and protection of cortical bone are found and validated in clinical trials. The fluoride experience may reflect an inherent problem with stimulators of bone formation. Unless the agent is able to stimulate bone formation de novo, that is, in the absence of preexisting bone structure, the effect will result in thickening of preexisting trabeculae in the cancellous bone without regeneration of supporting horizontal structures. The resulting bone will be mechanically inferior. In addition the thick trabeculae may be subject to internal remodeling with cavities inside the structures further decreasing bone quality.

Parathyroid Hormone

Chronic elevation of parathyroid hormone such as in primary hyperparathyroidism increases bone turnover and results in bone loss, primarily from cortical bone. In contrast, intermittent administration increased bone density in the spine (about 10% a year), but decreased it in appendicular cortical skeleton. Some, though incomplete improvement in the cortical bone status and calcium balance followed the addition of calcitriol to the regimen. The beneficial effect on the spine vanished after the first year of treatment.

The paradox of dual effect of parathyroid hormone, the stimulation of bone formation by a hormone that primarily stimulates bone resorption, has been resolved in vitro. In animal bone intermittent application of the hormone stimulates the osteoblasts to produce one of the major growth factors, insulin-like growth factor I, which stimulates osteoblastic action and bone formation. Continuous presence of the hormone results in the typical stimulation of osteoclastic resorption and inhibition of bone formation.

The formation-stimulating property of parathyroid hormone was demonstrated recently in women with postmenopausal osteoporosis. The patients received estrogens until bone density stabilized (1 year or more), and then injections of human parathyroid hormone (1–34 segment, 400 U daily) were added. Parathyroid hormone in combination with estrogen increased vertebral bone density by 10% in 18 months over controls on estrogen only. There was no adverse effect on cortical bone, including the femoral neck.

The use of parathyroid hormone is in the experimental stage of pilot studies and obviously not ready for clinical application. Still it shows one of the possible approaches to resolve the major problem of management of osteoporosis, that is, the lack of a safe agent that would restore bone mass by stimulating bone formation. Interestingly both fluoride and parathyroid hormone act as targeted (on bone) agents that exert their beneficial action by interaction with local growth factors such as insulin-like growth factor and transfoming growth factor β. This approach obviates the unwelcome effects of growth factors (such as hypoglycemia) administered systemically.

Prevention and Perspectives

At the present time, for the majority of osteoporotic patients the bone loss is irreversible except for a small and transient gain related to remodeling space. A patient presenting in her eighth decade of life with spinal deformity, severe reduction of bone mass, and evidence of low bone turnover is a candidate for mild physical therapy, judicious use of bracing, and pain management. The only approved agents besides supplemental calcium and vitamin D are antiresorptives unlikely to affect low turnover bone.

A better understanding of the pathogenesis of low bone mass and its irreversibility should make us realize the importance of prevention. Prevention of osteoporosis starts in childhood because the first determinant of bone mass is its peak value. The peak bone mass (at the approximate age of 35 years) is under genetic control, which accounts for 80% of variance. Recent studies identified a genetic marker, a variant of vitamin D (calcitriol) receptor gene, to be associated with low peak bone mass and biochemical evidence of high bone turnover. If confirmed we may have a reliable way to predict osteoporosis risk before low bone mass develops.

The full potential of peak bone mass is probably not reached in the average population because of environmental factors. Therefore the measures for the earliest prevention of osteoporosis start in childhood with adequate (apparently higher than recommended) calcium intake and physical activity. Low physical activity is interconnected with calcium intake also in young adults: it decreases the energy output, and to prevent overweight the young woman tends to reduce caloric intake and with it the calcium supply. Relevant information on separate effects of calcium and physical activity follows. Calcium supplements in children (to increase daily calcium intake from 1000 to 1600 mg) increase the mineral content of the skeleton by 5%. In addition, above average (customary) physical activity adds another 7% to 10% over the bone mass achieved with lower than average activity. The calcium intake data above contrast with the most recent recommendation of 1200 mg daily for adolescents. Bone mass continues to increase into the third decade, long after completion of longitudinal bone growth. In healthy young women the average increment in the spine bone mass is 6% per decade. High calcium intake (2100 mg daily) increases the increment to 16% per decade, the highest physical activity to 8% per decade, each factor independently of the other.

In adulthood past 30 years the prevention is centered on adverse effects of smoking, low physical activity, low calcium intake, alcohol abuse and specific drugs, and hormonal preparations. Prompt treatment of diseases known to affect bone mass (secondary osteoporosis) is necessary. This includes early ovarian failure, amenorrhea of top athletes, and the menopausal state. The decision to treat postmenopausal women with estrogen or other antiresorptive agents has to take her bone mineral status and bone turnover into consideration. In the elderly in addition to the measures above the prevention of falls is of primary importance, including frequent review of prescription and over-the-counter medication, eyesight improvement, mechanical support (quad canes, walkers), and environment adjustment (slippery floor, furniture clutter, night lights). Hip padding is cumbersome but it is proved as an efficient measure.

Since the first studies on bone mass quantitation by metacarpal cortical thickness measurement on radiograms, age-related bone loss has been accepted as an inevitable physiologic phenomenon (see Fig 29.1). However, recent clinical studies on effects of osteotropic drugs occasionally fail to demonstrate bone loss in untreated controls, usually on moderate calcium supplements only. An average life span less than 50 years and a high incidence of cardiovascular deaths were probably considered inevitable at some time, too. It is possible that implementation of protective measures against osteoporosis risk factors in an acceptable form (to educated population) will reduce if not abolish the age-related bone loss.

Development of effective osteotropic agents that will stimulate bone formation de novo and thus restore the architectural integrity of cancellous and endosteal cortical bone will be probable based on local stimulation of cytokines and growth factors in a manner similar to that described in fluoride and parathyroid hormone actions. No such agent appears imminent. Safe antiresorptive agents are the closest next development in bone protection (e.g., in temoporary disuse, surgical stress, immunosuppression etc.).

Before all this happens, the slogan "know your bone mass and your bone turnover" should be equally important as analogous slogans in hypertension and serum cholesterol. At the present time interested individuals and organizations should try to convice governmental agencies about the usefulness of bone density measurement.

SUGGESTED READINGS

Monographs

Avioli LV, ed. The osteoporotic syndrome. Detection, prevention, and treatment. 2nd ed. Orlando, FL: Grune & Stratton, 1987.

Eriksen EF, Axelrod DW, Melsen F. Bone histomorphometry. New York: Raven Press, 1994.

Favus MJ, ed. Primer on the metabolic bone diseases and disorders of mineral metabolism. 2nd ed. New York: Raven Press, 1993.

Nordin BEC, Need AG, Morris HA, eds. Metabolic bone and stone disease. Edinburgh: Churchill Livingstone, 1993.

Riggs DL, Melton LJ III, eds. Osteoporosis. Etiology, diagnosis, and management. New York: Raven Press, 1988.

Recent Reviews

Consensus Development Conference. Diagnosis, prophylaxis and treatment of osteoporosis. Am J Med 1993;94:646–647.

Delmas PD, ed. Osteoporosis: who should be treated? Am J Med 1995;4.

Johnson CC, Melton LJ III, Lindsay R, Eddy DM. Clinical indications for bone mass measurements. J Bone Mineral Res 1989;4(suppl 2).

Kanis JA, ed. Osteoporotic vertebral fracture. Bone 1992:13(suppl 2).

Lindsay R, Meunier PJ, eds. Can we make osteoporosis a disease of the past? Osteoporos Int 1994;4(suppl 1).

Sherman S, Heany RP, Parfitt AM, et al., eds. NIA Workshop on Aging and Bone Quality. Calcif Tissue Int 1993;53(suppl 1).

Third International Symposium on Osteoporosis, Research Advances and Application. March 2–5,1994. Abstracts.

CHAPTER 30

OSTEOARTHRITIS

Gene L. Watterson, Jr.,
Larry W. Moreland

Demographics

Osteoarthritis (OA), also known as osteoarthrosis or degenerative joint disease, is a condition characterized by progressive degeneration of articular cartilage, proliferative osseous changes, and clinical features of joint pain, limitation of motion, and deformity. It is the most common of the arthritic disorders, affecting over 50 million patients in the United States alone (1,2). As a result of the debility that can result from the disease and associated prevalence, OA exerts a major socioeconomic impact.

Prevalence

A strong association of the occurrence of OA with increasing age has been demonstrated in most study populations. Although uncommon in age groups under 25 years, it is manifest to some degree in approximately 60% of persons older than age 35, and almost ubiquitously above age 65. Radiographic features of OA have been noted in over 90% of patients at the eighth decade of life.

Additionally, the prevalence of the disease differs between genders. When all age groups are considered, OA appears to affect men and women equally. A greater prevalence is seen among men below age 45, and among women after age 55 (3–5). The frequency of symptomatic and severe disease is increased among women (6). Gender may additionally affect the distribution of joint involvement. First carpometacarpal, proximal and distal interphalangeal, and knee joint disease is more common in women, whereas metacarpophalangeal and hip joint involvement are present more often in men.

Associations

Obesity

The evidence linking obesity and OA is most clear in involvement of the knee (7–9). In other load-bearing joints such as the hips the association is less clear. Interestingly, OA of the hands also appears to be more common among obese patients (10). One hypothesis regarding the etiopathogenesis of OA suggests that biomechanical factors such as excessive joint loading might tend to potentiate the disease process (Fig 30.1). The fact that obesity is a risk factor for involvement of non–weight-bearing joints may indicate that other mechanisms are also involved. Some observations suggest that obesity developing at a younger age may be predictive of OA in later life.

Repetitive/Occupational Stress

Data suggest a possible link between OA and repetitive or increased biomechanical stress, as might be associated with various occupations or sport activities. Evidence supporting such associations is seen in studies involving coal miners, farmers, and dock workers, where an increased incidence of OA was noted relative to control groups (11–14). Additionally, predominant involvement of the right hand among right hand-dominant women working in a weaving factory has been noted (15).

The role of sports participation as a risk factor for the development of early or more severe OA is less clear. Sports and exercise-associated joint injury, resulting in structural damage to supporting ligaments, musculature, and cartilage, has been linked to

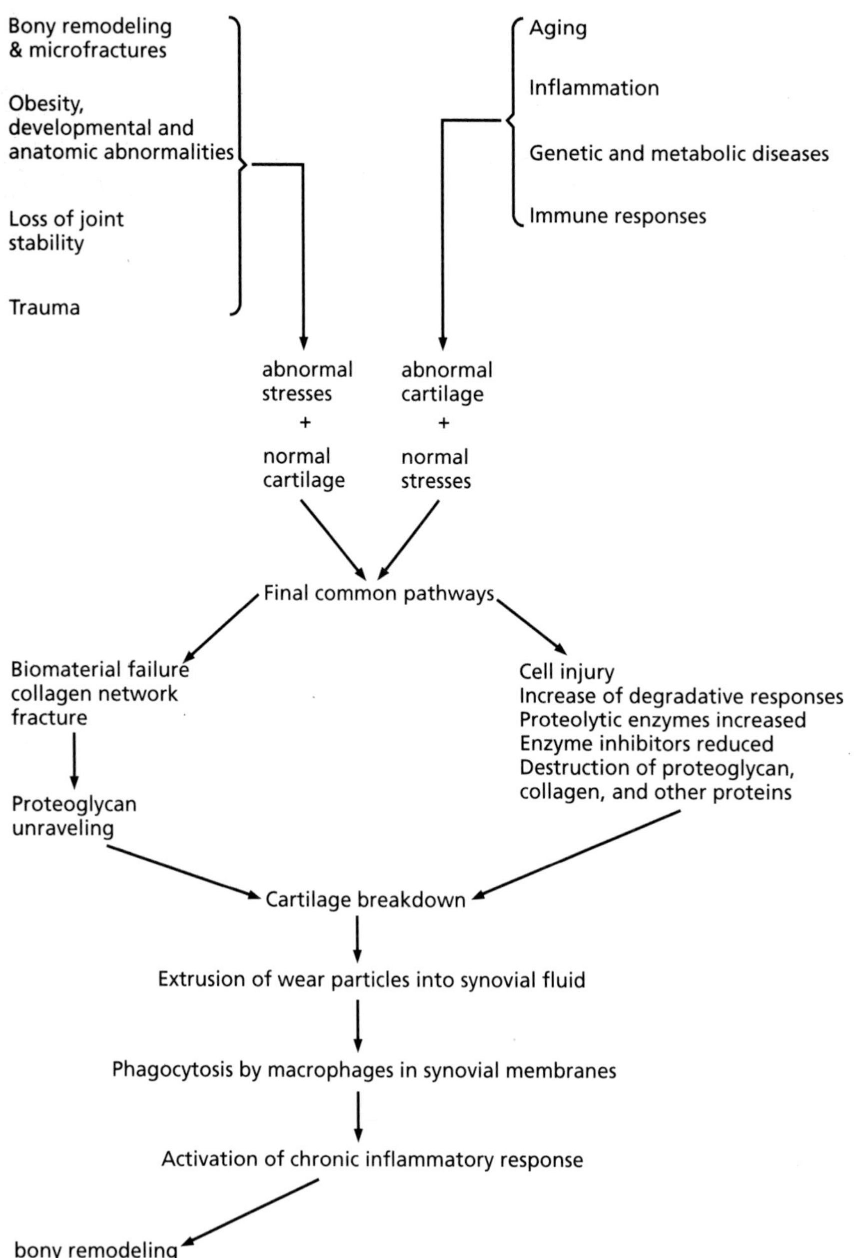

Fig 30.1 Etiopathogenic factors in osteoarthritis. *(Reproduced by permission from Howell DS. Etiopathogenesis of osteoarthritis. In: McCarty DJ, ed. Arthritis and allied conditions. 11th ed. Philadelphia: Lea & Febiger, 1989:1596.)*

more rapid articular degeneration (9). However, in the absence of trauma, athletic participation is a less conclusively defined precipitant.

Bone Density

Increased bone mineralization has exhibited a positive correlation with the development of OA (16). This association has been seen both among study populations and patients with the congenital condition osteopetrosis (17). In contrast, among patients with diminished bone density, the incidence of OA appears to be decreased (6). This inverse relationship has been hypothesized to arise due to an enhancement in the ability of less dense subchondral bone to absorb peak mechanical stresses. Secondarily suggested by this hypothesis is an explanation for the increased incidence of OA in obese patients among whom bone mineralization is often increased (18).

Genetic Associations

Recent studies identifying a linkage between the development of primary generalized osteoarthritis and a gene coding for type II procollagen provide evidence that heritable factors may play a role in the pathogenesis of the disease. Among the families studied, a single base substitution in this gene was associated with early cartilage degeneration and mild chondrodysplasia (19–21).

Further evidence supporting a genetic predisposition for the disease is found in patients with inherited crystal deposition diseases such as familial chondrocalcinosis. Deposition of calcium pyrophosphate dihydrate (CPPD) crystals in the hyaline cartilage of these individuals is associated with a higher incidence of osteoarthritic joint degeneration (22).

Classification

Osteoarthritis may present as either a primary (idiopathic) disease or as a secondary process associated with a variety of conditions (Table 30.1). The primary form of the disorder, or *primary generalized OA*, displays a predilection for the knees, hips, first metatarsophalangeal and metacarpophalangeal joints, and interphalangeal joints. Axial skeletal involvement is also common. A variant form of primary disease, *inflammatory OA*, most frequently appears in middle-aged women. It is characterized by painful episodic inflammatory changes principally of the interphalangeal joints of the hands. Long-standing recurrent inflammatory disease may result in considerable deformity or ankylosis. Radiographically, these joints may display erosions, typically of the more central aspect of the articular surface. Accordingly, the term *erosive OA* has been used to denote this subset. *Diffuse idiopathic skeletal hyperostosis* (DISH, Forestier's disease) is a form of primary OA defined chiefly by characteristic radiographic changes in the spine. Most typically, a pattern of ossification denoted "flowing calcification" is present along the anterolateral aspects of affected vertebral elements. These changes often result in a spine that radiographically resembles the "bamboo spine" of ankylosing spondylitis. It is generally possible to differentiate the disorder from ankylosing spondylitis by clinical means as well as radiographic criteria. In contrast to ankylosing spondylitis, sacroiliac and intervertebral disc involvement is absent. Most commonly DISH involves the thoracic

Table 30.1 Classification of Osteoarthritis

- Primary (idiopathic)
  - Peripheral joints
  - Spine
    - Apophyseal joints
    - Intervertebral joints
  - Subsets
    - Generalized osteoarthritis
    - Erosive inflammatory osteoarthritis
    - Diffuse idiopathic skeletal hyperostosis
    - Chondromalacia patellae
- Secondary
  - Trauma
    - Acute
    - Chronic (occupational, sports)
  - Underlying joint disorders
    - Local (fracture, infection)
    - Diffuse (rheumatoid arthritis)
  - Systemic metabolic or endocrine disorders
    - Ochronosis (alkaptonuria)
    - Wilson's disease
    - Hemochromatosis
    - Kashin-Beck disease
    - Acromegaly
    - Hyperparathyroidism
  - Crystal deposition disease
    - Calcium pyrophosphate dihydrate (pseudogout)
    - Basic calcium phosphate (hydroxyapatite-octacalcium phosphate-tricalcium phosphate)
    - Monosodium urate monohydrate (gout)
  - Neuropathic disorders (Charcot joints)
    - Tabes dorsalis
    - Diabetes mellitus
  - Intra-articular corticosteroid overuse
  - Miscellaneous
    - Bone dysplasia (multiple epiphyseal dysplasia; achondroplasia)
    - Frostbite

Reproduced by permission from Moskowitz RW. Clinical and laboratory findings in osteoarthritis. In: McCarty DJ, Koopman WJ, eds. Arthritis and allied conditions. 12th ed. Philadelphia: Lea & Febiger, 1993:1736.

spine. However, cervical and lumbar segments may also be affected. Additionally, extra-axial DISH may affect the appendicular skeleton at the calcaneus, olecranon process, patella, and sites of ligamentous and tendinous insertion in the pelvis.

Secondary OA may result from previous local trauma, congenital articular abnormalities, multiple endocrine and metabolic disorders, crystal deposition disease, and various other conditions associated with nonspecific alterations in joint architecture (see Table 30.1 and Fig 30.1). Mechanical factors resulting in joint incongruities, as found in trauma (occupational, Charcot arthropathy, meniscal surgery, fracture) or congenital skeletal anomolies (slipped femoral capital epiphysis, multiple epiphyseal dysplasia) are known causes of secondary OA. Metabolic and endocrine disorders such as hemochromatosis, ochronosis (alkaptonuria), Wilson's disease, lysosomal storage disorders, acromegaly, hypothyroidism, hyperparathyroidism, and Paget's disease of bone (osteitis deformans) are also known causes of secondary OA. All of these disorders, with the exception of storage disorders and osteitis deformans, are also linked to CPPD crystal deposi-tion disease, a disorder of intrasynovial crystalline deposition. CPPD crystal deposition disease, along with other crystalline arthropathies such as gout and hydroxyapatite-induced arthropathy, are themselves recognized causes of secondary OA. Inflammatory joint disorders of both infectious and noninfectious causes may lead to secondary osteoarthritic degeneration. Septic arthritis due to bacterial, mycobacterial, and fungal agents can result in the development of secondary OA as a consequence of microbial and host–response cartilage degradation. Autoimmune inflammatory arthropathies such as rheumatoid arthritis often result in similar changes predominately involving the hips, knees, and shoulders after several years of active disease.

Pathology

The characteristic articular changes noted in OA likely represent nonspecific pathologic responses to multiple forms of injury. A hallmark of the disease is that it is a degenerative process involving articular cartilage. The associated pathologic and radiographic findings are attributable to these degenerative changes or to reparative processes occurring in response to injury. In the initial stages of the disease thickening of the diseased cartilage, regarded as a likely consequence of increased proteoglycan synthesis and water content, has been observed (22). As the disease progresses, degenerative alterations in the cartilaginous architecture including flaking, fissuring, and erosion develop. The latter changes may progress to confluency, resulting in large denuded areas on the articular surface. The exposed underlying bony surfaces, through repetitive loaded contact, become sclerotic or eburnated. Eventually, reactive osseous proliferation may occur with subsequent production of higher density bone. Such new bone formation, when occurring at the joint margins, confers the appearance of spurs or osteophytes. Cystic changes often develop within the subarticular bone in regions devoid of articular cartilage. These lesions are hypothesized to arise as a result of focal bony necrosis or uneven channeling of force into the subchondral area. Microfracturing of the subchondral region may also occur as a result of these abnormalities in load distribution within the joint.

Etiopathogenesis

The underlying mechanisms that culminate in cartilage degeneration in OA are not completely understood. In general terms, biomechanical factors, congenital and acquired alterations in macromolecular structural proteins and inflammatory processes all may play important roles in the etiopathogenesis of the disease (see Fig 30.1).

Presently, two putative pathways are postulated in the pathogenesis of OA. One hypothesis suggests that underlying alterations in articular cartilage, as is seen in the previously described point mutation in type II collagen, predispose toward early structural failure. Similarly, acquired changes in the cartilaginous matrix associated with such processes as CPPD crystal deposition may result in premature degeneration. In this scheme, osteoarthritic changes develop as a consequence of injury sustained by defective cartilage under conditions of normal biomechanical stress.

In contrast, a second theory invokes direct physical injury to the chondrocyte as the primary inciting pathogenic factor. These damaged cells subsequently release a multiplicity of proteolytic enzymes that act on structural matrix proteins (Fig 30.2). Metalloproteinases such as stromelysin, collagenase, and gelati-

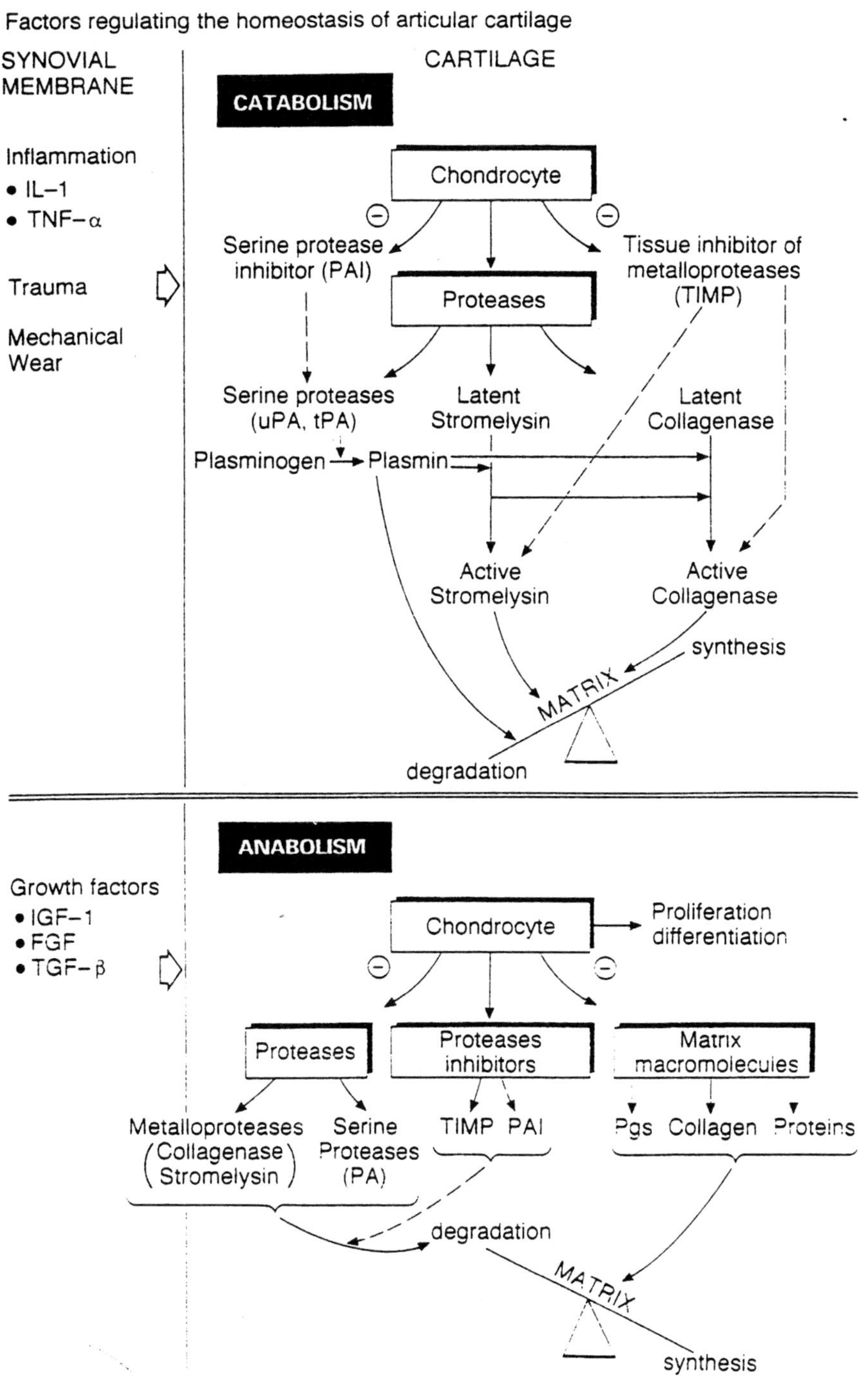

Fig 30.2 Factors regulating the homeostasis of articular cartilage. *(Reproduced by permission from Howell DS, Pellietier J. Etiopathogenesis of osteoarthritis. In: McCarty DJ, Koopman WJ, eds. Arthritis and allied conditions. 12th ed. Philadelphia: Lea & Febiger, 1993:1725.)*

nase, which are found in articular cartilage, exhibit matrix substrate specificity. Stromelysin has demonstrated in vitro activity at the hyaluronate binding region of proteoglycan (23–25). This enzyme also plays a role in the activation of collagenase, a proteolytic enzyme that requires processing following secretion to attain full activity (26). Collagenase additionally undergoes cleavage and initial activation through the action of serine proteinases such as plasmin (27,28). The fully potent enzyme affects degradation of type II collagen through proteolysis at a single substrate locus. Gelatinase, a metalloproteinase with lesser known function in cartilage degradation, may possess specificity for collagen previously cleaved by collagenase. Thiol proteinases, including cathepsin B, have also been implicated as agents involved in the digestion of matrix macromolecules. Cathepsin B may possess degradative activity for both proteoglycans and collagen. Additionally, evidence exists that this enzyme is involved in metalloproteinase activation (29). In addition to the noted examples, other unidentified or less characterized proteinases could also be responsible for early cartilage failure.

Through moderation of these catabolic enzymatic pathways, proteinase inhibitors could play an important part in reducing concomitant cartilage degradation. The tissue inhibitors of metalloproteinase (TIMP), TIMP 1 and TIMP 2, noncovalently but irreversibly bind and inactivate metalloproteinase substrate enzymes (30–32). Plasminogen activator inhibitor 1 (PAI-1) has demonstrated potent inhibition of tissue plasminogen activator (tPA) (33,34). tPA, a serine proteinase, is an enzyme that may be prominently involved in the activation of this cascade of cartilage-digesting proteinases. Cytokines have demonstrated a variety of effects on the metabolism of articular cartilage. Interleukin-1 (IL-1) has been found to exert stimulatory effects on stromelysin, collagenase, gelatinase, tPA, TIMP 1, and PAI-1 in both in vitro and in vivo studies. Additionally, this cytokine has been implicated as an inhibitory factor to proteoglycan and collagen synthesis (35–37). Tumor necrosis factor-α (TNF-α) similarly has exhibited the ability to stimulate metalloproteinase and plasminogen activator production. Although further investigation is needed to define the relevance of these findings to OA, a role for cytokines in the pathogenesis of OA likely exists. Growth factors, through anabolic effects on cartilage metabolism, potentially provide a means of counterbalancing the catabolic pathways stimulated by TNF-α and IL-1. Transforming growth factor-β has been shown to stimulate PAI-1 and TIMP-1 synthesis (38). Further studies support the ability of this factor to inhibit collagenase transcription while enhancing collagen production in synovial cells (39).

These models for degradative pathways in OA are largely based on in vitro studies. Although suggestive that enzymatic degradation and intrinsic alteration of articular cartilage are potentially important elements in the etiopathogenesis of the disease, the clinical significance of these observations has yet to be established.

Clinical Features

To a large extent, the clinical features associated with OA depend on the joints involved. The clinical manifestations of OA may vary from mono- or oligoarticular involvement to more extensive and diffuse disease (Table 30.2). Although the disease displays a predilection for weight-bearing joints such as the hips and knees, OA also involves non–weight-bearing joints such as the hands. The joints in the hand most frequently affected include the proximal and distal interphalangeal and first carpometacarpal joints. Involvement of the latter joints is characteristic of the disease. Persons so affected may experience focal tenderness of the base of the thumb both with movement and inactivity. Proximal and distal interphalangeal joint disease, when associated with regional osteophyte development, gives rise to the clinical findings of Bouchard's and Heberden's nodes, respectively (Fig 30.3). These nodular bony changes, easily detectable with inspection and palpation of the joints, may be of considerable value diagnostically. Development of chronic flexion deformities and medial or lateral deviation of the distal phalanges is often noted. Primary OA generally spares the metacarpophalangeal joints. However, in secondary OA involvement of these joints is more common.

Hip involvement in OA, which may develop insidiously, can result in considerable debilitation. Initial symptoms of pain localized in the groin, medial thigh, or lateral aspect of the hip are commonly noted. However, in some instances, pain may be experienced in the buttocks or knees along the distributions of the sciatic and obturator nerves. For this reason, suspicion of hip disease should be maintained during evaluation of pain in these regions. Additionally, during examination of the hip, a significant decline in range of motion may be appreciated. With progressive degeneration, ambulation and weight bearing may become severely compromised.

Similarly, OA of the knee can be a significant source of pain and functional incapacitation. Characteristically, stiffness and pain with motion or joint loading

Table 30.2 Clinical Profiles of Osteoarthritis

Factor	Characteristics and Occurrence
Age	Usually advanced; symptoms uncommon before age 40, unless due to secondary cause
Joint involvement	Commonly, distal interphalangeal, proximal interphalangeal, first carpometacarpal, hip, knee, first metatarsophalangeal joints, and lower lumbar and cervical vertebrae; rarely, metacarpophalangeal, wrist, elbow, or shoulder joints, except after trauma
Joint effusion	Little or none
Onset	Usually insidious
Systemic manifestations	Rare
True bony ankylosis	Uncommon
Symptoms	Pain on motion (early); pain at rest (later); pain aggravated by prolonged activity, relieved by rest; localized stiffness of short duration ("gelling") relieved by exercise; possibly painful muscle spasm; limitation of motion; "flares" associated with crystal-induced synovitis
Signs	Localized tenderness; crepitus and cracking on motion; mild joint enlargement with firm consistency from proliferation of bone and cartilage; synovitis (less common), gross deformity (later)

Reproduced by permission from Moskowitz RW. Clinical and laboratory findings in osteoarthritis. In: McCarty DJ, Koopman WJ, eds. Arthritis and allied conditions. 12th ed. Philadelphia: Lea & Febiger, 1993:1740.

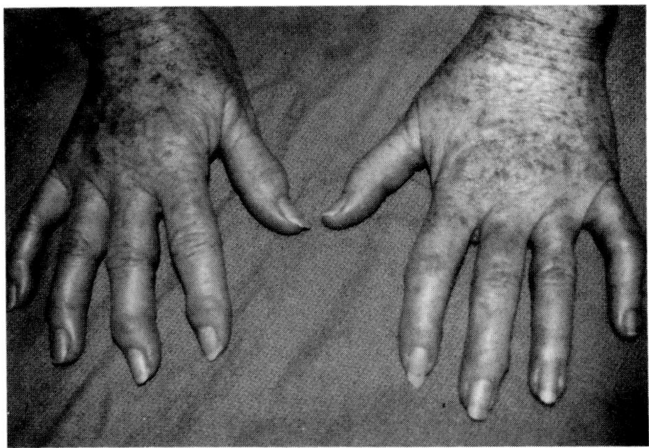

Fig 30.3 Typical changes involving the hands in a patient with primary osteoarthritis. Note the nodular lesions involving the distal interphalangeal joints (Heberden's nodes).

are early symptoms. At this stage, rest typically ameliorates the joint tenderness. However, inactivity may precipitate stiffness in a manner similar to the "gelling" phenomenon seen in various inflammatory arthropathies. With further degeneration of the knee joint, more indolent pain that is unrelieved by rest is common. On examination, chronic changes such as genu varus (bowleg deformity) may be apparent by inspection. Tenderness and diminished range of motion may be noted with active and passive movement. Palpation frequently reveals discernable crepitus, joint effusion, or uncommonly synovitis.

Osteoarthritis frequently involves the spine. Either the apophyseal or intervertebral disc articulations may be affected. However, spinal OA properly refers to typical changes occurring in the diarthroidal apophyseal joints. Common symptoms associated with spinal disease include regional stiffness, pain, and crepitus. Additionally, a variety of neurologic symptoms often develop in these patients. Osteophytic changes in the apophyseal joints may result in neuroforaminal stenosis with subsequent symptoms suggestive of radiculopathy such as pain, paresthesia, and weakness. Degenerative changes occurring within the intervertebral disc articulations (degenerative disc disease), can also result in a nerve root impingement syndrome concurrent with loss of the intervertebral joint spaces.

Additionally, osteophytes arising more posteriorly may result in apposition against the cord with concomitant compression. Examination may reveal diminished regional range of motion, tenderness, crepitus, muscular spasm, sensory and motor deficits, and abnormal deep tendon reflexes.

Laboratory Findings

No specific abnormalities are characteristic of OA on the laboratory examination. Serologic data including rheumatoid factor and antinuclear antibody are negative (Table 30.3). In suspected or defined cases of secondary OA, other supportive or exclusionary laboratory data may be indicated for evaluation of a concomitant process. When CPPD crystal deposition disease or chondrocalcinosis is identified, additional studies should be performed including serum ferritin, iron, iron-binding capacity, thyroid-stimulating hormone, and calcium. Other studies are indicated as dictated on clinical grounds.

Arthrocentesis typically yields noninflammatory joint fluid. Grossly, such fluid is nonturbid, straw-colored or yellow, and normal in viscosity. Microscopic examination of osteoarthritic synovial fluid usually reveals a paucity of inflammatory cells. In most instances, fewer than 2000 leukocytes/μL are noted. However, in cases of crystal-induced arthritis (e.g., CPPD disease), larger numbers of leukocytes may be noted. Synovial aspiration further affords evaluation for the presence of a crystalline arthropathy through plane polarized microscopy of the obtained fluid.

Radiographic Findings

Radiographic imaging can be useful in OA in both establishing the diagnosis and planning surgical intervention. In general, the information gained from plain radiographs is not augmented significantly by other imaging techniques. In most cases, if radiologic findings are present, they are evident on these studies (see

Table 30.3 Laboratory and Radiologic Findings in Primary Osteoarthritis

Laboratory Tests	Results
Erythrocyte sedimentation rate	Usually normal
Routine blood counts	Normal
Rheumatoid factor	Negative
Antinuclear antibody	Negative
Serum calcium, phosphorus, alkaline phosphatase, serum protein electrophoresis	Normal
Synovial fluid analysis	Good viscosity with normal mucin clot; modest increase in leukocyte number
	Presence of fibrils and debris (wear particles)
Radiologic Findings	**Causes**
Narrowing of joint space	Articular cartilage ulceration
Subchondral bone sclerosis (eburnation)	New bone formation
Marginal osteophyte formation	Proliferation of cartilage and bone
Bone cysts and bony collapse	Subchondral microfractures
Gross deformity with subluxation and loose bodies	Ligamentous laxity as a result of mechanical forces

Reproduced by permission from Moskowitz RW. Clinical and laboratory findings in osteoarthritis. In: McCarty DJ, Koopman WJ, eds. Arthritis and allied conditions. 12th ed. Philadelphia: Lea & Febiger, 1993:1748.

Table 30.3; Figs 30.4 through 30.6). Joint space loss or narrowing is a common, early, and prominent feature. In many cases of significantly symptomatic OA, mild diminution in the joint space is the sole finding in an involved joint. Primary OA typically results in an asymmetric pattern of narrowing. By contrast, secondary disease is often characterized by more uniform narrowing in the joint spaces. These changes may culminate in a "bone on bone" appearance in advanced disease. Changes in the juxtaarticular bone such as subchondral sclerosis and cyst formation are also noted frequently in OA. Bony sclerosis typically occurs in areas in which articular cartilage is most denuded. Periarticular cysts are often up to several centimeters in diameter. Osteophytes, quite characteristic of the disorder, appear as bony spurs of variable size arising from the margins of osteoarthritic joints. Osteophytic changes develop in both the primary and secondary forms of OA. Ankylosis infrequently occurs in association with inflammatory OA. When present, the hands and spine are the most frequent sites of involvement.

In addition to these abnormalities, it is important to note the absence of several features. In contrast to the juxtaarticular osteopenia seen in some inflammatory arthropathies such as rheumatoid arthritis and systemic lupus erythematosus, bone mineralization in OA is not characteristically altered. Additionally, marginal or periarticular erosions, also a feature of rheumatoid arthritis are absent. Erosive changes are sometimes present in inflammatory OA, but in a more central distribution within the joint. In the interphalangeal joints of the hands, this erosive pattern has been denoted as the "seagull" sign (see Fig 30.4). The combination of proliferative new bone and erosions, displayed on plain hand films in erosive OA, should not be confused with the pattern of abnormalities characteristic of psoriatic arthritis. In the latter condition, osteophytes are distinctly absent and erosive changes develop at the joint periphery.

Other imaging techniques such as scintigraphy, computed tomography scanning (CT), and magnetic resonance imaging (MRI) are helpful in specific clinical circumstances. In cases in which OA appears to be a more generalized process associated with diffuse arthralgic or bony pain, skeletal survey with multiple plain films and bone scanning should be considered to rule out other arthropathies or osseous pathology.

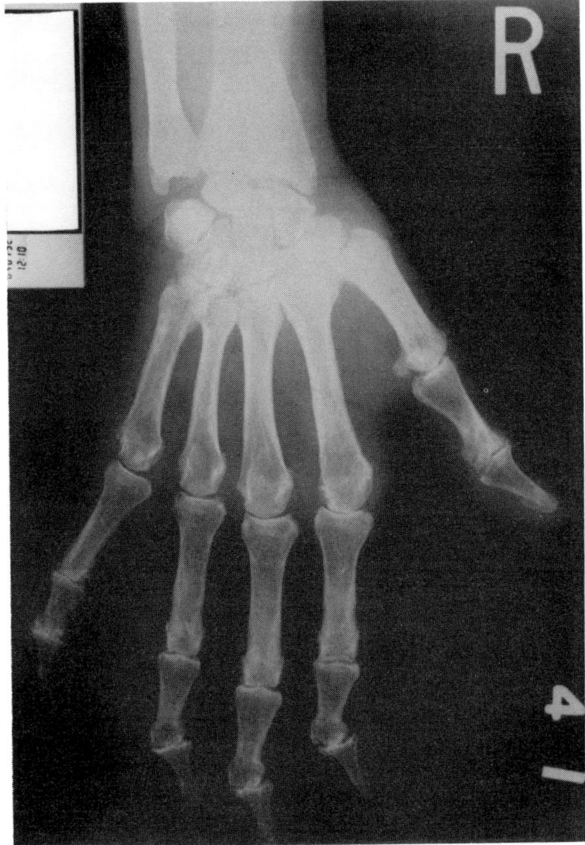

Fig 30.4 Hand radiograph in a patient with erosive osteoarthritis. Note the characteristic central erosive pattern of the distal interphalangeal joints ("seagull sign"). Also apparent are more general findings of joint space narrowing, subchondral sclerosis, periarticular cysts, and osteophytes.

MRI is often useful in distinguishing early avascular necrosis from OA. This condition, a concomitant of multiple precipitating factors (exogenous corticosteroids, Cushing's syndrome, Gaucher disease, alcoholism, trauma, others) is characterized by articular pain in the face of minimal plain radiographic changes in the early stages. Less common disorders that can present with some similar features to OA, such as Charcot arthropathy, pigmented villonodular synovitis, and synovial chondromatosis are more effectively identified by CT scanning or MRI. Alternatively, in the latter two disorders, arthrography is often useful in securing the correct diagnosis. CT and MRI scanning also play a major role in the evaluation of OA of the spine. These modalities are especially important in

A

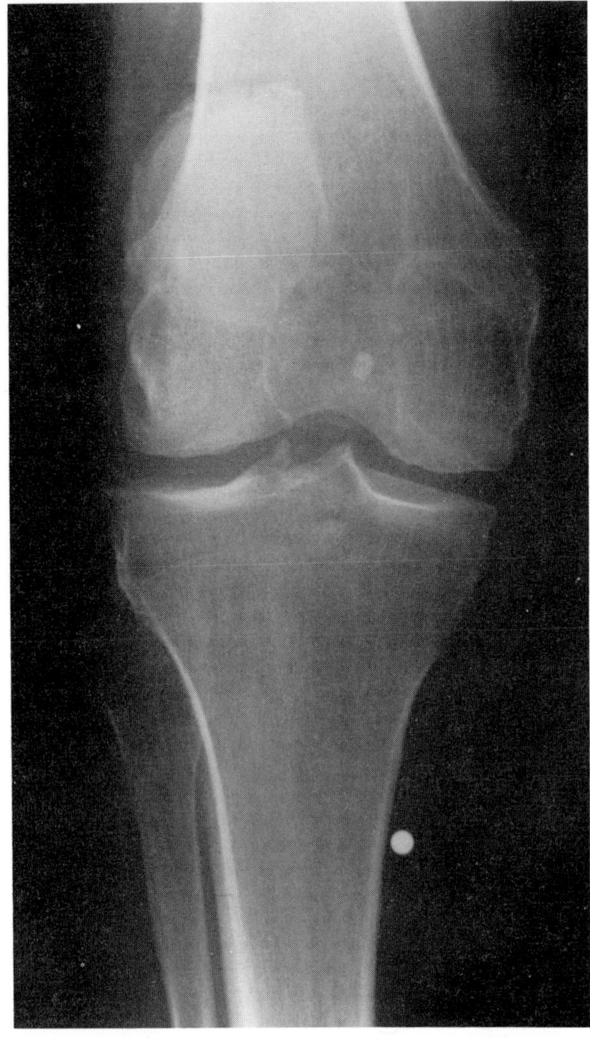

B

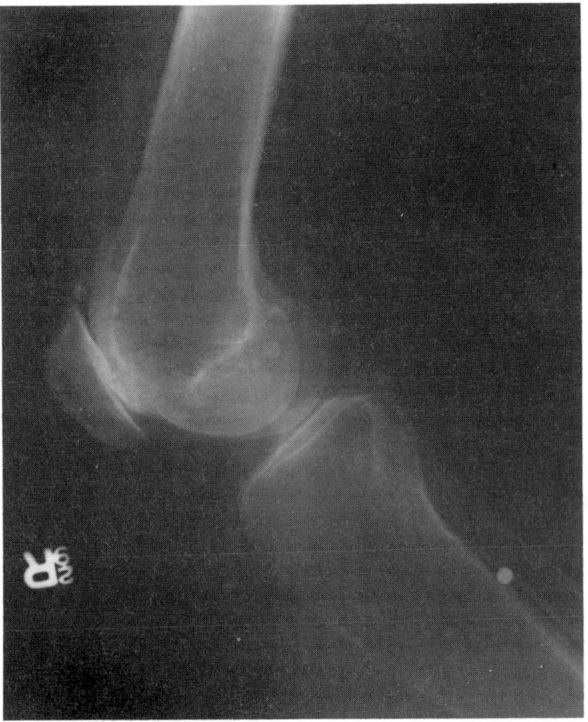

Fig 30.5 Osteoarthritis of the knee associated with calcium pyrophosphate dihydrate (CPPD) crystal deposition disease. *A*, Chondrocalcinosis appearing as curvilinear radiodensities in the lateral tibiofemoral joint space. Osteophytes and subchondral bony sclerosis are also apparent. *B*, Lateral view shows diminished patellofemoral joint space typical of CPPD crystal deposition disease.

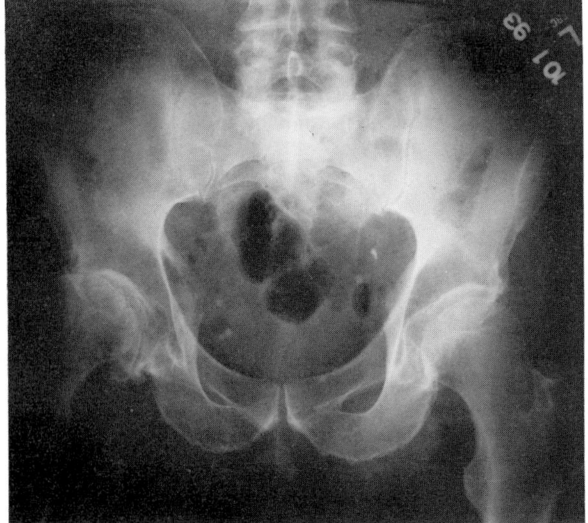

Fig 30.6 Osteoarthritis of the hip. Non-uniform joint space loss with typical superolateral migration of the femoral head. Osteophytes and subchondral sclerosis are also present.

clarifying the origin of radiculopathic or cord compression syndromes.

Treatment

Among the objectives to be considered in the treatment of OA, amelioration of pain and preservation of functional capacity figure prominently. Although the disease frequently presents as a superimposed process in patients debilitated by concurrent health issues, a significant number otherwise possess few medical problems. Along this spectrum, a rational therapeutic scheme may have a favorable impact on the quality of life of those affected to variable degrees.

Treatment of OA commonly requires a multimodal approach to significantly benefit the patient. In some cases, achieving adequate pain relief is sufficient to restore the patient to a nearly normal level of functioning. Most typically, except in milder or earlier disease, a component of recalcitrant or recurrent pain remains despite reasonable medical management. For this reason, patient education is important to convey the potentially indolent and chronically painful nature of this irreversible disease. Some patients adapt more easily to the sequelae of OA when their expectations become more realistic in this regard. In other patients, considerable debility remains after achieving suitable analgesia, due to chronic structural changes in the joints. It is incumbent on the clinician, in cooperation with the patient, to evaluate the effect of this functional decline in the context of the demands of lifestyle.

Physical Medicine

Physical therapy is an important adjunct in the treatment of OA in achieving pain reduction, maintaining range of motion, and improving muscular strength. Modalities that apply heat to affected joints and associated soft tissues often reduce pain and stiffness temporally. For this reason,the application of heat is often the initial modality used in physical therapy sessions. Alternatively, cryotherapy may effect greater symptomatic relief in some patients. Supervised and graded range-of-motion exercises of the hip and knee facilitate ambulation by reducing or preventing flexion contractures in load-bearing joints. Muscle strengthening and low-impact aerobic exercises help to counteract deconditioning that often accompanies long-standing and severe arthrosis. Repetitive joint motion through a large arc, however, should be performed judiciously or avoided to prevent escalating pain and inflammation. Isometric contractions have been advocated as an effective alternative means of building muscular strength in the quadriceps group without inflicting undue stress on the knee. Physical therapy often provides an effective venue for equipping patients with appropriate assistive appliances such as canes, walkers, and splints, and for developing facility in using them.

Medical Intervention

Due to the chronic and irreversible nature of the disorder, medical treatment of OA is necessarily palliative. However, in many cases, excellent and durable symptomatic relief is gained from drug therapy. The primary aim of pharmacologic treatment is attainment of an adequate degree of analgesia. The importance of this goal should not be minimized because achieving even a moderate degree of pain relief can markedly influence a patient's quality of life. Development of an effective therapeutic regimen is, in many cases, a matter of experimentation with various agents and escalation of treatment as dictated by therapeutic response. Some patients require little medication other than periodic analgesics for acute exacerbations of pain, In others, regular dosing with anti-inflammatory agents and analgesics, or intermittent intra-articular corticosteroid injections may be tried with varying degrees of success for more intractable pain.

Analgesics

A simple nonnarcotic analgesic represents a reasonable initial agent in many patients. Acetaminophen can be an effective drug when used alone or in combination with other medications. A further advantage of this drug is a relative paucity of associated toxicity at recommended therapeutic dosages. Narcotic analgesics provide temporal relief from pain but are associated with such adverse effects as physiologic dependence, constipation, and clouding of the sensorium. Care should particularly be exercised in using these drugs in elderly patients among whom these effects may be potentiated. Nevertheless, a role exists for judicious use of such agents as propoxyphene, codeine, and hydrocodone on an intermittent basis as a complement to other components of the treatment regimen.

Nonsteroidal Anti-inflammatory Drugs

The use of nonsteroidal anti-inflammatory drugs (NSAIDs) should be considered in patients who are nonresponsive to simple analgesics such as acetaminophen. In particular, these agents may prove efficacious when inflammatory changes are noted. Frequently, the most effective agent for a given patient is determined by therapeutic trial. Should a particular drug yield suboptimal symptomatic relief, it is reasonable to try another. Additionally, cost may be a factor in selecting a drug. Many elderly patients on fixed incomes find the cost of a prescribed NSAID to be prohibitive.

Aspirin, the prototypical NSAID, and other salicylates (magnesium choline salicylate, salsalate, diflunisal, meclofenamate) are also frequently used. Aspirin is advantageous to use in that it is among the least expensive alternatives in treatment of OA. Intolerance militates against the use of this agent in many patients.

Multiple toxicities are associated with this group of drugs. Mucosal irritation of the upper gastrointestinal tract results in esophagitis, gastritis, or development of frank ulceration. Patients at a higher risk of developing NSAID-induced gastrointestinal ulcers include women over 60 years of age and those with a prior history of ulcers or other serious concomitant medical illnesses. Hepatocellular injury, a less frequent form of NSAID-induced toxicity, is often reversible on withdrawal of the offending agent. Clinically, elevation of hepatic transaminases is the most frequently noted expression of liver toxicity. Abnormal renal function, evidenced by elevation in serum creatinine and diminished creatinine clearance, may arise through inhibition of prostaglandin-mediated renal perfusion. This effect is most pronounced under conditions that diminish renal blood flow such as hypovolemia. For these reasons, NSAIDs should be used with caution in geriatric patients.

Corticosteroids

Systemic corticosteroids are contraindicated in the treatment of OA. However, a role exists for the use of intra-articular injection of these agents. Although the relief obtained is often transient, it may be of sufficient duration and degree to significantly benefit the patient symptomatically. Joints most often injected include the knees and shoulders. Although individual injections are generally well tolerated and safe, repetitive and frequent injections may result in more rapid cartilage degeneration. Intra-articular corticosteroids are probably best regarded as palliative interventions to be infrequently used for the alleviation of acute painful exacerbations of OA.

Surgical Intervention

Among the various modalities used in the treatment of OA, surgery perhaps carries the greatest potential to significantly ameliorate the debilitating and painful effects of advanced disease. This is primarily attributable to refinement in the surgical techniques and appliances used in total joint replacement. In addition to arthroplasty, other surgical procedures such as arthroscopy, osteotomy, and arthrodesis have been useful in management of the disease as well. The potential benefits derived from such interventions must be weighed against the possibility of deleterious outcomes such as prosthesis failure, local sepsis, and persistent functional incapacitation.

General indications for surgical intervention include intractable pain despite reasonable medical management, significant joint deformity or instability, and functionally restrictive joint range of motion. These criteria are by no means absolute, but should be viewed in the context of how they actually affect the functional capacity of the patient. Furthermore, the adequacy of a patient's level of functioning is best judged in reference to the demands of lifestyle.

Arthroscopic procedures may be helpful in debridement of severely degenerative joints. Joint lavage, shaving of the chondral surfaces, and removal of loose bodies are performed with minimal morbidity through use of the arthroscope. The therapeutic efficacy of chondral surface abrasion is somewhat unclear, however. Patients often experience diminished pain and symptoms of joint locking after arthroscopy.

Osteotomy corrects the malalignment that results from asymmetric degeneration within the diseased joint. This procedure, generally performed on hips or knees, involves excision of regional bone to bring about better joint congruence. In the knee, removal of a wedge of bone from the proximal tibia and occasionally from the distal femur often reduces an existing varus or valgus deformity. Hip osteotomies similarly involve excision of sections of intertrochanteric bone to alleviate problems with biomechanical alignment. These surgeries are conservative interventions in that joint prosthesis procedures can be subsequently performed in either case if necessary.

Arthrodesis, or surgical joint fusion, is an effective means of alleviating chronic pain and stabilizing an unstable joint. However, these benefits are achieved at the expense of joint mobility. In weight-bearing joints, fusion procedures should be reserved for patients in whom prosthesis failure might be predicted due to vigorous activities involving the target joint. Arthrodesis should be avoided in load-bearing joints when the disease significantly affects the contralateral joint.

Arthroplasty, or joint replacement, can attenuate pain without sacrificing range of motion appreciably. Joint prosthesis procedures are especially noted for the former positive outcome. However, the degree to which functional disability improves after arthroplasty is somewhat more variable. Such factors as preoperative flexion contractures or extreme deconditioning may severely hinder the usefulness of these procedures. Nevertheless, arthroplastic surgery remains a major means by which patients with advanced OA are able to achieve relief from recalcitrant pain and functional impairment. Common operative sites include the knees, hips, and carpometacarpal joint of the thumb. Elbow and shoulder prostheses exist, but are less commonly used.

REFERENCES

1. Mankin HJ, Brandt KD, Shulman, LE. Workshop on etiopathogenesis of osteoarthritis: proceedings and recammendations. J Rheumatol 1986;13:1130–1160.

2. Peyron JG, Altman RD. The epidemiology of osteoarthritis. In: Moskowitz RW, Howell DS, Goldberg VM, Mankin HJ eds. Osteoarthritis: diagnosis and management. Philadelphia: WB Saunders, 1992:15–38.

3. Mikkelsen WN, Duff IF, Dodge HJ. Age and sex specific prevalence of radiographic abnormalities of the joints of the hands, wrist, and cervical spine of adult residents of Tecumseh, Michigan, community health study area, 1962–1965. J Chronic Dis 1970;23:151–159.

4. Jurmain RD. Stress and the etiology of osteoarthritis. Am J Phys Anthropol 1977;46:353–366.

5. Acheson RM, Collart AB. New Haven survey of joint diseases. XVII. Relationship between some systemic characteristics and osteoarthrosis in a general population. Ann Rheum Dis 1975;34:379–387.

6. Silberberg R, Thommasson R, Silberberg M. Degenerative joint disease in castrate mice. II. Effect of orchioectomy at various ages. Arch Pathol 1958;65:442–444.

7. Lawrence JS, Sebo M. The geography of osteoarthritis. In: Nuki G, ed. The aetiopathogenesis of osteoarthrosis. England: Pittman Medical Publishing, 1981: 155–183.

8. Anderson JJ, Felson DT. Factors associated with osteoarthritis of the knee in the first national Health and Nutrition Examination Survey (HANES I): evidence for an association with overweight, race, and physical demands of work. Am J Epidemiol 1988;127:179–189.

9. Davis MA, Ettinger WH, Neuhaus JM, et al. The association of knee injury and obesity with unilateral and bilateral osteoarthritis of the knee. Am J Epidemiol 1989;130:278–288.

10. Kellgren JH, Lawrence JS. Osteoarthrosis and disk in an urban population. Ann Rheum Dis 1958;17:388–397.

11. Louyot P, Savin R. La coxarthrose chez l'agriculteur. Rev Rhum Mal Osteoartic 1966;33:625–632.

12. Pommier L. Contribution a l'etude de la coxarthrose chez l'agriculteur. Profil clinique et etiologique. A propos de 245 dossiers de coxarthrose chirurigicale. These Med, University of Tours, Tours, France, 1977.

13. Schlomka G, Schroter G, Ocherwal A. Uber der bedeutung der beruflischer Belastung fur die entsehung der degenerativen Gelenkleiden. Z Gesamte Inn Med 1955;10:993.

14. Partridge REH, Duthie JJR. Rheumatism in dockers and civil servants: a comparison of heavy manual and sedentary workers. Ann Rheum Dis 1968;27: 559–568.

15. Hadler NM, Gillings DB, Imbus HR, et al. Hand structure and function in an industrial setting. Influence of three patterns of stereotyped repetitive usage. Arthritis Rheum 1978;21:210–220.

16. Foss MVL, Byers PD. Bone density, osteoarthrosis of the hip, and fracture of the upper end of the femur. Ann Rheum Dis 1972;31:259–264.

17. Milgram JW. Osteopetrosis. A morphological study of twenty-one cases. J Bone Joint Surg 1974; 56A:587–591.

18. Slemenda CW, Hui SL, Williams CJ, et al. Bone mass and arthropometric measurements in adult females. Bone Miner 1990;11:101–109.

19. Knowlton RG, Katzenstein PL, Moskowitz RW, et al. Genetic linkage of a polymorphism in the type II collagen gene (COL2A1) to primary osteoarthritis associated with a mild chondroplasia. N Engl J Med 1990;322:526–530.

20. Palotie A, Vaisanen P, Ott J, et al. Predisposition to familial osteoarthritis linked to type II collagen gene. Lancet 1989;1:924–927.

21. Moskowitz RW, Pun Y, Lei ST, Haqqi TM. Arg→Cys mutation in COL2A1 defines a new subset of osteoarthritis. Arthritis Rheum 1992:35:S35.

22. Adams ME, Brandt KD. Hypertrophic repair of canine articular cartilage in osteoarthritis after anterior cruciate ligament transection. J Rheum 1991;18:428–435.

23. Martel-Pelletier J, Pelletier JP, Malemud CJ. Activation of neutral metalloprotease in human osteoarthritic knee cartilage: evidence for degradation in the core protein of sulfated proteoglycan. Ann Rheum Dis 1988;47:801–808.

24. Campbell IK, Roughley PJ, Mort JS. The action of human articular cartilage metalloproteinase on proteoglycan and link protein. Similarities between products of degradation in situ and in vitro. Biochem J 1986; 237:117–122.

25. Tyler JA. Chondrocyte-mediated depletion of articular cartilage proteoglycans in vitro. Biochem J 1985;225:493–507.

26. Murphy G, Cockett MI, Stephens PE, et al. Stromelysin is an activator of procollagenase: a study with natural and recombinant enzymes. Biochem J 1987;248:265–268.

27. Woessner JF Jr. Matrix metalloproteinases and their inhibitors in connective tissue remodelling. FASEB J 1991;5:2145–2154.

28. Nagase H, Enghild JJ, Suzuki K. Stepwise activation mechanisms of the precursor of matrix metalloproteinase 3 (stromelysin) by proteinases and (4-aminophenyl) mercuric acetate. Biochemistry 1990;29: 5783–5789.

29. Eeckhout Y, Vaes G. Further studies on the activation of procollagenase, the latent precursor of bone collagenase. Effects of lysosomal cathepsin B, plasmin and kallikrein, and spontaneous activation. Biochem J 1977;166:21–31.

30. Morales TI, Kuettner KE, Howell DS, Woessner JF. Characterization of the metalloproteinase inhibitor produced by bovine articular chondrocyte cultures. Biochim Biophys Acta 1983;760:221–229.

31. Dean DS, Woessner JF Jr. Extracts of human articular cartilage contain an inhibitor of tissue metalloproteinases. Biochemistry 1984;218:277–280.

32. Campbell EJ, Cury JD, Lazarus CJ, Welgus HG. Monocyte procollagenase and tissue inhibitor of metalloproteinases. Identification, characterization and regulation of secretion. J Biol Chem 1987;262:15862–15868.

33. Pavia M, Towle CA, Treadwell BV. IL-1 activated chondrocytes synthesize an inhibitor of plasminogen activator. Trans Orthop Res Soc 1990;15:238. (Abstract).

34. Ghosh P, Collier S, Andrews J. Synovial membrane-cartilage interaction-the role of serine proteinase inhibitors in interleukin-1 mediated degradation of articular cartilage. J Rheumatol 1987;14:122–124.

35. Benton H, Tyler JA. Inhibition of cartilage proteoglycan synthesis by interleukin-1. Biochem Biophys Res Commun 1988;154:421–428.

36. Tyler JA. Articular cartilage synthesis: a decreased number of normal proteoglycan molecules. Biochem J 1985;227:869–878.

37. Saklatavala J. TNF-α stimulates resorption and inhibits synthesis of proteoglycan in cartilage. Nature 1986;322:547–549.

38. Overall CM, Wrana JL, Sodek J. Independent regulation of collagenase, 72 kDa progelatinase and metalloendoproteinase inhibitor expression in human fibroblasts by transforming growth factor-beta. J Biol Chem 1989;264:1860–1869.

39. Lafyatis R, Thompson NL, Remmers EF. Transforming growth factor-production by synovial tissues from rheumatoid patients and streptococcal cell wall arthritic rats: studies on secretion by synovial fibroblast-like cells and immunohistologic localization. J Immunol 1989;143:1142–1148.

CHAPTER 31

RHEUMATOID ARTHRITIS

S. Louis Bridges, Jr.

Rheumatoid arthritis is a chronic systemic disease that primarily affects synovial-lined diarthrodial joints. The term rheumatoid arthritis was introduced into the medical literature by Sir Alfred B. Garrod in 1859. Archaic terms for this condition include rheumatic gout, arthritis deformans, chronic atrophic arthritis, and infectious rheumatoid arthritis. The use of these terms illustrates the nosologic difficulties surrounding the diseases we now refer to as rheumatoid arthritis, gout, rheumatic fever, osteoarthritis, and septic arthritis. Because of these misunderstandings, the American Rheumatism Association (now American College of Rheumatology) did not officially sanction use of the term rheumatoid arthritis until 1941 (1).

Rheumatoid arthritis is a common disorder, affecting an estimated 1% of the adult population in the United States (2). This disease appears to affect individuals of all races and ethnic groups worldwide. As is true of most autoimmune diseases, it is two to three times more common in women than men (2). Its peak incidence is in women aged 30 to 60 years, but onset in elderly patients may occur as well (3).

Diagnosis and Presentation

Symptoms of rheumatoid arthritis include joint pain, swelling, and stiffness, often accompanied by fatigue and malaise. Occasionally, patients have fever and weight loss in addition to other constitutional symptoms. Published diagnostic criteria (4) emphasize polyarticular symmetric swelling of the small joints of the hands and feet (Table 31.1), but this pattern may not be evident in some individuals until symptoms have been present for weeks or months. The symmetry of joint involvement refers to groups of joints, such as metacarpophalangeal (MCP), proximal interphalangeal (PIP), or metatarsophalangeal (MTP), rather than individual joints. The onset of symptoms is usually insidious; however, symptoms may develop abruptly, even overnight (5,6). In as many as 20% of patients, the disease onset may be monarticular, later progressing to polyarticular (7). The most commonly involved joints at the time of initial presentation are those of the fingers and wrists (2) (Table 31.2).

Differential Diagnosis

Long-standing severe rheumatoid arthritis with its typical deformities, laboratory, and radiographic findings is not a diagnostic challenge. However, a multitude of clinical conditions may resemble rheumatoid arthritis in its early stages. A cursory overview of the most common diseases included in the differential diagnosis of early rheumatoid arthritis follows.

Osteoarthritis, especially if it affects the small joints of the hands, may be confused with rheumatoid arthritis. Chapter 30 discusses osteoarthritis in detail. The distribution and appearance of affected joints are often helpful in differentiating osteoarthritis and rheumatoid arthritis. Frequently affected in rheumatoid arthritis but rarely in primary osteoarthritis are the carpal joints, the MCP joints, the second through fifth MTP joints, and the ulnohumeral (elbow) and glenohumeral (shoulder) joints. Involvement of the lumbar spine, carpometacarpal joints of the thumbs, and bony swelling of the distal interphalangeal joints (Heberden's nodes) or proximal interphalangeal joints (Bouchard's nodes) are characteristic of primary osteoarthritis. Both osteoarthritis and rheumatoid arthritis may affect the hip or knee. Characteristic radiographic abnormalities of rheumatoid

Table 31.1 The American Rheumatism Association 1987 Revised Criteria for the Classification of Rheumatoid Arthritis

Criterion	Definition
1. Morning stiffness	Morning stiffness in and around the joints, lasting at least 1 hr before maximal improvement
2. Arthritis of three or more joint areas	At least three joint areas simultaneously have had soft-tissue swelling or fluid (not bony overgrowth alone) observed by a physician. The 14 possible joint areas are right or left PIP, MCP, wrist, elbow, knee, ankle, and MTP joints
3. Arthritis of hand joints	At least one area swollen (as defined above) in a wrist, MCP, or PIP joint
4. Symmetric arthritis	Simultaneous involvement of the same joint areas (as defined in 2) on both sides of the body (bilateral involvement of PIPs, MCPs, or MTPs is acceptable without absolute symmetry)
5. Rheumatoid nodules	Subcutaneous nodules, over bony prominences, or extensor surfaces, or in juxta-articular regions, observed by a physician
6. Serum rheumatoid factor	Demonstration of abnormal amounts of serum rheumatoid factor by any method that has been positive in <5% of normal control subjects
7. Radiographic changes	Radiographic changes typical of rheumatoid arthritis on posteroanterior hand and wrist radiographs, which must include erosions or unequivocal bony decalcification localized in or most marked adjacent to the involved joints (osteoarthritis changes alone do not qualify)

For classification purposes, a patient shall be said to have rheumatoid arthritis if he or she has satisified at least four of these seven criteria. Criteria 1 through 4 must have been present for at least 6 weeks. Patients with two clinical diagnoses are not excluded.

MCP, metacarpophalangeal; MTP, metatarsophalangeal; PIP, proximal interphalangeal
Reproduced by permission from Arnett FC, Edworthy SM, Block DA, et al. The American Rheumatism Association 1987 revised criteria for the classification of rheumatoid arthritis. Arthritis Rheum 1988;31:315–324.

Table 31.2 Joints Involved in Rheumatoid Arthritis

	PERCENTAGE INITIALLY INVOLVED			PERCENTAGE ULTIMATELY INVOLVED
	Right	Left	Bilateral	
Metacarpophalangeal	65	58	52	87
Wrist	60	57	48	82
Proximal interphalangeal	63	53	45	63
Metatarsophalangeal	48	47	43	48
Shoulder	37	42	30	47
Knee	35	30	24	56
Ankle	25	23	18	53
Elbow	20	15	14	21

Other joints affected by rheumatoid arthritis are not tabulated here.
Reproduced by permission from Harris ED Jr. Clinical features of rheumatoid arthritis. In: Kelley WN, Harris ED Jr, Ruddy S, Sledge CB, eds. Textbook of rheumatology. Philadelphia: WB Saunders, 1993:874–911.

arthritis (see below), the presence of serum rheumatoid factor, and inflammatory joint effusions are also helpful in differentiating rheumatoid arthritis from osteoarthritis.

Systemic lupus erythematosus (SLE) also has features in common with rheumatoid arthritis (see Chapter 32). Characteristic features such as skin rash and nephritis, and the presence of specific subsets of antinuclear antibodies such as anti-DNA and anti-Sm antibodies often help differentiate SLE from rheumatoid arthritis. Sera of 15% to 35% of patients with rheumatoid arthritis are positive on screening for fluorescent antinuclear antibodies (8).

Polymyalgia rheumatica, a symptom complex of aching and stiffness, is commonly seen in older women, and may present with symptoms indistinguishable from those seen in rheumatoid arthritis (9). The most commonly symptomatic areas are the neck, lower back, and muscles of the shoulders, upper arms, and thighs. Occasionally patients with polymyalgia rheumatica have mild synovitis. The erythrocyte sedimentation rate (ESR) is usually elevated to at least 40 mm/hr by the Westergren method. The symptoms of polymyalgia rheumatica usually respond dramatically to low-dose corticosteroids (prednisone 10–20 mg/day) or nonsteroidal anti-inflammatory drugs (NSAIDs). NSAIDs can be given to patients who do not have additional features of giant cell (temporal) arteritis.

Fibromyalgia or fibrositis is seen with great frequency in the U.S. population. As many as 90% of patients are women (10). Diffuse nonarticular pain is a universal complaint and defines the syndrome. Often patients state that they hurt over their entire bodies. Arthralgias, fatigue, and poor sleep often accompany fibromyalgia. Patients with fibromyalgia have tender trigger points, but they do not have objective evidence of joint swelling and the serum rheumatoid factor is negative.

Many infectious processes can mimic rheumatoid arthritis. Rubella, parvovirus B19, and hepatitis B are the most common viruses that may cause arthralgias or arthritis (11). Usually the joint symptoms manifested in these syndromes are transient and self-limited, which explains the requirement that symptoms be of at least 6 weeks' duration for the diagnosis of rheumatoid arthritis.

Septic arthritis should be one of the first considerations in patients who present with acute onset monarticular arthritis, especially if fever is present. Migratory polyarthritis may precede the development of septic arthritis. Gram-positive organisms such as *Staphylococcus aureus* or streptococci, and gram-negative cocci such as *Neisseria gonorrheae* are the most frequent causes of infectious arthritis among adults (12). Disseminated gonococcal infection should be considered in sexually active women who present with polyarthritis and fever. Patients with this condition often have tenosynovitis, fever, and papular or pustular skin lesions, but a minority have genitourinary symptoms (13). Synovial fluid is usually grossly purulent, often with white cell counts more than 50,000/μL, but the Gram stain and culture are positive in only about 25% of cases. Cultures should be obtained from the cervix, rectum, pharynx, and blood. Tests such as the ESR and C-reactive protein are not sufficiently sensitive or specific to diagnose or exclude septic arthritis.

The clinical picture of polyarticular gout may resemble rheumatoid arthritis (14), but gout is rare in premenopausal women (15). The pathognomonic abnormality of gout is the presence of monosodium urate crystals in synovial fluid or tophi. Monosodium urate crystals are typically needle shaped and examination using polarized, compensated microscopy reveals negative birefringence. Patients with gout are hyperuricemic although serum uric acid levels may be normal during an acute attack. Rheumatoid factor may be found in the sera of 5% to 30% of patients with gout and no evidence of rheumatoid arthritis (16,17). Concomitant gout and rheumatoid arthritis is much less common than would be expected from prevalence data of these two common illnesses (2).

Calcium pyrophosphate dihydrate (CPPD) crystal deposition disease, a common disease of the elderly, is also included in the differential diagnosis of rheumatoid arthritis. About 5% of patients with CPPD crystal deposition disease have symptoms in multiple joints, with attacks resembling rheumatoid arthritis (18). Chondrocalcinosis on radiographs is characteristic, but not absolutely necessary for the diagnosis of CPPD crystal deposition disease. The most common sites of chondrocalcinosis are the symphysis pubis, wrist, knee, and hip. Pseudogout, an acute mono- or polyarticular arthritis, is characterized by positively birefringent CPPD crystals in synovial fluid of affected joints.

Seronegative spondyloarthropathies include ankylosing spondylitis, Reiter's syndrome, psoriatic arthritis, reactive arthritis, and the arthritis of inflammatory bowel disease. These diseases, which are associated with the HLA B27 gene, may sometimes be confused with rheumatoid arthritis (19). In general, these diseases are less prevalent among women than is rheumatoid arthritis. Axial symptoms, such as back pain, and asymmetric oligoarticular arthritis, especially of the lower extremities, and lack of rheumatoid factor are clues to the diagnosis of seronegative spondyloarthropathies. Radiographs of the pelvis reveal characteristic changes of sacroiliitis such as narrowing and sclerosis of the joints. Late in the disease, there may be total loss of joint space, with fusion (ankylosis). Reiter's syndrome is characterized by inflammatory eye disease, oral ulcerations, urethritis, or characteristic skin lesions, such as keratoderma blennorrhagicum. Individuals with Reiter's syndrome rarely present with all of these findings simultaneously.

Lyme disease is most commonly found in parts of the northeastern, midwestern, and western United States (20). It is caused by the spirochete *Borrelia burgdorferi* and is carried by the deer tick *Ixodes dammini*. The characteristic skin rash, erythema chronicum migrans, begins as a macule or papule at the site of the tick bite. Erythema often extends outward over a period of days. The arthritis of Lyme disease can resemble rheumatoid arthritis but is usually asymmetric and involves large joints more than small joints. Other clinical findings in Lyme disease may include meningoencephalitis, cranial nerve palsies, and carditis. False-positive, usually low titer, antibodies against *B. burdorferi* are a common problem because of methodologic variation in serologic tests (20). Therefore, it is prudent to test only those patients in whom there is reasonable suspicion for the disease, that is, patients with a clinical picture compatible with Lyme arthritis who have been in an endemic area.

Carcinoma polyarthritis is an inflammatory arthritis seen, albeit rarely, in association with malignancy, most often breast or ovarian carcinoma, or lymphoid malignancies such as non-Hodgkin's lymphoma (21).

Patients with hypothyroidism may have a noninflammatory, nonerosive arthropathy, but this presentation is rare.

Etiology and Pathogenesis

Although it has been under intensive investigation for many years, the etiology of rheumatoid arthritis remains unknown. Current theories postulate that antigen(s), either exogenous or endogenous, trigger the disease among persons with genetic susceptibility. Multiple infectious organisms have been investigated as possible causative agents. These include bacteria (e.g., mycoplasma, streptococci, and mycobacteria), and viruses (e.g., rubella, parvovirus, retroviruses, and Epstein-Barr virus) among others. Despite circumstantial suggestions, there is no definitive evidence of a causative association between rheumatoid arthritis and any pathogenic organism.

Immunologic Abnormalities

Figure 31.1 is a simplified scheme of some of the complex cellular interactions and humoral events thought to be important in the pathogenesis of rheumatoid arthritis. Antigen-presenting cells display processed peptide antigens within the groove of class II major histocompatibility complex (MHC) molecules on their cell surfaces. Helper T lymphocytes recognize the antigen and the class II MHC molecule through T-cell receptors and associated CD4 molecules on their cell surfaces. These T lymphocytes become activated and secrete cytokines and stimulate B lymphocytes to produce antibodies (22).

Macrophages generate large amounts of growth factors and cytokines that participate in the inflammatory response in synovium (23). Interleukin (IL)-1, IL-6, IL-8, granulocyte–macrophage colony-stimulating factor (GM-CSF), tumor necrosis factor (TNF)-α, interferon-γ (IFN-γ), and transforming growth factor (TGF)-β likely participate in the inflammatory response characteristic of rheumatoid arthritis. These cytokines and growth factors often have pleiotropic effects on cells involved in rheumatoid arthritis. Among other effects, IFN-γ, TNA-α, and IL-1 can upregulate expression of endothelial adhesion molecules such as intercellular adhesion molecule-1 (see Fig 31.1). Adhesion molecules facilitate adherence of cells of the immune system to endothelial cells through interaction with cell surface molecules such as lymphocyte function-associated antigen-1 (LFA-1). After adhering to the endothelial surface, the cells migrate through the vessel to sites of inflammation. Cartilage

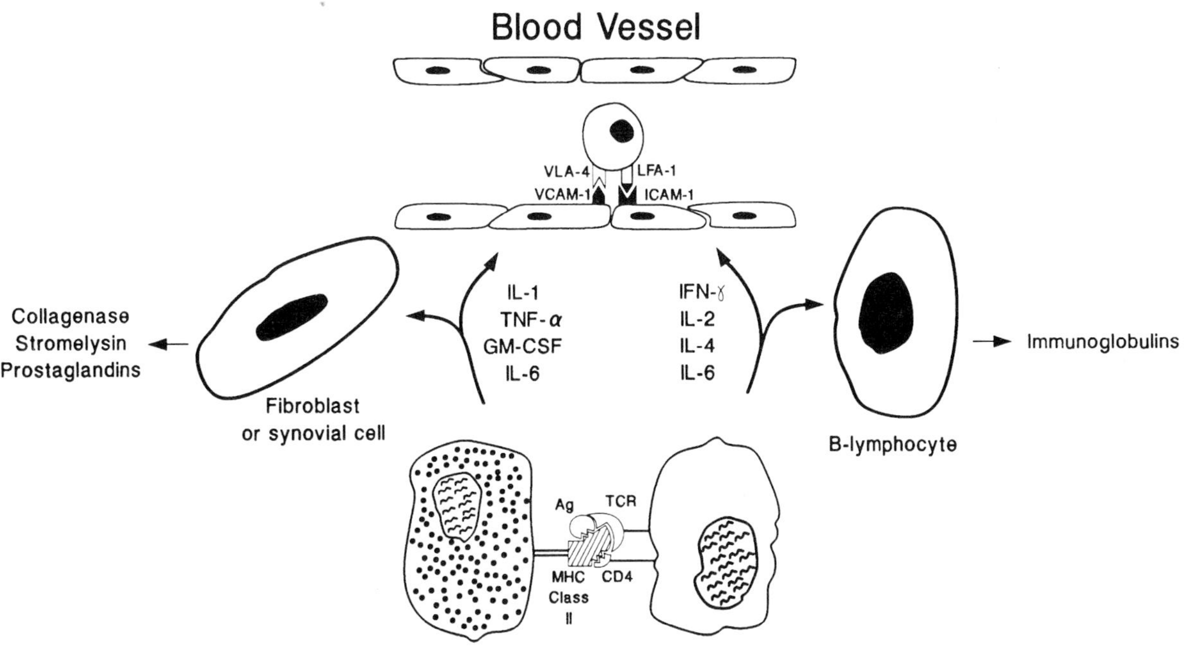

Fig 31.1 Overview of the cellular and humoral pathways implicated in the pathogenesis of rheumatoid arthritis. IL, interleukin; TNF-α, tumor necrosis factor-α; GM-CSF, granulocyte-macrophage colony-stimulating factor; IFN-γ, interferon-γ; Ag, antigen; TCR, T-cell receptor; MCH, major histocompatibility complex; VLA-4, very late antigen-4; VCAM-1, vascular adhesion molecule-1; LFA-1, lymphocyte function-associated antigen-l; ICAM-1, intercellular adhesion molecule-1. *(Reproduced by permission from Moreland LW, Heck LW Jr, Sullivan W, et al. New approaches to the therapy of autoimmune diseases: rheumatoid arthritis as a paradigm. Am J Med Sci 1993;305:40–51.)*

destruction is mediated in part by proteinases such as collagenase, stromelysin, elastase, and cathepsin G, which are secreted by fibroblasts and neutrophils.

Synovial Pathology

Normally one to three cell layers thick, the synovial membrane serves primarily to remove cellular debris from the joint space and to lubricate the joint by producing small amounts of synovial fluid. In rheumatoid arthritis, synovial tissue undergoes lymphocytic infiltration and microvascular changes. Adhesion molecules play an important role in the migration of inflammatory cells into synovial tissue. Eventually, the synovium becomes infiltrated with large numbers of lymphocytes, predominantly CD4-positive T lymphocytes. Structures resembling the germinal centers normally found in spleen and lymph nodes may be seen in rheumatoid arthritis synovial tissue. These lymphoid aggregates may produce immunoglobulin at levels approaching that of a lymph node (24). A significant proportion of the antibodies produced have rheumatoid factor activity. The precise role of rheumatoid factor in the pathogenesis of rheumatoid arthritis is unclear. However, rheumatoid factors can form immune complexes that deposit in the cartilage of affected joints and are capable of activating the complement system. The inflamed synovial tissue proliferates and eventually forms granulation tissue referred to as pannus. Pannus erodes into cartilage and subchondral bone and may lead to total destruction of the joint.

In addition to the lymphocytic infiltration of the synovial tissue, there is also hyperplasia of the connective tissue cells, referred to as mesenchymoid transformation (25). This abnormality, along with the finding that synovitis can exist without lymphocytes in the synovial tissue, implies that there is a nonimmunologic component to rheumatoid arthritis (26).

Genetic Susceptibility

The genes of the MHC loci have been extensively characterized with regard to their role in the pathogenesis of rheumatoid arthritis. Particular class II MHC haplotypes are associated with the presence or severity of rheumatoid arthritis. The DR4 subtypes Dw4 (*DRB*0401*), Dw14 (*DRB1*0404*), and Dw15 (*DRB1*0405*) and DR1 molecules associated with rheumatoid arthritis share amino acid sequence homology in the third hypervariable region of the β chain, suggesting the presence of a susceptibility epitope (27). The presence of HLA-DR4 susceptibility haplotypes has been reported to give a relative risk of about four to five times that of individuals without these haplotypes (28). HLA-DR alleles may also affect disease severity because individuals with rheumatoid arthritis who bear two susceptibility alleles are more likely to have severe disease and extra-articular manifestations than heterozygous individuals (29).

The Neuroendocrine System

The endocrine system, central nervous system, and immune system have complex interactions that may have implications with regard to the rheumatic diseases (30). For example, Lewis rats, which are susceptible to streptococcal cell wall-induced inflammatory arthritis, have a defect in hypothalamic production of corticotropin-releasing hormone (31). The observation that women are more commonly affected than men has prompted many investigations into the relationship between sex hormones and rheumatoid arthritis. Some investigators have found that the use of oral contraceptives protects individuals from developing rheumatoid arthritis, whereas others observed no such beneficial effect (32,33). Nulliparity may be a risk factor for developing rheumatoid arthritis although this finding is also controversial (34).

Further circumstantial evidence that hormonal factors are important in the pathogenesis of rheumatoid arthritis is the observation that pregnancy often ameliorates the disease, first reported by Dr. Philip Hench at the Mayo Clinic in 1938 (35). It is likely that gestational changes in the levels of progesterone, cortisol, and prolactin influence disease activity. However, a recent study found that women whose rheumatoid arthritis improves during pregnancy frequently have fetuses with MHC class II alloantigens that differ from their own (36). Improvement in disease activity may be related to displacement of self-peptides by foreign fetal peptides derived from paternal haplotypes.

Silicone Breast Implants

Although there has been a great deal of publicity about the possible link between silicone breast implants and autoimmune diseases, no data support the hypothesis that silicone breast implants are implicated in the initiation or perpetuation of rheumatoid a rthritis. However, because of the high prevalence of both rheumatoid arthritis and history of augmentation mammoplasty among young women, there are patients with silicone breast implants who have bona fide rheumatoid arthritis.

Clinical Manifestations

The defining abnormality on physical examination is synovitis, ranging from mild (minimal synovial thickening) to severe (tender, erythematous, swollen joints with boggy synovial tissue). The pattern of joint involvement is usually helpful in differentiating rheumatoid arthritis from other types of arthritis because most often there is symmetric involvement of the small joints of the hands and feet. Joints frequently involved during the course of rheumatoid arthritis are listed in Table 31.2. In addition to those listed, the hip and cervical spine are often involved. Thoracic and lumbosacral spine involvement is rare. Other affected joints include cricoarytenoid, temporomandibular, sternoclavicular, and rarely the manubriosternal joint.

Although rheumatoid arthritis is a disease primarily of joints, contiguous anatomic structures such as bursae, tendons, ligaments, and muscles may be painful or inflamed as a result of joint disease. Nerve entrapment syndromes such as carpal tunnel syndrome or tarsal tunnel syndrome are common. The risk of osteoporosis and fractures is higher among patients with rheumatoid arthritis who have never been treated with corticosteroids than in the general population.

Chronic inflammation of a joint may lead to loss of normal anatomic landmarks and relationships (deformities), partial or complete loss of range of motion (flexion contractures), or bony fusion (ankylosis).

Deformities of the hands and wrists and associated muscle atrophy are common and may have a significant impact on the patient's ability to perform activities of daily living. Damage to the collateral ligaments of the small joints may lead to flexion deformities of the distal interphalangeal (DIP) joint and concomitant hyperextension of the PIP joint, referred to as swan-neck deformities (Fig 31.2). Ulnar deviation of the fingers may occur in rheumatoid arthritis (see Fig 31.2), but may also be seen in diverse conditions such as SLE and Parkinson's disease. Subluxation of the MCP joints (see Fig 31.2) may result in a significant decrease in functional ability. Boutonnière deformities are characterized by hyperextension of the DIP joints and flexion of the PIP joints. The so-called Z deformity of the thumb is sometimes seen late in the course of the disease. It consists of subluxation of the carpometacarpal joint, flexion of the MCP joint, and hyperextension of the interphalangeal joint. Persistent synovitis in the wrist may lead to rupture of the extensor tendons, most commonly of the fourth and fifth digits, with resultant inability to extend these fingers. Tenosynovitis of the flexor tendon sheaths is less common. Joint deformity does not always correlate with functional ability because some patients with severe deformities can perform activities of daily living with surprising dexterity.

The glenohumeral joint of the shoulder is frequently involved, as are surrounding structures, including the rotator cuff, supraspinatus and biceps tendon, and subacromial and subdeltoid bursae. Radiographs may reveal erosions or subluxation of the humeral head superiorly. Pain and subsequent voluntary limitation of movement may lead to muscle atrophy or adhesive capsulitis. The elbow is a common site for flexion contractures, rheumatoid nodules, and olecranon bursitis.

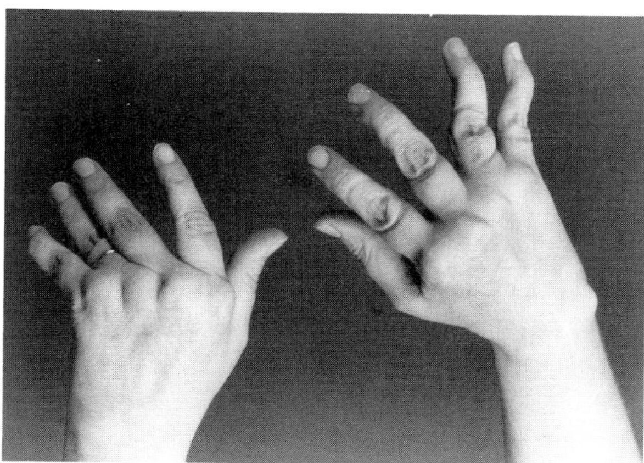

Fig 31.2 Characteristic deformities of the hand in long-standing rheumatoid arthritis. There is ulnar deviation of the fingers of both hands. Significant swelling of the metacarpophalangeal joints is present, along with subluxation of the metacarpal heads. Swan-neck deformities are best seen in the right ring and little fingers. (See accompanying radiographs, Fig 31.3.)

Involvement of the hip joint typically produces pain in the groin region or the buttocks. Occasionally the pain of hip arthritis radiates to the knees, so radiographs of the pelvis may be useful in patients with long-standing disease who have knee pain and normal knee radiographs. There is often pain on active or passive movement, especially internal rotation. With long-standing disease, there may be flexion contractures or markedly decreased range of motion. With destruction of the joint, there may be medial migration of the femoral head into the pelvis, referred to as protrusio acetabuli. Osteonecrosis of the hips should be a diagnostic consideration, especially if the patient has been treated with corticosteroids. Trochanteric bursitis is frequently seen and is characterized by an abnormal degree of tenderness over the greater trochanter of the femur.

Involvement of the knee joint is common. Small effusions in the knee are usually detectable by the bulge sign. This is performed by pushing synovial fluid from the normally concave area medial to the patella, then milking the fluid back into the area from the area lateral or superior to the patella. With large effusions, the patella may be ballotable. Valgus deformity of the knee with associated loss of cartilage in the lateral compartment is common. Radiographs of the knees should be performed with the patient standing because in non-weight-bearing views cartilage loss may be underestimated. Flexion contractures of the knees are a common problem. They are sometimes seen in conjunction with flexion contractures of the hips. Popliteal swelling may be the result of a ruptured popliteal synovial cyst, referred to as a Baker's cyst. Synovial fluid may track down into the calf and be confused with deep vein thrombosis. Popliteal cysts are usually diagnosed by ultrasonography. Treatment consists of percutaneous arthrocentesis with injection of intra-articular corticosteroids. When symptomatic and refractory, synovectomy is required.

The foot may be everted as a result of chronic

arthritis of the subtalar joint. Involvement of the MTP joints frequently causes significant pain in the feet. Hammer or cock-up deformities of the toes represent dorsal subluxation, and as a consequence, the metatarsal heads are displaced toward the plantar surface of the foot. Hallus valgus may lead to overlapping of the second and third toes over the great toe.

Rheumatoid arthritis affects the synovial joints in the cervical spine. The patient may be asymptomatic or may complain of pain in the occipital area, the neck, or headache; symptoms do not necessarily correlate with radiographic changes. Severe disease may cause atlantoaxial subluxation as a result of disruption of the ligaments that normally stabilize these two vertebrae. Most commonly, there is anterior displacement of the C1 vertebra (atlas) on the C2 vertebra (axis), although lateral or vertical displacement may also occur. The odontoid process may be eroded by pannus and migrate superiorly to protrude through the foramen magnum and impinge on the medulla. Signs of cervical myelopathy typically include spasticity, hyperreflexia, upgoing toes, and sensorimotor deficits.

Extra-articular Manifestations

Although rheumatoid arthritis affects joints predominantly, significant morbidity and mortality may result from extra-articular involvement. The most common of these manifestations are listed in Box 31.1.

Box 31.1 Extra-articular Manifestations of Rheumatoid Arthritis

- Rheumatoid nodules
- Rheumatoid vasculitis
- Ophthalmologic
  - Keratoconjunctivitis sicca
  - Episcleritis
  - Scleritis
- Pulmonary
  - Pleural effusion
  - Interstitial lung disease
- Cardiac
  - Pericardial effusion
- Hematologic
  - Felty's syndrome

Rheumatoid Nodules

Rheumatoid nodules are present in up to 35% of patients with established rheumatoid arthritis. As many as 90% of patients with rheumatoid nodules are rheumatoid factor positive; only 5% to 6% of seronegative patients have nodules. Most often nodules appear on the extensor surfaces of the elbows, forearms, and hands, but can also form in the eye, lungs, heart, and central nervous system. The most common nodular skin lesions confused with rheumatoid nodules are gouty tophi. The diagnosis of a tophus is confirmed by examining a small amount of aspirated material for monosodium urate crystals. The characteristic histologic pattern of rheumatoid nodules is central necrosis surrounded by palisading fibroblasts and infiltrates of chronic inflammatory cells. Biopsy of a rheumatoid nodule is seldom needed for diagnostic purposes except when it occurs in the lung (see below). Surgical removal of rheumatoid nodules is not usually successful because they often recur. However, if a nodule is in a particularly bothersome location or is unusually large, patients may opt for removal.

Vasculitis

Rheumatoid vasculitis, a rare complication of rheumatoid arthritis, is characterized histologically by panarteritis (2). Most commonly, rheumatoid vasculitis occurs in male patients with severe erosive arthritis and high titers of rheumatoid factor. There is a wide spectrum of clinical findings in rheumatoid vasculitis (37). Mild sensory neuropathy or sensorimotor neuropathy, such as foot drop, are common in patients with rheumatoid vasculitis. Cutaneous manifestations include splinter hemorrhages of the digits, palpable purpura (leukocytoclastic vasculitis), ulceration, and gangrene of the digits. Involvement of the lungs (alveolitis) or the bowel may occur. Pericarditis may occur as part of the spectrum of rheumatoid vasculitis, but may also occur in patients with rheumatoid arthritis without vasculitis.

Ocular Manifestations

Keratoconjunctivitis sicca is common, with dryness, burning, redness of the eyes, and photophobia as the most frequent complaints. Inflammation of the lacrimal glands is the underlying problem; the glands are often enlarged and may eventually atrophy. Keratoconjunctivitis sicca in conjunction with xerostomia (dry mouth) in the context of established rheumatic disease is referred to as secondary Sjögren's syndrome. Xerostomia is less common than xerophthalmia; symptoms are soreness of the mouth, dryness, and difficult mastication. Accelerated dental caries and tooth loss may result. Episcleritis, manifested by redness, usually causes only mild discomfort, is self-limited, and generally does not require treatment. Nodules histologically resembling rheumatoid nodules may be present in the eye. Scleritis, which occurs less frequently than episcleritis, is often painful; its complications can lead to decreased vision. Necrotizing scleritis without inflammation may lead to thinning of the sclera or perforation into the anterior chamber of the eye (scleromalacia perforans).

Pulmonary Manifestations

Both pleural and parenchymal lung disease are associated with rheumatoid arthritis. Pleural effusions are not often diagnosed clinically but are frequently recognized at autopsy. Pleural fluid is usually exudative in nature and has a low glucose level (usually 10 to 50 mg/dL) (2). Interstitial lung disease may cause a reticulonodular pattern on chest radiographs. On pulmonary function tests, a restrictive defect and decreased diffusion capacity may be reported. Although uncommon, single or multiple rheumatoid nodules may form in the lung parenchyma, appearing as pulmonary nodules on chest radiographs. These should be biopsied in patients with risk factors for bronchogenic carcinoma or if there is reason to suspect infections such as cryptococcosis.

Cardiac Manifestations

Like pleural effusions, pericardial effusions are often noted on autopsy, but they are not a common clinical problem. Constrictive pericarditis and cardiac tamponade have been reported. Myocarditis, endocarditis, and cardiac arrhythmias are rare consequences of rheumatoid arthritis. Coronary arteritis leading to myocardial infarction has also been reported.

Hematologic Manifestations

Normochromic normocytic anemia almost always accompanies rheumatoid arthritis and in general reflects disease activity. There appear to be several factors that contribute to this anemia, including iron deficiency, ineffective erythropoiesis, and impaired response to erythropoietin (2,37). Serum iron levels are often low. Because ferritin is an acute phase reactant, a normal or high ferritin level does not rule out the presence of iron deficiency. The most reliable method of assessing iron stores is examination of bone marrow stained for iron, but this is not usually clinically indicated. Concomitant iron deficiency and vitamin B_{12} and folate deficiency may be seen, with a normal mean cell volume. The anemia of rheumatoid arthritis generally improves when the disease is treated successfully. Thrombocytosis is a nonspecific finding that correlates with inflammatory disease and is seen frequently in patients with active synovitis.

Felty's syndrome is defined as the triad of rheumatoid arthritis, neutropenia, and splenomegaly. Lymphocyte counts are usually normal. Patients may have frequent infections, but not as often as one might expect given the degree of neutropenia. Patients are usually rheumatoid factor positive, and many have antinuclear antibodies to histones or antineutrophil cytoplasmic antibodies.

Laboratory Findings

Some of the more commonly noted laboratory abnormalities found in patients with rheumatoid arthritis are listed in Box 31.2.

Rheumatoid Factor

Rheumatoid factors are antibodies that react against the Fc region of immunoglobulin G. These autoantibodies are present in the serum of 75% to 80% of patients with rheumatoid arthritis, but they are also found among normal individuals and patients with chronic infectious or inflammatory diseases (38,39). The major categories of illness associated with rheu-

Box 31.2 Laboratory Abnormalities Commonly Seen in Patients with Rheumatoid Arthritis

Rheumatoid factor
Elevated erythrocyte sedimentation rate
Normochromic normocytic anemia
Thrombocytosis
Hypoalbuminemia

matoid factor production are rheumatic diseases and other chronic inflammatory diseases, chronic bacterial infections, acute viral illnesses, parasitic diseases, and hypergammaglobulinemic states (Table 31.3).

The most commonly used method of measurement of rheumatoid factor is the latex fixation test. However, many large clinical laboratories use nephelometry, with results reported in international units. The specificity of the rheumatoid factor assay for rheumatoid arthritis is relatively high among highly selected patient populations, such as patients followed in rheumatology practices. Among the general population, however, the specificity is lower. False-positive rates among patients over 75 years of age range from 2% to 25% (8). These findings suggest that the rheumatoid factor assay is best used in patients with a clinical picture that resembles rheumatoid arthritis. Testing for rheumatoid factor should not be done as a screening procedure. Repeated testing among patients with low pretest probability of disease likely increases the chances of a false-positive result (40).

Table 31.3 Diseases Associated with Elevated Serum Rheumatoid Factor

Rheumatic Diseases
Rheumatoid arthritis
Sjögren's syndrome
Systemic lupus erythematosus
Scleroderma
Mixed connective tissue disease
Chronic Bacterial Infections
Subacute bacterial endocarditis
Leprosy
Tuberculosis
Syphilis
Lyme disease
Viral Diseases
Rubella
Cytomegalovirus
Infectious mononucleosis
Influenza
Acquired immunodeficiency syndrome
Parasitic Diseases
Trypanosomiasis
Malaria
Schistosomiasis
Chronic Inflammatory Diseases
Sarcoidosis
Periodontal disease
Pulmonary interstitial disease
Chronic liver disease
Mixed Cryoglobulinemia
Hypergammaglobulinemic Purpura

Sources: Adapted from Schrohenloher RE, Koopman WJ. Rheumatoid factor. In: McCarty DJ, Koopman WJ, eds. Arthritis and allied conditions. Philadelphia: Lea & Febiger, 1993:861–876. Carson DA. Rheumatoid factor. In: Kelley WN, Harris ED Jr, Ruddy S, Sledge CB, eds. Textbook of rheumatology. Philadelphia: WB Saunders, 1993:155–163.

High titers of rheumatoid factor may have prognostic importance among both normal individuals and those with rheumatoid arthritis. In a large longitudinal study of Pima Indians, high titers of rheumatoid factor were associated with increased risk of the subsequent development of rheumatoid arthritis (41). Patients with rheumatoid arthritis who have high titer rheumatoid factor tend to have more severe joint disease and extra-articular manifestations (38).

Erythrocyte Sedimentation Rate

Patients with active rheumatoid arthritis usually, but not always, have elevations in the ESR. As with the rheumatoid factor assay, the ESR is nonspecific because many infectious and inflammatory processes may cause an abnormally elevated ESR (42). In general, the ESR and other acute phase reactants, such as C-reactive protein, reflect disease activity, and seldom provide information that cannot be obtained on history and physical examination.

Synovial Fluid Analysis

Arthrocentesis of affected joints to provide synovial fluid for analysis is often helpful in excluding other types of arthritis. Tests that are sometimes useful on synovial fluid of patients for whom the diagnosis of rheumatoid arthritis is not clearly established include Gram stain and bacterial culture (to rule out infectious arthritis), examination by polarized and nonpolarized light microscopy for crystals (to rule out gout or other crystal-induced arthropathies), and cell count (to allow classification as noninflammatory, inflammatory, or septic fluid). Other tests such as glucose and protein are not helpful. The synovial fluid in rheumatoid arthritis is typically inflammatory, is usually translucent or opaque in appearance, and contains a minimum of 2000 leukocytes/μL (mostly neutrophils) (43). The synovial fluid leukocyte count in active rheumatoid joint effusions often exceeds 2000/μL, but joints with complete cartilage loss may have noninflammatory effusions (<200/μL). Routine analysis of synovial fluid is seldom useful in patients with established, chronic rheumatoid arthritis for whom crystal-induced arthropathy or septic arthritis is not suspected.

Radiographic Findings

Radiographs of the hands and feet are often helpful in the diagnosis of rheumatoid arthritis; radiographs of larger joints are less specific. Early in the disease, nonspecific periarticular soft-tissue swelling and juxta-articular osteopenia may be all that are noted. However, erosive changes, most often in the hands and wrists (Fig 31.3) or feet may be seen early in aggressive disease (44). Common sites for erosions in the hands are shown in Figure 31.4. Early target in the feet include the MTP and PIP joints. Erosions tend to start at the medial and lateral margins of the small joints

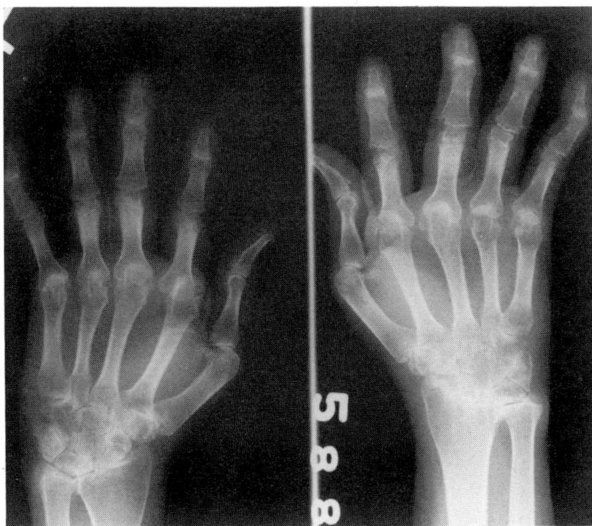

31.3 Radiographic abnormalities characteristic of long-standing rheumatoid arthritis. Juxta-articular osteopenia is present. There is subluxation of all the metacarpal heads and cartilage loss in the radiocarpal and carpometacarpal joints. Marginal erosions are best seen in the proximal interphalangeal joints of the right long and ring fingers. The ulnar styloid processes are eroded and there is soft-tissue swelling most notable in the area of the metacarpophalangeal joints. (See accompanying photographs, Fig 31.2.)

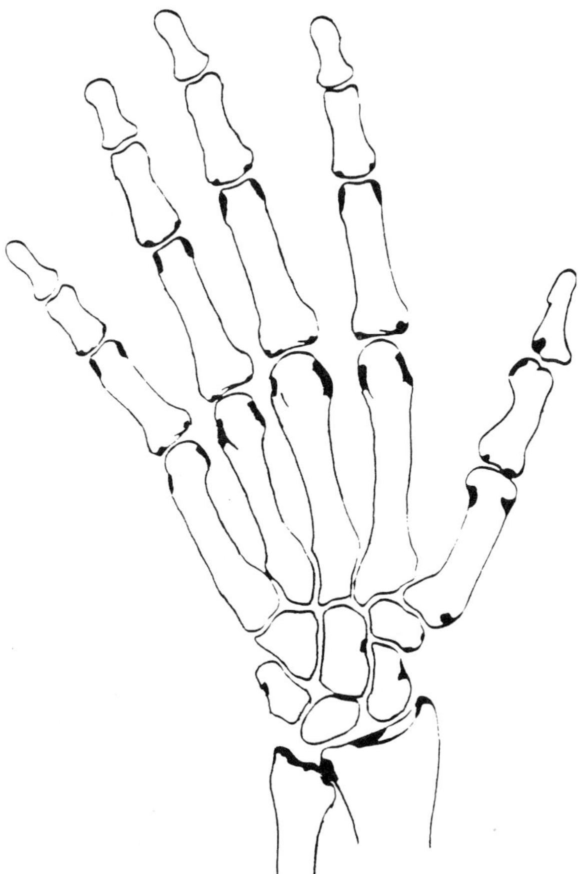

Fig 31.4 Schematic representation of the bones of the hand and wrist. Frequent sites of early erosion in rheumatoid arthritis shaded in black. *(Reproduced by permission from Genant HK. Radiology of the rheumatic diseases. In: McCarty DJ, ed. Arthritis and allied conditions. 11th ed. Philadelphia: Lea & Febiger, 1985: 88–100.)*

because there is no articular cartilage underlying the synovium at the margins of the joints, thus making the bone more susceptible to erosion. In contrast to osteoarthritis, there is usually uniform loss of joint space and no osteophyte formation. Chronic rheumatoid arthritis often leads to subluxations of the phalanges (see Figs 31.2 and 31.3). Ankylosis or complete joint destruction represent the last stage of long-standing rheumatoid arthritis.

Inflammation of the synovial joints of the cervical spine may lead to atlantoaxial subluxation. Initial evaluation of patients suspected of having atlantoaxial subluxation should include lateral radiographs of the cervical spine taken during flexion and extension of the neck. Significant anterior subluxation is usually defined as greater than 3 mm distance between the anterior aspect of the odontoid process of the axis and the posterior arch of the atlas on flexion views. Magnetic resonance imaging may be indicated to determine if there is impingement of the spinal cord or nerve roots.

Treatment

The short-term goals of treatment are to relieve pain and to prevent loss of joint function. Long-term treatment goals include averting the disability, morbidity, or mortality accompanying rheumatoid arthritis. Because the clinical pattern of rheumatoid arthritis is variable, markers that reliably predict the course of the disease and allow stratification of patients according to disease severity would be helpful to clinicians; at present, there are no such parameters. Thus, clinicians use their overall assessment of clinical, radiologic, and laboratory findings to individualize therapeutic regimens. All patients with rheumatoid arthritis should be educated about the disease and the medications used to treat it because this may improve the patient's compliance and attitude toward this chronic illness.

Pharmacologic Management

The goal of pharmacologic treatment is to abrogate the abnormal inflammatory response in affected tissues with the hope of preventing joint destruction. Over 20 years ago, a pyramidal approach was proposed to guide treatment of rheumatoid arthritis. Basic therapy included education of the patient, rest, psychosocial support, and the use of NSAIDs. Progressively more potent (but also more toxic) medications, the disease-modifying antirheumatic drugs (DMARDs), were tried sequentially, beginning with antimalarials and gold salts (45). In recent years, however, several rheumatologists have advocated a more aggressive approach to treatment (46–48). These physicians recommend starting several agents simultaneously early in the course of the disease. As the synovitis improves, medications are sequentially discontinued. The rationale underlying this approach is that significant joint damage occurs in the first 2 years after diagnosis, and that there is a paucity of evidence supporting success of less aggressive treatment strategies. Despite these arguments, however, these aggresive therapeutic approaches have not been widely accepted by rheumatologists.

Nonsteroidal Anti-inflammatory Drugs and Other Analgesics

Aspirin has been used to treat inflammatory conditions since the eighteenth century (48). Aspirin and other NSAIDs have analgesic, antipyretic, and anti-inflammatory effects. NSAIDs are thought to exert their effect largely by inhibiting cyclooxygenase, an enzyme that oxidizes arachidonic acid to prostaglandins, which serve as important mediators of the inflammatory response. Because of the substantial side effects of aspirin, nonacetylated salicylates and nonsalicylate NSAIDs were developed with the goal of providing similar benefit but less toxicity. Nonacetylated salicylates include salsalate and choline magnesium trisalicylate. A rapidly growing number of nonsalicylate NSAIDs are available. Some of these include diclofenac, diflunisal, etodolac, flurbiproben, ibuprofen, indomethacin, ketoprofen, meclofenamate, nabumetone, naproxen, oxaprozin, piroxicam, sulindac, and tolmetin. There is some variability in the mechanisms of action and side effect profiles of these medications, but in general they are similar.

Although they were designed to provide benefits of aspirin with fewer adverse effects, NSAIDs unfortunately cause substantial morbidity and mortality. The most common toxicities are gastrointestinal and include bleeding, peptic ulcer disease, and dyspepsia. Nonacetylated salicylates may be less likely to cause gastic ulceration. Using omeprazole or histamine H_2-receptor antagonists to prevent NSAID-induced duodenal ulcers or misoprostol to prevent gastric ulcerations may provide some benefit, but the long-term efficacy and cost effectiveness of these strategies are unclear at present. Other side effects of NSAIDs are hepatotoxicity as manifested by elevated liver function test results and renal insufficiency secondary to decreased renal perfusion. Chronic use of NSAIDs should be avoided, if possible, in patients at high risk of complications from gastrointestinal ulceration, especially elderly individuals, patients taking anticoagulants, and those with a history of peptic ulcer disease.

Management of the chronic pain associated with rheumatoid arthritis is often difficult. Acetaminophen may be used in conjunction with NSAIDs to relieve pain. If patients require more potent analgesics, low doses of drugs with the least potential for dependency should be tried.

Corticosteroids

One of the seminal observations in the history of rheumatoid arthritis is the discovery of the beneficial effects of adrenal hormones by Hench and colleagues at the Mayo Clinic in 1949 (49). Some experts recommend using corticosteroids as a bridge to span the time from initiation of remittive drug therapy to the time its effects are seen (48). Others, however, do not recommend use of systemic corticosteroids at all because of side effects and lack of prevention of joint destruction (50). A recent study showed that low-dose prednisone may increase risk of side effects such as gastrointestinal bleeding, cataract formation, infection, or fracture, in a dose-dependent fashion (51).

Despite the potential side effects, low-dose prednisone is commonly prescribed for the treatment of rheumatoid arthritis. A dose of 5.0–7.5 mg prednisone given once daily or once every other day may provide symptomatic relief. Prednisone is usually given in the morning, to coincide with the normal circadian pattern of physiologic cortisol release. The use of periodic intramuscular corticosteroid injections or pulse doses of dexamethasone should be avoided because these can potentially lead to recurrent flare-ups as the effect of the drug decreases.

Intra-articular corticosteroids are often helpful in management, particularly among patients with one or two joints that are particularly symptomatic. Injection of a corticosteroid preparation such as methylprednisolone acetate or triamcinolone hexacetonide plus lidocaine can provide temporary and sometimes sustained relief (52). Joints often injected include the shoulder (glenohumeral joint), elbow, wrist (radiocarpal), knee, subtalar, and ankle (tibiotalar). As much synovial fluid as possible should be removed to allow the corticosteroid preparation to be maximally concentrated within the joint. Contraindications to intra-articular steroids include unstable joints, osteonecrosis, and infectious arthritis. Arthrocentesis can generally be performed safely in patients taking anticoagulants if a small-bore needle (22 gauge or smaller) is used, manipulation of the needle is minimized, and pressure is held over the puncture wound for at least 5 minutes. Patients with rheumatoid arthritis who have active involvement of only one joint should probably have synovial fluid Gram stain and culture to rule out infectious arthritis before corticosteroids are injected. Repeated injections into a particular joint should be avoided because evidence suggests it may accelerate degenerative changes. In general, the adverse effects from intra-articular corticosteroid injections, including infection, are rare if careful sterile technique is used.

Disease-Modifying Antirheumatic Drugs

The DMARDs (also known as slow-acting antirheumatic drugs) are commonly used in the treatment of patients with rheumatoid arthritis. There are no universally reliable markers to help physicians decide when to start DMARDs. However, controlling inflammation early in the course of the disease may prevent long-term damage to the joints.

Hydroxychloroquine: The antimalarial drug hydroxychloroquine is useful in the treatment of rheumatoid arthritis. It is less likely to be efficacious than gold or methotrexate but is generally safe (48). Routine laboratory tests are not necessary, so the overall costs are lower than with other DMARDs. Therapy is begun at a dose of 200 mg twice a day. A response is most often seen within 2 to 6 months. Gastrointestinal side effects and skin rashes have been reported, but the most worrisome side effects involve the eye. Fortunately these problems are rare and permanent visual loss can be avoided by early detection. Retinopathy may first present as visual field scotomata. Corneal deposits may be observed but are usually benign and reversible. It is recommended that patients treated with hydroxychloroquine undergo ophthalmologic examinations at 6- to 12-month intervals and that they stop the drug if they experience any unusual visual symptoms.

Gold Compounds: Parenteral gold salts have been used in the treatment of rheumatoid arthritis for many years. The most commonly used forms are aurothioglucose and gold sodium thiomalate. Patients are given an initial dose of 10 mg IM and observed for an idiosyncratic reaction. The dose is increased to 25 mg the next week, then to 50 mg a week thereafter. Lack of efficacy cannot be reliably assessed until the patient has received approximately 1 gm, which usually takes about 5 to 6 months. If the patient has a good response, the gold is continued at a dose of 50 mg weekly. After several months of successful treatment, the dose can be tapered to 50 mg every 2 to 3 weeks, according to the patient's response. Side effects of gold include skin rash, which is usually pruritic, and ulcers of the mucous membranes. Proteinuria is common, but usually readily reversible if detected early. Thrombocytopenia, leukopenia, and aplastic anemia can be a consequence of chrysotherapy, but fortunately they are rare. Complete blood counts and dipstick tests of urine for protein should be performed weekly before each injection. The drug should be discontinued permanently if it appears to be the cause of leukopenia or thrombocytopenia.

Oral gold (auranofin) was designed to provide benefits similar to parenteral gold. Unfortunately, results of treatment have been disappointing and side effects, especially diarrhea, are common.

Methotrexate: Methotrexate has been used extensively to treat malignancy and psoriasis. The Food and Drug Administration approved it for use in the treatment of rheumatoid arthritis in 1988. In long-term studies, methotrexate has been shown to be efficacious and generally safe for use in patients with rheumatoid arthritis (53). Doses of 5.0–25.0 mg are given PO, SQ, or IM once a week. Patients may split the oral dose into two divided doses if nausea is a problem. The injectable form of methotrexate is well absorbed if taken orally in fruit juice or other suitable vehicle (54) and is substantially cheaper than tablets.

The use of methotrexate to treat rheumatoid arthritis appears to be limited more by toxicity than by lack of efficacy (55). Hepatic abnormalities (fatty infiltration, fibrosis, and cirrhosis) were first reported among patients taking antifolates for psoriasis. Patients with rheumatoid arthritis, however, appear to have a low risk of significant liver disease, estimated at about 1/1000 patients treated for 5 years (56). The natural history of methotrexate-induced liver abnormalities is unclear because some patients who continue to receive methotrexate have improvements in liver histology on subsequent biopsy.

The American College of Rheumatology has recently published guidelines for monitoring for potential liver toxicity in patients on methotrexate (57). Patients should be counseled to abstain from ethanol use. Pretreatment liver biopsies should be considered for patients with a history of significant ethanol use or underlying liver disease. Recommended monitoring includes measurement of serum alanine aminotransferase, aspartate aminotransferase, and albumin at 4- to 8-week intervals during therapy. Consistent elevation of liver function tests should prompt consideration of liver biopsy to rule out hepatic damage.

Other potential adverse effects of methotrexate therapy include bone marrow suppression, ulceration of the oral mucosa, and nausea. Complete blood counts should be ordered once a month to detect bone marrow suppression, which usually resolves after the medication is discontinued. Severe life-threatening bone marrow toxicity is very uncommon in patients on low-dose weekly methotrexate, but when present, should be treated with folinic acid (leucovorin). Because methotrexate is excreted through the kidneys and renal dysfunction can result in unacceptably high plasma levels, serum creatinine should be measured every 2 months. Evidence suggests that side effects may be avoided by concomitant treatment with folic acid (1 mg daily) with no loss of efficacy (58).

Sulfasalazine: Sulfasalazine, a conjugate of a salicylate and a sulfonamide, has been used to treat many inflammatory diseases, including inflammatory bowel disease, rheumatoid arthritis, ankylosing spondylitis, Reiter's syndrome, and psoriatic arthritis. The two major categories of toxicities include those that are dose related, such as nausea and vomiting, headache, hemolytic anemia, and methemoglobinemia, and those more suggestive of hypersensitivity reactions, such as aplastic anemia and skin rashes. Renal disease from sulfasalazine has also been reported. Patients are usually started on a dose of 500 mg daily, with a maximum dose of 2–3 gm daily. Complete blood counts and urinalyses should be obtained one or two times monthly at the beginning of therapy, and less often later in the course if the patient tolerates the medication well. Patients with glucose-6-phosphate dehydrogenase deficiency appear to be more likely to develop hemolytic anemia than those with normal enzyme levels.

Other DMARDs: D-Penicillamine, azathioprine, cyclosporin A, and other drugs have been used in the treatment of rheumatoid arthritis. D-Penicillamine has side effects similar to gold compounds, but it has also been associated with the development of autoantibodies such as anticentromere and antihistone antibodies.

Rarely, patients treated with D-penicillamine have been reported to develop antibodies against acetylcholine receptors and basement membranes, resulting in clinical myasthenia gravis and Goodpasture's syndrome, respectively. There are numerous rare side effects of D-penicillamine. Azathioprine is useful in the treatment of rheumatoid arthritis, but potential side effects are substantial; cytopenias and hepatic toxicity are relatively common. Whether azathioprine leads to increased risk of malignancy is controversial. Cyclosporin A has been shown to be effective but is limited by its nephrotoxicity.

Combination Therapy: Multiple permutations of remittive agents have been used in the treatment of rheumatoid arthritis, mostly of patients for whom multiple medications used singly have been ineffective. Lack of data from controlled trials preclude routine recommendation of particular combinations of DMARDs for refractory rheumatoid arthritis.

Biologic Agents and the Future of Treatment of Rheumatoid Arthritis

Recent advances in understanding rheumatoid arthritis at the molecular level have led to changes in therapeutic strategies. Numerous biologic agents are under investigation. These therapies are directed against particular cell surface molecules, cytokines, or receptors that are thought to participate in the perpetuation of the disease (59). Monoclonal antibodies directed against the CD4 molecule (found on helper T cells), TNF-α, and intercellular adhesion molecule-1 as well as soluble IL-1 receptors, IL-1 receptor antagonist, diphtheria-IL-2 fusion toxin, and others are currently being tested (59). Long-term safety and efficacy data are not available at present, but hopefully these agents will provide another avenue for therapeutic intervention.

Nonpharmacologic Management

Psychosocial Issues

Many psychosocial issues surround chronic illnesses such as rheumatoid arthritis. Patients are often fearful of becoming deformed, disabled, or dependent on others. Addressing these issues may help allay fears. Depression and frustration are common among patients, especially those with severe or refractory disease. Pain, fatigue, and altered self-image may have detrimental effects on the patient's sexuality (60).

Nutrition

Patients with rheumatoid arthritis may have protein calorie malnutrition. Difficulty with cooking due to pain or deformity in the hands or to lack of mobility may contribute to this problem. Hypoalbuminemia is common and usually correlates with disease activity. Dietary deficiencies of pyridoxine (vitamin B_6), folic acid, zinc, and magnesium have been reported (61). Although many diets have been purported to be beneficial for rheumatoid arthritis, most have not been scientifically evaluated (62).

Physical and Occupational Therapy

Physical and occupational therapy have an important role in the management of rheumatoid arthritis. Physical therapists may help alleviate pain by using hydrotherapy, diathermy, massage, and ultrasound to affected joints, tendons, or bursae. Stretching and range-of-motion exercises may help maintain joint mobility and function. Joint mobilization may help correct flexion contractures. Routine exercise is often helpful in terms of maintaining patients' functional status (63). Water exercise is especially helpful because pressure on weight-bearing joints is significantly reduced. Walking devices such as canes, crutches, and walkers may assist patients significantly in their activities of daily living. Orthotics, such as shoe inserts or metatarsal bars, may provide symptomatic relief.

Occupational therapists can provide patients with assistive devices useful for dressing, cooking, and housework and other activities of daily living. Instruction on joint protection and conservation of energy are often helpful. Intensive inpatient rehabilitation may provide short-term benefit for some patients with severe rheumatoid arthritis. Inpatient rehabilitation is costly, however, and its cost effectiveness has yet to be proven.

Orthopedic Surgery

Despite the best efforts of physicians to suppress inflammation and preserve normal function of joints, patients often require referral to orthopedic surgeons. Synovectomy, the removal of inflamed synovial tissue, may provide relief of symptoms and improvement of function, especially among patients with severe proliferative synovitis of a particular joint. Development of the technology for total joint replacement of the hip and knee represents one of the major advances in this century for therapy of the rheumatic diseases. Severe pain, destruction of cartilage, and limited function are indications for knee or hip replacement. Results of joint replacement of the shoulder, elbow, wrist, and ankle are generally less satisfactory than hip and knee replacement.

Sometimes joint fusion may be a better option than joint replacement. Such is the case with the ankle, where triple arthrodesis of the subtalar, talonavicular, and calcaneocuboid joints can provide significant pain relief while maintaining normal alignment and only moderate loss of range of motion.

As mentioned previously, patients with severe erosive disease and complaints of neck or occipital pain may have cervical spine involvement. Such patients for whom surgical procedures are being considered should have evaluation for possible cervical spinal cord compression because of the risk of spinal cord injury during intubation for general anesthesia. Refractory neck or occipital pain with documented impingement on the spinal canal should lead to a consideration of fusion of the cervical spine.

Unconventional Therapies

Anecdotal reports of benefit from the use of unproven therapies abound in the lay press. Such remedies include nutritional supplements, vitamins, minerals, venoms, herbal preparations, topical agents such as dimethyl sulfoxide, and many others (64). Patients are willing to try these therapies because conventional treatments are often expensive, have side effects, and are not curative. Reports of success from nontraditional remedies are attributable in part to the episodic nature of rheumatoid arthritis. Spontaneous improvements and exacerbations are common among rheumatoid arthritis patients. Many patients in placebo-controlled groups of therapeutic trials have improvement of disease, highlighting the need for controlled trials for adequate evaluation of therapeutic interventions.

Prognosis

Some patients with rheumatoid arthritis may have prolonged clinical remissions beginning within the first year of disease (2). Published criteria for remission include morning stiffness of less than 15 minutes' duration; the absence of fatigue, joint pain, tenderness, or pain on motion; the absence of soft-tissue swelling in joints or tendons sheaths; and a normal ESR (65). After a year of sustained disease, such remissions are rare. A substantial proportion of patients with rheumatoid arthritis have progressive disease that may eventually lead to joint destruction. Patients with seronegative rheumatoid arthritis appear to have a slightly better prognosis than those with seropositive rheumatoid arthritis. Patients who are positive for rheumatoid factor tend to have more aggressive synovitis and are more likely to develop extra-articular manifestations such as nodules and vasculitis.

Decreased survival of patients with rheumatoid arthritis has been consistently documented and appears to be related to severity of the disease (66). Attributable causes of death in rheumatoid arthritis generally reflect those seen in the general population. Premature deaths from cardiovascular disease, infectious disease, and other causes unrelated to rheumatoid arthritis may in fact be the result of physical disability and psychosocial factors associated with this chronic illness, although this has not been proven.

Referral to a Rheumatologist

Patients with rheumatoid arthritis are often managed by primary care physicians and rheumatologists working together. Because rheumatoid arthritis is associated with an increase in morbidity and mortality, referral to a rheumatologist should occur as early in the course of the disease as possible (67). Primary care physicians help with managing comorbid conditions and monitoring for drug side effects, often through screening for abnormal results of laboratory tests. Rheumatologists can provide primary care physicians with assistance in directing long-term care. Specifically, they can assess prognosis and institute treatment with DMARDs, determine the need for referrals to physical therapists or orthopedic surgeons, and perform intra-articular corticosteroid injections.

REFERENCES

1. Short CL. Rheumatoid arthritis: historical aspects. J Chron Dis 1959;10:367–387.

2. Harris ED Jr. Clinical features of rheumatoid arthritis. In: Kelley WN, Harris ED Jr, Ruddy S, Sledge CB, eds. Textbook of rheumatology. 4th ed. Philadelphia: WB Saunders, 1993:874–911.

3. McCarty DJ. Clinical picture of rheumatoid arthritis. In: McCarty DJ, Koopman WJ, eds. Arthritis and allied conditions. 12th ed. Philadelphia: Lea & Febiger, 1993:781–809.

4. Arnett FC, Edworthy SM, Block DA, et al. The American Rheumatism Association 1987 revised criteria for the classification of rheumatoid arthritis. Arthritis Rheum 1988;31:315–324.

5. Jacoby RK, Jayson MIV, Cosh JA. Onset, early stages, and prognosis of rheumatoid arthritis: a clinical study of 100 patients with 11 year follow-up. Br Med J 1973;2:96–100.

6. Fleming A, Crown JM, Corbett M. Early rheumatoid disease. 1. Onset. Ann Rheum Dis 1976;35:357–360.

7. Fallahi S, Halla JT, Hardin JG. A reassessment of the nature of onset of rheumatoid arthritis. Clin Res 1983;31:650A. Abstract.

8. Shmerling RH, Liang MH. Evaluation of the patient: B. Laboratory evaluation of the rheumatic diseases. In: Schumacher HR Jr, Klippel JH, Koopman WJ, eds. Primer on the rheumatic diseases. 10th ed. Atlanta, GA: Arthritis Foundation, 1993:64–66.

9. Hunder GG, Goronzy J, Weyand C. Is seronegative RA in the elderly the same as polymyalgia rheumatica? Bull Rheum Dis 1994;43(1):1–3.

10. Yunus MB, Masi AT. Fibromyalgia, restless legs syndrome, periodic limb movement disorder, and psychogenic pain. In: McCarty DJ, Koopman WJ, eds. Arthritis and allied conditions. 12th ed. Philadelphia: Lea & Febiger, 1993:1383–1405.

11. Mangi RJ. Viral arthritis—the great masquerader. Bull Rheum Dis 1994;43(1):5–6.

12.Schmid FR. Principles of diagnosis and treatment of bone and joint infections. In: McCarty DJ, Koopman WJ, eds. Arthritis and allied conditions. 12th ed. Philadelphia: Lea & Febiger, 1993:1975–2001.

13. Goldenberg DL. Gonococcal arthritis and other neisserial infections. In: McCarty DJ, Koopman WJ, eds. Arthritis and allied conditions. 12th ed. Philadelphia: Lea & Febiger, 1993:2025–2033.

14. Talbott JH, Altman RD, Yu T-F. Gouty arthritis masquerading as rheumatoid arthritis or vice versa. Semin Arthritis Rheum 1978;8:77–114.

15. Turner RE, Frank MJ, Van Ausdal D, Bollet AJ. Some aspects of the epidemiology of gout: Sex and race incidence. Arch Intern Med 1960;106:400–406.

16. Wallace SL, Robinson H, Masi AT, et al. Preliminary criteria for the classification of the acute arthritis of primary gout. Arthritis Rheum 1977;20:895–900.

17. Kozin F, McCarty DJ. Rheumatoid factor in the serum of gouty patients. Arthritis Rheum 1977;20:1559–1560.

18. Ryan LM, McCarty DJ. Calcium pyrophosphate crystal deposition disease; pseudogout; articular chondrocalcinosis. In: McCarty DJ, Koopman WJ, eds. Arthritis and allied conditions. 12th ed. Philadelphia: Lea & Febiger, 1993:1835–1855.

19. Reveille JD. The spondyloarthropathies. In: Ball GV, Koopman WJ, eds. Clinical rheumatology. Philadelphia: WB Saunders, 1986:164–182.

20. Rahn DW, Malawista SE. Lyme disease. In: McCarty DJ, Koopman WJ, eds. Arthritis and allied conditions. 12th ed. Philadelphia: Lea & Febiger, 1993:2067–2079.

21. Caldwell DS, McCallum RM. Rheumatologic manifestations of cancer. Med Clinics North Am 1986;70:385–417.

22. Panayi GS, Lanchbury JS, Kingsley GH. The importance of the T cell in initiating and maintaining the chronic synovitis of rheumatoid arthritis. Arthritis Rheum 1992;35:729–735.

23. Arend WP. Mediators of inflammation B. Growth factors and cytokines in the rheumatic diseases. In: Schumacher HR Jr, Klippel JH, Koopman WJ, eds. Primer on the rheumatic diseases. 10th ed. Atlanta, GA: Arthritis Foundation, 1993:46–50.

24. Smiley JD, Sachs C, Ziff M. In vitro synthesis of immunoglobulin by rheumatoid synovial membrane. J Clin Invest 1968;47:624–632.

25. Fassbender HG. Rheumatoid arthritis. In: Fassbender HG, ed. Pathology of rheumatic diseases. New York: Springer-Verlag, 1975:79–210.

26. Koopman WJ, Gay S. Do nonimmunologically mediated pathways play a role in the pathogenesis of rheumatoid arthritis? Rheum Dis Clin North Am 1993;19:107–122.

27. Gregersen PK, Silver J, Winchester R. The shared epitope hypothesis: an approach to understanding the molecular genetics of susceptibility to rheumatoid arthritis. Arthritis Rheum 1987;30:1205–1213.

28. Stasny P. Association of the B-cell alloantigen DRw4 with rheumatoid arthritis. N Engl J Med

1978;298:869–871.

29. Weyand CM, Hicok KC, Conn DL, Goronzy JJ. The influence of HLA-DRB1 genes on disease severity in rheumatoid arthritis. Ann Intern Med 1992;117: 869–871.

30. Cash JM, Wilder RL. Neurobiology and inflammatory arthritis. Bull Rheum Dis 1992;41(5):1–3.

31. Sternberg EM, Young WS III, Bernardini R, et al. A central nervous system defect in biosynthesis of corticotropin-releasing hormone is associated with susceptibility to streptococcal cell wall-induced arthritis in Lewis rats. Proc Natl Acad Sci, USA 1989;86:4771–4775.

32. Wingrave SJ, Kay CR. Reduction in incidence of rheumatoid arthritis associated with oral contraceptives. Lancet 1978;1:569–571.

33. Hernandez-Avila M, Liang MH, Willett WC, et al. Exogenous sex hormones and the risk of rheumatoid arthritis. Arthritis Rheum 1990;33:947–953.

34. Wilder RL. Rheumatoid arthritis: A. Epidemiology, pathology, and pathogenesis. In: Schumacher HR Jr, Klippel JH, Koopman WJ, eds. Primer on the rheumatic diseases. 10th ed. Atlanta, GA: Arthritis Foundation, 1993:86–89.

35. Hench PS. The ameliorating effect of pregnancy on chronic atrophic (infectious rheumatoid) arthritis, fibrositis, and intermittent hydrarthrosis. Proc Staff Meet Mayo Clin 1938;13:161–167.

36. Nelson JL, Hughes KA, Smith AG, et al. Maternal-fetal disparity in HLA class II alloantigens and the pregnancy-induced amelioration of rheumatoid arthritis. N Engl J Med 1993;329:466–471.

37. Bacon PA. Extra-articular rheumatoid arthritis. In: McCarty DJ, Koopman WJ, eds. Arthritis and allied conditions. 12th ed. Philadelphia: Lea & Febiger, 1993:811–840.

38. Schrohenloher RE, Koopman WJ. Rheumatoid factor. In: McCarty DJ, Koopman WJ, eds. Arthritis and Allied Conditions. 12th ed. Philadelphia: Lea & Febiger, 1993:861–876.

39. Carson DA. Rheumatoid factor. In: Kelley WN, Harris ED Jr, Ruddy S, Sledge CB, eds. Textbook of rheumatology. 4th ed. Philadelphia: WB Saunders, 1993:155–163.

40. Lichtenstein MJ, Pincus T. How useful are combinations of blood tests in "rheumatic panels" in the diagnosis of rheuamtic disease? J Gen Intern Med 1988;3:435–442.

41. Del Puente A, Knowler WC, Pettitt DJ, Bennett PH. The incidence of rheumatoid arthritis is predicted by rheumatoid factor titer in a longitudinal population study. Arthritis Rheum 1988;31:1239–1244.

42. Sox HC Jr, Liang MH. The erythrocyte sedimentation rate: guidelines for rational use. Ann Intern Med 1986;104:515–523.

43. Gatter RA. A practical handbook of joint fluid analysis. Philadelphia: Lea & Febiger, 1984.

44. Brower AC. Rheumatoid arthritis. In: Arthritis in black and white. Philadelphia: WB Saunders Company, 1988:137–165.

45. Williams HJ. Rheumatoid arthritis: C. Treatment. In: Schumacher HR Jr, Klippel JH, Koopman WJ, eds. Primer on the rheumatic diseases. 10th ed. Atlanta, GA: Arthritis Foundation, 1993:96–99.

46. Wilske KR, Healey LA. Remodeling the pyramid—a concept whose time has come. J Rheumatol 1989;16:565–567. Editorial.

47. McCarty DJ. Suppress rheumatoid inflammation early and leave the pyramid to the Egyptians. J Rheumatol 1990;17:1115–1118. Editorial.

48. Harris ED Jr. Treatment of rheumatoid arthritis. In: Kelley WN, Harris ED Jr, Ruddy S, Sledge CB, eds. Textbook of rheumatology. 4th ed. Philadelphia: WB Saunders, 1993:912–923.

49. Hench PS, Kendall EC, Slocumb CH, Polley HF. The effect of a hormone of the adrenal cortex (17-hydroxy-11-dehydrocorticosterone: compound E) and of pituitary adrenocorticotropic hormone on rheumatoid arthritis. Proc Staff Meet Mayo Clin 1949;24:181–197.

50. McCarty DJ. Treatment of rheumatoid arthritis. In: McCarty DJ, Koopman WJ, eds. Arthritis and allied conditions. 12th ed. Philadelphia: Lea & Febiger, 1993:877–886.

51. Saag KG, Koehnke R, Caldwell JR, et al. Low dose long-term corticosteroid therapy in rheumatoid arthritis: an analysis of serious adverse effects. Am J Med 1994;96:115–123.

52. McCarthy GM, McCarty DJ. Intrasynovial corticosteroid therapy. Bull Rheum Dis 1994;43(3):2–4.

53. Weinblatt ME, Weissman BN, Holdsworth DE, et al. Long-term prospective study of methotrexate in the treatment of rheumatoid arthritis: 84-month update. Arthritis Rheum 1992;35:129–137.

54. Jundt JW, Browne BA, Fiocco GP, et al. A comparison of low dose methotrexate bioavailability: oral solution, oral tablet, subcutaneous, and intramuscu-

lar dosing. J Rheumatol 1993;20:1845–1849.

55. Alarcón GS, Tracy IC, Blackburn WD Jr. Methotrexate in rheumatoid arthritis: toxic effects as the major factor in limiting long-term treatment. Arthritis Rheum 1989;32:671–676.

56. Walker AM, Funch D, Dreyer NA, et al. Determinants of serious liver disease among patients receiving low-dose methotrexate for rheumatoid arthritis. Arthritis Rheum 1993;36:329–335.

57. Kremer JM, Alarcón GS, Lightfoot RW Jr, et al. Methotrexate for rheumatoid arthritis: suggested guidelines for monitoring liver toxicity. Arthritis Rheum 1994;37:316–328.

58. Morgan SL, Baggott JE, Vaugh WH, et al. The effect of folic acid supplementation on the toxicity of low dose methotrexate in patients with rheumatoid arthritis. Arthritis Rheum 1990;33:9–18.

59. Moreland LW, Heck LW Jr, Sullivan W, et al. New approaches to the therapy of autoimmune diseases: rheumatoid arthritis as a paradigm. Am J Med Sci 1993;305:40–51.

60. Liang MH. Psychosocial management of rheumatic diseases. In: Kelley WN, Harris ED Jr, Ruddy S, Sledge CB, eds. Textbook of rheumatology. 4th ed. Philadelphia: WB Saunders, 1993:535–543.

61. Kremer JM. Nutrition and rheumatic diseases. In: Kelley WN, Harris ED Jr, Ruddy S, Sledge CB, eds. Textbook of rheumatology. 4th ed. Philadelphia: WB Saunders, 1993:484–497.

62. Panush RS. Arthritis, food allergy, diets, and nutrition. In: McCarty DJ, Koopman WJ, eds. Arthritis and allied conditions. 12th ed. Philadelphia: Lea & Febiger, 1993:1139–1146.

63. Galloway MT, Jokl P. The role of exercise in the treatment of inflammatory arthritis. Bull Rheum Dis 1993;42(1):1–4.

64. Panush RS. Is there a role for diet or other questionable therapies in managing rheumatic disease? Bull Rheum Dis 1993;42(4):1–4.

65. Pinals RS, Masi AF, Larsen RA. Preliminary criteria for clinical remission in rheumatoid arthritis. Arthritis Rheum 1981;24:1308–1315.

66. Pincus T, Callahan LF. Early mortality in RA predicted by poor clinical status. Bull Rheum Dis 1992;41(4):1–4.

67. Hochberg MC. Editorial: influencing mortality outcomes in RA. Bull Rheum Dis 1992;41(4):4–5.

CHAPTER 32

SYSTEMIC LUPUS ERYTHEMATOSUS

W. Winn Chatham

Systemic lupus erythematosus (SLE) is a systemic inflammatory disease that may affect multiple organs. The disease predominantly affects women, with a female-male ratio of disease prevalence of approximately 5:1 (1). Manifestations of SLE may initially develop over the age of 50 but most commonly present in women between the ages of 15 and 40. The prevalence is variable, dependent to a large extent on the racial constituency of the population. Estimates of SLE prevalence in populations of black women in the United States approach 1 in 250, whereas the prevalence in white women is much lower, approximating 1 in 4000 (2,3). Relative to non-Hispanic white women, SLE appears to be more prevalent among Hispanic and Asian women (3,4). The etiology of SLE generally remains unknown, but there is a strong familial aggregation of disease prevalence and several genetic risk factors for development of SLE have been identified. However, a significant percentage of patients with SLE have no identifiable familial or genetic risk factors for development of the disease, suggesting the disease may be triggered by a variety of mechanisms.

Clinical Features

Constitutional Symptoms

Fatigue is commonly a presenting feature of SLE and may be present in the absence of other disease manifestations. Patients typically complain of inability to perform work tasks or daily living activities without frequent rest periods or naps during the day. Fatigue often improves during treatment with corticosteroids or antimalarials, and may be a sensitive indicator of a pending exacerbation of disease activity.

Fever is frequently present during flares of disease activity and may be the sole presenting feature. Elevations in temperature above 38.8°C (102°F) attributable to disease activity are not uncommon, but the presence of fever in a patient with SLE always requires a diligent search for associated infection. Infectious complications are a major cause of mortality in patients with SLE, even among patients not treated with steroids or other immunosuppressive measures (5).

Despite the relative inactivity imposed by fatigue symptoms, up to two thirds of patients report weight loss during the months antedating diagnosis of SLE (6). Increased catabolism due to systemic inflammation likely accounts for weight loss because anorexia is not commonly reported. Weight loss may be particularly pronounced in patients with myositis.

Articular and Musculoskeletal Features

Arthritis affecting the peripheral joints is the most common disease manifestation of SLE, occurring at some time in over 80% of patients studied, regardless of the age at onset of disease (7,8). Articular symptoms are also one of the most common presenting symptoms, both in young women and in women over the age of 50 who present with SLE. Joint symptoms are typically symmetric, most commonly involving the proximal interphalangeal, wrist, metacarpophalangeal (MCP), and knee joints. The shoulders, hips, elbows, ankles, and metatarsal joints are less frequently involved. Axial (cervical/lumbar/sacroiliac) joints are rarely affected by SLE.

The arthritis in SLE patients usually does not produce the radiographic appearance of bony erosions characteristic of patients with advanced rheumatoid arthritis. However, erosions may occasionally be seen in the MCP joints, and radiographic evidence of significant cartilage loss may develop in chronically swollen joints.

Tenosynovitis is reported to occur in up to 8% of patients, typically involving extensor tendons of the forearms and lower legs. Inflammation of tendon sheaths is characterized by focal pain and swelling exacerbated by passive manipulation of the involved tendons. It is important to remember that tenosynovitis commonly occurs due to other factors, including overuse syndromes and infections. The acute onset of tenosynovitis in a sexually active woman should always bring to mind to the possibility of disseminated gonococcal infection. In a small minority of patients, chronic periarticular inflammation involving tendons and ligamentous structures adjacent to the MCP joints may eventuate in ulnar deviation of the MCP joints or swan-neck deformities. Patients with SLE may also develop subcutaneous nodules, typically found over extensor surfaces. These lesions are histologically indistinguishable from those seen in rheumatoid arthritis and often resolve during treatment for other disease manifestations (5,9).

Osteonecrosis or avascular necrosis is a complication of SLE, which may present as joint or extremity pain. Osteonecrosis in lupus patients most commonly occurs in the proximal humerus, proximal or distal femur, proximal or distal tibia, or in the talus. A major risk factor for the development of osteonecrosis in patients with SLE is treatment with moderate to high doses of corticosteroids (10,11). The presence of antiphospholipid antibodies may also be a risk factor for development of osteonecrosis, even in the absence of treatment with corticosteroids (11). Osteonecrosis should be considered in patients presenting with pain in the shoulder, groin or anterior thigh, knee, or ankle that is not otherwise explained by synovitis or other periarticular disorders. The diagnosis is best confirmed with magnetic resonance imaging of the involved joint; this modality reliably reveals evidence of osteonecrosis weeks or months before changes detected by routine radiographs and reveals findings much more specific than those detected by radionuclide bone scans.

Cutaneous Manifestations

Following articular symptoms, skin rashes comprise the next most common disease manifestation of SLE (7,8). Cutaneous lesions in SLE are quite variable, ranging from macular rashes to necrotic ulcers. Erythematous rashes are the most frequent cutaneous lesion, appearing predominantly (but not exclusively) on sun-exposed areas of the face, neck, arms, and upper torso. Although sunlight frequently triggers many of the erythematous rashes seen in SLE, cutaneous lesions may appear without antecedent sun exposure.

The typical appearance of malar erythema (butterfly rash) on the maxillary areas of the face and bridge of the nose is often the initial objective manifestation of SLE, antedating other physical findings. Its appearance in some patients may be quite subtle and intermittent; other patients may have a much more pronounced rash with significant subcutaneous edema. Conditions such as seborrhea or acne rosacea may result in a similar appearance, but the tendency for the malar erythema of SLE to spare the nasolabial fold may be a helpful distinguishing feature. The malar rash of SLE usually heals without residual scarring or changes in skin pigmentation.

Photosensitivity is a common feature of SLE; in addition to skin rashes, patients often report significant constitutional symptoms such as fever, fatigue, or nausea after sun exposure. Rashes after sun exposure are usually macular or maculopapular, but may have an urticarial or bullous component. With the exception of the unusual occurrence of bullous lesions, photosensitive rashes are transient, often lasting no more than a day or two. However, even in patients whose rash persists for several weeks, most lesions resolve without scarring or permanent changes in pigment.

Diffuse, maculopapular erythematous rashes occurring on the extremities and torso (sun exposed as well as non-sun exposed) may also be seen in a subset of SLE patients having antibodies to the Ro (SS-A) antigen (12). Many of these patients comprise a subset of patients with SLE who do not have demonstrable antinuclear antibodies (ANA) in their sera (13,14). Identification of pregnant women with antibodies to SS-A/Ro antigen is important because of the association of these antibodies with fetal cardiac conduction abnormalities (15).

Discoid skin lesions are more chronic and frequently leave residual scarring and pigment changes. These lesions begin as well demarcated papules that evolve through an erythematous and edematous phase into hyperkeratotic lesions. The lesions eventually undergo atrophy, with loss of pigmentation centrally and hyperpigmentation at the margins of the lesion. Their distribution is similiar to other rashes seen in SLE, commonly occurring on the malar area, torso, and proximal upper extremities; however, discoid lesions may also appear on the scalp and ears. Discoid skin lesions may be the sole manifestation of SLE for decades, with some patients never developing other disease manifestations.

Alopecia is present to some extent in over 50% of patients at disease onset (7,8). Hair loss may be diffuse or (less commonly) patchy and may occur in the absence of other identifiable scalp lesions. Except for areas of the scalp with discoid lesions, hair loss during periods of disease activity is usually not permanent.

Vascular lesions are a common pathologic finding in SLE and may result in a variety of cutaneous manifestations. Vasculitic lesions resulting in tender, indurated papules most commonly appear on the fingertips and extensor surfaces of the forearms and may ulcerate. Nonulcerating lesions may appear on the palms and soles. Cutaneous vasculitis in patients with SLE may also present as purpura, splinter hemorrhages beneath the nail beds, or as nail fold infarcts. Vasculopathy involving deeper, subcutaneous arterioles may result in a lacy, reticular pattern over the distal upper and lower extremities (livedo reticularis).

Tender, erythematous nodules on the extremities may also occur as a result of nonsuppurative nodular panniculitis (lupus profundus). Although panniculitis is uncommon in SLE, it may be a presenting feature of the disease, antedating other disease manifestations by several years (16). These lesions may ulcerate and frequently result in residual scarring and induration.

Oral Mucosal Lesions

Oral ulcers frequently occur in SLE. Patients may report painful lesions occurring on the buccal mucosa, tongue, or mucosa of the lips. However, painless lesions involving the hard or soft palate occur commonly and may not be appreciated unless they are looked for. Inspection of the hard palate for mucosal lesions often provides a useful diagnostic clue to the presence of SLE in a young woman presenting with arthralgias or otherwise unexplained skin rash. Hard palate lesions may range in appearance from small, scattered areas of erythema to geographic hyperpigmented areas covering the entirety of the palate.

Renal Disease

Nephritis is one of the more serious complications of SLE and has historically been associated with lower survival. However, earlier recognition of patients with nephritis and improvements in management may be effecting improved survival in this subset of patients. Accordingly, an essential component of the care of any patients with SLE is frequent assessment for signs of nephritis such as elevation in blood pressure, proteinuria, hematuria, or increase in the serum creatinine level.

The pathologically defined categories of lupus nephritis most commonly used are those defined by the World Health Organization (WHO) (17). WHO class I refers to patients for whom no lesions can be identified by light, immunofluorescent, or electron microscopy. Such a finding at renal biopsy is unusual in a patient with SLE because abnormalities ranging from subepithelial deposits of immunoglobulin and complement to proliferative glomerular lesions are present in the vast majority of patients with SLE studied with renal biopsy or at autopsy.

Mesangial disease (WHO class II) is characterized by subepithelial and/or mesangial deposits of immunoglobulin and complement, with (class IIB) or without (class IIA) focal proliferative glomerular lesions. Varying degrees of proteinuria and hematuria may be present in patients with this lesion, but renal insufficiency is uncommon. A significant number of patients noted to have mesangial disease with only subepithelial deposits at biopsy have been followed for years without development of clincally apparent renal disease. Patients with focal proliferative nephritis (WHO class III) typically have mild to moderate proteinuria with hematuria, often in association with other significant systemic disease manifestations. Mild renal insufficiency (manifest by decreased creatinine clearance) is often present. Patients initially noted to have either mesangial lesions with subendothelial deposits or focal proliferative lesions may later develop diffuse proliferative disease with accompanying deterioration in renal function (18).

Patients with diffuse proliferative nephritis (WHO class IV) typically present with heavy proteinuria, renal insufficiency, and hematuria, often with red cell casts in the urine. Histologically, cellular proliferation is present in over 50% of glomeruli, often with cellular crescents enveloping the glomeruli. Electron microscopy typically reveals extensive subepithelial, mesangial, and subendothelial deposits. The presence of antibodies to double-stranded DNA in significant titer, low levels of serum complement components C3 and C4, and a low CH50 often correlate with the presence of active nephritis in this group of patients.

Membranous nephritis (WHO class V) is typically associated with moderate to heavy proteinuria and nephrotic syndrome. Although not present initially, renal insufficiency often develops in the absence of immunosuppressive therapy. The lesions of membranous lupus nephritis are histologically indistinguishable from those of idiopathic membranous glomerulonephritis. Serologic abnormalities such as low complement levels or antibodies to DNA are often absent if extrarenal manifestations of SLE are not present.

In addition to glomerular disease, patients with SLE may also develop interstitial and renal tubular disease (6,19,20). Interstitial disease is most commonly seen in patients with diffuse proliferative nephritis, but histologic evidence of immune complex interstitial disease has been noted in the absence of severe glomerular lesions (6). Some patients have evidence of renal tubular acidosis, but such patients frequently have accompanying evidence of Sjögren's syndrome (19).

The clinical presentation of patients with lupus nephritis does not always correlate with the pathologic lesions present on biopsy (21,22). Patients presenting with moderate proteinuria may have membranous disease or evolving diffuse proliferative disease. Factors unrelated to SLE such as drug-induced (nonsteroidal anti-inflammatory drugs [NSAIDs]) decreases in glomerular filtration or interstitial disease may also account for renal dysfunction and abnormalities of the urinary sediment.

Although renal biopsy is not uniformly recommended for all patients with clinical evidence of nephritis, in selected patients the information provided by renal biopsy may be useful in establishing the cause of deteriorating renal function and formulating the optimal treatment plan. Biopsy may be particularly useful in determining if progressive renal insufficiency in a given patient is associated with active glomerular inflammation and not progressive glomerular scarring and tubular atrophy. In such cases, aggressive immunosuppressive therapy is likely to be of benefit; however, should a biopsy in this setting reveal significant scarring and tubular atrophy (high chronicity index), the risk of toxicity associated with immunosuppressive therapy would likely outweigh any potential benefits of salvaging renal function.

Pleuropericardial Disease

Serositis involving the pleura or pericardium occurs in up to 50% of SLE patients at some time during the course of their disease (7,8). Pleuritic pain often occurs in the absence of radiographic evidence of pleural effusion or audible pleural friction rub. Fluid obtained by thoracentesis is typically exudative; the cellularity is variable, but neutrophils are the predominant cell type. Lupus erythematosus cells may be present in the pleural fluid of lupus patients and are most readily found when examining Wright-stained cytospin preparations of pleural fluid.

Pericarditis is most often manifest by pericardial rub, with or without chest pain. As is the case for pleural disease, pain or presence of a rub frequently occurs in the absence of significant pericardial fluid accumulation identifiable by echocardiography. Although chronic, adhesive pericarditis may occur in patients with SLE, pericardial tamponade is uncommon (23).

Lung Disease

Parenchymal lung disease in patients with SLE may occur as an acute pneumonitis or as a chronic interstitial process (24,25). Acute pneumonitis typically presents as dyspnea with or without accompanying cough, fever, or chest pain. Chest radiographs usually reveal diffuse acinar infiltrates; although unilateral involvement may occur, the infiltrates predominantly involve the basilar segements of both lung bases. Acute pneumonitis occurring as a consequence of disease-related alveolitis may be accompanied by a component of alveolar hemorrhage (26). It should be recognized that acute pneumonitis in patients with SLE most commonly occurs as a consequence of infection; accordingly, a thorough diagnostic evaluation including bronchoscopy or lung biopsy to exclude possible infectious processes should be undertaken in lupus patients presenting with signs of pneumonitis. Acute alveolitis not due to infection in patients with SLE may be rapidly fatal and requires prompt treatment with high-dose corticosteroids. Patients may fully recover without residual scarring or pulmonary dysfunction, whereas others may develop chronic infiltrates with persistent impairment in gas exchange.

Chronic interstitial lung disease may develop in patients with lupus in the absence of antecedent acute pneumonitis. The presenting features are usually exertional dyspnea with bibasilar infiltrates on chest radiographs. Pulmonary function testing most often reveals a restrictive ventilatory defect with impaired diffusion capacity.

Cardiovascular Disease

Although much less common than pericarditis, myocardial inflammation resulting in congestive heart failure may occur (27). In addition to congestive cardiomyopathy, inflammatory lesions may cause myocardial conduction disturbances including sinus arrest, atrioventricular block, or bundle branch block (28). Myocardial infarction may occur as a consequence of accelerated atherosclerosis of coronary vessels or, less commonly, as a result of coronary arteritis (29). Patients treated with long-term steroids are particularly at risk for coronary artery disease; several studies have demonstrated a direct correlation between the dose and duration of steroid therapy and symptomatic coronary artery disease (30,31).

A variety of cardiac valvular disorders have been reported in patients with SLE, resulting in symptomatic stenotic or regurgitant lesions (32). In the presteroid era, up to a third of lupus patients studied at autopsy had evidence of verrucous lesions on valve leaflets or chordae tendineae (Libman-Sacks lesions). These lesions often are of little significance clinically, but they may serve as a nidus for bacterial seeding of the valve resulting in bacterial endocarditis. Thrombi associated with Libman-Sacks lesions may enlarge significantly, resulting in valve dysfunction or peripheral arterial embolization. In the past decade, there have been a number of lupus patients reported with large thrombi on the valve leaflets, many of whom also have significant titers of antibody to phospholipid (33). Acute valvular inflammation resulting in severe regurgitant lesions in the absence of valvular thrombi has also been reported (32). Valve replacement has been undertaken with success for all of these lesions, but the operative mortality rates are significant (32,34).

Gastrointestinal Features

Inflammatory lesions and mucosal ulceration may occur throughout the intestinal tract. Patients with esophageal ulcers often present with dysphagia. Mucosal ulceration of the stomach, small bowel, or colon may be complicated by bleeding or perforation (35). Mucosal ulcers that perforate are often associated with mesenteric arteritis; involvement of medium to large vessels may result in bowel infarction (36). Vascular inflammation of mucosal venules may occur and may be associated with a protein-losing enteropathy and ascites (37). Ascites may also occur in lupus patients as a result of a sterile peritonitis.

Although abdominal pain in lupus patients is most often due to non–SLE-related conditions, the onset of acute abdominal pain in patients with active disease involving other organ systems should prompt consideration of bowel vasculitis with impending infarction or perforation. In these patients, immediate surgical exploration is indicated in the presence of local peritoneal signs or subdiaphragmatic free air. In the absence of such signs, mesenteric angiography may yield signs of arteritis. If blood is present in the stool, endoscopic evaluation of the colon may confirm the presence of mucosal ulceration.

Hepatobiliary manifestations of SLE include acalculous cholecystitis and hepatitis (38,39). Elevation in serum transaminase values are not uncommon during periods of disease activity. Liver biopsies obtained from lupus patients with persistent liver function abnormalities have revealed varied lesions including acute hepatitis, granulomatous hepatitis, chronic active hepatitis, cholestasis, and cirrhosis (40). The relationship between SLE activity and the development of these lesions is uncertain.

Autoimmune chronic hepatitis is a disorder seen predominantly in young or middle-aged women that may have a number of extrahepatic manifestations commonly seen in patients with SLE, including erythematous rashes, fever, pleuropericarditis, and interstitial lung disease. Autoantibodies, including antinuclear and antismooth muscle antibodies, are frequently present. Controversy exists as to whether these patients constitute a subset of patients with SLE or a distinct diagnostic entity (autoimmune or "lupoid" hepatitis). Presently, such distinctions have little therapeutic significance because most of these patients respond favorably to corticosteroids.

Elevations in serum amylase concentration, with or without accompanying signs or symptoms of pancreatitis, may be seen during periods of disease activity. Although treatment with high doses of corticosteroids may induce pancreatitis, elevations in serum amylase or lipase levels have been reported in patients with active SLE not treated with steroids. Severe pancreatitis resulting in death has been reported in patients with active lupus; autopsy findings in some of these patients have revealed necrotizing arteritis within the pancreas (41).

Neuropsychiatric Manifestations

Disorders of the central as well as peripheral nervous system may occur in patients with SLE. Central nervous system (CNS) dysfunction may present as an organic brain syndrome manifest by seizures, delirium, or coma. Acute psychosis may be another presenting feature of CNS lupus. Focal deficits resulting in limb paresis or chorea occur less commonly. A variety of pathologic lesions have been identified in association with CNS lupus, including cerebral inflammation, focal arterial thrombosis, and diffuse or focal vasculitis (42–44).

Identification of the pathologic process giving rise to organic brain or stroke syndromes antemortem in lupus patients is often difficult if not impossible to ascertain. Cerebrospinal fluid findings may be normal or may reveal only minimal elevations in protein or cellularity. With the exception of identifying areas of old infarction, computed tomography (CT) scans of the brain are of minimal value. Magnetic resonance imaging is a senstive indicator of focal cerebral inflammation, but the role of this modality in the evaluation and management of patients with possible neuropsychiatric manifestations of SLE is still evolving. Inflammatory lesions involving cranial nerves may result in optic neuritis or cranial nerve palsies (45). Although uncommon, acute transverse myelitis with paraplegia may occur as a consequence of vasculitis or thrombosis of spinal arteries (46). The presence of antiphospholipid antibodies may be a risk factor for transverse myelitis in patients with SLE (47). Examination of the cerebrospinal fluid in patients with neurologic findings of leptomenigeal or spinal cord inflammation characteristically reveals a mild to moderate pleocytosis with elevated protein levels and low glucose.

Mononeuritis multiplex with combined motor/sensory deficits of peripheral nerves may occur as a consequence of focal inflammation involving perineuronal blood vessels. Patients with SLE may also develop a diffuse sensory or combined motor/sensory neuropathy.

Headache syndromes occur commonly in lupus patients. Frontal headaches may be due to episcleritis or sinus infection. Patients with acute headache and meningismus may have a sterile meningitis due to SLE activity or infections. Ibuprofen or other NSAIDs may also induce an aseptic meningitis syndrome in patients with SLE (48). Hypertension complicating steroid therapy or renal disease may be another common cause of headache requiring prompt therapy. Migraine syndromes may herald flares of disease activity and often respond to therapy with corticosteroids. Diffuse headache may be the initial manifestation of intracranial vasculitis. Otherwise unexplained, nonfocal headache in immunosuppressed patients requires investigation for opportunistic pathogens such as *Cryptococcus neoformans.*

Hematologic Abnormalities

Anemia, leukopenia, or thrombocytopenia may occur alone or in combination at any time during the course of SLE. Anemia may occur as a consequence of hemolysis or marrow dysfunction. Patients with autoimmune hemolytic anemia usually have a positive direct Coombs' test with IgG antibodies on the erythrocyte surface mediating the hemolysis, resulting in anisocytosis and spherocytes on the peripheral blood smear. Hemolysis may also occur as a consequence of diffuse vasculitis with microangiopathy, resulting in schistocytes on the peripheral blood smear. Reticulocytosis, elevations in serum lactic dehydragenase level, or diminution in serum haptoglobin concentration may accompany immune or microangiopathic hemolysis. Impaired erythrocyte production due to autoimmune responses to red cell precursors in the marrow, relative folic acid deficiency in patients with chronic hemolysis, or the marrow-suppressing effects of chronic inflammation are other potential causes of anemia in patients with SLE.

Leukopenia, particularly lymphopenia, is frequently present at disease onset and may be a clue to early diagnosis in patients presenting with multisystem disease, unusual skin rashes, or arthritis of unknown cause. Although leukocytosis may occur during periods of disease activity, particularly in patients taking corticosteroids, lupus patients with elevations in their white blood cell count more frequently have underlying bacterial infection.

Thrombocytopenia in lupus patients is most often mediated by antibodies adherent to platelets; diminution or absence of megakaryocytes in the marrow due to drugs or autoimmune responses directed toward megakaryocytic cell lines occurs much less frequently. Other conditions associated with increased consumption of circulating platelets may also cause thrombocytopenia in lupus patients. Patients with severe vasculitis may present with a thrombocytopenic syndrome virtually indistinguishable from that seen in patients with thrombic thrombocytopenic purpura. Patients with significant titers of antiphospholipid antibodies (see below) may also develop mild to moderate thrombocytopenia, but the mechanism whereby these antibodies effect a diminution in the platelet count remains to be elucidated. Thrombocytopenia appears to be a significant marker for earlier than expected mortality because its occurrence has been correlated with decreased survival (49).

Bleeding disorders unrelated to thrombocytopenia may occur as a consequence of antibodies to clotting factors; deficiency of factor VIII has been the most common acquired factor deficiency reported in SLE (50). Antibodies to clotting factors may result in either diminished levels of the factor (due to clearance of the resulting immune complexes) or impaired function of the factor. In either case, a bleeding diathesis may occur.

Antibodies to phospholipid components of thromboplastin may result in an in vitro phenomenon of prolongation of the partial thromboplastin time. The presence of a serum factor resulting in prolongation of the partial thromboplastin time was initially observed in patients with SLE and was therefore referred to as the "lupus anticoagulant." Patients with these antibodies may also develop a mild to moderate thrombocytopenia. Rather than developing a bleeding diathesis, patients with antiphospholipid antibodies are at increased risk for arterial thrombosis. Other clinical associations include recurrent late first and early second trimester miscarriages, livedo reticularis, and cardiac valve thrombosis (51). Antibodies to phospholipid may also account for the false-positive serologic tests for syphilis seen in some patients with SLE. Antiphospholipid antibodies and the clinical syndrome associated with their presence may be seen in patients with or without SLE.

Autoantibodies and Other Laboratory Features

SLE is associated with the presence of autoantibodies, most commonly having specificity for nuclear antigens (ANA). ANA are present in over 95% of patients with SLE. Laboratories that report the presence of ANA typically indicate the presence of one or more nuclear staining patterns in the immunofluorescent assays used—homogeneous, speckled, nucleolar, or peripheral (rim) patterns. These staining patterns reflect the specificity of the ANA present in patients' sera. The titer of ANA yielding a given staining pattern may vary depending on the cellular substrate in the assay used to detect ANA.

The ANA that yield a homogeneous staining pattern react primarily with nuclear histones. These antibodies are less disease specific than ANA yielding other staining patterns, occurring often in otherwise normal elderly individuals as well as in patients with drug-induced lupus or other rheumatic diseases. ANA yielding a speckled pattern of immunofluorescence are somewhat more disease specific for SLE but may also be seen in patients with rheumatoid arthritis, polymyositis, Sjörgen's syndrome, or scleroderma. A nucleolar pattern of staining may occasionally be seen in patients with SLE but is more commonly seen in patients with scleroderma, polymyositis, or overlap syndromes. ANA that yield a peripheral/rim pattern of staining are seen relatively infrequently but correlate strongly with the presence of antibodies to double-stranded DNA (dsDNA) and are seen almost exclusively in patients with SLE.

Antibodies to dsDNA

Using other immunologic techniques such as radioimmunoassay (RIA), enzyme-linked immunosorbent assay (ELISA), immunoelectropharesis, or immunodiffusion, the specificity of ANA can be further characterized to render more useful diagnostic information. Antibodies to dsDNA or single-stranded DNA (ssDNA) can be quantitated using ELISA or RIA techniques. Antibodies to dsDNA have the highest specificity for SLE and may be present in the sera of the 5% of lupus patients who do not have demonstrable ANA by conventional immunofluorescence techniques; antibodies to ssDNA are less disease specific. Anti-dsDNA are of particular interest because their presence tends to correlate with the development of nephritis (52).

Antibodies to Sm/nRNP

Immunodiffusion techniques have facilitated the identification of disease-specific antibodies having specificity for RNA-protein antigens. Antibodies to one such antigen, Sm, are highly specific for SLE and levels of these antibodies may correlate with disease activity. Patients with high titers of antibody to another RNA–protein complex, nRNP tend to have clinical features overlapping those seen in SLE, scleroderma, and polymyositis.

Table 32.1 Autoantibodies Commonly Prevalent in Systemic Lupus Erythematosus (SLE) and Other Disorders

Antibody	Diseases
ANA	SLE, rheumatoid arthritis, Sjögren's syndrome, polymyositis, scleroderma, chronic hepatitis, thyroiditis
anti-DNA	SLE
anti-Sm	SLE
anti-RNP	SLE, overlap syndromes (mixed connective tissue disease)
anti-Ro/SS-A	Sjögren's syndrome, SLE
anti-La/SS-B	
anti-centromere	Scleroderma (CREST variant), SLE
anti-histone	Drug-induced lupus, SLE
anti-tRNA synthetase (Jo-1)	Polymyositis (with interstitial lung disease)
Rheumatoid factor	Rheumatoid arthritis, Sjögren's syndrome, SLE, infectious illnesses (bacterial endocarditis, parvovirus)

CREST, calcinosis, Raynaud's (phenomenon), esophageal (dysfunction), sclerodactyly, telangiectasia

Antibodies to SS-A(Ro)/SS-B(La)

Antibodies to the RNA-protein antigens SS-A(Ro) and SS-B(La) are of clinical interest because one or both of these antibodies are seen in the majority of lupus patients who do not have detectable ANA (13,14). Anti-SS-A antibodies are also frequently seen in patients with Sjögren's syndrome. A subset of lupus patients who develop recurrent erythematous eruptions on the upper torso, face, and proximal extremities (subacute cutaneous lupus erythematosus) frequently have antibodies to SS-A. The presence of antibodies to SS-A is of particular importance in women of childbearing age because these antibodies are invariably present in the sera of mothers bearing infants with complete heart block and likely play a role in the pathogenesis of fetal cardiac conduction abnormalities (15,53).

Other autoantibodies that are more commonly associated with other rheumatic diseases may occasionally be identified in the sera of patients with SLE (Table 32.1). These antibodies often occur in patients with clinical features overlapping those seen in disorders with which the antibody is more commonly associated.

Complement Levels

Serum complement levels, as measured by assays for C3, C4, or total hemolytic complement (CH50), are often depressed in patients with SLE and may correlate with disease activity in a given individual patient. The CH50 may be depressed irrespective of disease activity in patients with inherited deficiency of C1q, C1r, C1s, C2, C3, or C4, all of which have been associated with development of SLE. For patients without inherited complement deficiency, following the C3, C4, and CH50 may be useful in determining disease activity.

Etiology and Pathogenesis

The primary pathologic findings of SLE in organs throughout the body are inflammation, immune complex deposition, and varying types of vasculopathy. Evidence of acute and chronic inflammation may be found in the pleura, pericardium, peritoneum, joint synovia, pulmonary parenchyma, or renal tubules. Skin and kidney biopsies frequently reveal the presence of immunoglobulin deposits (IgA, IgM, or IgG) as well as complement at the dermal–epidermal junction or along the glomerular basement membrane, respectively. The vascular lesions noted on biopsy specimens or at autopsy can be found in any organ and include necrotizing arteritis of small- to medium-sized vessels, nonnecrotizing vasculitis characterized by lymphoid infiltrates around small arterioles or venules, or occlusive lesions with venous or arterial thrombosis.

A number of immunologic disturbances are present in SLE, most notably the production of autoantibodies. Whether a given autoantibody identified in SLE patients plays a pathophysiologic role in the disease or represents an epiphenomenon of tissue injury and immune dysfuction remains controversial. Antibodies to DNA are likely pathogenic because dsDNA–anti-dsDNA complexes and ssDNA–anti-ssDNA immune complexes have been implicated in the pathogenesis of lupus nephritis (54). The high correlation between antibodies to SS-A(Ro) and neonatal lupus suggests a likely pathogenic role for these antibodies as well, but a role for the majority of other ANA in triggering tissue injury remains to be established (53).

Homozygous deficiencies in the early components of complement, including C1q, C1r/s, C2, or C4 confer significant risk for development of SLE (55). Because these proteins are required for complement fixation to immune complexes, processing and clearance of immune complexes may be impaired in patients deficient in these components of complement. In addition, the genes coding for C1q/r/s, C2, and C4 are closely linked to HLA determinants regulating immune responses. Whether SLE develops in patients with complement deficiency because of an associated impairment in handling of immune complexes or because of linkage to an as yet unidentified immune response gene that governs disease susceptibility remains to be determined.

Because a significant number of patients with SLE have no identifiable deficiency in the expression of complement proteins, other genetic factors likely contribute to disease susceptibility. HLA haplotyping studies of lupus patients indicate that certain subspecificities of the class II molecules DR2 and DR3 are associated with SLE, but these associations have varied with the population group studied (56). Rather than conferring disease susceptibility, immune responses governed by HLA class II molecules more likely regulate the specificities of autoantibodies generated by individuals with SLE (57). Recent studies in the MRL mouse, a murine model of SLE, indicate that the SLE-like disease in these mice occurs as a consequence of defects in the *fas* gene regulating apoptosis of autoreactive T cells (58). The relevance of these findings with the murine *fas* gene to human patients with SLE is uncertain, but failure to delete autoreactive T cells could account for the large numbers of autoantibodies and polyclonal B cell activation characteristic of SLE.

The peak incidence of SLE in women during the time period between late adolescence and menopause suggests that sex hormones may influence the development or course of SLE. The observation that some patients experience mild flares of disease activity during the days preceding menses has also suggested a role for sex hormones in modulating disease activity. A role for sex hormones in regulating the development of inflammatory disease is supported by the NZB/NZW mouse model of lupus in which the disease is more severe in female mice and is favorably altered when female mice are treated with androgens. However, in other murine models of lupus (MRL/l and BXSB mice), severity of disease is equivalent or greater in male mice. Furthermore, recent studies indicate the frequency of SLE flares among pregnant women with lupus is no greater than the frequency of disease flares among age- and disease severity-matched women with lupus who are not pregnant (59,60). These considerations suggest that sex hormones have a limited role in modulating disease activity in SLE.

A number of drugs, most notably procainamide and hydralazine, are capable of triggering syndromes clinically indistinguishable from SLE. Drug-induced lupus syndromes are usually milder than idiopathic SLE and occur with the same frequency among men and women. The presenting manifestations are usually arthritis and pleuropericarditis, with renal disease and CNS disease noted only rarely in patients with drug-induced lupus. ANA are present in moderate to high titer, usually with specificity for nuclear histones. Phenothiazines and several of the anticonvulsants have also been implicated in the development of drug-

Box 32.1 Drugs Most Commonly Associated with Drug-induced Lupus Syndrome

Well established inducers
- hydralazine
- procainamide
- isoniazid
- chlorpromazine
- methyldopa

Less well established, but possible inducers
- phenytoins (diphenylhydantoin)
- carbamazepine
- primidone
- ethosuximide
- chlorthalidone
- D-penicillamine
- methylthiouracil, propylthiouracil
- quinidine
- tolazamide
- griseofulvin
- sulfonamides
- tetracyclines

induced lupus; a role for other drugs (Box 32.1) is less certain.

Diagnosis and Assessment

A diagnosis of SLE should be considered in any patient presenting with malar erythema, serositis, recurrent oral ulcers, unexplained leukopenia or thrombocytopenia, proteinuria, inflammatory arthritis, or other persistant erythematous rash. Rashes or arthralgia associated with significant morning stiffness or synovial swelling are the symptoms most commonly prompting patients with SLE to seek medical attention. The diagnosis of SLE rests primarily on clinical features elicited from the history and physical examination. Evaluation of the hematologic profile and urinalysis may also help to establish a diagnosis of SLE.

The American College of Rheumatology has developed clinical and laboratory criteria for a diagnosis of SLE (Table 32.2). These criteria were designed primarily to ensure accurate diagnoses for lupus patients enrolled in clinical studies or therapeutic intervention trials. At the time initial symtoms of disease or laboratory abnormalities are noted, patients with evolving SLE may not have sufficient clinical or laboratory manifestations to establish a diagnosis of SLE by these criteria. Such a scenario not uncommonly occurs when patients present with new onset of an erythematous rash, arthritis, or proteinuria in association with a significant titer of ANA. Provided other diagnostic considerations have been appropriately ruled out, such patients are usually managed as though these initial presenting features represent active SLE.

Evaluation of patients with suspected SLE should include a complete history with particular attention to medication history, family history of rheumatic disease, articular symptoms, presence of photosensitivity, Raynaud's symptoms, and sicca symptoms. A throrough physical examination should be performed with careful inspection of the entire skin and scalp for occult rash or discoid lesions as well as the oral cavity for asymptomatic buccal, lingual, or hard palate ulcers. The presence of arthritis may be manifest only by subtle abnormalities in wrist or elbow joint range of motion. Chest and cardiac examination should be performed routinely to detect the presence of pleuropericarditis, parenchymal lung disease, or valvular dysfunction. Abdominal examination may reveal hepatomegaly or splenomegaly. Enlargement of cervical, axillary, or inguinal lymph nodes may be present at disease onset or during significant flares of disease activity.

Initial laboratory evaluation should include a complete blood count with differential, urinalysis, and chemistry profile including creatinine and liver function tests. Evaluation of the peripheral blood smear for signs of hemolysis as well as a Coombs' test should be performed for patients with anemia. Because antibodies to Sm antigen and dsDNA are relatively disease specific for SLE, confirmation of the presence of these antibodies may help to confirm the presence of SLE when the clinical diagnosis is uncertain. Documenting the presence of antibodies to dsDNA may also identify patients at increased risk for renal disease. Measurement of serum C3, C4, and CH50 are useful in identifying patients with inherited complement deficiency and may also be of use in following the activity of renal disease in some patients. Assays for antiphospholipid antibodies should be obtained for patients with thrombocytopenia or a history of recurrent miscarriage.

Table 32.2 The 1982 Revised Criteria for Classification of Systemic Lupus Erythematosus

Criterion	Definition
1. Malar rash	Fixed or raised erythema, flat or raised, over the malar eminences, tending to spare the nasolabial folds
2. Discoid rash	Erythematous raised patches with adherent keratotic scaling and follicular plugging; atrophic scarring may appear in older lesions
3. Photosensitivity	Skin rash as a result of unusual reaction to sunlight, by patient history or physician observation
4. Oral ulcers	Oral or nasopharyngeal ulceration, usually painless, observed by a physician
5. Arthritis	Nonerosive arthritis involving two or more peripheral joints, characterized by tenderness, swelling, or effusion
6. Serositis	a. Pleuritis—convincing history of pleuritic pain or rub heard by a physician or evidence of pleural effusion *or* b. Pericarditis—documented by electrocardiogram or rub or evidence of pericardial effusion
7. Renal disorder	a. Persistant proteinuria >0.5 gm/day or >3+ if quantitation not performed *or* b. Cellular casts—may be red cell, hemoglobin, granular, tubular, or mixed
8. Neurologic disorder	a. Seizures—in the absence of offending drugs or known metabolic derangements, e.g., uremia, ketoacidosis, or electrolyte imbalance *or* b. Psychosis—in the absence of offending drugs or known metabolic derangements, e.g., uremia, ketoacidosis, or electrolyte imbalance
9. Hematologic disorder	a. Hemolytic anemia *or* b. Leukopenia—<4000/μL total on two or more occasions *or* c. Lymphopenia—<1500/μL on two or more occasions *or* d. Thrombocytopenia—<100,000/μL in the absence of offending drugs
10. Immunologic disorder	a. Positive lupus erythematosus cell preparation *or* b. Anti-DNA: antibody to native DNA in abnormal titer *or* c. Anti-Sm: presence of antibody to Sm nuclear antigen *or* d. False-positive serologic test for syphilis known to be positive for at least 6 months and confirmed by *Treponema pallidum* immobilization or fluorescent treponemal antibody absorption test
11. Antinuclear antibody	An abnormal titer of ANA by immunofluorescence or an equivalent assay at any point in time and in the absence of drugs known to be associated with "drug-induced lupus" syndrome

The proposed classification is based on 11 criteria. For the purpose of identifying patients in clinical studies, a person shall be said to have systemic lupus erythematosus if any 4 or more of the 11 criteria are present, serially or simultaneously, during any interval of observation.

Although laboratory tests for ANA or other autoantibodies may assist in confirming a clinical diagnosis, a diagnosis of SLE cannot be established solely on the basis of autoantibody test results. The presence of ANA among otherwise healthy individuals is not uncommon, particularly in the elderly. Individuals who are found to have high titers of ANA (≥1:640) but lack other clinical features of SLE may be at increased risk for later development of SLE or other rheumatic diseases such as rheumatoid arthritis, Sjögren's syndrome, or scleroderma. Counseling of such individuals should include reassurance that they may never develop rheumatic disease, but some education regarding the presenting signs and symptoms of these disorders is prudent because early diagnosis can improve long-term outcomes in rheumatic disease.

Management

The heterogeneity of clinical features and pathologic lesions found among patients with SLE dictates that management be highly individualized. General measures applicable to all patients with SLE include patient and family education regarding the various disease manifestations and how the disease may have an impact on the patient's lifestyle. Patient recognition of the chronicity of the disease and its potential to involve virtually any organ system may increase compliance with keeping regular follow-up appointments and reporting early symptoms of disease activity. Although emphasis on the potential seriousness of the disease is important, patients with predominantly cutaneous and articular symptoms in the absence of renal or other visceral disease can be reassured of a near normal life expectancy.

Recognition that fatigue is experienced by the majority of patients, often in the absence of other obvious disease manifestations, is an important concept to stress with patients and their families. A 1 hour mid-afternoon rest period is often quite helpful in managing fatigue symptoms. Regular exercise is important to maintain overall muscle conditioning, but vigorous exercise should be curtailed during periods of increased disease activity. Although not all patients with SLE experience photosensitivity, patients with a history of having exacerbation of skin rash, fever, or other constitutional complaints following sun exposure should use high SPF (≥20) sunscreens and use attire that minimizes exposure to ultraviolet light.

Patients with SLE are no less prone to develop medical problems experienced by patients without SLE and should be managed accordingly. Although activity of SLE should be considered as a potential cause of symptoms such as cough, fever, or abdominal pain, a previous diagnosis of SLE should not preclude consideration of other disorders potentially causing such symptoms. Patients with lupus are at increased risk for infections, even when not taking corticosteroids or other immunosuppressive drugs. The presence of fever in a patient with lupus always requires careful evaluation for infection. Even in the presence of obvious lupus-related disease manifestations, the attending clinician should not be disuaded from looking for concurrent infection because infection may trigger disease activity.

Because of the morbidity and mortality associated with infections in patients with SLE, routine immunizations against influenza and pneumococcus are highly recommended. Studies to date indicate that these immunizations are effective and do not trigger disease activity in patients with SLE (61,62).

Although no disease-specific intervention has been identified for the treatment of SLE, a variety of anti-inflammatory and immunosuppressive treatments have been identified as useful in managing specific disease manifestations. Because the course of disease is highly unpredictable, often with spontaneous remissions of disease activity, re-evaluation of the need for pharmacologic agents or other immunosupressive measures should be undertaken frequently in a given patient.

Mucocutaneous Problems

Skin rashes in SLE are often transient, not requiring therapy. Flares of malar erythema commonly occur in the absence of other significant disease manifestations; in such instances cosmetic preparations to cover the erythema is the only advisable treatment. Persistent skin eruptions associated with visceral disease or significant constitutional symptoms such as fever usually respond to moderate doses of corticosteroids (equivalent of 10–30 mg prednisone daily). Steroids are also recommended as initial treatment for patients with bullous or ulcerating lesions. Recurrent bullous, ulcerative, or discoid skin lesions frequently respond favorably to antimalarial agents such as hydroxychloroquine. Although an occasional patient may experience mild symtoms of gastric irritation, antimalarial drugs are generally well tolerated.

Symptomatic mouth ulcers will usually respond to a brief (5- to 10-day) course of steroids, the equivalent of 15–20 mg prednisone daily usually being sufficient. Improvement in the frequency and severity of mouth ulcers may be seen in patients treated with antimalarial drugs.

Patients taking chronic antimalarial therapy require periodic (every 6 month) ophthalmologic evaluation to monitor for retinal toxicity. Retinal toxicity is uncommon with the doses of hydroxychloroquine typically used in management of SLE (400 mg/day or less). With early detection, the retinal changes usually resolve with discontinuation of the drug; however, permanent visual damage may occur if the drug is not withdrawn once early signs of toxicity become apparent.

Arthritis

Synovitis in lupus patients can usually be succesfully managed with judicious use of an NSAID. NSAIDs should be used with caution in patients with significant renal disease. Some lupus patients may develop an aseptic meningitis with use of NSAIDs, most notably ibuprofen. For patients with joint swelling not responding to an NSAID or who are unable to use an NSAID, low doses of prednsione (5–10 mg/day) are frequently efficacious in managing the arthritis associated with SLE. Hydroxychloroquine may also be useful in the long-term managment of lupus-related synovitis.

Pleuropericarditis

Serositis symptoms often respond to anti-inflammatory doses of any of the NSAIDs. Patients with demonstrable pleural or pericardial effusion not responding to an NSAID may require treatment with moderate or even high doses of corticosteroids to alleviate pain or symptomatic fluid accumulation.

Hemolytic Anemia and Thrombocytopenia

Hemolytic anemia or thrombocytopenia due to autoantibodies bound to the respective blood elements usually responds to corticosteroids. A 5-day course of IV γ-globulin or a single IV dose of vincristine (1–2 mg) or cyclophosphamide (200–300 mg) is often successful in reversing cytopenias not responding promptly to corticosteroids. Hemolysis and thrombocytopenia due to microangiopathy may require more aggressive measures directed toward the vasculopathy, including plasma exchange or higher doses of cyclophosphamide. Leukopenia is common in lupus patients and in the absence of dangerously low neurtrophil counts or other disease manifestations requires no treatment. Severe leukopenia with absolute neutrophil counts less than 1000 μl requires further investigation to rule out sepsis or autoantibodies directed against granulocytes or granulocyte precursors.

Nephritis and Other Visceral Manifestations

Left untreated, visceral disease due to SLE may result in significant morbidity and mortality. Accordingly, prompt and aggressive treatment with immunosuppressive measures is often required for patients presenting with nephritis, pneumonitis, vasculitis, or acute organic brain syndromes attributable to active SLE. Initial treatment of these disease manifestations includes high-dose corticosteroids given parenterally, usually the equivalent of 1–2 mg methylprednisolone per kilogram. Higher, daily 500–1000-mg "pulse" therapy with IV methylprednisolone given over 48 to 72 hours is often used for patients presenting in extremis with severe multisystem organ involvement, or patients presenting with flares of nephritis accompanied by rapidly evolving renal insufficiency.

Although potentially toxic, cyclophosphamide may be very useful in the management of lupus patients with severe nephritis, vasculitis, or thrombocytopenia. Long-term follow-up studies of patients with lupus nephritis indicate that relative to patients treated with steroids alone or in combination with azathioprine, the most favorable outcomes were seen in cohorts treated with monthly IV cyclophosphamide (63). The risk of hemorrhagic cystitis and serious bone marrow supression may be minimized when cyclophosphamide is administered as a monthly IV dose. However, the efficacy of monthly IV cyclophosphamide remains to be established for patients with gut or neurologic lesions such as mononeuritis multiplex or transverse myelitis due to necrotizing arteritis.

Accordingly, daily oral cyclophosphamide (2–3 mg/kg per day) is still recommended as an adjunct to steroid therapy for patients with these particular disease manifestations.

The major predictable side effect of cyclophosphamide is marrow suppression; mucositis of the urinary tract is less common but may be severe. Regardless of the route of administration, frequent monitoring of blood counts and urinalysis is required when patients are treated with this drug. Patients should be advised that cyclophosphamide may induce sterility and amenorrhea, which may be permanent. Less predictable is a small but well established increased risk of subsequent malignancy in patients treated with cyclophosphamide. Patients should be advised of this risk, but with the proviso that the mortality associated with failure to adequately treat their disease likely exceeds the risk of developing a subsequent fatal malignancy.

Azathioprine may be useful as a steroid-sparing agent in patients with myositis, nephritis, organic brain syndromes, or other disease manifestations requiring prolonged treatment with moderate to high doses of corticosteroids. Given the undesirability of treating patients with daily high doses of corticosteroids beyond 4 to 6 weeks, addition of azathioprine may be useful in patients for whom disease activity cannot be controlled with every other day or lower daily corticosteroid therapy. The major side effects of azathioprine are bone marrow suppression and hepatotoxicity; accordingly, periodic monitoring of blood counts and liver enzymes is recommended for patients treated with azathioprine.

Contraception and Pregnancy in Patients with SLE

Pregnancy is generally well tolerated by lupus patients if their disease is quiescent at the time of conception. For patients with active disease or nephritis, pregnancy is likely to be problematic and contraceptive measures are recommended. Given the attendant risk of uterine infection, intrauterine devices are generally not recommended for patients with SLE. Oral contraceptives may be used, but the lower estrogen-containing preparations are preferred. Barrier methods rather than oral contraceptives should be used by patients with severe hypertension or a history of arterial or venous thrombosis.

For lupus patients who become pregnant, careful clinical and laboratory monitoring for disease activity extending through the peripartum period is essential. Proteinuria, skin rashes, arthritis, and thrombocytopenia are the complications most commonly reported in published series of pregnant SLE patients. Flares in disease activity are just as likely to occur during the first, second, or third trimester of pregnancy, or during the postpartum period. In addition to routine monthly assesments of blood pressure, weight, and uterine growth, attention should also be directed toward the presence of any skin rash, mucosal ulcers, or synovitis at the time of each visit. Laboratory evaluation should include monthly urinalysis and complete blood count. Baseline measurements of the CH50 and antibodies to dsDNA are also recommended, with follow-up of these parameters at the middle of the second and third trimesters for patients with known renal disease.

Lupus patients with previous renal disease commonly develop worsening of proteinuria during pregnancy, but the clinical course for patients with inactive nephritis is usually uncomplicated. Complications of pre-eclampsia, hypertension, or deterioration in renal function are more likely to occur in patients with active nephritis at the time of conception. The development of hypertension and proteinuria during pregnancy often poses the difficult question of whether the disturbances in renal function are due to a flare of lupus nephritis or pre-eclampsia. A significant decrease in the CH50 or the presence of hematuria (in the absence of infection) are suggestive of active nephritis. Some investigators have observed that serum levels complement activation products, particularly the alternative pathway product Ba, are frequently elevated in lupus patients experiencing a flare of nephritis during pregnancy (64). Elevated levels of these complement split products occurring in association with a low CH50 may differentiate a flare of lupus nephritis from pre-eclampsia.

Flares in disease activity during pregnancy can be managed with judicious use of corticosteroids with minimal effects on the fetus. Prednisone or methylprednisolone are most commonly used because these steroid compounds are not readily transported into the fetal circulation. Decisions regarding use of anti-inflammatory and immunosuppressive drugs other than corticosteroids in lupus patients who become pregnant must be individualized. Although no untoward fetal effects have been noted in published reports of pregnant patients treated with hydroxychloroquine, the safety of using this drug during pregnancy has not been established and patients are generally advised to discontinue its use during pregnancy. Whether to discontinue azathioprine in patients with active disease who become pregnant is problematic because stopping the drug in such patients may result in further exacerbation of disease activity. Studies with limited numbers of patients treated with azathioprine during the course of pregnancy indicate successful outcomes without evidence of teratogenicity (65,66). Because the safety of azathioprine use during pregnancy remains to be firmly established, patients with inactive disease who desire to become pregnant should consider stopping the drug before planned conception. Provided liver function tests are monitored periodically, salicylates can be used safely but should be discontinued several weeks before anticipated delivery to avoid labor or bleeding complications.

Patients with a history of recurrent miscarriage occurring beyond 8 to 10 weeks' gestation should be evaluated for the presence of antiphospholipid antibodies. The mangement of patients with a history of recurrent miscarriage and documented antiphospholipid antibodies remains controversial. Varying combinations of low-dose aspirin, daily prednisone (20–60 mg/day), twice daily SQ heparin administration (5000–15,000 U), and azathioprine have been used with varying degrees of success (67,68). Because many patients noted to have these antibodies never develop thrombotic complications, no treatment is recommended for patients who have not experienced miscarriage beyond the late first trimester of pregnancy. For similar reasons, screening pregnant lupus patients who have not experienced previous miscarriage or thrombosis for the presence of antiphospholipid antibodies is not necessary.

Patients with antibodies to SS-A (Ro antigen) are at risk for development of fetal or neonatal lupus syndrome. Features of this syndrome include development of cardiac conduction abnormalities, including complete heart block, myocarditis with heart failure, and pleural/pericardial effusions. A diffuse erythematous rash or cytopenias may be present at birth, persisting several months into infancy. The disease is likely mediated by maternal IgG autoantibodies transported across the placenta. Neonatal lupus is usually a self-limited syndrome although the development of complete heart block is usually permanent. Serial ultrasound examinations to look for the presence of fetal heart block or heart failure is recommended for mothers known to have antibodies to SS-A. Improvement in fetal pleuropericardial effusions and ascites associated with the syndrome after treatment of the mother with dexamethasone has been reported (69).

Breast-feeding

The primary concerns of lactating women with SLE relate to exposure of the infant to medications. Factors related to drug solubility and long elimination half-life may contribute to accumulation of drugs in breast milk. Ibuprofen is a reasonable choice for lactating mothers needing an NSAID because only small amounts have been noted to accumulate in breast milk. High-dose salicylates, NSAIDs with long half-lives, and hydroxychloroquine are best avoided. Because steroids including prednisone have been demonstrated to enter breast milk, lactating mothers requiring corticosteroid therapy are best advised to avoid nursing their infants for 3 to 4 hours after steroid ingestion whenever possible (70).

Prognosis

The prognosis with regard to survival for the majority of patients with SLE is quite favorable. Although the presence of renal disease or thrombocytopenia has historically been associated with decreased survival, survival among SLE patients with renal disease has significantly improved in recent decades. For patients without significant renal involvement or a history of thrombocytopenia, the long-term survival is comparable to that of age-matched women without SLE.

In most reported series of patients with SLE, the leading causes of mortality among patients with SLE are sepsis and complications of coronary atherosclerosis. Both of these complications have been linked to extent and duration of corticosteroid use, thus emphasizing the need for judicious and probationary use of these medications. The relative contributions of chronic steroid treatment and chronic vascular injury to development of atherosclerosis in patients with SLE remain undefined, but these observations emphasize the need for minimizing other coronary risk factors in patients with lupus. Recent studies suggest that use of hydroxychloroquine may favorably alter high-density lipoprotein levels and the premature development of atherosclerosis in patients with SLE (71). Whether low-dose aspirin might also have a favorable impact on the development of symptomatic atherosclerotic vascular disease in patients with SLE has not been determined.

REFERENCES

1. Maddock RK. Incidence of systemic lupus erythematosus in age and sex. JAMA 1965;191:149–150.

2. Fessel WJ. Systemic lupus erythematosus in the community: incidence, prevalence, outcome, and first symptoms; the high prevalence in black women. Arch Intern Med 1974;134:1027–1035.

3. Siegel M, Lee SL. The epidemiology of systemic lupus erythematosus. Semin Arthritis Rheum 1973;3:1–54.

4. Samanta A, Roy S, Feehally J, Symmons DP. The prevalence of diagnosed systemic lupus erythematosus in whites and Indian Asian immigrants in Leicester city, UK. Br J Rheumatol 1992;31:679–682.

5. Ropes MW. Systemic lupus erythematosus. Cambridge: Harvard University Press, 1976:13–118.

6. Rothfield N. Clinical features of systemic lupus erythematosus. In: Kelly WN, Harris ED, Ruddy S, Sledge CB, eds. Textbook of rheumatology. 2nd ed. Philadelphia: WB Saunders, 1986:1070–1097.

7. Ballou SP, Khan MA, Kushner I. Clinical features of systemic lupus erythematosus. Differences related to race and age of onset. Arthritis Rheum 1982;25:55–60.

8. Hochberg MC, Boyd RE, Ahearn JM, et al. Systemic lupus erythematosus: a review of clinico-laboratory features and immunogenetic markers in 150 patients with emphasis on demographic subsets. Medicine 1985;64:285–295.

9. Hahn BH, Yardley YH, Stevens MB. Rheumatoid nodules in systemic lupus erythematosus. Ann Intern Med 1970;72:49–58.

10. Zizic TM. Osteonecrosis. Curr Opin Rheumatol 1991;3:481–489.

11. Asherson RA, Liote F, Page B, et al. Avascular necrosis of bone and antiphospholipid antibodies in systemic lupus erythematosus. J Rheumatol 1993;20:284–288.

12. Gilliam JN, Sontheimer RD. Systemic lupus erythematosus and the skin. In: Lahita RG, ed. Systemic lupus erythematosus. New York: John Wiley & Sons, 1992:657–682.

13. Fessel WJ. ANA-negative systemic lupus erythematosus. Am J Med 1978;64:80–86.

14. Gladman DD, Chakmers A, Urowitz MB. Systemic lupus erythematosus with negative LE cells and antinuclear factor. J Rheumatol 1978;5:142–147.

15. Scott JP, Maddison PJ, Taylor PV, et al. Connective tissue disease, antibodies to ribonucleoprotein, and congenital heart block. N Engl J Med 1983;309:209–212.

16. Winkelmann RK. Panniculitis and systemic lupus erythematosus. JAMA 1970;211:472–475.

17. Churg J, Sobin LH. Renal disease. Classification and atlas of glomerular disease. New York: Igaku-Shoin, 1982:127–149.

18. Ginzler EM, Nicastri AD, Chun-Juo C, et al. Progression from mesangial and focal to diffuse nephritis. N Engl J Med 1974;291:693–696.

19. Graninger WB, Steinberg AD, Meron G, Smolen JS. Interstitial nephritis in patients with systemic lupus erythematosus: a manifestation of concomitant Sjögren's syndrome? Clin Exp Rheumatol 1991;9:41–45.

20. Bretjens JR, Sepulueda M, Baliah T, et al. Interstitial-immune complex nephritis in patients with systemic lupus erythematosus. Kidney Int 1975;7:342–350.

21. Gladman DD, Urowitz MB, Cole E, et al. Kidney biopsy in SLE. I. Clinical-morphologic evaluation. Q J Med 1989;272:1125–1133.

22. Schwartz MM, Lan SP, Bernstein J, et al., and the Lupus Collaborative Study Group. Role of pathology indices in the management of severe lupus glomerulonephritis. Kidney Int 1992;42:743–748.

23. Kahl LE. The spectrum of pericardial tamponade in systemic lupus erythematosus. Arthritis Rheum 1992;35:1343–1349.

24. Mathay RA, Schwarz MI, Retty TL, et al. Pulmonary manifestations of systemic lupus erythematosus: review of 12 cases of acute lupus pneumonitis. Medicine 1975;54:397–409.

25. Lawrence EC. Systemic lupus erythematosus and the lung. In: Lahita RC, ed. Systemic lupus erythematosus. New York: John Wiley & Sons, 1992:731–746.

26. Churg A, Franklin W, Chan KL, et al. Pulmonary hemorrhage and immune complex deposition in the lung: complications in a patient with systemic lupus erythematosus. Arch Pathol Lab Med 1980;104:388–391.

27. Stevens MB. Systemic lupus erythematosus and

the cardiovascular system. In: Lahita RC, ed. Systemic lupus erythematosus. New York: John Wiley & Sons, 1992:707–718.

28. Bhartu S, de la Fuente DJ, Kallen RJ, et al. Conduction system in systemic lupus erythematosus with atrio-ventricular block. Am J Cardiol 1975;35:299–304.

29. Bonfiglio TA, Bolfi RE, Hangstrom JWC. Coronary arteritis and myocardial infarction due to lupus erythematosus. Am Heart J 1972;83:153–158.

30. Buckly BH, Roberts WC. The heart in systemic lupus erythematosus and the changes induced in it by corticosteroid therapy. Am J Med 1975;58:243–364.

31. Petri M, Perez-Gutthann S, Spence D, Hochberg MC. Risk factors for coronary artery disease in patients with systemic lupus erythematosus. Am J Med 1993;93:513–519.

32. Straaton KV, Chatham WW, Revielle JD, et al. Clinically significant valvular heart disease in systemic lupus erythematosus. Am J Med 1988;85:645–650.

33. Chartash EK, Lans DM, Paget SA, et al. Aortic insufficiency and mitral regurgitation in patients with systemic lupus erythematosus and the antiphospholipid syndrome. Am J Med 1989;86:407–412.

34. Dajee H, Hurley EJ, Szarnicki RJ. Cardiac valve replacement surgery in systemic lupus erythematosus. A review. J Thorac Cardiovasc Surg 1983;85:718–726.

35. Zizic TM. Gastrointestinal manifestations. In: Schur PH, ed. The clinical management of SLE. Orlando, FL: Grune & Stratton, 1983:153–166.

36. Rothfield NF. Systemic lupus erythematosus: clinical aspects and treatment. In: McCarty DJ, Koopman WJ, eds. Arthritis and allied conditions. 12th ed. Philadelphia: Lea & Febiger, 1993:1155–1178.

37. Heck LW, Alarcon GS, Ball GV, et al. Pure red cell aplasia and protein losing enteropathy in a patient with systemic lupus erythematosus. Arthritis Rheum 1985;28:1059–1061.

38. Newbold KM, Allum WH, Downing R, et al. Vasculitis of the gall bladder in rheumatoid arthritis and systemic lupus erythematosus. Clin Rheumatol 1987;6:287–289.

39. Mayer LF, Salomon P. Gastrointestinal manifestations of systemic lupus erythematosus. In: Lahita RC, ed. Systemic lupus erythematosus. New York: John Wiley & Sons, 1992:747–760.

40. Runyon BA, LaBroque DR, Anuras S. The spectrum of liver disease in systemic lupus erythematosus. Report of 33 histologically proved cases and review of the literature. Am J Med 1980;69:187–194.

41. Reynolds JC, Inman RD, Kimberly RP, et al. Acute pancreatitis in systemic lupus erythematosus: report of 20 cases and a review of the literature. Medicine 1982;61:25–32.

42. Johnson RT, Richardson EP. The neurological manifestations in systemic lupus erythematosus. Medicine 1968;47:337–369.

43. Zvaifler NJ, Bluestein HG. The pathogenesis of central nervous system manifestations of systemic lupus erythematosus. Arthritis Rheum 1982;25:862–866.

44. Ellis SG, Verity MA. Central nervous system involvement in systemic lupus erythematosus. A review of neuropathologic findings in 57 cases, 1955–1957. Semin Arthritis Rheum 1979;8:212–221.

45. Bluestein HG. Neuropsychiatric disorders in systemic lupus erythematosus. In: Lahita RC, ed. Systemic lupus erythematosus. New York: John Wiley & Sons, 1992:639–656.

46. Warren RW, Kredich DW. Transverse myelitis and acute central nervous system manifestations of systemic lupus erythematosus. Arthritis Rheum 1984;27:1058–1060.

47. Lavelle C, Pizarro S, Drenkard C, et al. Transverse myelitis: a manifestation of systemic lupus erythematosus strongly associated with antiphospholipid antibodies. J Rheumatol 1990;17:34–37.

48. Hoppmann RA, Peden JG, Ober SK. Central nervous system effects on nonsteroidal anti-inflammatory drugs. Aseptic meningitis, psychosis, and cognitive dysfunction. Arch Intern Med 1991;151:1309–1313.

49. Reveille JD, Bartolucci A, Alarcon GS. Prognosis in systemic lupus erythematosus. Negative impact of increasing age at onset, black race, and thrombocytopenia, as well as causes of death. Arthritis Rheum 1990;33:37–48.

50. Laurence J, Nachman R, Wong JEL. Hematologic aspects of systemic lupus erythematosus. In: Lahita RC, ed. Systemic lupus erythematosus. New York: John Wiley & Sons, 1992:771–806.

51. Harris NE, Khamushta MA, Hughes GRV. Antiphospholipid antibody syndrome. In: McCarty DJ, Koopman WJ, eds. Arthritis and allied conditions. 12th ed. Philadelphia: Lea & Febiger, 1993:1201–1212.

52. Emlen W, Pisetsky DS, Taylor RP. Antibodies to DNA. A perspective. Arthritis Rheum 1986;29:1417–1426.

53. Alexander E, Buyon JP, Provost TT, Guarnieri T.

Anti-Ro/SS-A antibodies in the pathophysiology of congenital heart block in neonatal lupus syndrome, an experimental model. Arthritis Rheum 1992;35:176–188.

54. Fournie GJ. Circulating DNA and lupus nephritis. Kidney Int 1988;33:487–497.

55. Agnello V. Complement deficiency states. Medicine 1978;57:1–23.

56. Scherak O, Smolen JS, Mayr WR. HLA-DRw3 and systemic lupus erythematosus. Arthritis Rheum 1980;23:954–956.

57. Griffing WL, Moore SB, Luthra HS, et al. Associations of antibodies to native DNA and HLA-DRw3. A possible major histocompatibility complex-linked human immune response gene. J Exp Med 1980;152:319s–325s.

58. Wu J, Zhou T, He J, Mountz JD. Autoimmune disease in mice due to integration of an endogenous retrovirus in an apoptosis gene. J Exp Med 1993;178:461–468.

59. Urowitz MB, Gladman DD, Farewell VT, et al. Lupus and pregnancy studies. Arthritis Rheum 1993;36:1392–1397.

60. Lockshin MD. Pregnancy does not cause systemic lupus erythematosus to worsen. Arthritis Rheum 1989;32:665–670.

61. Williams GW, Steinberg AD, Reinertsen JL, et al. Influenza immunization in systemic lupus erythematosus. Ann Intern Med 1978;88:729–734.

62. Klippel JH, Karsh J, Stahl NI, et al. A controlled study of pneumococcal polysaccharide vaccine in systemic lupus erythematosus. Arthritis Rheum 1979;22:1321–1325.

63. Austin HA, Klippel JH, Balow JE, et al. Therapy of lupus nephritis. Controlled trial of prednisone and cytotoxic drugs. N Engl J Med 1986;314:614–619.

64. Buyon JP, Tamerius J, Ordorica S, et al. Activation of the alternative pathway accompanies disease flares in systemic lupus erythematosus during pregnancy. Arthritis Rheum 1992;35:55–61.

65. Ostensen M. Treatment with immunosuppressive and disease modifying drugs during pregnancy and lactation. Am J Reprod Immunol 1992;28:148–152.

66. Ramsey-Goldman R, Mientus JM, Kutzer JE, et al. Pregnancy outcome in women with stystemic lupus erythematosus treated with immunosuppressive drugs. J Rheumatol 1993;20:1152–1157.

67. Many A, Pauzner R, Carp H, et al. Treatment of patients with anti-phospholipid antibodies during pregnancy. Am J Reprod Immunol 1992;28:216–218.

68. Buchanan NM, Khamashta MA, Morton KE, et al. A study of 100 high risk lupus pregnancies. Am J Reprod Immunol 1992;28:192–194.

69. Chua S, Ostman-Smith I, Sellers SS, Redman CW. Congenital heart block with hydrops fetalis treated with high-dose dexamethasone; a case report. Eur J Obstet Gynecol Reprod Biol 1991;42:155–158.

70. Needs CJ, Brooks PM. Antirheumatic medication during lactation. Br J Rheumatol 1985;24:291–297.

71. Petri M, Lakatta C, Madger L, Goldman D. Effect of prednisone and hydroxychloroquine on coronary artery disease risk factors in systemic lupus erythematosus: a longitudinal data analysis. Am J Med 1994;96:254–259.

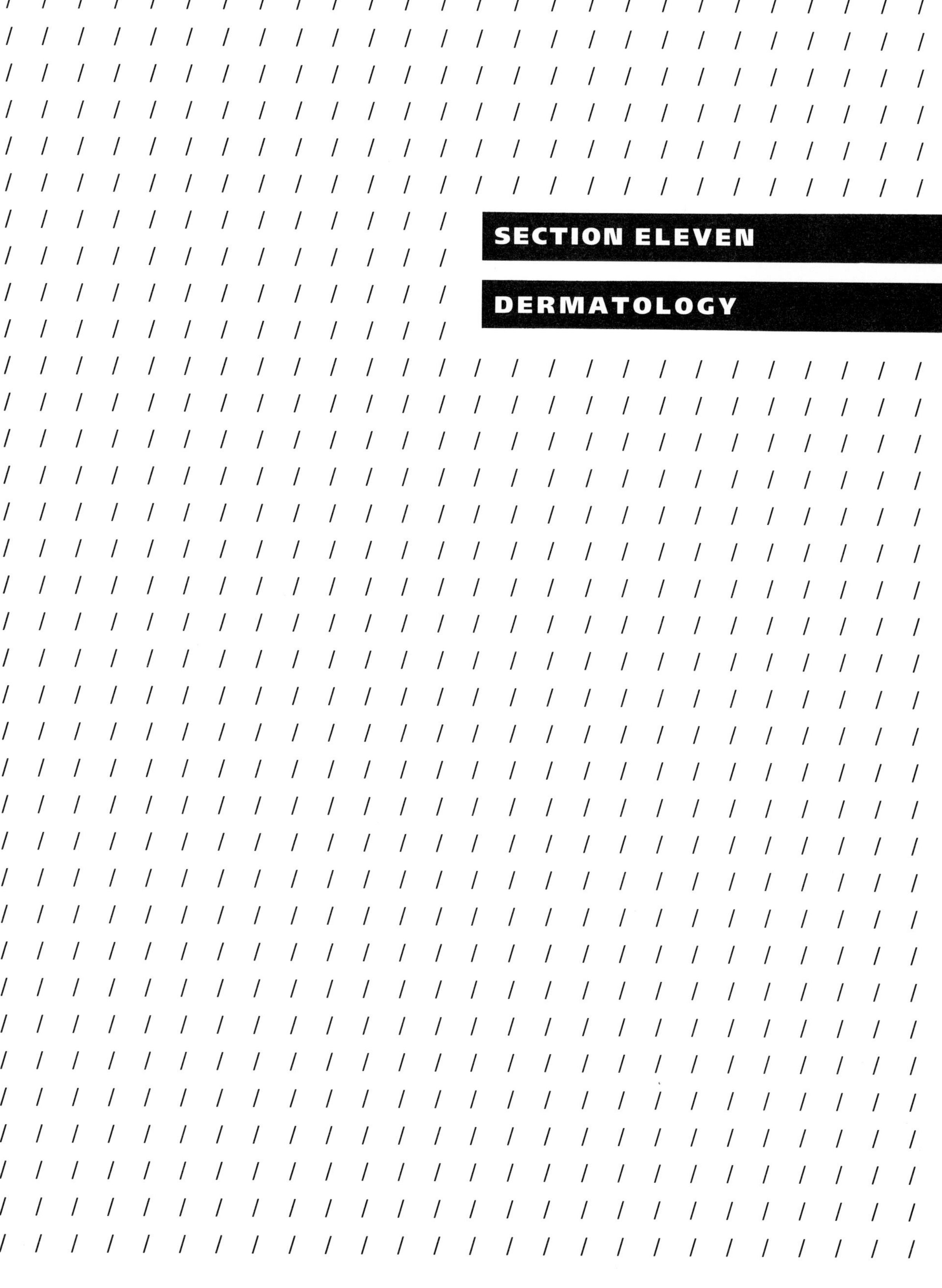

SECTION ELEVEN

DERMATOLOGY

CHAPTER 33

COMMON SKIN DISEASES

Jane McClure Blaum

Acne

Acne is a common, often inflammatory, disorder of sebaceous follicles that affects, in varying degrees of severity, the majority of people during their second and third decades. However, people ranging in age from infancy to late middle age may be afflicted. The disorder is rarely physically, but often emotionally, symptomatic.

Pathophysiology

The pathogenesis of acne appears to be multifactorial, involving four main factors: abnormal follicular keratinization, increased sebum production (which is hormonally mediated), proliferation and metabolic activity of *Propionibacterium acnes*, and inflammation. It is a disease of hair follicles with prominent associated sebaceous glands known as sebaceous follicles, which are found in acne-prone areas such as face, mid-chest, and upper back. Before puberty, these follicles are small and their associated glandular structures are undeveloped. With the onset of puberty, androgenic hormones stimulate enlargement of the follicles, as well as the development and function of associated sebaceous glands.

The earliest changes in the development of an acne lesion occur in the epithelium of the hair follicle where, for reasons unknown, keratinization is altered resulting in thickening of the stratum corneum. Excessive shedding of the stratum corneum into the follicular lumen ensues, with partial or complete occlusion of the lumen, accumulation of sebum and bacteria, and the formation of a closed comedo (whitehead). An open comedo (blackhead) results when the follicular orifice dilates sufficiently to reveal the keratinaceous plug. The comedo is the precursor lesion for all acne. It is the rupture of the comedo and the dermal inflammatory response thereto that result in the inflammatory acne lesion. The severity and depth of the inflammatory response determine the clinical appearance of the inflammatory acne lesion. Upper dermal inflammation results in the formation of a pustule, whereas deeper inflammation results in an inflammatory papule or nodule/cyst.

Under the influence of androgenic hormones, sebaceous glands produce sebum, a mixture of lipids consisting primarily of triglycerides, wax esters, and squalene. *P. acnes*, an anaerobic pleomorphic diphtheroid bacillus that is part of the normal flora of the sebaceous follicle, produces lipases, which hydrolyze the triglycerides in sebum, producing most of the free fatty acids found on the skin. Free fatty acids may be involved in the production of noninflammatory or inflammatory acne lesions although their role is not clear. *P. acnes* also produces substances that are chemotactic for polymorphonuclear leukocytes. These leukocytes release hydrolases, which may damage the follicular wall, resulting in rupture. Extrusion of follicular contents, including keratin, bacteria, and hair fragments, into the dermis results in a dense inflammatory infiltrate consisting of both leukocytes and foreign body giant cells. Therefore, the metabolic activity of *P. acnes* appears to play a major role in the production of inflammatory acne lesions.

The primary role of androgenic hormones in the development of acne is felt to be through stimulation of sebaceous gland activity. The androgen with the greatest metabolic influence on the hair follicle is dihydrotestosterone, which is produced locally by the action of the enzyme 5α-reductase. In women there is often poor correlation between circulating androgen levels and the presence of acne, a fact that is not well understood but may be accounted for by local factors such as increased 5α-reductase activity, increased numbers of androgen receptors, or increased sensitivity of androgen receptors. Some women with acne have measurable hyperandrogenemia, which may be of ovarian or adrenal origin, in rare instances produced by underlying tumors.

Other factors occasionally involved in the genesis of acne include occlusion/friction ("acne mechanica"), cosmetics/oils ("acne cosmetica"), and some drugs.

Clinical Considerations

The onset of acne (Fig 33.1) usually temporally coincides with puberty although acne sometimes begins much later. The severity of acne tends to decrease with age, and in most people affected the disorder has resolved by the late teens or early twenties. Occasionally, acne persists into the fourth and fifth decades. Approximately 80% of people with acne, and 96% of people with severe acne, are between the ages of 15 and 44 (1). Acne is generally more severe in men, and even severe acne usually has a shorter course in women. Acne most commonly affects the face (with sparing of the periorbital area), upper chest, and back. A patient may have both inflammatory and noninflammatory lesions. Lesions may vary in size, severity, and number even in different sites on the same patient. Disease of similar severity and morphology in different patients may respond quite differently to the same therapy.

Efforts have been made to classify acne lesions with some uniformity (2). Lesions are classified fundamentally as either noninflammatory or inflammatory.

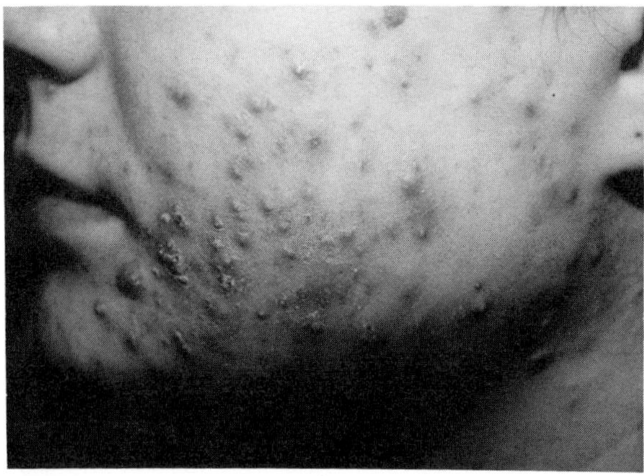

Fig 33.1 Acne. Severe nodulocystic acne in a young woman.

Noninflammatory lesions are comedones, closed (whiteheads) or open (blackheads), which represent dilated plugged follicles with orifices of different sizes. Inflammatory lesions may be papules, pustules, or nodules/cysts (⩾5 mm in size), and are termed mild, moderate, or severe based on the number of lesions present.

There are several well-recognized subsets of acne. *Acne conglobata* is a form of severe nodulocystic acne, often with sinus tract formation, primarily involving the face, trunk, and upper extremities of adult men. *Acne fulminans* refers to severe nodulocystic ulcerative acne primarily of the trunk, most often affecting adolescent boys, often accompanied by fever, arthralgias, myalgias, leukocytosis, elevated erythrocyte sedimentation rate, and osteolytic bone lesions. The *follicular occlusion triad* is the occurrence in a patient of acne conglobata, hidradenitis suppurativa, and dissecting cellulitis of the scalp.

Subsets of acne implicating a precipitant include *acne cosmetica* (cosmetic-related), *pomade acne* (associated with the use of scalp oils, appearing primarily as comedones of forehead and hairline, more common in blacks), *acne mechanica* (occlusion/friction-related under athletic gear, usually papulopustular), and *occupational acne* (associated with various industrial agents such as coal tar and petroleum oil, including chloracne secondary to halogenated hydrocarbon exposure, often exhibiting large comedones). Drugs implicated in the induction of acne include topical, systemic, and inhaled corticosteroids (3), androgenic steroids, oral contraceptives containing high levels of progestins, hydantoins, lithium, iodides/bromides, and isoniazid. Neonatal acne is probably due to maternal–fetal transplacental transfer of androgens resulting in sebaceous gland stimulation, is primarily comedonal, has its onset in the first 2 to 3 months of life, and spontaneously resolves in the course of a few months.

Postinflammatory pigmentary changes are common in the aftermath of acne lesions. Acne scars may either be atrophic (depressed with sloping edges, or "ice pick" with steep sides) or hypertrophic. Scarring is unpredictable and may follow either severe or mild disease.

Differential Diagnosis

The differential diagnosis includes rosacea (which does not have comedones); other folliculitides of bacterial, dermatophyte, or *Demodex* origin; perioral dermatitis; and, in men, pseudofolliculitis from ingrown hairs.

Laboratory Evaluation

Laboratory evaluation for diagnostic purposes is seldom necessary although occasionally bacterial or fungal cultures or microscopic examination of pustule contents can assist in distinguishing acne from other forms of folliculitis.

Hormonal evaluation of women with acne is variably productive, possibly because hormonal pathology may be operative at the level of the follicle, rather than systemically. However, such an evaluation may be productive in women with severe acne and should certainly be performed when signs of androgen excess (acne, hirsutism) are associated with oligomenorrhea, to rule out the presence of significant underlying disease. Women with associated mild-to-moderate slowly progressive hirsutism and regular menses require less extensive evaluation because this is not characteristic of an androgen-secreting tumor (4). Prepubertal children with severe or persistent acne should also be evaluated. Hormonal evaluation may include assessment of luteinizing hormone, follicle-stimulating hormone, prolactin, dehydroepiandrosterone sulfate, total and free testosterone, sex hormone-binding globulin, 17-hydroxyprogesterone, and cortisol, as indicated by historical and clinical findings (5).

Management

Acne often persists for years. With the exception of isotretinoin, treatment probably does not significantly shorten the course of the disease. Treatment does, however, reduce the severity of the disease and the likelihood of scarring. Therapy focuses on reducing numbers of *P. acnes* organisms, inhibiting sebum production, and decreasing follicular hyperkeratosis. Response to therapy is often delayed, so that it is advisable to continue a particular course of therapy for approximately 3 months before considering changes. The therapeutic approach should be individualized, depending on lesion morphology, severity, and distribution. Teratogenicity and other adverse fetal effects limit treatment options for pregnant women with acne (6).

The most widely used topical agents are benzoyl peroxide preparations, tretinoin (*trans*-retinoic acid) preparations, and topical antibiotics. Benzoyl peroxide has antibacterial activity but may also have some keratolytic properties. It is available in various vehicles in concentrations ranging from 2.5% to 10.0% (some of which are available without prescription), and is intended for application once or twice a day. Side effects include irritation and, rarely, allergic contact dermatitis. Patients should also be informed that it may bleach hair and clothing. Tretinoin is especially effective for comedones, inhibiting their formation and eliminating those present, due to its suppression of hyperkeratosis and thinning of the stratum corneum. Chemically, it is a vitamin A-related substance (retinoid). Tretinoin is available in cream, gel, and liquid forms ranging in concentration from 0.025% to 0.5%, and is applied at bedtime. It is important to note that the gels are more potent than the creams, irrespective of the concentration, and the liquid is the most potent preparation. Treatment for approximately 3 months is required for obvious improvement. The most common side effects are irritation, erythema, and scaling although these subside after several weeks of therapy. Occasionally, there is an initial flare of inflammatory acne, but this, too, subsides with continued application. Some patients experience photosensitivity, due to the thinning of the stratum corneum. Benzoyl peroxide and tretinoin may inactivate each other and should not be applied simultaneously although benzoyl peroxide may be applied in the morning and tretinoin in the evening. The most commonly prescribed topical antibiotics are clindamycin and erythromycin, which are most effective for papular and pustular lesions. They are available in a variety of vehicles, including solutions, lotions, and gels, and are applied once or twice a day. Side effects are uncommon but include vehicle-associated stinging, allergic contact dermatitis, and rare reports of transdermal absorption of clindamycin sufficient to cause pseudomembranous colitis. Resistant *P. acnes* occasionally develops with usage spanning months to years. Topical antibiotics are often used in conjunction with tretinoin or benzoyl peroxide.

Oral agents include antibiotics and isotretinoin (13-*cis*-retinoic acid). Oral antibiotics are indicated for extensive inflammatory acne unresponsive to topical preparations and for truncal acne that is usually less responsive to topical products. The most commonly used oral antibiotics are tetracycline and erythromycin, both of which are antibacterial and, by inhibiting polymorphonuclear leukocyte chemotaxis, anti-inflammatory. Because it is safe, effective, and inexpensive, tetracycline is probably the drug of choice, the exception being its contraindication in pregnant women and children 8 years of age or younger. Appropriate initial dosages are 250 mg–500 mg twice a day, with eventual tapering of the dose to the lowest maintenance dose required for control. Side effects include gastrointestinal complaints (especially nausea), photosensitivity, vulvovaginal candidiasis, allergy, pseudotumor cerebri, and esophageal ulceration (particularly if taken at bedtime). There is some concern that oral antibiotics may interfere with the absorption of oral contraceptives. The absorption of tetracycline is adversely affected if taken with food, dairy products, iron supplements, or aluminum-, calcium-, or magnesium-containing antacids. Laboratory abnormalities include an elevation of blood urea nitrogen and, rarely, elevated liver enzymes. Various protocols have been recommended in the past for routine laboratory monitoring of patients receiving long-term antibiotic therapy for acne. However, some data suggest that, in young healthy patients, routine laboratory studies are generally unremarkable, and perhaps laboratory monitoring should be performed only in those at increased risk for an adverse drug reaction (such as patients with renal insufficiency) or those who actually develop symptoms (7). Other often effective oral antibiotics include minocycline, doxycycline, clindamycin, and trimethoprim-sulfamethoxazole. The development of antibiotic resistance occurs but is not common. A potential complication of the prolonged administration of oral antibiotics is the overgrowth of gram-negative organisms, with the development of gram-negative folliculitis. This should be considered in a patient who becomes unresponsive to previously effective therapy.

Isotretinoin, an oral vitamin A analogue, is indicated for severe, usually scarring, nodular or cystic acne unresponsive to other therapy. Because of the potentially severe and extensive side effects of the drug, patients for whom this is a therapeutic consideration probably merit referral to a dermatologist for discussion of alternative therapeutic options, risks, and benefits, and monitoring throughout therapy. Isotretinoin works primarily by causing involution of sebaceous glands and decreasing keratinocyte proliferation and, hence, keratotic plugging of follicles; however, it also has some anti-inflammatory properties. Initial dosages are 0.5–1.0 mg/kg per day, taken over a period of 4 to 5 months (depending on response). Some patients require more protracted courses or additional courses (8,9). Isotretinoin is a powerful teratogen, and pregnancy is absolutely contraindicated while therapy is in progress and for at least 1 month following cessation of the drug. Side effects include an initial acne flare, blepharoconjunctivitis, xerophthalmia, alopecia, epistaxis secondary to drying of nasal mucosa, cheilitis, xerosis, asteatotic dermatitis, photosensitivity, diminution in night vision, the development of exuberant granulation tissue, arthralgias, myalgias, headaches, liver function abnormalities, pseudotumor cerebri, hypertriglyceridemia, hypercholesterolemia, flaring of inflammatory bowel disease, depression, diffuse idiopathic skeletal hyperostosis, and, in children, premature closure of the epiphyses. Laboratory monitoring, in addition to an assessment of pregnancy status, includes a baseline complete blood count, chemistry profile, and lipid screen, with reassessment at intervals thereafter.

Additional therapeutic interventions include the use of systemic corticosteroids for severe flares of cystic acne, comedo expression, intralesional injections of corticosteroids into cysts, and superficial peels (especially for comedonal and superficial acne). In women, hormonal interventions intended to decrease androgen-stimulated sebum production and, hence, improve acne, include the administration of antiandrogens such as spironolactone, estrogens in the form of oral contraceptives, and low-dose dexamethasone.

Choice of treatment for acne scars depends on severity and morphology, but options include dermabrasion, scar excision, punch elevation, punch grafting, chemical peels, and the dermal injection of fat or collagen.

Molluscum Contagiosum

Molluscum contagiosum is a benign self-limiting (in immunocompetent hosts) cutaneous viral infection which, in the past, was most commonly seen in children or as a sexually transmitted disease (STD) in adults. Currently, however, the disease is also frequently seen in individuals infected with human immunodeficiency virus (HIV) and, occasionally, in other immunocompromised patients.

Pathophysiology

The molluscum contagiosum virus is a double-stranded DNA virus of the Pox virus family (*Poxviridae*) and is one of the largest viruses known. Infected cells fill with intracytoplasmic viral inclusions known as molluscum bodies or Henderson-Patterson bodies. Because the virus is as yet unculturable in vitro, the pathogenesis is incompletely understood. The molluscum contagiosum virus has the most limited tissue tropism of any poxvirus, replicating only in human epidermis (10). Viral replication causes epidermal hyperplasia, resulting in the clinical papule, and it has been suggested that the presence of an epidermal growth factor-like gene within the viral genome may explain the proliferative nature of the skin lesions (10).

The virus may be transmitted by close personal contact or fomites and is often spread on a given individual by autoinoculation (as opposed to hematogenous or lymphatic spread [11]). Abrasions, in some instances microscopic, including in the case of autoinoculation those generated by scratching, probably provide access for the virus to the epidermis. Infection is not associated with viremia, and, perhaps due to its confinement to the epidermis, results in limited, if any, host immune response (10). However, the increased incidence and persistence of molluscum contagiosum infection in immunocompromised hosts implies a role for cell-mediated immunity in the disease.

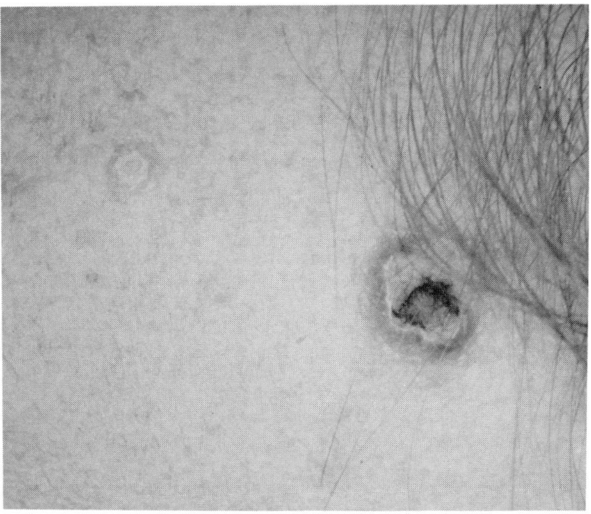

Fig 33.2 Molluscum contagiosum. Giant atypical molluscum on the face of a patient with acquired immunodeficiency syndrome (AIDS). Also note smaller, more typical umbilicated lesion.

Clinical Considerations

The skin lesions of molluscum contagiosum (Fig 33.2) are usually 2- to 5-mm, dome-shaped, skin-colored shiny translucent papules, often with a central indentation (umbilication) filled with an expressible plug (containing epidermal cells filled with viral inclusion bodies). The incubation period is estimated to range from 2 weeks to 6 months (12).

There are three epidemiologic patterns of infection (13). The first, infection in children, is a self-limiting disease involving face, trunk, and extremities, transmitted by direct skin contact. The virus may be transmitted to a child in the setting of sexual abuse. However, widespread lesions are common in childhood infection, including groin area involvement, so the presence of such lesions may not be sufficient to evoke concern in the absence of other indications of sexual abuse. The second pattern is that of an STD in adults, with lesions occurring on the genitalia, buttocks, lower abdomen, and upper thighs. Third, molluscum contagiosum infection may occur in the setting of local or systemic immunosuppression. Patients with atopic dermatitis or those using topical corticosteroids are at risk presumably due to cutaneous immunosuppression. Systemic immunosuppression, particularly associated with HIV infection, may result in molluscum infection that is either venereal (with extensive genital area involvement) or nonvenereal (with extensive facial or truncal lesions). The face is a particularly common site of involvement in AIDS patients, in whom the lesions may be large ("giant"), multiple, and poorly responsive to therapy.

Molluscum lesions may occur anywhere on the skin but are unusual on palms, soles, or in the mouth. Periorbital lesions are especially common in children, who may have an associated conjunctivitis (12). Autoinoculation frequently occurs, as evidenced by clustered and sometimes linearly arrayed lesions. Viral lesions are usually asymptomatic but may be pruritic (with associated excoriations) and may be tender if traumatized or inflamed. Patients sometimes develop an associated eczematous dermatitis. Excoriated lesions may develop a secondary bacterial infection.

In immunocompetent hosts, untreated individual lesions usually spontaneously regress in 2 months (although they sometimes persist up to 5 years), and an untreated episode of infection generally resolves in 6 to 9 months (12). Reinfection is not common.

Differential Diagnosis

A single molluscum contagiosum lesion of the face in an adult may easily be confused with a basal cell carcinoma, leading to an unnecessary invasive procedure. The differential diagnosis may also include keratoacanthoma, wart, and, if inflamed or traumatized, abscess or furuncle.

Laboratory Evaluation

When small papules typical of molluscum contagiosum are present, histologic or cytologic evaluation is unnecessary. When diagnostic uncertainty exists, contents expressed from a lesion's central umbilication may be examined under a microscope for the presence of molluscum bodies. Atypical lesions may require biopsy for diagnosis.

Management

Because the natural history of molluscum infection in normal hosts is eventual spontaneous resolution, therapeutic intervention is not absolutely necessary. However, as new lesions often continue to appear and siblings, schoolmates, caretakers, or sexual contacts are at risk of infection, therapy is frequently initiated. Therapeutic options include: removal of the core from the umbilicated center of the lesions with a sharp instrument (this may be done at home with a toothpick), curettage with or without electrodessication (a process poorly tolerated by young children), liquid nitrogen cryotherapy (variably tolerated by children), trichloroacetic acid application, cantharidin (blistering agent) application, and topical tretinoin (especially the strong gel formulation, applied at home with a toothpick). Caution should be exercised in the treatment of eyelid lesions because all of the aforementioned interventions entail some ophthalmologic risk, particularly when attempted on uncooperative children. It is reasonable to leave eyelid lesions alone, awaiting spontaneous resolution. Caustic or blistering agents should be used with caution, if at all, on facial or genital lesions in general. More than one treatment session is often required. If secondary bacterial infection exists, a topical or oral antibiotic may be indicated, and the presence of an associated eczematous dermatitis may require therapy with a mild topical corticosteroid. While therapy is in progress, patients or parents should be counseled regarding ways to decrease the risk of transmission until the infection has resolved, including avoidance of sharing towels or washcloths, contact activities, and swimming pools.

Molluscum contagiosum infection may present a significant therapeutic problem in immunocompromised patients, particularly HIV-infected patients. In this setting, the infection is often not curable and may even be poorly containable.

Pityriasis Rosea

Pityriasis rosea is an acute self-limited inflammatory skin eruption of unknown etiology that usually results in oval scaly patches primarily of the trunk and proximal extremities.

Pathophysiology

Although a variety of causes of the eruption have been suggested, the etiology of pityriasis rosea is as yet unknown. The most widely accepted explanation is that pityriasis rosea is a viral exanthem. However, antibody titers of numerous known viruses have been examined in conjunction with the eruption, without documentation of a consistent viral association. Circumstantial evidence supporting an infectious etiology includes reports of occasional patients in whom there seems to have been a temporal association between an antecedant upper respiratory tract infection and the eruption, some reports of intrahousehold spread, a few reports of small epidemics, some reports of laboratory abnormalities in association with the eruption, and the fact that a single episode of pityriasis rosea seems to confer immunity (14). Histology reveals a lymphohistiocytic inflammatory infiltrate, but the pathophysiology, as the etiology, is not currently understood.

Clinical Considerations

The lesions of pityriasis rosea are usually asymptomatic although occasional patients complain of pruritus. The eruption is more common during fall and winter months. There is no sex predilection. The disease may

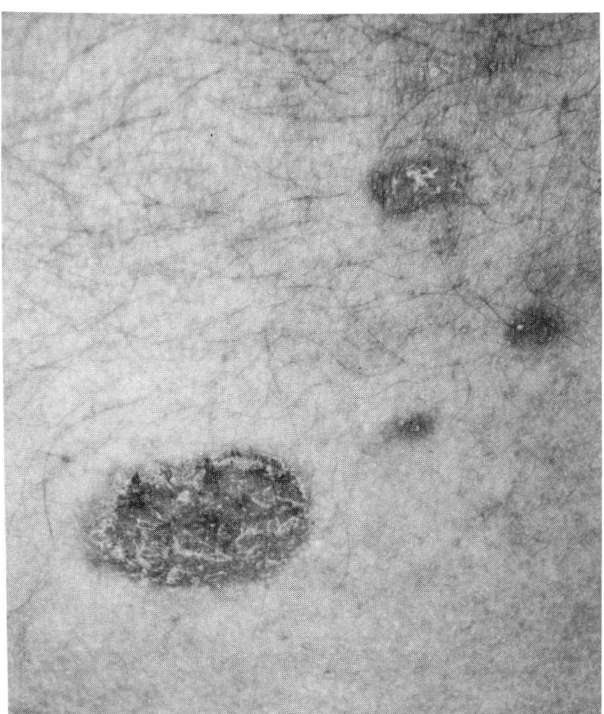

Fig 33.3 Pityriasis rosea. Large herald patch can be seen in association with three smaller typical oval lesions with central scale.

occur at any age, but the majority of cases occur in adolescents and young adults.

The first sign of disease is often the so-called herald patch (Fig 33.3), which is a 2- to 5-cm erythematous scaly patch, sharply marginated, most frequently occurring on the trunk or neck. Although the herald patch is usually a single lesion, rare patients may have multiple herald patches. A herald patch does not necessarily occur, and estimates of its frequency of occurrence vary widely. One recent study documented the presence of a herald patch in 28 of 50 patients with pityriasis rosea (15). The time interval between the appearance of the herald patch and the more widespread eruption ranges from hours to weeks, most commonly 1 to 2 weeks.

The generalized eruption consists of oval pink lesions with central fine scale, oriented along skin tension lines. Other morphologies may occur, including a papular variant (more common in children and black patients), a vesicular variant (more common in children), and a rare hemorrhagic variant. Anatomic sites most often involved are trunk, neck, and proximal extremities. Children are more likely than adults to have involvement of face, hands, and feet. Although patients are seldom examined for oral lesions, oral mucosal involvement has been reported in as many as 16% of patients with pityriasis rosea when patients were consistently examined for such, usually consisting of asymptomatic erosions or ulcerations (15).

The average duration of the eruption is 6 weeks (with new lesions developing for 2 weeks, persistence of a stable eruption for approximately 2 weeks, followed by gradual resolution) although it may persist for 3 months or more. Recurrences of pityriasis rosea may occur but are uncommon and generally single.

Differential Diagnosis

Other diagnostic considerations for the herald patch include dermatophytosis and nummular eczema. For the more generalized eruption of pityriasis rosea, differential diagnostic possibilities include guttate psoriasis, secondary syphilis (which may also have associated oral lesions), tinea versicolor, pityriasis lichenoides, erythema annulare centrifugum, viral exanthem, and drug eruption. Of note, a variety of drugs can produce a pityriasis rosea-like eruption, among them gold, captopril, clonidine, barbiturates, metronidazole, D-penicillamine, and istretinoin (14).

Laboratory Evaluation

There is no specific diagnostic test for pityriasis rosea, and the diagnosis is made clinically. However, when diagnostic uncertainty exists, a potassium hydroxide preparation or fungal culture may be indicated to exclude the possibility of dermatophytosis, and serology may be required to rule out the presence of secondary syphilis. A skin biopsy is rarely necessary for diagnosis.

Management

For patients who are experiencing pruritus, topical or oral antipruritics may be symptomatically helpful although they will not alter the course of the disease. Topical antipruritics include low- to medium-potency topical corticosteroids (low potency only in children), pramoxine, and menthol/phenol preparations (although topical phenol should not be used by pregnant women). More intense pruritus may require oral antihistamines. Ultraviolet B phototherapy may reduce the pruritus and hasten resolution of pityriasis rosea in some patients. Systemic corticosteroids are seldom indicated, but they may be a therapeutic consideration for patients with extensive symptomatic disease and will suppress the eruption.

Rosacea

Rosacea is a common, predominantly facial, inflammatory dermatosis that occurs in a series of phases encompassing a spectrum of cutaneous findings ranging from flushing, erythema, and telangiectasia to papules and pustules, to ocular lesions, to (rarely) rhinophyma.

Pathophysiology

The etiology of rosacea is unknown and, because the disease is multiphasic, it may be that the etiology differs for different stages. Evidence supporting rosacea as primarily a vascular disorder includes the fact that flushing is almost invariably the first component of rosacea to become apparent, patients with rosacea are especially prone to physiologic flushing, some patients with flushing secondary to other disease processes (including carcinoid tumor and mastocytosis) have been reported with other cutaneous features of rosacea, rosacea often occurs in women after the age of 35 (when the frequency of hormonally induced flushing is increased), and patients with rosacea seem statistically more prone to have migraine headaches (16). A role for ultraviolet light-induced dermal connective tissue damage leading to vessel distention (as opposed to, or predisposing to, active vasodilatation) is suggested by the typical facial distribution of the disease, its predominance in people with fair skin, and the almost uniformly associated histologic finding of solar elastosis.

With respect to the papulopustular component of rosacea, which is a later manifestation of the disease and occurs in a minority of patients, a role (albeit controversial) has been suggested for the *Demodex* mite. Although the mite is a normal commensal of hair follicles and sebaceous glands, several studies have documented the presence of significantly increased numbers of mites in the skin appendages of rosacea patients, especially those with the papular/pustular stage and corticosteroid-induced rosacea (17–19). Whether the presence of excessive numbers of these mites is etiologic (either by mechanically obstructing the follicle or by engendering the inflammatory perifollicular immune response seen histologically) or simply opportunistic is unknown.

The etiology and pathogenesis of the rarest manifestation of rosacea, the sebaceous gland and connective tissue hypertrophy of the nose known as rhinophyma, are also unknown.

Clinical Considerations

Rosacea (Fig 33.4) is characterized by a range of skin findings, only some of which may be present in a given individual, including flushing, persistent erythema, telangiectasia, facial edema, papules, pustules, ocular lesions, and rhinophyma. The disease usually involves the nose, cheeks, forehead, and chin, sometimes extending to the lateral neck and presternal chest. People with fair complexions are more commonly affected although black patients can develop rosacea. More women than men experience the early stages of rosacea, and yet, rhinophyma occurs predominantly in men. The usual age of onset is 30 to 50 years, and the process tends to be chronic and recurrent although not necessarily progressive.

Rosacea may be viewed as occurring in four stages (20) even though, again, the majority of patients do not ever experience the later stages of the disease. The first stage is intermittent flushing, stimulated by stress, extremes of temperature change, spicy or hot foods or drinks, and alcohol. Flushing may eventuate in persistent erythema. The second stage is telangiectasia, which

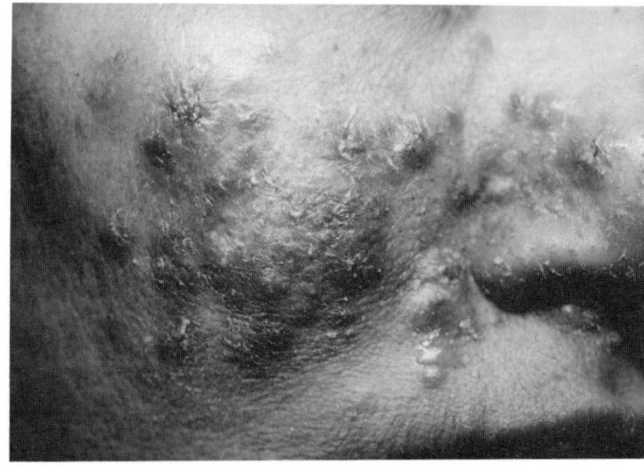

Fig 33.4 Rosacea. Extensive inflammatory papules and pustules of acne rosacea in a middle-aged woman.

develops over the same areas involved with flushing. Telangiectasia over the cheeks is usually fine, but often results in larger caliber vessels over the nose. In most patients, the disease halts at this stage. However, a minority will develop the third stage, known as acne rosacea, which consists of inflammatory papules and pustules. Very few patients, overwhelmingly men, develop the final stage of rosacea, rhinophyma. Rhinophyma is diffuse, sometimes nodular, thickening and distortion of the skin of the nose due to hypertrophy of sebaceous glands and connective tissue. Patients with rhinophyma often have large telangiectases, which may be confined to the nose, and may have flushing confined to the nose.

Ocular involvement is common and most often consists of blepharitis and conjunctival hyperemia although other reported ocular findings include sties, chalazia, superficial punctuate keratopathy, episcleritis, iritis, and corneal neovascularization (20).

Regular protracted use of potent fluorinated topical coticosteroids on the face may result in skin findings indistinguishable from rosacea, which may flare dramatically with subsequent attempts to discontinue the corticosteroids.

Differential Diagnosis

Facial flushing is not unique to rosacea, occurring in association with a number of underlying neoplasms, mastocytosis, thyroid disease, menopause, and a variety of other conditions (21). Persistent facial erythema may occur in the setting of topical corticosteroid abuse, as well as seborrheic dermatitis and lupus erythematosus. Diagnostic considerations for facial papules and pustules include acne vulgaris, topical corticosteroid withdrawal, tinea facei, perioral dermatitis, *Demodex* folliculitis, and contact dermatitis. Rarely, unusual infectious processes or neoplasms may mimic rhinophyma.

Laboratory Evaluation

When facial flushing occurs in the setting of other clinical signs or symptoms suggestive of systemic disease, laboratory evaluation is indicated as appropriate for the underlying disease suspected. Persistent facial erythema suggestive of lupus erythematosus may merit assessing an antinuclear antibody titer. A potassium hydroxide preparation of pustule contents (or associated scale) may be necessary to rule out facial dermatophytosis. Rarely, biopsy may be required for diagnostic clarification.

Management

There is no very effective treatment for flushing and early erythema. The avoidance of facial irritants and precipitants and exacerbants of flushing and the use of sunscreens may be helpful. Menopausal flushing may respond to low doses of oral clonidine. Topical 1% hydrocortisone cream used twice a day is sometimes useful in decreasing erythema and inflammation, but more potent topical steroids should never be used. Telangiectases may respond to electrical or laser destruction.

First-line therapy for inflammatory papules and pustules is generally considered to be oral antibiotics, specifically tetracycline (with an initial dose of 500 mg twice a day until lesions subside, after which the dose can be gradually reduced). Other oral antibiotics sometimes used include minocycline, metronidazole, erythromyin, and trimethoprim-sulfamethoxazole. Isotretinoin can be effective (22), but it has significant potential side effects. Furthermore, it is a potent teratogen, requiring effective contraception when used by women of reproductive capacity. Topical therapy is usually more effective for maintenance of remission than for treatment of active inflammatory lesions. Rosacea has a high relapse rate without maintenance therapy. Topical metronidazole gel, topical erythomycin and clindamycin preparations, and sulfur-containing creams may be used twice a day. Mild (0.025%) topical tretinoin cream applied at bedtime may be beneficial (although it may also be irritating and may, in some, actually cause angiogenesis, worsening the telangiectatic component of rosacea), as well as topical benzoyl peroxide products. Ocular rosacea often requires continual therapy with an oral antibiotic such as tetracycline.

Reduction of rhinophymatous tissue may be accomplished by surgical shave, carbon dioxide laser surgery, electrosurgery, or dermabrasion.

Scabies

Cutaneous infestation with the *Sarcoptes scabiei* mite results in an intensely pruritic dermatosis that may be confused clinically with a number of other skin diseases. However, once suspected, the diagnosis is easily confirmed.

Pathophysiology

The human scabies mite, *Sarcoptes scabiei var. hominis*, has no animal reservoir and is an obligate parasite, usually living no more than 24 to 36 hours without host contact. Human beings are occasionally infested with animal-specific scabies species, particularly *Sarcoptes scabiei var. canis* contracted from puppies, but these mite species cannot reproduce on human hosts and their infestations are self-limited. Human scabies is primarily transmitted by direct personal contact. Contact with infested clothing, bedclothing, or furniture is a much less common source although may be more significant when the index person has the crusted variant of the disease (carrying a mite population numbering in the hundreds of thousands). The average individual with scabies harbors less than a dozen live adult mites at any one time.

The female mite is fertilized on the skin surface, then burrows into the stratum corneum while the male mite remains on the surface. In the stratum corneum, the female mite deposits eggs from which larvae emerge, travel to the skin surface, pass through a nymphal form, then become adult mites. The female mite lives longer than the male, approximately 5 weeks.

In an individual with no previous mite infestation, no signs or symptoms of infestation are apparent for several weeks. The individual has to become sensitized to mite antigens and generate a cell-mediated immune response to the antigens, before disease becomes evident in the form of an intense inflammatory cutaneous reaction. In a patient already sensitized by a previous infestation, signs and symptoms may occur in 24 hours. The specific antigens responsible for the immune response are not well characterized. The lymphohistocytic infiltrate seen histologically consists primarily of T-helper cells (23). Scabietic nodules may be the result of locally persistent antigen that provokes an ongoing immune response.

An episode of scabies does not confer complete immunity, and reinfestation may occur. Crusted scabies tends to occur in people with compromised cell-mediated immunity.

Clinical Considerations

The most salient feature of scabies is severe pruritus, which is often nocturnal. Skin lesions (Fig 33.5) may have a variety of morphologies, including burrows (which are pathognomonic), papules (the most common morphology), pustules, vesicles, bullae, nodules, and urticarial lesions, all of which may be obscured by excoriations. Lesions are most commonly found on finger and toe webs, areolae, penis, axillae, lower buttocks, and around the waistline. In adults, facial involvement is uncommon. Burrows are especially common in interdigital areas, are threadlike in diameter and may be as long as 10 mm in length. Nodules are most common on male genitalia and in the axillae and may persist for months despite therapy. Secondary bacterial infections are common.

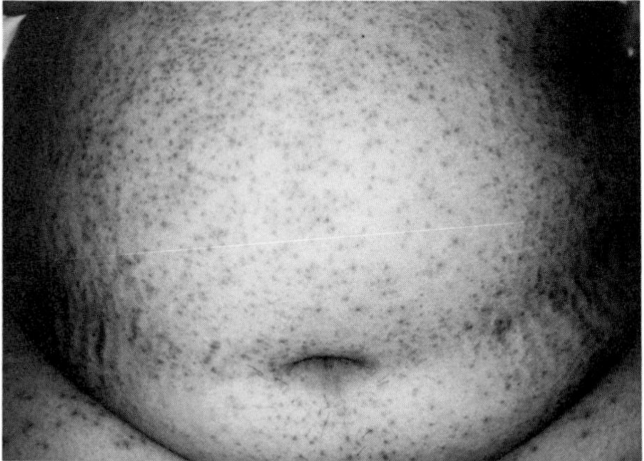

Fig 33.5 Scabies. Widespread pruritic papules in a pregnant woman.

Infants and children with scabies often differ from adults in their presentation and lesional distribution (24) although the disease is just as intensely pruritic. They may be infested for as long as 2 months before showing signs of disease. The lesions are often generalized, including face, palms, and soles, with vesicopustules being especially common on palms and soles. Excoriations and impetiginization are frequently seen.

Crusted (Norwegian) scabies (Fig 33.6) occurs most often in immunosuppressed and institutionalized individuals. Affected people are highly contagious due to the tremendous numbers of mites present, but they seem to experience minimal pruritus. The excessive numbers of mites and minimal pruritus may be due to a diminished host response. Affected individuals often have hyperkeratosis, especially of hands and feet, crusted plaques, and dystrophic nails with subungual debris.

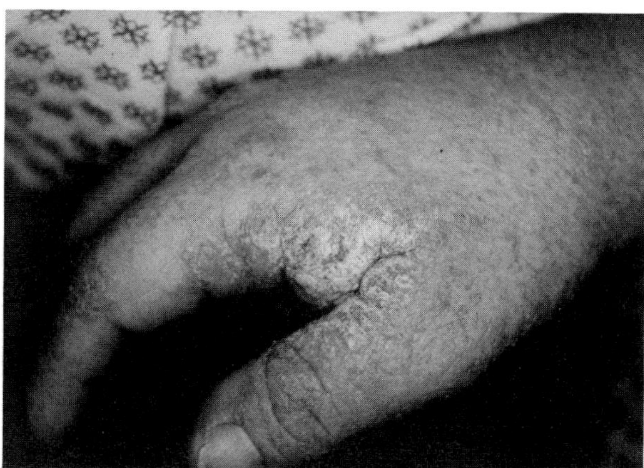

Fig 33.6 Scabies. Crusted (Norwegian) scabies, with hyperkeratotic crusting of web spaces, in an institutionalized young woman with Down syndrome.

Differential Diagnosis

The differential diagnosis in adults includes other bites, folliculitis, neurodermatitis, and dermatitis herpetiformis. In pregnant women, herpes gestationis and pruritic urticarial papules and plaques of pregnancy must be considered. Diagnostic considerations in infants and children include insect bites, recurrent impetigo, miliaria, acropustulosis of infancy, atopic dermatitis, and seborrheic dermatitis. The differential diagnosis of crusted scabies includes drug eruption, xerosis, psoriasis, contact dermatitis, and seborrheic dermatitis.

Laboratory Evaluation

Lesional scrapings performed with a No. 15 blade and mineral oil may reveal the diagnostic mites, ova, or feces. The best yield is from new nonexcoriated lesions, especially burrows, and the more lesions that are scraped, the better the chance of a positive result.

Management

Treatment of an individual with scabies involves four aspects: elimination of the mites, management of the associated pruritus, treatment of patient contacts, and decontamination of fomites. If secondary infection exists, antibiotic therapy may be required, as well.

The scabicide of choice for adults and children is permethrin 5% cream (25) because it is efficacious and has a low potential for toxicity. However, it is not approved for use in infants less than 2 months of age or in pregnant or lactating women. A single overnight application (8 to 12 hours) is usually sufficient although a second overnight application may be performed 1 week later. Treatment of crusted scabies often requires multiple applications. Adults should apply the cream from neck to toes; however, children's scalps and faces should be treated, as well. Side effects are uncommon and mild and include stinging or burning on application. The drug is poorly absorbed and rapidly metabolized and has no known systemic side effects. Because the cream's preservative is formaldehyde, the potential for allergic contact dermatitis exists. Treatment failures may result from inadequate application, and patients should be instructed to apply the cream between fingers and toes, in the groin area, umbilicus, and intergluteal cleft, and beneath nails (which should be trimmed). The treatment of choice for infants less than 2 months of age or pregnant or lactating women is precipitated sulfur 5% to 10% in petrolatum, applied nightly for three successive nights, washing off just before reapplication. Although there are no reports of toxicities with this preparation, it is messy to apply, stains clothing, and has an unfortunate odor.

Lindane 1% lotion is another scabicide that is applied in a manner similar to permethrin 5% cream and probably has a similar cure rate (26). However, transcutaneous absorption can be significant, neurotoxicity may result, and the drug cannot be used in infants, young children, and pregnant or lactating women. There also may be some lindane-resistant disease (27). Another available scabicide is crotamiton cream although it probably is not highly effective.

Pruritus may persist for 2 weeks or more after eradication of mites. Both oral antihistamines and topical corticosteroids are helpful in managing pruritus although nothing stronger than 1% hydrocortisone should be used on the skin of children. Postscabietic nodules may linger for months, but eventually spontaneously resolve.

Household members and others with close personal contact should be treated, and clothing and bedclothing should be washed in hot water and detergent.

Seborrheic Dermatitis

Seborrheic dermatitis is an extremely common skin condition characterized by the formation of greasy scale, sometimes with associated erythema, often with associated pruritus, of characteristic anatomic sites, most notably scalp and face.

Pathophysiology

Increasing evidence suggests that the yeast *Pityrosporum ovale* is the etiologic agent of seborrheic dermatitis although, because *P. ovale* is part of the normal skin flora found in asymptomatic patients, the precise role of the organism is difficult to define (28,29). Supportive evidence includes the findings that there are increased numbers of organisms at involved sites, there is a correlation between the density of *P. ovale* organisms and the severity of seborrheic dermatitis, seborrheic dermatitis responds to antifungal therapy in a manner that correlates with a decrease in the number of organisms, and reintroduction of the organism to the scalp results in recrudescence of disease (29). Not all studies confirm these findings, however (30).

An association between sebaceous gland activity and seborrheic dermatitis has long been noted because, with the exception of infantile seborrheic dermatitis ("cradle cap"), the disease is generally not present in prepubertal individuals, and the most common sites of involvement (face, scalp, upper trunk) are those with increased sebum production. This may indirectly support the pityrosporal association in that *P. ovale* is lipophilic, its colonization of human skin begins at puberty (temporally associated with increased sebaceous gland activity), and some studies indicate that the greatest numbers of organisms are found in those same sites of increased sebum production and highest incidence of seborrheic dermatitis (29).

A neurologic component has been suggested, but never explained, to account for the noted increased incidence and severity of seborrheic dermatitis in patients with some neurologic disorders, including Parkinson's disease. Immunologic parameters have also been investigated, particularly in light of the frequency and severity of the disease in HIV-infected patients. The HIV association is as yet unexplained, other than the suggestion that *P. ovale* may be an opportunistic pathogen in this setting. There has been no consistent documentation of even selective immunodeficiency in normal hosts with seborrheic dermatitis, and it may be that the absolute numbers of *P. ovale* present are not as important as other immunologic or local factors that participate in the transformation of the organism from a commensal to a pathogen.

Clinical Considerations

The anatomic sites most often involved with seborrheic dermatitis are scalp ("dandruff") and face. The presternal area, especially in men, and the interscapular area are frequently involved, and, occasionally, disease occurs in axillae and groins. Seborrheic dermatitis affects men more frequently than women, is rare before puberty (except for the infantile form), and may worsen in the fall and winter. The process is often pruritic, especially when involving the scalp, and may be exacerbated by heat. The disease tends to be chronic, with intermittent flares.

Seborrheic dermatitis of the scalp usually manifests as noninflammatory perifollicular scale although more severe disease may be inflammatory. Facial seborrheic dermatitis is characterized by erythema with overlying greasy scale, especially of nasolabial folds, eyebrows, glabella, and the frontal hairline. Hair-bearing areas of the face may be involved in men with beards or mustaches. Malar areas are sometimes affected in a butterfly pattern mimicking lupus erythematosus. Seborrheic dermatitis frequently involves the ears, including concha, external auditory meatus, and posterior auricular folds, and may be complicated by otitis externa. Eyelids may be affected in the form of blepharitis.

Seborrheic dermatitis is especially common in neurologic patients, nursing home patients, and HIV-infected patients. In HIV-infected patients, the disease may be severe and inflammatory, even mimicking psoriasis, sometimes involving the face while sparing the scalp, and tends to worsen with progressive immunocompromise.

Infantile seborrheic dermatitis has its onset in the first 3 months of life and is characterized by thick yellow scale with or without inflammation, primarily involving the vertex of the scalp. The process usually is nonpruritic. Although the disease is generally confined to the scalp, it may involve the diaper area or other intertriginous areas and rarely becomes generalized. Infantile seborrheic dermatitis usually resolves in approximately 1 month, and its relationship to adult seborrheic dermatitis, if any, is not clear.

Differential Diagnosis

Seborrheic dermatitis of the scalp may be severe enough to resemble psoriasis (an entity sometimes referred to as sebopsoriasis), although psoriasis does not commonly involve the face, and patients with psoriasis of the scalp often have typical psoriatic lesions elsewhere. The presence of inflammatory papules or pustules may help distinguish the facial erythema of rosacea from that of seborrheic dermatitis. Other diseases that may manifest as facial erythema and scale include allergic contact dermatitis, photocontact dermatitis, lupus erythematosus, and a rare form of pemphigus known as pemphigus erythematosus. Seborrheic dermatitis-like drug eruptions have been reported with a number of agents, including cimetidine, methyldopa, and penicillamine.

In infants, diseases that may mimic seborrheic dermatitis include atopic dermatitis, psoriasis, and, rarely, histiocytosis X, certain enzyme and nutrient deficiencies, and immunodeficiency states.

Laboratory Evaluation

The diagnosis of seborrheic dermatitis is made clinically, seldom requiring laboratory evaluation. Rarely, concern regarding lupus erythematosus may prompt obtaining antinuclear antibody serology, and considerations of pemphigus erythematosus may necessitate a skin biopsy for histology and direct immunofluorescence studies.

Management

Effective management of seborrheic dermatitis of the scalp may be accomplished through the frequent use of shampoos containing a variety of agents with antipityrosporal activity, including selenium sulfide, zinc pyrithione, salicylic acid, sulfur, coal tar, and ketoconazole (31). Ketoconazole shampoo may be used twice weekly and left on the scalp for 5 to 10 minutes before rinsing; it may be more effective than selenium sulfide or zinc pyrithione (32). The addition of a low-to-mid potency corticosteroid solution for daily use on the scalp may enhance control and further diminish pruritus and scale. Seborrheic dermatitis of the face and other sites ususally responds well to 1% hydrocortisone cream or 2% ketoconazole cream applied twice daily. Ongoing treatment is generally required because the disease frequently recurs with cessation of therapy.

Infantile seborrheic dermatitis often responds to topical 2% ketoconazole cream or shampoo (with gentle scrubbing to remove scales) and topical 1% hydrocortisone cream. Seborrheic dermatitis in HIV-infected patients may be difficult to control.

Tinea Versicolor

Tinea versicolor is a superficial fungal infection, usually involving the trunk and upper arms, which results in slightly scaly patches of skin that are either hypopigmented or hyperpigmented.

Pathophysiology

Controversy exists concerning the name of the causative organism, with investigators referring to the organism as *Malassezia furfur*, *P. ovale*, or *Pityrosporum orbiculare*. *Pityrosporum* is now probably the more commonly used name, and the *Pityrosporum* species may be polymorphic forms of the same organism (33). The *Pityrosporum* organism in yeast form is felt to be part of normal hair follicle flora, but conversion to hyphal form results in spread on to the skin surface and clinical disease (34). The change from yeast to hyphal form is influenced by several factors, including pregnancy, oral contraceptives, Cushing's disease, systemic corticosteroid therapy, diabetes, immunosuppression, and hyperhidrosis (33). The fungus is lipophilic, which accounts for the usual postpubertal onset of clinical disease (increased sebaceous gland activity). Clinical disease occurs with increased frequency in warm humid climates. Clinical disease is not contagious, perhaps signifying the importance of host factors. There is as yet no clear immunologic explanation for the predisposition of some people for recurrent disease.

Clinical Considerations

Tinea versicolor occurs most commonly in young adults, with the postpubertal increase in incidence felt due to enhanced sebaceous gland activity. Disease may occur in children, however, especially in tropical climates.

Skin lesions (Fig 33.7) are often pink or light brown initially but may become hypopigmented. The lesions are usually asymptomatic although occasional patients complain of pruritus. The most common site of involvement is the upper trunk, but involvement of the upper arms is not uncommon. Facial involvement may be more common in black individuals.

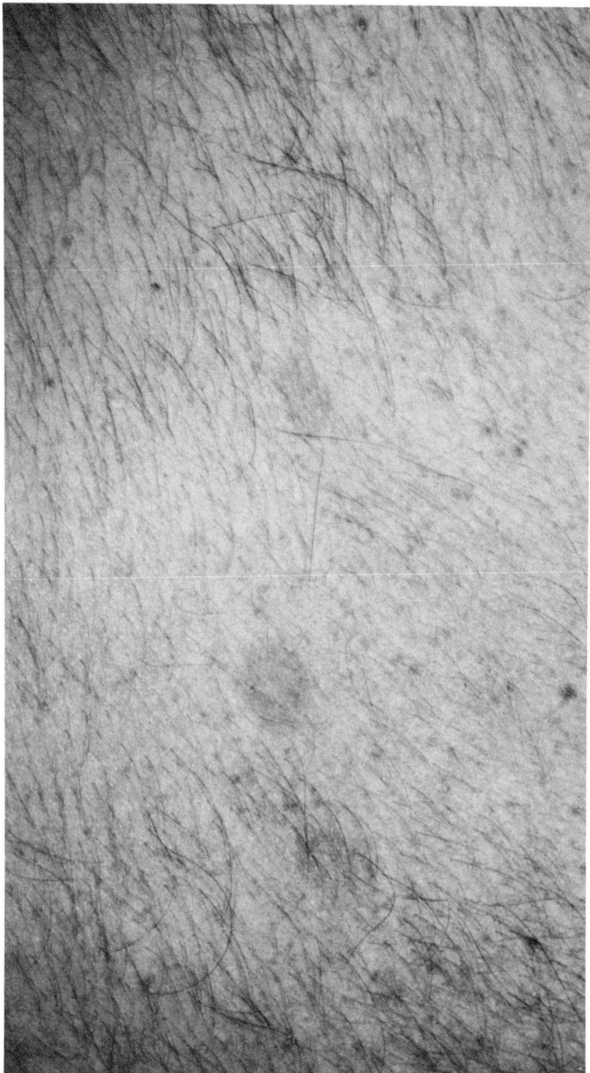

Fig 33.7 Tinea versicolor. Rather subtle, slightly scaly hyperpigmented patches on a man's trunk.

Differential Diagnosis

The differential diagnosis of tinea versicolor may include vitiligo, pityriasis alba, pityriasis rosea, dermatophytosis, seborrheic dermatitis, and secondary syphilis.

Laboratory Evaluation

The clinical presentation of tinea versicolor is usually sufficiently distinctive that laboratory evaluation is not required for diagnosis. If diagnostic clarification is needed, physician-performed microscopic evaluation of potassium hydroxide-treated scale gently scraped from involved areas will reveal multiple short thick hyphae and round budding yeasts, present in varying proportions. Because of its lipid nutrient requirements, the *Pityrosporum* organism is not culturable on standard mycologic media. Wood's lamp evaluation of skin lesions may reveal yellow fluorescence.

Management

A variety of topical agents will effectively treat tinea versicolor, including selenium sulfide suspension (applied daily for 5 to 15 minutes, for 1 to 2 weeks), zinc pyrithione (found in a number of shampoos, applied nightly for 5 to 10 minutes, for 2 weeks), salicylic acid preparations (3% to 6%, applied overnight for 1 to 2 weeks), propylene glycol solution (applied once or twice daily for 1 to 2 weeks), retinoic acid cream (applied twice a day for 1 to 2 weeks), and a variety of topical antifungal preparations applied twice a day for 2 weeks (including tolnaftate, haloprogin, ciclopirox olamine, clotrimazole, miconazole, ketoconazole, and econazole). All of these topical agents are effective if used for an adequate duration. However, it is important to inform patients that pigmentary changes resolve much more slowly than the actual fungal infection, over a period of weeks to months.

Systemic therapy is effective although seldom required. The organism does not respond to oral griseofulvin therapy. A variety of treatment regimens using oral ketoconazole have been successful, including a single 400-mg dose (35). Ketoconazole, an imidazole antifungal that interferes with the synthesis of ergosterol, the major lipid comprising fungal cell walls, reaches the stratum corneum rapidly through eccrine sweat ducts. However, its use entails a small but present risk of significant hepatotoxicity, and its safety in pregnancy has not been established. Itraconazole, a triazole antifungal, has also been reported effective (36), but with safety issues not unlike those of ketoconazole.

Recurrences are common with any treatment. Maintenance prophylactic therapy with sulfur- or zinc pyrithione-containing soaps may be helpful in decreasing the frequency of recurrences.

Xerosis

Dry skin is a common complaint, and the condition increases in frequency and severity with age. However, patients often incorrectly equate scaly skin of any etiology, from seborrheic dermatitis to postinflammatory desquamation, with dry skin.

Pathophysiology

Although convention defines xerosis as scaly skin resulting from dehydration of the stratum corneum, the pathogenesis appears to be far more complex than this and is incompletely understood. Terminal differentiation of the epidermis results in formation of the stratum corneum, the layer of dead corneocytes overlying and protecting the living epidermis. An integral part of this process is the continuous loss, or desquamation, of corneocytes from the skin surface. Xerosis is the result of abnormalities of corneocyte desquamation, with the accumulation of grossly visible clumps of corneocytes (scales) on the surface of the skin. The cause of the abnormal desquamation is multifactorial, but is essentially the result of abnormal degradation of corneocyte adhesive elements, including desmosomes and lipids. The hydrolytic enzymes involved in the degradation of corneocyte adhesive structures require an aqueous environment, but the relative contributions of stratum corneum lipids, desmosomes, and other structural components to the process are not well understood (37).

Clinical Considerations

Xerosis (Fig 33.8) may be generalized or occur in patches but most commonly occurs on anterior tibial areas, forearms, and hands. It is especially common in the elderly ("senile xerosis") and is often worse during winter months presumably related to decreased ambient humidity. Also at risk are people with occupations that expose them to overcleansing or degreasing of their skin, including those with occupations requiring frequent handwashing (physicians, dentists, nurses), those with exposures to solvents, and those with frequent soap/detergent exposures (such as homemakers and dishwashers). Xerotic skin is often pruritic and is probably the most common cause of pruritus in the elderly. Severe xerosis can progress to asteatotic eczema, with superficial reticulate cracking known as eczema craquele. Drugs that may precipitate or exacerbate xerosis include oral retinoids and cholesterol-lowering agents.

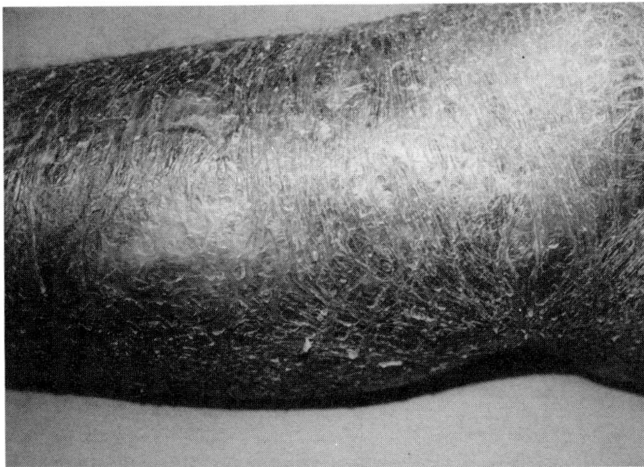

Fig 33.8 Xerosis. Extensive scale of unusually severe xerosis on a patient's lower extremity.

Differential Diagnosis

Other diagnostic considerations for skin with fine scale include ichthyosis vulgaris, atopic dermatitis, and contact dermatitis. Patches of finely scaling skin may represent nummular eczema or dermatophytosis.

Laboratory Evaluation

Laboratory evaluation is seldom required. Scaly patches resembling dermatophytosis may merit microscopic examination of scales in a potassium hydroxide preparation. Because xerosis may accompany hypothyroidism, patients with other signs or symptoms of thyroid dysfunction should undergo an assessment of thyroid function.

Management

The primary intervention in the treatment of xerosis is the frequent use of emollients, which mainly act by remaining on the skin surface and diminishing flaking. However, when applied immediately after bathing, emollients may also reduce water loss from the hydrated stratum corneum. In general, heavier (greasier) emollients are more effective, but they may not be cosmetically acceptable. Ointments such as petrolatum, therefore, are effective, with creams and lotions being less effective. α-Hydroxy acids such as pyruvic, lactic, and glycolic acids, as well as ammonium lactate lotion (5% and 12%), act by decreasing corneocyte adhesion with resultant thinning of the stratum corneum and are often useful in the management of xerosis. Urea creams (10% to 20%) may also be helpful. Possible side effects of heavy emollients include miliaria and folliculitis. With respect to all topical preparations, the potential for allergic contact dermatitis exists, especially from preservatives and fragrances. α-Hydroxy acids often sting on initial application.

Additional preventive measures for xerosis-prone skin include humidification of ambient air, reduction in the frequency of bathing (with use of the coolest water tolerable), and minimization of exposure to soaps, detergents, and solvents.

In patients with severe xerosis and associated eczematous changes, topical corticosteroids may initially be helpful in rapidly reducing inflammation and pruritus.

REFERENCES

1. Stern RS. The prevalence of acne on the basis of physical examination. J Am Acad Dermatol 1992;26:931–935.

2. Pochi PE, Shalita AR, Strauss JS, et al. Report of the Consensus Conference on Acne Classification. Washington, DC, March 24 and 25, 1990. J Am Acad Dermatol 1991;24:495–500.

3. Monk B, Cunliffe WJ, Layton AM, Rhodes DJ. Acne induced by inhaled corticosteroids. Clin Exper Dermatol 1993;18:148–150.

4. Rittmaster RS. Hyperandrogenism—what is normal? N Engl J Med 1992;327:194–196.

5. Sperling LC, Heimer WL. Androgen biology as a basis for the diagnosis and treatment of androgenic disorders in women. II. J Am Acad Dermatol 1993;28:901–916.

6. Rothman KF, Pochi PE. Use of oral and topical agents for acne in pregnancy. J Am Acad Dermatol 1988;19:431-442.

7. Driscoll MS, Rothe MJ, Abrahamian L, Grant-Kels JM. Long-term oral antibiotics for acne: is laboratory monitoring necessary? J Am Acad Dermatol 1993;28:595–602.

8. Layton AM, Cunliffe WJ. Guidelines for optimal use of isotretinoin in acne. J Am Acad Dermatol 1992;27:S2–S7.

9. Stainforth JM, Layton AM, Taylor JP, Cunliffe WJ. Isotretinoin for the treatment of acne vulgaris: which factors may predict the need for more than one course? Br J Dermatol 1993;129:297–301.

10. Buller RM, Palumbo GJ. Poxvirus pathogenesis. Microbiol Rev 1991;55:80–122.

11. Epstein WL. Molluscum contagiosum. Semin Dermatol 1992;11:184–189.

12. Highet AS. Molluscum contagiosum. Arch Dis Child 1992;67:1248–1249.

13. Buntin DM, Roser T, Lesher JL Jr, et al. Sexually transmitted diseases: viruses and ectoparasites. Committee on Sexually Transmitted Diseases of the American Academy of Dermatology. J Am Acad Dermatol 1991;25:527–534.

14. Parsons JM. Pityriasis rosea update: 1986. J Am Acad Dermatol 1986;15:159–167.

15. Vidimos AT, Camisa C. Tongue and cheek: oral lesions in pityriasis rosea. Cutis 1992;50:276–280.

16. Wilkin JK. Rosacea: pathophysiology and treatment. Arch Dermatol 1994;130:359–362.

17. Bonnar E, Eustace P, Powell FC. The *Demodex* mite population in rosacea. J Am Acad Dermatol 1993;28:443-448.

18. Forton F, Seys B. Density of *Demodex folliculorum* in rosacea: a case-control study using standardized skin-surface biopsy. Br J Dermatol 1993;128:650–659.

19. Sibenge S, Gawkrodger DJ. Rosacea: a study of clinical patterns, blood flow, and the role of *Demodex folliculorum*. J Am Acad Dermatol 1992;26:590–593.

20. Rebora A. Rosacea. J Invest Dermatol 1987;88(3 suppl):56S–60S.

21. Mooney E. The flushing patient. Int J Dermatol 1985;24:549–554.

22. Ertl GA, Levine N, Kligman AM. A comparison of the efficacy of topical tretinoin and low-dose oral isotretinoin in rosacea. Arch Dermatol 1994;130:319–324.

23. Cabrera R, Agar A, Dahl MV. The immunology of scabies. Semin Dermatol 1993;12:15–21.

24. Paller AS. Scabies in infants and small children. Semin Dermatol 1993;12:3–8.

25. Anonymous. Permethrin for scabies. Med Lett Drug Ther 1990;32(813):21–22.

26. Schultz MW, Gomez M, Hansen RC, et al. Comparative study of 5% permethrin cream and 1% lindane lotion for the treatment of scabies. Arch Dermatol 1990;126:167–170.

27. Purvis SP, Tyring SK. An outbreak of lindane-resistant scabies treated successfully with permethrin 5% cream. J Am Acad Dermatol 1991;25:1015–1016.

28. Rebora A, Rongioletta F. The red face: seborrheic dermatitis. Clin Dermatol 1993;11:243–251.

29. Bergbrant IM, Faergemann J. The role of *Pityrosporum ovale* in seborrheic dermatitis. Semin Dermatol 1990;9:262–268.

30. Ashbee HR, Ingham E, Holland KT, Cunliffe WJ. The carriage of *Malassezia furfur* serovars A, B and C in patients with pityriasis versicolor, seborrheic dermatitis and controls. Br J Dermatol 1993;129:533–540.

31. McGrath J, Murphy GM. The control of seborrhoeic dermatitis and dandruff by antipityrosporal drugs. Drugs 1991;41:178–184.

32. Van Cutsem J, Van Gerven F, Fransen J, et al. The in vitro antifungal activity of ketoconazole, zinc pyrithione, and selenium sulfide against *Pityrosporum* and their efficacy as a shampoo in the treatment of experimental pityrosporosis in guinea pigs. J Am Acad Dermatol 1990;22(6 Pt 1):993–998.

33. Borelli D, Jacobs PH, Nall L. Tinea versicolor: epidemiologic, clinical, and therapeutic aspects. J Am Acad Dermatol 1991;25(2 Pt 1);300–305.

34. Rezabek GH, Friedman AD. Superficial fungal infections of the skin. Diagnosis and current treatment recommendations. Drugs 1992;43:674–682.

35. Rausch LJ, Jacobs PH. Tinea versicolor and prophylaxis with monthly administration of ketoconazole. Cutis 1984;34:470–471.

36. Delescluse J. Itraconazole in tinea versicolor: a review. J Am Acad Dermatol 1990;23(3 Pt 2):551–554.

37. Rawlings AV, Scott IR, Harding CR, Bowser PA. Stratum corneum moisturizaiton at the molecular level. Prog Dermatol 1994;28:1–12.

CHAPTER 34

SKIN CANCERS

Patricia Mercado

Photodamage and Skin Cancer

Skin cancer is the foremost cutaneous concern of the dermatologic patient. Current trends of patient education have brought in many patients for evaluation of changing skin lesions. This is a response to the spiraling increase in the incidence of skin cancer. The rate of development is so rapid that one in six Americans will develop a skin cancer. Potentially disfiguring or fatal, skin cancer deserves prompt recognition and treatment. Full body skin examinations from the scalp to the toes should be included as part of any comprehensive physical examination.

Photodamage

Photodamage is the leading causative agent in the development of skin cancer. The primary source for photodamage is solar radiation. Sunlight emits a wide range of electromagnetic radiation including infrared, visible, and ultraviolet spectra. The only radiation that remains clinically important are those rays that penetrate the ozone layer and reach the earth's surface. The two radiation bands that fit this description are ultraviolet A radiation (UVA) and ultraviolet B radiation (UVB).

UVB Radiation

This type of radiation encompasses the wavelength spectrum of 290 to 320 nm. This shorter length, higher energy fraction of ultraviolet radiation is substantially absorbed by the ozone layer. Any loss of the earth's protective ozone layer will increase the transmission of UVB. UVB is absorbed primarily by the epidermis. The transferred energy is expressed by erythema and sunburn. After sun exposure, erythema is noted in 2 to 6 hours with the peak damage after 15 to 24 hours. This is the "sunburn" spectrum.

UVA Radiation

Ultraviolet A radiation is a longer wavelength with a spectrum of 320 to 400 nm. Virtually no UVA is absorbed by the ozone layer. This is the spectrum of ultraviolet radiation that is promoted in the tanning salons. The energy of this radiation is absorbed in the dermis where the damage is directed to collagen, elastic tissue, and the vasculature. The long-term effects of this radiation are clinically evident as photodamage. The ability of UVA to cause structural damage to DNA in the form of cross-linkage, strand breakage, dimer formation, and free radical formation is well described. In animals, UVA is carcinogenic. UVA tanning followed by sunbathing potentiates the damage caused by solar radiation. UVA is the "wrinkle" spectrum.

Charactistics of Photodamage

Photodamage is the effect of repeated phototrauma. Repeated episodes of sunburn result in textural changes and mottled hyperpigmentation. Lentigines, freckles, and telangiectasias are further evidence of photodamage. If no protective measures are instituted, fine wrinkling followed by a sallow complexion and further laxity of the skin result. It is in this background that actinic keratoses, basal carcinomas, and squamous cell carcinomas arise.

Susceptibility to photodamage may be influenced by numerous factors. Skin type, age, genetic disorders of pigmentation or DNA repair, photosensitive disease states, immunosuppressed states and medications can affect one's vulnerability.

Geographic location, altitude, and seasonal variation all affect the intensity of the sun. Those locales closer to the equator and at higher altitudes experience more intense UVB radiation. Incidence rates of melanoma are higher closer to the equator. Epidemiologic studies incriminate UVB as the most important environmental factor in the pathogenesis of melanoma. Summer sun is stronger than the winter sun. Cloudy days, shade and umbrellas offer little protection for the beach enthusiast. The clouds offer little protection because they reduce ultraviolet radiation by only 20% to 40%. Sand and water will reflect up to 85% of the solar rays.

Photoprotection

Sunscreen with an SPF of 15 or greater will filter 92% of the UVB radiation and so offer protection for most users. The SPF, or sun protection factor, relates to UVB protection only. Most sunscreens only partially protect from UVA. The physical blockers that contain titanium dioxide or zinc oxide will protect against the UVA spectrum as well. These are only limited by their lack of cosmetic appeal. Similarly, window glass blocks all UVB and almost half of UVA radiation. Tinted automobile glass is, therefore, unnecessary in most circumstances.

Protective clothing in the form of tight knit weave shirts, pants, and hats will block most UVB and all UVA. The average T-shirt has the equivalent of an SPF 5. Wet clothing loses most of its protective effect. Commercial photoprotective clothing with a tested SPF of 30 or greater is now available. These items can be indispensable to your most photosensitive patients.

Avoidance of sun exposure between the hours of 10 AM and 1 PM is important, especially for children and adolescents.

Avoidance of tanning booths, which potentiate the effects of solar radiation, should also be encouraged.

Actinic Keratoses

This is the most common premalignant lesion that the practicing physician will encounter. When it degenerates into a malignancy, timely intervention becomes necessary.

Its clinical presentation is subtle and slow. A palpable difference in the skin texture with the sensation of sandpaper is the first appreciable change. Color alteration follows with the appearance of reddish, brown macules. Actinic keratoses are usually asymptomatic but may be noted to burn or sting. Sun-exposed areas of the face, arms, upper chest, and back are the sites most commonly affected.

Treatment options include cryodestruction, chemical destruction, or surgical destruction. Cryosurgery is one of the preferred methods of treating actinic keratoses. The cryogen of choice is liquid nitrogen (−195.8°C). Liquid nitrogen spray, probes, or cotton-tipped applicators are used in cryosurgery. Topical chemotherapy with 5-fluorouracil or masoprocol remains the most efficient way to treat numerous lesions. Treatment with 5-fluorouracil is more effective than masoprocal in treating actinic keratoses but has a higher incidence of irritation. This may preclude its use in some patients. Masoprocal is an effective alternate in this situation. Chemical peels using trichloracetic acid should be reserved for the patient who does not respond to a therapeutic course of the above agents. Surgical intervention is unnecessary unless the diagnosis is in doubt. Lesions that are larger than 1.0 cm should be suspect for malignancy. A biopsy, rather simple destruction, should be performed.

Primary prevention of actinic photodamage remains the mainstay of reducing actinic keratoses and skin cancer in the long term. Thompson and colleagues (1) clearly demonstrated that regular sunscreen use does reduce the development of actinic keratoses. Proper sun protective measures on a daily basis are an important step on the road to prevention.

Basal Cell Carcinoma

The most common, malignant neoplasm in the general population is basal cell carcinoma (BCC). Approximately two thirds of these lesions are found on sun-exposed surfaces; the remaining one third are found on more sun-protected areas. The incidence of this neoplasm has increased with the popularity of sunbathing and outdoor recreation. Patients are now presenting at a younger age with actinic damage and BCC.

Pathogenesis

The most common factor in the etiology of BCC is ultraviolet radiation, with UVB exposure correlating best with the incidence of skin cancer. Cumulative exposure over 20 to 30 years is required for tumor development. Damage to DNA either through cross-linking or oxidation is thought to be the primary mechanism of carcinogenesis. With aging, the ability to repair damaged DNA declines, placing that age group at a higher risk. X-rays, burns, areas of chronic trauma, and immunosuppression may also predispose to BCC but these are much more often associated with the development of squamous cell carcinoma.

Presentation

A gelatinous, papule with rolled borders, central umbilication or ulceration, and surface telangiectasia is the hallmark of this tumor. Plate 7 illustrates the typical topography of this lesion. Located on the head and neck, it is asymptomatic until it ulcerates. Bleeding or oozing is a common presenting complaint. Differential diagnoses include seborrheic keratoses, sebaceous hyperplasia, and trichoepitheliomas.

Treatment is primarily surgical. Electrodesiccation and curettage or primary excision are the most common treatments. Certain locations as the inner canthus or preauricular areas overlie embryonic planes and should be handled with caution. Invasion to deeper underlying structures and perineural invasion complicate the treatment protocols. Moh's microscopic surgery is often used to eradicate tumors in these locations. This procedure involves a step-wise excision where frozen sections of all edges are checked for tumor involvement and any positive areas are removed until all margins are free of involvement. Moh's surgery demands on-site tissue processing and slide interpretation. The disadvantages are the high cost, the length, and tediousness of the procedure, and the low availability of Moh's surgeons.

Superficial, Multicentric Basal Cell Carcinoma

A shiny, red macule on the face or trunk is often spotted because of its light reflex. This tumor can be either smooth and shiny or slightly scaly. If blue or black pigment is present on the periphery, the diagnosis is easier to confirm. This variant of BCC can be very small in diameter or cover large areas of skin totaling several centimeters. A slow-growing tumor, the superficial BCC expands radially. It may have serpiginous or geographic patterns in its larger sizes.

Differential diagnoses include actinic keratoses, Bowen's disease, or superficial spreading melanoma. The presence of pigment should narrow the differential to a pigmented BCC or a melanoma. If melanoma is a concern, a full-thickness excision or a punch biopsy of larger lesions is indicated. If the diagnosis is not in doubt, treatment should be simple and inexpensive. This is a superficial tumor that is confined to the epidermis. These lesions can be completely treated by tangential excisions, electrodesiccation, and curettage. To minimize recurrences, these tumors need to be treated beyond the clinically apparent margin.

Sclerosing or Morpheaform Basal Cell Carcinoma

This variant of BCC is difficult to diagnose and difficult to treat. It is often overlooked because of its innocuous appearance. The lesion presents as a slowly expanding, flesh colored or white plaque that is completely asymptomatic. It will usually occur on sun-exposed surfaces. It is often confused with morphea. Any change in the integrity or the substance of the skin or the presence of scarlike tissue without a reason for a white scar should be suspect.

A punch or incisional biopsy is necessary to confirm the diagnosis. Histologically, the tumor has no connection to the epidermis. This is a dermal process in which strands of basaloid tumor cells are intertwined with thickened collagen bundles. Extension of the tumor is centrifugal with aggressive invasion of hair follicles and nerves.

Treatment should be aggressive. Surgical excision with wide and deep margins is often necessary because the boundaries of this tumor type cannot be visualized. Referral to a Moh's surgeon is often warranted in this situation so that the tumor may be removed with the aid of intraoperative frozen sections. This becomes especially important in areas where tissue conservation is critical.

Treatment

Many different therapeutic strategies have been used to treat the different types of BCC. No one therapy is suited to all. Treatment should be individualized and chosen based on a thorough knowledge of the treatment modality, its complications, recurrence rates, and cosmetic results. The most commonly used treatments for BCC are curettage–electrodesiccation, primary excision, Moh's microscopic surgery, and irradiation.

The curettage–electrodesiccation method is an excellent choice for BCC less than 6 mm in diameter on any site. Lesions greater than 6 mm found on low-risk areas such as the neck, trunk, and extremities can also be treated with high cure rates. In experienced hands, 5-year recurrence rates will range from 3.3% in the low-risk sites regardless of size to 4.5% for small lesions treated in the high-risk areas of the central face.

Surgical excision offers good to excellent cosmetic results with similar high cure rates to the curettage method in the same group of smaller tumors. Lesions of intermediate size, 6 to 9 mm, found on the head and neck can be effectively treated with a 95% cure rate.

Radiation therapy is effective for small and intermediate primary tumors on the head and neck as well as for recurrent BCCs. Overall, the cosmetic result is not as good as surgical treatment. Therefore, this modality is often used for the older patient who cannot tolerate a surgical procedure.

Moh's microscopic surgery or wide local excisions should be used for large, invasive BCC. Moh's microscopic surgery is especially useful in the sclerosing or morpheaform variants of BCC where the tumor margins are clinically indistinct. Recurrent tumors in high-risk areas of the nose, ocular, or aural areas and those that demonstrate perineural invasion are best handled by an expert trained in this specialty.

Finally, patient follow-up is important. The greatest risk for recurrences of treated BCCs is within 5 years. During that interval, these patients are also at increased risk for development of new BCCs.

Squamous Cell Carcinoma

Squamous cell carcinoma (SCC) is the second most common skin cancer. Unlike BCC, this carcinoma has a clear propensity for metastases. A lesion that arises from actinically damaged skin has an estimated risk of 3% to 5% for metastases, whereas mucocutaneous lesions carry a risk of 11%. When the SCC arises from an old burn, ulcer, or site of chronic injury, the risk increases dramatically to 10% to 40%. It is this biologic behavior that makes early treatment so important.

Presentation

The classic presentation of invasive SCC is that of a man in the seventh decade of life who presents with a tender, red papule or an asymptomatic, keratinous growth in a sun-exposed area, especially the head and neck (Plates 8 and 9). A nonhealing ulceration or an enlarging crusted lesion should also trigger a response to biopsy (Plate 10). Large SCCs (Plate 11) should be evaluated for local lymph node involvement. The differential diagnosis of SCC is broad because there is no single presentation. The eczema that does not respond to therapy, the ulcer that does not heal, and the wart that arises on a sun-exposed site of an adult should all be suspect.

Pathogenesis

Photodamage from solar radiation is generally accepted as the major contributor to the etiology of SCC. The incidence of SCC increases with increased sun exposure. Other forms of radiation including ionizing and x-rays have been reported to cause these lesions as well. Psoralen and UVA, a phototherapy treatment used in psoriasis, has been associated with an increased risk of developing SCC. Chemical factors such as coal tar derivatives and arsenic have also been implicated in inducing a small number of these lesions. All of the agents described can have an additive effect or work as cofactors in the genesis of SCC, but solar radiation clearly has the dominant role. Immunosuppressed renal and heart transplant patients as well as patients with lymphoproliferative diseases are at increased risk for SCC in actinically damaged areas.

Treatment

Treatment should be tailored to the individual patient based on tumor size, location, etiology, and degree of histologic differentiation.

Small, primary SCC of actinically damaged skin can be managed with a number of different surgical modalities. Electrodesiccation and curettage, radiation, cryosurgery, and conservative excision have all been used with good results. Moh's microscopic surgery can be especially useful for recurrent tumors. Cure rates correlate best with the degree of tumor differentiation and the size of the lesion. Adequate surgical excisions should be obtained to demonstrate clear pathologic margins.

Mucocutaneous tumors and larger SCCs should be treated more aggressively with either large margins or with Moh's microscopic surgery. Patients with poorly, differentiated tumors or tumors extending into the deep dermis or subcutaneous tissue should be monitored for metastases. Lymph node removal is indicated only if the nodes are clinically enlarged.

Bowen's Disease

Bowen's disease is a clinically recognizable, SCC in situ. It may occur in sun-exposed or sun-protected areas of the body. Asymptomatic, it can expand radially up to several centimeters before it is diagnosed (Plate 12). It is a red, scaly, solitary patch that is often confused with psoriasis or eczema. Multiple lesions of Bowen's disease in sun-protected areas in conjunction with palmar and plantar keratoses may signify chronic arsenic ingestion. When Bowen's disease affects the glans penis, scrotum, or vulva, it appears as a red, velvety, plaque and is often asymptomatic. This clinical variant is called erythroplasia of Queyrat. The differential diagnosis for this lesion includes a candida balanitis, psoriasis, lichen planus, and fixed drug eruption.

Treatment

Treatment of this condition starts with the recognition that you are dealing with a neoplastic rather than an inflammatory condition. After a biopsy to confirm the diagnosis, treatment remains primarily surgical. Electrodessication and curettage will eliminate this superficial process with a minimum of tissue destruction.

Bowenoid Papulosis

This is a banal-appearing skin lesion of the external genitalia of men and women that histologically is a SCC in situ. The typical patient is a young adult in the third or fourth decade of life who presents with multiple lesions ranging in size from 2 mm to confluent plaques over 1 cm. Men and women are equally affected. These lesions have been described not only on the penile shaft and vulva but also on the perineum, perianal area, scrotum, and inner thigh.

The differential diagnosis includes condyloma acuminata, seborrheic keratoses, verrucae, or epidermal nevi.

The pathogenesis of these lesions is felt to be viral in origin with human papillomavirus 16 being the most common DNA retrieved using DNA hybridization techniques.

Treatment of these in situ carcinomas should be conservative but complete. Electrodesiccation and curettage, cryosurgery, and Moh's microscopic surgery have all been used. Radical procedures such as vulvectomy or penectomy are not indicated for these lesions. Some investigators recommend cytologic screening on female patients with bowenoid papulosis and close follow-up.

Keratoacanthoma

A keratoacanthoma is a common, dramatic squamous neoplasm of the skin that arises quickly and painfully causing great consternation (Plate 13). This type of neoplasm has been described as benign with the potential for malignant transformation. However, the locally destructive nature of this tumor and reports of metastases should weigh the scales in favor of early intervention.

This tumor will present on the sun-exposed areas, especially the head, neck, and dorsum of the hand in fair-skinned individuals. Men are affected twice as frequently as women. A painful pink papule that doubles in size over several weeks, it evolves into a "volcano"-shaped pink nodule with a central, keratinous plug (see Plate 13). The lesion may remain stationary with gradual involution over several months or it may continue to expand at an alarming rate causing extensive local destruction. Initially, the lesion may be confused with a hypertrophic actinic keratosis, a verruca, or a warty dyskeratoma. In the more mature lesion, BCC and SCC are in the differential.

Although there is controversy over the classification of keratoacanthoma as a benign or malignant tumor, there is no disagreement over treatment. Early, complete removal should be affected to minimize local tissue involvement by the tumor and thereby obtain a better cosmetic result.

Radiation therapy has been used successfully in doses of 600 to 1000 rads. This modality should be used for the patient who is unable to undergo surgery or for lesions that are too large to resect in a cosmetically important location.

Chemotherapy is primarily used for treatment of aggressive keratoacanthomas or multiple keratoacanthomas. Intralesional 5-fluorouracil or bleomycin have been used for giant or aggressive keratoacanthomas or in difficult surgical areas such as the nose, ear, lip, or nail bed. The physician should be familiar with all of the consequences of these chemotherapeutic agents before embarking on treatment.

Cutaneous Malignant Melanoma

Cutaneous malignant melanoma is a lethal disease of the young and middle-aged adult. Its incidence has increased exponentially over the last two decades. Genetic factors and environmental factors play a role in the development of melanoma. Sunlight, especially UVB, remains the single most important environmental factor in the etiology of melanoma. Intermittent solar exposure, rather than simple cumulative exposure, has been found to have a more significant impact on the development of melanoma. A case controlled study by Lew and colleagues has linked blistering sunburns in childhood and adolescence to increased rates of melanoma later in life (2). Early detection and prevention through physician and patient education remain our most effective tools to combat the disturbing mortality rates of malignant melanoma.

Presentation

The "ABCDs" of diagnosis (Plate 14) remain the cornerstone for evaluating the patient with pigmented lesions:

A for Asymmetry
B for Border irregularity or notching
C for Color variegation
D for Diameter greater than 6 mm

The average adult will typically have 10 to 40 nevi scattered over the body. Any change in size, shape, or color should alert the physician.

The profile of the "high-risk" patient is a blond or red-haired person who demonstrates significant freckling and gives a history of three or more blistering sunburns during childhood. A positive family history of malignant melanoma is a strong single risk factor. Parents and offspring of melanoma patients are at a 12-fold increase of risk for the disease (3).

Precursor Lesions

Most melanomas arise de novo but approximately 20% are associated with a preexisting nevus. Pigmented lesions that have a known increased association with melanoma are congenital nevi and dysplastic nevi as described in the dysplastic nevus syndrome.

The incidence of congenital nevi in the newborn has been estimated at 1%. Most of these lesions are small or medium sized. The propensity for these smaller congenital nevi to develop melanoma is controversial. The giant congenital nevus (≥20 cm), however, has a clearer risk for developing melanoma. The lifetime risk for developing melanoma in these patients has been placed at 6%. Unfortunately, these nevi are also much more difficult to remove because of the larger surface area involved.

The dysplastic nevus syndrome patient is one who demonstrates the following three features: 1) more than 100 moles, 2) at least one mole 8 mm or larger, and 3) at least one mole with "atypical" features. It is this patient who is at an increased lifelong risk for developing melanoma (4). A single dysplastic nevus, not found in the setting of the dysplastic nevus, should be evaluated on its own merit and should not be included in this high-risk category.

In summary, any patient over age 40 who presents with a growing, pigmented lesion or a "new" mole merits further evaluation either through biopsy or complete excision.

Classification

Cutaneous malignant melanoma has been divided into four major categories of clinical presentation that have different characteristics.

Superficial spreading melanoma is the most frequently recognized and diagnosed variant. Inherent in its title is the fact that it is a "superficial" melanoma. It remains in situ or confined to the epidermis while advancing radially. Development into an invasive malignant melanoma is usually noted clinically by the appearance of papules, nodules, or induration. Sun-exposed sites, such as the backs of men and legs of women, are its preferred location.

Nodular melanoma is a tumor that has entered a vertical growth phase and so, presents with a papular or nodular component. This is the second most common form of melanoma, but it carries a more grave prognosis. Some authors would argue that this represents a more end-stage disease state.

Acral-lentiginous melanoma is a flat, irregular macule of the palms, soles, or nail beds. It is typically found in blacks, Hispanics and Orientals and is biologically aggressive. Discoloration of the proximal nail fold in association with a linear streak of the nail (Hutchinson's sign) is highly suggestive of subungual melanoma (Plate 15).

Lentigo maligna (Plate 16) is an in situ malignant

melanoma on sun-damaged skin. Described as "Hutchinson's melanotic freckle" around the turn of the century, this lesion is a slow-growing melanoma that is typically seen on the face of the elderly with the peak occurring in the seventh decade of life. It starts as an uneven lentigo that evolves slowly over years often reaching sizes of up to 10 cm.

Differential Diagnoses

Melanomas must be differentiated from other colored lesions such as pigmented BCCs, seborrheic keratoses, and hemangiomas. Amelanotic melanomas are often misdiagnosed because of the lack of color. These lesions are often pink to flesh colored and have no special site of predilection. All pigmented lesions deserve close inspection and a biopsy if there are the warning signs of melanoma. Biopsies before definitive surgical extirpation are warranted in large lesions so that unnecessary procedures can be avoided.

Pathogenesis

The biologic behavior of malignant melanoma is poorly understood. Melanocytes originally arise from neural crest tissue during fetal development and migrate to the skin and other visceral locations. The malignant transformation appears to begin within the epidermis. As long as the neoplasia is confined above the basement membrane, the malignancy is curable. Once that physiologic barrier is breached, metastasis can result.

Work-up

The ABCDs of diagnosis should be a guide in the decision for biopsy. If the diagnosis is suspect, the most appropriate biopsy is a conservative, full-thickness excision. If the lesion is too large and the diagnosis is in doubt, a photograph of the intact lesion should precede a punch or incisional biopsy. The biopsy should be obtained through the thickest or darkest portion of the lesion. If clinical suspicion is high for melanoma, a shave or needle biopsy is contraindicated because the ability to stage the tumor may be lost.

Once the diagnosis of melanoma is established, a comprehensive, physical examination, including a complete skin examination, should follow. Particular attention should be directed to other pigmented lesions, regional lymphatics, and a review of high-risk organ systems, that is, the respiratory, gastrointestinal, central nervous, musculoskeletal, and genitourinary systems. A complete blood count, chemistry screen, urinalysis, and chest x-ray may be obtained. Symptoms of weight loss, malaise, bone pain, and headaches should prompt further investigation for metastasis.

Staging: Measurement of the vertical thickness of the melanoma microscopically from the top of the stratum granulosum to the deepest penetration in the dermis has become a standard approach in prognosticating survival. The New York University Melanoma Cooperative Group evaluated 1130 consecutive patients with malignant melanoma and divided them into lesion thicknesses of: zero to 0.75 mm, 0.76 to 1.69 mm, 1.70 to 3.59 mm, and 3.60 mm and larger. The respective 5-year survival rates for those thicknesses were 99%, 94%, 81%, and 49%, respectively. Similarly, the 10-year survival rates were 98%, 89%, 67%, and 43%, respectively (5). The single prognostic factor that correlated most directly with prognosis was tumor thickness. Other factors that have been noted to influence survival are the site of the melanoma, patient gender, evidence of tumor regression, and mitotic rate.

Site: In general, patients with lesions on the head and neck, trunk, hands, and feet have a poorer prognosis. Lesions on the forearms and legs have a better than average prognosis.

Gender: Male and female patients initially have no difference in survival the first 2 years after diagnosis. However, several studies note a more favorable survival for women at 10 years. The reason for this difference remains unexplained.

Regression: Regression, or an immunologic host response directed against melanoma cells, is generally felt to be a favorable feature. However, tumors with regression of 70% to 80% or more with a lesion width greater than 10 mm were at an increased risk of metastases. After diagnosing a thin melanoma, the presence and extent of regression should be made to determine an accurate prognosis.

Mitosis: The number of mitoses noted on histologic examination correlates inversely with prognosis. By multiplying the lesion thickness by the number of mitoses per square millimeter, a mitotic index is obtained. Kopf and colleagues found that for lesions with a mitotic index greater than 18, a 23% survival rate was noted as compared with a survival rate of 85% for those with an index less than 18 (6).

Conclusion: Although multiple factors are used to assess a patient's survival, only lesion thickness remains a constant element of analyses. Proper staging ultimately relies on a full-thickness biopsy specimen where the entire lesion can be visualized histologically.

Treatment: The definitive treatment for melanoma is surgical. A wide, deep excision is performed. Surgical margin size remains controversial but the trend is toward narrower margins with a range of 1 to 3 cm. Elective regional lymph node dissection remains controversial but is being studied in the intermediate thickness stage 1 melanomas.

Regular postoperative follow-up is important because of the risk of metastases and the increased lifelong risk of a second primary cutaneous melanoma. Specific treatment modalities of advanced disease is beyond the scope of this chapter, but new strategies of radiation therapy, chemotherapy, and immunotherapy are being investigated.

REFERENCES

1. Thompson SC, Jolley D, Marks R. Reduction of solar keratoses by regular sunscreen use. N Engl J Med 1993;329:1147–1151.
2. Lew RA, Sober AJ, Cook, N, et al. Sunexposure habits in patients with cutaneous melanoma: a case control study. J Dermatol Surg Oncol 1983;9:981–986.
3. Duggleby W, Stoll H, Priore R, et al. A genetic analysis of melanoma—polygenic inheritance as a threshold trait. Am J Epidemiol 1981;114:63–72.
4. Tiersten A, Grin C, Kopf A, et al. Prospective follow-up for malignant melanoma in patients with atypical-mole (dysplastic-nevus) syndrome. J Dermatol Surg Oncol 1991;17:44–48.
5. Friedman RJ, Rigel DS, Kopf AW, et al. Cancer of the skin. Philadelphia: WB Saunders, 1991.
6. Kopf AW, Gross DF, Rogers GS, et al. Prognostic index for malignant melanoma. Cancer 1987;59:1236–1241.

SUGGESTED READINGS

Clark D. Cutaneous micrographic surgery. Otolaryngol Clin North Am 1993;26:185–202.

Clark W, Mihm M. Lentigo maligna and lentigo-maligna melanoma. Am J Pathol 1969;55:39–67.

Dobak J, Liu F. Sunscreens, UVA, and cutaneous malignancy: Adding fuel to the fire. Int J Dermatol 1992;31:544–548.

Haydon R. Cutaneous squamous carcinoma and related lesions. Otolaryngol Clin North Am 1993;26:57–71.

Hoffman SJ, Yohn JJ, Norris DA, et al. Cutaneous malignant melanoma. Curr Prob Dermatol January/February 1993;V:7–41.

Jacobs G, Rippey J, Altini M. Prediction of aggressive behavior in basal cell carcinoma. Cancer 1982;49:533–537.

Koh H. Cutaneous melanoma. N Engl J Med 1991;325:171–182.

Lewis G, Tyring S, Wagner R. Possible role of adjuvant therapy for thin malignant melanoma. Cutis 1992;50:377–379.

Rhodes AR, Silverman RA, Harrist TJ, Melski JW. A histologic comparison of congenital and acquired nevomelanocytic nevi. Arch Dermatol 1985;121:1266–1273.

Ronan S, Eng A, Briele H, et al. Thin malignant melanomas with regression and metastases. Arch Dermatol 1987;123:1326–1330.

Roy M, Wagner R. Prevention of primary cutaneous malignant melanoma: increasing cure rate in the 1990's Cutis 1992;50:365–351.

Schwartz R. Keratoacanthoma. J Am Acad Dermatol 1994;30:1–19.

Silverman M, Kopf A, Grin C, et al. Recurrence rates of treated basal cell carcinomas, part 1: overview. J Dermatol Surg Oncol 1991;17:713–718.

Silverman M, Kopf A, Grin C, et al. Recurrence rates of treated basal cell carcinomas, part 2: curettage-electrodesiccation. J Dermatol Surg Oncol 1991;17:720–726.

Silverman M, Kopf A, Grin C, et al. Recurrence rates of treated basal cell carcinomas, part 3: surgical excison. J Dermatol Surg Oncol 1992;18:471–476.

Silverman M, Kopf A, Grin C, Bart R, Levenstein M. Recurrence rates of treated basal cell carcinomas, part 4: x-ray therapy. J Dermatol Surg Oncol 1992;18:549–554.

Studniberg H, Weller P. PUVA, UVB, psoriasis, and nonmelanoma skin cancer. J Am Acad Dermatol 1993;29:1013–1022.

Taylor CR, Stern RS, Leydon JJ, Gilchrist BA. Photoaging/photodamage and photoprotection. J Am Acad Dermatol 1990;22:175.

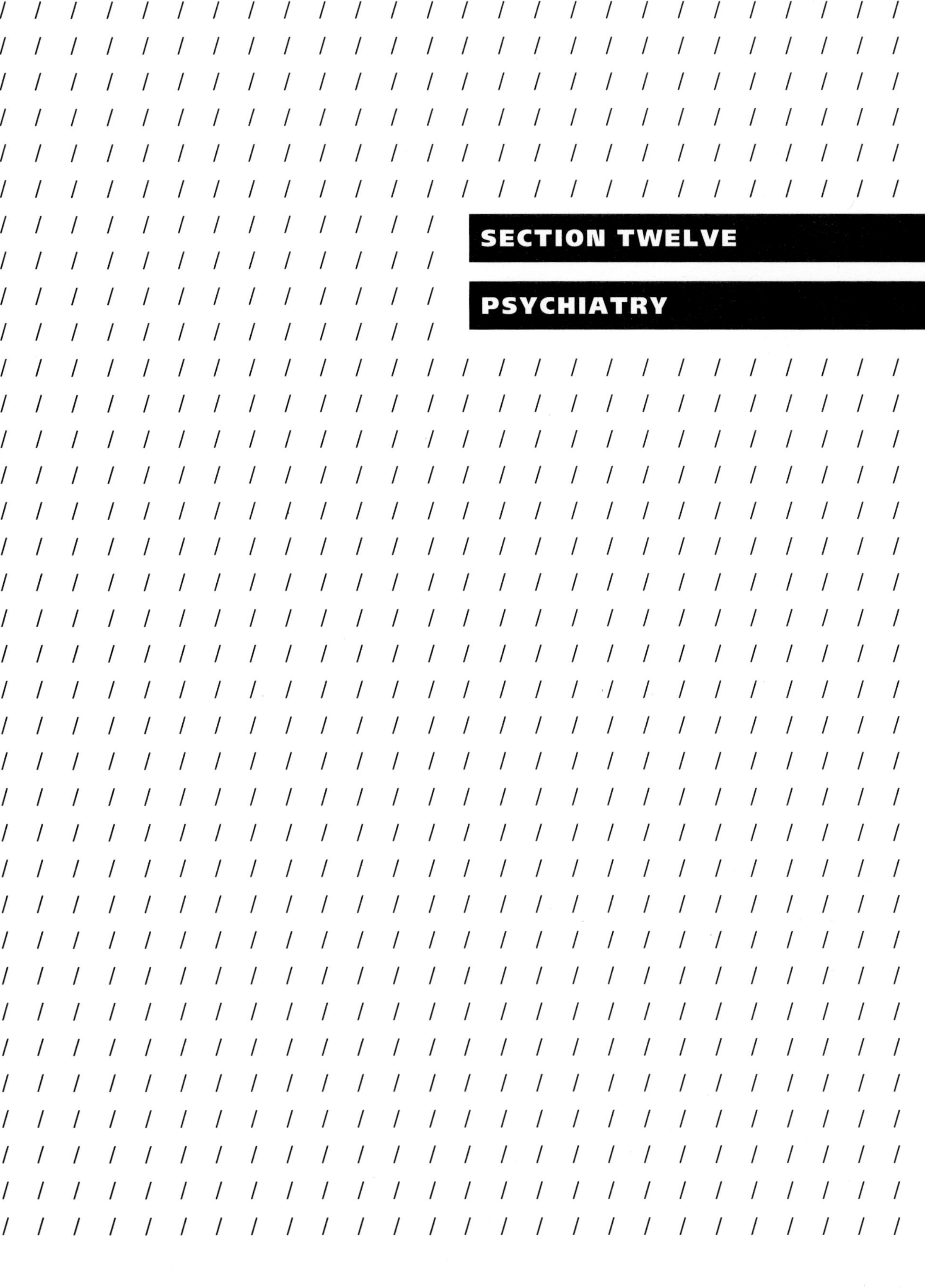

SECTION TWELVE

PSYCHIATRY

CHAPTER 35

PREMENSTRUAL SYNDROME

Shambhavi Chandraiah

The association of physical and psychological symptoms with the menstrual cycle has been recorded since Hippocrates time. However, in 1931, Frank (1), a gynecologist, labeled premenstrual symptoms as premenstrual tension. Over the years, this condition has received varying names reflective often of the current understanding of the symptom constellation, association with menses, or presumed etiology. These names have included premenstrual syndrome (PMS), premenstrual tension syndrome, perimenstrual syndrome, menstrually related mood disorders, late luteal phase dysphoric disorder, and premenstrual dysphoric disorder. The latter ones emphasize the affective symptoms.

The primary research in this area has been broadly in the gynecologic/psychological fields with some differing emphasis on symptom importance and presentation. As a result of the varying definitions used, early research is particularly hard to compare. Despite advances in understanding this condition, the exact etiology is still unclear. It has been demonstrated that premenstrual symptoms are not necessarily caused by the hormonal milieu of the late luteal phase (2). That the reproductive neuroendocrine axis is involved is recognized by the abolition or decrease of symptoms with suppression/cessation of ovulation. The efficacy of psychotropics in diminishing some of the psychiatric symptoms suggests neurotransmitter involvement. In addition, psychological or environmental factors, such as past or current stress or genetic vulnerability, may also play a role in the presentation of symptoms in some but not all individuals. Kindling (repeated low level stimuli evoking a response) or entrainment of other medical/psychiatric conditions to the menstrual cycle manifesting in PMS symptoms has also been proposed (3).

In this chapter on PMS the emphasis is on the common presentation and clinical treatment with an overview of the various major proposed etiologic theories that provide a rationale for some of the proposed treatments.

Clinical Features

Premenstrual syndrome consists of a cyclic occurrence of physical and psychological symptoms that present in the luteal phase starting at ovulation or later and diminishes over the course of menses with then a symptom-free, postmenses “week” (in the follicular phase). The most common physical symptoms of PMS are bloating of the abdomen, hands, or feet; breast tenderness/swelling; increased appetite with cravings for salt or sugar; headaches and backaches; fatigue; and sleep changes. Common psychiatric symptoms are mood swings (within hours or minutes), irritability or anger, anxiety, depression, and feeling overwhelmed or out of control (Box 35.1). Also about 10% to 15% of women, actually have positive premenstrual symptoms (e.g., euphoria, increased energy, etc.) (4). Some women may experience a transient euphoria in the postmenses week—it is unclear whether this is secondary to relief from distressing premenstrual symptoms or due to biologically mediated changes. Some women have symptoms for 1 to 2 days around ovulation with resolution and subsequent recurrence of premenstrual symptoms closer to menses. Some premenstrual symptoms may occur to a mild degree in the majority (80%) of women (defined as molimina) at some time during their reproductive years. However, PMS is considered to represent the small percentage of women, approximately 5% to 10%, whose symptoms create significant impairment or interference with

Box 35.1 PMS Symptoms

Common Somatic Symptoms

Bloating (hands, feet, abdomen)
Breast tenderness/swelling
Cravings for salt/sugar
Increased appetite
Headache
Backache
Fatigue
Sleep ↑ or ↓

Common Psychobehavioral Symptoms

Mood swings
Irritability
Anger
Depression
Anxiety
Overwhelmed/out of control feelings
Crying spells
Decreased interest
Lowered work/school performance or efficiency
Social avoidance

Other Symptoms

Clumsiness
Decreased concentration
Generalized aches/pains
Libido ↑ or ↓
Transient suicidal ideation
Physical aggressiveness
Decreased self-esteem

work, home, or social activities. A recently adopted definition within the psychiatric literature with emphasis on the mood symptoms of PMS is shown in Table 35.1 (5).

Epidemiologic studies show that although 20% of women may seek evaluation or treatment for PMS symptoms, only about 2% regularly miss work due to their symptoms (6). PMS is most common in the third and fourth decades of a woman's life but can occur at any time from puberty to menopause. Some triggers that may precipitate symptoms are pregnancy, tubal ligation, oral contraceptive use, or stress. Symptom severity may vary from cycle to cycle and symptoms may remit spontaneously for months or years. Of interest, premenstrual symptoms have been noted cross-species in zoo-contained chimps and gorillas as well as cross-culturally—with the chief complaint differing between cultures, for example, more headaches in Nigerians and more psychiatric symptoms in Americans (7). PMS can occur more frequently within female members of a family with studies showing greater monozygotic than dizygotic concordance (8) and symptom correlation in mother–daughter diads (9).

Evaluation

A medical, gynecologic, and psychiatric history and examination are relevant to rule out or identify alternate or concurrent conditions to PMS (Box 35.2). Although no specific laboratory tests are indicated to diagnose PMS, common tests like hemoglobin, thyroid-stimulating hormone, and fasting blood sugar levels may allow detection of possible other etiologies of patient's symptoms. Hormonal assays can be used primarily to detect if ovulation has occurred in any given cycle because the presence or severity of PMS symptoms appear linked to the occurrence of ovulation. Elevated, decreased, or unchanged levels of ovarian hormones/steroids have been reported in earlier studies, as have changes in various other hormones, steroids, or neurotransmitters. However, a well designed study comparing women with confirmed PMS to normal controls showed no differences in levels of leutenizing hormone (LH), follicle-stimulating hormone, prolactin, progesterone, estradiol, testosterone, estradiol-binding globulin, dihydrotestosterone sulfate, dihydrotestosterone, and cortisol during any menstrual phase (10). Nevertheless, it may be variation of hormonal levels over the cycle (not just in the premenstruum) that may have a regulatory/etiologic role in the causation of symptoms rather than basal hormonal levels. Specific biochemical markers have not been clearly identified for PMS although increased thyroid abnormalities (11), possible serotonergic deficiency (12), and others have been proposed.

Differential Diagnosis

Physical conditions that can mimic PMS include endometriosis, ovarian cysts or fibroids, breast cancer, thyroid abnormality, subclinical diabetes mellitus,

Table 35.1 Diagnostic Criteria for Late Luteal Phase Dysphoric Disorder*

A. In most menstrual cycles during the past year, symptoms in B occurred during the last week of the luteal phase and remitted within a few days after onset of the follicular phase. In menstruating females, these phases correspond to the week before, and a few days after, the onset of menses. (In nonmenstruating females who have had a hysterectomy, the timing of luteal and follicular phases may require measurement of circulating reproductive hormones.)

B. At least five of the following symptoms have been present for most of the time during each symptomatic late luteal phase, at least one of the symptoms being either (1), (2), (3), or (4):
1. marked affective lability, e.g., feeling suddenly sad, tearful, irritable, or angry
2. persistent and marked anger or irritability
3. marked anxiety, tension, feelings of being "keyed up" or "on edge"
4. markedly depressed mood, feelings of hopelessness, or self-deprecating thoughts
5. decreased interest in usual activities, e.g., work, friends, hobbies
6. easy fatigability or marked lack of energy
7. subjective sense of difficulty in concentrating
8. marked change in appetite, overeating, or specific food cravings
9. hypersomnia or insomnia
10. other physical symptoms, such as breast tenderness or swelling, headaches, joint or muscle pain, a sensation of "bloating," weight gain

C. The disturbance seriously interferes with work or with usual social activities or relationships with others.

D. The disturbance is not merely an exacerbation of the symptoms of another disorder, such as Major Depression, Panic Disorder, Dysthymia, or a Personality Disorder (although it may be superimposed on any of these disorders).

E. Criteria A, B, C, and D are confirmed by prospective daily self-ratings during at least two symptomatic cycles. (The diagnosis may be made provisionally prior to this confirmation.)

*DSM, 4th edition, Proposed criteria changes the name to premenstrual dysphoric disorder.
Reproduced by permission from American Psychiatric Association. Diagnostic and statistical manual of mental disorders. 3rd ed., revised. Washington, DC: American Psychiatric Association, 1987.

Box 35.2 General Principles of Evaluation and Treatment of PMS

1. Initial visit—medical/psychiatric history and physical/gynecologic examination ± relevant laboratory tests to rule out other medical problems, e.g., hemoglobin and thyroid-stimulating hormone; stress management and education; prescribe PMS diet, exercise, and daily PMS logs for two cycles.
2. Second visit—review PMS daily logs; if significant confirmed PMS, consider treatment options based on major symptoms
3. Third visit—review treatment efficacy; modify treatment if needed and continue treatment at least 6 mo

anemia, or abnormalities in the hypothalamic-pituitary-adrenal axis. Psychiatric disorders that must be included in the differential diagnosis are anxiety, depression, personality disorder, and substance abuse. More importantly, most medical and psychiatric illnesses may exacerbate premenstrually, notably migraines, epilepsy, asthma, acne, panic attacks, and depression.

Diagnosis

Reporting of PMS symptoms may be biased by retrospective recall, that is, patients may more easily recall symptoms as occurring related to the monthly menses than as occurring at other times of the cycle or unrelated to the cycle. Alternatively, these ratings may reflect a patient's preconceptions of the premenstruum as being always a negative experience (13). Only about 50% of women who complain of premenstrual symptoms have confirmation of the association of their symptoms to the premenstruum when prospective daily PMS logs are used (14,15). Thus current standard practice is to use daily logs of PMS symptoms over at least two prospective, symptomatic cycles to confirm the diagnosis although a provisional diagnosis can be made based on history. A variety of such logs exist in the literature and in clinical practice and include the Visual Analog Scale, a 100-mm line rating a few common PMS symptoms (15); the Daily Rating Form, a 21-item 6-point rating scale (16); the Calendar of Premenstrual Experiences (17); and the Prospective Record of the Impact and Severity of Premenstrual Symptoms (18). I have developed a one-sheet 36-item daily symptom severity log (DSSL) that allows prospective assessment of the severity and impact on lifestyle of specific common PMS symptoms, as well as life stresses or medication usage during the cycle (Fig 35.1). National Institute of Mental Health 1983 conference criteria require at least a 30% PMS symptom change from pre- to postmenses to diagnose PMS, but clinically if the premenstrual pattern is confirmed and the impact on occupational or social functioning is at least moderate, a diagnosis of PMS can be made. In addition, various retrospective questionnaires or scales exist with cut-off scores that can be used to make a provisional diagnosis of PMS. The premenstrual tension syndrome rating scales have patient-rated (Fig 35.2) (19), and observer-rated versions for subjective and objective assessment of symptoms in the luteal and follicular phases of the cycle. The Premenstrual Assessment Form (20) is a thorough but lengthy 95-item initial questionnaire of PMS symptoms. The original Moos Menstrual Distress Questionnaire (21) rates 47 PMS symptoms. The simplicity of any assessment form ensures more accurate compliance.

Women without confirmation of typical PMS often have other psychiatric conditions aggravated in the premenstruum or unrelated to the cycle (Fig 35.3). Some may have other medical conditions as the etiology of their symptoms. In other women, symptoms may be of insufficient severity to meet the narrow criteria for PMS especially with respect to serious lifestyle interference. A high prevalence (20% to 80%) of lifetime psychiatric illness in women with complaints of premenstrual symptoms has been recurrently reported, in particular, major mood disorders (40% to 80% lifetime history) (22). This may suggest an increased risk for development of PMS in women with affective disorders and visa versa. Endicott's group found a 60% prevalence of premenstrual depression in women with a history of affective disorder (16) and an 80% lifetime history of premenstrual depression (14). Other associated risks linked to the reproductive cycle may be postpartum depression, hormonally induced mood changes, and menopausal depression.

Common Proposed Etiologies and Treatments of PMS

Theories of the etiology of PMS (Box 35.3) have at times developed through retrospective hypothesizing based on efficacy of certain treatments and their known biochemical effect in vitro or in vivo. Although numerous etiologies (often explaining only some of the symptoms of PMS) or treatments of PMS have been proposed, only the common old and new theories that have been noted in the literature are reviewed here.

Pyridoxine Deficiency

A pyridoxine (vitamin B_6) deficiency hypothesis has been proposed based on this vitamin's role as a cofactor in the conversion of tryptophan to neurotransmitters such as serotonin, dopamine, and noradrenaline, which modulate mood states including depression, aggression, anxiety, among others. As well, dopamine has an antagonistic action on prolactin, which could potentially cause breast symptoms. However, no specific deficiency of B_6 has been identified in PMS women (23). Double-blind studies of pyridoxine's efficacy in doses of usually 50–200 mg/day in the luteal phase or throughout the cycle have largely been negative (24), with any apparent benefit likely secondary to placebo response or a nonspecific benefit throughout the cycle. Also there have been reports of peripheral neuropathy with long-term, higher doses (usually $\geqslant$100 mg/day) (25). Thus, a role for pyridoxine in the treatment of premenstrual symptoms is hard to support currently. However, pyridoxine at 50–100 mg/day, has been shown to improve depression in oral contraceptive users, where estrogen's role in decreasing pyridoxine may have a role in inducing the depression (26).

PREMENSTRUAL SYNDROME DAILY SYMPTOM SEVERITY LOG (PMS DSSL)

Name: ______________________

ID #: ______________________

Grading of Symptoms
0-none 1-minimum 2-mild 3-moderate 4-severe 5-extreme

Cycle Day	1 *	2	3	4	5	6	7	8	9	10	11	12	13	14	15	16	17	18	19	20	21	22	23	24	25	26	27	28	29	30
Date																														
Weight																														
BBT																														
Anger/ Irritablity																														
Anxiety/ "On Edge"																														
Depression/ Hopelessness																														
Overwhelmed/ Out of Control																														
Mood Swings																														
Decreased Interest																														
Sleep Changes																														
Fatigue/ Decreased Energy																														
Concentration Difficulty																														
Appetite Changes/ Food Cravings																														
Breast Pain/ Swelling																														
Bloating																														
Headache/Joint or Muscle Pain																														
Work/School/ Home/Activity Interference																														
Social Activities Interference																														
Relationship Interference																														
Other Symptoms																														
Comments																														

* First Day of Period Note M for Menses   BBT = Basal Body Temperature   Developed on DSM criteria, S. Chandraiah, M.D.

Fig 35.1 Daily rating log of the severity of premenstrual symptoms.

SELF-RATING SCALE FOR PREMENSTRUAL TENSION SYNDROME

Name: Date: Cycle Day:

Instructions: The following questions are concerned with the way you feel or act today (i.e. typical premenstrual "bad" day or typical premenstrual "good" day)

Please answer all questions by circling YES or NO as indicated.

1. Do you find yourself avoiding some of your social commitments? YES NO
2. Have you gained 5 or more pounds during the past week? YES NO
3. Is your coordination so poor that you are unable to use kitchen utensils, garden tools or unable to drive? YES NO
4. Do you feel more angry than usual? YES NO
5. Do you avoid family activities and prefer to be left alone? YES NO
6. Do you doubt your judgement or feel that you are prone to hasty decisions? YES NO
7. Do you feel more irritable than usual? YES NO
8. Is your efficiency diminished? YES NO
9. Do you feel tense and restless? YES NO
10. Do you feel a marked change in your sexual drive or desire during the last week? YES NO
    If YES, is it *increased* or *decreased*?
11. Are your present physical symptoms causing so much pain and discomfort that you are unable to function? YES NO
12. Have you recently cancelled previously scheduled social activities? YES NO
13. Do you feel as if you were unable to relax at all? YES NO
14. Do you feel confused? YES NO
15. Do you suffer from painful or tender breasts? YES NO
16. Do you have an increased desire for specific kinds of food (e.g. cravings for candy, chocolate, etc.)? YES NO
17. Do you scream/yell at family members (friends, colleagues) more than usual?
    Are you "short-fused"? YES NO
18. Do you feel sad, gloomy, and hopeless most of the time? YES NO
19. Do you feel like crying? YES NO
20. Do you have difficulty completing your daily household/job routine? YES NO
21. Was there a marked changed in your sexual drive with definite change in your sexual behavior during the last week? YES NO
22. Do you find yourself being more forgetful than usual or unable to concentrate? YES NO
23. Do you happen to have more "accidents" with your daily housework/job (cut fingers, break dishes, etc.)? YES NO
24. Have you noticed significant swelling of your breasts and/or ankles and/or bloating of your abdomen? YES NO
25. Does your mood change suddenly without obvious reason? YES NO
26. Are you easily distracted? YES NO
27. Do you think that your restless behavior is noticeable by others? YES NO
28. Are you clumsier than usual? YES NO
29. Are you obviously negative and hostile towards other people? YES NO
30. Are you so fatigued that it interferes with your usual level of functioning? YES NO
31. Do you tend to eat more than usual or at odd irregular hours (sweets, snacks, etc.)? YES NO
32. Do you become more easily fatigued than usual? YES NO
33. Is your handwriting different (less neat than usual)? YES NO
34. Do you feel jittery or upset? YES NO
35. Do you feel sad or blue? YES NO
36. Have you stopped calling or visiting some of your best friends? YES NO

Total Score

Fig 35.2 Self-rating scale for PMS. Score one for each "yes." Scores greater than 14 on a premenstrual day and less than 5 on a postmenstrual day suggest moderately severe PMS. (*Adapted by permission from Steiner M, Haskett RF, Carroll BJ. Acta Psychiatr Scand 1980;62:187–188. © 1980 Munksgaard International Publishers Ltd., Copenhagen, Denmark.*)

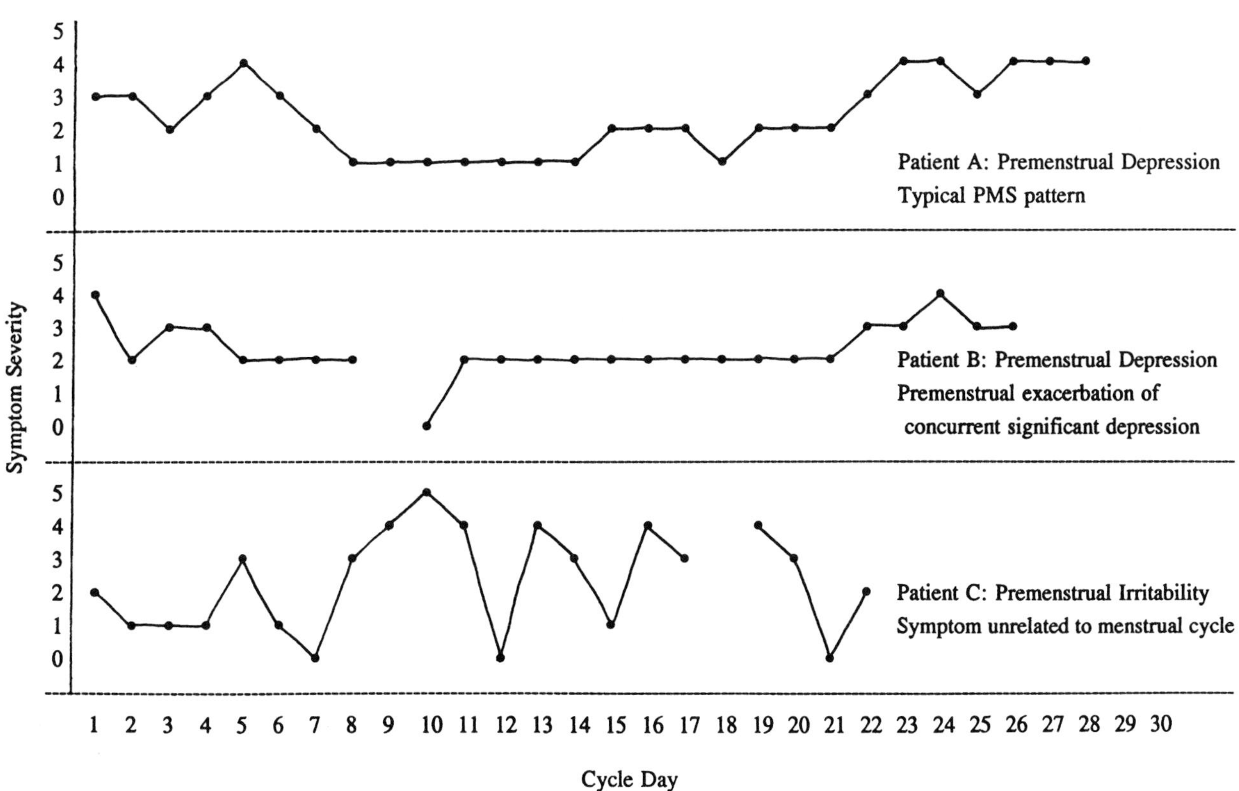

Fig 35.3 Graphic representation of *one* major premenstrual symptom in three different patients.

Box 35.3 Major Theories of Etiology of PMS

- Vitamin B_6 deficiency
- Prostaglandin deficiency
- Prostaglandin excess
- Prolactin excess
- Fluid retention
- Hypoglycemia
- Progesterone deficiency/estrogen excess
- Endogenous opiate withdrawal
- Serotonin deficiency
- Psychiatric

Prostaglandin Deficiency

This theory (27) proposes a deficiency of γ-linoleic acid, an essential fatty acid that is a precursor of prostaglandin E_1. Prostaglandin E_1 attenuates the effects of prolactin and may thus have a role in premenstrual symptoms, especially breast symptoms. Treatments to correct this deficiency include use of Evening Primrose Oil that contains 9% γ-linoleic acid using doses of about 4 gm/day, usually throughout the cycle. However double-blind studies have shown variable results with this agent, with efficacy more in European studies or particularly for the breast symptoms of PMS (24).

Prostaglandin Excess

This theory (28) proposes that an increase in prostaglandin levels premenstrually may result in a variety of symptoms including pain, edema, and thirst. Double-blind crossover, placebo-controlled studies of prostaglandin inhibitors, namely, mefenamic acid 500 mg three times a day or sodium naproxen 550 mg twice daily, used in the luteal phase have shown efficacy for largely pain symptoms (e.g., abdominal cramps, headaches, backaches, and other aches) (29). Some general decrease in depression and irritability has been reported, especially with mefenamic acid. However, it is possible that the improvement in mood is due to relief of the pain symptoms.

Prolactin Excess

This theory has been postulated partly based on prolactin's role in breast symptoms and potentially fluid retention. However, no differences with respect to prolactin levels in PMS patients versus normal patients has been found (10). Double-blind placebo-controlled studies using bromocriptine (a prolactin antagonist) at doses of 1.25–7.50 mg daily or twice daily doses in the luteal phase have shown efficacy for treatment of primarily breast pain (30).

Fluid Retention

Various agents have been considered to have a role in fluid retention including dietary excess, altered capillary permeability, and hormonal level changes (i.e., a primary or secondary role of aldosterone, estrogen, progesterone, prolactin, dopamine, or vasopressor). Aldosterone levels have not been found to be significantly different between normal and PMS women (31). Premenstrual increase in capillary filtration has been found, which may be the cause of localized fluid redistribution (32). Controlled studies of diuretic use in the luteal phase have shown variable results with generally efficacy in decreasing weight gain/bloating symptoms and possibly some benefit on psychological symptoms. The most commonly studied agent has been spironolactone at 100 mg/day premenstrually (24).

Hypoglycemia

Premenstrual symptoms of increased appetite, craving for sweets, fatigue, headache, shakes, and dizziness are similar to those seen in patients with hypoglycemia, resulting in this hypothesis. Conflicting reports regarding decreased glucose tolerance and insulin resistance in normal women in the luteal phase has been reported (33,34). "Hypoglycemia" symptoms associated with low normal blood glucose in PMS women versus normals has been reported, suggesting that PMS women may be more sensitive to the same glucose levels (35). A PMS diet low in refined sugar, high in complex carbohydrates and frequent, smaller meals is suggested to combat this relative hypoglycemia (Box 35.4).

Appetite Changes

Increased caloric (especially carbohydrate) intake and increased depression in PMS women versus normals during the late luteal phase has been reported (36). Decreased depression, fatigue, and tension was noted with consumption of a carbohydrate-rich, protein-poor (to increase tryptophan absorption and thus potentially brain serotonin) evening meal in the late luteal phase as compared to controls (36).

Box 35.4 Diet for PMS

1. Avoid refined sugars, e.g., sugar, cookies, ice cream, and regular soda.
   Increase complex carbohydrates, e.g., vegetables, whole grain breads and cereals.
   Eat five to six smaller meals/snacks.
   These changes may minimize highs and lows of blood sugar, which may affect mood swings.
2. Avoid caffeine because this may increase breast symptoms, anxiety, irritability, and insomnia.
3. Decrease salt intake to minimize fluid retention.
4. Decrease red meat in diet and keep total protein intake low (1/5 of total calories).

Exercise

Aerobic activity has been reported to help premenstrual symptoms possibly by release of endorphins (decreasing pain) and catecholamines (decreasing depression). Aerobic exercise may also improve circulatory capacity, which may decrease fluid retention. In a large survey of students decreased premenstrual symptoms of anxiety, depression, and headache was noted in women who exercised aerobically versus women who conducted resistance exercises only or controls (37). Another study found that increasing aerobic activity in previously sedentary women by running several times a week over 6 months led to decreased breast and fluid retention symptoms versus sedentary controls (38). Some women may have menstrual cycle changes, that is, shortened luteal phase or anovulation as a result of strenuous aerobic exercise.

Progesterone Deficiency/Estrogen Excess

An imbalance of estrogen and progesterone, with increased estrogen secondary to decreased renal excretion, was proposed by Frank in 1931 (1). A relative progesterone deficiency (in the luteal phase) theory continues to be promulgated by Katherina Dalton of Great Britain. A recent study by Schmidt and colleagues (2) showed that truncation of the luteal phase with thus an early onset of the follicular phase still resulted in occurrence of PMS symptoms, suggesting that events earlier in the cycle may be responsible for PMS symptoms or that an alternate etiology may be the cause. Further, no consistent changes between normal versus PMS women with respect to a variety of reproductively related hormones have been found (10). Double-blind, placebo-controlled studies of progesterone (29) administered generally as a 200–400-mg rectal or vaginal suppository in the luteal phase have not shown efficacy. Only one report using 300 mg/day oral micronized progesterone showed improvement in a few PMS symptoms but has not been replicated. Local (fungal infections) and serious systemic side effects (such as menstrual irregularities and hepatic changes) can result from continued progesterone use. Therefore, it should not be used as a treatment for PMS.

Oral Contraceptives

High-dose estrogen (200 μg transdermal patch every day or 100-mg SQ implant) (39), progesterone (daily oral medroxyprogesterone 15 mg or 400 mg IM every month depot) (40), or danocrine or gonatotropin-releasing hormone (GnRH) agonists (adminstered throughout the cycle) abolish ovulation and dramatically decrease or eliminate PMS symptoms, suggesting that ovulation plays a role in PMS etiology. However, although oral contraceptives that contain varying estrogen/progesterone combinations may suppress ovulation and thus potentially eliminate PMS symptoms, the effect of the cyclic combination extrinsic hormones themselves may initiate or aggravate many women's PMS symptoms. Nevertheless, oral contraceptives can be tried and may be helpful for a small subgroup of women among those who need PMS treatment and contraception. No consistent effect in treatment of PMS symptoms has been noted with various types of oral contraceptives that contain estrogen or progesterone combinations (41).

Androgens

Androgens at higher continuous doses (e.g., danocrine 400 mg/day) cause anovulation by decreasing production of sex steroids at target organs by influencing the hypothalamic-pituitary-gonadal system and may thus improve physical or psychological PMS symptoms. However, masculinizing side effects and altered serum lipid profiles are major adverse effects for women, precluding long-term use of these agents for PMS treatment. Double-blind, placebo-controlled studies have shown that daily danocrine of 200–400 mg/day significantly improves PMS symptoms including depression, anxiety, and breast pain (29). Low-dose danocrine at 100–200 mg/day when used daily or in the luteal phase has fewer side effects, but more women ovulate with it and thus efficacy is less.

Gonadotropin-Releasing Hormone Agonists

The GnRH agonists abolish ovulation by binding the LH-releasing receptors for long periods of time and preventing ovarian stimulation. This improves symptoms in the majority of PMS women generally by the second or third month of treatment. In essence, a medical menopause is created with its attendant side effects, of which the most serious long-term ones are osteoporosis and coronary artery disease. Recent studies have added estrogen or estrogen/progesterone combinations to the GnRH agonist and shown relief of the menopausal side effects, but some decrease in the effectiveness of premenstrual symptom relief may occur (42). Generally 400 μg intranasal buserelin spray daily has been studied for up to 6 months (43). A recent open trial of leuprolide has shown efficacy in significantly decreasing physical and affective PMS symptoms to follicular phase levels (44). Monthly depot GnRH treatment modalities cannot be considered long-term treatment options due to the side effects and cost.

Endogenous Opiate Withdrawal

It has been postulated that PMS symptoms may be due to more intense endogenous opiate exposure in the early luteal phase followed by rapid withdrawal (as estrogen levels decrease premenstrually) resulting in symptoms of depression, fatigue, sweet cravings, and constipation in the early premenstruum, with irritability and anxiety occurring in the late premenstruum (45). Significantly lower luteal peripheral β-endorphin concentrations in PMS patients than in controls has been shown (46). Also, in PMS women, luteal phase endorphin concentration has been found to be lower than in the follicular phase (46), which is the converse of what has been noted in normal women. A 6-month double-blind, placebo-controlled crossover study of naltrexone (an oral opiate antagonist) given to 20 PMS women as 25 mg PO twice daily over three cycles showed that naltrexone significantly decreased concentration problems, negative affect, and behavioral changes in PMS women with side effects of nausea, decreased appetite, and dizziness (47).

Serotonin Deficiency Theory

Due to the occurrence of premenstrual depression as a symptom in many women with PMS, monoamine neurotransmitter deficiencies (as seen in major depression) have been sought in PMS women. Current biochemical and clinical support for a possible serotonin deficiency in PMS women exists. Whole blood concentrations of 5-hydroxytryptamine (5-HT) and platelet uptake of 5-HT are decreased in the luteal phase of women with PMS (48). Also, double-blind, placebo-controlled studies of selective serotonin reuptake inhibitors, notably fluoxetine at 20 mg (49,50) and clomipramine at 25–75 mg (51) throughout the cycle have shown efficacy in diminishing PMS symptoms especially depression. Also, one recent study of low-dose clomipramine administered as 25–75 mg in the luteal phase has been shown to help premenstrual symptoms with lower side effects (51). One study of buspirone (a serotonin partial agonist) showed overall benefit when used as 25 mg during the luteal phase (52) but has not been replicated.

Psychiatric Theories and Treatment

Theories

Early psychological papers suggested that women with premenstrual complaints had rejection of feminine psychosexual role (53), sexual repression (53), conflicted mother–daughter relationships (54), or traumatic menarche experiences (54). Subsequently increased neuroticism (55) and marital distress (56) were reported, but many of these earlier studies were conducted in women with complaints of PMS not necessarily confirmed PMS. Social indoctrination against menses has been noted to play a role in how negatively one views menses or attaches negative symptoms to the premenstruum (57). Increased accidents (58) and exacerbations of psychological and medical illness premenstrually may suggest increased sensitivity to physical and psychological changes during the premenstruum. Increased lifetime history of psychiatric disorder, particularly depression, in women with PMS has been recurrently shown (22) with suggested increased vulnerability to affective illness in these PMS women (14).

Treatment

Psychotropic treatments have recently received more attention. Similarities in cyclical occurrence of mood symptoms in PMS, such as in manic depressive illness, resulted in trials of lithium treatment; however, controlled studies have shown no greater efficacy of lithium carbonate in treating PMS symptoms (41). Three double-blind, placebo-controlled studies of alprazolam administered in the luteal phase at doses of 0.25–0.50 mg three times a day have shown significantly greater benefit in PMS women versus controls, especially for anxiety, irritability, and mild depression (59,60), whereas one did not (61). Recent studies of antidepressants targeted especially at the depressive symptoms of PMS have generally been of the serotonergic agents and are discussed in a previous section.

Short-term weekly support groups, relaxation therapy, and cognitive therapy (62) may all be helpful in decreasing premenstrual symptoms; however, replication of benefit of these therapies in a controlled format do not yet exist. Individual or family therapy for intrapsychic or family issues may be relevant for significant related neurotic or personal problems.

Other Treatment Theories

Other treatments that have been studied include light therapy (63), sleep deprivation (64), calcium supplementation (65), antibiotic treatment (66), and allergy shots (67).

Treatment

A multitude of treatments have been suggested for PMS (Table 35.2). However, many earlier studies of treatment are marred by methodologic problems including lack of placebo-controlled groups, use of retrospectively diagnosed PMS patients, or use of patients with *perimenstrual* not just premenstrual symptoms. Although most open studies show favorable response, perhaps because of the reported 20% to 90% placebo response in this population, efficacy of

Table 35.2 PMS Treatment

Symptom	Options	Approximate Cost
Self-help	PMS diet and exercise, education/support stress management	–
Pain symptoms	naproxen sodium or mefenamic acid in luteal phase	$30–80
Breast symptoms	bromocriptine in luteal phase	$45
Fluid retention	spironolactone in luteal phase	$5
Anxiety/irritability	alprazolam in luteal phase	$35
Depression	fluoxetine, daily	$70
Multiple severe symptoms	± oral contraceptive	$20
	–depo-medroxy-progesterone, every 3 mo	$50
	–danocrine daily	$160
	GnRH agonist–nafarelin, nasal spray, daily	$100
	leuprolide, depot, monthly	$375

double-blind placebo-controlled studies is limited to a few modalities of treatment generally targeted at symptom relief.

General Management

Validation of the existence of the syndrome and education of the patient regarding the benign and intermittent premenstrual nature of the symptoms and its natural course are important. Specific suggestions for decreasing life stress, especially at premenstrual times, such as avoiding scheduling stressful meetings if possible during premenstrual times and dietary changes and regular aerobic exercise throughout the cycle (see Box 35.2), may provide adequate symptom relief for some women and allow a sense of control over their symptoms and treatment.

Physical Symptoms

For primarily pain symptoms (e.g., headaches, backaches, and general aches), the prostaglandin inhibitors, sodium naproxen or mefenamic acid used for 7 to 14 days premenstrually are most helpful. (The Food and Drug Administration only recommends use of 7 days of mefenamic acid due to risks of potential hematologic, renal, and neurologic toxicity.) These agents may improve some mood symptoms also. Side effects are gastrointestinal distress, nausea, diarrhea, and rash. For major breast swelling/tenderness symptoms, bromocriptine is helpful. Side effects include nausea, vomiting, diarrhea, and syncope. Alternatively danocrine in the luteal phase can be used. For documented, distressing bloating/fluid retention symptoms (generally $\geqslant$5 lb weight gain from pre- to postmenses), spironolactone (a potassium-sparing diuretic) in the luteal phase may be considered, if dietary sodium restriction is not adequate. However, most women who complain of bloating do not have documented weight gain–rather their symptoms may be secondary to redistribution of fluid to sites in the abdomen, breast, or peripheral limbs. Administration of diuretics then could cause a relative dehydration and possible iatrogenic cyclic edema by activation of the renin–angiotensin–aldosterone system.

Psychological Symptoms

For predominant symptoms of anxiety or irritability, alprazolam during the symptomatic days (generally 7 to 14 days before menses and 1 to 5 days of menses) can be used. Sedation may be a side effect. Due to the potential risk of withdrawal seizures, tapering alprazolam over the 3 to 5 days of menses has been recommended but this is probably not necessary due to the intermittent nature of the use of alprazolam and very little likelihood of development of physiologic or psychological dependency when the drug is used at low doses for 2 weeks at a time. It must be emphasized that patients must be advised and monitored regarding use of alprazolam at other times of the cycle or for other reasons (e.g., transient insomnia or life stressors because then dependency risks increase). For significant depressive symptoms, fluoxetine as a morning dose can be used. Due to the 4- to 6-week delay in achieving therapeutic effect, fluoxetine should be continued throughout the cycle. Nausea, insomnia, and nervousness may be side effects.

Combined and Severe Symptoms

For women with physical or psychological symptoms of PMS and especially those who also want contraception, a trial of oral contraceptives can be used and may be effective for some women. However, some women have worsening of PMS symptoms with any cyclic estrogen/progesterone combination pill. Daily oral medyoxyprogesterone may be more effective in such women, but irregular bleeding can be a problem. For those few women with severe symptoms not responsive to the above modalities, a 6-month trial of suppression of ovulation using either a GnRH agonist (daily intranasal spray or IM depot) or high-dose daily danocrine can be diagnostic and therapeutic. Apart from providing symptom relief for several months it is possible that the PMS symptoms will undergo a spontaneous remission after this period of time, because the natural course of PMS symptoms is to ebb and tide. Obviously inducing such a medical menopause is not a long-term treatment solution for PMS. Surgical treatment via hysterectomy and oophorectomy would also induce a menopause with potential long-term need for hormone replacement therapy with estrogen.

Referral to Other Clinicians

One may wish to refer certain patients for further work-up or specialized evaluation and treatment depending on the specialty of the clinician who first sees the patient (e.g., family physician, internist or psychiatrist). These patients might include those with newly identified medical problems such as thyroid abnormalities, diabetes mellitus, nonmenstrually related headaches, or other gynecologic problems that may warrant further specialized evaluation with appropriate testing and subsequent treatment. If major premenstrual psychological complaints or if psychological symptoms not restricted to the premenstruum are present, one may wish to refer these patients to a psychiatrist for further evaluation, which may include psychological testing, blood work, and treatment with psychotropics or psychotherapy.

Natural History of the Disease

The natural course of PMS is usually marked by exacerbation and remission of symptoms often related to reproductive or psychological events during the reproductive years. Some women may have persistence of symptoms throughout the reproductive years with increased severity of symptoms over time. At menopause, if hormone replacement therapy is initiated with estrogen alone PMS symptoms do not occur. However, if the hormone therapy regimen includes estrogen as well as cyclical progesterone to prevent hypertrophy of the endometrium of the uterus, a recurrence of premenstrual-type symptoms may occur (68).

Long-Term Management of PMS

Due to the intermittent nature of the symptom presentation, long-term treatment may not be necessary. However, in women with persistent, severe premenstrual symptoms a variety of options can be considered. As indicated in the treatment section, long-term use of luteal phase antiprostaglandins, bromocriptine, or continuous oral contraceptives may not have as major negative sequelae as daily danocrine or GnRH agonists. Newer selective serotonin reuptake inhibitor antidepressants are unlikely to cause any major long-term side effects and therefore may be the drugs of choice for treatment of significant mood symptoms of PMS. Because mood symptoms often have the most negative impact on patients' lives, treatment of these symptoms often allows them to cope with other annoying premenstrual physical symptoms.

REFERENCES

1. Frank RT. The hormonal causes of premenstrual tension. Arch Neurol Psychiatry 1931;26:1053–1057.

2. Schmidt PJ, Nieman LK, Grover GN, et al. Lack of effect of induced menses on symptoms in women with

premenstrual syndrome. N Engl J Med 1991;324:1174–1179.

3. Rubinow DR, Schmidt PJ. Models for the development and expression of symptoms in premenstrual syndrome. Psychiatr Clin North Am 1989;12:53–68.

4. Stewart DE. Positive changes in the premenstrual period. Acta Psychiatr Scand 1989;79:400–405.

5. American Psychiatric Association. Diagnostic and statistical manual of mental disorders. 3rd ed., revised. Washington, DC: Author, 1987.

6. Johnson SR. The epidemiology and social impact of premenstrual symptoms. Clin Obstet Gynecol 1987;30:367–376.

7. Janiger O, Riffenburgh R, Kersh R. Cross cultural study of premenstrual symptoms. Psychosomatics 1972;13:226–235.

8. Dalton K. Incidence of the premenstrual syndrome in twins. Br Med J 1987;295:1027–1028.

9. Widholm O. Dysmenorrhea during adolescence. Acta Obstet Gynecol Scand Suppl 1979;87:61–66.

10. Rubinow DR, Hoban MC, Grover GN, et al. Changes in plasma hormones across the menstrual cycle in patients with menstrually related mood disorder and in control subjects. Am J Obstet Gynecol 1988;158:5–11.

11. Roy-Byrne PP, Rubinow DR, Hoban MC, et al. TSH and prolactin responses to TRH in patients with premenstrual syndrome. Am J Psychiatry 1987;144:480–484.

12. Halbreich U, Tworek H. Altered serotonergic activity in women with dysphoric premenstrual syndromes. Int J Psychiatry Med 1993;23:1–27.

13. Ruble DN. Premenstrual symptoms: a reinterpretation. Science 1977;197:291–292.

14. Endicott J, Halbreich U. Clinical significance of premenstrual dysphoric changes. J Clin Psychiatry 1988;49:486–489.

15. Rubinow DR, Roy-Byrne P, Hoban MC, et al. Prospective assessment of menstrually related mood disorders. Am J Psychiatry 1984;141:684–686.

16. Endicott J, Halbreich U. Retrospective reports of premenstrual depressive changes: factors affecting confirmation by daily ratings. Psychopharmacol Bull 1982;18:109–112.

17. Mortola JF, Girton L, Beck L, Yen SS. Diagnosis of premenstrual syndrome by a simple, prospective, and reliable instrument: the calendar of premenstrual experiences. Obstet Gynecol 1990;76:302–307.

18. Reid RL. Premenstrual syndrome. Curr Probl Obstet Gynecol Fertil 1985;8:1–57.

19. Steiner M, Haskett RF, Carroll BJ. Premenstrual tension syndrome: the development of research diagnostic criteria and new rating scales. Acta Psychiatr Scand 1980;62:229–240.

20. Halbreich U, Endicott J, Schacht S, Nee J. The diversity of premenstrual changes as reflected in the premenstrual assessment form. Acta Psychiatr Scand 1982;65:46–65.

21. Moos RH. The development of a menstrual distress questionnaire. Psychosom Med 1968;30:853–867.

22. Chandraiah S, Levenson JL, Collins JB. Sexual dysfunction, social maladjustment, and psychiatric disorders in women seeking treatment in a premenstrual syndrome clinic. Int J Psychiatry Med 1991;21:189–204.

23. Mira M, Stewart PM, Abraham SF. Vitamin and trace element status in premenstrual syndrome. Am J Clin Nutr 1988;47:636–641.

24. Steinberg S. The treatment of late luteal phase dysphoric disorder. Life Sci 1991;49:767–802.

25. Parry GJ, Bredesen DE. Sensory neuropathy with low dose pyridoxine. Neurology 1985;35:1466–1468.

26. Adams PW, Wynn V, Seed M. Vitamin B_6, depression and oral contraception. Lancet 1974;2:516–517.

27. Horrobin DF. The role of essential fatty acids and prostaglandins in the premenstrual syndrome. J Reprod Med 1983;28:465–468.

28. Budoff PW. Use of prostaglandin inhibitors in the treatment of PMS. Clini Obstet Gynecol 1987;30:453–464.

29. Smith S, Schiff I. The premenstrual syndrome—diagnosis and management. Fertil Steril 1989;52:527–543.

30. Andersch B. Bromocriptine and premenstrual symptoms: a survey of double blind trials. Obstet Gynecol Surv 1983;38:643–646.

31. O'Brien PMS, Craven D, Selby C, Symonds EM. Treatment of premenstrual syndrome by spironolactone. Br J Obstet Gynecol 1979;86:142–147.

32. Tollan A, Oian P, Fadnes HO, Maltau JM. Evidence for altered transcapillary fluid balance in women with the premenstrual syndrome. Acta Obstet Gynecol Scand 1993;72:238–242.

33. Toth EL, Suthijumroon A, Crockford PM, Ryan EA. Insulin action does not change during the menstrual cycle in normal women. J Clin Endocrinol Metab 1987;64:74–80.

34. Valdes CT, Elkind-Hirsch KE. Intravenous glucose tolerance test-derived insulin sensitivity changes during the menstrual cycle. J Clin Endocrinol Metab 1991;72:642–646.

35. Reid RL, Greenaway-Coates A, Hahn PM. Oral glucose tolerance during the menstrual cycle in normal women and women with alleged premenstrual "hypoglycemic" attacks: effects of naloxone. J Clin Endocrinol Metab 1986;62:1167–1172.

36. Wurtman JJ, Brzezinski A, Wurtman RJ, Laferrere B. Effect of nutrient intake on premenstrual depression. Am J Obstet Gynecol 1989;161:1228–1234.

37. Timonen S, Procopè B. Premenstrual syndrome and physical exercise. Acta Obstet Gynecol Scand 1971;50:331–337.

38. Prior JC, Vigna Y. Conditioning exercise and premenstrual symptoms. J Reprod Med 1987;32:423–428.

39. Watson NR, Studd JW, Savvas M, et al. Treatment of severe premenstrual syndrome with oestradiol patches and cyclical oral norethisterone. Lancet 1989;2:730–732.

40. Reid RL. Psychological aspects of menstruation: premenstrual syndrome. In: Carr BR, Blackwell RE, eds. Textbook of reproductive medicine. East Norwalk, CT: Appleton & Lange, 1993:409–426.

41. Harrison W, Sharpe L, Endicott J. Treatment of premenstrual symptoms. Gen Hosp Psychiatry 1985;7:54–65.

42. Mortola JF, Girton L, Fischer U. Successful treatment of severe premenstrual syndrome by combined use of gonadotropin-releasing hormone agonist and estrogen/progestin. J Clin Endocrinol Metab 1991;72:252A–252F.

43. Hammarback S, Backstrom T. Induced anovulation as treatment of premenstrual tension syndrome: a double-blind cross-over study with GnRH-agonist versus placebo. Acta Obstet Gynecol Scand 1988;67:159–166.

44. Freeman EW, Sondheimer SJ, Rickels K, Albert J. Gonadotropin-releasing hormone agonist in treatment of premenstrual symptoms with and without comorbidity of depression: a pilot study. J Clin Psychiatry 1993;54:192–195.

45. Reid RL, Yen SSC. Premenstrual syndrome. Am J Obstet Gynecol 1981;139:85–104.

46. Chuong CJ, Coulam CB, Kao PC, et al. Neuropeptide levels in premenstrual syndrome. Fertil Steril 1985;44:760–765.

47. Chuong CJ, Coulam CB, Bergstralh EJ, et al. Clinical trial of naltrexone in premenstrual syndrome. Obstet Gynecol 1988;72:332–335.

48. Taylor DL, Mathew RJ, Ho BT, Weinman ML. Serotonin levels and platelet uptake during premenstrual tension. Neuropsychobiology 1984;12:16–18.

49. Stone AB, Pearlstein TB, Brown WA. Fluoxetine in the treatment of late luteal phase dysphoric disorder. J Clin Psychiatry 1991;52:290–293.

50. Wood SH, Mortola JF, Chan Y, et al. Treatment of premenstrual syndrome with fluoxetine: a double-blind, placebo-controlled crossover study. Obstet Gynecol 1992;80:339–344.

51. Sundblad C, Hedberg MA, Eriksson E. Clomipramine adminstered during the luteal phase reduces the symptoms of premenstrual syndrome: a placebo-controlled trial. Neuropsychopharmacology 1993;9:133–145.

52. Rickels K, Freeman E, Sondheimer S. Buspirone in treatment of premenstrual syndrome. Lancet 1989;1:777.

53. Fortin JN, Wittkower ED, Kalz F. A psychosomatic approach to the premenstrual tension syndrome: a preliminary report. Can Med Assn J 1958;79:978–981.

54. Shainess N. A re-evaluation of some aspects of femininity through a study of menstruation. A preliminary report. Compr Psychiatry 1961;2:20–26.

55. Taylor JW. Psychological factors in the aetiology of pre-menstrual symptoms. Aust N Z J Psychiatry 1979;13:35–41.

56. Clare AW. Psychiatric and social aspects of premenstrual complaint. Psychol Med Monogr Suppl 1983;4:1–58.

57. Parlee MB. Stereotypic beliefs about menstruation: a methodological note on the Moos menstrual distress questionnaire and some new data. Psychosom Med 1974;36:229–240.

58. Patel S, Cliff KS, Machin D. The premenstrual syndrome and its relationship to accidents. Public Health 1985;99:45–50.

59. Smith S, Rinehart JS, Ruddock VE, Schiff I. Treatment of premenstrual syndrome with alprazolam: results of a double-blind, placebo-controlled, randomized crossover clinical trial. Obstet Gynecol 1987;70:37–43.

60. Harrison WM, Endicott J, Nee J. Treatment of premenstrual dysphoria with alprazolam: a controlled study. Arch Gen Psychiatry 1990;47:270–275.

61. Schmidt PJ, Grover GN, Rubinow DR. Alprazolam in the treatment of premenstrual syndrome: a dou-

ble-blind, placebo-controlled trial. Arch Gen Psychiatry 1993;50:467–473.

62. Morse CA, Dennerstein L, Farrell E, Varnavides K. A comparison of hormone therapy, coping skills training, and relaxation for the relief of premenstrual syndrome. J Behav Med 1991;14:469–489.

63. Parry BL, Berga SL, Mostofi N, et al. Morning versus evening bright light treatment of late luteal phase dysphoric disorder. Am J Psychiatry 1989;146:1215–1217.

64. Parry BL, Wehr TA. Therapeutic effect of sleep deprivation in patients with premenstrual syndrome. Am J Psychiatry 1987;144:808–810.

65. Thys-Jacobs S, Ceccarelli S, Bierman A, et al. Calcium supplementation in premenstrual syndrome: a randomized crossover trial. J Gen Intern Med 1989;4:183–189.

66. Toth A, Lesser ML, Naus G, et al. Effect of doxycycline on premenstrual syndrome: a double-blind randomized clinical trial. J Int Med Res 1988;16:270–279.

67. Atton-Chamla A, Favre G, Goudard JR, et al. Premenstrual syndrome and atopy: a double-blind clinical evaluation of treatment with a gamma-globulin/histamine complex. Pharmatherapeutica 1980;2:481–486.

68. Hammarback S, Backstrom T, Holst J, et al. Cyclical mood changes as in the premenstrual tension syndrome during sequential estrogen-progestagen postmenopausal replacement therapy. Acta Obstet Gynecol Scand 1985;64:393–397.

CHAPTER 36

DEPRESSION

Carl A. Houck

Depression is a common psychiatric problem in women that may lead to numerous complications. It is often underdiagnosed and may present in forms appearing to be physical illness, leading to diagnostic confusion and possibly unnecessary medical procedures. In obstetrics and gynecology, as in any primary care specialty, depressed patients are unavoidable. The physician who recognizes depression in his or her patients and either treats or refers for treatment these patients is not only performing a compassionate service but is also reducing the serious consequences of untreated depression.

Definition

In essence, depression is an abnormal sadness or disinterest in life. It is classified in the American Psychiatric Association's *Diagnostic and Statistical Manual, Fourth Edition* (*DSM-IV*) as a mood disorder (1). The capacity to feel sad is part of being human, and indeed not feeling sad in some contexts may indicate a psychiatric problem. However, sadness becomes pathologic when it is especially intense, frequent, enduring, disruptive, or unassociated with any apparent cause.

Importance of Depression

Depression is a disorder that deserves vigilant diagnosis and aggressive treatment because it is common, causes significant psychosocial disability, and causes psychological and emotional pain as intense as any physical pain. Two national epidemiologic studies have shown the prevalence of depression. The Epidemiologic Catchment Area Study in 1984 and the National Comorbidity Survey (NCS) in 1994 revealed that depression is one of the most common psychiatric disorders (2,3). The NCS discovered that 17% of people surveyed had a history of major depression at some time in their lives, and 10% had a major depression within the preceding year. Furthermore, depression has been shown to be a disorder that strikes women more often than men. In the NCS, women were 1.7 times more likely than men to have ever had a major depression (4).

The impact on social functioning is another reason depression is important. Depression may seriously interfere with one's role as a spouse, parent, student, or worker. Marital discord, infidelity, separation, or divorce may result. Occasionally child neglect or child abuse may develop because of depressive irritability and hostility. Students may have great difficulty paying attention, studying, and passing tests because of depressive lack of concentration. Workers may be frequently late, absent from work, inefficient, or unproductive because of depressive lack of energy and lack of motivation. Troubles working with others or with management may arise, sometimes leading to outbursts of rage or violence. The most important reason depression should be addressed is the risk of lethality associated with depression. The most publicized risk is suicide, but another risk that is gaining increasing attention is murder. These psychosocial dysfunctions make depression a costly national problem. In examining the costs of direct medical, psychiatric, and pharmacologic treatment, plus the costs of mortality from suicide, plus the costs of depressive inability to perform at work, it has been estimated that depression costs our nation approximately $44 billion yearly (5).

Finally, depression causes great suffering. Many patients, if given the hypothetical choice of living with a physical illness or living with depression, would choose to live with the physical illness. This is evidence of the unbearable suffering depression may create and the great trouble patients have coping with depression. Treating depression not only improves the patient's role functioning but leads to a happier and more peaceful life.

Importance to the Obstetrician-Gynecologist

Some aspects of depression make it of special importance to the obstetrician-gynecologist. Depression may interfere significantly in obstetric-gynecologic practice (Box 36.1). Perhaps the most problematic interference is noncompliance. The depressed woman does not value life as much as the healthy woman and consequently there is less motivation to care for herself medically. Doctor's recommendations may be ignored, prescriptions may be unfilled, medicines may be taken improperly, appointments may be missed, and tests or procedures may be refused. The depressed woman may have difficulty in relating interpersonally with the physician, leading to poor communication and behavior, a weakened doctor–patient relationship, and aggravation of noncompliance. The lack of medical cooperation and self-care is especially serious during the prenatal period when strict compliance is vital to fetal development. Noncompliance may be worsened when the depressed woman begins using alcohol or illegal drugs to combat the depression, a very common scenario.

Depression can create problems during the postpartum period. The same lack of motivation and interest in self and others that may lead to noncompliance may lead to poor mothering and a disturbed infant–mother relationship, with neglect of the infant in serious cases. Spouses may also be neglected, leading to marital discord and a volatile environment for the newborn.

The physical symptoms that are often prominent in depression and are often the woman's presenting complaint may create problems for the obstetrician-gynecologist in either of two ways. First, these physical symptoms may affect the obstetric or gynecologic health of the woman. For example, weight loss during depression may be significant and enough to endanger fetal development. Appetite changes, especially lack of appetite, may cause the woman to eat an insufficiently balanced diet to support the fetus. Second, these physical complaints may also frequently create diagnostic confusion for the obstetrician-gynecologist. Numerous physical symptoms may bring the patient to the physician, including headaches, fatigue, vague chest, abdominal or pelvic pain, sexual symptoms, or dyspareunia or menstrual irregularities. Each of these presentations may reflect either depression, a known coexisting medical disease, or an occult medical disease, and the physician must struggle with the diagnostic meaning of these symptoms and the dilemma of how far to proceed in searching for physical explanations for them. With tremendous pressures on physicians to allocate diagnostic tests efficiently and cost effectively, this diagnostic confusion arising from depressive somatic symptomatology becomes an important impact of depression on obstetric-gynecologic practice.

Overdose is a risk with depressed patients and will present the obstetrician-gynecologist with problems. Overdose during early pregnancy is harmful to both mother and fetus. Treatments used to counteract the pharmacologic effects of the overdosed drugs may have risks to the mother or fetus. A patient who overdoses may also put the obstetrician-gynecologist in medicolegal jeopardy.

Box 36.1 How Depression May Interfere in Obstetric-Gynecologic Practice

Noncompliance

Failing to take medicines properly
Missed appointments
Refusal to accept diagnostic tests

Diagnostic Confustion Created By

Depression presenting as obstetric-gynecologic illness
Depression coexisting with obstetric-gynecologic illness
Doctor shopping and polypharmacy
Self-treatment with alcohol or other substances

Disruptive Behaviors

Leaving against medical advice
Stresses in the doctor–patient relationship
Overdose

Role of the Obstetrician-Gynecologist in Recognizing Depression

The obstetrician-gynecologist often plays a crucial role in diagnosing and treating depression. Depressed women frequently consult their obstetrician-gynecologists first for help with depression before they consider seeing psychiatrists. A woman may have seen her obstetrician-gynecologist for many years before becoming depressed and naturally turns initially to this trusted physician for relief. Regrettably, psychiatrists are still often feared or viewed skeptically by many patients, while these same attitudes are generally not present toward nonpsychiatrists. By choice or default, the obstetrician-gynecologist often has the best chance of helping a depressed woman.

Symptoms of Depression

Depression is a broad syndrome with many symptoms, clustered into different types of disorders, and with variable expressions of the same disorder in different patients (1,6,7). The symptoms of depression may be grouped into emotional, cognitive, vegetative, and behavioral symptoms (Box 36.2).

Box 36.2 Symptoms of Depression

Emotional	**Vegetative**
Sadness	Sleep changes
Disinterest	Appetite changes
Anger	Poor energy
Irritability	Poor sex drive
Bitterness	Crying
Emptiness	
Boredom	
Cognitive	**Behavioral**
Cynicism	Agitation
Pessimism	Withdrawal from friends, family, activities
Self-hatred	Marital discord, adultery, divorce
Self-criticism	School failure
Hopelessness	Job difficulties–absenteeism, conflicts, inefficiency
Helplessness	Child neglect or abuse
Suicidal thoughts, wishes, plans	Juvenile delinquency
Poor memory or concentration	Self-neglect of medical care
	Suicide or suicide attempt
	Murder or violence

Emotional Symptoms

The cardinal symptom of depression is sadness. This emotion is the one patients usually describe, but different patients will describe it differently. Patients may report feeling blue, down, down in the dumps, gloomy, despondent, mopey, lonely, unhappy, unloved, unwanted, melancholy, or myriad other terms conveying the essential theme of sadness. It is important to note, however, that emotions other than sadness are felt and in some patients these may be the presenting or prominent emotions. Some patients may report apathy, boredom, or disinterest, whereas others may report lack of pleasure, fun, or excitement as emotional symptoms of depression. They may also report anger, irritability, bitterness, or resentment. Emotional symptoms are central in depression and are considered essential in the DSM-IV to making the diagnosis of depression. There is, rarely, a patient who appears clearly depressed but denies emotional symptoms, no matter how persistently probed. This phenomenon has been called *masked depression* (8).

Cognitive Symptoms

Cognitive symptoms are those that reflect abnormalities in thoughts, beliefs, attitudes, memory, concentration, and learning. One's thoughts and beliefs about life and oneself are often significantly changed by depression. The depressed woman is likely to focus inordinately on problems and worries. Some depressed women worry virtually constantly. Patients may report believing they are worthless, useless, terribly sinful, or bad. They may see themselves as unwanted by others or unwelcome in the world. They may be plagued by excessive, pathologic guilt, dwelling on minor failures or transgressions as if these were monumental, unforgivable, or evidence of unworthiness. Guilt may be present about current behavior or past behavior, sometimes decades ago. The person may not respond to reassurance from others and cannot be talked out of the irrational beliefs. The guilt may become delusional. Because of their sense of failure, inadequacy, and unworth, patients have an attitude of self-hatred or excessive self-criticism. The attitude becomes pessimistic and negative. People may not be trusted and others' motives and actions may be viewed cynically. Self-esteem is usually low in depression. Patients lack pride and self-confidence and often blame themselves readily. Women may find it difficult to escape poor relationships because of a depressive lack of confidence. Patients may view things as hopeless, believing that they will never recover, and view themselves as helpess, unable to extricate themselves from the depressed state. Hopelessness is a serious and ominous symptom because it is often fertile ground for the development of suicidal thinking that all too often culminates in an actual suicide.

Suicidal thoughts may be fleeting and easily disavowed or may be frequent and intense. The patient may believe suicide is the only escape from her distress, or she may entertain the idea but banish it because of strong religious faith or the unwillingness to leave her children motherless. The suicidal thinking may take the form of thoughts only, of wishes for it, or as frank plans to carry out the thoughts or wishes. Suicide may be seen as an imminent option or as a distant, future possibility that may be chosen if needed at that time. Some patients are not willing to try suicide but will engineer circumstances so that death appears to be the certain outcome. For example, a woman with a breast lump may ignore it, hoping that it will progress beyond treatment.

Thoughts of homicide or revenge, rather than thoughts of suicide, may predominate in some depressed patients (9,10). The patient may believe she has been wronged and deserves justice. A potentially dangerous situation may arise if the depressed woman is in a relationship with an abusive spouse, who may be targeted in these homicidal thoughts.

Other cognitive symptoms arise when higher cortical functions are affected. Depressed patients often have problems remembering, concentrating, and learning. They may describe their thinking as foggy, clouded, disorganized, confused, or distracted. Concentrating becomes difficult, so reading, writing, and studying are impeded. In severe cases even simple tasks become too trying. Planning may become impossible. Schoolwork, housework, and job duties suffer. Decisions become hard because of inability to plan and diminished motivation. Often the patient procrastinates on key decisions until events decide themselves, sometimes worsening the patient's troubles. The memory problem may become so prominent, especially in the elderly woman, that it appears that the patient has a dementia (a loss of memory and intellectual skills without a loss of attention). This phenomenon is called *depressive pseudodementia.*

Vegetative Symptoms

Basic body, or vegetative, functions may be altered in depression. One hypothesis of this phenomenon is that these changes result from depressive alteration in hypothalamic function. Sleep is almost always affected by depression, appearing as either poor quality of sleep or insufficient quantity of sleep. Most patients report insomnia with depression, complaining of early, middle, or late insomnia. Early or initial insomnia is inability to fall asleep easily, requiring in some patient several hours before sleep onset. Middle insomnia is trouble maintaining sleep after falling asleep. Patients may awaken frequently or may awaken for a considerable time before finally falling asleep again. They may arise and do things around the house. The sleep may be punctuated by stressful dreams or frank nightmares. During the periods of wakefulness, the woman is likely to report dwelling on worries and problems. Late or terminal insomnia occurs at the end of sleep and is an inability to sleep as late as desired. The patient complains of awakening spontaneously, sometimes several hours before the intended wake-up time, without being able to return to sleep for its completion. Even when able to sleep adequate time, patients often report their sleep is unrefreshing, waking up tired before the day starts. In a less common variant, patients may report hypersomnia, or sleeping too much. Arising from sleep becomes a struggle, and sleep may be viewed as a retreat from a painful existence. These patients may have problems performing adequately at work. Even though depressed patients with hypersomnia sleep excess hours, they usually still complain of poor quality of sleep.

Appetite is often altered in depression. Patients predominantly complain of decreased appetite, but some complain of increased appetite. With decreased appetite, food is no longer enjoyed in mild cases and may be abhorred in more severe cases. Patients may have to be pushed to eat enough. With increased appetite, patients often report eating more but not enjoying the food they eat. As a consequence of altered eating, weight changes. Patients may lose or gain huge amounts of weight: 50 to 100 lb in severe cases. The appetite and weight changes may simulate physical disease such as cancer or endocrine disease.

Libido, or sexual drive, is another vegetative function often changed in depression. Patients generally lose their previous level of interest in sex, and sex may be seen as a nuisance, in milder cases, to a dreaded ritual, devoid of any pleasurable activity in more depressed women. Numerous psychosocial consequences may occur when the sexual partner fails to understand compassionately that the sexual problems are from depression, not other problems.

Fatigue is another common symptom of depression, which may or may not be accompanied by lack of motivation. The fatigued woman complains of a lack of physical energy sufficient to carry out her usual daily activities. Occasionally patients may appear to be overactive and may appear to have plenty of energy, but usually when probed these patients still report poor energy. The excess activity represents agitation rather than pleasant, productive energy.

Crying is often present in depression. The woman may cry easily or frequently and may cry without clear precipitant. She may be unable to explain how she feels or what the crying is about. On the other hand, she may be overly sensitive and cry at the slightest offense from others. Although crying is often seen as a hallmark of depression, this association is not pathognomonic. Many patients with depression never cry, sometimes saying that they are "too depressed to cry." Conversely, crying may be the result of many conditions other than depression, including normal, healthy crying.

Behavioral Symptoms

Depression may create behavioral disturbances to a subtle or drastic degree. Probably the most common behavioral change is social withdrawal. Patients quit visiting friends and family, and interacting with others becomes unnatural and burdensome. When this affects the spouse, marital discord may result, which further aggravates the depression. Patients may drop out of school, church, hobbies, clubs, and even work because of depressive withdrawal. Although less common than withdrawal, suicide is the most important behavioral consequence of depression. Statistically, women tend to attempt suicide by overdosing or mixing alcohol with sedative-hypnotics. The suicidal behavior may be only a mild gesture, but it should always be taken seriously and probed carefully by the obstetrician-gynecologist. Other behavioral consequences that have been described previously include neglect of medical care, child neglect or abuse, marital arguments, separation, adultery, divorce, alcohol or drug abuse, and homicide or homicide attempts.

Types of Depression

Not all depression is alike. The DSM-IV recognizes several forms of depression, characterized by differences in symptom content, course, and etiology (Box 36.3). The most well known kind of depression is major depression, but the nonpsychiatrist should remember that other forms exist because treatments vary from type to type, and the need for psychiatric referral is greater in some types than in others.

Organic Depression

Organic depression is depression that is caused by a physical agent. Common examples of depressogenic agents are corticosteroids, hypothyroidism, and stroke (Box 36.4). The depression is hypothesized to develop in reaction to the primary disease's affect on the mood-regulating areas of the central nervous system (CNS). This kind of depression is seen frequently in primary care practices such as obstetrics-gynecology (11,12). The physical agent that is etiologic may be anatomic (e.g., frontal lobe brain tumor) or physiologic (e.g., hypocalcemia). The agent may arise within the CNS (e.g., multiple sclerosis) or may arise outside the CNS (e.g., hypothyroidism). In addition, many external agents, including medicines, toxins, and street drugs may induce a secondary organic depression. The symptoms induced may be only mild and sporadic or may be very intense and persistent, resembling a severe major depression. Suicidal ideation may also occur with this form of depression.

All other forms of depression are conceptualized as nonorganic. Physical signs of depression may be present, and some neurochemical changes have been measured, but these forms of depression are consid-

Box 36.3 Types of Depression

Diagnostic Type	Characteristics
Organic depression	Occurs secondary to a known or strongly presumed organic agent Common in medically sick women Should always be suspected
Major depression	Intense depression with numerous symptoms Suicide risk often high
Dysthymic depression	A low-grade, chronic, festering depression Must be present at least 2 yr to diagnose Often present since childhood or adolescence
Bipolar depression	Depression in a manic-depressive woman
Cyclothymic depression	Essentially a milder form of bipolar depression Often missed because patients sense mood hills and valleys as normal
Adjustment depression	Clearly reactive, situational depression after a stress May be intense for a short time, but usually improves quickly in a healthy woman If intensity persists for 2 weeks, consider major depression to have developed

Box 36.4 Common Organic Etiologies of Depression

Medicines

Oral contraceptives
Corticosteroids
Antihypertensives
Levodopa
Cimetidine
Metoclopramide
Disulfiram
Barbiturates
Chemotherapeutics

Withdrawal States

Amphetamine and other stimulants
Cocaine

Endocrine Diseases

Hypothyroidism
Cushing's syndrome
Addison's disease
Hypo- or hyperparathyroidism

Neurologic Diseases

Cerebrovascular accidents
Parkinson's disease
Huntington's disease
Multiple sclerosis

Infections

Acquired immunodeficiency syndrome
Influenza
Mononucleosis
Hepatitis
Epstein-Barr virus

Other Medical Conditions

Pancreatic cancer
Carcinoid syndrome
Systemic lupus erythematosus
Pernicious anemia

ered nonorganic because no clearly identifiable physical disease state produced the syndrome.

Major Depression

Major depression is a significant, persistent depression with a rich symptom cluster that includes depressed mood or disinterest plus a minimum of at least four other depressive symptoms. This disorder significantly affects a patient's functioning and is experienced as a daily or near-daily disturbance. Suicidal risk is higher with this form of depression. Symptoms must be present for at least 2 weeks to diagnose this type of depression.

Variants of Major Depression

A melancholic depression is a subtype of major depression in which vegetative symptoms are marked, there is characteristic early morning awakening, and the depression is severe and virtually constant. A psychotic depression is one in which a patient feels both depressed and shows evidence of psychosis, usually appearing as a delusion with depressive content. For example, the psychotically depressed woman may believe sincerely and unalterably that she should be tortured because she is worthless or that she has been the cause of everyone's misfortunes. Seasonal depression occurs when symptoms develop during only certain seasons, especially the winter. It is more common in the northern latitudes where winter sunshine is scarce.

Dysthymic Depression

Dysthymic disorder is more chronic, low grade, and intermittent than major depression. Patients have many depressive symptoms, but they are felt less intensely and less often than in major depression. Patients often report stretches of depression-free "good days" lasting a few days. Suicidal risk may be present but in most patients is less of a risk than in major depression. A minimum of 2 years of this pattern of symptoms is required before the diagnosis can be made. Most patients with dysthymic depression report chronic depressive symptoms ever since childhood or adolescence.

Bipolar Depression

Bipolar depression occurs in patients with bipolar disorder (manic-depressive disorder) who undergo a mood shift into depression. The depression is generally intense and may be indistinguishable from a major depression. Suicidal risk is high and may continue if the patient shifts into the manic mood. Bipolar depression may develop quickly and often recurs. The diagnosis may be missed if it is not known that the patient is bipolar or if a history of previous mania is missed.

Cyclothymic Depression

Cyclothymia is a form of depression in which patients experience mild, sporadic depressive symptoms at times and mild periods of elevated, euphoric mood (hypomania) at other times. It can be conceptualized as a milder form of bipolar disorder. Because it less often leads to psychosocial dysfunction, and patients may actually enjoy their hypomanic periods, this condition is often not experienced by patients as abnormal and consequently is underdiagnosed.

Adjustment Disorder with Depression

Adjustment depression occurs when a patient experiences depression in reaction to an identifiable, bothersome change in life. Almost anything significant may be a stressor disturbing enough to trigger depression in some people. Common examples include obstetric or gynecologic illness, pregnancy, delivery, abortion, divorce, marital discord, job stress, getting fired, conflicts with children or relatives, school troubles, or changing locations. Adjustment depression may initially be intense, but the psychologically healthy person should recover within a few days to a few months. Suicidal risk may be very high soon after the stressor but generally subsides once equilibrium is restored. The disorder initially may look like major depression, and if it continues to persist for 2 weeks with this intensity, most psychiatrists would consider it to have evolved into a major depression. People vary in their susceptibility to this condition, and the obstetrician-gynecologist should never presume that because the stress may seem benign to the physician then it cannot be stressful to the patient.

Depression Not Otherwise Classified

This cumbersome term is used to recognize that patients with mood disorders are complex and do not always conform to the previously described forms of depression. This form of depression is also called atypical or nonspecific depression. Depressive symptoms are present, and clearly cause either subjective distress or objective dysfunction, but are not abundant or persistent enough to be considered one of the other forms of depression.

Postpartum Depression

The term "postpartum depression" is a general descriptive term for any depression appearing in the postpartum period. The exact type of depression may be any of the DSM-IV varieties of depression previously reviewed. Depending on the symptoms present, their frequency, and duration, the depression may be classified as an adjustment depression, major depression, bipolar depression, or atypical depression. A postpartum depression is a clinically important depression that causes some dysfunction, to be distinguished from the postpartum "maternity blues," which are common but do not create any significant psychosocial dysfunction (13). Some recent studies have shown that depression in the postpartum period is no more prevalent than depression in nonpregnant women (14). Numerous possible etiologies for depression in this setting have been proposed. Biologic variables, including low progesterone, low estrogen, or high prolactin, as well as psychosocial variables, such as family support and life stressors, have been studied (15). However, no variables unique to the postpartum period have been shown to cause depression.

Depression in Different Age Groups

In the elderly woman, depression often presents with prominent physical complaints. The patient may not clearly describe depressed mood, and relatively greater importance of the family's report is necessary. In the adolescent, behavioral changes are typical of depression. The teenager may not report depression, but poor sleep, poor school performance, and withdrawal from friends and previously enjoyed activities may suggest depression. A variation is the hostile, delinquent teenager who expresses depression as aggressive acts toward property or others. The child often expresses depression almost entirely by changes in appearance and behavior, with a sad look, less activity, and less playfulness.

Etiologies of Depression in Women

There is no single, uniform cause of depression in all women. In any given patient, occasionally there may be one cause, but the more common situation is that several forces converge to result in depression. These forces are usually classified as biologic, psychological, or social. Biologic forces include not only biologic agents that may secondarily induce an organic depression, as discussed previously (see Box 36.4), but also any genetic predisposition to depression. Psychological forces are characteristic styles of thinking about life, attitudes, expectations, and beliefs that may invite depression. For example, a woman who has an excessive, unhealthy need to be the center of attention may suffer a severe blow to this pathologic need if rejected by her husband, and she may develop a severe depression. Other psychological forces are various developmental changes in life (e.g., growing up, getting married, growing old). Many of the surgeries performed on women have the potential to carry special psychological meaning to the patient and may spawn a depression. Hysterectomy, mastectomy, abortion, and deforming gynecologic operations may profoundly sadden women and result in clinical depression. Social forces are unavoidable and are those influences on mood that arise from a woman's participation in various relationships. The woman may simultaneously be a member of a family, with relationships with each family member, a member of a place of work, and a member of one or more other social bodies, such as hobby clubs, civic organizations, or political parties. In some women, there are covert relationships, including being part of an adulterous relationship or part of a crime or drug organization. Various disappointments or emotional injuries in a woman's social relationships may be enough to trigger depression.

Depression is more common in women than men. This differential occurrence has been noted in numerous epidemiologic studies. Proposed explanations have consisted of hormonal differences between men and women, differences in sociocultural roles, and differences in psychological development. Altered levels of some brain neurotransmitters have been associated with depression. The two neurotransmitters most studied are norepinephrine and serotonin. Although far from proven, the biogenic amine hypothesis contends that lowering of these neurotransmitters causes depression and normalizing them improves depression. There is much supportive evidence for this hypothesis, and current clinical antidepressant drugs increase levels of norepinephrine or serotonin or both while they relieve depression.

Differential Diagnosis

Several disorders or conditions may appear to be depression but are not (Box 36.5). For the obstetrician-gynecologist, chief among these is physical disease, which may be already known or may be occult. Cancer patients may lose weight and appetite, become fatigued, lose sex drive, and sleep poorly and appear depressed when they are not. Patients in acute or chronic pain may not be depressed but may show many of the symptoms of depression.

Normal fluctuations in mood are not considered pathologic and should not be treated. Only when mood changes are significantly distressing, lasting, or create dysfunction should they be judged abnormal.

Grief also is not considered pathologic. The grieving woman will show many symptoms of depression, but to grieve is considered human and does not indicate a problem. The line between normal grieving and depression is fuzzy, and experts disagree on where it should be drawn. Severe or prolonged psychosocial dysfunction, marked vegetative disturbances, significant change in self-esteem, or suicidal wishes are generally accepted as inconsistent with a simple, healthy

Box 36.5 Differential Diagnosis of Depression

Normal fluctuations in mood
Grief
Medical illnesses
Anxiety conditions
Schizophrenia and other psychotic conditions
Organic mental disorders
Alcohol or substance abuse
Personality disorders

grief reaction and therefore indicate the presence of a depression that needs treatment.

Anxiety disorders may resemble depression. Anxiety disorders share many symptoms in common with depression, including weight changes, fatigue, and insomnia. However, in anxiety disorders the predominant mood is one of fear, apprehension, and avoidance rather than sadness or disinterest.

Many patients with schizophrenia and other psychoses appear to be depressed. The flat affect, poor sleep, lack of motivation, and social withdrawal that accompany schizophrenia may lead to a misdiagnosis of depression.

Patients with some organic mental disorders may mistakenly appear depressed. In dementia, patients may show insomnia, poor energy, and blunted or labile affect. Patients with organic personality syndrome may show apathy, disinterest, or social withdrawal. Occasionally patients with delirium are socially withdrawn, do not sleep, and appear depressed. Alcohol or substance abuse may present as an apparent depression. Alcohol or other substances frequently alter sleep, appetite, mood, or behavior.

Personality disorders sometimes masquerade as depression. The paranoid, schizoid, schizotypal, or avoidant patient generally is withdrawn. The obsessive-compulsive personality is often emotionally constricted, which may be interpreted as depression. The passive-aggressive person may be resentful, sulky, contrary, and complaining, all of which may look like depression. These symptoms indicate enduring, innate character styles of relating to the environment rather than inner experiences of depression.

Coexistence of Depression and Other Psychiatric Disorders

Not only do other disorders often present to the clinician as apparent depression, but also other disorders and depression often coexist. It is common for women struggling with other disorders to lose morale and lose hope and become secondarily depressed. For example, a woman whose main problem is panic anxiety disorder may become depressed over her inability to control her panic attacks. A woman with a personality disorder may lead such a chaotic, unsatisfying lifestyle that depression develops to complicate the clinical picture. Depression may coexist with any of the psychiatric disorders discussed in the differential diagnosis section. Women with coexisting psychiatric conditions should be referred for psychiatric evaluation.

Diagnosis

The diagnosis of depression is a clinical process made after a psychiatric interview with the patient (16–18). Presently no laboratory tests or procedures reveal the presence, severity, or type of depression. The dexamethasone suppression test, which generated some initial excitement a decade ago as a possible reliable biologic test for depression, has many false-positive and false-negative results and now has only very limited use in the diagnostic process.

The interview should begin with as much privacy as possible. Other people in the room should be asked to leave because the patient may be embarrassed or reluctant to reveal personal information about inner feelings, sex drive, work performance, and other private matters in the presence of them. However, if the patient's immediate safety from suicidal impulses is a risk, privacy should be sacrificed.

The obstetrician-gynecologist should conduct the interview gently and with adequate time to elicit useful information. Sitting down is a simple maneuver that conveys caring and interest to the patient. Although it may be difficult in busy obstetric-gynecologic practices, the physician should be prepared to spend much more time with the depressed patient than with the average patient.

The patient may or may not spontaneously report depressed mood. If it is reported, the physician should acknowledge it and begin elaborating its intensity; frequency; duration; associated symptoms such as sleep, appetite, or energy changes; and any identifiable precipitants. If it is not reported spontaneously, but suspected, the physician may elicit it by asking general questions such as "How have you been emotionally lately?", "How has your mood been?", or "Besides your physical health, how has your emotional health been?" An occasional depressed patient may not respond to questions that focus on mood, sadness, blueness, and other terms for dysphoric emotions. These patients may have trouble recognizing and describing their emotions or may have a depression in which not sadness but rather disinterest and social withdrawal predominate. Consequently, it is vital for the physician to push the patient and ask questions in a variety of ways using alternate terms if depression is suspected.

The physician should not be misled by how the patient looks. Not all depressed patients look depressed. Some patients are able to conceal the depression in social settings. Unless there is reason to suspect the credibility of the patient's report, the physician should base the diagnosis on the patient's description of herself, rather than only on her appearance.

Always ask about suicide and homicide with any depressed patient, regardless of how minor the depression is. The question may be phrased in many ways, including "Have you felt so bad that you've wanted to end your life?" or "Have you been so upset that you've wanted to hurt anyone else?"

The best diagnostic evidence is the patient's own report, but this is sometimes either unavailable or of dubious value. In patients suspected to be depressed but unable to give a reliable history, the physician may need to interview collateral sources of information. Husbands, wives, other relatives, supervisors, or friends may be able to provide enough collateral evidence of depression to make the diagnosis. If the patient is hospitalized, talking with nurses taking care of her may reveal behavioral evidence of depression.

If collateral sources are interviewed, the principle of patient confidentiality must be strictly obeyed. Any information a patient provides is confidential and should never be discussed with anyone else not directly providing care for the patient, unless the patient agrees. This extends to even husbands, children, and other family members. Always write in the chart that the patient gave permission to talk with others. The exception to the rule of confidentiality is when someone's life could be at risk: the patient's own life if she is suicidal or someone else's life if she is homicidal.

The Problem of Diagnosing Depression in the Medically Sick Woman

When interviewing a woman with suspected depression who is also medically sick, the physician must decide whether symptoms are arising from the medical illness or from depression. For example, consider a woman with advanced ovarian cancer and some evidence of depression. Is the presence of weight loss part of the cancer effects or part of a depression? And if the patient is not sleeping well, perhaps because of pain at night, should that be counted as a manifestation of depression? These questions are important because most psychiatrists consider the number of depressive symptoms present as the best indicator of the need for an antidepressant medicine: more symptoms indicate a greater need for and potential benefit from medicine. Some authorities have suggested excluding some symptoms as diagnostically valid in the medically ill, whereas others have suggested modifying diagnostic criteria in these patients. However, the obstetrician-gynecologist, in an effort to preserve diagnostic simplicity and maximize the recognition of depression, should avoid trying to determine the exact origin of symptoms suggesting depression. If characteristic depressive symptoms are reported, they should be accepted as indicators of a depression. This approach may include women who are not seriously depressed, but in the nonpsychiatric setting it has value and is justified because it will err on the side of overdiagnosis rather than underdiagnosis (19).

Diagnosing Organic Depression

After interviewing and observing the patient, and others if necessary, the obstetrician-gynecologist should try to discern what kind of depression is present, especially if treatment will be started. The first and most important diagnostic step is to consider the possibility of an organic depression (Box 36.6). To diagnose an organic depression, the clinician should determine

Box 36.6 Diagnosing Organic Depression

Depressive symptoms are present.

An organic agent (or agents) is present that has been associated with causing depression.

The depressive symptoms and organic agent are linked temporally.

The physician judges that the organic agent is the cause of the depression rather than another cause (although in some patients both organic and non-organic causes are judged to be present).

that three conditions are present. The first is the presence of an organic agent or agents that may be the cause of the depression (see Box 36.4). Next, the clinician should temporally connect the onset of the etiologic agent with the appearance of the depression. For example, a woman who begins cimetidine and shortly thereafter becomes depressed is more likely to have an organic depression than is a woman who has been on cimetidine for 10 years but only recently became depressed. Finally, the physician must judge that the organic agent, rather than psychosocial stressors, is the cause of the depression. For example, a woman who began cimetidine recently but also experienced a painful divorce recently may have an organic depression, a nonorganic situational depression, or elements of both.

Diagnosing Major Depression

If an organic depression can be ruled out, then the kind of nonorganic depression present can be determined. The depressive symptoms reported or elicited should be scrutinized to see if they constitute a major depression. Major depression should be carefully ruled in or out because, besides organic depression, it is the depression that the obstetrician-gynecologist may have the greatest opportunity for treating without referral to a psychiatrist. The DSM-IV provides criteria that establish the minimum number and kind of symptoms that should be present to issue a diagnosis of major depression (Table 36.1). These criteria are useful in serving as a diagnostic guide and maintaining uniformity in diagnosing major depression among different physicians.

Table 36.1 Synopsis of DSM-IV Criteria for Major Depression

1. For at least 2 weeks the patient has had:
   Either a. depressed mood
   or
   b. lost of interest or pleasure
   Plus at least four of these:
   c. appetite disturbance–usually loss, sometimes increase
   d. weight loss or gain
   e. sleep disturbance–usually insomnia, sometimes hypersomnia
   f. psychomotor activity disturbance–either agitation or retardation
   g. lack of energy–fatigue
   h. sense of worthlessness or pathologic guilt
   i. inability to concentrate or make decisions
   j. thoughts of death or suicide or attempts
2. The depressed syndrome is not:
   a. a normal grief reaction
   b. part of another psychiatric disorder, e.g., schizophrenia
   c. an organic depression

Treatment

When treatment is suggested to a depressed woman, the first step the obstetrician-gynecologist faces is to decide who should treat her. Different physicians will have different interests in and tolerances of treating depressed patients, but every physician should urge the patient to accept treatment from some source. Many patients will refuse treatment, but for those who accept, the rates of success are relatively high.

There are three established strategies for the treatment of depression: biologic methods, psychosocial methods, and behavioral methods (20). Biologic treatment includes antidepressant medicines, antidepressant adjuncts, and electroconvulsive therapy. Psychosocial treatment includes psychotherapy and changes in one's social relationships. Behavioral methods include various techniques to diminish negative thoughts or moods and reinforce more positive ones. All of these strategies except antidepressant medicines are beyond the expertise of the average obstetrician-gynecologist and will not be described further. A psychiatrist evaluating a woman and planning a treatment program for her would examine the origins, content, and context of her depression and organize a plan from these treatment options.

Antidepressant Medicines

The treatment method that the obstetrician-gynecologist can become proficient in using is antidepressant medicines. This is fortunate because of the proven efficacy of these drugs, the increasing number of drugs available, the increasing ease of prescribing these newer drugs, the increasing safety and improving side effect profile of the drugs, and the large number of patients who are willing to try a medicine but refuse any other psychiatric treatment. The treatment of depression and need for antidepressant medicines vary with the kind of depression diagnosed. If an organic depression is diagnosed, the depression may remit if the causative agent can be identified and removed. For example, an organic depression secondary to hypothyroidism may resolve if the hypothyroid state is detected and corrected. Unfortunately, in some women the offending agent cannot be removed easily or quickly, and in others the depression persists even after the agent is removed. These patients need evaluation for symptom intensity and incapacitation and may need antidepressant medicine treatment.

The treatment of major depression almost always uses antidepressant medicines as a prominent part of the treatment plan, and many studies have proven the usefulness of these drugs in major depression (21). In other forms of depression, the use of antidepressant medicines is either more complex, less prominent, or unnecessary. In bipolar depression, antidepressant medicines should be used cautiously, generally in combination with a mood-stabilizer agent (e.g., lithium) to prevent precipitation of a manic episode. In dysthymic depression the efficacy of antidepressant medicines is less well studied but may be worth trying if the woman consents, especially with the safer medicines available now. The treatment of a simple adjustment depression does not include antidepressant medicines as a rule because this syndrome is either mild or short lived.

Approximately 20 drugs available in the United States are marketed as antidepressants. They may be classified as the tricyclics, the nontricyclics, the serotonin-selective agents, the norepinephrine-serotonin reuptake inhibitors, the monoamine oxidase inhibitors, and the psychostimulants (Table 36.2). The monoamine oxidase inhibitors and psychostimulants require special expertise and will not be discussed here. All other antidepressants, on the other hand, may be used quite effectively by obstetrician-gynecologists. Amitriptyline, a tricyclic, was for many years the "gold standard" among antidepressants. Newer drugs developed since amitriptyline generally are safer and have fewer or more tolerable side effects. These newer antidepressants increase the breadth of patients who can be safely treated in primary care and relieve the nonpsychiatrist of much of the worry of prescribing these drugs.

Therapeutic Effectiveness

All of the antidepressants are equally effective at relieving depression if used correctly. No antidepressant has been shown to have a therapeutic advantage in relieving symptoms faster or for a greater number of patients. These drugs relieve depression in 60% to 80% of patients who try them. Nonresponders may still improve with other methods of treatment.

Side Effects

Where the drugs differ clinically is not in overall effectiveness but in side effects (Table 36.3). Tricyclics tend to cause anticholinergic side effects that result from blockade of cholinergic neuron receptors. The symptoms that result include dry mouth, blurred vision, difficulty urinating, constipation, and forgetfulness or confusion. These side effects are so common and pharmacologically predictable that if a patient denies any of them, even on modest doses, the physician should question her compliance with the drug. These side effects are often mild and may improve or disappear with time, but for many patients they are insurmountably uncomfortable and lead to drug discontinuation. The most dangerous side effects from tricyclics are cardiovascular problems, which greatly limit their use. Tachycardia and conduction delay are fairly common but benign in healthy patients without heart disease. More serious side effects are orthostatic hypotension and cardiac arrhythmias. Orthostatic hypotension may be especially hazardous in the

Table 36.2 Antidepressant Medicines: Classification

COMMONLY USED IN OBSTETRICS-GYNECOLOGY			
Tricyclics	Nontricyclics	Serotonin-Selective Reuptake Inhibitors	Norepinephrine-Serotonin Reuptake Inhibitors
amitriptyline imipramine doxepine nortriptyline desipramine	trazodone bupropion	fluoxetine sertraline paroxetine	venlafaxine

RARELY USED IN OBSTETRICS-GYNECOLOGY	
Monoamine Oxidase Inhibitors	Psychostimulants
phenelzine tranylcypromine	methylphenidate dextroamphetamine

elderly woman and may lead to syncope or falls. Tricyclics slow cardiac conduction, lengthening the PR and QRS intervals on the electrocardiogram. These prolongations may present a danger for women with second-degree heart block or bundle branch block. The rhythm effects of tricyclics resemble the type 1A antiarrhythmic drugs (quinidine) and may reduce premature ventricular contractions. However, after a myocardial infarction, these drugs should be avoided because of the altered electrophysiology of the injured heart and the risk of inducing an arrhythmia. Tricyclics commonly cause drowsiness, which may be severe. They may cause a tremor, weight gain, or sexual side effects, including decreased desire or anorgasmia. Other less common side effects include seizures, precipitation of mania, and delirium. The tricyclics vary in their side effect profile. The triad of amitriptyline, imipramine, and doxepin share the tendency to produce strong anticholinergic side effects, relatively strong orthostatic hypotension, and strong sedation. These side effects are generally less frequent or milder with nortriptyline and desipramine. The tricyclics are contraindicated in patients with narrow-angle (closed-angle) glaucoma, certain cardiovascular conditions, constipation, and urinary retention.

The nontricyclics are a heterogeneous group of drugs that include trazodone and bupropion. Trazodone is very sedating but has few cardiac effects and is generally accepted as safe for use in cardiac illness. It also has no anticholinergic potential. Bupropion is not sedating and in fact may be stimulating to patients. It has no anticholinergic properties or cardiovascular side effects and does not cause weight gain. However, it may cause seizures at a higher rate than other antidepressants and care should be used in prescribing it. It is contraindicated in women with a known seizure disorder or a medical condition that increases the risk of a seizure, such as recent brain trauma. It is also contraindicated in women with bulimia.

The serotonin-selective reuptake antidepressants are fluoxetine, sertraline, and paroxetine. The name indicates their neurochemical mechanism of action: they selectively increase the availability of the neurotransmitter serotonin without affecting norepinephrine. These drugs have similar side effect profiles. They may cause nausea, sometimes with vomiting, headache, decreased sexual desire, anxiety, or sleep changes, either insomnia or hypersomnia. They do not cause anticholinergic side effects, weight gain, or cardiovascular problems. A problem that has been recognized with this class of drugs is that they inhibit the hepatic cytochrome system and may lead to elevated levels of other drugs depending on that system for degradation. There have been reports of toxic drug–drug interactions as a result. Sertraline is reported to have the least cytochrome inhibition, but the obstetrician-gynecologist should consider this potential carefully when prescribing any of these agents.

Venlafaxine is also free of anticholinergic, sedative,

Table 36.3 Antidepressant Medicines: Common Side Effects

Tricyclics	Nontricyclics	Serotonin-Selective Agents	Norepinephrine-Serotonin Reuptake Inhibitors
Dry mouth	trazodone	Nausea	Nausea
Blurry vision	Drowsiness	Headache	Drowsiness
Constipation	Dry mouth	Nervousness	Dizziness
Difficulty urinating	Dizziness	Insomnia	Nervousness
Increased pulse	Headache		
Orthostatic hypotension			
Drowsiness	bupropion		
Weight gain	Nervousness		
	Dry mouth		
	Insomnia		
	Headache		
	Nausea		
	Constipation		
	Tremor		

or serious cardiovascular side effects (22). Its common side effects are nausea, drowsiness, dry mouth, and dizziness, all of which are usually mild. It has also been associated with dose-dependent elevation of blood pressure, and blood pressure of a patient on venlafaxine should be measured at each visit. Venlafaxine is not highly bound to plasma proteins as with other antidepressants and does not inhibit the hepatic cytochrome enzymes responsible for the metabolism of many drugs. Consequently, venlafaxine has less potential for unpredictable drug–drug interactions than many antidepressants.

Overdose

The obstetrician-gynecologist, like any physician treating depressed patients with these medicines, must weigh the risk of a potential overdose. Depressed patients often try suicide with the very drugs used to help them. Tricyclics are dangerous or fatal in overdose. The newer agents are less dangerous and rarely fatal if taken alone, which is a huge advance in the drug treatment of depression.

Use During Pregnancy and Postpartum

Although it is advisable to avoid any psychotropic use during pregnancy, the risk of a severe untreated depression versus the risk of fetal exposure must be considered in deciding whether or not to use an antidepressant. Relative to other psychotropic drugs, tricyclic antidepressants are considered fairly safe to prescribe in pregnancy (23). There is no known tendency of these drugs to cause fetal abnormality although it cannot be recommended that they be used routinely in the first trimester. Newer antidepressants have not been in service long enough to generate any reliable safety information for use in pregnancy. There have been no fetal developmental problems reported yet, but the physician is again advised to carefully weigh all the risks when deciding whether or not to use these newer antidepressants. Antidepressants present in a delivering mother may affect the neonate. Tachycardia, heart failure, myoclonus, seizures, cyanosis, respiratory distress, irritability, and urinary retention may result. The cautious approach is to discontinue drugs for at least 2 weeks before anticipated delivery. If the obstetrician does not want to use an antidepressant, then psychotherapy may be of help. Electroconvulsive therapy also has been used safely during pregnancy. Antidepressants are secreted in the mother's milk, but the consequences of infant exposure are not known.

Prescribing Principles

Once the obstetrician-gynecologist has decided that a patient's depression may respond to an antidepressant medicine, the next step is to decide which one to use and to discuss the rationale of the medicine with the patient (Table 36.4). The patient should be informed of the purpose of the medicine and of the potential for side effects. She should be told about the delayed onset

Table 36.4 Antidepressant Medicines: Principles of Use

Diagnose correctly
  Rule out another psychiatric disorder presenting as depression
  Determine likelihood of antidepressant medicine response–best for major depression

Screen out medical contraindications and weigh risks of using versus risks of not using. Choose on basis of:
  Least disruptive, most advantageous side effects
  Patient response to particular drug in past
  Family history of response to drug in past

Generally start with low dose and increase slowly, especially in the elderly

Monitor for side effects and compliance

Weigh suicide risk
  Treat as inpatient in high-risk patients
  Outpatient acceptably safe in lower-risk patients, but
    Give small supplies of medicine
    Get family to keep and give medicine

Educate patient thoroughly
  Tell patient of possible side effects
  Inform about advantages–speed recovery
  Emphasize need for compliance and regular schedule dosing
  Tell patient they will not work as PRN medications
  Tell patient of delayed therapeutic onset–no "overnight miracles"
  Tell patient of need to commit to 6 to 12 months of treatment

of therapeutic effect (about 2 to 3 weeks in most patients, but up to 6 to 8 weeks in some slow responders) and the critical importance of taking the medicine on schedule rather than sporadically. She should be told not to increase doses when previous doses are missed. Finally, any questions the patient asks must be adequately answered.

Patients may reveal biases and prejudices against psychiatric medicines during the discussion of starting treatment, and it is important to address these adequately (Box 36.7). The woman may have taken an antidepressant previously and had a bad experience. She may have known someone else, often a relative, who had an unsatisfactory treatment experience. She may have heard overly critical media reports about problematic cases. She may have a resistance to the idea of using a psychiatric drug for help because of a fear of addiction or a feeling of humiliation. When these obstacles to treatment are addressed before beginning treatment, the doctor–patient relationship is generally strengthened, the chances of compliance are increased, and the chances of recovery from depression are increased.

The pharmacologic rationale for the selection of the

Box 36.7 Obstacles to Treatment

Before Treatment

Stigma of being a "psych case"
  Shame, family pressure
Misinterpretation, exaggeration of doctor's message:
  "I'm not crazy!"
Fear of psychiatric medicines and other treatments
  Movie stereotype
    "One Flew Over the Cuckoo's Nest"
  Past experience with treatments
    Personal experience–side effects
    Family or friends
Religious influence
  "You don't need that dope . . . just trust God!"

During Treatment

All of above issues plus constant risk of noncompliance

best antidepressant medicine for a patient is based on identifying the most prominent symptoms present that need prompt relief, predicting the drug's expected pharmacologic actions, including side effects, that may be helpful to or intolerable to the patient, and screening for any medical contraindications that may restrict the use of a particular antidepressant. Also important are the patient's previous experience, if any, with the drug and the expense of the drug. A target symptom is one that causes the patient significant dysfunction or distress. Insomnia, fatigue, weight loss, and poor concentration are symptoms that patients complain loudly about or cause significant dysfunction. Antidepressant selection should address these symptoms. An anticipated side effect from a given antidepressant may be intolerable in one patient but may be used advantageously in another patient with different depressive symptoms. For example, a patient who is greatly distressed by insomnia may benefit from a more sedating antidepressant. A patient who has lost weight may benefit from one that stimulates appetite and leads to weight gain. On the other hand, a patient who is already sluggish and oversleeping should not be placed on an antidepressant that is predictably sedating.

The physician must ensure that there are no medical contraindications to antidepressant use. The patient should be asked about heart disease, glaucoma, increased seizure risk, and the possibility of being pregnant. She should be asked about any conditions that may be aggravated by the anticholinergic potential of tricyclics, including preexisting urinary retention or constipation. She should be asked about liver or renal disease that may affect the metabolism or excretion of these drugs. The possibility of drug–drug interactions should be considered. Measuring baseline pulse and blood pressure and reviewing a pretreatment electrocardiogram are important, especially if a tricyclic will be prescribed.

Three other prescribing principles are crucial, but often neglected, in treating depression to a successful resolution. Compliance should be repeatedly and vigilantly monitored, the drug must be increased to an adequate level, and the dose must be continued at an adequate level for an adequate time. Most authorities recommend that, once a patient commits to an antidepressant, she continue it for 6 to 12 months before stopping it. Some patients require even longer treatment. If possible, withdrawal should be tapered over 2 to 4 weeks rather than abrupt.

Dosing Guidelines

If possible, the drug dosage should be started at low, introductory doses (Table 36.5). Also if possible, the drug dosage should be increased gradually for those drugs that need titration over a wide dosage range. Both of these strategies may diminish the risk of side effects. For example, in a healthy young woman, nortriptyline might be started at 25 mg at bedtime and increased to 50 mg at bedtime after 3 or 4 days and then to 75 mg at bedtime after another 3 or 4 days.

Among the tricyclics, nortriptyline may offer the most advantages in obstetrics and gynecology. Its side effects are similar to those of amitriptyline but usually much more tolerated. One large advantage in using nortriptyline in medical contexts is that its serum level can be monitored. It has an accepted therapeutic window of 50 to 150 ng/mL. No other antidepressant has a well established serum level therapeutic range. This feature allows the obstetrician-gynecologist to treat depressed patients with a greater degree of confidence in dosing accuracy. It also allows the monitoring of compliance. Because of the altered physiology of the woman during pregnancy, and the value of knowing reliably the level of antidepressant present in the body, nortriptyline may be the optimal antidepressant to use during pregnancy.

Trazodone, because of a relatively short half-life, should be given in divided doses, although some psychiatrists give it as a single dose once the depression has improved. Of all the antidepressants, trazodone has the highest allowable upper dosage limit, 600 mg/day, but this should be prescribed only after careful titration as an inpatient. Most patients will be helped in the range of 200–400 mg/day. Nonpsychiatrists often underprescribe trazodone because one of its side effects, drowsiness, often appears even at small doses. If this occurs, the physician probably should switch to another antidepressant that can be titrated up to a therapeutic level.

Bupropion has special dosing titration guidelines designed to introduce the drug gradually in divided doses and minimize the risk of a seizure. In a healthy young woman, the initial dose should be 100 mg twice a day. It may be increased to 300 mg/day in three divided doses but only on the fourth day. If it is

Table 36.5 Antidepressant Medicines: Dosing Parameters

Generic Name	Brand Name	Dosage Range (mg)	Typical Dose (mg)	Safety in Overdose
amitriptyline	Elavil	50–300	150	Dangerous
imipramine	Tofranil	50–300	150	Dangerous
doxepin	Sinequan	50–300	150	Dangerous
nortriptyline	Pamelor	25–150	75	Dangerous
desipramine	Norpramin	50–300	150	Dangerous
trazodone	Desyrel	150–600	300	Usually safe
bupropion	Wellbutrin	150–450	300	Usually safe
fluoxetine	Prozac	20–80	20	Usually safe
sertraline	Zoloft	50–200	50	Usually safe
paroxetine	Paxil	20–50	20	Usually safe
venlafaxine	Effexor	75–375	150	Usually safe

increased further, no single dose should be greater than 150 mg, and the maximum daily dosage is 450 mg/day.

Dosing of the serotonin-selective drugs is relatively simple. The usual starting doses of fluoxetine, sertraline, and paroxetine are, in order, 20, 50, and 20 mg daily. Because they may cause insomnia or stimulation as side effects, most authorities recommend starting them in the morning. If the less common side effects of drowsiness or lethargy occur, the dose can be switched to night.

Venlafaxine should be prescribed in divided doses because of its short half-life. Treatment in a healthy young woman should begin at 75 mg daily in divided doses of 37.5 mg twice a day. The physician should wait 2 weeks and reassess the woman for therapeutic versus side effects. The dose then may be increased to 150 mg daily, in divided doses of 50 mg three times a day or 75 mg twice a day.

Dosing in Special Populations

In general, starting doses should be lower and dose increases should be slower in both the elderly woman and the medically sick woman with depression. These special populations often have physiologic alterations that alter the pharmacokinetics of the antidepressants and lead to greater uncertainty of response with a given dose. Side effects, antidepressant toxicity, or drug–drug interactions with other concurrent medicines are more likely in these populations and may have more serious consequences than in the younger, healthy woman. Varying degrees of hepatic or renal impairment may be present that require dose adjustment.

The need to adjust dosage is most important with the tricyclics because the elderly and the medically sick may be extremely sensitive to the anticholinergic, cardiovascular, and sedative potential of these drugs. Trazodone and bupropion also should be started at lower doses. The serotonin-selective antidepressants are less a concern, but if time permits, it is probably wise to begin these also at lower doses. Venlafaxine currently is considered safe to start in the elderly at usual doses, but the safest approach with all antidepressants is to start at one fourth to one half usual doses. Divided rather than single doses are often better tolerated in these populations.

Impact of the Depressed Woman on the Obstetrician-Gynecologist

A depressed patient may be difficult to treat, and some physicians may develop emotional or behavioral reactions to depressed patients that adversely affect judgment and hinder good treatment. The physician may react with anger, frustration, detachment, or overzealousness in attempting to treat the depressed woman. These emotions may lead to inadequate, excessive, or illogical treatment. When this happens the important point to remember is that it should be recognized, addressed, and resolved, usually by referral to another physician.

Mistakes in Treating Depression

If the obstetrician-gynecologist accepts the task of treating a depressed woman, there are many potential errors to avoid (Box 36.8). The physician should not inadvertently reinforce any obstacles the patient may present to treatment, including fear, shame, or bias against receiving treatment. The physician must be certain that depression is indeed the main emotional problem rather than another condition. The physician should give the patient an adequate dose of an antidepressant medicine for an adequate time and must search for noncompliance if the patient fails to respond. Finally, the physician must try diligently to persuade the patient to accept psychiatric referral if the patient fails to respond to an adequate drug trial.

Psychiatric Referral

Women vary widely in their willingness to accept referral to a psychiatrist, but for those who are reluctant, the obstetrician-gynecologist can play a key role in facilitating the referral (Box 36.9). Probably the most important step in persuading the patient to accept referral is to have a positive, hopeful attitude (Box 36.10). If the physician sounds skeptical, then the patient will probably feel this way, too. The physician may be able to provide the patient with hope, which is often absent in depression. Although successful treatment of any patient is not guaranteed, it is not misleading patients to state that they have a very high chance of successful treatment.

The physician may also be able to decrease the patient's shame or fear. Patients can be told that they are not alone or unique in feeling depressed, which is a belief that many depressed patients acquire. Patients can be told that their depression is considered an ill-

Box 36.8 Common Mistakes in Treating Depression

Antitherapeutic attitude—reinforcing patient's fear, shame, bias

Incorrect medicine—using anxiolytics instead of antidepressants

Insufficient dose of antidepressant

Adequate dose but insufficient duration of treatment

Failing to adjust dose of some antidepressants for age

Overlooking patient's noncompliance

Box 36.9 Guidelines for Referral

When the obstetrician-gynecologist prefers not to treat the patient

When treatment has been tried but has failed

When the depression is especially intense or dangerous
- Suicidal depression
- Psychotic depression

When the depression coexists with another psychiatric condition

When the physician develops an emotional response to the patient that may interfere with treatment

When the patient requests referral

Box 36.10 Persuading the Patient to Accept Referral

The physician's attitude is important! If the physician sounds skeptical, the patient will probably feel this way, too.

The physician can:
- Decrease patient's shame
  - "What you're feeling happens to a lot people."
- Decrease patient's fear
  - "The psychiatrist is another doctor who may want to try a medicine to help you feel better."
- Mention past successes
  - "I've referred other people in the past and they got better."
- Instill hope and optimism
  - "With the right treatment, almost everyone eventually feels better."

ness, as deserving of treatment as any physical illness. Patients can be told that the psychiatrist is another physician with special expertise working within the medical community, which may decrease fear. If the obstetrician-gynecologist has referred patients in the past, and the patients were treated successfully, this can be mentioned to emphasize the potential for recovery.

Conclusion

Depression is a disorder of mood with other accompanying vegetative, cognitive, and behavioral symptoms. There are different kinds of depression, with major depression the most common and important to the obstetrician-gynecologist. Major depression may be disabling, distressing, and sometimes deadly. Psychiatry has developed good treatments for depression if the patient accepts them. The obstetrician-gynecologist will have abundant opportunities to treat depressed women or facilitate their referral to a psychiatrist.

REFERENCES

1. Frances A, First MB, Pincus HA, Widiger TA, eds. Diagnostic and statistical manual. 4th ed. Washington, DC: American Psychiatric Association, 1994.

2. Regier DA, Myers JK, Kramer M, et al. The NIMH Epidemiologic Catchment Area Program. Arch Gen Psychiatry 1984;41:934–941.

3. Kessler RC, McGonagle KA, Zhao S, et al. Lifetime and 12-month prevalence of DSM-III-R psychiatric disorders in the United States. Arch Gen Psychiatry 1994;51:8–19.

4. Kessler RC, McGonagle KA, Swartz M, et al. Sex and depression in the National Comorbidity Survey I: lifetime prevalence, chronicity and recurrence. J Affective Disord 1993;29:85–96.

5. Greenberg PE, Stiglin LE, Finkelstein SN, Berndt ER. The economic burden of depression in 1990. J Clin Psychiatry 1993;54:405–418.

6. Hirschfeld RMA, Goodwin FK. Mood disorders. In: Talbott JA, Hales RE, Yudofsky SC, eds. The American Psychiatric Press Textbook of psychiatry. Washington, DC: American Psychiatric Press, 1988: 403–441.

7. Hamilton M. Mood disorders: clinical features. In: Kaplan HI, Sadock BJ, eds. Comprehensive textbook of psychiatry. 5th ed. vol I. Baltimore: Williams & Wilkins, 1989:892–913.

8. Lesse S. The masked depression syndrome-results of a seventeen-year clinical study. Am J Psychother 1983;37:456–475.

9. Fava M, Anderson K, Rosenbaum JF. "Anger attacks": possible variants of panic and major depressive disorders. Am J Psychiatry 1990;147:867–870.

10. Rosenbaum M. The role of depression in couples involved in murder-suicide and homicide. Am J Psychiatry 1990;147:1036–1039.

11. Cohen-Cole SA, Brown FW, McDaniel JS. Assessment of depression and grief reactions in the medically ill. In: Stoudemire A, Fogel BS, eds. Psychiatric care of the medical patient. New York: Oxford University Press, 1993;53–69.

12. Cassem NH. Depression. In: Cassem NH, ed. Massachusetts General Hospital handbook of general hospital psychiatry. 3rd ed. St. Louis: Mosby-Year Book 1991:237–268.

13. Harris B. Maternity blues. Br J Psychiatry 1980;136:520–521.

14. O'Hara MW, Zekoski EM. Postpartum depression: a comprehensive review. In: Kumar R, Brockington IF, eds. Motherhood and mental illness. vol 2. London: Wright, 1988:17–63.

15. Robinson GE, Stewart DE. Postpartum disorders. In: Stewart DE, Stotland NL, eds. Psychological aspects of women's health care. Washington, DC: American Psychiatric Press, 1993:115–138.

16. MacKinnon RA, Yudofsky SC. The psychiatric evaluation in clinical practice. Philadelphia: JB Lippincott, 1986:1–33.

17. Halleck SL. Evaluation of the psychiatric patient: a primer. New York: Plenum Medical Book, 1991:53–110.

18. Shea SC. Psychiatric interviewing: the art of understanding. Philadelphia: WB Saunders, 1988:138–192.

19. Cohen-Cole SA, Stoudemire A. Major depression and physical illness: special considerations in diagnosis and biologic treatment. Psychiatr Clin North Am 1987;10:1–17.

20. American Psychiatric Association. Practice guideline for major depressive disorder in adults. Am J Psychiatry 1993;150(suppl):1–26.

21. Gelenberg AJ, Bassuk EL, Schoonover SC. The practitioner's guide to psychoactive drugs. 3rd ed. New

York: Plenum Medical Book, 1991:23–87.

22. Montgomery SA. Venlafaxine: a new dimension in antidepressant pharmacotherapy. J Clin Psychiatry 1993;54:119–126.

23. Stewart DE, Robinson GE. Psychotropic drugs and electroconvulsive therapy during pregnancy and lactation. In: Stewart DE, Stotland NL, eds. Psychological aspects of women's health care. Washington, DC: American Psychiatric Press, 1993:71–95.

CHAPTER 37

ALCOHOL AND DRUG ADDICTIONS

Norman D. Huggins

Alcohol and drug addictions are referred to in the *Diagnostic and Statistical Manual of Mental Disorders* (DSM-IV) (1) as substance-related disorders, and substances are referred to as drugs of abuse, medications, or toxins. Specific criteria were developed by the American Psychiatric Association to describe and diagnose the various substance-related disorders. The term *substance-related disorders* will be restricted to those substances that are psychoactive. *Psychoactive substances* are defined as substances that alter mood or feeling states. Psychoactive substances that induce pleasurable feelings or lessen unpleasant feelings tend to be used more frequently and repeatedly by the chemically dependent woman.

Substance-related disorders follow a common course, usually initiated with experimental use of the psychoactive substance then progression to abuse and finally to dependency. *Psychoactive substance use* is defined as a reversible substance-specific syndrome due to the recent ingestion of a substance that causes significant maladaptive behavioral or psychological change due to the substance effects on the central nervous system (CNS). The psychoactive substance produces an acute state of intoxication. *Psychoactive substance abuse* is defined as the recurrent use of a substance in a manner that differs from generally approved medical or social practices and in such a manner that endangers health and social or occupational functioning, and continued use despite combined problems caused by use of the substance. *Psychoactive substance dependency/addiction* is defined as a syndrome manifested by an overwhelming desire or compulsion to continue taking a substance in such a manner to produce a state of periodic or chronic intoxication (impairment), inability to decrease or stop use of the substance (loss of control), a tendency to increase the dosage (tolerance), a daily need for the substance to feel normal (physical/psychological dependence), and continued use of the substance despite the detrimental effects the substance causes to the individual and society. The term psychoactive substance will be used interchangeably with drugs and alcohol; the term addiction will be used interchangeably with chemical dependency.

These definitions of psychoactive substance use, abuse, and dependency are generally accepted by health care providers working in the specialty of addiction medicine and substance abuse. There is disagreement regarding whether or not psychoactive substance dependence/chemical dependence/addiction is a disease process or a behavioral problem. An ailment is more likely to be considered a disease when a physician's intervention is necessary for treatment; otherwise, it is not considered a disease process. If the cause or course of the condition appears to be primarily under the control of the individual then it is thought to be a moral or behavioral problem. If on the other hand, the cause and course of the condition is primarily beyond the control or the intention of the individual, it is more acceptable to call that condition a disease. There is little agreement as to the etiology of chemical dependency/addiction. Multiple theories attempt to explain the cause or causes of chemical dependency but as of yet no single theory is generally accepted (2).

Etiology

Researchers have identified several factors involved in the initiation and perpetuation of psychoactive substance use including genetic, familial, environmental, occupational, cultural, psychological, and biologic. The relative contributions of these risk factors vary among individuals. Factors associated with the initial use of a psychoactive substance differ from factors associated with continued or progressive use. There are individual differences and variations in response to psychoactive substances. The substance effect and pattern of usage are the result of complex interactions among biologic, psychological, sociocultural, family, and environmental variables. Women are differentially at risk for psychoactive substance use and making the transition from use to abuse to dependency. Studies on the etiology of drug use and abuse have identified several risk factors: genetic, psychological, and peer and environmental.

Genetic Risk Factors

Studies demonstrate an apparent genetic inheritance of an unspecified substance-induced response (3). Some individuals experience more euphoria from alcohol than do others. This factor is believed to be under genetic control. Euphoria is a positive reinforcer; people who experience the most euphoria are the ones most likely to use and continue using the substance. Alcohol may be more reinforcing in genetically susceptible individuals. There is a wide range of innate variations in response to alcohol, and this response may be genetically influenced. Some individuals feel the "drug effect" more intensely than others—both the positive euphoriant effects and the negative dysphoriant effects. Drug effects vary greatly depending on the physiology and psychology of the person taking them. Susceptibility to a particular substance may be partly inherited (under genetic control) or it may reflect psychosocial influences or both.

Psychological/Psychiatric Risk Factors

Studies using clinical populations of chemically dependent patients consistently demonstrate high levels of psychopathology (4). Female patients tend to have high levels of anxiety, depressive symptoms, and lower-self esteem. Individuals tend to have a personal preference for a particular substance, the "drug of choice." This preference is the result of the drug's psychoactive effects interacting with the unique personality and behavioral patterns of the individual. This interaction between drug effect and personality predisposes the individual to becoming dependent on a particular drug. Some substances produce changes in personality that are enduring. If these changes are valued by the individual the probability of continued use will be increased. Some behaviors, which appear to be self-destructive, might be aimed at achieving secondary gains that are highly valued by the individual and not recognized by an outside observer. Continued use is influenced by the user's perception of how well the substance satisfies specific needs.

Peer and Environmental Risk Factors

The attitudes and behavior of others regarding substance use is a strong influence on the individual's initial use of the substance. Initiation and continuation of usage are supported by peer group involvement. Peers also provide role models of drug users who have not experienced negative consequences from their drug usage. Association with drug-using peers is a strong and consistently reported finding for predicting drug abuse and addiction. An important factor in initiating drug usage is the degree of access to the substance (drug availability). The availability of substances, easy access to substances, prevailing attitudes of significant others, and the acceptability of substance use perceived within the woman's social network make it easier for a woman to use drugs. Many women who have an initial experience with a specific psychoactive substance do not become repetitive users and many who do become repetitive users do not become addicted. The cause for each stage is different. Different women may be influenced by different situations, producing different behavioral effects. The same behavior may have different causes in different people. What stimulates one woman to engage in substance usage may not stimulate another. Every woman is different and must be accessed individually.

Theories of Addiction

The more risk factors a woman has, the more at risk she is to becoming addicted to substances. A single isolated risk factor has little significance in predicting why women begin taking drugs, escalate to abusing drugs, and progress to addiction. Every psychoactive substance user is not an abuser and every psychoactive substance abuser does not become dependent. The 1991 National Household Survey on Drug Abuse reported that 5 million childbearing women aged 15 to

44 reported they had used an illicit drug at least once during the month prior to the survey and 3.3 million of these women reported that one of the drugs they used was cocaine. Most women who use alcohol and other psychoactive substances (prescription drugs) and illicit drugs (heroin, cocaine, marijuana, etc.) never develop an addiction to these substances. Why is it that some women become chemically dependent and others do not? What separates the user from abuser and the abuser from the addict? What makes a woman susceptible to becoming addicted to psychoactive drugs? Many theories are proposed. The three most advocated theories of psychoactive chemical dependency are biogenetic disease, psychodynamic, and behavioral learning.

Biogenetic Disease Theory

According to this theory, chemical dependency is a primary disease process, which is inherited. The disease is chronic, progressive, and fatal if not treated. The clinical course is identifiable and predictable. The process of addiction appears to be linked to changes in the biochemistry of the individual who uses chemicals. The neurochemical changes can bring about tolerance, dependence, and withdrawal symptoms. A physiologic defect causes chemical dependence and the addiction is initiated when the chemical is used by individuals with a genetic predisposition. The individual must stop all intake of the substance. This means that a dependent person cannot drink or use drugs socially. Treatment is directed toward achieving total abstinence from all psychoactive substances.

Psychodynamic Theory

Chemical dependency is a syndrome caused by some underlying psychological conflict. When the conflict exists, it causes abnormal behaviors that become symptoms by which the presence of the psychological conflict can be recognized. The nature of the psychological conflict is responsible for the chemical dependency. Chemical dependency occurs either as symptoms of another primary mental disorder or as a coping mechanism for deficits in psychological structuring or functioning. The chemically dependent woman uses psychoactive substances to medicate symptoms of other mental disorders such as anxiety or depression. The use of psychoactive substances acts as medication to treat, the underlying condition. Treatment using psychotherapy and pharmacotherapy is directed toward resolving the underlying psychological conflict.

Behavioral Learning Theory

Chemical dependency is caused by learning maladaptive behaviors and habits. The woman learned inappropriate and ineffective ways of coping with life's experiences. Use of psychoactive substances is considered maladaptive behavior and can be reversed by relearning more appropriate behavior. Treatment is directed toward teaching new behaviors and unlearning maladaptive behavior.

Theory Acceptance

The numerous theories being voiced provide a means to conceptualize psychoactive substance dependency. They allow clinicians to predict the clinical course of the condition, treatment needs of the patient, and prognosis. The biogenetic disease theory of psychoactive substance dependence is the theory officially advocated and accepted by the American Psychiatric Association, the American Medical Association, the World Health Organization, the American Public Health Association, the National Council on Alcoholism, and the American Society of Addiction Medicine. According to this biogenetic disease theory, the etiology of biologic factors are considered to be important. The psychoactive substance abuser is viewed as someone who is suffering from an illness caused by the disease of chemical dependency itself. The primary symptom of the disease is considered to be an irreversible loss of control over the substance. Without complete abstinence the disease is regarded as being progressive and often fatal. The major treatment is to focus on psychoactive substance dependence as the primary problem rather than focusing on moral weakness, lack of self-control, or lack of psychological stability. The biogenetic disease theory conceptualizes addiction as a primary, progressive relapsing, chronic but treatable disease with biologic, psychological and sociocultural components. It is important that clinicians be aware of the various theories of addiction and be flexible enough to use the advantages each offers. Psychoactive substance dependency appears to have multiple causes and therefore, it is a multifactorial biopsychosocial illness. The clinician needs to be aware of multiple treatment approaches to individualize treatment according to the individual woman's needs.

Presentation

Women are frequently portrayed in pharmaceutical advertisements. A common theme in these advertisements is that a woman should not suffer from allergies, asthma, muscle cramps, menstrual cramps, colds, diarrhea, insomnia, or any other physical discomfort when relief is available with the use of their pharmaceutical product. Women are the major consumers of over-the-counter medications and are also prescribed more medications by their personal physicians than are men. Women's usage of illicit psychoactive substances and prescriptions has been increasing at an alarming rate. Women's prescription psychoactive substance usage has been and remains very high. Women tend to obtain psychoactive substances from several sources, the two primary ones being physicians and drug dealers. The drug dealers provide both prescription pharmaceutical psychoactive substances, which have been obtained illegally, and illicit drugs such as cocaine, heroin, amphetamines, cannabis, methylenedioxyamphetamine (MDA), and D-lysergic acid diethylamide (LSD). Physicians provide pharmaceutical psychoactive substances. Female psychoactive substance users generally find it easier to obtain prescription psychoactive drugs from physicians because women are believed to have more medical problems and it is acceptable for them to seek medical attention.

Women routinely present with multiple complaints that are commonly treated with prescription psychoactive medications. The treating physician unsuspectingly prescribes medications that tend to perpeputate or exacerbate the underlying psychoactive substance disorder. Physical health concern is the most common reason for psychoactive substance-dependent women to seek medical attention. They complain of multiple physical and emotional symptoms as well as problems experienced in daily living. These women are physically ill more often than nonaddicted women and they frequently seek medical attention. They may not be consciously aware that the psychoactive substance is the source of their ailments and complaints. They may be too ashamed or embarrassed to report psychoactive substance use to the physician. The physician's failure to recognize psychoactive substance use problems in women during the early stages of the disease process results in symptomatic treatment of the complaints with prescription psychoactive medications, thus perpetuating or creating additional psychoactive substance dependency without interrupting the underlying disease process. These women often use prescription psychoactive substances to hide the addiction. Because women view taking prescription medications as being acceptable, their psychoactive substance dependency is likely to have progressed farther before it is diagnosed and treated.

Early diagnosis and intervention are the most effective means of reducing the mental and physical complications associated with the disease of psychoactive substance dependency. Failure to identify the disease of psychoactive substance dependency often allows women to maintain a lifestyle that places them at risk for contacting serious disease. They suffer with an increased incidence of anxiety, depression, infections of the gynecologic and urinary systems, infection with human immunodeficiency virus, anemia, sexually transmitted diseases, hepatitis type B, hypertension, diabetes, colitis, gastritis, sleep disturbance, dysmenorrhea, toxemia, and pre-eclampsia. They are also at greater risk for cervical and uterine malignancies and have a high incidence of unplanned pregnancies and dental problems. Their lifestyles cause them to neglect health and nutrition. Minor health problems are often neglected until they progress to serious life-threatening conditions. Definitive treatment becomes more difficult and less successful.

There is no "typical woman substance abuser." She presents in all shapes and sizes, from all segments of society, from all racial and ethnic groups, and from all socioeconomic levels. The psychoactive substance-dependent woman rarely appears at the physician's office or hospital with a primary complaint of drug addiction. She presents with multiple subjective complaints or symptoms resulting from use of the substance, directly caused by the substance or complications secondary to the substance. Presenting complaints must be differentiated from the specific substance used and possible medical condition unrelated to psychoactive substance use.

On first appearance, the psychoactive-dependent woman presenting with physical ailments may be indistinguishable from the nonsubstance-abusing woman. She is likely to present in a sober state with no obvious signs of being addicted. She may have or have had a bonafide complaint for which the psychoactive substance was prescribed. She may have a past medical history of a painful ailment, which has been unresponsive to treatment; however, the current appropriate physical examination is usually normal. She usually presents with symptoms of depression and extreme anxiety with acting out behavior, loss of emotional control, weeping, and a dramatic display of symptoms. Diagnosing the psychoactive-dependent woman after one visit is often difficult. The physician must assess the patient over a period of time to obtain as much information as possible. No single symptom or even a few can identify the psychoactive substance-dependent woman. Only when several of these symptoms are present together with a psychosocial history and the physician observes an increasing number of signs and symptoms suggesting that psychoactive substances are responsible for disrupting the life of the female patient is the physician then able to diagnose the disease of psychoactive substance dependence. A primary identifying sign that is always present is that the use of the psychoactive substance has become a disruptive factor in the woman's life.

Psychoactive substance-dependent women are not characterized by specific signs and symptoms; however, they exhibit common characteristics. They are most likely to have been doctor shopping and report feeling dissatisfied with previous doctors or her personal physician is unavailable. They primarily seek prescription drugs for their personal use. The most desired prescription drugs are opiate-derivative analgesics, benzodiazepines, barbiturates, and amphetamines. They often give a history of being allergic to less potent psychoactive substances, thus limiting the physician's selection to the potent psychoactive substances. They often report being successfully treated with a specific psychoactive substance in the past but cannot recall the specific name of the medication. They describe the drug in detail, thus indirectly providing the physician with the name of the psychoactive substance they desire.

They possess more than a general knowledge of psychoactive substances and are well versed in clinical terminology. They present with a ready made diagnosis and monopolize the interview to discourage specific questions. They frequently complain of a painful ailment and they frequently telephone the physician requesting pain medication or sedatives, frequently obtain medications from associate physicians during the primary physician's absence, frequently misuse medication, attempt to obtain refills of psychoactive medications early, and report loss of prescriptions or medications. They fail to keep follow-up appointments; they are often absent from work on Mondays and Fridays and request medical verification of illness and return-to-work slips. They tend to come from dysfunctional families, have experienced physical abuse or sexual abuse, and have family disruption due to chronic family illness, parental death, or parental conflict. They maintain strong ties with family of origin, relying on their mother for support. Often they exhibit poor interpersonal skills, have few social support systems, and are more likely to cope alone. They are less likely to use social strategies to cope with unpleasant emotions and experience difficulty in relating to other women. They experience much higher levels of stress than nondrug-using women and have a negative self-concept as a single parent with one or more dependent children. Terminated marriages through divorce or separation are common. Low level of education, lack of financial resources, living alone, and higher levels of stress in responsibility for children contribute to their substance dependency. They tend to neglect personal grooming and hygiene and present with unexplained cuts, abrasions, and bruises and cigarette burns in clothing. They exhibit minimal facial expression and use a flat tone of voice, always crying, self-pitying, filled with unreasonable anger and hostility, and supersensitive. They are unable to maintain stable employment or friendships.

All of these are signs that something is seriously wrong in a woman's life and use of psychoactive substances may be the cause. The woman may have strong denial of suffering with a psychoactive substance dependence. The physician's early diagnosis of medical consequences of psychoactive substance dependence may be useful in motivating the woman to accept treatment. She may be less likely to conceal information and may become ready to accept that use of psychoactive substances has caused her to lose control of her life.

Psychoactive substances tend to cause psychiatry symptoms consistent with their pharmacologic properties: acute use of stimulants causes signs and symptoms that can be seen in mania, anxiety, panic, delirium, and delusional disorders. Chronic stimulant usage can result in fatigue, disturbances in sleep, depressed mood, and suicidal ideation. Drug effects vary greatly depending on the individual's physical and mental state at the time she ingests the drug, the social setting in which the drug was ingested, the substance used, the substance purity and dosage, duration of substance effects, frequency of usage, degree of tolerance to the substance, concurrent use of other substances, presence of underlying medical or psychological problems, route of administration, and prior substance abuse experience. Reaction to psychoactive substances presents some of the most complex diagnostic and treatment issues to clinicians. Diagnosis requires knowledge of the pharmacology properties of psychoactive substances as well as an understanding of the various physical and behavioral reactions that occur. When the physician observes an increasing number of risk factors and signs and symptoms suggestive of a psychoactive substance disorder, he or she should consult with a specialist in the field of addiction. Women psychoactive substance abusers require treatment services that address their addiction as well as their unique personal problems.

Classification of Psychoactive Substances

Substances discussed in this section are limited to drugs that effect the brain by inducing a pleasurable sensation, euphoria, altering mood and behavior. These substances are commonly abused by women. The psychoactive substances are grouped into categories based on their usual effects induced at usual dosages and their clinically revelant properties. The most prominent effects are emphasized and observations are made on the responses most likely to occur. All substances are capable of inducing different effects when administered at different dosages. Many drug effects are dose related. The drug has one set of effects when one amount is consumed and quite different effects if four times the initial amount is consumed. Substances that share similar clinical properties are placed into the same group. If one substance in a group is physically addicting, it is very likely that other substances within the group are also physically addicting. If two substances within the group are taken at the same time, they are likely to potentiate the effects of each other, resulting in a potential overdose.

Some psychoactive drugs when taken in toxic amounts may induce effects characteristic of substances in another group. For example, opiate analgesics taken in sufficient quantity can cause CNS depression. Cocaine when taken in sufficient quantity can cause hallucinatory experiences. MDA in usual dosage can cause both CNS stimulation and altered sensory perception. Some psychoactive substances such as phencyclidine (PCP) process properties from several different groups. PCP is a dissociative anesthetic that causes mind–body dissociation anesthesia, psychomotor stimulation, and hallucinations. Psychoactive substances commonly abused by women are grouped into one of these categories:

Central nervous system stimulants
Central nervous system depressants
Opiate analgesies
Hallucinogens

Central Nervous System Stimulants

These psychoactive substances stimulate the brain. Frequently prescribed CNS stimulants are cocaine HCl, phenmetrazine (Preludin), methylphenidate (Ritalin), phentermine (Ionamin), diethylpropion (Tenuate, Tepanil), mazindol (Sanorex), pemoline (Cylert), and dextroamphetamine (Biphetamine, Dexedrine). Over-the-counter less potent CNS stimulants include beverages containing caffeine (cocoa, coffee, tea, soft drinks), tobacco (nicotine), chocolate (*Theobroma cacao*), propylhexedrine (Benzedrex inhaler), Oxymetazoline HCl (Afrin Nasal Spray), phenylephrine HCl (Neo-Synephrine), Phenylpropanolamine (Dexatrim), ephedrine (Efedron), and pseudoephedrine sulfate (Afrinol). Illicit CNS stimulates include crack cocaine, methoxylated amphetamines, MDMA, MDA, STP, XTC, ecstacy, among others. The methoxylated amphetamines are substances with stimulant and hallucinogenic properties. They have a tendency to activate latent genitiourinary tract infection in women. CNS stimulants produce euphoria, a sense of well-being, increased energy, and mental alertness. At low dosage sexual desire is enhanced but as the dosage increases and use becomes chronic, sexual desire is inhibited and women have difficulty achieving orgasm. Tolerance and psychological dependency develop rapidly. The withdrawal syndrome consists of depression, irritability, lassitude, anxiety, mood swings, hypersomnia, hyperphagia, suicidal ideation, and a strong desire to use the stimulant again. There can be a dysphoric state with intense feelings of boredom, which can last for months. Urinalysis can usually detect the substance 24 to 72 hours after last use although no specific laboratory abnormalities are directly caused by CNS stimulants. Treatment for both the acute intoxicated state and withdrawal syndrome is supportive and symptomatic; medication is rarely needed.

Central Nervous System Depressants

These psychoactive substances reduce brain activity. Commonly prescribed CNS depressants are benzodiazepines (Xanax, Valium, Ativan, Klonipin, etc.), barbituates (Amytol, Nembutal, Seconal, etc.), muscle relaxants (Parafon, Forte, Soma, etc,), and over-the-counter preparations containing alcohol, antihistamines, scopolamine, or bromides (Nervine, Sominex, Unisom, Sleep-EZE, Excedrin P.M., etc.). These over-the-counter preparations are generally taken in amounts 5 to 10 times the recommended dosage. The acute effects caused by CNS depressants include euphoria, tranquility, loss of inhibitions, gregariousness, slurred speech, unsteady gait, and relaxation. Some individuals exhibit progressive and violent behavior. CNS depressants are generally taken orally; tolerance and physical dependency develop quickly. Abruptly stopping or suddenly reducing the dosage consumed can result in a withdrawal syndrome characterized by postural hypotension, coarse rhythmic intention tremors, hyperreflexia, anxiety, agitation, insomnia, clammy skin, dilated pupils, muscle weakness, weak and rapid pulse, hallucinations, delirium, and convulsions. The CNS depressant withdrawal syndrome can be life-threatening and inpatient treatment is generally required to withdraw these CNS depressants. Inhalants (nitrous oxide, amylnitrate, butylnitrate) and household products (hair spray, nail polish remover, lighter fluid, liquid paper) all contain volatile hydrocarbon and chlorohydrocarbon chemicals with CNS depressant properties. The intoxication from these substances is similar to other CNS depressants. Adult women seldom abuse these substances; they tend to be more frequently abused by adolescent girls.

Alcohol is the primary CNS depressant abused by women. Women tend to mix alcohol with other drugs more frequently than men (5,6) and often consume alcohol in secret or in the privacy of their home. Women become problem drinkers at a much later age than do men. Women suffer more negative effects from alcohol than do men because of their different physiology (7). A given amount of alcohol will produce higher blood alcohol levels in a woman than in a man because women have a lower percentage of body water content that do men. A woman can absorb up to 30% more alcohol into her blood than a man of the same weight consuming the same amount of alcohol. Women risk developing liver disease at an earlier age and after a shorter period and lower level of alcohol consumption than men.

Laboratory tests are available to identify altered organ functioning caused by excessive alcohol consumption. These simple blood tests can be used to identify recent heavy drinking (women consuming five or more drinks per day). The laboratory test γ-glutamyltranspeptidase (GGT) is one of the most frequently used blood tests for the evaluation of heavy alcohol intake. GGT levels are elevated following repetitive heavy alcohol consumption. Similar results are likely to be observed for other liver function tests such as aspartate aminotransferase and alanine aminotransferase. The average size of the red blood cell is likely to be increased in women who consume large amounts of alcohol. The mean corpuscular volume (MCV) is often elevated. The combination of elevated GGT and MCV is believed to identify 91% of alcoholics in the general medical population. These laboratory tests are useful in identifying women with heavy acute and chronic alcohol consumption.

Opiates/Analgesics

These psychoactive substances suppress pain. Frequently prescribed natural opiates are morphine and codeine, synthetic opiate derivatives; hydrocodone (Hycodan, Loritab), dihydromorphine (Heroin), and synthetics; meperidine (Denerol), methadone (Dolophine), propoxyphene (Darvon), and pentazocine (Talwin). Opiate analgesics are generally taken orally; however, chronic users sometimes inject the opiates IV. Opiates are desired for the "rush," which is most intense when the opiate is injected IV. The rush is described as an intense pleasurable sensation similar to a total body orgasm, as sense of well-being and euphoria, complete relaxation, mental tranquility, and drowsiness. Tolerance and physical dependency develop rapidly with prolonged use of opiates. A withdrawal syndrome begins 8 to 12 hours after the last dosage. The initial withdrawal symptoms are similar to those of a common cold—rhinorrhea, lacrimation, perspiration, slightly elevated temperature, and dilated pupils sluggishly reactive to direct light. Symptoms increase in severity 48 to 72 hours after the last dosage and include symptoms similar to dysentery—diarrhea, abdominal cramps, weakness, nausea, vomiting, muscle and joint pain, insomnia, muscle twitches, and piloerection. If untreated the opiate withdrawal syndrome will gradually subside in 7 to 14 days. Inpatient treatment is necessary for administering medications to ameliorate the withdrawal syndrome. No specific laboratory tests identify opiate abusers.

Hallucinogens

These psychoactive substances alter sensory perception and induce intense emotional feelings. Commonly abused hallucinogens include LSD, PCP, psilocybine, ibogaine, peyote, and mescaline. Hallucinogens are taken orally; usually periodically chronic repetitive use is rare. Tolerance develops rapidly to the effects of LSD, mescaline, psilocybine and PCP, which is one reason hallucinogens are not taken continually. Hallucinogens induce a state of relaxation, euphoria, distortions of surroundings and body image, sensation of floating in space, vivid hallucinatory experiences involving all sensory organs, and a feeling that certain visual perceptions can be seen and heard. This phenomenon is called synesthesia. Hallucinogens do not produce physical dependency. Treatment involves supportive and symptomatic therapy for the undesirable symptoms or panic reaction associated with "bad trips." The environmental setting, personality of the woman, and personal expectations determine if the hallucinogenic effects will be positive or negative.

The second most frequently abused illicit psychoactive substance is Δ-tetrahydrocannabinol (THC, marijuana), which is classed as an hallucinogen. Marijuana is usually smoked. It produces a dreamlike state of relaxation, sense of well-being, loss of inhibitions, and changes in the perception and sense of time. Marijuana impairs short-term memory and performance of tasks that require concentration and coordination. In susceptible women, marijuana can produce adverse effects characterized by acute panic reaction and psychosis. Marijuana with a low concentration of THC is well tolerated but forms of marijuana with highly concentrated THC can induce hallucinatory experiences similar to the other hallucinogens.

Treatment

Women are underrepresented in substance abuse treatment programs. An estimated 10 million American adult women currently experience problems directly related to the disease of psychoactive substance dependency, however, very few are currently in treatment. Several factors have been identified as being barriers to treatment.

1. Women are ashamed and guilty over their drug and alcohol use and tend to conceal their use of psychoactive substances. They tend to drink alcohol and take other drugs alone, often in the privacy of the kitchen or bedroom.
2. Women fail to seek treatment for psychoactive substance abuse because of the negative moralistic attitude of physicians toward chemically dependent women.
3. Because of social prejudices against excessive alcohol and drug use by women, they tend to drink alone and away from other people and tend to combine sedatives and tranquilizers with alcohol.
4. Women often use prescription drugs to hide their usage of other drugs. Prescription drugs are prescribed by a physician and are socially acceptable. Women view taking prescription drugs as being acceptable. They conceal the use of such medications unless specifically asked because they do not feel they are harmful.
5. Lack of financial resources, responsibility for child care, fear of losing custody of children if discovered to be chemically dependent are also factors.
6. Women are identified as being responsible for taking care of others and many families oppose the women entering treatment because it disrupts their lives. Many women feel guilty about seeking treatment.

Traditional treatment programs have used services and techniques that were developed primarily for the treatment of men. Women entering treatment are different from men. Women experience a great deal more guilt and shame than do men and frequently enter treatment with feelings of rejection and abandonment plus guilt over neglecting their children. Women are hypersensitive to the attitudes of the counselors. These women often have been victims of incest, sexual abuse, and physical abuse. Women feel more isolated and their social support systems are more limited than those of men. Treatment programs must remove these perceived barriers to treatment. Treatment should be individualized and matched to meet the specific needs of the individual woman.

Treatment counselors must use dual diagnosis models and be experienced in treating depression, anxiety, and survivors of physical abuse, sexual abuse, and incest. The treatment program must have an atmosphere in which the woman can discuss the environment in which she lives and to which she may return on completion of treatment. Basic services necessary for comprehensive treatment of addicted women should include child care, medical care, family therapy, marital therapy, vocational counseling, job placement, legal assistance, psychological and psychiatric services, and therapy for sexuality and intimacy problems. Women often experience a variety of problems that either antecede substance use or directly result from substance usage. These problems must be addressed for treatment to be successful.

REFERENCES

1. American Psychiatric Association. Diagnostic and statistical manual. 4th ed., revised. Washington, DC: Author, 1994. This is a handbook for the classification of mental illness. Formulated by the American Psychiatric Association, it was first issued in 1952. It correlates closely with the World Health Organization International Classification of Disease (ICD), which is the WHO's official list of disease categories subscribed to by all WHO member nations. DSM-IV is the current 1994 edition.

2. Kirk J, Brown MD, Blow FC, et al. Treatment implications of chemical dependency models, an integrative approach. J Subst Abuse Treat 1989;6:147–157.

3. Lettieri DJ, Sayers M, Pearson HW, eds. Theories on drug abuse, selected contemporary perspectives. National Institute on Drug Abuse Research Monograph Series, 30, March 1980.

4. Colten ME. A comparison of heroin addicted and nonaddicted mothers. Their attitudes, beliefs and parenting experiences. Heroin addicted parents and their children. Washington, DC: National Institute on Drug Abuse, U.S. Government Printing Office, 1980.

5. Beckman DP, Mulford H. Women and men problem drinkers, sex differences in parents served by Iowa's community health center. J Stud Alcohol 1977;38:1624–1639.

6. Knupfer G. Problems associated with drunkenness in women, some research issues, special population issues. National Institute on Alcohol Abuse and Alcoholism. Alcohol and Health Monograph No. 4, 1982.

7. Frezza M, DiPadova C, Pozzato G, et al. High blood alcohol levels in women: the role of decreased gastric alcohol dehydrogenase activity and first-pass metabolism. N Engl J Med 1990;322:95–99.

CHAPTER 38

EATING DISORDERS

Richard E. Blackwell

The eating disorders are typified by patients with anorexia nervosa and those women afflicted with bulimia. However, patients with eating disorders often present to the gynecologist with psychogenic amenorrhea. This category includes individuals with body weight disturbance, exercise-related menstrual dysfunction and stress-related disorders. Because these conditions to some degree mimic each other and present with similar laboratory findings, they will be discussed along with the eating disorders. The patient with psychogenic amenorrhea or an eating disorder will rarely present to the gynecologist with this complaint. These individuals usually request evaluation of their amenorrhea or are attempting to achieve pregnancy. However, the bulimic woman will frequently present seeking diuretics or cathartics under the guise of another diagnosis. Unfortunately, there exists a cult in our society that worships thinness and exercise (1). This idealized body habitus is expressed in fashion, entertainment, art, and literature. Along with this comes a career, success, and sexuality. All of these factors have an impact in dealing with the psychogenic amenorrheic patient because unfortunately weight (percent body fat), stress, and exercise all have a major impact on ovulation. Deviating from ideal body weight by about 15% produces menstrual dysfunction or subtle infertility problems. Often one sees irregular cycles; however, one may encounter the "short luteal phase" or long follicular phase, the family of "dysfolliculogenesis syndromes." These variances of "normal" make individuals subfertile. This is confirmed by the studies of Bates and colleagues who studied women who were either over- or underweight and brought them to within a standard deviation of ideal body weight. He achieved an astounding 73% pregnancy rate with no other management (2). The impact of body weight deviation is perhaps greater at the lower end of the scale than the upper. Patients probably have more tolerance for obesity than "pseudostarvation"; therefore, a drop in body weight produces a marked compromise in reproductive function. If one adds to this some element of tubal disease such as minimal endometriosis or an occult male factor, these women may be practicing contraception unintentionally or intentionally by keeping their body weight below normal. The extreme condition in the patient with anorexia nervosa or a marathon runner may be obvious. However, not all anorectic women are emaciated. One sees many anorectoid personalities present to the office who are trim and appear to be in a relatively good state of nutrition. However, they share many characteristics with the anorectoid patient and this family of disorders should always be suspected in the patient with an inappropriate height-weight ratio or in young girls with delayed puberty.

Anorexia Nervosa

Anorexia nervosa has a long history. In 1687, Richard Morton described a 17-year-old girl (with nervous consumption). "I did not remember that did ever in all my practice see one that was conversant with the living so much wasted with the greatest degree of consumption (like a skeleton, only clad with skin), yet there was no fever, but on the contrary, a coolness of the whole body. . . ." Similar patients were described by other historical figures such as Gull and Simpson. In fact, Sheehan's syndrome was at one time thought to be the same as anorexia nervosa and it took years to differentiate the two syndromes. Freund believed that anorectics maintain their lean body state in an attempt to avoid the expression of sexuality. The Germans call anorexia nervosa leanness passion of puberty (pubertätsmagersucht). Likewise, anorexia nervosa was thought to be a form of hysterical neurosis and, in fact, the French word is anorexie hysterique. In the modern era it was suggested that genetic tendency and environmental and nutritional factors were involved in the overall disease process. Dr. Hilde Bruch wrote the definitive book on the description and management of anorexia (3). In her book the condition was described as arising in teenagers who lose 25% of body weight and acquire disorder eating attitudes. First, patients with anorexia nervosa deny they are ill, fail to recognize their nutritional needs, and have a paralyzing sense of ineffectiveness. They hoard food like a miser with gold; many of them are in fact employed in the food processing business or fields related to nutrition. They have no apparent other psychological problems and no medical illnesses that can account for the condition. In the differential diagnosis of anorexia nervosa, one must consider cancer, hypothalamic problems, various endocrine disorders such as Addison's disease, hyperthyroidism, functional disorders like depression, schizophrenia, chronic wasting diseases like tuberculosis, and Crohn's disease. Anorexia tends to occur almost always in females; however, male athletes have been described with anorexia nervosa (4). The patients may be purely anorectic or may have a bulimic phase. That is, not all anorectics vomit and starvation may be the primary process. Amenorrhea occurs virtually in almost all female patients and it occurs before women lose weight indicating a psychic component. When they regain their weight most of them do not restart their periods (5). However, most anorectics are amenable to treatment with ovulation induction with drugs such as Pergonal or a gonadotropin-releasing hormone (GnRH) pump unless they are extremely wasted (6). These women become pregnant quite easily because they have resting ovaries, respond readily to these medications, and they can carry pregnancies successfully to term.

The diagnostic criteria for anorexia nervosa (Box 38.1) include fear of obesity, body image disturbance, loss of 25% body weight, and refusal to attempt to gain weight. On physical examination, patients have hypotension, hypothermia, bradycardia, cachexia, bradypnea, parotid gland enlargement, peripheral edema secondary to hypoalbuminemia, increased body hair, and hypercarotenemia (Box 38.2).

Box 38.1 Diagnostic Criteria

Fear of obesity
Body image disturbance
Loss of 25% body weight
Refusal to attempt weight gain

Box 38.2 Physical Findings

Hypotension
Hypothermia
Bradycardia
Cachexia
Bradypnea
Parotid enlargement
Peripheral edema (second-degree hypoalbuminemia)
Increased body hair
Hypercarotinemia

Box 38.3 lists laboratory findings in patients with anorexia. A patient with suspected anorexia nervosa should be evaluated with a luteinizing hormone (LH) and follicle-stimulating hormone (FSH) level. These patients will be found to have a prepubertal level with an inverted LH/FSH ratio. They will have low estradiol levels, altered LH pulses, and an altered GnRH response with FSH rising greater than LH. The response to thyroid-releasing factor (TRF) may be altered, reverse T_3 will be elevated as will corticoids. Growth hormone will generally be increased, T_3 and T_4 decreased, dehydroepiandrosterone (DHEA) and dehydroepiandrosterone sulfate (DHEAS) decreased, and antidiuretic hormone (ADH) regulation altered. No normal pulses of LH will occur during the sleep cycle and anorectic patients demonstrate a loss of pulse frequency as they gain and lose weight (7). During the weight gain process, the LH/FSH ratio will become equal then mimic the polycystic ovary pattern with the LH being markedly elevated above the FSH before returning to a normal relationship with LH levels slightly greater than FSH. Likewise, anorectic patients will have a return of their nocturnal pulses and establishment of a

Box 38.3 Laboratory Findings in Patients with Anorexia Nervosa

Follicle-stimulating hormone and luteinizing hormone decreased with inverted ratio
Gonadotropin-releasing hormone increased
Cortisol normal or increased
T_3, T_4 decreased, reverse T_3 increased
Dehydroepiandrosterone and dehydroepiandrosterone sulfate decreased
Estrogen and 17β-estradiol decreased
Antidiuretic hormone regulation altered

normal pattern as they gain and lose weight just as though they were passing puberty. Anorectic women in fact have LH pulses; however, arcuate nucleus dysfunction results in a change in pulse frequency that yields the patterns described above (8).

Treatment of Anorexia Nervosa

Anorectics require prompt medical attention because a significant number of them pass into the chronic phase and death can occur from cardiovascular failure. These individuals need to be treated with a high-calorie diet; sometimes hospitalization and hyperalimentation are needed. Occasional neuroleptic medication is used for acute intervention and psychiatric assistance should be sought. Anorectic patients by and large do not respond to group therapy and do better with a classic analytical approach. The therapy for these patients involves a team approach with gynecologist, bariatrician, and psychiatrist being involved because the etiology of anorexia probably involves early experiences, innerpsychic conflicts, and familial and social problems. Results of the treatment of the anorectic show that 50% achieve a normal weight and 50% to 70% menstruate yet cycles are irregular, 20% show some improvement, 20% are unchanged by therapy, 5% become obese, and 6% die (Box 38.4) (9,10).

Box 38.4 Outcome of Treatment of Anorexia Nervosa

50% achieve normal weight
20% improve
20% are unchanged
5% become obese
6% die
50% to 75% menstruate, yet cycles are irregular

Bulimia

Bulimia is an extremely common disorder. The name bulimia is derived from the Greek meaning ox hunger. Most of these patients do not present with menstrual dysfunction; however, there are a tremendous number of bulimic individuals in the population. It has been estimated that a third of college freshmen have experienced the problem and many women report some episode of bulimia during their lifetime (11,12). Bulimics are binge eaters, and they tend to have food preferences, their favorites being ice cream, cookies, pastries, and popcorn with butter. They gorge then vomit; their eating is usually done alone and it is generally hidden. The termination of the binge usually involves vomiting and these women may vomit dozens of times a day. They may present with an esophageal laceration (Mallory-Weiss tear). They may present to the emergency room vomiting blood and oral examination will show loss of tooth enamel. Although bulimics attempt to control their weight and often seek diuretics and cathartics, they usually fluctuate no more than 10 lb. This probably is the reason that their menstrual function is generally not disturbed. As opposed to the patient with anorexia nervosa, they are usually aware that they have some disturbance in thinking and eating behavior (13). Unfortunately, bulimics are frequently polydrug abusers and they tend to take a great many diet pills and recreational drugs. In addition, alcoholism can be a problem. Many of them have criminal records and are caught shoplifting because their eating habits can often cost $100 a day; therefore, they steal food.

Bulimics often manifest in late high school and college. This is a time when young women are under intense social pressure from both peers and family. Patients suffering from bulimia, once diagnosed, respond to individual psychotherapy or group therapy. Further, fluoxetine HCl (Prozac) has just been approved by the Food and Drug Administration for the treatment of bulimia and this has been used in numerous foreign countries for the treatment of this disorder (14). Finally, at times it is necessary to hospitalize the bulimic patient, not so much for control of the eating problem but to separate her from family and social pressures.

Body Weight and Menstrual Function

One needs about 22% body fat to menstruate. Menarche occurs at about 48 kg (106 lb) and undernourishment in individuals such as ballet dancers delays menses. If women lose 10% to 15% of their body weight, problems occur in menstrual function and this often happens in dieters who exercise. Often inadequate precursors cannot be synthesized because essential amino acids are not consumed in adequate quantities (15). In addition, changes in catechol estrogen metabolism occur with starvation. Estrone metabolism changes and 2-hydroxyestrone is produced (16). Further, the thyroid produces a reversed T_3 to keep from burning body mass and there is a change in sex hormone-binding globulin (17,18). The metabolic clearance of steroids is also altered by the change in body weight.

Stress and Menstrual Function

Stress interferes with menstrual function through a different mechanism. When the stressful state is entered, the hypothalamus produces corticotropin-releasing factor (CRF). CRF acts on the corticotrophs of the pituitary to generate adrenocorticotropic hormone (ACTH). The pro-opiomelantocortin is acted on by CRF to generate a variety of products including ACTH, clip components, and various endorphins and enkeflins. These compounds act through numerous receptors to affect dopamine metabolism and prolactin, which both interfere with menstrual function (19). In addition to these indirect pathways, CRF directly affects GnRH as does its feedback product cortisol (20). These are the probable mechanisms by which stress affects reproduction. Stress by itself probably produces no absolute deleterious effect unless carried to extreme. However, when stress interacts with low body weight and exercise, such as in the young ballet dancer, alterations in pubertal progression and menstrual dysfunction occur (21).

Exercise and Menstrual Function

The impact of strenuous exercise on menstrual function is somewhat difficult to separate from the effects of low body weight with altered fat-lean mass ratio and stress. Nevertheless, strenuous physical fitness in women has been increasing, not only in the area of competitive athletics, but through individual training such as aerobics and step exercises. Regular strenuous exercise leads to a variety of menstrual dysfunctions, delay in puberty or menarche, luteal phase defect, and variations of dysfolliculogenesis (22). The incidence of dysfunction is probably related to type of exercise, psychic factors, intensity of exercise, body composition, diet, and level of stress. Nearly 60% of women olympians will show some form of menstrual dysfunction regardless of the type of event in which they participate. However, long distance runners appear to have the greatest incident of dysfunction with approximately 50% showing amenorrhea at the training level of 70 miles per week (23). Swimmers, on the other hand, show only a 12% incidence with a similar amount of training (24). It should be noted, however, that amenorrhea can occur in the absence of weight loss; for instance, basketball players may not menstruate when training as they alter their fat-lean mass ratio. On the other hand, injury to athletes may result in a return of menstruation without an appreciable change in body weight or in fat-lean mass ratio. There appears to be an association between increasing frequency of amenorrhea with decreasing body fat (calculated total body water divided by body weight).

Strenuous exercise induces defects in GnRH secretion, and aberrant LH pulse frequency and amplitude have been observed (25). One also sees hypercortisolism, which may result in an impact on GnRH secretion. There is a significant reduction in serum T_3 and T_4, TSH is not elevated; however, the response to TRH is blunted (26). β Endorphins, growth hormone, prolactin, melatonin, epinephrine, and norepinephrine are all activated within minutes of the onset of exercise. Likewise, LH secretion is increased as is testosterone. These changes result in many beneficial effects including alteration of the age-associated increased serum lipids, altered insulin resistance, decreased incidence of cardiovascular disease, and retardation of bone loss (27). Further, there appears to be a decreased incidence of breast cancer in women who exercise regularly. Plasma high-density lipoprotein levels increase and low-density lipoprotein levels decrease, and amenorrheic women have lower levels of plasma apolipoprotein B than sedentary women. Unfortunately, amenorrheic athletes have lower apolipoprotein A1 levels, which negate part of this beneficial effect.

Because exercise-induced menstrual dysfunction is not technically a disease, the primary care physician should counsel these women about both its positive and negative effects. Many of these women are obviously hypoestrogenic, and this will result in alteration in bone structure, vaginal and bladder blood flow, and mood. It is suggested that these women be offered estrogen replacement therapy either in the form of an oral contraceptive agent or with estrogen/progestogen. It is also suggested the calcium supplementation at 1500 mg/day (2 Tums tablets) be administered as well. At times, however, the physician will find that this group of patients is highly refractory to medical therapy. This is reminiscent of the control issue that is often seen with patients with variations of anorexia nervosa. Therefore, the best tool that the physician has at his or her disposal is extensive education and counseling.

REFERENCES

1. Pugliese MT, Lipshitz F, Grad G, et al. Fear of obesity: a cause of short stature and delayed puberty. N Engl J Med 1983;309:513–518.
2. Bates GW, Bates SR, Whitworth NS. Reproductive failure in women who practice weight control. Fertil Steril 1982;37:373–378.
3. Bruch H. Anorexia nervosa and its differential diagnosis. J Nerv Ment Dis 1965;141:555–566.
4. Yates A, Leehay K, Shisslak CM. Running: an analogue of anorexia. N Engl J Med 1983;308:251–255.
5. McArthur JW, Johnson L, Hourihan J, Alonso C. Endocrine studies during the refeeding of young women with nutritional amenorrhea and infertility. Mayo Clin Proc 1976;51:607–615.
6. Braat DD, Schoemaker R, Schoemaker J. Life table analysis of fecundity in intravenously gonadotropin-releasing hormone-treated patients with normogonadotropic and hypogonadotropic amenorrhea. Fertil Steril 1991;55:266–271.
7. Boyar RM, Katz J, Finkelstein JW, et al. Anorexia nervosa immaturity of the 24-hour luteinizing hormone secretory pattern. N Engl J Med 1974;219:861–865.
8. Genazzani AD, Petraglia F, Fabbri G, et al. Evidence of luteinizing hormone secretion in hypothalamic amenorrhea associated with weight loss. Fertil Steril 1990;54:222–226.
9. Crisp A. Therapeutic outcome in anorexia nervosa. Can J Phys 1981;26:232–235.
10. Hsu L. Outcome of anorexia nervosa: a review of the literature (1954–1978). Arch Gen Psychiatry 1980;37:1041–1046.
11. Stangler R, Printz A, DSM III. Psychiatric diagnosis in a university population. Am J Psychiatry 1980;137:937–940.
12. Mitchell J, Pyle R. The bulimic syndrome in normal weight individuals: a review. Int J Eating Dis 1982;1:61.
13. Pyle R, Mitchell J. Bulimia, a report of 34 cases. J Clin Psychiatry 1981;42:460–464.
14. Bray GA. Use and abuse of appetite supplement drugs in the treatment of obesity. Ann Intern Res 1993:119(7 pt 2);707–713.
15. Gross H, Lake L, Ebert M, et al. Catecholamine metabolism in primary anorexia nervosa. J Clin Endocrinol Metab 1979;49:805–809.
16. Fishman J, Boyar RM, Hellman L. Influence of body weight on estradiol metabolism in young women. J Clin Endocrinol Metab 1975;41:989–991.
17. Miyai K, Yamamto T, Azukizawa M, et al. Serum thyroid hormones and thyrotropin in anorexia nervosa. J Clin Endocrinol Metab 1975;40:334–338.
18. Moshang T, Utiger R. Low triiodothyronine euthyroidism in anorexia nervosa. In: Vigasky RA, ed. Anorexia nervosa. New York: Baven Press, 1977:236–270.
19. Liu JH. Anovulation of CNS origin: functional and miscellaneous causes. In: Carr RB, Blackwell RE, eds. Textbook of reproductive medicine. East Norwalk, CT: Appleton & Lange, 1993:281–295.
20. Olster D, Ferin M. CRH inhibits gonadotropin secretion in the ovariectomized rhesus monkey. J Clin Endocrinol Metab 1987;65:262–267.
21. Frisch R, Wyshak G, Vincent L. Delayed menarche and amenorrhea in ballet dancers. N Engl J Med 1980;303:17–19.
22. Cumming DC, Rebar RW. Exercise and reproductive function in women. Am J Ind Med 1983;4:113–125.

23. Sangorn C, Martin B, Wagner W. Is athletic amenorrhea specific in women. Am J Obstet Gynecol 1982;143:859–861.

24. Veldhuis JD, Evans WS, Demus LM, et al. Altered neuroendocrine regulation of gonadotropin secretion in women distance runners. J Clin End Met 1985;61:557–563.

25. Genazzani AD, Petraglia F, Fabbri G, et al. Evidence of luteinizing hormone secretion in hypothalamic amenorrhea associated with weight loss. Fertil Steril 1990;54:222–226.

26. Loucks AB, Laughlin G, Yen SSC. Thyroid hormone deficiency in women athletes. Submitted for publication.

27. Lamon-Fava S, Fisher EC, Nelson ME, et al. Effect of exercise and menstrual cycle status on plasma lipids, low density lipoprotein particle size, and apolipoproteins. J Clin Endocrinol Metab 1989;68:17.

CHAPTER 39

SLEEP DISORDERS

G. Vernon Pegram, Robert L. Yuspeh,
Virginia H. Pascual, Robert C. Doekel

Sleep is a behavior that occurs as a fundamental part of one's natural cycling pattern of sleep and wakefulness. A more detailed consideration of the sleep–wakefulness cycle, using an electroencephalograph (EEG) analysis, reveals that mammalian behavior involves three distinct, readily identifiable behavioral states: wakefulness, non–rapid eye movement (NREM) sleep, and rapid eye movement (REM) sleep. If the fragile balance among these three behavioral states is altered by environmental change, psychological disturbance, pharmacologic agents, or physical disease, a person begins to report the result of the fluctuations in terms that we refer to as symptoms of sleep disorders. These complaints range from too much wakefulness (insomnia) to too much sleepiness (hypersomnia), thus representing the extremes of the imbalance of the sensitive sleep–wakefulness cycle.

Complaints of problems with sleep are among the most common medical complaints in our society. In fact, approximately 35% of all adults report experiencing insomnia at some time during the previous year, and half of these persons perceive their problem as serious (1). Add to this statistic the number of adults who have obstructive sleep apnea, narcolepsy, and other neurologic disorders of excessive somnolence, as well as the many millions with circadian rhythm disorders and parasomnias, and it becomes apparent that at least 40% of all adults experience some type of sleep disorder (2).

This chapter provides a brief update on the basic and applied knowledge concerning the sleep–wakefulness mechanisms and reviews the major sleep disorders and present current approaches to their treatment and management.

Normal Sleep

Sleep Architecture

Over the past 40 years research has revealed that sleep consists of two distinct states: REM sleep and NREM sleep. REM sleep is characterized on a psychological level by dreaming and on a physiologic level by cortical activation (a mixed frequency, low-voltage EEG pattern), bursts of extraocular and middle ear muscle activity, variability of heart and respiratory rates, activity-induced atonia of major antigravity and locomotor muscles, and increased cerebral blood flow. In a normal adult, 20% to 25% of each sleep period is spent in REM sleep. REM sleep may be described as consisting of a highly active brain in an immobilized body. As a result of this paradoxical phenomenon, REM is often referred to as paradoxical sleep.

Based on relatively distinguishable EEG brain wave patterns, NREM sleep is subdivided into four stages. Stage 1 is a brief transitional stage between wakefulness and sleep. It is characterized by a low-voltage, mixed frequency EEG pattern and accounts for approximately 5% of the total sleep period. Stage 2, which is characterized by the presence of sleep spindles (EEG waves of brief duration in the range of 12 to 14 cps) and K-complexes (a well-delineated negative sharp wave immediately followed by a sharp component), usually constitutes 40% to 55% of total sleep in the young adult. Stages 3 and 4, referred to as delta sleep, are characterized by moderate and large numbers of delta-frequency slow waves, respectively. Most of stage 3 and 4 sleep occurs during the first 1 to 3 hours of sleep and usually comprises 15% to 25% of total sleep in healthy young adults.

One can conceive of NREM sleep as being organized according to depth. Specifically, stage 1 is the lightest sleep, and stage 4 is the deepest state, as determined by both arousal and threshold mechanisms and the appearance of the EEG. However, REM sleep does not fit into this organizational design. The arousal threshold is usually higher in REM sleep than in NREM sleep, and resting muscle potential is lower during REM sleep. Thus, REM sleep is neither light sleep nor deep sleep but a different kind of sleep (3).

Nocturnal normal sleep is cyclic, with four or five cycles per sleep period. As healthy adults fall asleep, they enter stage 1, then stage 2, and finally stages 3 and 4. After a person sleeps for approximately 90 minutes, the first REM sleep occurs. This interval may be longer in some normal sleepers and older adults, but it is significantly shorter only during abnormal clinical and experimental conditions (4,5). Subsequent to a brief (5 to 15 minute) REM period, the NREM–REM cycle begins again and is repeated throughout the sleep period. The first REM periods are apt to be shorter, whereas later REM periods may last as long as 20 to 40 minutes. Thus, the majority of REM sleep occurs in the last third of the sleep period.

Neuroanatomic/Neurochemical Foundations of Sleep

Current research indicates that control of NREM sleep likely resides in circuits ranging from the area around the solitary tract of the medulla through the dorsal raphe nucleus to the basal forebrain area. The sleep-inducing areas are opposed by the ascending reticular activating system and the posterior hypothalamus, which promote wakefulness (2,6). Thus, according to Brezinova and colleagues (7) and Monnier and Gaillard (8) it appears as though two systems exist: a system that promotes sleep and another that promotes wakefulness. These researchers hypothesize that for sleep to occur, the system controlling wakefulness must subside for the weaker sleep system to dominate.

Research presently indicates that the brain stem, forebrain, and cerebellum are all involved in the structure, timing, and dream imagery of REM sleep (2). More specifically, this author implicates the lateral portions of the nucleus reticularis pontis oralis (RPO) and adjacent nuclei of the pons as being the brain regions most critical for REM sleep.

Finally, a number of neurochemicals are believed to play a role in sleep and its stages. For instance, acetylcholine appears to be involved in eliciting and maintaining REM sleep and 5-hydroxytryptamine (5-HT) found in serotonergic neurons, appears to play a role in sleep–wake cycling. More specifically, serotonergic neurons have inhibitory effects on REM sleep, and their rate of activity appears to be at their very lowest levels during sleep (6).

The Effects of Age on Sleep

Sleep stages and sleep cycles are markedly altered by various changes affecting the individual (e.g., stress, many drugs). However, the one common and inevitable change in sleep is produced by the aging process. Although most human sleep data have come from young adults, an increasing number of studies have revealed that EEG wave forms and sleep architecture change significantly with age (9–12). For example, newborns' total sleep time averages about 14 to 18 hours per 24 hours, half of which may be spent in REM sleep. Young adults spend approximately 16 hours awake and 8 hours asleep, with only 1.5 to 2.0 hours being REM sleep. As adults enter middle age and old age, stages 3 and 4 often decrease significantly, and sleep becomes progressively more fragmented, with brief arousals and longer periods of wakefulness. Despite these remarkable changes, REM sleep percentages remain relatively constant after the first 2 to 3 years of life.

Individual Sleep Needs

Individual differences in total sleep time are highly variable, and the acceptable range seems to be remarkably wide. The average healthy adult requires nearly 8 hours of sleep per 24 hours. However, some healthy adults require only 4 hours or less per 24 hours, whereas others require 10 to 12 hours to feel sufficiently rested. Individual variability is also found in the amount of time spent in each stage, but this pattern in each individual tends to be stable from night to night.

Effects of Sleep Deprivation

Although for obvious reasons extended total sleep deprivation cannot be studied in human beings, observations of short-term deprivation indicate that an insufficient amount of sleep has a slight effect on task performance the following day (13). Hauri (2) elaborated on these results stating that for most of the short-term tasks that are usually tested, one can gather reserves after a sleepless night. However, mood, performance of creative or monotonous tasks, sleepiness, and vigilance appear to worsen after one sleepless night. After 2 to 3 days of sleep deprivation, "microsleeps" of a few seconds' duration start to intrude into wakefulness, resulting in inattentiveness. Thus, performance deteriorates further, even when the person's motivation is high. As sleep deprivation continues, microsleeps become longer and more frequent. Consequently, after 10 days, an EEG cannot determine whether a person is awake or asleep, even when performing functions that occur while awake (e.g., walking) (2).

When sleep ensues on the first night after prolonged wakefulness, delta sleep increases; REM sleep rebound may come later in the same sleep period or be more pronounced on the second or third night. Even after 10 days of sleep deprivation, two to three nights of extended sleep will usually return a healthy volunteer to normal sleep patterns (14). Similarly, Rechtschaffen, Bergmann, & Everson (15) report that human beings tolerate sleep loss more easily than rats do. Finally, if subjects are deprived specifically of slow-wave or REM sleep, pressure to restore that particular phase of sleep increases (2).

Circadian Systems

Circadian rhythms are defined as any group of biologic rhythms that approximate a 24-hour schedule (6). Circadian rhythms are evidenced in a variety of biologic systems (16) including sleep (11). Furthermore, these rhythms have been assessed through a variety of manual and psychophysiologic measures (16–20). This work has suggested that light is the primary influence in synchronizing the various biologic cycles as a result of the rotations of the planet (2). In this way, light serves as a zeitgeber (time-giver). This system has been more actively explored in recent years and appears to involve brain areas in and around the suprachiasmatic nucleus (6,21,22).

In addition, a hormone that is very important when discussing the circadian system is melatonin. This hormone referred to by some as the hormone of darkness is synthesized and secreted during darkness and is usually undetectable during daylight (23). The linkage between melatonin levels and the circadian system has made it a marker of the circadian system (24). In fact, some reports have suggested that melatonin infusion may reset the circadian clock (25).

In addition to light, a major variable within the circadian system is body temperature. In healthy adults, sleep onset occurs as the temperature falls, and this decrease in temperature continues to fall until the early morning hours (2). Furthermore, the duration of NREM sleep and REM sleep appears to be associated to the circadian cycle, with most REM sleep occurring close to the nadir of the temperature cycle. For example, studies have shown that the temperature clock will drive sleep patterns in the absence of light (21). In fact, body temperature continues to rise until late afternoon, except for a decrease that typically occurs in early afternoon and is usually associated with sleepiness.

Sleep Disorders in Women

Previous literature has indicated that women have a higher rate of sleep disturbances across all age ranges (26,27). This is likely due to women possessing several different physiologic states that have been demonstrated to cause sleep disturbances such as pregnancy and the postpartum period, as well as menstruation and the menopause. Thus, the following discussion will focus on sleep disorders and their relationship to pregnancy and menopause.

Sleep and Pregnancy

The hormonal, psychological, and social changes that occur during pregnancy significantly influence sleep patterns (28). Furthermore, these changes are more likely to occur during the third trimester of pregnancy and to be caused by physiologic discomfort (29).

Polysomnography has demonstrated that sleep patterns vary during pregnancy (28,30). For example, during the first trimester of pregnancy, women tend to complain of being sleepy and to take more naps and sleep for longer periods during the day. During the second trimester, sleep tends to return to normal. However, during the third trimester, sleep is characterized by difficulty falling asleep, as well as many nocturnal awakenings. Furthermore, marked suppression of sleep time is noted that does not return to baseline levels until several weeks postpartum. Likewise, stage 4 sleep is reported to be significantly diminished compared with that of controls (30) and with baseline recordings taken at 4 months postpartum (31). Thus, it is hypothesized that hormonal changes (e.g., estrogen, progesterone, thyroid) may be responsible for these alterations (30).

Following parturition, sleep is reported to worsen. For instance, on the first postpartum night women are reported to spend significantly more time awake and have a minimal amount of sleep (28,30). According to Karacan and Williams (28), sleep disturbances significantly diminish by the third postpartum night, and sleep patterns return to normal approximately 2 to 3 weeks after parturition. However, a few cases have been reported in which slow-wave sleep (stage 4) and total sleep time did not return to normal until 4 to 6 weeks postpartum. It is this significant drop in stage 4 sleep during late pregnancy or a delay or failure in its complete return that is suggested to increase a woman's susceptibility to emotional disturbance.

There have been several reports describing sleep disturbances as an important symptom indicating the likelihood of postpartum emotional disturbance (28,32,33). For example, postpartum depression is characterized by dysphoria along with transitory irritability, sadness, and crying spells. Furthermore, women who are affected have obsessional thoughts, which often prevent them from falling asleep. Consequently, they do not receive enough sleep and present with cognitive and emotional disturbances similar to sleep-deprived individuals (28,34).

In contrast, another disorder reported by Berlin (35) is associated with slow-wave sleep during pregnancy. More specifically, this author described sleepwalking in a woman during pregnancy who had suffered from this condition during childhood.

Pulmonary function and gas exchange during pregnancy are affected by both mechanical and hormonal changes. Such changes could hypothetically lead to hypoxemia or hypoventilation during sleep, whereas other changes might prove protective (36). For example, pulmonary restriction can be observed during pregnancy when the progressive enlargement of the uterus increases intra-abdominal pressure, thus pushing the diaphragm up into the thorax and increasing the work of breathing (37). However, maternal oxygenation has been reported to be healthy in sleeping pregnant women (38). Furthermore, the number and duration of apneas and hypopneas are significantly reduced, presumably as a result of a 10-fold increase in progesterone during pregnancy (39,40), which is known to increase alveolar ventilation by increasing tidal volume (41,42).

However, there have been several case reports of sleep apnea during pregnancy. For example, Joel-Cohen and Schoenfeld (43) reported data on three obese women who were snorers and clinically diagnosed as having sleep apnea. Although polysomnography was not available, fetal monitoring indicated significant acidosis and heart rate changes related to apneic episodes. In addition, a study of eight pregnancies in similarly obese snoring patients with a diagnosis of sleep apnea found intrauterine growth retardation in all eight cases (44). Thus, in some patients with major risk factors, there appears to be evidence that sleep apnea does occur during pregnancy and may have negative ramifications for the fetus (36). Despite this, Conti and colleagues (45) reported a case of a pregnant woman given a clinical diagnosis of sleep apnea who had a normal infant at delivery.

Several treatments have been used in pregnant women with sleep apnea. The most commonly used medication is progesterone, which is already present in high physiologic concentrations during pregnancy (36). The tricyclic antidepressant protriptyline has also been used. Although the mechanism of action of this drug is unclear, it may include a reduction in REM sleep as well as an increase in upper airway muscle tone (36). However, fetal malformations, lethargy, urinary retention, and withdrawal symptoms have been reported in neonates whose mothers received tricyclic antidepressants, and their safe use in pregnancy has not been established (46). Thus, in light of these problems with at least some medications, the most commonly recommended form of therapy for sleep apnea is nasal continuous positive airway pressure (CPAP). However, despite its use during pregnancy, several concerns are raised including decreasing cardiac output and placental blood flow as a consequence of increasing intrathoracic pressure or compression of the inferior vena cava because of increasing intra-abdominal pressure (36). Nevertheless, successful use of nasal CPAP during pregnancy has been described (47,48) and appears to be the treatment of choice for significant sleep apnea during pregnancy (36).

Menstrual-Associated Sleep Disorder

Menopause is characterized by low levels of estrogen and elevated gonadotropins (luteinizing hormone and follicle-stimulating hormone). These hormonal changes result in vasomotor flashes, which disrupt sleep by causing frequent nocturnal awakenings (49–52), thus resulting in significant fatigue (53). Furthermore, Shaver and colleagues (54) reported that women who experience hot flashes tend to have lower sleep efficiencies and longer REM latencies than non-symptomatic women.

Treatment studies have provided further evidence of the central role of gonadal hormones in perimenopausal sleep disturbances (26). For example, Thomson and Oswald (55) reported that estrogen treatment decreased the number and duration of episodes and wakefulness in menopausal women. Moreover, after 2 months of estrogen treatment, patients experienced a longer sleep period, as well as an increase in REM sleep, likely the result of an increase in sleep duration because REM periods are known to become longer toward the end of the night. Similarly, Schiff and associates (56) reported that women taking estrogen display a shorter sleep onset latency and significant REM increase. In fact, estrogen decreased sleep onset latency with a magnitude comparable to that seen with sleeping aids. However, in contrast to sleeping pills, estrogen increased the amount of REM sleep.

It is proposed that the hormonal status of premenopausal women protects them against the development of sleep-disordered breathing through the effect of progesterone on the maintenance of oxygen saturation during sleep (57) and as a result induces a better arousal response (58). Despite this, there is now good evidence that menopause places women at risk for sleep apnea that is approximately equal to that for men (59–61). With regard to treatment of sleep apnea in postmenopausal women, trials of medroxyprogesterone have failed to show a statistically significant decrease in the number of apneas during sleep (62–64). However, Pickett and associates (65) reported that the combined administration of estrogen and progestin significantly decreased the number of sleep-disordered breathing episodes. In addition, the duration of hypopneas also decreased leading these researchers to conclude that the presence of progestin and estrogen may be involved in protecting premenopausal women against sleep-disordered breathing.

Fibromyalgia Syndrome

Fibromyalgia syndrome (FMS), also commonly known as fibrositis, is a rheumatologic disorder frequently seen in women. FMS can significantly disrupt sleep and for this reason is a common cause of insomnia among women. FMS manifests itself as diffuse aches in large groups of muscles and has been defined as myalgia without myositis. Pressure points are also characteristic of this disorder. Fibromyalgia is commonly associated with a phenomenon known as alpha intrusion in which the brain waves normally associated with wake (alpha) are noted to be interspersed in all sleep stages (66). These patients frequently have the sensation that their sleep is not refreshing and alpha intrusion is thought to account for this. This phenomenon has been suggested to be related to low serotonin levels and to low estrogen levels (67) and to be exacerbated by stimulants such as caffeine and nicotine. Sleep deprivation itself, specifically delta sleep loss, has been demonstrated to cause fibromyalgia-like symptoms in otherwise healthy subjects. Antidepressants in low doses, especially amitriptyline (Elavil) and related compounds such as cyclobenzaprine (Flexeril) have been shown to be effective in not only reducing the alpha intrusion, but also improving the muscle aches and the restfulness of sleep.

Dysautonomia

Also common, but certainly not exclusive to women, is the compendium of symptoms known as dysautonomia. As discussed briefly with anxiety disorders, these symptoms are often associated with mitral valve prolapse. Specifically, these include daytime fatigue, insomnia (especially difficulty initiating and maintaining sleep), palpitations, chest pain, migraine headaches, irritable bowel syndrome, and tingling in hands and feet. Furthermore, there is significant overlap with this disorder and panic disorder and both seem to respond to similar therapy. Initially, reassurance is important, for the patient's anxiety to the symptoms only exacerbates many of these symptoms. Nonpharmacologic measures are important and are sufficient in correcting milder cases. These include total abstinence from caffeine, avoidance of refined sugar, adequate volume intake, and daily aerobic exercise. β Blockers and calcium channel blockers in low doses are often successful in relieving the cardiac symptoms. Low-dose benzodiazepines are also effective generally with such compounds as the longer acting clonazepam (Klonopin) being successful in relieving some of the panic disorder, as well as the insomnia. Antispasmodic agents are sometimes necessary for total correction of the irritable bowel symptoms. There is no specific EEG abnormality or other identifiable disruption of sleep that is able to be objectively seen on overnight polysomnography in this disorder. For a more detailed discussion of this disorder, the reader is referred to Chapter 8.

Primary Sleep Disorders

Sleep Apnea Syndromes

Sleep apnea, whether it produces a complaint of excessive daytime sleepiness or insomnia, is a serious and potentially life-threatening disorder. Clinical features characteristic of this disorder include excessive daytime sleepiness, nocturnal insomnia, morning headaches, noisy snoring, abnormal motor activity during sleep, intellectual and personality changes, sexual impotence, systemic hypertension, pulmonary hypertension, cor pulmonale, heart failure, and polycythemia (68,69).

Apnea is operationally defined as the cessation of air flow lasting at least 10 seconds. Several important clinical subtypes of sleep apnea syndromes are identified. These include upper airway obstructive sleep apnea, central sleep apnea, mixed apnea, pickwickian syndrome, and sudden infant death syndrome. Although sleep apnea can appear from infancy to old age, it occurs more commonly in modestly obese men over 40 years of age (70). More recently, Young and colleagues (71) estimated that 9% of women and 24% of men meet the minimal diagnostic criteria for the sleep apnea syndrome. These findings led these authors to conclude that the prevalence of undiagnosed sleep-disordered breathing is high among men and is much higher than previously suspected among women, and moreover, that undiagnosed sleep-disordered breathing is associated with daytime hypersomnolence.

Sleep apnea appears to be much more common in men. In fact, a recent review indicated that 94% of patients evaluated at the Stanford Sleep Disorders Clinic were male (68). Similarly, Hauri (72) reports that men outnumber women by a ratio of 10:3 in cases of apnea.

Clinically, snoring is an important clue. The characteristic loud, pharyngeal snoring, interspersed with snorting, appears as the first clinical symptom in most patients. This symptom can even be seen as early as preschool or elementary school age. The continuous snoring pattern can be interrupted by as many as several hundred apneic periods per night. These apneic episodes usually last 10 to 180 seconds. Accompanying the apneic episodes are abnormal movements ranging from small movements of the hands or feet to large flailing movements involving the entire upper and lower limbs. If the patient is awakened suddenly, he or she may appear confused and disoriented (73).

Most often, the presenting complaint is excessive daytime sleepiness. In fact, daytime drowsiness may be so severe that patients fall asleep while eating, but they are especially susceptible during monotonous situations such as driving, attending meetings, reading, or watching television. Various studies have suggested that 32% to 74% of apnea patients have had one or more automobile accidents attributed to drowsiness at the wheel (74).

Personality changes resulting in reactive depression, abnormal outbursts of emotion, episodes of jealousy and suspicion, irrational behavior, and sudden impotence are also symptoms that may develop secondary to the sleep apnea syndrome. Morning headaches are also frequently observed in association with sleep apnea (73).

The definitive diagnostic test for sleep apnea syndrome is an all-night polysomnogram. Polysomnography is a complex evaluation of a patient during sleep that involves assessment of the central nervous system. In the case of sleep apnea, polysomnography also includes assessment of respiratory and cardiac function with the use of a pulse oximeter, nasal and oral respiratory thermistors, measures of respiratory effort, and electrocardiogram (ECG), in addition to the standard EEG measurements. Finally, it is essential to determine which subtype of sleep apnea the patient has because the treatment varies accordingly.

Although sleep apnea can be suspected on the basis of a careful history and physical examination, a myriad of associated symptoms can result in diagnostic confusion. Thus, it is mandatory to confirm the diagnosis with an all-night polysomnogram because therapeutic indications depend on 1) the predominant type of sleep apnea, 2) the degree of disability, and 3) the severity of sleep-related cardiovascular symptoms. The presence of other clinical problems is significant as well.

For central sleep apnea, no definitively effective therapeutic approach has been found. However, improvement has been reported with a carbonic anhydrase inhibitor (acetazolamide) (75), as well as with medroxyprogesterone and chlorimipramine (5). Fortunately central sleep apnea occurs rather infrequently.

Clearly, the most effective treatment for obstructive sleep apnea is nasal CPAP, which acts as a pneumatic splint to prevent collapse of pharyngeal tissues (2). Most patients undergoing this treatment report an improvement or a return to normal sleep, alertness, endocrine function, and mood (76). The primary reasons for treatment failure are nasal obstruction, dryness, excessive nasal secretions when CPAP is used, and inability of the patient to tolerate the mask (2).

At this time the level of CPAP must be determined in a laboratory while the patient is sleeping. This gives the technician the advantage of observing and adjusting in small increments the level of CPAP. As patients begin to feel more alert, obese CPAP patients appear to find it easier to lose weight (77). In fact, a 20% weight loss will enable the patient to decrease the level of CPAP required.

If a patient presents with an obstructive sleep apnea due to an anatomic defect, surgical correction may be the treatment of choice. In some cases, significant weight loss can decrease the incidence and severity of apneic periods. However, when the apnea is life-threatening, the most immediate and effective treatment is a tracheostomy to bypass the upper airway obstruction during sleep (68). The results of this procedure are often dramatic, with marked improvement in the patient's symptoms within the first few days of surgery.

The diagnosis and treatment of sleep apnea is attracting much attention from a variety of disciplines. Thus, a variety of other treatments have been tested and are proving beneficial for certain types of apnea. Examples of advances in this field include mandibular osteotomy in patients with retrognathism (78), uvulopalatopharyngoplasty for patients with large soft palates (79–81), the use of protriptyline for certain patients with upper airway obstruction (82), treatment with maxillomandibular advancement surgery (83), and the use of a nocturnal tongue-retaining device for patients with obstructive sleep apnea (84).

Narcolepsy

Narcolepsy is a syndrome of unknown origin that is characterized by excessive daytime sleepiness, disturbed nocturnal sleep, and pathologic manifestations of REM sleep. The most typical REM sleep manifestations include cataplexy (to be described later), and sleep onset REM periods. However, sleep paralysis (the inability to move any muscles when falling asleep but especially on awakening) and hypnogogic hallucinations (dreamlike experiences difficult to distinguish from reality that occur when falling asleep) may also be present (85–87). A relatively small number of patients experience all four manifestations of the disorder, known as the narcoleptic tetrad.

The manifestations of excessive daytime sleepiness include inappropriate and irresistible sleep episodes, amnesic periods, and often severe drowiness. However, narcoleptics do not sleep more than normal individuals (85). Their problem is principally the uncontrollable nature of their sleepiness. Excessive daytime sleepiness is usually the earliest manifestation of narcolepsy. Symptom onset typically occurs between the teen years and the third decade of life. The majority of narcoleptic patients appear to experience excessive daytime sleepiness before the age of 20 (88,89) although a study by Billiard, Besset, and Cadilhac (90) found the median age of onset to be 22 years of age. Excessive daytime sleepiness tends to worsen over time, often resulting in social embarrassment and employment difficulties (4,5).

Cataplexy seems to be a more prevalent symptom in narcolepsy (i.e., approximately 70%) than either sleep paralysis or hypnogogic hallucinations. This troubling symptom is usually triggered by an emotional stimulus such as anger or excitement and is characterized by a sudden but reversible loss of skeletal muscle tonus lasting as briefly as a few seconds to as long as 30 minutes. Cataplexy is thought to result from the inhibition of alpha and gamma motor systems (91) and can subsequently result in patients having abnormal perception and proprioception (92). The muscles most affected are those of the jaw, neck, and knees. The attack may range in severity from a feeling of slight weakness to involvement of the entire voluntary musculature. Extraocular muscles are usually uninvolved, and the patient usually continues to breathe, although he or she may express some difficulty breathing during an attack. Furthermore, patients are apparently awake and are aware of their surroundings during the episodes. Patients with narcolepsy–cataplexy usually experience from one to four cataplectic attacks daily, but the frequency may vary widely. Consequently, patients may learn to self-impose restrictions on their activities or emotions and are apt to present clinically as somewhat depressed or apathetic.

A patient presenting with the chief complaint of excessive daytime sleepiness who also has a history of cataplexy is strongly suspected of having narcolepsy. However, a definitive diagnosis can only be made with an overnight polysomnogram to exclude other sleep disorders that might artifactually produce short sleep latencies or sleep onset REM periods on the multiple sleep latency test (MSLT) performed in a sleep laboratory the following day. This test consists of repeated measures of sleep latency in controlled nap situations. *Sleep latency* is defined as the time between the point at which an individual tries to sleep and the point at which EEG patterns of sleep first develop. This multiple nap procedure reveals that narcoleptics consistently fall asleep more readily than do control subjects and are more likely to exhibit sleep onset REM periods (21,90). It is recommended that a MSLT study be conducted after the patient has been free of stimulant medication, hypnotics, alcohol, and psychotropic medication for at least 2 weeks.

Treatment of the narcoleptic patient depends on the patient's symptoms and previous history of treatment. Although pharmacologic interventions are not the ideal solution to narcolepsy, there are cases in which the use of stimulant medication, such as dextroamphetamine, methylphenidate, or pemoline is indicated for excessive daytime sleepiness (85,86). However, some patients with narcolepsy may not respond well to stimulant treatment, primarily because of side effects and the development of tolerance. In such cases, it is sometimes beneficial to alternate stimulants every few weeks to prevent tolerance. The tolerance to stimulant medications is unlikely when patients come off medication on weekends. In addition, some patients have responded well to low doses of stimulants in combination with scheduled brief naps during the day, whereas others have responded positively to scheduled naps alone. Cataplectic attacks usually respond well to divided doses of imipramine (25–100 mg/day). This dose may also effectively control sleep paralysis and hypnogogic hallucinations (93). Some success in treating cataplexy has also been achieved with protriptyline (94) propranolol (95), γ-hydroxybutyrate (96), and fluoxetine (97).

One area of therapeutic need that is often neglected pertains to the psychological effect of narcolepsy. Although there is no evidence that narcolepsy is psychogenic, it can seriously affect the patient's ability to cope with stress and is often harmful to personal relationships. Thus, by clearly explaining the sleep disorder to family members, some of the stress and anxiety that is elicited by the nature of the illness can be reduced.

Periodic Limb Movement Disorder

Also known as nocturnal myoclonus, patients with periodic leg movements of sleep (PLMS) usually have pronounced jerks in one or both legs. These jerks, or twitches, may be accompanied by flexion at the ankle, knee, and hip. If the jerking is pronounced enough, it will arouse the patient. The leg movements are confined to sleep and are generally not seen while awake. The myoclonic jerks usually occur every 20 to 40 seconds and last approximately 1.5 to 4.0 seconds (98). Several hundred leg movement episodes may occur during the night, with most occuring during NREM rather than REM sleep.

Complaints of frequent arousals during sleep and aching leg muscles are common. Furthermore, because PLMS may "lighten" sleep and interfere with deep restorative sleep, patients are often chronically fatigued and may exhibit symptoms of depression. Thus, PLMS can be associated with both insomnia and hypersomnia. However, at this point it is not possible to conclude that PLMS actually causes insomnia or hypersomnia (99,100). Moreover, there is an increasing tendency to refer to this disorder as periodic movements in sleep (PMS) to distinguish it from myoclonus associated with epilepsy (99).

Currently, the most effective treatment for PLMS is carbidopa/levodopa (Sinemet, 25–100 mg) or Sinemet CR. In addition, clonazepam has been shown to be effective in treating PLMS (0.5–1.0 mg at bedtime). In more severe cases a number of other medications have been used including propoxyphene, codeine, hydrocodone, oxycodone, and methadone.

Restless Legs Syndrome

Periodic leg movements of sleep frequently coexist with restless legs syndrome (101,102) although the latter may occur independently. This syndrome is so bizarre that patients often have difficulty describing the problem. Usually they say they feel as if there is something crawling inside their legs. This sensation appears to occur approximately every hour or two during wakefulness as well as during sleep. Apparently, moving about or stretching alleviates the symptoms. Thus, during sleep periods, patients must get out of bed and walk around or take a hot bath before they can go back to sleep. Similar to sleep apnea, the effects of this problem result in a sleep pattern characterized by a marked reduction of delta (or deep) sleep, as well as excessive daytime sleepiness.

The physician can establish if restless legs syndrome or PLMS is related to complaints of insomnia by directly inquiring about the twitching in the patient's legs while the patient is asleep or falling asleep. The bed partner's input is often helpful. To firmly establish a diagnosis of restless legs syndrome (and PLMS) nocturnal and daytime recording from the left and right anterior tibialis muscles is necessary. A clue in differentially diagnosing between the two disorders is that patients suffering from restless legs syndrome exhibit twitching during waking, whereas those suffering from PLMS exhibit twitching exclusively during sleep. Particular emphasis should be placed on whether or not the patient is awakened by the twitching.

Current evidence suggests that approximately one third of all cases of restless legs syndrome are genetically transmitted (103). Moreover, the disorder appears to be transmitted as an autosomal dominant trait (103,104).

As with PLMS, a variety of pharmacologic agents including anticonvulsants, benzodiazepines, antidepressants, central nervous system stimulants, opiates, and levodopa have been proposed in the treatment of restless legs syndrome (101). In particular, clonazepam (99,105–107), codeine, and propoxyphene have been remarkably effective (108). Despite their effectiveness one must be careful in prescribing these medications because of their addictive potential.

The Parasomnias

The most commonly encountered parasomnias include sleepwalking (somnambulism), sleep terrors, and sleeptalking. These disorders are most commonly observed in children (109). In all three of these disorders the symptoms usually begin during the first third of the night. More specifically, partial arousals from delta (or deep) sleep occur creating the episodes (73,110). All three disorders are seen more often in relatives of children with these disorders than in relatives of children without the disorder (109). Finally, although these disorders are not usually associated with psychopathology in children, the occurrence of them in adults, particularly sleepwalking and sleep terrors can frequently be associated with psychopathology (111,112).

An additional parasomnia that has received a significant amount of attention is REM sleep behavior disorder (113). Also known as loss of REM sleep atonia (114), this rare disorder is characterized by the dreams of REM sleep being acted out. Moreover, there is often a predominance of active behavior. Typically, the limbs are moved about as if they were being used for the activity and the individual may punch or kick as if struggling with an imagined assailant (110). Polysomnographic studies have demonstrated the emergence of these behaviors during REM sleep, a stage during which most voluntary muscles normally exhibit atonia (109). Most patients afflicted with this disorder are middle-aged or elderly, which is in contrast to the more common parasomnias, which are more common in children. Although the etiology remains unclear, the possibility of a neurologic basis is supported by the presence of olivopontocerebellar degeneration, as well as acute polyradiculitis and delirium tremens in some affected patients (113,115,116).

Finally, enuresis during sleep is a common problem that affects approximately 5% to 17% of children. Although not technically classified as a parasomnia, many people refer to it as such because it occurs during sleep. Bedwetting may occur at any time during the night but is more common in the first third of the night.

Typically, parasomnias that are common in children do not require treatment. However, an evaluation for underlying psychopathology and subsequent psychiatric treatment should be instituted in older adolescents and adults who manifest these primarily childhood disorders, particularly sleepwalking and sleep terrors (110). For example, positive results have been reported with relaxation training and hypnosis (117,118). In addition, benzodiazepines may be appropriate in some situations such as when an afflicted child sleeps away from home. Apparently, the effect of benzodiazepines is not due to their slow-wave suppressant effects but may be due to their impairment of arousal (110).

The disturbing manifestations of REM behavior disorder can be effectively controlled with clonazepam (113,119) Furthermore, desipramine has also been reported to benefit selected patients. However, this tricyclic antidepressant is not well tolerated in the elderly. In additon to pharmacologic interventions, it is important to provide patients with a safe bedroom environment. This can be accomplished by removing furniture with glass and sharp edges, securing doors and windows, and installing padding if necessary (110).

Insomnia

Insomnia is typically defined as the chronic inability to obtain the amount of sleep that a person needs for optimal functioning and well-being. This may include difficulty falling asleep, brief awakenings during the night, awakening too early, or feeling unrefreshed after a night's sleep. Furthermore, insomnia is not a disease, but rather a symptom that may be associated with organic disease (e.g., hyperthyroidism), psychiatric illness such as depression, underlying sleep disorder (e.g., sleep apnea, nocturnal myoclonus, gastroesophageal reflux), or the patient's lifestyle (120–123).

The following is a brief description of many of the various specific diagnoses of insomnia.

Adjustment Sleep Disorder: Acute insomnia may arise from a number of sudden changes in life. These may include medical, surgical, or traumatic conditions; sleeping in any new environment; personal stress and anxiety (e.g., bereavement); or disturbances of biologic rhythms such as jet lag or shift work. Acute forms of insomnia typically respond to the passage of time, patient education, or the judicious use of hypnotics.

Insomnia Associated with Psychological Disorders: Varying degrees of depression, anxiety, and concern about physical well-being are common in patients with insomnia. For example, Hauri (2) reported that emotional and psychiatric problems appear to be the source of many insomnia-like sleep disturbances. In addition, insomniacs evidence more psychophysiologic disorders than do good sleepers (124,125) especially when measured on a psychometric test such as the Minnesota Multiphasic Personality Inventory (MMPI). Kales and colleagues (125) found that insomniacs, when compared to controls, had a significantly higher mean value on those clinical scales that reflect anxiety and depression. These authors suggested that sleep maintenance appeared to be more closely associated with severe psychopathologic states (e.g., schizophrenia), whereas sleep latency appeared to be more closely related to anxiety and neurotic conditions.

Hypnotic-Dependent Sleep Disorder: Pharmacologic factors must always be evaluated in patients with insomnia. Dependence on, tolerance to, and withdrawal from hypnotic agents themselves may be major factors in the complaints of some insomniac patients (126). Alcohol is a particularly important issue concerning insomnia because it is the most commonly used self-medication for insomnia. Generally, alcohol may shorten sleep onset time, but it also disrupts and fragments sleep when used in excess or on a chronic basis (122,127).

Insomnia Associated with Medical Disorders: Insomnia has been reported as a chief complaint in a number of medical conditions including thyroid dysfunction, pain, central nervous system disorders, and cardiovascular disorders (128). Thus, a thorough medical history, physical examination, and appropriate laboratory examinations must be included in the evaluation of chronic insomniac patients. Moreover, coexisting medical conditions and treatments must be considered while planning treatment for other types of insomnia. For example, hepatic or renal insufficiency may predispose certain patients to toxic reactions when taking hypnotics (129).

Insomnia Associated with Sleep Apnea: Unsatisfactory nocturnal sleep can be a complaint of a person with sleep apnea. More importantly, the routine administration of hypnotic drugs to patients presenting with sleep apnea may be life-threatening (130). Many hypnotics have been shown to produce obvious central nervous system depression, thus worsening the sleep disorder (131).

Insomnia Associated with Periodic Limb Movement Disorder or Restless Legs Syndrome: The closely associated periodic leg movements and restless legs syndrome present clinically in a person who cannot maintain sleep and suffers from brief arousals throughout the sleep period.

Sleep State Misperception: Some patients may exaggerate their sleep difficulties. The extreme case is that of the patient who complains of insomnia but exhibits no objectively demonstrable sleep problem in the sleep laboratory. In addition, this category includes the "short sleeper," who apparently requires less sleep than the average person (e.g., 3 to 5 hours) to feel rested and function effectively. In this case, simply making the patient aware of individual differences in sleep requirements may ease the patient's concern over the apparent problem.

In conclusion, while some insomnias are due to somatic factors, many persistent insomnias seem to be especially learned habits of poor sleep, with conditioning and internal arousal playing important roles. With conditioned insomnia, the stimuli and rituals surrounding sleep have preceded poor sleep so many times that they themselves can trigger frustration and insomnia. On the other hand, with internal arousal insomnia, the patient's desperation to sleep causes increased arousal and an inability to relax, thus leading to insomnia.

Treatment of Insomnia

Treating insomnia requires a careful medical and psychiatric evaluation. When the differential diagnosis of insomnia is not clear on the basis of a clinical evaluation, an overnight polysomnogram including complete recording of the EEG, electro-oculogram, electromyogram, respiration, and ECG may be recommended.

Whenever possible, treatment of insomnia should focus on a specific illness or underlying cause. Thus, the treatment plan will vary from person to person and may include psychological support, a change in life patterns, or a change in environment; at other times it may involve psychotherapy or behavioral therapy. Furthermore, treatment is sometimes aimed at a specific medical condition that causes pain or discomfort. In a large majority of cases, insomnia is best treated without hypnotic medication.

When medication is required, it is frequently an antidepressant, antipsychotic, or other medication intended to treat specific underlying conditions rather than a hypnotic aimed at the symptom of inability to sleep. However, there are times when a benzodiazepine is appropriate. These include transient situational insomnia, in which it is understood by both patient and physician that medication is being used for a brief period of time and will gradually be withdrawn. Fortunately, there are a number of short-acting benzodiazepines from which to choose. In addition, periods of sleep difficulty associated with hospitalization and surgery or other clearly defined medical conditions are also good reasons for short-term use of hypnotics. Despite this, one of the drawbacks relating to hypnotic efficacy is the belief that most sedative-hypnotic drugs do not retain their sleep-inducing effectiveness for more than a few nights (122,132,133). However, in recent years more testing of sedative-hypnotic agents have shown efficacy for as long as 3 months or longer. In fact, some clinicians treat chronic insomnia by using long-acting hypnotics every second or third night. In addition, zolpidem tartrate (Ambien) is a new nonbenzodiazepine hypnotic agent that has been shown to be effective in the treatment of short-term insomnia. In fact, studies have shown zolpidem to decrease the time it takes to fall asleep (sleep onset usually within 30 minutes of ingestion) and increases total sleep time. Furthermore, patients' normal sleep physiology is maintained (134–138).

Pharmacologic factors must always be evaluated in the patient with insomnia. Dependence on, tolerance to, and withdrawal from hypnotic agents themselves may be major factors in the complaint of some insomniac patients. In fact, some of these patients appear to improve once they have ended their dependence on hypnotics. Nevertheless, it is imperative to withdraw these drugs slowly under careful supervision to avoid the dangers of serious withdrawal symptoms, including convulsions.

Recommendations offered to patients that may be helpful with managing their insomnia include: 1) establishing rigid times of going to bed and, especially, of arising; 2) eliminating daytime naps; 3) recognizing that bed is a place for sleep (and sexual activity) but not for wakefulness, reading, eating, watching television, worrying, letter writing or any other activity; 4) getting out of bed and occupying oneself until ready to return to sleep if one cannot go to sleep or cannot return to sleep on awakening; 5) establishing a program of daytime exercise, which tends to promote nocturnal sleep; 6) engaging in evening activities conducive to relaxation, including hobbies, rest, hot baths, drinking warm milk, and so forth; and 7) avoiding stimulants all day, including caffeine.

More specifically, caffeine is a stimulant found in appreciable amounts in tea and coffee, as well as in many over-the-counter medications including pain killers and appetite suppressants. Although smaller doses of caffeine improve overall mental functioning, larger doses may impair performance and disturb sleep. Caffeine leads to increased wakefulness and drowsy sleep and reduced slow-wave sleep and total sleep time (139).

As an alternative, various behavioral therapy techniques have recently been studied and have been found to be successful in treating insomnia (121,140–142). These methods are likely to be most effective when insomnia is suspected to be the result of maladaptive learning and conditioning. Methods that have shown some efficacy in the treatment of insomnia include progressive relaxation, electromyographic biofeedback, autogenic training, systematic desensitization, and stimulus control therapy. However, due to the time commitment involved in these therapies, a health care team approach is usually more practical. Moreover, exploration should be made of greater use of social workers, counselors, nurses, and physician's assistants, along with a clinical psychologist in the formation of health care teams.

Disorders of the Circadian Rhythm

Sleep disorders of this nature have to do with internal circadian rhythms being properly entrained to the 24-hour cycling of the planet, and usual bedtime hours must be properly located within the individual's circadian rhythm (2). Many disorders of the sleep–wake schedule arise from mismatches between the patient's internal circadian rhythms and society's timetables. Consequently, patients with these disorders sleep soundly, but not at the preferred times.

Time Zone Change Syndrome

After a flight across three or more time zones, people may experience a variety of symptoms including daytime fatigue, gastrointestinal distress, headaches, tired muscles, moodiness, poor psychomotor coordination, or reduced cognitive skills (143,144). These symptoms result from a conflict between the person's internal timing system and the displaced external time cues that normally guide it (2). There are three components to jet lag: 1) external desynchronization in which the external and internal clocks are misaligned (e.g., the body wants to sleep, but the person needs to be awake). Continued exposure to the new time cues will gradually resolve the problem; 2) internal desynchronization has to do with the relationship among manifestations of the various bodily rhythms (e.g., core temperature, hormonal secretion, and sleep–wake centers). Each rhythm adjusts at a different pace, some lingering more than others; and 3) sleep loss that is the resulting common complaint (2).

The direction of the flight and the number of time zones crossed are the two variables that determine the severity of jet lag. The internal clocks of most individuals can tolerate variations of up to about 2 hours from their innate rhythm (2). However, as the circadian rhythm shortens with age (e.g., to 24 hours or less), many people notice that it gets easier to fly eastward and gradually more difficult to fly westward (145–147).

The most efficient countermeasure to jet lag is exposure to bright light (i.e., outdoor) at the destination. The person should be outside and moving in the bright light when the body wants to sleep at times inappropriate to the new destination. In addition, physical activity can also be helpful (e.g., walking). Other anticipatory steps people can take include gradually shifting all social and clock cues to the new time (e.g., meals, light/dark, sleep/wake) while still at home (2). Finally, short-acting benzodiazepines (e.g., temazepam, triazolam) have been shown to produce high quality sleep after extensive shifts in sleep schedules or after time zone transitions (148,149). However, caution should be observed because of potential side effects in some individuals and the known rebound effects of these drugs when they are discontinued (150).

Shift Work Sleep Disorder

The primary problem shift workers encounter is their attempt to restructure their personal circadian clocks while living in a world where all the chemical, physical, and social cues around them are designed for a different orientation (151). As a result, mood, well-being, and performance efficiency are apt to be disrupted by circadian rhythm disarray. Furthermore, factors within the individual, such as medical and mental health, as well as those associated with the workplace (e.g., the sequence and timing of rotating shifts) contribute to ineffective performance (2).

Education seems to be the first step in dealing with the problems of shift work. Of particular importance is teaching shift workers what is actually happening to their bodies and how to use sleep hygiene and Zeitgeber manipulation to their advantage (2,151). In addition, the application of light at appropriate times can reset the circadian clocks. Increasing the light levels under which shift workers work and darkening the places where they sleep have provided significant gains in adaptation, with clear improvement in both the quality of sleep and productivity during working hours. Furthermore, domestic and social factors play a significant role. Thus, it is essential to protect the shift worker from socially common interruptions of new daytime sleep patterns and protect both workers and family members from the social isolation that may develop as a result of shift work (151). Moreover, it may be worthwhile for shift workers to wear dark wraparound sunglasses when going home to ensure that they do not get a bright light stimulus when they are getting ready to sleep (2). Finally, the use of sedative-hypnotics is almost always inadvisable because the development of tolerance and dependence is likely.

Sleep Disorders Associated with Psychiatric Disorders

Psychiatric problems and insomnias often present together and, in fact, often potentiate each other. Furthermore, some clinicians believe that psychological stress interferes more with the process of falling asleep than with the subsequent sleep. However, this is not usually the case in middle-aged and older patients, who often fall asleep quite easily, even under significant psychological stress, only to wake up early (2).

Depression

In general, disturbed sleep serves as a diagnostic sign in patients with depression because it is so common. More specifically, sleep in depression is characterized by long sleep latencies, many awakenings during the night, early morning awakenings, low delta sleep, and shortened REM latencies, as well as a significant amount of REM sleep early in the night (152).

Any sleep disturbance associated with depression should initially be addressed by treating the underlying affective disorder. A trial of antidepressant medication may be a reasonable first step (2). However, recent assessments of psychotherapy suggest that sleep is likely to improve as other depressive symptoms abate (153). In addition, efficacious interventions include deprivation of REM sleep, total sleep deprivation, partial sleep deprivation (e.g., restricting sleep to the first half of the night), and phase advancement of the sleep–wake cycle (e.g., designating sleep hours as 6 PM to 2 AM) (109). Furthermore, when compliance with these sleep manipulations is not possible, combinations that have been reported to be of benefit include lithium with partial sleep deprivation (154) and clomipramine with total sleep deprivation (155).

Anxiety Disorders

Anxiety disorders are psychiatric disorders characterized by anxiety and agitation, in addition to avoidance behavior in some individuals. Patients with these disorders generally have difficulty falling asleep, frequent and long awakenings from sleep, a decreased amount of delta sleep, as well as relatively long REM latencies compared to sleep in depression (2).

Insomnia is often associated with anxiety disorders, keeping patients from being able to confront the underlying psychiatric issues while symptoms continue. Appropriate treatment can include psychotherapy, behavior therapy, and, in some cases, pharmacotherapy. However, medication should be viewed as part of a therapeutic program, not as the only treatment (2).

Another condition that causes a significant amount of dysautonomia resulting in sleep disturbances is mitral valve prolapse syndrome. More specifically, this condition can create a significant amount of anxiety including sleep panic attacks (156) and difficulty maintaining sleep (157). Pharmacologically, effective treatment has been demonstrated with a variety of medications including alprazolam, verapamil, clonopin, and phenobarbital (12). In addition, modifications in diet including eliminating caffeine and sugar, and reducing fat consumption has been shown to be of benefit. Exercise and fluid replacement have also been shown to be an important component in the control of the symptoms of mitral value prolapse (157).

Personality Disorders

Patients with these psychiatric disorders often have predominant anxiety, fear, and preoccupations, as well as racing thoughts that may keep them awake. Furthermore, these patients often are diagnosed with another disorder (e.g., substance abuse/dependence) that may affect sleep negatively.

Treatment of these patients tends to be difficult because of the numerous issues they bring to therapy, as well as their reluctance often to remain in treatment. Thus, the focus of treatment should be on the most acute issues.

Alcoholism

Patients with alcoholism commonly report sleep disturbances. Typically, the sleep of these individuals is fragmented, shallow, and shortened. Many recovering alcoholics experience insomnia and objective sleep disturbances for many years. These problems with sleeping often predispose patients to renew drinking. Research has also shown alcoholics to have significant and persistent circadian rhythm disturbances (158–160).

Currently, no specific therapies have been discovered to successfully treat sleep disturbances in alcoholics. Furthermore, these patients are susceptible to cross-addiction to other CNS depressants (e.g., benzodiazepines). However, the use of light therapy, as well as general sleep hygiene principles may be of some benefit (2).

Sleep Disorders Associated with Dementia

Dementia is an organically produced impairment that disrupts higher cortical functions. Moreover, many patients with dementia experience moderate to severe sleep disturbances. For example, Vitiello and Prinz (161) report that patients in the later stages of Alzheimer's disease have significant losses in REM sleep, as well as breakdown of the sleep–wake circadian rhythm resulting in a significant amount of sleep occurring during the day. However, these authors note this daytime sleep is of poor quality consisting primarily of stages 1 and 2 sleep. Thus, this daytime sleep does not compensate for the nighttime loses of slow-wave sleep and REM sleep experienced by patients.

Treating sleep disturbances in these patients is rather difficult. However, families need to be encouraged to try to minimize the napping behavior of the patient in an attempt to try and consolidate sleep into the night. Vitiello and Prinz (161) state this may have the effect of somewhat lessening the amount of nocturnal disruption of sleep that accompanies progression of the disease. Moreover, exposure to bright light may help strengthen the circadian rhythm and avoid the "sundowning" syndrome (2).

REFERENCES

1. Mellinger GD, Balter MB, Uhlenhuth EH. Insomnia and its treatment: prevalence and correlates. Arch Gen Psychiatry 1985;42:225–232.

2. Hauri PJ. Current concepts: the sleep disorders. Kalamazoo, MI: Upjohn, 1992.

3. Hartmann E. What we know about sleep. Medical Times 1979;107:36–47.

4. Pegram GV, Hyde P, Weiler D. Sleep and its disorders: an overview. Alabama Journal of Medical Sciences 1980;17:147–155.

5. Pegram GV, Connell BE, Gnadt J, Weiler D. Neu-

ropsychology and the field of sleep and sleep disorders. In Filskov SB, & Boll TJ, eds. Handbook of clinical neuropsychology. Vol II. New York: John Wiley & Sons, 1986:426–492.

6. Carlson NR. Physiology of behavior. Boston: Allyn and Bacon, 1994.

7. Brezinova V, Oswald I, Loudon J. Two types of insomnia: too much waking or not enough sleep. Br J Psychiatry 1975;126:439–445.

8. Monnier M, Gaillard JM. Biochemical regulation of sleep. Experientia 1980;36:21–24.

9. Bliwise DL. Sleep in normal aging and dementia. Sleep 1993;16:40–81.

10. Bonnet MH, Arand DL. Sleep loss in aging. Clinics in geriatric medicine. 1989;5:405–420.

11. Webb WB. Sleep as a biological rhythm. Paper presented at the annual meeting of the Southern Sleep Society, Memphis, TN, 1984.

12. Wooten V. Medical causes of insomnia. In Kryger MH, Roth T, Dement WC, eds. Principles and practice of sleep medicine. Philadelphia: WB. Saunders, 1994:509–522.

13. Morgan BB. Effects of continuous work and sleep loss in the reduction and recovery of work efficiency. Am Ind Hygi Assoc J 1974;35:13–20.

14. Williams HL, Karacan I, Hirsch CJ. Electroencephalography (EEG) of human sleep: Clinical applications. New York: John Wiley & Sons, 1974.

15. Rechtshaften A, Gilliland MA, Bergman BM, Winter JB. Physiological correlates of prolonged sleep deprivation in rats. Science 1983;221:182–184.

16. Aschoff J, Wever R. Human circadian rhythms: a multioscillatory system. Fed Proc 1976;35:2326–2332.

17. Kokkoris CP, Bradlow H, Czeisler CA, et al. Long-term ambulatory temperature monitoring in a subject with hypernycthermal sleep-wake cycle disturbance. Sleep 1978;1:177–190.

18. Lowenstein O, Lowenfeld IE. The sleep-waking cycle and pupillary activity. Ann N Y Acad Sci 1964;17:142–156.

19. Mitler MM. The multiple sleep latency test as an evaluation for excessive somnolence. In Guilleminault C, ed. Sleeping and waking disorders: indications and techniques. Menlo Park, CA: Addison-Wesley.

20. Weitzman ED. Sleep and its disorders. Annu Rev Neurosci 1981;4:381–417.

21. Czeisler CA, Kronauer RE, Mooney JJ, et al. Biologic rhythm disorders, depression, and phototherapy: a new hypothesis. Psychiatr Clin North Am 1987;10:687–709.

22. Monk TH. Circadian rhythms. Clin Geriatr Med 1989;5:331–346.

23. Kryger MH, Roth R, Carskadon M. Circadian rhythms in humans: an overview. In: Kryger MH, Roth T, Dement WC, eds. Principles and practice of sleep medicine. Philadelphia: WB Saunders, 1994:301–308.

24. Shanahan TL, Czeisler CA. Light exposure induces equivalent phase shifts of the endogenous circadian rhythms of circulating plasma melatonin and core body temperature in men. J Clin Endocrinol Metab 1991;73:227–235.

25. Lewy AJ, Sacks RL. The dim light melatonin onset as a marker for circadian phase position. Chronobiol Int 1989;6:93–102.

26. Mauri M. Sleep and the reproductive cycle: a review. Health Care for Women International 1990;11:409–421.

27. National Commission on Sleep Disorders Research. Wake up America: a national sleep alert. Vol. I. United States Department of Health and Human Services, 1993.

28. Karacan I, Williams RL. Current advances in theory and practice relating to postpartum syndromes. Psychiatry and Medicine 1970;1:307–328.

29. Schweiger MS. Sleep disturbance in pregnancy. A subjective survey. Am J Obstet Gynecol 1972;114:879–882.

30. Karacan I, Heine W, Agnew HW Jr, et al. Characteristics of sleep patterns during late pregnancy and the postpartum period. Am J Obstet Gynecol 1968;101:579–586.

31. Anders TF, Rolffwarg HP. The relationship between infant and maternal sleep. Psychophysiology 1968;5:227–228.

32. Kales A, Kales JD. Evaluation and treatment of insomnia. New York: Oxford University Press, 1984.

33. Steiner M. Psychobiology of mental disorders associated with childbearing. Acta Psychiatr Scand 1979;60:449–464.

34. Dalton K. Postnatal depression. In: Depression after childbirth. New York: Oxford University Press, 1980:22–25.

35. Berlin RM. Sleepwalking disorders during pregnancy: a case report. Sleep 1988;11:208–210.

36. Feinsilver SH, Hertz G. Respiration during sleep in pregnancy. Clin Chest Med 1992;13:637–644.

37. Weinberger SE, Weiss ST, Cohen WR. State of the art: Pregnancy and the lung. Am Rev Res Dis 1980;121:559–581.

38. Brownwell LG, West P, Kryger MH. Breathing during sleep in normal pregnant women. Am Rev Respir Dis 1986;133:38–41.

39. Jaffe RB, Josimovich JB. Endocrine physiology of pregnancy. In: Danford DN, Obstetrics and gynecology New York: Harper & Row, 1977:286–298.

40. Lyons HA. Centrally acting hormones and respiration. Pharmacological Therapy 1978;2:743–751.

41. Mischell DR, Davajan V. Reproductive endocrinology, infertility, and contraception. Philadelphia: FA Davis, 1979.

42. Yannone, ME. McCurdy JR, Goldfein A. Plasma progesterone levels in normal pregnancy, labor, and the puerperium. Am J Obstet Gynecol 1968;101:1058–1061.

43. Joel-Cohen SH, Schoenfeld A. Fetal response to period sleep apnea: a new syndrome in obstetrics. Eur J Obstet, Gynecol Reprod Biol 1978;8:77–81.

44. Schoenfeld A, Ovadia Y, Neri, A. Obstructive sleep apnea (OSA)—implications in maternal-fetal medicine. A hypothesis. Med Hypothses 1989;30;51–54.

45. Conti M, Izzo V, Muggiasca ML. Sleep apnea syndrome in pregnancy: a case report. Eur J Anaesthesiol 1988;5:151–154.

46. American Society of Hospital Pharmacists. American hospital formulary service drug information. Bethesda, MD: 1989:1115.

47. Charbonneau M, Falcone T, Cosio MG. Obstructive sleep apnea during pregnancy: therapy and implications for fetal health. Am Rev Respir Dis 1991; 144:461–463.

48. Kowell J, Clark G, Nino-Murcia G. Precipitation of obstructive sleep apnea during pregnancy. Obstet Gynecol 1989;74:453–455.

49. Campbell S, Whitehead M. Estrogen therapy and the post-menopausal syndrome. Clin Obstet Gynecol 1977;4:31.

50. Erlik Y, Tataryn IV, Meldrum DR. Association of waking episodes with menopausal hot flashes. JAMA 1981;245:1741.

51. Meldrum DR. Treatment of hot flashes. In: Mischell DR, ed. Menopause: physiology and pharmacology. Chicago: Year Book Medical Publishers, 1987:141–148.

52. Ravnikar VA, Schiff I, Regestein QR. Menopause and sleep. In Buchsbaum HJ, ed. The menopause. New York: Springer-Verlag, 1983:161–171.

53. Anderson E, Hamburger S, Lin JH, Revar RW. Characteristics of menopause women seeking assistance. 1987.

54. Shaver J, Biblin E, Lentz M, Lee K. Sleep patterns and stability in perimenopausal women. Sleep 1988; 11:556–561.

55. Thomson I, Oswald I. Effect of estrogen on the sleep, mood, and anxiety of menopausal women. Br Med J 1977;2:1317–1319.

56. Schiff I, Regestein Q, Tulchinsky D, Ryan KJ. Effects of estrogen on sleep and psychological state of hypogonadal women. JAMA 1979;242:2405–2407.

57. Kopelman PG, Apps MC, Cope T, Empey DW. The influence of menstrual status, body weight, and hypothalamic function on nocturnal respiration in women. J Royal Coll Physicians Lond 1985;19:243–247.

58. Guilleminault C, Quera-Salva M, Partinen M, Jamieson A. Women and the obstructive sleep apnea syndrome. Chest 1988;93:104–109.

59. Block AJ, Boysen PG. Wynne JW, Hunt LA. Sleep apnea, hypopnea, and oxygen desaturation in normal subjects: a strong male predominance. N Engl J Med 1979;300:513–517.

60. Kreis P, Kripke DP, Ancoli-Israel S. Sleep apnea: a prospective study. West J Med 1983;139:171–173.

61. Phillipson EA. State of the art: control of breathing during sleep. Am Rev Respir Dis 1978;118:909–939.

62. Block AJ, Wynne J, Boysen P, et al. Menopause, medroxyprogesterone, and breathing during sleep. Am J Med 1981;70:506–510.

63. Hensley M, Saunders N, Stohl K. Medroxyprogesterone treatment of obstructive sleep apnea. Sleep 1980;3:441–446

64. Orr W, Imes N, Martin R. Progesterone therapy in obese patients with sleep apnea. Arch Int 1979;139:109–111.

65. Pickett CK, Regensteiner JG, Woodard WD, et al. Progestin and estrogen reduce sleep-disordered breathing in postmenopausal women. J Appl Physiol 1989;66:1656–1661.

66. Moldavsky H, Scarisbrick P, England R. Musculoskeletal systems and non-REM sleep disturbance in patients with "fibrositis syndrome" and healthy subjects. Psychosom Med 1975;37:341–351.

67. Waxman J, Zatzkis SM. Fibromyalgia and menopause: examination of the relationship. Postgrad Med 1986;80:165–171.

68. Guilleminault C. Obstructive sleep apnea: a review. Psychiatr Clin North Am 1987;10:607–621.

69. Shepard JW. Cardiopulmonary consequences of obstructive sleep apnea. Mayo Clin Proc 1990;65:1250–1259.

70. Smirne S, Franceschi M, Zamproni P, et al. Prevalence of sleep disorders in an unselected inpatient population. In: Guilleminault C, Lugaresi E, eds. Sleep/wake disorders: natural history, epidemiology and long-term evolution. New York: Raven Press, 1983:61–72.

71. Young T, Palta M, Dempsey J, et al. The occurrence of sleep-disordered breathing among middle-aged adults. N Engl J Med 1993;328:1230–1235.

72. Hauri PJ. Evaluating disorders of initiating and maintaining sleep (DIMS). In: Guilleminault C, ed. Sleep and waking disorders: indications and techniques. Menlo Park, CA: Addison-Wesley, 1982;225–244.

73. Kovacevic-Ristanovic R, Nausieda PA. Sleep disorders. In Weiner WJ, Goetz CG, eds. Neurology for the non-neurologist. Philadelphia; JB Lippincott, 1989:271–286.

74. Findley LJ. Automobile driving in sleep apnea. Sleep and Respiration 1990;57:337–345.

75. White DP, Zwillich CW, Pickett CK, et al. Central sleep apnea: improvement with acetazolamide therapy. Arch Intern Med 1982;142;1816–1819.

76. Sullivan CE, Grunstein RR. Continuous positive airway pressure in sleep-disordered breathing. In: Kryger MH, Roth T, Dement WC, eds. Principles and practice of sleep medicine. Philadelphia: WB. Saunders, 1994;694–705.

77. Harman EM, Wynne JW, Block AJ. The effect of weight loss on sleep-disordered breathing and oxygen desaturation in morbidly obese men. Chest 1982;82:291–294.

78. Kuo PC, West RA, Bloomquist DS, McNeil RW. The effects of mandibular osteotomy in three patients with hypersomnia sleep apnea. Oral Surg 1979;48:385–392.

79. Shepard JW, Olsen KD. Uvulopalatopharyngoplasty for treatment of obstructive sleep apnea. Mayo Clin Proc 1990;65:1260–1267.

80. Silvestri R, Guilleminault C, Simmons FB. Palatopharyngoplasty in the treatment of obstructive sleep apneic patients. In: Guilleminault C, Lugaresi E, eds. Sleep/wake disorders: natural history, epidemiology and long-term evolution. New York: Raven Press, 1983:163–170.

81. Stevenson EW, Turner GT, Sutton FD, et al. Prognostic significance of age and tonsillectomy in uvulopalatopharyngoplasty. Laryngoscope 1990;100:820–823.

82. Clark RW, Schmidt HS, Schaal SF, et al. Sleep apnea treatment with protriptyline. Neurology 1979;29:1287–1292.

83. Waite PD, Wooten V, Lachner J, Guyette RF. Maxillomandibular advancement surgery in 23 patients with obstructive sleep apnea. J Oral Maxillofac Surg 1989;47:1256–1261.

84. Cartwright RD, Samuelson CF, Weber S, et al. A mechanical treatment for obstructive sleep apnea: the tongue retaining device. Sleep Res 1980;9:188. Abstract.

85. Mitler MM, Nelson S, Hajdukovic, R. Narcolepsy: diagnosis, treatment, and management. Psychiatr Clin North Am 1987;10:593–606.

86. Richardson JW, Frederickson PA, Lin SC. Narcolepsy update. Mayo Clin Proc 1990;65:991–998.

87. Zarcone V. Narcolepsy. N Engl J Med 1973;288:1156–1166.

88. Guilleminault C, Wilson RA, Dement WC. A study on cataplexy. Arch Neurol 1974;31:255-261.

89. Kales A, Cadieux RJ, Soldatos CR, et al. Narcolepsy-cataplexy: I. Clinical and electrophysiological characteristics. Arch Neurol 1982;39:164–168.

90. Billiard M, Besset A, Cadilhac J. The clinical and polygraphic development of narcolepsy. In: Guilleminault C, Lugaresi E, eds. Sleep/wake disorders: Natural history, epidemiology and long-term evolution. New York: Raven Press, 1983.

91. Mitler M, Orem J, Dement WC. Cataplexy in dogs I: patterns of tendon reflex and H-reflex suppression. Sleep Res 1976;5:49.

92. Mitler MM, Gujavarty KS. Narcolepsy: when to suspect it and how to help. Consultant 1982;22:215–224.

93. Dement WC. Narcolepsy—not as rare as we believed! Medical Times 1979;107:51–55.

94. Schmidt HS, Clark RW, Hyman P. Protriptyline: an effective agent in the treatment of the narcolepsy-cataplexy syndrome and hypersomnia. Am J Psychiatry 1977;134:183–185.

95. Kales A, Cadieux RJ, Soldatos C, Tjiauw-Ling T. Successful treatment of narcolepsy with propranolol: a case report. Arch Neurol 1979;36:650–651

96. Broughton R, Mamelak M. The treatment of narcolepsy-cataplexy with nocturnal gamma-hydroxybutyrate. Can J Neurol Sci 1979;6:1–6.

97. Langdon N, Bandak S, Shindler J. Fluoxetine in the treatment of cataplexy. Sleep 1986;9:371.

98. Adams RD, Victor M. Principles of neurology. New York: McGraw-Hill, 1985.

99. Coleman RM, Blinise DL, Sajben N, et al. Epidemiology of periodic movements during sleep. In: Guilleminault C, Lugaresi E, eds. Sleep/wake disorders: natural history, epidemiology and long-term evolution. New York: Raven Press, 1983:87–98.

100. Vgontzas AN, Kales N, Bixler EO, Vela-Bueno A. Sleep disorders related to another mental disorder (nonsubstance/primary): a DSM-IV literature review. J Clin Psychiatry 1993;54:256–259.

101. Krueger BR. Restless legs syndrome and periodic movements of sleep. Mayo Clin Proc 1990;65;999–1006.

102. Lugaresi G, Cirignotta F, Zucconi M, et al. Good and poor sleepers: An epidemiological survey of the San Marino population. In: Guilleminault C, Lugaresi E, eds. Sleep/wake disorders: Natural history, epidemiology and long-term evolution New York: Raven Press, 1983:1–12.

103. Boghen D, Peyronnard JM. Myoclonus in familial restless legs syndrome. Arch Neurol 1976;33:368–370.

104. Montagna P, Coccagna G, Cirignotta F, Lugeresi E. Familial restless legs syndrome: long-term follow-up. In Guilleminault C, Lugaresi E, eds. Sleep/wake disorders: natural history, epidemiology and long-term evolution. New York: Raven Press, 1983:231–236.

105. Ohanna N, Pelad R, Rubin AE, et al. Periodic leg movements in sleep: effect of clonazepam treatment. Neurology 1985;35:408–411.

106. Oshtory MA, Vijayan N. Clonazepam treatment of insomnia due to sleep myoclonus. Arch Neurol 1980;15:234–239.

107. Pelad R, Lavie P. Double-blind evaluation of clonazepam on periodic leg movements in sleep. J Neurol, Neurosurg Psychiatry 1987;50:1679–1681.

108. Kavey N, Hening W, Walters A, et al. Treatment of restless legs and periodic movements in sleep with opioids. Sleep Research 1985;14:177. Abstract.

109. Doghramji K. Sleep disorders: a selective update. Hosp Community Psychiatry 1989;40:29–40.

110. Thorpy MJ, Glovinsky PB. Parasomnias. Psychiatr Clin North Am 1987;10:623–639.

111. Kales JD, Kales A, Soldatos, CR. Night terrors: clinical characteristics and personality patterns. Arch Gen Psychiatry 1980;37:1413–1417.

112. Kales A, Soldatos CR, Caldwell AB. Sleepwalking. Arch Gen Psychiatry 1980;37:1406–1410.

113. Schenck CH, Bundie SR, Patterson AL. Rapid eye movement sleep behavior disorder: a treatable parasomnia affecting older adults. JAMA 1987;257:1786–1789.

114. Dogrhamji K, Connell TA, Gaddy JR. Loss of REM sleep atonia: three case reports. Sleep Research 1987;16:327.

115. Quera Salva MA, Guilleminault C. Olivo-ponto-cerebellar degeneration, abnormal sleep, and REM sleep without atonia. Neurology 1986;36:576–577.

116. Gross MM, Goodenough DG, Tobin M. Sleep disturbances and hallucinations in the acute alcoholic psychoses. J Nerv Ment Dis 1966;142:493–514.

117. Reid WH. Treatment of somnambulism in military trainees. Am J Psychiatry 1975;29:101–105.

118. Hurwitz TD, Mahowald MW, Schenck CH, et al. A retrospective outcome study and review of hypnosis as treatment of adults with sleepwalking and sleep terror. J Nerv Men Dis 1991;179:228–233.

119. Schenck CH, Mahowald MW. Polysomnographic, neurologic, psychiatric, and clinical outcome report on 70 consecutive cases with REM sleep behavior disorder (RBD): sustained clonazepam efficacy in 89.5% of 57 treated patients. Clev Clin J Med 1990;57:S9–S23.

120. Erman MK. Insomnia. Psychiatr Clin North Am 1987;10:525–539.

121. Hauri PJ, Esther MS. Insomnia. Mayo Clin Proc 1990;65:869–882.

122. Mendelson WB Pharmacotherapy of insomnia. Psychiatr Clin North Am 1987;10:555–563.

123. Mendelson WB. Insomnia and related sleep disorders. Psychiatr Clin North Am 1993;16:841–851.

124. Hauri P. Behavioral treatments of insomnia. Medical Times 1979;107:36–47.

125. Kales A, Caldwell A, Bixler EO, et al. Further evaluation of MMPI findings in insomnia: comparison of insomniac patients and normal controls. Sleep Research 1978;7:189. Abstract.

126. Morin CM. Insomnia: psychological assessment and management. New York: Guilford Press, 1992.

127. Zarcone VP. Sleep hygiene. In: Kryger MH, Roth T, Dement WC, eds. Principles and practice of sleep medicine. Philadelphia: WB Saunders, 1994:542–548.

128. Williamson DA, Barker SE, Vernon-Guidry S. Psychophysiological disorders. In Van Hasselt & Hersen, eds. Advanced abnormal psychology. New York: Plenum Press, 1994:373–384.

129. Wengel SP, Burke WJ, Ranno AE, Roccaforte WH. Use of benzodiazepines in the elderly. Psychiatric Annals 1993;23:325–331.

130. Hartmann E. The sleeping pill. New Haven, CT: Yale University Press, 1978.

131. Fredrickson PA, Richardson JW, Esther MS, Siong-Chi L. Sleep disorders in psychiatric practice. Mayo Clinic Proceedings, 1990;65:861–868.

132. Bernstein JG. Handbook of drug therapy in psychiatry. Littleton, MA: PSG Publishing, 1988.

133. Julien RM. A primer of drug action. New York; W.H. Freeman, 1992.

134. Merlotti L, Roehrs T, Koshorek G. The dose effects of zolpidem on the sleep of healthy normals. J Clin Psychopharmacol 1989;9:9–14.

135. Oswald I, Adam K. A new look at short-acting hypnotics. In: Sauvaret JP, Langer SZ, Morselli PL, eds. Imidazopyridines in sleep disorders. New York: Raven Press, 1988.

136. Sharf MB, Mayleben DW, Kaffeman M. Dose response effects of zolpidem in normal geriatric subjects. J Clin Psychopharmacol 1991;52:77–83.

137. Vogel G, Sharf M, Walsh J. Effects of chronically administered zolpidem on the sleep of healthy insomniacs. Sleep Res 1989;18:80. Abstract.

138. Walsh JK, Schweitzer PK, Sugarman JL. Transient insomnia associated with a 3-hour phase advance of sleep time and treatment with zolpidem. J Clin Psychopharmacol 1990;10:184–189.

139. Nicholson AN, Bradley CN, Pascoe PA. Medications: effect of sleep and wakefulness. In: Kryger MH, Roth T, Dement WC, eds. Principles and practice of sleep medicine. Philadelphia: WB Saunders, 1994:364–372.

140. Knapp T, Downs D, Alperson J. Behavior therapy for insomnia: a review. Behavior Therapy 1976;7:614–625.

141. Ribordy SC, Denney DR. The behavioral treatment of insomnia: an alternative to drug therapy. Behav Res Ther 1977;15:39–50.

142. Shealy RC. The effectiveness of various treatment techniques on different degrees and durations of sleep-onset insomnia. Behav Res Ther 1979;17:541–546.

143. Loat CER, Rhodes EC. Jet-lag and human performance. Sports Med 1989;8:226–238.

144. O'Connor KA, Mahowald MW, Ettinger MG. Circadian rhythm disorders. In: Chokroverty S, ed. Sleep disorders medicine: basic science, technical considerations, and clinical aspects. Boston: Butterworth-Heinemann, 1994:369–379.

145. Dement WC, Seidel WF, Cohen SA, et al. Sleep and wakefulness in aircrew before and after transoceanic flights. Aviat Space Environ Med 1986;57(suppl 12):B14–B28.

146. Nicholson AN, Pascoe PA, Spencer MB. Sleep after transmeridian flights. Lancet 1986;1:1205–1208.

147. Preston FS. Further sleep problems in airline pilots on worldwide schedules. Aerospace Medicine 1973;44:775–782.

148. Nicholson AN, Pascoe PA, Spencer MB, et al. Nocturnal and daytime alertness of aircrew after transmeridian flights. Aviat Space Environ Med 1986;57(suppl 12):B43–B52.

149. Seidel WF, Endo S, Roehrs T. Treatment of a 12-hour shift of sleep schedule with benzodiazepines. Science 1984;224:1262–1264.

150. Graeber RC. Jet lag and sleep disruption. In: Kryger MH, Roth T, Dement WC, eds. Principles and practice of sleep medicine. Philadelphia: WB Saunders, 1994:463–470.

151. Monk TH. Shift work. In: Kryger MH, Roth T, Dement WC, eds. Principles and practice of sleep medicine. Philadelphia: WB Saunders, 1994:471–481.

152. Reynolds CF, Coble PA, Kupfer DJ. Depressive patients and the sleep laboratory. In Guilleminault C, ed. Sleeping and waking disorders: indications and techniques. Menlo Park, CA: Addison-Wesley, 1982:245–264.

153. Simons A, Murphy GE, Levine JL. Cognitive therapy and psychotherapy for depression. Arch Gen Psychiatry 1986;43:43–48.

154. Baxter LR, Liston EH, Schwartz JM. Prolongation of the antidepressant response to partial sleep deprivation by lithium. Psychiatry Res 1986;19:17–23.

155. Elsenga S, van den Hoofdakker RH. Response to total sleep deprivation and clomipramine in endogenous depression. J Psychiatr Res 1987;21:151–161.

156. Uhde TW, Roy-Byrne PP, Gillen JC. The sleep of patients with panic disorder: A preliminary report. Psychiatr Res 1984;12:251–259.

157. Frederickson L. Confronting mitral valve prolapse syndrome. San Marcos, CA: Avant Books, 1988.

158. Gross MM, Hastey JM. Sleep disturbances in alcoholism. In: Tarter RE, Suguman AA, eds. Alcoholism: interdisciplinary approaches to an enduring problem. Reading, MA: Addison-Wesley, 1976.

159. Imatoh N, Nakazawa Y, Ohshima H. Circadian rhythm of REM sleep of chronic alcoholics during alcohol withdrawal. Drug & Alcohol Dependence 1986;18:77–85.

160. Wolin SJ, Meilo NK. The effects of alcohol on dreams and hallucinations in alcohol addicts. Ann N Y Acad Sci 1973;215:266–302.

161. Vitiello MV, Prinz PN. Alzheimer's disease: sleep and sleep/wake patterns. Clin Geriatr Med 1987;5;289–299.

CHAPTER 40

PERSONALITY DISORDERS

Nathan Smith

Patients with personality disorders are a part of most physician's clinical practice. These patients, however, are more likely to be referred to as croaks, cranks, or hateful patients. They make up a large part of patients who are clinical management problems, treatment failures, and high users of medical care. They have an unusual ability to get under other people's skin. Because patients with personality disorders are often difficult to manage and physicians may not like them, these patients represent a challenge and a potential threat to their physicians. The challenge is to understand these patients better and to provide care that appropriately uses medical resources. The threat is that a lack of understanding of these patients may result in the physician neglecting the patient's genuine health care needs or overindulging the patient's needs. The goal of this chapter is to present a description of personality disorders with an emphasis on how these disorders may have an impact on the physician–patient relationship.

The Definition of Personality Disorders

Patients with personality disorders may present with symptoms of anxiety, depression, or substance abuse, which are common to a variety of psychiatric disorders. More often, the most dramatic evidence of the disorder is not found in the patient's presenting history, but is evident in how the patient relates to the physician and how the physician feels toward the patient. Escalating demands for attention from the physician by a patient in face of growing anger or loathing in the physician may be evidence of a patient with personality disorder.

The *Diagnostic and Statistics Manual of Mental Disorders, Third Edition-Revised* (DSM-III-R) of the American Psychiatric Association, the most popular classification of mental disorders, defines personality traits and personality disorders as follows:

> Personality *traits* are enduring patterns of perceiving, relating to, and thinking about the environment, and oneself, and are exhibited in a wide range of important social and personal contexts. It is only when *personality traits* are inflexible and maladaptive and cause either significant functional impairment or subjective distress that they constitute *Personality Disorders.* The manifestations of Personality Disorders are often recognizable by adolescence or earlier and continue throughout most of adult life, though they often become less obvious in middle or old age.

We all have personality traits. This may be illustrated by the different ways that people squeeze toothpaste from a tube of toothpaste. Some have the trait to press compulsively the toothpaste tube flat from the bottom up to the opening (and think this is the only way it should be done!), whereas others have the trait to press the toothpaste tube randomly along its length (not noticing nor having concern about how it should be done!). Although both of these traits are adaptive as a part of good dental hygiene, to refuse to brush one's teeth because one's spouse prefers to use a method of squeezing toothpaste from a toothpaste tube different from one's own would be suggestive of maladaptive inflexibility. Obviously, this alone would not indicate a personality disorder. It does illustrate how we all have traits that are potentially maladaptive in interpersonal relationships. Personality disorders are characterized by having combinations of traits that are inflexible and maladaptive and reflect the person's recent and long-term functioning since early adulthood, are present across time and a variety of situations, and lead to impairments in social or occupational functioning or subjective distress.

People with personality disorders often have difficulty regulating their anger or other strong emotion in an appropriate manner and also find it difficult to adapt to demands from the outside world, attempting instead to make the world adapt to them. Individuals with pneumonia or rheumatoid arthritis know they are sick and in pain. Individuals with personality disorders, on the other hand, are not likely to acknowledge they are in pain, now or in the future. The few who do recognize they have a problem are usually unable to do anything about their problem.

The DSM-III-R divides personality disorders into three clusters of related disorders. Box 40.1 lists the three clusters, the distinctive characteristics of the cluster, and the personality disorders in each cluster. The descriptions of personality disorders that follow are based on the DSM-III-R criteria. Of all the disorders in the DSM-III-R, personality disorders are the most debated and, in most cases, the least studied of the disorders in the DSM-III-R. Personality disorders, as chronic and long-standing conditions, also differ from the other psychiatric diagnoses, which are primarily episodic in nature.

Box 40.1 DSM-III-R Personality Disorder Clusters

DSM-III-R Clusters	Typical Characteristic	DSM-III-R Diagnoses
Cluster A	Odd or eccentric	Paranoid Schizoid Schizotypal
Cluster B	Dramatic, emotional or erratic	Antisocial Borderline Histrionic Narcissistic
Cluster C	Anxious or fearful	Avoidant Dependent Obsessive compulsive Passive aggressive

Causes of Personality Disorder

Although discussions of the pathogenesis of personality disorders are extensive, definitive comprehensive explanations are nonexistent. Trying to explain the origin and development of the patterns of how a person comes to perceive, relate to, and think about his environment and self invites many theoretical perspectives. Consistent findings on the causal factors are scanty and unreliable. As a consequence of the complex systemic context in which psychopathology originates and the lack of reliable data, a variety of approaches to understanding and explaining the pathogenesis of personality disorders have evolved. As a way of organizing the various approaches, personality may be divided into two components, temperament and character.

Temperament includes the domain of biology and includes the contribution of genes and other biologic processes to personality. These other biologic factors may include the presence of birth trauma or the occurrence of the following in childhood: physical illness, encephalitis, learning disabilities, signs of nonspecific neurologic dysfunction, or temporal lobe epilesy. Temperament may be thought of as representing nature's contribution to personality.

Character includes the domains of learning from upbringing and relationships and from cultural and social influences. Dynamic theorists have focused on the childhood experiences within the primary caregiving environment. Character may be thought of as representing the contribution of nurture to the development of personality. Although dynamic theorists provide vivid characterizations of personality disorders and plausible explanations for how personality disorders develop, there is almost a total absence of empiric data to support these explanations.

Cluster A Personality Disorders—Odd or Eccentric Disorders

The cluster A disorders share many features of schizophrenia and delusional disorder. The diagnosis of these personality disorders is not made if the defining symptoms occur only in the course of schizophrenia or delusional disorder.

Paranoid Personality Disorder

Description

Paranoid personality disorder is characterized by a person's long-standing and pervasive suspiciousness and mistrust of others. The actions of others are interpreted as deliberately demeaning and threatening. There is an expectation of being exploited and harmed by others. They focus on irrelevant details that confirm their suspicions and they have no appreciation for the broader context of life. People with paranoid personalities are unable to or do not accept responsibility for their own feelings. They attribute their feelings and motives to others and then question their loyalty and trustworthiness. They are often seen by others as humorless, unsentimental, guarded, defensive, secretive, stubborn, and scheming. They may be highly moralistic. Interpersonal relationships are strained by their difficulty in expressing warm feelings and their inability to tolerate feelings of dependence. They tend to generate fear and uneasiness in others. This disorder includes many of life's least attractive characters: the litigious grouch; various fanatics, bigots, and injustice collectors; pathologically jealous lovers.

Under stress, they may become delusional or express ideas of reference. If delusions are present they are transient.

Although occupational problems are common due to problems with authority figures and, in most cases, all relationships are impaired, they can on occasion be loyal, if not enjoyable patients.

Causes

The cause of this disorder is unknown. Adoption studies suggest a biologic relationship between chronic schizophrenia and this disorder. Psychoanalytic explanations suggest that this disorder is caused by the child, after being the object of the parent's irrational and overwhelming rage, adopting the parent's style and projecting irrational and overwhelming rage onto others.

Epidemiology

The prevalence of paranoid personality disorder is not known. It is more commonly diagnosed in men than women.

Differential Diagnosis

Among disorders in the differential diagnosis are two Axis I (DSM-III-R disorders), or major psychiatric disorders, delusional disorder and schizophrenia. These two disorders both differ in that they have prominent symptoms of delusions or hallucinations, which are absent in paranoid personality disorder. People with paranoid personality share problems developing close relationships and poor occupational performance with antisocial personality disorder. The latter is distinguished by its history of lifelong antisocial behavior. People with borderline personality disorder may show paranoid features, but their overinvolved, chaotic relationships contrast with the paranoid's aloofness and distance from others.

Treatment

Treatment requires a professional and straightforward manner on the part of the caregiver. Paranoid people are suspicious of others, leading them to assign ill-intentioned motives to others. Under stress, paranoid people can become threatening. The caregiver must set limits on any threatening behavior and take whatever action necessary to maintain the patient's and the caregiver's safety.

Because of the nature of the disorder, patient's with paranoid personality are difficult to engage in treatment. Individual psychotherapy is the treatment of choice because patients with this disorder do not tolerate the confrontation of group therapy or the directive techniques of behavior therapy. There are no studies on the use of pharmacologic agents in this disorder. Clinical experience is that these patients are often reluctant to accept medications for treatment.

Schizoid Personality Disorder

Description

Schizoid personality disorder has been called the disorder of lighthouse keepers. The disorder is characterized by pervasive and lifelong social isolation and restricted range of emotional experience and expression. There is a lack of desire for and enjoyment of close relationships. Because of this, and a lack of social skills, men rarely marry. Women may passively accept dating and marriage. Their sex life may exist only in fantasies. Although they prefer to be loners, often resulting in occupational difficulties, they may be successful in isolated or abstract jobs most people would find difficult to tolerate. Usually there is difficulty in acknowledging the experience of or the expression of anger. Other people may see them as aloof, self-absorbed, emotionally cold, or socially awkward. Although they may appear self-absorbed and distracted, they demonstrate no loss in their ability to organize reality. This disorder may be found in the community of street people as well as in the halls of academia, as mathematicians or astronomers, or in other work situations that involve working in social isolation.

Causes

The importance of heredity in the development of this disorder is unclear, though there is speculation that genetic factors play a role. The feature of introversion seems to be highly heritable. By retrospective report the childhoods of patients with this disorder are bleak and lacking in emotional warmth. No prospective longitudinal studies have been conducted to study this.

Epidemiology

Although the prevalence of this disorder is unknown and it rarely presents in mental health clinics, it is likely overrepresented in certain jobs that require social isolation. The sex distribution in the general population is unknown, but it is diagnosed more commonly in men in the psychiatric clinical setting.

Differential Diagnosis

The differential diagnosis includes schizophrenia, in which patients may also be aloof. Schizoid personality disorder lacks the problems with reality testing prominent in schizophrenia. People with schizotypal personality disorder may avoid social interaction, but this is due to excessive social anxiety not indifference to social relationships. Also, schizotypal personality disorder is distinguished by its peculiarities in perception and communication. The social isolation of avoidant personality disorder is due to fear of rejection. With paranoid personality disorder the person may seem odd and aloof, much as in schizoid personality disorder. The distinguishing features in the former is the prominent paranoid ideation.

Treatment

Treatment of schizoid personality disorder is primarily individual psychotherapy although some patients may, in time, find group therapy useful. Behavioral therapy may be useful for some patients with the treatment focused on developing the ability to engage in progressively more socially involved behavior. There are no formal studies of pharmacologic agents used to treat this disorder and little in terms of primary symptomatology to suggest a particular psychopharmacologic agent would be useful.

Schizotypal Personality Disorder

Description

Schizotypal personality disorder has manifestations peculiar enough to catch the attention of most observers. This disorder is characterized by a pervasive pattern of unconventional thoughts, appearance, and behavior as well as deficits in interpersonal relationships. Peculiarities of thought include magical thinking and ideas that other people, events, or objects in the environment have particular and unusual meaning specifically for that person (that a statement on the evening newscast is about them). These people may have eccentric behavior or appearance such as talking to themselves or dressing oddly or being unkempt. Speech may be difficult to understand due to unusual use of words or metaphors or it may be vague or inappropriately abstract. To most people these people appear strange and aloof. They usually avoid close relationships, in part, because they are unable to enjoy the reward of close relationships but experience much of the distress accompanying relationships. There are few ways in which they can take on common cultural roles but may find a place in subcultural roles in religious cults. This disorder is sometimes complicated by anxiety and varying degrees of depression.

Causes

There is evidence of increased cases of this disorder in biologic but not adoptive relatives of chronic schizophrenics suggesting a link with schizophrenia. There is little known about the environmental factors that may contribute to the development of this disorder.

Epidemiology

The prevalence is reported to be 3% in the general population. The sex ratio is unknown.

Differential Diagnosis

The differential diagnosis for this disorder includes schizophrenia, residual type. The distinguishing feature is a history of psychotic symptoms in the active phase of schizophrenia, whereas less severe, transient symptoms may occur in schizotypal personality disorder. Social avoidance may be seen in schizotypal, schizoid, and avoidant personality disorders. There are no oddities in behavior, thinking, perception, or communication present in the latter two disorders. Frequently patients with this disorder meet criteria for borderline personality disorder. In these instances both diagnoses are made.

Treatment

Treatment of this disorder is usually individual psychotherapy. Initiating a relationship is often challenging and the role of treatment is typically supportive in nature. Most studies of pharmacologic treatment suggest a modest benefit from the use of low-dose antipsychotic medications. Symptoms most likely to benefit from this treatment are depression, anxiety, derealization, and social isolation. High-dose fluoxetine was found to be helpful for depressive symptoms in an open trial to a small group of patients with schizotypal or mixed schizotypal and borderline disorder.

Cluster B—Dramatic, Emotional, and Erratic Personality Disorders

Antisocial Personality Disorder

Description

Antisocial personality disorder is associated with criminality but is not synonymous with criminality because this disorder involves a range of behaviors including but also extending beyond criminality. With this disorder there is a long continuous and chronic history of antisocial behavior that begins before adulthood. The range of adult antisocial acts may include inability to sustain work, failing to conform to social norms regarding person and property rights, failing to honor financial obligations, being irritable and aggressive toward others, being irresponsible as a parent, having little regard for the truth, and having reckless regard for one's own or others' safety. Sexual promiscuity is common. There is a general lack of remorse about the harm they cause to others, rather they may feel justified in their uncivil and destructive acts. To those observing the person with this disorder, these people appear to lack anxiety and their behavior often seems without purpose. There, however, is nothing to suggest delusions or other evidence of loss of touch with reality. In presenting to physicians they may initially appear to be colorful or seductive. If they feel challenged they may become manipulative and threatening. Substance abuse is a commonly associated disorder. This disorder has tremendous social morbidity. People with this disorder make up much of the population of jails and prisons and fill many places on welfare roles.

Causes

Evidence suggests that both environmental and genetic factors play a role in the development of this disorder. The most critical environmental factor seems to be sustained childhood deprivation of consistent emotional ties with any significant person. Parents who are inconsistent and impulsive often themselves have this disorder. The evidence for genetic factors come from studies that show that having a father with this disorder or alcoholism is a powerful predictor of having antisocial personality disorder as an adult. This holds true whether or not the father was present in the child's life. Other environmental factors which, contrary to what one might think, are not significant predictors for developing this disorder include living in a high crime neighborhood, social class, having bad associates, or being a member of a deviant subgroup.

There appears to be a modest relationship between hyperactivity, attention-deficit disorder, and soft clinical neurologic signs in childhood and the development of antisocial personality disorder in adulthood.

Epidemiology

The prevalence of antisocial personality disorder is estimated to be less than 1% in American women and around 3% in American men.

Differential Diagnosis

Important considerations in a differential diagnosis include psychoactive substance abuse and the other personality disorders. Psychoactive substance abuse and antisocial personality disorder are both diagnosed if both disorders began in childhood and continued in to adulthood. If the antisocial behavior is secondary to the adult development of substance abuse, the diagnosis of antisocial personality disorder is not made. As indicated above, both antisocial and borderline personality disorder are commonly diagnosed in the same person. A manic episode may have antisocial behavior as a feature, but such behavior is clearly episodic, not chronic. As noted above, antisocial personality disorder is not simply criminality. It is a disorder that severely impairs all areas of a person's life resulting in poor occupational and social performance and inability to maintain intimate interpersonal relations. All of these behaviors may manifest themselves within the bounds of the law. On the other hand, many people who commit criminal acts are in the other areas of their lives supportive of and responsible to their families and community institutions and would not be diagnosed with antisocial personality disorder by the DSM-III-R criteria.

Treatment

Treatment of antisocial disorder requires that there be actual control over the behavior and acknowledgement by the patient that he or she is responsible for his or her behavior. Control requires a locked or highly controlled setting. Although individual therapy may be used, peer support groups are likely to be more effective. The antisocial patients may be charming in time of need, but having someone protect them from the consequences of their behavior (legal charges, jail sentences,) will only potentiate the behavior.

Borderline Personality Disorder

Description

Of all the personality disorders, borderline personality disorder has received the most notoriety in recent years. The notion of "fatal attractions," familiar to both lay persons and professionals, is associated with this disorder. Characterized by a pervasive pattern of instability of mood, interpersonal relationships, and self-image, this disorder is the most studied and in many ways the most difficult personality disorder with which health professionals deal. Because of the nature of this disorder, it may present in seemingly contradictory ways. If seen in times between crises, the patient may appear to have unexceptional affect. On investigation they will usually reveal a history of periods of intense anxiety, anger, depression, chronic feelings of emptiness and boredom, and a history of recurrent self-damaging behavior. In times of crisis these people may present as argumentative, irritable, impulsive, and demanding. They may behave in ways that attempt to make others responsible for their problems.

Many caregivers find themselves engaged in inappropriate efforts to rescue these patients. Examples of inappropriate rescue behaviors range from giving the patient money to having sexual relations with the patient as a form of "therapy." Caregivers may engage in unusual behaviors due to their own vulnerabilities and the tendency of the person with borderline personality disorder to develop intense and ultimately unstable relationships. The caregiver is initially caught up in an overidealized relationship only later to be devalued as the intensity of the relationship becomes unbearable for the person with borderline personality disorder. The person with borderline personality disorder then may respond with rage as well as threats and acts of litigation.

Patients with borderline personality disorder have a low tolerance for being alone and will often engage in frantic and torturous efforts to have a relationship, preferring this to feelings of loneliness. Problems with self-image and identity are manifested by uncertainty about sexual orientation, goals for life, and what types of friends and lovers to pursue.

Recurrent suicidal acts and self-mutilation may be a part of the disorder. These behaviors may serve one or more purposes including an attempt to manipulate other people, a response to overwhelming anger, or as a way to counteract feelings of numbness and depersonalization (a way to feel "real" again). Overwhelming feelings of anger and frustration may lead to other impulsive acts including drug abuse or sexual promiscuity.

Cause

Most theorists have suggested a constitutional role in the development of this disorder. Affective instability and inability to tolerate anxiety are two commonly offered factors. Family studies of patients with borderline disorder demonstrate an increased prevalence of non-bipolar depression in first-degree relatives suggesting a vulnerability to faulty affect regulation. Psychoanalytic theorists posit that disturbances in the mother–child relationship in early childhood can leave children with a poorly developed sense of self and render them extremely sensitive to separations from significant others. Recent studies have revealed a high frequency of childhood physical and sexual abuse in adults with borderline personality disorder.

Epidemiology

Borderline personality disorder is more commonly diagnosed in women than in men at a rate of about 2:1. There is inadequate information to determine the prevalence of this disorder in the general population. People with borderline personality disorder may be overrepresented in medical clinics and mental health settings.

Differential Diagnosis

This disorder may be complicated by major depression, dysthymia, or psychoactive substance abuse. It is not uncommon for persons with borderline personality disorder to meet criteria for one or more other personality disorders, commonly histrionic, antisocial, or schizotypal.

Treatment

Treatment of borderline personality disorder requires a knowledgeable caregiver. In recognition that fears of both closeness and distance from others underlie the patient's instability of relationships, a middle ground approach between underinvolvement and excessive closeness should be sought in the helping relationship. Individual psychotherapy is the treatment of choice. The psychotherapy may be frequent and aimed to explore how the patient relates to the other people in his or her life, particularly the therapist. Another school of therapy takes a more practical approach and focuses on improving occupational performance and stabilizing interpersonal relationships. Group therapy may be a useful adjunct or a primary treatment modality. Groups provide an effective setting for peer confrontation of manipulative behavior.

Although borderline personality disorder is not effectively treated by pharmacologic agents alone, evidence suggests that the disorder responds to some medications even in absence of Axis I disorders. The benefits of low doses of antipsychotic medications are best documented. Therapeutic effects are typically broad based including improvement of depressed mood, anxiety, suicidal behavior, and psychotic symptoms. Of the antidepressants, fluoxetine has shown benefit in open trials and tricyclics have shown little promise; monoamine oxidase inhibitors show promise in patients with marked mood reactivity and rejection sensitivity. Carbamazepine has demonstrated some benefit for behavioral dyscontrol. Benzodiazepines other than alprazolam have not been systematically studied in this population. In the study of treatment with alprazolam, alprazolam was associated with increased suicidality and behavioral dyscontrol, although two patients seemed to respond positively. Many clinicians believe the use of benzodiazepines can be problematic in this disorder and that they should be used cautiously, if at all.

Histrionic Personality Disorder

Description

Histrionic personality disorder is characterized by a pervasive pattern of flamboyant emotionality and behavior that brings attention to the person. The term histrionic has been used in our culture as a term of disapproval, especially regarding women. The term histrionic may be used to describe a normal personality style that is characterized by warmth, imagination, and intuition, which may prove effective in certain vocations. People with histrionic personality disorder are impaired in their relationships in that they constantly seek praise or approval, may be inappropriately sexually seductive in appearance or behavior, may be overly concerned about physical attractiveness, or give evidence of being uncomfortable when not the center of attention. Expressions of emotions are often exaggerated or are rapidly shifting and shallow. Speech may be impressionistic and vague. Relationships may be strained by a low tolerance for frustration and delayed gratification. They often impress others as being superficial and flirtatious. Interpersonal relationships are often stressed and disrupted by inconsistent and labile emotions and intense dependency needs.

In clinical encounters behavior is usually well mannered and eager to please. Speech may be colorful but vague. There may be exaggerated gestures or dramatic displays of emotion. When pressed to talk about the emotions displayed, the response may be one of surprise or anger as they deny the emotion.

Causes

The causes of histrionic personality disorder are unknown. This disorder, antisocial personality disorder, and somatization disorder commonly occur in the same families but their relationship is not clear.

Epidemiology

The prevalence of histrionic personality disorder as defined by DSM-III-R criteria is unknown. In clinical settings, women are more frequently diagnosed with this disorder than men. This may, in part, be due to the sex role bias of the criteria because men with similar presentations may be seen as having antisocial or narcissistic personality disorder.

Differential Diagnosis

The differential diagnosis includes somatization disorder, a disorder in which physical complaints without apparent physical disorder are the central elements. The complaints are often presented in dramatic, vague, or exaggerated manner consistent with features of histrionic personality disorder. These two disorders often occur together. Although borderline personality disorder has some of the same features as this disorder, histrionic personality lacks the pervasive sense of emptiness and identity disturbance of borderline personality disorder. Antisocial personality disorder may be distinguished from histrionic by the dependent qualities in the interpersonal relationships of histrionic personality disorder. Narcissistic personality disorder shares the quality of excessive self-centeredness. The difference is that with narcissistic personality disorder the core issue related to self-centeredness is self-esteem, whereas in histrionic personality disorder the issue is dependency. Dependent personality disorder is characterized by excessive dependence but without the exaggerated emotions of histrionic personality disorder.

Treatment

Treatment for histrionic personality disorder is insight-oriented psychotherapy. Both individual and group psychotherapy are used as primary treatments. Pharmacologic studies in this disorder are lacking. Some patients with mood lability and rejection sensitivity do not meet the diagnostic criteria for borderline disorder but do meet the criteria for histrionic personality disorder. These patients are likely to benefit from monoamine oxidase inhibitors as well as similar patients with borderline personality disorder.

Narcissistic Personality Disorder

Description

Narcissistic personality disorder is characterized by a pervasive pattern of grandiosity (in fantasy or behavior), hypersensitivity to the evaluation of others, and a lack of empathy. Like histrionic, narcissistic is a commonly used term in our culture. It has a variety of meanings ranging from self-centeredness to having healthy self-love. Narcissistic personality disorder is marked by a severe impairment in maintaining a realistic concept of one's own self-worth. People with this disorder have a sense of grandiose self-importance, grandiose fantasies, and require attention and admiration from those around them. The grandiosity is characterized by an exaggerated sense of superiority, uniqueness, or having special talents. This grandiosity or specialness may play out in exploiting others to achieve one's own ends, exaggerating one's achievements, or expecting unusually special treatment. They have expectations of themselves that are unrealistic and feel helpless and inadequate when they fail to meet this standard. Issues around self-esteem lead to a vulnerability to criticism (with feelings of shame, worthlessness, emptiness, or inappropriate rage), seeking attention and admiration (as reinforcement of shaky self-esteem), and being preoccupied with feelings of envy (when self-esteem is shaken by the perception that others are more successful). Interpersonal relationships are strained by the emotional distance created by a sense of being unique and having special problems understandable only by other special people as well as a lack of empathy. These people are often experienced by others as moody, oversensitive to criticism, insensitive to the feelings of others, or as having unreasonable expectations of others. Impairment by this disorder is variable. In the right occupational niche, their grandiosity may fuel an unrelenting drive for success with positive results while, at the same time, they are unable to engage in meaningful love relations.

Causes

No particular genetic or environmental factors have been demonstrated to cause this disorder.

Epidemiology

The prevalence and sex ratio are unknown. The diagnosis appears to be made more commonly in men than in women in clinical settings.

Differential Diagnosis

The differential diagnosis include the other cluster B personality disorders and obsessive compulsive personality disorder. Antisocial personality disorder causes much greater impairment in work settings and is characterized by more actively exploitive behavior and impulsiveness. With narcissistic disorder the person either does not recognize the violations of social norms or else sees himself or herself as due special treatment. Borderline personality disorder may be distinguished by their less stable sense of identity, greater emotional lability, and greater tendency to impulsive self-destructive behaviors. They appear to be emotionally needy, whereas people with narcissistic disorder appear to be self-sufficient. In histrionic personality disorder there is evidence of dependency on others and the emotional tone tends to be warm and playful, contrasted to the self-sufficiency and cold emotional tone of narcissistic disorder. Patients with obsessive compulsive personality disorder share the tendency to set high standards and a drive for perfection. For obsessive compulsive personality disorder this serves to maintain a sense of control and competency, whereas the person with narcissistic disorder claims perfection to maintain an idealized self-image. Patients with narcissistic personality disorder are vulnerable to dysthymia and major depression.

Treatment

Treatment is usually individual or group psychotherapy. The goal of therapy is for the patient to develop a more realistic understanding of themselves and others as neither perfect not worthless. There are no controlled studies of pharmacologic interventions.

Cluster C—Anxious, Fearful, Introverted Personality Disorders

Avoidant Personality Disorder

Description

Avoidant personality disorder is characterized by extreme sensitivity to rejection. This is evidenced by social discomfort, fear of negative evaluation, and timidity. There is hypersensitivity to potential criticism or rejection, avoidance of interpersonal contact, and unwillingness to be involved with others without great assurance of acceptance. Because of these qualities, the person may live a socially withdrawn life. In social situations the person may be reluctant to speak out of fear he or she will say something inappropriate or he or she may fear being embarrassed by a display of anxious behavior such as blushing. The person with avoidant personality disorder desires human relationships with warmth and affection. The fear of rejection by others is a barrier to achieving this. They may appear uncertain and lacking in self-confidence to others. When speaking about themselves they are usually self-effacing. Impairment of social relations is significant. If they marry they are likely to marry some one with similar qualities. In occupational activities they may pass up opportunities for advancement to avoid increased social interaction or assuming more authority.

Causes

The causes are unknown, but it is assumed that socialization and temperament play important roles in the causes.

Epidemiology

The prevalence of avoidant personality disorder is undetermined in the general population. It is suspected to be relatively common. The male-female ratio is thought to be close to 1:1 or to be slightly more frequent in women.

Differential Diagnosis

The differential diagnosis includes schizoid personality disorder, social phobia, and agoraphobia. In schizoid personality disorder the social isolation is a result of there being little desire for social interaction and in contrast to avoidant personality, there is a lack of sensitivity to criticism. Social phobia is an anxiety disorder that is usually experienced in specific socially demanding situations that are avoided. It is not a fear of most, if not all, social relationships as in avoidant personality disorder. Agoraphobia is also an anxiety disorder characterized by the fear of being in certain places or situations that results in either restricted travel or need for a companion for travel.

Treatment

Treatment is usually individual psychotherapy. Some patients are able to benefit from group psychotherapy; however, most patients tend to find this too threatening. The goal of therapy is for the patient to learn to tolerate the struggles of developing relationships.

Dependent Personality Disorder

Description

Dependent personality disorder is characterized by a pervasive pattern of dependent and submissive behavior. These people experience themselves as very needy and attempt to get others to assume responsibility for their lives. Out of a need for attachment they may agree with people regardless of the truth of a matter or they may pursue demeaning activities. Lack of a sense of attachment to another may result in difficulty initiating a task or result in feelings of helplessness. On the other hand, they may be able to perform burdensome tasks for someone else. Fears of abandonment and sensitivity to criticism inhibit expressions of aggressive emotions and increase vulnerability to abusive relationships. An abusive relationship may be endured to avoid the emotional devastation that comes when relationships end. These people appear to others to be clingy and needy. Impairment in occupational functioning increases with escalating need for independent activities. In some service occupations they may perform adequately. Social relationships are limited to the few people on whom the person is dependent. Anxiety and major depression are commonly associated with this disorder.

Causes

No studies have produced useful information about the cause of this disorder. Most theories are psychosocial in nature and emphasize early childhood experiences. One theory says that parents may subtly give their children the message autonomous behavior is bad and will lead to abandonment.

Epidemiology

The prevalence of this disorder is not known, though it is thought to be relatively common. In clinical settings, it is more often diagnosed in women.

Differential Diagnosis

The differential diagnosis for dependent personality disorder is difficult because dependent traits are present in many psychiatric diagnoses. Some important diagnoses to consider are agoraphobia, and schizoid, borderline, and histrionic personality disorders. With agoraphobia there may be an intense dependence on another person, but this dependence tends to be related to particular experiences of travel from home or some other particular experience. The passivity and lack of initiative that may be present in schizoid personality disorder are common to dependent personality disorder. The distinguishing factors are the social isolation and lack of emotional attachment of schizoid personality disorder. Borderline personality disorder shares an intensity of attachment and fears of abandonment with dependent personality disorder. The emotional lability and self-destructive behavior of borderline personality disorder are not present in dependent personality disorder. The dependence of histrionic personality disorder is not necessarily a drive for attachment to a few individuals as in dependent personality disorder but rather a shallow emotional activity attuned to receiving approval from a range of people they may encounter.

Treatment

Treatment is individual or group psychotherapy. The goal is to help patients to identify their own abilities and self-worth and to see the importance of taking responsibility for their own lives.

Obsessive Compulsive Personality Disorder

Description

Obsessive compulsive personality disorders are characterized by a pervasive pattern of perfectionism and inflexibility. The term obsessive compulsive is also used to describe a personality style that may be normal and highly effective. Although as a personality style this may allow a person to focus intensely and productively on a task, in obsessive compulsive personality disorder there is a level of perfectionism and indecisiveness that is disabling in that it inhibits productivity due to overly strict, self-imposed standards. By unreasonable insistence on doing things a particular way and by preoccupation with details and orderliness people with this disorder alienate others. Life for these people offers little pleasure with its preoccupation with details and rumination over trivial matters, excessive devotion to work, and restricted ability to express tender and warm feeling. Stinginess and unexplained attachment to worthless objects may be present. To others, people with this disorder appear to be dull, stiff, indecisive, and overscrupulous. Emotional tone is typically constricted, yet at times they may appear anxious or depressed. Because many of the traits of this disorder are valued in our culture, this disorder of all personality disorders is least likely to be seen as bad behavior. This disorder can be severely incapacitating occupationally, but the level of function overall tends to be better than other personality disorders. People with this disorder, in contrast to those with most other personality disorders, are often aware that they suffer. They may acknowledge their role in a marital difficulty or be aware that their life is not satisfying.

This disorder may be complicated by dysthymia, major depression, or hypochondriasis.

Causes

Obsessive compulsive personality disorder is more common among family members of probands with obsessive compulsive personality disorder than in the general population. The contribution of genes versus environment is unknown. The classic psychoanalytic theory linking this disorder with toilet training has not been supported by empiric studies.

Epidemiology

The prevalence of obsessive compulsive disorder is not known. It is thought to be a relatively common personality disorder and appears to be more common in men.

Differential Diagnosis

Obsessive compulsive disorder, an anxiety disorder, is distinct from obsessive compulsive personality disorder. Obsessive compulsive disorder is characterized by obsessions that are recurrent, persistent thoughts, or impulses that are perceived as intrusive and are distressing (the fear of contamination from anything one touches) and compulsions, repetitive and seemingly purposeful behavior performed in response to an obsession or according to certain rules (washing one's hands to remove the contamination). The rituals of this disorder are senseless and distressing. In contrast the rituals and sameness of obsessive compulsive personality disorder are purposeful and satisfying. Both obsessive compulsive personality disorder and schizoid personality disorder have the qualities of constricted emotional range and value work over relationships. People with schizoid personality disorder are satisfied to remain socially isolated and aloof, but those with obsessive compulsive personality disorder tend to engage others socially.

Treatment

Treatment is either individual or group psychotherapy. As noted above, people with obsessive compulsive personality disorder are more likely than people with other personality disorders to acknowledge they suffer and may seek help on their own. The goal of therapy is to help the patient identify and experience feelings. At the heart of the disorder are issues of control, which can hinder the development of an effective therapeutic relationship.

Passive Aggressive Personality Disorder

Description

Passive aggressive personality disorder is characterized by a pervasive pattern of passive resistance to demands for adequate social and occupational performance. This resistance may be expressed indirectly by procrastination, shirking responsibility, stubbornness, deliberate inefficiency, or forgetfulness. There may be inability to appropriately evaluate one's own efforts or to respond positively to appropriate feedback.

The name of this disorder incorporates a psychodynamic assumption that the observed passive behavior is a reflection of unspoken aggression. Clearly, the social context and the perspective of the observer of the behavior is critical for making this diagnosis. Civil disobedience in face of horrible social deprivation may be regarded by some as saintly and by others as masochistic. To some it may be martyrdom, to others treason.

Interpersonal relationships in occupational and personal realms are impaired by the tension generated by failing to do one's share of work. Commonly, people with this disorder find fault with the very people they depend on and continue to engage in the relationship despite the difficulties. Because they are more bound to resentment than any other emotion they find little enjoyment in life. Others experience people with passive aggressive personality disorder as manipulative or punitive.

This disorder is often complicated by dysthymia, major depression, and alcohol abuse or dependence.

Causes

There have been no prospective studies of the causes of this disorder. Given the nature of the traits of the disorder, some theorists speculate that early childhood experiences play a primary role. They suggest that parents are assertive in dealings with the child yet they inhibit or punish the normal assertiveness of the child and only grudgingly and partially meet the dependency needs of the child. The child learns to put on the appearance or being polite and well-mannered while expressing anger by punishing the oppressor with inefficiency.

Epidemiology

No good data exist on the prevalence or sex ratio of this disorder.

Differential Diagnosis

The passive aggressive mechanism of passive aggressive personality disorder may be seen in many other personality disorders. This creates some problems with differential diagnosis. Compared to borderline and histrionic personality disorders, passive aggressive personality disorder tends to be less labile, flamboyant, and directly aggressive.

Treatment

Treatment is either individual or group psychotherapy. The goal is to help these patients understand how they put others in a bind by holding them to unreasonable demands with anything but acquiescence to the demand seen as rejection. The covert anger and aggression must be carefully confronted and explored.

Final Thoughts on Treatment and the Course of Personality Disorders

Even though people with personality disorders rarely seek psychiatric care on their own, they are a part of most general medical practice settings. Evidence for the personality disorder may be lacking until a crisis arises in the course of treatment or in the patient's life outside the physician–patient relationship. In others instances the patient and physician have a difficult interpersonal relationship from the outset. In either instance the patient is often managed without psychiatric intervention commonly because the patient refuses referral or the physician has the skills to effectively manage the patient. Other presenting problems that may be indicative of personality disorder include chronic depression, anxiety, substance abuse, suicidal behavior, self-abusive and self-mutilative behavior, poor compliance with treatment for chronic or acute medical problems, excessively demanding behavior, inappropriate and intense anger, persistent seductive behavior, inability for the patient to respect reasonable interpersonal boundaries (excessive gifts, excessive interest in the physician's personal life), or problems with conflict among nursing and support staff around the care of the patient (the patient devalues some staff and idealizes others).

There is little systematically gathered information on the natural history of personality disorders. It has been observed that borderline disorders tend to improve and stabilize in their forties. There is other evidence that, with age, many individuals mature out of personality disorder.

When to Refer

Suicidal, homicidal, self-abusive, or self-mutilative behavior requires a referral to a psychiatrist or other qualified mental health care professional. The physician should be mindful about the safety of the patient as well as his or her own safety. Suicide is often attempted with the medications prescribed by physicians. Prescriptions for patients who are at increased risk of suicide should be limited in quantity when possible. Drug and alcohol abuse are associated with a number of personality disorders and should involve consultation by a psychiatrist or addictionologist.

Major depression and generalized anxiety disorder may be comorbid with various personality disorders and may be refractory or only partially responsive to standard pharmacologic therapies. Psychiatric referral should be pursued for evaluation and treatment of these disorders.

Patients with personality disorders are vulnerable to involvement in physically, sexually, and emotionally abusive relationships either as victims, perpetrators, or both. Referrals for counseling, support, and other interventions should be made to social service agencies or psychotherapists. Perpetrators should be reported as required by local laws and regulations.

Personality disordered patients may have significant problems with noncompliance with medical treatment. If this is persistent or seriously endangering the patient's health, psychiatric evaluation may be useful.

Once these patients are engaged in psychiatric treatment, especially psychotherapy, they may at some time devalue the psychiatrist or therapist. The referring physician should acknowledge the patient's concern and at the same time continue to support the patient's involvement in therapy.

It is difficult to assess the cost or effectiveness of treatment of personality disorders. By definition these are chronic disorders that have significant morbidity. Aggressive treatment of comorbid depression and substance abuse may decrease social and economic costs. Psychotherapy is not covered or is poorly covered by most health insurance plans. This adds another barrier to engaging patients in potentially beneficial therapy.

Suggested Readings

American Psychiatric Association. Diagnostic and statistical manual of mental disorders. 3rd ed., revised. Washington, DC: Author, 1987.

Cowdry RW, Gardner DL. Pharmacotherapy of borderline personality disorder. Arch Gen Psychiatry 1988;45:111–119.

Gitlin MJ. Pharmacotherapy of personality disorders: conceptual framework and clinical strategies. J Clin Psychopharmacol 1993;13:343–353.

Gutheil TG. Borderline personality disorder, boundary violations, and patient-therapist sex: medicolegal pitfalls. Am J Psychiatry 1989;146:597–602.

John C, Schwenk TL, Roi LD, Cohen M. Medical care and demographic characteristics of 'difficult' patients. J Fam Pract 1987;24:607–610.

Liebowitz MR, Stone MJ, Turkat D. Treatment of personality disorders. In: Frances AJ, Hales RE, eds. American Psychiatric Press review of psychiatry. Vol. 5. Washington, DC: American Psychiatric Press, 1986:356–391.

Perry JC, Vaillant GE. Personality disorders. In: Kaplan HI, Sadock BJ, eds. Comprehensive textbook of psychiatry/V. 5th ed. Vol. 2. Baltimore: Williams & Wilkins, 1989:1352–1387.

Vaillant GE. The wisdom of the ego. Cambridge: Harvard University Press, 1993.

Waldinger RJ. Fundamentals of psychiatry. Washington, DC: American Psychiatric Press, 1986.

Widiger TA, Frances AJ. Personality disorders. In: Talbott JA, Hales RE, Yudofsky SC, eds. American Psychiatric Press textbook of psychiatry. Washington, DC: American Psychiatric Press, 1988:621–648.

CHAPTER 41

ANXIETY DISORDERS

John L. Shuster

Anxiety, when used as a clinical term, refers to a number of mental syndromes and disorders that are characterized by feelings of fear, worry, tension, self-doubt, apprehension, uneasiness, or threat. The anxiety disorders are among the most common mental disorders in the general population, especially among women. Disorders in this category include panic disorder, agoraphobia, simple phobia, social phobia, obsessive compulsive disorder, post-traumatic stress disorder, and generalized anxiety disorder.

Prevalence of Anxiety Disorders

Mental disorders, including the anxiety disorders, are prevalent in the United States. Epidemiologic samples from the general population give widely varying estimates of prevalence. Some published surveys, without criterion-based, standardized diagnostic instruments to identify cases, have estimated a prevalence of mental disorders as high as 81.5% (1). This is almost certainly an overestimate, although results of recent, well designed studies estimate an overall lifetime prevalence of mental disorder as high as 48% (2,3).

Anxiety disorders are important causes of suffering in women. Overall, mental disorders, as defined in the American Psychiatric Association's *Diagnostic and Statistical Manual of Mental Disorders* (DSM) (4,5) are about equally common in men and women (2,3). Among the exceptions to this rule, however, are the anxiety disorders. As illustrated in Table 41.1, a number of the specific anxiety disorders (e.g., panic disorder, agoraphobia, simple phobia, social phobia, generalized anxiety disorder), as well as anxiety disorders in general, are more common in women than in men. Less is known about the prevalence and sex ratio of the other anxiety disorders although obsessive compulsive disorder seems to occur in men about as often as in women (4).

An estimated 30.5% of all women will suffer from an anxiety disorder at some time during their lives (see Table 41.1). The 12-month prevalence of anxiety disorders among women is an estimated 22.6%, illustrating the persistence of these disorders. Much of the morbidity related to anxiety is attributable to phobias. However, the more pervasive and disabling of these disorders (i.e., panic disorder, obsessive compulsive disorder, post-traumatic stress disorder) are also fairly common. For example, approximately 5% of American women will meet diagnostic criteria for panic disorder at some time in their lives.

Anxiety Disorders in the Primary Care Setting

Recognition and treatment of anxiety disorders is an important function of the primary care physician. The majority of patients with mental disorders never receive any kind of treatment (6,7). Among patients receiving treatment for mental disorders, many more receive this care from their primary care doctor than from psychiatrists (6,7). Among patients in a primary care practice, as many as 25% may have a mental disorder and approximately 5% may suffer from one of the anxiety disorders (8).

Unfortunately, primary care physicians may miss the diagnosis of a mental disorder, including the anxiety disorders, as much as half the time (9,10). Underrecognition is largely responsible for the fact that approximately 71% of all mental disorders in the United States go untreated (2), as illustrated in Table

Table 41.1 Anxiety Disorders: Prevalence and Rates of Treatment

DISORDER	PREVALENCE (%)						CASES RECEIVING ANY TREATMENT (%)
	Women		Men		Total		
	12 mo	Lifetime	12 mo	Lifetime	12 mo	Lifetime	
Any anxiety disorder	22.6	30.5	11.8	19.2	17.2	24.9	32.7
Panic disorder	3.2	5.0	1.3	2.0	2.3	3.5	58.8
Agoraphobia	3.8	7.0	1.7	3.5	2.8	5.3	—
Simple phobia	13.2	15.7	4.4	6.7	8.8	11.3	31.1
Social phobia	9.1	15.5	6.6	11.1	7.9	13.3	31.1
Generalized anxiety disorder	4.3	6.6	2.0	3.6	3.1	5.1	—
Obsessive compulsive disorder	—	—	—	—	2.1	—	45.1

Adapted by permission from Regier DA, Narrow WE, Rae DS, et al. The de facto US mental and addictive disorders service system: Epidemiologic Catchment Area prospective 1-year prevalence rates of disorders and services. Arch Gen Psychiatry 1993;50:85–94. Adapted by permission from Kessler RC, McGonagle KA, Zhao S et al. Lifetime and 12-month prevalence of DSM-III-R psychiatric disorders in the United States: results from the National Comorbidity Study. Arch Gen Psychiatry 1994;51:8–19. Copyright 1994, American Medical Association.

41.1. Nearly 70% of all anxiety disorders go untreated. Even panic disorder, which is an obvious diagnosis in many cases, is only treated about 60% of the time. These figures do not reflect whether the treatments given were adequate or effective.

A combination of factors is probably responsible for the underrecognition of anxiety and other mental disorders in the primary care setting. First of all, primary care patients may have less severe (i.e., more subtle) mental disorders as a group than those patients who initially present to psychiatrists (7). In addition, patients suffering from mental disorders, especially anxiety and mood disorders, often present with primarily somatic complaints (7). Patients may not recognize their anxiety symptoms, or they may be reluctant to discuss mental symptoms with their physician. Primary care physicians may have difficulty fitting a thorough screening diagnostic assessment for mental disorders into a very busy schedule. Finally, some primary care physicians may not have the training and experience necessary to accurately screen for mental disorders.

A number of documents and instruments aimed at helping the primary care physician recognize and treat mental disorders have been developed. One of the most practical of these is the PRIME-MD, an instrument for the primary care evaluation of mental disorders (11). Based on DSM criteria, the PRIME-MD includes a brief (26 yes-or-no items) patient questionnaire for screening. Each item on the questionnaire, if answered in the affirmative, serves as a trigger for one of the diagnostic modules. The modules contain standardized questions to assist in the diagnosis of one of five categories of mental disorder commonly seen in primary care practice (mood disorders, anxiety disorders, alcohol use disorders, eating disorders, and somatoform disorders). The PRIME-MD is designed to be administered quickly; its designers estimate that each evaluation requires only 5 to 10 minutes. Unfortunately, the brevity necessary to achieve this kind of time efficiency is accomplished by limiting the number of disorders included in some of the modules. In the anxiety module, the PRIME-MD contains specific screens for panic disorder and generalized anxiety disorder. Other anxiety disorders might still be easy to miss using this instrument.

Clinical practice guidelines for mental disorders should also be helpful to the primary care physician. The American Psychiatric Association has already published guidelines for treatment of major depression (12) and eating disorders (13). More guidelines, including guidelines for the treatment of anxiety disorders, will be published in the near future. Specific guidelines for the treatment of depression in the primary care setting have also been recently published (14).

A General Approach to the Diagnosis of Anxiety

Recognizing and diagnosing anxiety disorders is challenging, especially for the nonpsychiatric physician. The situation is further complicated by the need to sort out causes of anxiety symptoms unrelated to formal anxiety disorders. Most patients who complain of feeling anxious or nervous will not meet full diagnostic criteria for a *DSM* anxiety disorder. This is not surprising because any problem that causes distress can lead to the clinical symptoms of anxiety. A systematic approach to evaluating a patient's complaint of anxiety, as outlined in Box 41.1, is helpful. The psychiatric classification of anxiety symptoms unrelated to a formal anxiety disorder is illustrated in Box 41.2.

Box 41.1 A General Approach to the Diagnosis of Anxiety Disorders

1. Routinely screen for symptoms of anxiety disorders.
2. Consider causes of anxiety unrelated to a formal anxiety disorder because treatment and prognosis differ with different causes of anxiety:
   - Emotions aroused by stress, anger, fear, grief, reasonable worry, or interpersonal problems
   - General medical and pharmacologic causes of anxiety
   - Mental disorders other than anxiety disorders
   - Personality disorders
3. Once these alternatives have been considered, formal anxiety disorders should be ruled out.
4. Remember that the etiology of anxious symptoms is usually multifactorial. A comprehensive diagnostic approach with a biopsychosocial focus is most helpful.

Box 41.2 Classification of Anxiety Unrelated to a Formal Anxiety Disorder

Anxiety disorder due to a general medical condition (i.e., secondary to physical disorders, medication side effects, or drug interactions)

Other Axis I mental disorders

- Depression
- Delirium
- Dementia
- Impulse control disorders (e.g., trichotillomania)
- Psychotic disorders
- Sleep disorders
- Somatoform disorders (e.g., somatization disorder, hypochondriasis, body dysmorphic disorder)
- Substance-related disorders (e.g., substance abuse, dependence, intoxication, withdrawal)
- Substance-related anxiety disorders

Personality disorders

- Avoidant
- Borderline
- Dependent
- Paranoid
- Schizoid

Others

- Adjustment disorder with anxiety
- Caffeine anxiety disorder
- V codes (e.g., relational problems, bereavement, phase of life problems, acculturation problems, religious or spiritual problems, problems related to physical or sexual abuse)

Recognize Anxiety Symptoms

Obviously, a key to accurate diagnosis of anxiety symptoms is the recognition of anxiety symptoms. In cases where anxiety is the patient's chief complaint, or when anxiety produces obvious discomfort or dysfunction, little skill or effort is required to determine that anxiety may be a significant problem. In most cases, however, anxiety is more subtle and will have to be screened for in a review of symptoms. Even then, some patients may deny or fail to recognize anxiety in themselves. Anxiety may present as a physical complaint (e.g., cardiac symptoms in a patient with panic disorder). It is often helpful to use common synonyms for anxiety—such as worry, tension, nervousness, or panicky feelings. Some patients will initially feel more comfortable discussing anxiety symptoms in these less clinical terms.

Consider Nonclinical Causes of Anxiety

Many causes of anxiety symptoms are unrelated to anxiety disorders as defined by the DSM criteria. Anger, fearfulness, grief, interpersonal problems, or occupational stress commonly lead to anxious feelings. Some patients may present with anxiety related to worries that are reasonable but would be troubling to anyone. Interpersonal conflicts (with spouse, children, other relatives, friends, coworkers) may be similarly problematic. These real-life situations can occur in the setting of formal anxiety disorders (and, in fact, predictably complicate these disorders when present). However, the presence of a DSM diagnosis is not necessary for life stresses to produce symptoms that mimic a full-blown anxiety disorder. A large proportion of life stressor-related anxiety would be most accurately diagnosed using a "V code," the DSM term for conditions that are not mental disorders but are often the focus of psychiatric treatment (these DSM numeric codes begin with the letter V) (4).

Uncomplicated anxiety reactions secondary to life stresses can be differentiated from anxiety disorders on symptomatic grounds. The former are often limited to a vague, although sometimes intense, feeling of anxiety or tension and do not meet diagnostic criteria for a formal anxiety disorder. Additionally, patients with anxiety disorders often have personal and family histories of their disorder. Most of the diagnostic guidelines for anxiety disorders include symptom severity and duration criteria to differentiate these disorders from transient, stress-related anxiety.

Although these anxiety complaints are often temporary and self-limiting, symptomatic treatment is indicated when distress due to anxiety is substantial. Individuals who suffer from such nondiagnostic anxiety symptoms for an extended period of time (or in a repetitive pattern) may benefit from a referral for psychotherapy aimed at the underlying cause of the anxiety symptoms.

Consider General Medical Causes of Anxiety

Before beginning treatment for any mental disorder, including the anxiety disorders, causative general medical conditions should be ruled out (Table 41.2). The evaluation of anxiety is an opportunity to diagnose a primary medical condition or drug side effect. Misdiagnosing one of these conditions as a primary anxiety disorder obviously leaves the patient at risk of complications from the undiagnosed condition. In addition, anxiolytic treatment is less likely to be of benefit in the presence of an untreated physical cause. Poor response to treatment should be considered another opportunity to search for underlying general medical causes before embarking on further courses of anxiolytic treatment.

Clues to an underlying general medical cause include presence of a known anxiogenic medical condition or administration of a known anxiogenic medication (see Table 41.2). Late-life onset of anxiety symptoms, sudden onset of new anxiety symptoms, or lack of family history of anxiety symptoms should also raise the clinician's index of suspicion that anxiety symptoms may be secondary. An atypical symptom pattern or course is another signal of a possible general medical cause.

Consider Other Mental Disorders as Causes of Anxiety

The symptoms of anxiety may be seen in a number of mental disorders other than the anxiety disorders. Symptomatic treatment is often helpful, but treatment of the primary mental disorder often relieves anxiety symptoms more effectively in these cases than primary anxiolytic treatment.

Depressive disorders, particularly major depres-

Table 41.2 General Medical Causes of Anxiety

Cardiovascular	Angina
	Arrhythmias
	Congestive heart failure
	Coronary artery bypass surgery
	Hypovolemia
	Mitral valve prolapse
	Myocardial infarction
	Severe hypertension
	Valvular disease
Drug-related	Anticholinergic medications
	Antidepressants (early in treatment)
	Antihypertensives
	Antipsychotics—and some antiemetics such as metoclopramide, prochorperazine, and promethazine—(akathisia)
	Antiretrovirals
	Bronchodilators
	Caffeine
	Cyclosporine
	Steroids
	Stimulants
	Yohimbine
Endocrine/Metabolic	Carcinoid
	Cushing's syndrome
	Hyperkalemia
	Hyperthermia
	Hyperthyroidism
	Hypothyroidism
	Hypocalcemia
	Hypoglycemia
	Hyponatremia
	Menopause
	Pheochromocytoma
	Premenstrual syndrome
Neurologic	Collagen vascular disease
	Dementia
	Encephalopathies (delirium)
	Epilepsy, especially partial complex seizures
	Huntington's disease
	Intracranial mass lesions
	Multiple sclerosis
	Postconcussive syndrome
	Vestibular dysfunction
	Wilson's disease
Pulmonary	Asthma
	Chronic obstructive pulmonary disease
	Hyperventilation syndrome
	Pneumonia
	Pneumothorax
	Pulmonary edema
	Pulmonary embolism
Other	Anaphylaxis
	Anemia
	Porphyria
	Vitamin deficiency diseases
	Withdrawal states

Adapted from information appearing in *The New England Journal of Medicine* by permission from Rosenbaum JF. The drug treatment of anxiety. N Engl J Med 1982;306:402. Adapted by permission from Raj AB, Sheehan DV. Medical evaluation of the anxious patient. Psychiatr Ann 1988;17:177.

sion, are very commonly comorbid with anxiety disorders (3,4,8). Panic attacks are often seen during depressive episodes. Depressive symptoms such as worry, psychomotor agitation, sleep inhibition, poor concentration, and ruminative or self-deprecatory thoughts are easily mistaken for anxiety. Sometimes, the distinction can be difficult, even for an experienced psychiatrist. Fortunately, most depressive and anxiety disorders commonly respond to antidepressants. Depressive disorders are discussed in Chapter 36.

Delirium, also called encephalopathy or acute confusional state, can mimic many other mental disorders, including anxiety disorders. Delirium is a neuropsychiatric disorder caused by diffuse cerebral dysfunction and is typically seen in the inpatient setting during a serious physical illness. Its sudden onset, clouding of consciousness, and waxing-waning pattern distinguish it from other mental disorders. Although symptomatic treatment of anxiety secondary to delirium is often helpful, treatment of the underlying medical cause is required.

Dementia may be mistaken for anxiety, especially early in the course of the dementing process. At this stage, the patient may be aware of a progressive loss of cognitive functioning yet retain enough intact function to maintain fairly normal appearances. The fear and anxiety aroused by this condition may be the only apparent symptom. Later in the course, anxiety or agitation may add to the suffering of the dementing patient (or complicate care), but dementia is seldom mistaken for primary anxiety. Issues pertinent to aging, including dementia, are discussed more fully in Chapter 42.

Patients who suffer from psychotic disorders, such as schizophrenia, schizophreniform disorder, and delusional disorder, may exhibit prominent anxiety symptoms at any time during the course of their illness. The differential diagnosis may be particularly difficult, though, during the prodromal phase of the first psychotic break. The withdrawal, apprehension, and anxiety commonly seen during the prodrome may lead to a mistaken initial diagnosis of primary anxiety disorder; progression to full psychotic symptoms usually clarifies the diagnosis. Patients with primarily paranoid symptoms may have their wariness and interpersonal distancing mistaken for anxiety, as well.

Somatoform disorders, characterized by a pattern of physical symptoms in the absence of a demonstrable physical cause and the presence of a known (or presumed) psychological cause, should also be considered in the differential diagnosis of anxiety. Patients with disorders in this category exhibit anxiety regarding their physical condition. Somatization disorder (more common among women) should be considered when the patient presents with a vague and confusing pattern of physical symptoms, superimposed on a chronic pattern of such presentations and a feeling that she is "sickly." Hypochondriasis (more common among men) should be considered when the patient presents with an often unshakeable conviction that he has a specific disease, arousing a great deal of fear and anxiety. Body dysmorphic disorder is diagnosed when the patient is preoccupied with some imagined or exaggerated defect in physical appearance.

Substance-related disorders should always be considered in the evaluation of anxiety symptoms. This is especially true because substance-related disorders are the only category of mental disorder more common than anxiety disorders, especially among men (2,3). DSM-IV (5) includes a number of new diagnostic categories for substance-induced anxiety disorders. Substances of abuse may produce anxiety during episodes of intoxication (as with cocaine, other stimulants, and hallucinogens) or withdrawal (as with alcohol or sedative-hypnotics). Patients who are anxious as a result of a formal anxiety disorder or another mental disorder may use alcohol or illicit substances to self-medicate their anxiety. Anxious patients should always be screened for substance use, especially alcohol. The CAGE questions are a quick and useful diagnostic screen (17), although clinicians should be careful not to destroy the diagnostic utility of the CAGE questions by preceding them with comments that make the patient defensive about his or her drinking (18). Substance-related disorders are discussed more fully in Chapter 37.

Other mental disorders may present with symptoms of anxiety. Sleep disorders (see Chapter 39) may present with anxious symptoms due to disruption in the amount or quality of sleep. This differential diagnosis is especially important because anxiolytic medications (e.g., benzodiazepines) can exacerbate some of the sleep disorders (e.g., sleep apnea). The impulse control disorders, especially trichotillomania, commonly have anxiety as a prominent feature. In fact, trichotillomania has much in common with obsessive compulsive disorder (an anxiety disorder), including response to some of the same medications (19). A maladaptive or excessive reaction to an identifiable psychosocial stressor of less than 6 months' duration would be diagnosed as an adjustment disorder. If the predominant symptomatic manifestation is anxiety, nervousness, worry, or jitteriness, the best diagnosis would be adjustment disorder with anxiety (or anxious mood) (4,5).

The anxiogenic effects of caffeine are worthy of consideration in any patient who complains of anxiety. The relationship between excessive caffeine ingestion and anxiety has been well understood for several years. It now appears that even modest amounts of caffeine also have substantial anxiogenic effects, especially in those individuals who suffer from an anxiety disorder (20). Furthermore, interruption of regular ingestion of caffeinated beverages, as little as 1 to 2 cups of coffee per day, can precipitate caffeine withdrawal, with headache, malaise, and gastrointestinal distress (21). Given this information, it is reasonable to advise all patients who complain of anxiety to taper themselves off caffeine. They should be further instructed to proceed slowly with the taper to avoid precipitating a caffeine withdrawal episode (which often induces the patient to resume regular caffeine use).

Consider Personality Disorders as Causes of Anxiety

When anxiety symptoms present as a component of a long-standing pattern of maladaptive and inflexible response to stresses, a personality disorder should be considered. Anxiety is a common feature of some of the personality disorders, including borderline personality disorder, dependent personality disorder, paranoid personality disorder, schizoid personality disorder, and, most notably, avoidant personality disorder.

Avoidant persons exhibit a pervasive pattern of social discomfort, low self-confidence, rejection sensitivity, easy embarrassment, and timidity that leads to avoidance of potentially embarrassing (or potentially rewarding) situations. Although they crave affection and acceptance, avoidant individuals are typically unable to risk enough contact with others to achieve these goals. Some data suggest that some avoidant personality traits (i.e., behavioral inhibition) are genetically linked to anxiety disorders (22). Personality disorders are more fully discussed in Chapter 40.

Comprehensive Diagnostic Assessment

It is most common for more than one plausible diagnostic explanation to remain at the end of the initial evaluation. In such instances, provisional diagnoses should be labeled as such until they can be ruled out. Patients with anxiety complaints or anxiety disorders typically have a number of factors contributing to their symptoms. An individual's anxiety symptoms may be the result of a complex mixture of interpersonal stresses, an inherited biologic predisposition to anxiety, an avoidant characterologic style, and side effects of alcohol, caffeine, and prescription drugs. Each factor may play an important role in initiating, maintaining, or exacerbating the anxiety symptoms. Obviously, a comprehensive, biopsychosocial approach to evaluation and diagnosis is most likely to lead to an effective treatment plan.

The Anxiety Disorders

Once all the other causes of anxiety have been considered (and, if possible, ruled out), the formal anxiety disorders are considered. The anxiety disorders and an overview of their treatment are outlined in Table 41.3.

Panic Disorder

Panic attacks, sudden and rapidly progressive periods of intense fear and discomfort, are seen in a number of mental disorders. A typical panic attack is brief (lasting only a few minutes), but the intense distress these episodes arouse may cause profound suffering related to dread of recurrent attacks. In a full-symptom panic attack, at least four of the following symptoms develop during the course of the attack: dyspnea, dizziness or faintness, palpitations or tachycardia, trembling or shaking, diaphoresis, choking sensations, nausea or abdominal distress, depersonalization or derealization, paresthesia, hot flashes or chills, chest pain or discomfort, fear of dying, or fear of going crazy or losing control (4). Panic episodes that do not include at least four of these symptoms are referred to as limited-symptom panic attacks.

Panic disorder is diagnosed when panic attacks occur, in the absence of an identifiable general medical cause, either four times in a given 4-week period or once with at least 1 month of persistent fear of having another attack (4,5). At least some of the attacks must be spontaneous (i.e., not a phobic pattern of anxiety in response to a particular stimulus). Patients with panic disorder are usually able to describe the onset of their first (or first few) attacks in vivid detail, and often interpret the sudden onset of physical symptoms and intense fearfulness as a sign of impending death. It is common for patients with panic disorder to present to primary care physicians or cardiologists with complaints suggesting angina pectoris or myocardial infarction (27). Although its natural course is variable, panic disorder can become chronic and quite disabling if left untreated.

Pharmacologic treatment is usually required to block the recurrence of panic attacks in panic disorder (23,24). Benzodiazepines and antidepressants are effective and are most commonly used. Initial treatment should include benzodiazepines (whether or not antidepressants are coprescribed) because benzodiazepines, in adequate doses, can give almost immediate relief from panic episodes. Additionally, beginning treatment of anxiety with an antidepressant may temporarily increase the intensity of the target symptoms, a complication that can be alleviated or prevented by benzodiazepine coadministration. Once the antidepressant medication has had time to take effect, the

Table 41.3 The Anxiety Disorders

Disorder	Description	Specific Treatment
Panic disorder	Recurrent unexpected panic attacks (not due to a general medical cause) that cause worry, concern, or a behavioral change of at least 1 mo duration. Commonly complicated by agoraphobia (4,5).	Blockade of panic attacks with benzodiazepines and/or antidepressants. Behavioral or cognitive therapy for phobic anxiety (23,24).
Agoraphobia	Anxiety about being in places or situations from which escape might be difficult or embarrassing, or in which help might not be available if panic symptoms develop (4,5).	Same as panic disorder (23).
Simple phobia (specific phobia)	A persistent pattern of unreasonable or excessive fear in response to the presence or anticipation of a specific object or situation. No symptoms in the absence of the phobic stimulus (4,5).	Antidepressants; PRN use of benzodiazepines or β blockers. Behavioral therapy aimed at desensitization (23).
Social phobia (social anxiety disorder)	A persistent pattern of fear of one or more social performance situations characterized by exposure to unfamiliar people or the scrutiny of others. Fear of humiliation or embarrassment is a key feature. The person recognizes the fear as excessive or unreasonable. No symptoms in the absence of the phobic stimulus (4,5).	Same as simple phobia (23).
Obsessive compulsive disorder*	Recurrent intrusive or inappropriate nondelusional obsessions, which cause anxiety or distress. Attempts to suppress these obsessions are the rule because most of them are recognized as excessive or unreasonable. Compulsive behaviors are repetitively performed as an attempt to neutralize the distress caused by the obsessive thought (4,5).	Serotonergic antidepressants (e.g., fluoxetine, clomipramine). Monoamine oxidase inhibitors. Behavioral therapy aimed at symptom control (e.g., exposure, response prevention) (23,25).
Post-traumatic stress disorder*	Exposure to a potentially life-threatening event (usually unexpected) that evokes intense fear, helplessness, or horror. For at least 1 mo after the trauma, signs of re-experiencing the event, avoidance behavior, and increased arousal persist (4,5).	Prompt initiation of support, "debriefing." Psychotherapy (group or individual) aimed at recovery from trauma, adjustment to extraordinary life event, and regaining sense of safety (23,26).
Generalized anxiety disorder	Excessive worry and anxiety about a number of different items that are difficult to control, cause significant distress or impairment, and are present most of the time for at least 6 mo (4,5).	Benzodiazepines or buspirone. Behavioral (relaxation) therapy (23,24).
Anxiety disorder due to a general medical condition (organic anxiety disorder)	Prominent symptoms of any of the anxiety disorders that are judged to be etiologically related to a general medical condition and are the cause of a significant amount of distress or impairment (4,5).	Treat underlying general medical cause, if possible. Symptomatic medication treatment.
Anxiety disorder not otherwise specified (NOS)	Disorders that feature prominent anxiety or phobic avoidance yet do not meet the criteria for any specific anxiety disorder or another mental disorder. Commonly used as a provisional diagnosis for atypical anxiety states (4,5).	As indicated by the pattern of symptoms.

*Indicates disorders that should be referred to a psychiatrist or psychologist initially because specialized treatment modalities will likely be necessary as part of the initial treatment.

benzodiazepine can be tapered to discontinuation. Clonazepam and a high-potency tricyclic antidepressant (e.g., nortriptyline, desipramine), unless contraindicated, are good initial choices for the long-term treatment of panic disorder.

Agoraphobia

Agoraphobia (literally a "fear of the marketplace") is a pattern of avoidant, phobic behavior that often complicates panic disorder, but may been seen alone (4,5). Sufferers typically dread (and may go to great lengths to avoid) situations in which escape might be difficult or help unavailable if panic symptoms arise. This disorder can cause substantial social, interpersonal, and occupational impairment and, in extreme cases, agoraphobic individuals may be unable to leave the company of trusted others or the confines of their home. Recurrent panic attacks may lead individuals to interpret nonspecific or coincidental environmental stimuli as sources of danger to be avoided, even if desired activities or relationships must be sacrificed. Treatment of agoraphobic symptoms requires psychotherapy, usually with a behavioral or cognitive/behavioral approach (23,24). However, little progress is likely until panic attacks (if present) are controlled.

Simple Phobia (Specific Phobia)

Simple phobias (renamed specific phobias in DSM-IV [5]) are circumscribed fears and anxiety predictably and consistently related to contact with (or thoughts about) a specific object or situation (e.g., heights, air travel, bridges, dogs) (4,5). Exposure to the phobic stimulus may induce severe anxiety or even panic, but prominent anxiety symptoms do not occur except in association with the stimulus in uncomplicated simple phobia. The amount of anxiety evoked by the phobic stimulus is unreasonable or excessive, and this is recognized by the sufferer.

Management of this common disorder is usually achieved by simple avoidance of the phobic stimulus. However, when symptoms are severe or when avoidance is impractical (e.g., fear of air travel in a junior business executive whose career advancement depends on frequent business trips), more intensive treatment is indicated (23). Low-dose, PRN use of benzodiazepines, β blockers, or even alcohol taken just before exposure to the phobic stimulus are usually helpful, provided the patient will not be in a situation where the sedation produced by these agents would be dangerous. Behavioral therapy aimed at desensitization to the stimulus is also beneficial. Specific behavioral treatment programs may be available. For example, some commercial airline companies sponsor behavioral treatment programs for air travel phobia.

Social Phobia (Social Anxiety Disorder)

Social phobia (renamed social anxiety disorder in DSM-IV [5]) is the technical name for stage fright and other syndromes of anxiety related to social performance. The pattern of symptoms is similar to simple phobia, except that the anxiety is caused by situations involving exposure to unfamiliar people, the scrutiny of others, or perceived potential for embarrassment or humiliation (4,5). Like simple phobia, the amount of anxiety is recognized as unreasonable or excessive and prominent anxiety symptoms do not occur except in association with social performance situations.

Treatment is also similar to that for simple phobia (23). Propranolol in low doses (often as low as 20 mg) taken just before performance situations is often especially helpful. Patients should take at least one trial dose of the prescribed medication in the days before the anxiogenic event to make sure they will be able to tolerate the sedation these medications can cause. Otherwise, sedation may make the patient feel self-conscious or out of control during the event, paradoxically exacerbating the anxiety disorder the medication was intended to relieve.

Obsessive Compulsive Disorder

Obsessions are distressing, recurrent, persistent thoughts, impulses, or images that are more than just worries (4,5). These thoughts are intrusive and inappropriate, often purposeless, and lead to a significant amount of disability or distress. The patient recognizes these obsessions as excessive, unreasonable, and nonproductive products of her own mind, but she is usually unsuccessful in the inevitable attempts to suppress them. Compulsions are repetitive behaviors or mental acts the person feels driven to perform (4,5). They are usually performed in an attempt to provide at least temporary relief from the anxiety produced by the obsessions.

Obsessive compulsive disorder is not simply an extreme form of characterologic obsessiveness. Patients with obsessive compulsive disorder have obsessions or compulsions to such an extent that they interfere with social, occupational, or interpersonal functioning or are substantially time consuming (take more than an hour a day). Common symptomatic themes include obsessions about contamination (with compulsive handwashing or compulsions regarding bowel habits), safety (with compulsive checking of stove switches or door locks), and numbers (with compulsive counting).

Treatment begins with administration of a serotonergic antidepressant (23,25). Clomipramine (Anafranil) and fluoxetine (Prozac) are both indicated for the first-line treatment of obsessive compulsive disorder. Fluoxetine must usually be given in higher doses than when used for depression; 60–80 mg/day may be required. Monoamine oxidase inhibitors, though their safe use requires close adherence to dietary and pharmacologic restrictions, are also very effective treatments. Some behavioral therapy techniques, specifically exposure (desensitizing patients to feared obsessions) and response prevention (training patients to delay their compulsive responses), have also been shown to be beneficial in the treatment of obsessive compulsive disorder. The best response is usually obtained from a combination of antiobsessional medication and behavioral therapy.

Post-traumatic Stress Disorder

Emotional trauma of an intense, potentially life-threatening nature (e.g., rape, combat, natural disasters) may induce post-traumatic stress disorder. The inducing stresses are usually sudden, unexpected, and overwhelming. The traumatized person commonly feels terrified and helpless, but may feel numb or even dissociate during the trauma episode. Immediately after such an event, emotional distress is to be expected. Early provision of emotional support and comfort, as well as a chance to ventilate some of the intense feelings evoked by the trauma, may aid adaptation and prevent the development, or lessen the severity, of post-traumatic stress disorder.

The disorder is diagnosed when symptoms from three general categories (re-experiencing, avoidance, and arousal) persist for at least 1 month after the trauma and cause significant distress or impairment (4,5). Re-experiencing phenomena include intrusive daydreams, nightmares, or flashbacks of the event, which may induce a feeling that the event is actually recurring. Stimuli related to the event—thoughts, feelings, memories, returning to the scene of the trauma—are avoided. A general increase in arousal may result in an increased startle response, irritability, hypervigilance, sleep problems, or decreased concentration. In general, responsiveness is numbed and the patient may feel a sense of detachment or perceive her future as being foreshortened.

Treatment primarily involves psychotherapy, initiated as soon as possible (23,26). Chronic post-traumatic stress disorder becomes much more refractory to treatment. The focus of therapy is usually supportive, allowing ventilation and debriefing. The details of the traumatic event are empathically explored as a form of desensitization and to search for cognitive distortions (e.g., many victims of random violence feel that the event was somehow their fault). As therapy progresses, themes include adjustment to an extraordinary and (hopefully) isolated life event, integration of the overall experience into the patient's life, and recovery of normal functioning and a sense of safety. A number of psychopharmacologic agents have been studied for the treatment of the disorder or anecdotally reported to be helpful. At present, however, there is no clear drug of choice and the treatment of choice is clearly psychotherapy. Therefore, patients who develop post-traumatic stress disorder should be referred to an experienced mental health professional for treatment.

Generalized Anxiety Disorder

Generalized anxiety disorder is characterized by a pattern of excessive worry about a number of items that is difficult to control, causes significant distress or impairment, and is present more days than not for at least 6 months (4,5). These worries are complicated by at least three of the following: restlessness, fatigue, poor concentration, irritability, muscle tension, or sleep disturbance.

Treatment involves a combination of medication and therapy, especially relaxation techniques (23,24). Like panic disorder, antidepressants and benzodiazepines are usually helpful. Maintenance treatment with β blockers may provide relief, as well. Buspirone (BuSpar) seems to be more effective for the primary treatment of generalized anxiety disorder than for any other anxiety disorder. Although effective and nonhabituating, buspirone must be divided into at least three daily doses and has a substantial lag time (sometimes weeks) before the onset of beneficial effects. Worried anxiety may also be related to life problems, and this possibility should be explored, especially if pharmacotherapy is not providing relief.

Comorbidity

Psychiatric comorbidity adds another layer of complexity to the process of evaluating anxiety. Patients who have anxiety disorders may simultaneously suffer from other primary mental disorders (e.g., depression, alcohol dependence, personality disorders). In fact, such comorbidity is the rule, not the exception. The National Comorbidity Survey found that 79% of all reported lifetime mental disorders were comorbid with another mental disorder (3). Additionally, the minority of patients with the most comorbidity of mental disorders (14% of the sample population) accounted for nearly 90% of all the severe mental disorders detected in a 12-month period (3).

Box 41.3 A General Approach to the Treatment of Anxiety Disorders

1. Correct any contributory general medical conditions, if possible.
2. Educate the patient about the disorder and its treatment.
3. Intervene as early as possible, before anxiety disorders become more complicated (e.g., chronic post-traumatic stress disorder, panic disorder complicated by agoraphobia due to learned avoidance behavior).
4. Decide if initial referral to a specialist is indicated.
5. Provide support and encouragement.
6. Initiate specific treatments (e.g., medication, psychotherapy).
7. Consider referral of complicated cases or cases refractory to standard treatments.

Treating Anxiety: General Guidelines

The diagnosis of a specific anxiety disorder, taking the individual patient's biopsychosocial situation into account, ideally leads to a treatment plan tailored to that patient's needs. However, some general principles apply to the treatment of anxiety disorders, as outlined in Box 41.3.

First of all, the physician should search for (and correct, if possible) any underlying general medical causes of anxiety. This point bears repetition because many of the anxiety complaints patients present to their primary care physician will not be related to a formal anxiety disorder. Alternative explanations should be sought because symptomatic anxiolytic treatment in these cases is often unsatisfactory and can lull the physician into neglecting the search for specific and more helpful treatment strategies.

Education about the nature and course of anxiety disorders is essential (and often therapeutic in itself). Many undiagnosed anxiety disorder patients fear they are losing their minds, are in the early stage of a progressive neuropsychiatric deterioration, or are suffering from some vague but lethal physical disorder. Providing patients and families with factual information about anxiety disorders, their treatment, and their usual good response to treatment reduces anxiety and improves compliance. Patient education about anxiety disorders should be presented in an empathic but unapologetic manner. An anxiety disorder diagnosis is no reason for shame although the stigma attached to these and other mental disorders often compounds the suffering they cause.

Intervention (medication treatments or psychotherapy) should begin as soon as possible once a diagnosis of anxiety disorder is made. In all cases, treatment delay unnecessarily prolongs suffering. In some disorders, delay adversely effects eventual response to treatment and overall outcome. For example, post-traumatic stress disorder, if left untreated, may become chronic and treatment resistant. Untreated panic attacks may induce phobic avoidance of coincidental stimuli, possibly evolving into agoraphobia with its associated morbidity. Early control of uncomplicated panic disorder with medication may prevent such complications.

Generally, referring an anxious patient to a psychiatrist or other mental health professionals is best decided on a case-by-case basis. Most causes of anxiety can be effectively evaluated and treated by the primary care physician using a rational, systematic approach. With a few exceptions, formal anxiety disorders of mild to moderate severity are straightforward and can be well treated by the generalist. Referral should be considered for difficult or complicated cases, treatment-refractory cases, or any cases in which the experienced generalist feels less than comfortable managing the patient's anxiety complaint. Effective treatment of post-traumatic stress disorder requires referral to a specialist for psychotherapy. Most cases of obsessive compulsive disorder and complicated or chronic cases of panic disorder or phobias should be referred for comprehensive evaluation and treatment. Psychopharmacologic treatment of the pregnant patient (discussed below) is best undertaken in consultation with a psychiatrist.

Support and encouragement from the physician are crucially important aspects of the treatment of anxiety disorders. Many anxious patients have suffered with their disorders without hope of improvement. The patience to tolerate a slow, gradual recovery from the terror of panic attacks or the impairment of severe obsessive compulsive disorder may be in short supply. Complications or setbacks (e.g., improved but persistent symptoms, initial worsening of anxiety on antidepressants, comorbidity) may lead to discouragement. Without making false promises, the physician should show enthusiasm for treatment, give hope for improvement, and point out increments of progress.

Finally, specific pharmacologic and psychotherapeutic treatments, if indicated, should be initiated. Table 41.4 summarizes some practical information regarding anxiolytic drugs.

Treating the Anxious Pregnant Patient

None of the psychotropic drugs has been given approval by the Food and Drug Administration for use during pregnancy. As with other drugs, anxiolytics are ideally avoided during pregnancy, especially during the first trimester. However, in cases where the pregnant woman has a chronic or severe anxiety disorder, a difficult risk-benefit decision must be made. The morbidity of untreated anxiety, especially panic attacks (28), must be weighed against the potential teratogenicity of anxiolytic medications.

With the exception of lithium, which is associated with a low risk of cardiac defects such as Ebstein's anomaly in exposed fetuses, none of the psychotropic drugs are known to be teratogenic (29). There are reports associating benzodiazepine use with an increased risk of oral cleft abnormalities, but this association is controversial (29). Clonazepam, one of the benzodiazepines of choice for panic disorder, appears to have the lowest teratogenic potential in this drug class (29). Fluoxetine and tricyclic antidepressant use during pregnancy does not appear to increase the risk of major fetal malformations although both have been associated with a slightly increased rate of spontaneous abortion when used in the first trimester (30). Other psychotropics appear to be well tolerated (when indicated) in pregnancy although the long-term effects on central nervous system development in the exposed child, if any, are unknown.

Cohen and colleagues (29) recently published an overview of this topic with clinical guidelines for psychotropic drug use in the pregnant patient. For anxiety disorders, they recommend that female patients taking anxiolytic medications plan their pregnancies so medication changes (or discontinuation) and nonpharmacologic treatments can be planned before the first trimester. They suggest using tricyclic antidepressants as the anxiolytic of choice during pregnancy, with adjunctive cognitive/behavioral or supportive psychotherapy. They also recommend tapering patients off benzodiazepines before conception, if possible, or as early as possible in the pregnancy. Because all psychotropics are secreted in breast milk, new mothers who require treatment with anxiolytics should be discouraged from breast-feeding.

Summary

Anxiety disorders are common in the general population, especially among women. Fortunately, anxiety disorders generally respond well to treatment. Commonly seen in the primary care setting, more anxiety disorders are treated by generalists than specialists. A rational, systematic approach to the evaluation and treatment of anxiety can be helpful in improving the recognition, diagnosis, and treatment of anxiety disorders. Initial treatment by the primary care physician is usually effective, but complicated or treatment-refractory patients will benefit from referral to a specialist. Early referral is indicated for those patients in whom psychotherapy is the primary treatment or a necessary adjunct.

Table 41.4 Anxiolytic Drugs

Drug	Route(s)	Usual Starting Dose (mg)	Usual Maintenance Dose (mg)	Comments
Benzodiazepines				
alprazoloam (Xanax)	PO	0.5 three times a day	0.5–6.0/day*	Good for short-term use; habituation makes maintenance treatment and taper off of drug more problematic than drugs with longer half-lives.
clonazepam (Klonopin)	PO	0.5 twice daily	0.5–4.0/day*	Duration of action makes interdose breakthrough anxiety less likely than with shorter-acting agents.
lorazepam (Ativan)	PO, IM, IV	0.5–1.0 three times a day	1–10/day*	Especially useful in the setting of medical illness, due to multiple routes of administration; reliably absorbed by IM route; metabolism by glucuronidation without active metabolites.
Tricyclic antidepressants (TCAs)				
clomipramine (Anafranil)	PO	25 at bedtime	100–250/day	Especially useful for obsessive compulsive disorder.
desipramine (Norpramin)	PO	25 at bedtime	100–300/day	The least anticholinergic and the least sedating TCA.
imipramine (Tofranil)	PO	25 at bedtime	150–300/day	
nortriptyline (Pamelor)	PO	10–25 at bedtime	75–150/day	Therapeutic range of plasma levels is 50–150 ng/mL; least likely TCA to cause orthostasis.
Serotonin reuptake inhibitors (SRIs)				
fluoxetine (Prozac)	PO	5–20/day	5–20/day	Especially useful for obsessive compulsive disorder; very long half-life; available in liquid form.
sertraline (Zoloft)	PO	25/day	50–200/day	
paroxetine (Paxil)	PO	10/day	10–50/day	
Monoamine oxidase inhibitors (MAOIs)				
phenelzine (Nardil)	PO	15 twice daily	45–90/day*	Use as a first-line agent limited by numerous dietary and drug interactions that can lead to hypertensive crisis; may induce orthostasis.
tranylcypromine (Parnate)	PO	10 twice daily	30–60/day*	Same as phenelzine.
trazodone (Desyrel)	PO	50–100 at bedtime	150–400/day*	Very sedating; can cause orthostasis; has been associated with priapism.
buspirone (BuSpar)	PO	5 three times a day	15–60/day*	Not effective for panic attacks; best for generalized anxiety disorder, mild anxiety, or as an adjunct to other t reatments; has a lag time to onset of effect similar to antidepressants.
propranolol (Inderal)	PO	10–20 PRN	20–240/day*	Most useful as a PRN medication for phobias (e.g., social phobia), taken just before exposure to the phobic stimulus.
hydroxyzine (Vistaril)	PO, IM	25–50	50–400/day*	Useful for short-term, symptomatic treatment; may induce confusion in elderly or medically ill patients.
haloperidol (Haldol)	PO, IM, IV	0.5–1.0	1–4/day*	Used mostly in the inpatient setting and should not be used as a long-term maintenance treatment for anxiety due to the risk of developing movement disorders; helpful for extreme, disabling anxiety or fearfulness.

All doses should be initially lowered and advanced more cautiously in elderly patients or patients with any central nervous system degeneration or injury.
Benzodiazepines, propranolol, hydroxyzine, and haloperidol have quick onset of anxiolytic action. All others require days to weeks of maintenance treatment before anxiolytic effects can be expected.
TCAs, SRIs, MAOIs, and trazodone may transiently increase anxiety early in therapy. Downward adjustment and slow advancement of dose will usually alleviate these symptoms. Patients should be warned about this possibility in advance to maximize compliance.
* Given in divided doses.

REFERENCES

1. Srole L, Langner TS, Michael ST, et al. Mental health in the metropolis: the Midtown Manhattan Study. New York: McGraw-Hill, 1962.

2. Regier DA, Narrow WE, Rae DS, et al. The de facto US mental and addictive disorders service system: Epidemiologic Catchment Area prospective 1-year prevalence rates of disorders and services. Arch Gen Psychiatry 1993;50:85–94.

3. Kessler RC, McGonagle KA, Zhao S, et al. Lifetime and 12-month prevalence of DSM-III-R psychiatric disorders in the United States: results from the National Comorbidity Study. Arch Gen Psychiatry 1994;51:8–19.

4. American Psychiatric Association. Diagnostic and statistical manual of mental disorders, 3rd ed., revised. Washington, DC, 1987.

5. American Psychiatric Association: DSM-IV draft criteria. Washington, DC, 1993.

6. Regier DA, Goldberg ID, Taube CA. The de facto US mental health services system. Arch Gen Psychiatry 1978;35:685–693.

7. Schurman RA, Kramer PD, Mitchell JB. The hidden mental health network: treatment of mental illness by nonpsychiatrist physicians. Arch Gen Psychiatry 1985;42:89–94.

8. Barrett JE, Barrett JA, Oxman TE, Geber PD. The prevalence of psychiatric disorders in a primary care practice. Arch Gen Psychiatry 1988;45:1100–1106.

9. Freeling P, Rao BM, Paykel ES, et al. Unrecognised depression in general practice. Br Med J 1985;290:1880–1883.

10. Andersen SM, Harthorn BH. The recognition, diagnosis, and treatment of mental disorders by primary care physicians. Med Care 1989;869–886.

11. Spitzer RL, Williams JBW, Kroenke K, et al. PRIME-MD instruction manual. Roerig and Pratt Pharmaceuticals, 1993.

12. American Psychiatric Association. Practice guideline for major depressive disorder in adults. Am J Psychiatry 1993;150(suppl):1–29.

13. American Psychiatric Association. Practice guideline for eating disorders. Am J Psychiatry 1993;150:212–228.

14. Depression Guideline Panel. Depression in primary care. Vol. 1. Detection and diagnosis. Clinical Practice Guideline, No. 5. Rockville, MD: U.S. Department of Health and Human Services, Public Health Service, Agency for Health Care Policy and Research. AHCPR Publication No. 93-0550, 1993.

15. Rosenbaum JF. The drug treatment of anxiety. N Engl J Med 1982;306:401–404.

16. Raj AB, Sheehan DV. Medical evaluation of the anxious patient. Psychiatr Ann 1988;17:176–181.

17. Bush BB, Shaw S, Cleary P, et al. Screening for alcohol abuse using the CAGE questionnaire. Am J Med 1987;82:231–235.

18. Steinweg DL, Worth H. Alcoholism: keys to the CAGE. Am J Med 1993;94:520–523.

19. Swedo SE, Leonard HL, Rapoport JL, et al. A double-blind comparison of clomipramine and desipramine in the treatment of trichotillomania (hair pulling). N Engl J Med 1989;321:497–501.

20. Bruce M, Scott N, Shine P, et al. Anxiogenic effects of caffeine in patients with anxiety disorders. Arch Gen Psychiatry 1992;49:867–869.

21. Silverman K, Evans SM, Strain EC, et al. Withdrawal syndrome after the double-blind cessation of caffeine consumption. N Engl J Med 1992;327:1160–1164.

22. Rosenbaum JF, Biederman J, Gersten M, et al. Behavioral inhibition in children of parents with panic disorder and agoraphobia: a controlled study. Arch Gen Psychiatry 1988;45:463–470.

23. Reid WH, Balis GU, Wicoff JS, Thomasovic JJ. The treatment of psychiatric disorders. New York: Brunner/Mazel, 1988.

24. Tesar GE. Panic disorder and generalized anxiety disorder. In: Hyman SE, Jenike MA, eds. Manual of clinical problems in psychiatry. Boston: Little, Brown, 1990:71–86.

25. Jenike MA. Obsessive-compulsive and related disorders. In: Hyman SE, Jenike MA, eds. Manual of clinical problems in psychiatry. Boston: Little, Brown, 1990:86–94.

26. van der Kolk BA. Post-traumatic stress disorder. In: Hyman SE, Jenike MA, eds. Manual of clinical problems in psychiatry. Boston: Little, Brown, 1990:94–100.

27. Beitman BD, Mukerji V, Lamberti JW, et al. Panic disorder in patients with chest pain and angiographically normal coronary arteries. Am J Cardiol 1989;63:1399–1403.

28. Cohen LS, Rosenbaum JF, Heller V. Panic attack associated placental abruption: a case report. J Clin Psy-

chiatry 1989;50:266-267.

29. Cohen LS, Heller VS, Rosenbaum JF. Psychotropic drug use in pregnancy: an update. In: Stoudemire A, Fogel BS, eds. Medical psychiatric practice. Vol. 1. Washington, DC: American Psychiatric Press, 1991:615–634.

30. Pastuszak A, Schick-Boschetto B, Zuber C, et al. Pregnancy outcome following first-trimester exposure to fluoxetine. JAMA 1993;269:2246–2248.

SECTION THIRTEEN

AGING

CHAPTER 42

AGING

Donna M. Bearden, Sherron H. Kell, Linda G. Jones

Geriatric Considerations

Literature on the care of the aged is replete with references to the "graying of America." Certainly this demographic trend has its impact on the practice of medicine. The survival of many more people into old age has resulted in adult medicine focusing more on the care of the geriatric patient. It is not demographics, however, that have legitimized geriatrics as a practice entity. Geriatric medicine is legitimized because the diagnostic logic is different for the aged patient. Practice standards appropriate for adult medicine may not always recognize clinical implications for the care of the older patient, especially the old-old (those over age 80) or the frail elderly with their significant compromise in reserve capacity.

This chapter provides the physician with an overview of some practical considerations useful in making appropriate diagnostic and therapeutic decisions for the aged patient. Also included in this chapter are selected common illnesses among the elderly and the management approaches for those illnesses.

Special Considerations

A Scottish saying states that sick old people are sick because they are sick, not because they are old. Indeed, normal old age is usually characterized by good health and by far, the great majority of elders are functional, independent community dwellers. To assume that any illness presenting in the patient is due only to "old age" could lead to delayed treatment, resulting in progression of a once treatable underlying disease. The pursuit of a specific diagnosis and appropriate treatment is as important for the aged patient as for any other patient. Central to this pursuit must be diagnostic decisions based on distinguishing normal age-related physiologic changes from disease.

Rowe and Kahn have suggested that with normal aging there are two categories, successful aging and usual aging (1). Successful aging refers to those individuals who demonstrate few physiologic decrements that are due to aging alone. These people have greater physiologic capacity and lower risk of disease, which implies that there are preventable or reversible components to what was previously considered to be normal aging. In usual aging, the more common mode of aging, there are significant physiologic losses along with a substantially reduced reserve capacity.

Altered Presentation of Disease

There can be striking differences in how disease processes manifest themselves in older versus younger patients. In the elderly there is often a poor correlation—or even a noncorrelation—between presenting symptoms and the locus of disease. For example, presentation of myocardial infarction can be variable and may initially produce nonspecific changes such as confusion or shortness of breath rather than chest pain. Infection may be signaled by agitation, delirium, or other mental status changes as well, rather than by fever or leukocytosis.

Not only is the manifestation of disease typically altered in the elderly, but the natural history and presentation may be affected. Consider the following:

> While uncontrolled diabetes results in diabetic ketoacidosis in children and young adults, it frequently produces hyperosmolar nonketonic coma, with much higher blood glucose levels and little or no circulating ketones in the elderly. Instead of presenting with severe metabolic acidosis, polyuria,

and volume depletion, the elderly will be obtunded or in coma secondary to high blood osmolality (2, p. 308).

The clinical care of the elderly requires more than knowledge of specific disease states. Incorporated into diagnostic decisions must be an awareness of the progressive physiologic vulnerabilities of the aged patient.

Functional Assessment

With normal aging, a gradual decline in organ functional capacity results in a progressive decline in reserve. It is helpful to compare this decline to the shape of a curve with the old-old tapering to a significantly compromised reserve capacity. However, individuals do not age at the same rate but are heterogenous with respect to their physiologic function, their burden of illness, and any associated disability (3).

In the elderly, disease can present first or solely as functional loss. Health care providers, family members, and elders themselves should remember that deterioration of functional independence in active, previously unimpaired older patients can be an early and subtle sign of undiagnosed illness. When such functional impairments develop, quality of life may be preserved by rapid and thorough evaluation.

A systematic approach to assessment of functional ability—how well the aging patient functions independently in the environment—is a critical part of the geriatric medical history. The most commonly used tool to assess basic abilities considered necessary for a person to remain independent is the Katz Index of Activities of Daily Living (ADLs). The six ADLs are feeding, bathing, dressing, transferring, toileting, and continence (Table 42.1) (4). Inability to perform any one of these ADLs indicates that some level of assistance is required. Further, inabilities with ADLs have been shown to be an independent predictor of reduced survival (5), nursing home placement, and inadequate recovery after hip fracture (6).

The Instrumental Activities of Daily Living (IADLs) assess a higher level of function necessary for living independently in the community. Abilities assessed for IADLs include the ability to travel, shop, prepare meals, do housework, and handle finances. Disability in these activities indicates another level of

Table 42.1 Katz Index of Activities of Daily Living

	INDEPENDENT	
	Yes	No
1. Bathing (sponge bath, tub bath, or shower) Receives either no assistance or assistance in bathing only one part of body.	—	—
2. Dressing Gets clothes and dresses without any assistance except for tying shoes.	—	—
3. Toileting Goes to toilet room, uses toilet, arranges clothes, and returns without any assistance (may use cane or walker for support and may use bedpan/urinal at night)	—	—
4. Transferring Moves in and out of bed and chair without assistance (may use cane or walker)	—	—
5. Continence Controls bowel and bladder completely by self (without occasional "accidents")	—	—
6. Feeding Feeds self without assistance (except for help with cutting meat or buttering bread)	—	—
Total ADL score: ____ (Number of "yes" answers out of possible six)		

The patient's score is based on a scale of 0 to 6. Six represents the ability to perform all ADLs.
Source: Adapted by permission from Katz S, Downs TD, Cash HR, et al. Progress in the development of the index of ADL. The Gerontologist 1970;10(1):20–30.

frailty and vulnerability (4) with early functional loss often occurring in the areas of transportation and housework. Difficulties with IADLs may serve as a harbinger of a more significant functional decline.

Chronic Illness and Multiple Morbidities

Office visits for aged patients often involve a prolonged medical history, review of a regimen of multiple medications, a longer time to undress and dress, lengthy and vague complaints, difficulty establishing diagnoses, and less predictable outcomes of treatment. Add to this scenario a patient who is hard of hearing and it is easy to appreciate the challenges in providing care for the aging patient. Indeed, the ordinary elderly patient who comes to the physician's office is coping with multiple chronic diseases and is often partially treated, both of which may have a profound impact on the patient's quality of life.

As with any other age group, when cure is not possible, the reasonable therapeutic objective is improved or preserved function and the prevention of secondary complications. Successful management becomes the therapeutic emphasis when treating chronic conditions, which usually lead to activity limitation.

Vaccines in the Elderly

Because both acute and chronic disease tends to pose threats to independence, preventive measures can be of particular importance for the elderly. Preventive strategies such as regular exercise, sound nutrition, moderate alcohol intake, involvement in meaningful activities, and smoking cessation should be encouraged. The importance of screening and preventive care are discussed in Section 1 of this book. However, disease processes such as pneumonia are more prevalent in older than younger patients. They also result in increased morbidity and mortality among the elderly, and therefore their presentation and prevention are discussed below.

Influenza

Presentation and Vaccination

Influenza outbreaks occur yearly, usually between the months of October through March. The usual incubation period is 1 to 2 days, and patients who contract the virus usually present with the acute onset of fever, chills, mylagias, and cough. Headache and malaise are also common presenting symptoms. Fever usually lasts for 3 days, then subsides. Nasal discharge and a nonproductive cough are usually present at onsets, but become more predominant as systemic symptoms subside. Rhinorrhea typically resolves after 6 to 7 days, but the cough can persist for a longer period of time.

The prime method of preventing influenza is through vaccination. Table 42.2 lists groups recommended for vaccination. The vaccine should be administered in the fall of each year (usually September or October) to persons 65 years and older. Residents of nursing homes and all persons with chronic disorders of the cardiovascular or pulmonary system should also receive the vaccine. The vaccine is also recommended for adults with chronic metabolic disease including diabetes mellitus, renal dysfunction, hemoglobinopathies, or immunosuppression. Once administered, the vaccine takes 2 weeks to provide a protective effect, and vaccine effectiveness typically lasts 4 months after the date of administration.

Vaccine composition varies from year to year, based on the types isolated in the previous year's influenza outbreaks. In recent years, two influenza A subtypes have been included in the vaccine, and one influenza B subtype. In 1976, those vaccinated in the swine influenza immunization program had a higher rate of Guillain-Barré syndrome than those not vaccinated. This has not occurred, however, with other influenza vaccines (7).

Adverse reactions to the vaccine can be local or systemic. One third of persons receiving influenza vaccines will experience discomfort at the site of injection for up to 48 hours after administration. Of these, 5% may experience a more severe local reaction (8). Systemic reactions occur in 1% to 2% of older persons and can be toxic or allergic in nature. Toxic reactions generally consist of fever, malaise, and myalgia beginning 6 to 12 hours after vaccination and persisting 1 to 2 days (8). Immediate allergic reactions occur rarely and are most likely due to the presence of egg protein or preservative in the vaccine. Currently, the only known contraindication to influenza vaccination is allergy to eggs.

Chemoprophylaxis of Influenza

Protection against the influenza A virus can be augmented by the use of amantadine or rimantidine.

Table 42.2 Recommendations for Influenza Vaccination

Annual vaccination is recommended for the following persons or groups:

1. Groups at increased risk of influenza-related complications.
   a. Persons 65 years of age or older.
   b. All persons (adults and children) with chronic disorders of the cardiovascular or pulmonary system, including children with asthma.
   c. Residents of nursing homes or others with chronic illnesses.
   d. Adults and children with chronic metabolic disease (including diabetes mellitus), renal dysfunction, hemoglobinopathies, or immunosuppression, that required regular medical follow-up or hospitalization during the preceding year.
   e. Children and teenagers (6 mo to 18 yr) on long-term aspirin therapy, and therefore may be at risk of developing Reye's syndrome following influenza infection.
2. Groups potentially capable of transmission of influenza to high-risk individuals.
   a. Physicians, nurses, and other personnel (in hospital or outpatient settings) who have extensive contact with high-risk patients (e.g., primary care and certain specialty clinicians and staff of intensive care units).
   b. Providers of care to high-risk persons in the home setting (e.g., family members, visiting nurses, volunteer workers).
3. Any person wishing to reduce his or her chances of acquiring influenza infection.
4. Other special populations for whom the risk of influenza and its complications is less clear, but vaccine should be considered.
   a. Pregnant women with other risk factors for influenza or its complications.
   b. Persons infected with human immunodeficiency virus (HIV).
   c. Elderly or other persons with high-risk medical conditions traveling to foreign countries during periods when influenza activity is high.

Source: Prevention and control of influenza: part I. Vaccines. MMWR 1993;42(RR-6):1–14.

Amantadine has been the mainstay of chemical prophylaxis for years; however, rimantidine, a similar compound of the adamantine class, is also available for use. Both agents are effective against influenza A only and have no effect on influenza B viruses or other common viral pathogens that cause respiratory illness.

The Centers for Disease Control and Prevention recommend that these agents be used in following persons or circumstances:

1. To reduce spread of virus and maintain care for high-risk persons in the home, hospital, or institutional setting (by administration to unvaccinated persons responsible for care of high-risk patients) during outbreaks of influenza
2. As an adjunct to late vaccination in high-risk, persons
3. As an adjunct to vaccination in immunodeficient persons
4. In persons for whom influenza vaccine is contraindicated (e.g., those allergic to eggs)
5. To control outbreaks of influenza A caused by a variant strain not covered by the vaccine

Amantadine may also be considered for prophylaxis of otherwise healthy, unimmunized persons wishing to avoid influenza A illness (9).

Prophylaxis should be initiated as soon as the outbreak of influenza A is recognized and continued for the duration of influenza activity in the community (up to 90 days). When used as an adjunct to late vaccination, that is, for persons vaccinated after an outbreak of influenza in the area, amantadine or rimanditine should be given for the initial 2 weeks following vaccination. Finally, when used to reduce the severity or duration of symptoms of influenza, therapy with amantadine should be initiated within 24 to 48 hours of symptom onset and continued until 48 hours after signs and symptoms have resolved. The dose for both amantadine and rimantidine is 100 mg PO twice a day in younger patients; however, for those 65 and older, 100 mg/day is the recommended dose. Due to an increased risk of seizures, those with seizure disorders should receive a maximum dose of 100 mg/day. The dosage of both drugs must also be reduced in those with decreased renal function. The side effect profile of both agents includes insomnia, nervousness, and impaired concentration. The elderly generally do not tolerate the side effects well.

Pneumococcal Disease

Clinical Presentation

The bacterium, *Streptococcus pneumoniae*, is the most common secondary bacterial pathogen seen in influenza viral infections and is a major respiratory pathogen of the elderly. It is the most common community-acquired pneumonia and accounts for 40% to 60% of all cases of pneumonia in the elderly. Common comorbidities in older adults such as congestive heart failure, emphysema, cirrhosis, and malignancy increase the risk of death from pneumococcal disease. Other conditions such as alcoholism, splenic dysfunction, a history of splenectomy, and immunodeficiency syndromes also increase the risk of death from this disease (10).

Streptococcus pneumoniae is frequently carried in the upper respiratory tract of normal adults. Infections usually represent endogenous contamination of the respiratory tract due to impaired respiratory defense mechanisms such as a decreased gag reflex or cough. Because aspiration usually precedes the development of pneumonia, it often begins in the right middle or right upper lobe. After an incubation period of 1 to 3 days, clinical symptoms begin, heralded by a shaking chill or fever. Fevers of 38.8°C to 40.5°C (102°F to 105°F) occur. Rust-colored sputum is pathopnomonic for the disease. Pleuritic chest pain, usually severe, as well as anorexia, malaise, and weakness are seen. Examination reveals a toxic-appearing patient with signs of bronchopneumonia. A leukocytosis with left shift is usually found, but in the elderly leukopenia can be seen. A chest radiograph, Gram stain of the sputum, and sputum quelling reaction can confirm the diagnosis. Almost all elderly patients, particularly those with comorbidities, require hospitalization to monitor for hypoxemia and to maintain adequate fluid and electrolyte balance.

Pneumococcal Vaccine

The first commercial pneumococcal vaccine was released in 1978. It contained capsular polysaccharides of 14 different serotypes. In 1983, it was revised to contain 23 different capsular polysaccharides, which account for 90% of bacteremic infections in the United States. Pneumococcal vaccination is recommended for the following adults (11):

1. Those aged 65 years and older
2. Adults of all ages with long-term illnesses that are associated with a high risk of getting pneumococcal disease, including those with heart or lung diseases, diabetes, alcoholism, cirrhosis, or leaks of cerebrospinal fluid
3. Adults with diseases that lower the body's resistance to infections or who are taking drugs that lower the body's resistance to infections. Those with abnormal function or removal of the spleen, Hodgkins's disease, lymphoma, multiple myeloma, kidney failure, nephrotic syndrome or conditions such as organ transplantation should be vaccinated

Revaccination should be considered for the following groups:

1. Persons at highest risk of fatal pneumococcal infection such as persons with abnormal function or removal of the spleen, who received the original pneumococcal vaccine between 1977 and 1983, or who received the current vaccine 6 or more years ago
2. Other persons known to lose protection rapidly, such as persons with the nephrotic syndrome, kidney failure, or transplants, who received the current vaccine 6 or more years ago

Tetanus

Although tetanus is a rare disease in the United States, the majority of deaths seen annually are among those 65 and older. Therefore adults, even those above the age of 65, should continue to receive tetanus boosters every 10 years. Tetanus toxoid should always be used in conjunction with diphtheria toxoid to maintain immunity against both pathogens. Local reactions at the site of administration and fever are common adverse reactions to the booster.

Geriatric Syndromes

The remainder of this chapter describes the presentation and management of syndromes commonly seen in geriatric patients. Principals of drug prescribing in the elderly are reviewed. The management of patients presenting with lower extremity edema, falls, and dementia is also reviewed.

Drug-Prescribing Considerations for the Elderly

Geriatric patients consume 25% of all prescribed medications in the United States and large amounts of over-the-counter medications. Although pharmacologic therapy has improved the quality of life for many elderly patients, medication may also cause iatrogenic harm in older persons. As more is learned about geropharmacology, it is becoming increasingly clear that prescribing practices appropriate for younger patients must be altered for the elderly.

Polypharmacy

Polypharmacy, or polymedicating, in the elderly is associated with an increased risk of adverse drug reactions, drug interactions, noncompliance, and increased cost. Several factors contribute to polypharmacy in the elderly. Older patients have an increased incidence of chronic illness and may have multiple illnesses resulting in more frequent physician visits. Often, older patients may see more than one provider, each of whom may prescribe different medications. Misuse of medication may also occur because older persons may not understand dosing schedules or understand when to discontinue medications. The physician should thoroughly review all medications to avoid polypharmacy and misuse.

Although the word "polypharmacy" makes one think of a patient who takes multiple medications, an important truth is that even one unnecessary medication can place the older person at risk of an avoidable toxic reaction. Prescribing medications in the elderly should be done judiciously after careful consideration or a trial of nonpharmacologic therapy when appropriate.

Just as it is important to be cautious about polymedicating elderly patients, it is equally appropriate to mention underuse of medication. When the quality of life can be improved by the use of pharmacologic therapy, medications should not be withheld because of age. Even though older patients respond well to pharmacologic treatment of depression, physicians often underuse antidepressants in this age group.

Pharmacology and Aging

Understanding the impact of age-related physiologic changes on pharmacokinetics and pharmacodynamics is critical to drug prescribing in the elderly. The ability to excrete and metabolize medications, the distribution of drugs, and organ sensitivity to medications all change with age. The most important changes involve cardiovascular, central nervous system, renal and hepatic functions; body composition; tissue sensitivity to drugs; and baroreceptor reflex sensitivity (13).

Although the effect of aging on hepatic drug metabolism is variable, phase I metabolism (oxidation) is usually decreased, whereas phase II metabolism (conjugative) is usually unchanged. Therefore, drugs that undergo hepatic oxidation could result in increased plasma concentrations. Drugs affected by reduced efficiency of hepatic oxidation include benzodiazapines, nortriptyline, propranolol, quinidine, phenytoin, and warfarin. Because age-related changes in first-pass extraction are variable, dosage adjustments should be individualized.

Age-related changes in renal elimination are more predictable. Beginning with the fourth decade of life, there is 6% to 10% reduction of glomerular filtration rate and renal plasma flow every 10 years. Thus, by age 70, a person may have a 40% to 50% decrease in renal function, even in the absence of kidney disease (13). Measurement of creatinine clearance is useful in making dosing determinations, but it should not be the sole determinant. In general, drugs that are eliminated primarily by the kidneys should be given in reduced dosages or at less frequent intervals to avoid accumulation. Additionally, to further define dose requirements, therapeutic drug monitoring should be performed for toxic drugs with a low therapeutic index, including amioglycosides, lithium, digoxin, and procainamide (14). Table 42.3 describes drugs posing special risks in the elderly (14).

Because the elderly have proportionately more fat than lean tissue as compared to younger individuals, drug distribution is affected. A fat-soluble drug (e.g., diazepam) will be retained in the body longer in the

Table 42.3 Drugs Posing Special Risks in the Elderly

Drug	Special Considerations	Drug	Special Considerations
Amitriptyline	Most potent anticholinergic of all tricyclics. It can lead to confusion, orthostatic hypotension, dry mouth, blurred vision, urinary retention. Also the most sedating of all the tricyclics; can lead to confusion and unstable gait.	Long-acting benzodiazepines: diazepam, flurazepam, chlordiazepoxide	Half-lives are prolonged in the elderly up to as much as 4 days. They can lead to CNS toxicity such as confusion, oversedation, falls and fractures.
Antiemetics	These are phenothiazines and are anticholinergic and sedating. They may lead to confusion, orthostatic hypotension, blurred vision, falls, dry mouth, and urinary retention.	Narcotics	The elderly are more sensitive to all narcotics. Doses should be started low. The elderly are prone to constipation and all narcotics tend to constipate. Consider laxatives when narcotics are used.
OTC cold remedies	Most contain antihistamines, which are highly anticholinergic. They can lead to dry mouth, confusion, urinary retention, blurred vision, falls.	Diphenhydramine	Of all the medications used to induce sleep, diphenhydramine is the only one with anticholinergic side effects. It is rarely the drug of choice for older patients because it can lead to dry mouth, confusion, orthostatic hypotension, falls, and urinary retention.
Propoxyphene	Can lead to sedation and confusion.		

CNS, central nervous system; OTC, over the counter
Adapted by permission from Beers MH, Ouslander JG. Risk factors in geriatric drug prescribing: a practical guide to avoid problems. Drugs 1989;37:105–112.

elderly. A water-soluble drug (e.g., digoxin) will be present in increased concentrations, which may cause toxic effects.

Of all the body's systems, the central nervous system is the most sensitive to age-related changes. There is a reduction in the concentration of neurotransmitters and a decrease in the number of functional neurons. The action of stimulants is lessened, whereas the action of depressants is enhanced.

Adverse Drug Effects

"Any symptom in an elderly patient may be a drug side effect until proved otherwise" (15). Although this may be an overstatement, it defines a starting point for the evaluation of an older person. Indeed, many drugs that are usually safe in younger patients require close attention when used in the elderly. Age-related changes in pharmacokinetics and pharmacodynamics, multiple medications, severity of illness, and increased sensitivity to drug effects are among the risk factors for adverse drug reactions in the elderly. However, adverse drug effects in geriatric patients may be different in severity and presentation from those seen in younger patients and, therefore, may go unrecognized as an adverse drug effect and may even be treated with an additional medication.

Before prescribing new drugs, the physician should thoroughly review all medications the patient is taking, paying particular attention to any newly added drugs. Also, there should be a high index of suspicion of an adverse drug reaction if the patient is on a medication recently released for use. Often, the premarketing research in elderly patients is limited.

Prescribing Modifications

It is best to avoid medications with strong anticholinergic effects. Anticholinergic toxicity can be responsible for numerous symptoms. Because acetylcholine serves as a neurotransmitter in numerous key roles in both the parasympathetic and central nervous systems, its blockage can yield a host of problems including confusion, urinary retention with or without overflow, increased intraocular pressure, and constipation (15). Antihistamines are more likely to cause dizziness, sedation, and hypotension in older versus younger patients.

Benzodiazepines can have a depressant effect on the elderly. If prescribed, they should be given in low doses with small incremental increases until an effective and safe dose is reached. Agents with a long half-life should be avoided because they may result in an increased risk of falls and hip fractures in the elderly. Temazepam (Restoril), oxazepam (Serax), or low doses of alprazolam (Xanax) are preferred over longer-acting agents such as flurazepam (Dalmane).

Older persons use analgesic agents at a higher rate than younger patients. Acetaminophen is the preferred agent for noninflammatory pain. Although the hepatic metabolism of acetaminophen is often impaired in the elderly, dose adjustments are not necessary. For stronger pain relief, narcotic analgesics can be used cautiously. Older persons appear to be more sensitive to the pain-relieving effects of narcotics and therefore doses given to the elderly can initially be reduced.

For inflammatory pain, nonsteroidal anti-inflammatory drugs (NSAIDs) can be considered, but they must be used with extreme caution. When possible, they should only be used for short intervals of time, such as during arthritis flares. The response of the aged patient to NSAIDs is approximately the same as with younger individuals, but older patients are at a higher risk for NSAID-induced complications such as peptic ulcer disease and renal insufficiency.

Lower Extremity Edema

Evaluation of the patient with lower extremity edema begins with a search for the etiology of the edema. In most elderly patients, lower extremity edema will be secondary to venous insufficiency. Venous insufficiency refers to reverse blood flow in the veins secondary to inadequate venous valve function. The resulting venous hypertension can occur in the superficial or deep venous systems, or both. Superficial venous insufficiency occurs when the greater or lesser saphenous veins become incompetent, resulting in varicose veins. The disorder is more common in women and tends to be hereditary. Patients develop tortuous, dilated veins and lower extremity edema can occur.

Other potential causes of lower extremity or peripheral edema in elderly patients include congestive heart failure, the nephrotic syndrome, and hepatic cirrhosis. The patient's history will provide clues to the cause; the examination will help to confirm or deny suspicions.

History

Patients presenting with lower extremity edema should be questioned about the duration of the edema and any history of heart, liver, or kidney disease. A key question to ask is whether the edema resolves with elevation of the leg or with assuming the supine position for an extended period of time. Unilateral leg swelling that does not resolve could indicate a deep venous thrombosis, and the patient should undergo a Doppler ultrasound of the involved lower extremity. Lymphatic or venous obstruction at the pelvic level could also cause unilateral or bilateral leg swelling, and a pelvic ultrasound can screen for this.

The patient should also be questioned about swelling in other body parts such as the abdomen, face, or sacrum. Patients with advanced cirrhosis resulting in ascites and lower extremity edema typically complain of a swollen abdomen resulting in an increasing abdominal girth. Patients with heart failure present with classic symptoms of dyspnea on exertion, paroxysmal nocturnal dyspnea, and orthopnea.

Evaluation

The examination of the patient with lower extremity edema should include a pulmonary, cardiac, and abdominal assessment. In the patient with congestive heart failure, pulmonary rales and a gallop rhythm can often be heard. Jugular venous distention may also be evident. In patients with chronic right-sided heart failure, jugular venous distention and ascites can be present. Ascites can also be due to long-standing liver disease resulting in cirrhosis. In evaluating the patient for ascites, check for an increased abdominal girth, shifting dullness, and fluid wave. Ascites can be confirmed by an abdominal ultrasound.

Patients with the nephrotic syndrome rarely develop ascites. Likewise, jugular venous distention and pulmonary edema are absent. Patients with the nephrotic syndrome often present with periorbital edema and peripheral edema. A urinalysis should be checked in suspected cases and will demonstrate significant proteinuria.

Treatment

Patients with congestive heart failure, hepatic cirrhosis, and the nephrotic syndrome should be referred to an internist or appropriate subspecialist. Patients with venous insufficiency may need referral, but they can often be managed with simple conservative measures.

Many patients with varicose veins develop aching in the legs, which is exacerbated by increased hydrostatic pressure in the legs. This can include standing and activities that increase intra-abdominal pressure. Leg elevation and the use of elastic support stockings are needed to alleviate symptoms, by providing venous compression. Thromboembolic disease support hose can be purchased at most pharmacies. If more support is needed a Jobst stocking can be fitted to the patient and are readily available at medical supply stores.

Varicosities not responsive to conservative measures can be treated surgically, by ligation and stripping, or by injection. Surgery is usually reserved for varicosities involving the entire superficial system; injection with a sclerosing agent is indicated for more localized varicosities (16). According to Glover, absolute indications for surgical referral are 1) ulceration; 2) spontaneous bleeding from varicosities; and 3) significant thrombosis in varicosities (16). Relative indications for surgical referral include cosmesis and severe symptoms.

Deep Venous Insufficiency

Deep venous insufficiency is the result of incompetent valves in the deep venous system of the legs. Valve dysfunction over a large segment of a deep vein is usually the result of deep venous thrombosis. Therefore, the early diagnosis and treatment of deep venous thrombosis is the best preventive measure for deep venous insufficiency. Once recanalization of a thrombosed vein occurs, resulting incompetent valves lead to venous hypertension in the involved extremity. Chronic venous hypertension can result in increased capillary formation, extravasation of fibrin and blood cells, resulting in brownish discoloration of the lower extremities, due to hemosiderin deposition. Subcutaneous tissues become thick and firm, resulting in the so-called brawny edema. The thickening of the skin and tissues is called lipodermatosclerosis. With these changes patients become prone to the development of ulcers, which typically occur above the medial malleolus. Ulceration can result in pain and local infection or cellulitis.

The mainstay of treatment is to prevent the occurrence of edema and ulceration. For a minority of patients, venous reconstructive surgery can restore adequate venous flow and prevent the occurrence of complications. For most patients, however, conservative measures are all that is available. Prevention of edema is the most effective intervention to heal ulcers or prevent their occurrence. This is best accomplished through the use of external pneumatic compression devices, which are available for home use. Patients can be taught to use the devices for needed intervals on a daily basis. Often, 1 hour of use per day is adequate to control edema. Figure 42.1 shows a home compression device in use. The use of compression devices can be supplemented by having the patient wear fitted elastic stockings between compression treatments. Other conservative measures include counseling obese patients to lose weight, educating patients on the need to keep their legs elevated when possible, and reminding them to prevent trauma to the affected leg. If cellulitis occurs, hospitalization may be needed.

Falls

Falls are the leading cause of death from injury among those older than age 65. Approximately 30% of community-dwelling adults aged 65 and older will fall each

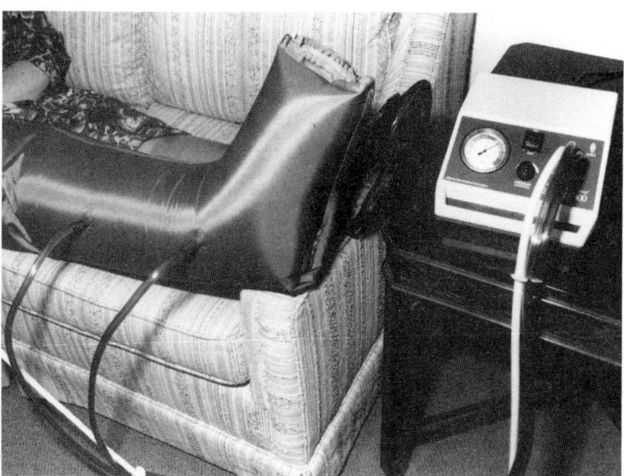

Fig 42.1 Example of pneumatic compression pump for home use.

year and 50% of those will fall repeatedly. There have been contradictory results as to whether older women fall more often than older men (17,18), but women appear to have a higher rate of both fracture and non-fracture injuries than men (19,20).

The rate of falls increases with age. More than half of all fatal falls involve those age 75 years and older, a group representing only 5% of the population (21). Although falling is more common among frail elderly persons, healthy elderly also fall, which would suggest that falling is not merely a marker for functional decline (17).

Aside from the risk of death, the consequences of falls include injury and the psychological trauma of fear of falling. Fortunately, most falls do not result in serious injury. Approximately 1% of falls result in a hip fracture, 5% result in other fractures, and another 5% result in serious soft-tissue trauma. Fifty percent of falls result in minor injury such as an abrasion or a contusion (17–19).

Hip fracture is the most common age-related fracture and is perhaps the most feared morbid outcome of a fall. Ninety percent of hip fractures occur as a result of a fall. Each year over 250,000 Americans suffer a hip fracture. Of these, 75% are women. Thirty-three percent of women who live to the age of 90 will have a hip fracture (22).

During a medical interview, geriatric patients may not volunteer that they have had a fall, feeling that falling is simply a part of growing old. Others may not recall the event due to cognitive difficulties, whereas some may fear that if they report falling, they may be placed in a nursing home. If the cause of the fall can be identified, a preventive strategy can be developed, which can minimize the risk of falling without compromising the mobility and functional independence of the older adult.

Multiple risk factors often interact to produce a fall. Biologic risk factors include musculoskeletal, neurologic, visual, auditory, cognitive, and proprioceptive abnormalities (23). Environmental risk factors include loose throw rugs, electrical cords and small objects that can be tripped over, dimly lit rooms, ill-fitting shoes, and surfaces with glare. Other predisposing risk factors include depression, postural hypotension, and medications. Most studies have shown that sedatives such as benzodiazepines, phenothiazines, and antidepressants increase the risk of falling, independent of the effect of the dementia or depression for which they are prescribed. The risk appears to be greater for the longer-acting sedatives. There is also an increased risk of falling among patients receiving four or more prescription medications. This risk appears to be independent of the diseases for which the medications are prescribed (17).

Table 42.4 lists the major causes of falls and their relative frequencies in seven studies of community-living adults. Falls related to so-called accidents, stemming from environmental hazards, caused the majority of falls. However, many falls attributed to accidents really stem from the interaction between identifiable environmental hazards and the patient's increased susceptibility to these hazards from the accumulated effects of age and disease (24).

Abnormal gait affects between 20% to 5% of persons over 65 (25). Postural control, speed of body-orienting reflexes, height of stepping, and muscle strength and tone all decrease with aging. These changes impair a patient's ability to avoid a fall after an unexpected trip or while reaching or bending (26). Abnormalities of proprioception occur on neurologic examination in 15% to 20% of elderly patients (27). After age 50, vibration and tactile sense both decrease significantly, especially in the lower extremities (28). These abnormalities result in a more cautious gait, a tendency to watch the feet while walking, and frequent missteps (29).

Drop attacks are defined as a sudden fall without loss of consciousness or dizziness and are reported

Table 42.4 Summary of Studies That Carefully Evaluated Elderly Persons After a Fall and Specified as "Most Likely Cause"

Cause of Falls	Community-Living Elderly (7 Studies; 2312 falls)
"Accident"/environment related	41% (23–53%)*
Gait/balance disorder, weakness	13% (2–29%)
Dizziness/vertigo	8% (0–19%)
Drop attack	13% (0–25%)
Confusion	2% (0–7%)
Postural hypotension	1% (0–6%)
Visual disorder	0.8% (0–4%)
Syncope	0.4% (0–3%)
Other specified causes[a]	17% (2–39%)
Unknown	6% (0–16%)

*Mean percentage calculated from the total number of falls in the studies reviewed. Ranges indicate the percentage reported in each of the studies. Percentages do not total 100% because some studies reported more than one cause per fall.
[a]This category includes arthritis, acute illness, drugs, alcohol, pain, epilepsy, and falling from bed.
Adapted from Rubenstein LZ, Josephson KR. Clinical research on falls in the nursing home. In: Rubenstein LZ, Wieland DW, eds. Improving care in the nursing home. Newbury Park: Sage Publications, 1993:216–240. Copyright © 1993 by Sage Publications. Reprinted by permission of Sage Publications, Inc.

as a cause of falls in up to 25% of community patients. Sudden head movement often brings on these attacks. This syndrome has been attributed to vertebrobasilar insufficiency although the exact etiology is probably due to diverse pathophysiologic mechanisms (24).

The sensation of dizziness is a common complaint among fallers and is often nonspecific. This description may reflect diverse etiologies such as cardiovascular disorders, postural hypotension, anxiety, hyperventilation, or medication side effects (24).

Once it has been established that a person has fallen, a complete evaluation is important. Acute injuries need to be evaluated first. Radiographs of the painful and injured areas are needed to assess for fractures. Sprains and soft-tissue injuries are common. If the patient reports a serious head injury, a head computed tomography scan without contrast is needed to rule out a subdural hematoma.

A thorough history of the fall event and precipitating factors is important in assessing the cause of the fall. Acute illnesses or exacerbations of chronic conditions can lead to falls. Falling is a well recognized nonspecific presentation for illnesses such as pneumonia, urinary tract infections, and congestive heart failure. Specific circumstances may give clues to the etiology: looking up or sideways (arterial or carotid sinus compression), loss of consciousness (syncope from an arrhythmia, aortic stenosis, or seizure), sudden rise from a lying or seated position (orthostatic hypotension), asymmetric weakness (stroke or transient ischemic attack), chest pain (myocardial ischemia or infarction) (26).

A careful physical examination after the fall may also give clues to etiology. You should check for orthostatic blood pressure changes; the presence of cardiac murmurs, arrhythmias, carotid bruits, nystagmus, focal neurologic signs, musculoskeletal weakness and abnormalities; visual and auditory losses; and cognitive problems. Blood tests are seldom helpful but a complete blood count, electrolytes and an electrocardiogram may yield abnormalities (26). When signs or symptoms suggest that further work-up or more expensive testing is necessary, a consult from the proper specialist may be necessary.

A referral to a physical therapist is appropriate if muscle weakness or gait instabilities are contributing to falling. Physical therapists can also assist in properly fitting the correct assistive device, such as a cane or walker. Some physical therapists make home visits and can identify environmental hazards that contribute to falls, such as cluttered floors and dimly lit rooms. Preventive measures can be suggested such as installing grab bars around bathtubs and toilets or securing stairway banisters.

A proper work-up for a fall can reveal otherwise undetected treatable abnormalities. Modifying risk factors for falls can prevent future morbidity and mortality in the elderly patients.

Dementia

Progressive intellectual decline is one of the most frightening problems faced by older adults. Although this problem was once thought to be a normal consequence of aging and termed "senility," this concept is no longer thought to be true. Serious difficulties with remembering and thinking (i.e., cognitive disorders) are not an inevitable consequence of growing old. Rather, cognitive problems are a symptom of a medical illness (30).

Although normal aging does not lead to serious cognitive impairment, complaints of failing memory are common with aging. Studies show that older persons' performances on tests of recent memory are reduced compared with those of younger subjects. However, these impairments are not extensive and older adults show no impairment on tests of general information, vocabulary, and immediate or remote recall (30).

Benign senescent forgetfulness is a syndrome that has been proposed to describe the mild impairment of memory that may accompany normal aging. It is characterized by an inability to recall certain parts of a remote experience, such as dates or names, while overall recall for the experience is intact. This syndrome is thought to be benign, in contrast to the cognitive deficits of dementing illnesses, because it is not rapidly progressive and does not affect survival or risk of institutionalization (30). Yearly neuropsychological testing can establish whether a dementing illness is present.

Most physicians can recognize the later stages of a dementing illness, but they are often unfamiliar with the presentation of an early dementia when the complaints are subjective and the patient's social skills are preserved (31). To make the diagnosis of dementia, the patient must have short- and long-term memory impairment, as well as a loss of other intellectual abilities that interfere with social or occupational functioning. Additionally, at least one of the following must be present:

- Impairment of abstract thinking
- Impaired judgment
- Personality change
- Other disturbances of higher cortical function, such as aphasia (disorder of language), apraxia (inability to carry out motor activities despite intact comprehension and motor function), agnosia (failure to recognize or identify objects despite intact sensory function), and constructional difficulty (e.g., inability to copy three-dimensional figures, assemble blocks, or arrange sticks in specific designs) (31)

Also, the above deficits must occur in a person who is not delirious. For instance, if a patient is suspected of being demented but was functioning well at work or at home just a week ago, this would be inconsistent with dementia and the patient would have to be evaluated for some acute cause, such as a delirium (31). Delirium and acute confusional states are associated with alterations in the level of consciousness, which lead to confusion and an inability to focus or to sustain attention. Delirium and acute confusional states usually last from hours to days, whereas, dementia persists for months or years (30).

Dementia occurs at all ages, but it increases with advancing age, so that the largest group of demented patients is in the older age groups (32). The prevalence of dementia has been estimated at less than 10% for individuals who are older than 65 and 15% to 20% by the age of 85 (33).

Dementia can be associated with at least 60 conditions (34). Based on etiology, dementia can be categorized as degenerative, vascular, infectious, toxic, or metabolic. Autopsy series suggest that 50% of dementias are due to Alzheimer's disease, 10% to 20% to multi-infarct dementia, and 10% to 20% to a combination of Alzheimer's disease and multi-infarct dementia (33).

Dementia is reversible in some cases. It is, therefore, essential to make the diagnosis of intellectual impairment as early as possible to screen for the reversible causes of dementia. Although estimates vary, many authorities have proposed that as many as 10% to 20% of persons with progressive intellectual deterioration have underlying reversible causes that can be diagnosed and treated (35). In some cases, a simple test may uncover a completely curable disorder such as B_{12} deficiency or hypothyroidism. In other cases such as multi-infarct dementia or neurosyphilis, intervention may modify the course of the illness, sparing the patient further morbidity without reversing the existing deficits. In Huntington's disease, treatment may lessen the symptoms without altering the course of the dementia. In Alzheimer's disease, tacrine, which is a cholinesterase inhibitor, is somewhat effective. Although 30% to 50% of patients with Alzheimer's disease exhibit some degree of cognitive improvement when taking tacrine, the underlying disease process continues. Evaluation of dementia may also reveal treatable medical complications, such as congestive heart failure, electrolyte imbalances, and urinary tract infections, or may uncover medication side effects that are worsening the patient's mental status or behavioral problems (36).

A medical history should be taken from the patient and from a caregiver or other person who is well acquainted with the affected person. It is important to establish a history of progressive deterioration and to identify tasks the patient can no longer perform adequately. The history often reveals abnormalities, including impaired memory and other cognitive functions, impaired activities of daily living, alterations in mood, and often delusions and hallucinations. Common complaints from the patient and caregivers include forgetfulness about appointments or errands; inability to find the way to an accustomed destination; inability to use money and instruments of daily living such as a telephone; deterioration in work or housework performance; difficulties in dressing, reading, and writing; and inability to recognize previously familiar persons (37).

A useful screening test for intellectual impairment is the Mini-Mental State Examination (MMSE), which can be easily administered in the physician's office in about 10 minutes (Table 42.5) (38–40). This test is scored from 0 to 30, with higher scores indicating better cognitive functioning. The following three cut-off levels classify the severity of cognitive impairment: 0 to

Table 42.5 Instrument for Folstein Mini-Mental State Examination

Maximum Score	Score	Item
		Orientation
5	( )	What is the (year) (season) (day) (month)?
5	( )	Where are we: (state) (country) (town) (hospital) (floor).
		Registration
3	( )	Name three objects: 1 second to say each. Then ask the patient all three after you have said them. Give 1 point for each correct answer. Then repeat them until he or she learns all three (for later checking).
		Attention and Calculation
5	( )	Serial 7s. Give 1 point for each correct. Stop after five answers. Alternatively spell "world" backward.
		Recall
3	( )	Ask for the three objects repeated above. Give 1 point for each correct.
		Language
9	( )	Show patient a pencil and watch, and ask for their names. (2 points) Follow a three-stage command: "Take a paper in your right hand, fold it in half, and put it on the floor." (3 points) Read and obey the following: "Close your eyes." (1 point) "Write a sentence." (1 point) "Copy a single design." (1 point) _______ Total score

The patient's score can range from 0 to 30.
Reproduced by permission from Lacks MS, Feinstein AR, Cooney LM, et al. A simple procedure for general screening for functional disability in elderly patients. Ann Intern Med 1990;112:699–706. Adapted and reprinted from Journal of Psychiatic Research, volume 12, Folstein MF, Folstein SE. Mini-mental state. A practical method for grading the cognitive state of patients for the clinician, 189–198, with kind permission from Elsevior Science Ltd, The Boulevand, Langford Lane, Kidlington OXS IGB, UK.

17 = severe cognitive impairment; 18 to 23 = mild cognitive impairment; 24 to 30 = no cognitive impairment (38). The MMSE contains items that assess orientation, registration, attention, calculation, recent recall, naming, repeating, understanding, reading, writing, and ability to draw or copy (37). If this test or other information leads one to believe that the patient may have intellectual deterioration, it may be necessary to refer the patient to a physician with a knowledge of and interest in dementia, such as a geriatrician or neurologist.

All patients with new-onset dementia should have several basic diagnostic studies. These studies include: complete blood cell count; electrolyte panel; screening metabolic panel; thyroid gland function tests; vitamin B_{12} and folate levels; syphilis tests; and, depending on the history, human immunodeficiency antibodies, urinalysis, electrocardiogram, and chest x-ray. When combined with a history and physical examination, the above tests may reveral reversible metabolic or endocrine deficiency and infectious states, whether causative or complicating. Depending on the history, other ancillary studies may be appropriate, such as computed tomography of the brain without contrast, electroencephalogram, and psychiatric and neuropsychological evaluation (32).

REFERENCES

1. Rowe JW, Kahn RL. Human aging: usual and successful. Science 1987;237:143–149.
2. Rowe JW, Schneider EL. Aging processes. In: Abrams WB, Berkow R, eds. Merck manual of geriatrics. Rahway, NJ: Merck & Co, 1990:303–308.
3. Ferri FF. Biology, epidemiology, and demographics of aging. In: Ferri FF, Fretwell MD. Practical guide to the care of the geriatric patient. St. Louis: CV Mosby, 1992:1–12.
4. Katz S, Downs TD, Cash HR. Progress in the development of the index ADL. Gerontologist 1970;1:20–30.
5. Lichtenstein MJ, Federspiel CF, Schaffner W. Factors associated with early demise in nursing home residents: a case control study. J Am Geriatr Soc 1985;33:315–319.
6. Katz S, Stoud MW. Functional assessment in geriatrics. A review of progress and directions. J Am Geriatric Soc 1987;37:267–271.
7. Prevention of control of influenza: part I: vaccines. MMWR 1993;42(RR-6):1–14.
8. Influenza prevention for 1993–1994. University of Alabama Hospital Drug Information Bulletin, Jackson A. Como, ed. 1993;27(10).
9. Prevention and control of influenza. MMWR 1992;41(RR-9):1–13.
10. Mufson M. *Streptococcus pneumoniae.* In: Mandell GL, Douglas RG, Bennett JE, eds. Principals and practice of infectious diseases. 3rd ed. New York: Churchill Livingstone, 1990:1539–1550.
11. Important information about pneumococcal disease and pneumococcal polysaccharide vaccine. U.S. Public Health Service Information Form, 9/1/89.
12. Beers M. Medication use in the elderly. In: Calkins E, Ford AB, Katz PR. Practice of geriatrics. 2nd ed. Philadelphia: WB Saunders, 1992:33–49.
13. Lowenthal DT. Clinical pharmacology. In: Abrams WB, Berkow R, eds. Merck manual of geriatrics. Rahway, NJ: Merck & Co, 1990:181–193.
14. Beers MH, Ouslander JG. Risk factors in geriatric drug prescribing: a practical guide to avoiding problems. Drugs 1984;37:105–112.
15. Avorn J, Gurwitz J. Principles of pharmacology. In: Cassel CK, et al., eds. Geriatric medicine. 2nd ed. New York: Springer-Verlag, 1990:66–76.
16. Glover JL. Diseases of the veins. In: Kelley WR, ed. Textbook of internal medicine. 2nd ed. Philadelphia: JB Lippincott, 1992:229–233.
17. Tinetti ME. Falls. In: Hazzard WR, Bierman EL, Blass JP, et al., eds. Principles of geriatric medicine and gerontology. 3rd ed. New York: McGraw-Hill, 1994: 1313–1320.
18. Tinetti ME, Speechley M, Ginter SF. Risk factors for falls among elderly persons living in the community. N Engl J Med 1988;319:1701–1707.
19. Sattin RW. Falls among older persons: a public health perspective. Annu Rev Public Health 1992;13:489–507.
20. Nevitt MC, Cummings SR, Kidd S, et al. Risk factors for recurrent nonsyncopal falls: a prospective study. JAMA 1989;261:2663–2668.
21. Baker SP, O'Neill B, Karpf RS, eds. Falls. In: The injury fact book. 2nd ed. New York: Oxford University Press, 1992:134–148.
22. Grisso JA, Kaplan F. Hip fractures. In: Hazzard WR, Bierman EL, Blass JP, et al., eds. Principles of geriatric medicine and gerontology. 3rd ed. New York: McGraw-Hill, 1994:1321–1327.

23. Zylke JW. As nation grows older, falls become greater source of fear, injury, death. JAMA 1990;263: 2021.

24. Rubenstein LZ, Josephson KR. Clinical research on falls in the nursing home. In: Rubenstein LZ, Wieland DW, eds. Improving care in the nursing home. Newbury Park: Sage Publications, 1993:216–240.

25. Sudarsky L. Geriatrics: gait disorders in the elderly. Current Concepts in Geriatrics 1990;322:1441–1446.

26. Rubenstein LZ. Falls. In: Yoshihawa TT, Cobbs EL, Brummel-Smith K, eds. Ambulatory geriatric care. Portland: CV Mosby, 1993:296–304.

27. Klawans HL, Tufo HM, Ostfeld AM. Neurologic examination in an elderly population. Dis Nerv Syst 1971;32:274–279.

28. Steiness I. Vibratory perception in normal subjects. Acta Med Scand 1957;158:315–325.

29. Caranasos GJ. Recognizing common gait disorders. Geriatric Consultant 1989;September/October:14–19.

30. Ramsdell JW, Rothrock JF, Ward HW, et al. Evaluation of cognitive impairment in the elderly. J Gen Intern Med 1990;5:55–64.

31. Jenike MA. Alzheimer's disease and other dementias. In: Jenike MA, ed. Geriatric psychiatry and psychopharmacology. Chicago: Year Book Medical Publishers, 1989:127–202.

32. Consensus Conference. Differential diagnosis of dementing diseases. JAMA 1987;258:3411–3416.

33. Geriatric syndromes, dementia. Beck JC, ed. Geriatrics review syllabus. Book 1. New York: American Geriatrics Society, 1991:117–128.

34. Skoog I, Nilsson L, Palmertz B, et al. A population-based study of dementia in 85-year-olds. N Engl J Med 1993;328:153–158.

35. Barry PP, Moskowitz MA. The diagnosis of reversible dementia in the elderly: a critical review. Arch Intern Med 1988;148:1914–1918.

36. Mahler ME, Cummings JL, Benson F. Treatable dementias. West J Med 1987;146:705–712.

37. McKhann G, Drachman D, Folstein M, et al. Clinical diagnosis of Alzheimer's disease: report of the NINCDS-ADRDA work group under the auspices of Department of Health and Human Services Task Force on Alzheimer's Disease. Neurology 1984;34:939–944.

38. Tombaugh TN, McIntyre NJ. The Mini-Mental State Examination: a comprehensive review. J Am Geriatr Soc 1992;40:922–935.

39. Lacks MS, Feinstein AR, Cooney LM, et al. A simple procedure for general screening for functional disability in elderly patients. Ann Intern Med 1990;112: 699–706.

40. Folstein MF, Folstein SE, McHugh, PR. "Mini-Mental State." A practical method for grading the cognitive state of patients for the clinician. J Psychiatr Res 1975;12:189–198.

INDEX

A
Abdominal examination
in hypertension, 27
in pneumonia, 164–165
Abdominal migraine, 388t
Abdominal obesity, 282–283, 286
Abdominal pain, 78, 180
in cholangitis, primary sclerosing, 187
in Crohn's disease, 193
in gallstones, 184
in irritable bowel syndrome, 180
in lupus erythematosus, 458
in ulcerative colitis, 194
Abortion, 17, 18
Abscess
of lung, differential diagnosis of, 166
of vulva, in inflammatory bowel disease, 197
Absorptiometry, dual energy, 410–411
Abuse
sexual
and borderline personality disorder, 579
molluscum contagiosum in, 479
of substances. *See* Substance abuse and addiction
Acebutolol in hypertension, 32t, 36
Acetaminophen
in elderly, 610
in headaches, 387, 392, 392t, 393
in osteoarthritis, 431
in pregnancy, 393
in rheumatoid arthritis, 446–447
Acetanilid in headaches, 387
Acetohexamide in diabetes mellitus, 270t
Acetylsalicylic acid. *See* Aspirin
Acidosis
diabetic ketoacidosis, 265, 266, 268, 271–272
renal tubular, in lupus erythematosus, 457
Acne, 475–478
nodulocystic, 475, 476, 476f
in pregnancy, 477, 478
rosacea, 483
Acral-lentiginous melanoma, Plate 15, 497
Actinic keratoses, 493
Acyclovir in chronic fatigue, 381
Addiction to alcohol and drugs, 538–546. *See also* Substance abuse and addiction
Adenoma
of adrenal gland, 305
of pituitary gland. *See* Pituitary gland, adenoma of
of thyroid gland, 252
Adjustment disorder, 591
with depression, 524, 529
insomnia in, 562
Adolescents. *See also* Children and infants
depression in, 525
hypertension in, 41, 41t
Adrenal gland
adenoma of, 305
in hirsutism, 302, 305
hyperplasia of, congenital, 305, 305f
in myxedema coma, 260, 261
α-Adrenergic agonists in allergic rhinitis, 362
β_2-Adrenergic agonists
in asthma, 127–129, 128t, 129t, 130
in emergency room care, 136, 137
exercise-induced, 136
nocturnal, 136
in pregnancy, 134
in chronic obstructive pulmonary disease, 145–146
side effects of, 127, 145–146
α-Adrenergic blockers in hypertension, 33t, 37
β-Adrenergic blockers
in angina pectoris, 88
in heart failure, 99
in hypertension, 32t-33t, 36–37
in hyperthyroidism, 245–246
in pregnancy, 257
and thyroid storm, 259
in migraine prevention, 395, 395t
in mitral valve prolapse syndrome/ dysautonomia, 108–109
side effects of, 36–37, 88, 246, 395
Adrenocorticotropic hormone in stress, 550
Aging, 603–617
Alzheimer's disease in, 4–5, 614–615
angina pectoris in, 88
bone changes in, 406–407, 408
and fracture risk, 406–407
in mass, 402–404, 403f
in remodeling, 405
calcium malabsorption in, 408
chronic illness and multiple morbidities in, 605
daily living activities in, 604t, 604–605, 615
dementia in, 4–5, 614–616
depression in, 521, 525
treatment of, 529–530, 534
diabetes mellitus in, 6, 603–604
drug-induced disorders in, 609–610
falls in, 612
drug therapy in, 608–610
with multiple drugs, 608
special risks in, 608, 609t
dyslipidemia in, 60–61
exercise in, 16
falls in. *See* Falls of elderly
functional assessment in, 604–605
gallbladder cancer in, 189
goiter in, sporadic, 254
hair growth in, 308
hearing loss in, 5
hypertension in, 3, 35, 40
and drug therapy, 38, 39, 40
lower extremity edema in, 610–611
melanoma in, 498
osteoarthritis in, 6, 431, 432
pneumococcal disease in, 607
pneumonia in, 163, 164, 165, 607
presentation of disease in, 603–604
rhinitis in, allergic, 362
sleep in, 554, 561
in menopause, 557
support network in, 19
tetanus boosters in, 607
thyroid disorders in, 6, 251
hyperthyroidism, 245, 247
myxedema coma, 259, 261
vaccinations in, 605–607
vision assessment in, 5
weight in, 6, 17
xerosis in, 489
Agoraphobia, 582, 593t, 594, 596
prevalence of, 586, 587t
AIDS. *See* HIV infection and AIDS
Airway disease, hyperactive, 119–138. *See also* Asthma
Airway obstruction
in asthma, 119
chronic. *See* Pulmonary disorders, chronic obstructive disease
differential diagnosis of, 122–123, 140
Albumin levels in hepatitis, 329
Albuterol
in asthma, 124, 127, 128t
nocturnal, 136
in pregnancy, 134
in lung cancer, 161
Alcohol use and alcoholism, 15, 16, 526, 538
blood pressure in, 26, 30
clinical presentation in, 541–543
gender differences in, 544
hypoglycemia in, 275, 276
laboratory tests in, 544
life expectancy in, 12, 13
lipid abnormalities in, 50
obesity in, 283
questionnaire on, 15, 591
risk factors in, 539
sleep disorders in, 562, 566
and theories of addiction, 539–541
treatment of, 545–546
Aldosteronism, hypertension in, 28, 28t
Allergy
to antibiotics in pneumonia, 172
asthmatic response in, 121, 121f, 126
fatigue in, chronic, 378
to influenza vaccine, 605

Allergy (*Continued*)
in mitral valve prolapse syndrome/ dysautonomia, 106
rhinitis in, 360–363
sinusitis in, 370
wheezing in, 123
Alopecia in lupus erythematosus, 456
Alprazolam
in anxiety disorders, 598t
in mitral valve prolapse syndrome/ dysautonomia, 109
in premenstrual syndrome, 512, 513–514
Alzheimer's disease, 4–5, 614–615
sleep disorders in, 566
Amantadine in influenza prophylaxis, 149, 605–607
Amaurosis fugax, 391
Amenorrhea
in anorexia nervosa, 548
in exercise, 550, 551
psychogenic, 547
Amiloride in hypertension, 31t, 32t, 35
Aminobutyric acid, and prolactin secretion, 293
Aminocaproic acid, 229
Aminophylline
in asthma, 128t, 137
in pregnancy, 135
in pulmonary edema, 97
5-Aminosalicylic drugs in inflammatory bowel disease, 197–198
Amiodarone, hypothyroidism from, 250
Amitriptyline
in depression, 529, 530, 530t, 534t
in elderly, 609t
in headaches, 389, 395
in migraine prevention, 395t, 395–396
side effects of, 530
Amlodipine
in angina pectoris, 88
in heart failure, 97, 99
in hypertension, 34t
Ammonium lactate in xerosis, 489
Amphetamines, 543
Amphotericin B in rhinitis, 360
Ampligen in chronic fatigue, 381
Amylase levels in pancreatitis, 184
Analgesic drugs
abuse of, 544–545
in elderly, 610
in headache, 392t, 392–393
in migraine prevention, 395t, 396
headache from, 389
in osteoarthritis, 431
Androgen-secreting tumors, 304–305
Androstenedione in hirsutism, 302, 305
Anemia, 205–212
in blood loss, 205, 208, 210, 213
drug-induced, 211t
iron deficiency in, 208, 209
of chronic disease, 209
clinical presentation of, 205
definition of, 205
differential diagnosis of, 206–212
drug-induced, 210, 211t
in hemoglobinopathies, 209
hemolytic, 205, 210, 211t
drug-induced, 211t
in lupus erythematosus, 459, 466
hypochromic, 206
microcytic, 206–210, 207f
iron deficiency, 206, 207–209
laboratory tests in, 206, 208, 208t
in lead poisoning, 209
in lupus erythematosus, 459, 466
macrocytic, 205, 210–212, 212f
megaloblastic, 211
microcytic, 205
hypochromic, 206–210, 207f
normocytic, 205
normochromic, 210, 210f
pathophysiology and classification of, 205–206
red blood cells in
decreased production of, 205, 210
increased loss or destruction of, 205, 210
morphology of, 205–206, 207t
in rheumatoid arthritis, 443
in thalassemia, 209
Aneurysms of abdominal aorta, 77
Angina, abdominal, 78
Angina pectoris, 83–90
clinical presentation of, 83–84
drug therapy in, 87–89
in elderly, 88
gender differences in, 83
history of patient in, 84, 85, 85t
laboratory tests in, 86–87, 87t
natural history of, 85
pathophysiology of, 84–85
physical examination in, 86
referral to specialist in, 89
stable, 83
unstable, 83–84, 85, 89
vasospastic or Prinzmetal's, 83, 86, 88
Angiography
in carotid artery disorders, 74, 391
in lower extremity vascular disease, 70, 71f, 72
magnetic resonance technique, 70, 71f, 74
Angioplasty
in carotid stenosis, 76f, 76–77
in subclavian artery occlusion, 72, 73f
Angiotensin-II, and prolactin secretion, 293–294
Angiotensin-converting enzyme inhibitors
in heart failure, 96–97
in hypertension, 33t, 38–39
and pulmonary edema, 96–97
side effects of, 39
Anisocytosis, 207t
Ankle
blood pressure at, compared to arm, 69f, 69–70
rheumatoid arthritis of, 436t, 441–442
treatment in, 447, 450
Ankylosis, 429
in rheumatoid arthritis, 445
in spondylitis, 423, 438
surgical, 433, 450
Anogenital papillomavirus infections, 313–323
Anorexia nervosa, 547–549
diagnostic criteria on, 548
treatment of, 549
Antibiotics
in acne, 477–478
in asthma, 135
in chronic obstructive pulmonary disease, 148
in diarrhea, 178
in inflammatory bowel disease, 195, 198–199
in myxedema coma, 261
in pneumonia, 164, 168, 168t, 170, 172
allergy to, 172
in elderly, 169t
in pregnancy, 173
in pregnancy, 135, 173
in rosacea, 483
in sinusitis, 368, 369
Antibodies
antithyroid, 243–244
to clotting factors, 225, 226
in lupus erythematosus, 460–461, 461t, 462
diagnostic criteria on, 463, 464t, 465
and pregnancy, 468
Anticholinergic drugs
in asthma, 129–130
in chronic obstructive pulmonary disease, 146
in elderly, 610
Anticoagulants, 233–234
lupus, 223, 225, 226, 232, 460
and pregnancy, 234–235
in pregnancy, 234, 235
in stroke prevention, 75
in venous thromboembolism, 79
Anticonvulsant therapy
hypothyroidism in, 250
lipid levels in, 52
Antidepressant drugs, 529–534
contraindications to, 533
dosage of, 533–534, 534t
in fibromyalgia, 556
nontricyclic, 529, 529t, 530, 531t
overdose of, 531
in pregnancy, 531, 533, 556
principles of therapy, 531–533, 532t
side effects of, 529–531, 531t
therapeutic effectiveness of, 529
tricyclic, 529, 529t, 531t
in anxiety disorders, 598t
in migraine prevention, 395t, 395–396
side effects of, 529–530, 531t
Antidiarrheal therapy, 178
Antiemetic drugs
in elderly, 609t
in headaches, 392t, 393
Antifibrinolytic agents, 229
Antihistamines
in allergic rhinitis, 361–362
in elderly, 610
side effects of, 362
in sinusitis, 368, 369
in vasomotor rhinitis, 363
Antihypertensive drug therapy, 30–41
dyslipidemia in, 51
in pulmonary edema, 96–97
Anti-inflammatory drugs
antiplatelet effect of, 227
in asthma, 127, 128t, 130
in chronic obstructive pulmonary disease, 147–148
in elderly, 610
in headaches, 392, 393, 396
and inflammatory bowel disease, 192, 193
interaction with other drugs, 35
in lupus erythematosus, 466
in osteoarthritis, 432
in polymyalgia rheumatica, 437
in rheumatoid arthritis, 446–447
toxicity of, 432, 446
Antimalarial drugs
in lupus erythematosus, 466
in rheumatoid arthritis, 447
Antioncogenes in lung cancer, 157
Antiplatelet agents
in angina pectoris, 88–89
in peripheral vascular disease, 71, 74
in stroke prevention, 74
Antiresorptive agents in osteoporosis, 415, 416f
Antirheumatic drugs, disease-modifying, 447–449
Antisocial personality disorder, 577–578
differential diagnosis of, 577–578, 580, 581
Antithrombin III, 219, 220t
deficiency of, 232
in disseminated intravascular coagulation, 231
Antithyroid antibodies, 243–244
Antithyroid drugs, 240, 246
in pregnancy, 257
in thyroid storm, 259
α_1-Antitrypsin deficiency, 141, 142, 143
Anxiety and anxiety disorders, 586–600

agoraphobia, 582, 593t, 594, 596
prevalence of, 586, 587t
classification of, 588
definition of, 586
diagnosis of, 588–592
comprehensive assessment in, 592
differential diagnosis of, 526, 589–591
and fatigue, chronic, 375, 378, 379
generalized, 593t, 595–596
prevalence of, 586, 587t
screening for, 587–588
medical causes of, 589, 590t, 593t
in mitral valve prolapse syndrome/dysautonomia, 105, 109, 566
obsessive compulsive disorder. *See* Obsessive compulsive disorder
panic disorders. *See* Panic disorders
in personality disorders. *See* Personality disorders, anxiety in
post-traumatic stress disorder, 593t, 595, 596
treatment of, 593t, 595, 596, 597
in pregnancy, 597
in premenstrual syndrome, 503, 510, 513, 513t
prevalence of, 586, 587t
in primary care setting, 586–588
referrals in, 595, 596, 597
simple phobia, 593t, 594
prevalence of, 586, 587t
sleep disorders in, 562, 565–566, 591
social phobia, 582, 593t, 594
prevalence of, 586, 587t
substance abuse and addiction in, 539, 540, 542, 591
symptoms in, 589
treatment of, 596–597, 598t
in post-traumatic stress disorder, 593t, 595, 596, 597
Anxiolytic medications, 591, 596, 598t
in pregnancy, 597
Aorta
abdominal
aneurysms of, 77
atherosclerosis of, 67, 77–78, 78f
discrete stenosis of, 78, 78f
coarctation of, in hypertension, 27, 28t
dissection of, 84, 86
Apnea, 558
sleep, 553, 558–559
insomnia in, 563
in menopause, 557
in obesity, 282, 285, 558
in pregnancy, 556–557
Apoproteins, 46, 47, 48
in hyperlipidemia, 48
measurement of, 47
Appendicitis, differential diagnosis of, 186
Appetite
in depression, 519, 521–522
in diabetes mellitus, 264
in obesity, 281
drugs suppressing, 288–289
and low calorie diet, 287
in premenstrual syndrome, 503, 510, 511, 512
Arcus senilis in familial hypercholesterolemia, 47
Arrhythmias
potassium serum levels in, 35
stroke in, 73, 74, 75
Arteries
atherosclerosis of, 66–78
of nasal cavity, 357
thrombosis of, 232–233
prevention of, 235
Arteriosclerosis, 66. *See also* Atherosclerosis
Arteritis, temporal, 437
headache in, 384, 390, 394
Arthritis
in cancer, 438
chronic atrophic, 435
deformans, 435
in gonococcal infection, disseminated, 348, 437
in inflammatory bowel disease, 438
in lupus erythematosus, 454–455, 463, 464t
management of, 466
in Lyme disease, 438
osteoarthritis, 421–434. *See also* Osteoarthritis
psoriatic, 429, 438
reactive, 438
rheumatoid, 435–453. *See also* Rheumatoid arthritis
septic, 435, 437
Arthrocentesis
in osteoarthritis, 428
in rheumatoid arthritis, 444, 447
Arthrodesis
in osteoarthritis, 433
in rheumatoid arthritis, 450
Arthroplasty
in osteoarthritis, 433
in rheumatoid arthritis, 450
Arthroscopy in osteoarthritis, 432
Asacol in inflammatory bowel disease, 198
Ascites, 95, 335
Aspergillus infection, nasal, 360
Aspiration
differential diagnosis of, 166
pneumonia in, 167
in pregnancy, 172
Aspiration biopsy of thyroid, 244, 247, 252–253, 254
Aspirin
in angina pectoris, 88–89
antiplatelet effect of, 216, 227
bleeding disorders from, 216
in headaches, 392t, 392–393
in migraine prevention, 395t, 396
in lupus anticoagulant and pregnancy, 234–235
in osteoarthritis, 432
in peripheral vascular disease, 71, 74
products containing, 216, 216t
in rheumatoid arthritis, 446
in stroke prevention, 74, 75
in thrombosis prevention, 235
Asthenia
and chronic fatigue, 373
and dysautonomia, 107
Asthma, 119–138
clinical presentation in, 121–126
compliance with therapy in, 127
definition of, 119
differential diagnosis of, 122–123, 139, 140
drug therapy in, 127–131, 128t, 129t
in breast-feeding, 135
cost of, 127
in emergency room, 136, 137
in nocturnal symptoms, 136
in pregnancy, 133–135
stepwise approach to, 130–131, 131f
economic impact of, 119, 127
emergency room care in, 126, 136–137
epidemiology of, 119–120, 120f
exercise-induced, 135–136
flow-volume loop in, 123f
history of patient in, 121–122
laboratory tests in, 124f, 124–125, 125f
mortality rate in, 120, 120f
nocturnal, 126, 136
pathophysiology of, 120–121, 121f
patient education in, 126–127, 131
physical examination in, 123–124
in pregnancy, 131–135
response to allergen exposure in, 121, 121f
risk factors in, 120
severity of, 125–126
and stepwise approach to drug therapy, 130–131, 131f
treatment in, 126–137
triggers in, 121, 122
avoidance of, 126
wheezing in, 122–123, 124
severity of, 125, 126
Atelectasis, differential diagnosis of, 166
Atenolol
in angina pectoris, 88
in hypertension, 32t, 36
Atherosclerosis, 66–78
of abdominal aorta, 67, 77–78, 78f
and alcohol use, 16, 50
coronary heart disease in. *See* Coronary heart disease
in diabetes mellitus, 61, 66–67, 265, 274
and estrogen therapy, 51, 60, 71, 73–74
lipid levels in. *See* Lipid levels, in atherosclerosis
of lower extremity, 66, 67–72
ankle brachial index in, 69f, 69–70
color return and venous filling time in, 69, 69t
embolism in, 68, 68f
gangrene in, 68, 68f
grading of elevation pallor in, 69, 69t
magnetic resonance angiography in, 70, 71f
management of, 70–72
stent placement in, 72, 72f
transcutaneous oximetry in, 70
in lupus erythematosus, 458, 468–469
premenopausal, 66–67
risk factors in, 4, 54, 54t, 66–67, 73–74
modification of, 70–71
and treatment goals, 55t
in smoking, 67, 71
of upper extremity, 66, 72–77
Atlantoaxial subluxation in rheumatoid arthritis, 445–446
Atopic disease, chronic fatigue in, 378
Atrial natriuretic factor, in mitral valve prolapse syndrome/dysautonomia, 114
Atropine
in chronic obstructive pulmonary disease, 146
in diarrhea, 178
Aura in migraine, 387, 388
Auranofin in rheumatoid arthritis, 448
Aurothioglucose in rheumatoid arthritis, 447
Autoantibodies in lupus erythematosus, 460–461, 461t, 462
Autoimmune disorders
cholangitis in, primary sclerosing, 188
Graves' disease in, 244
hepatitis in, 330
inflammatory bowel disease in, 191–192
lipid abnormalities in, 51
nose in, 365
thyroiditis in, 248–249, 254, 255–256
postpartum, 255–256
Autonomic nervous system, in mitral valve prolapse syndrome/dysautonomia, 104, 105
Autonomously functioning thyroid nodules, 247
Avascular necrosis in lupus erythematosus, 455
Avoidant personality disorder, 581–582
anxiety in, 581, 582, 592
differential diagnosis of, 576, 577, 581–582
Azathioprine
in inflammatory bowel disease, 199
in lupus erythematosus, 466, 467
and pregnancy, 468
in rheumatoid arthritis, 449

Azathioprine (*Continued*)
  side effects of, 467
Azithromycin in pneumonia, 168t, 170–171

B
Back pain
  in mitral valve prolapse syndrome/dysautonomia, 107
  in premenstrual syndrome, 503, 509, 513
Bacterial infections
  diarrhea in, 177
  inflammatory bowel disease in, 191, 198
  of nose, 358–360
  pneumococcal disease in, 149, 607
  pneumonia in. *See* Pneumonia
  septic arthritis in, 437
  sexually transmitted, 339, 340t
  sinusitis in, 366, 367, 368
    chronic, 369
  vaginosis in, 343, 344t, 344–345
Bacterial overgrowth in Crohn's disease, 195
Baker's cyst, 441
Balloon angioplasty in carotid stenosis, 76f, 76–77
Barium studies in ulcerative colitis, 194
Barrier contraceptive methods, 18, 341
Basal cell carcinoma of skin, 493–495
  clinical presentation of, Plate 7, 494
  sclerosing or morpheaform, 494
  superficial multicentric, 494
Basilar artery migraine, 388t
Basophilic stippling, 207t
Beclomethasone
  in allergic rhinitis, 362
  in asthma, 128t, 130
    in pregnancy, 134–135
Bed wetting, 562
Behavioral learning theory on psychoactive substance use, 540
Behavioral symptoms in depression, 522
Behavioral therapy
  in fatigue, chronic, 380
  in insomnia, 564
  in obesity, 286, 287
  in obsessive compulsive disorder, 595
Benazipril in hypertension, 33t, 39
Bendroflumethiazide in hypertension, 31t
Benzodiazepines
  in anxiety disorders, 598t
  in elderly, 609t, 610
Benzoyl peroxide in acne, 477
Benzthiazide in hypertension, 31t
Betaxolol
  in hypertension, 32t
  in mitral valve prolapse syndrome/dysautonomia, 109
Bile acid sequestrants in lipid-lowering therapy, 57t, 58–59
  in diabetes mellitus, 61
Bile acid therapy
  in cholangitis, primary sclerosing, 189
  in gallstones, 186
Bile ducts
  cancer of, 189–190
  common, calculi in, 183, 183f, 184, 185
    management of, 186
    in pregnancy, 187
  inflammation of, 183, 184, 185
    sclerosing, 187–189
Biliary tract disorders, 182–190
  cancer, 189–190
  diagnostic evaluation in, 184–185
  differential diagnosis of, 183
  in lupus erythematosus, 458
  in postcholecystectomy syndrome, 187
  sclerosing cholangitis, primary, 187–189
  treatment of, 185–186
Bilirubin levels in hepatitis, 329
Biogenetic disease theory on psychoactive substance use, 540
Biologic agents in rheumatoid arthritis, 449
Biopsy
  of bone, 413
  endometrial, in pelvic inflammatory disease, 347–348
  of liver, in hepatitis, 330
  pleural, in lung cancer, 157–158
  renal, in lupus erythematosus, 457
  in skin cancer, 494, 498
  of temporal artery, 390
  of thyroid gland, 244, 247, 252–253, 254
Bipolar depression, 524, 529
Birth control methods. *See* Contraceptive methods
Bisoprolol in hypertension, 32t
Bisphosphonates in osteoporosis, 417
Bitolterol in asthma, 127, 128t
Blastomycosis, 360
Bleeding
  anemia in, 205, 208, 210, 213
    drug-induced, 211t
    iron deficiency, 208, 209
  hemostasis in, 213
  subarachnoid, headache in, 385, 385t, 386, 390, 394
Bleeding disorders, 213–235
  acquired, 215–216
  causes of, 214–216
  congenital, 215
  in disseminated intravascular coagulation, 231
  drug-induced, 215, 216, 216t, 227
    in heparin therapy, 233
    in warfarin therapy, 234
  in hemophilia, 215, 224, 225, 228
  history of patient in, 213, 214
  laboratory tests in, 221–224
    and clinical approach, 224–229
  in lupus erythematosus, 460
  physical examination in, 216–217
  and pregnancy, 216, 218, 229, 230
  and prethrombotic conditions, 231–235
  symptoms of, 213–214
  treatment of, 229–231
    cost of, 229, 230
  in von Willebrand's disease, 215, 217, 223–224, 228–229
Bleeding time test, 223
Blindness
  in glaucoma, 5
  in temporal arteritis, 390
  transient, in amaurosis fugax, 391
Bloating symptoms in premenstrual syndrome, 503, 510, 513
Blood flow assessment, in peripheral vascular disease, 70
Blood gases, arterial. *See* Gases, arterial blood
Blood pressure
  ankle brachial index of, in peripheral vascular disease, 69f, 69–70
  diastolic, 3, 24t
    in hypertension, 3, 23, 24, 24t
  in headache, 385
  hypertension, 3, 23–43. *See also* Hypertension
  measurement of, 3, 23–24
  in mitral valve prolapse syndrome/dysautonomia, 107, 109
  in obesity, 28, 50, 282
    in weight loss, 286
  orthostatic hypotension
    in diabetes mellitus, 266
    in mitral valve prolapse syndrome/dysautonomia, 109
  systolic, 3, 24t
    in hypertension, 3, 23, 24, 24t
Blood supply of nasal cavity, 357
Blood tests in pneumonia, 165–166
Blue bloaters, 140, 142, 147
Body dysmorphic disorder, 591
Body mass index, 6, 278, 282
Bone. *See also* Musculoskeletal disorders
  age-related changes of, 406–407, 408
    in mass, 402–404, 403f
    in remodeling, 405
  biopsy of, 413
  density of, 410, 411–412
    in osteoarthritis, 422–423
  fatigue of, 407
  fragility of, 406–407
  marrow disease of, anemia in, 210
  osteoporosis of, 401–420
  radionuclide scan of, 413
  remodeling of, 404f, 404–406, 406f
    antiresorptive agents affecting, 415, 416f
  trabecular disconnectivity of, 405f, 407
  turnover of, 406, 406f
    assessment of, 412–413
    biochemical markers of, 412–413
Borderline personality disorder, 578–579
  anxiety in, 578, 592
  differential diagnosis of, 577, 579, 580
    and dependent personality disorder, 582
    and narcissistic personality disorder, 581
    and passive aggressive personality disorder, 584
Bouchard's nodes, 426, 435
Boutonnière deformity in rheumatoid arthritis, 441
Bowenoid papulosis, 318, 496
Bowen's disease, Plate 12, 496
Bowleg deformity in osteoarthritis, 427
Brachial artery
  blood pressure in, compared to ankle, 69f, 69–70
  pulse of, in hypertension, 27
Brachiocephalic disease, 72–77
  management of, 74–77
  noninvasive diagnostic techniques in, 74
Brain tumors
  depression in, 522
  headache in, 391
Branhamella infections, sinusitis in, 368
Breast
  cancer of, 8
  cysts of, 18
    in mitral valve prolapse syndrome/dysautonomia, 106, 108
  examination of, prolactin serum levels in, 295, 295f
  fibroadenoma of, 18
  fibrocystic disease of, 106
  in premenstrual syndrome, 503, 509, 510, 513, 513t
  self-examination of, 8
  silicone implants in, 440
Breast-feeding
  in anxiety disorders, 597
  in asthma, 135
  in depression, 531
  in hepatitis, 331
  in hyperthyroidism, 257
  in inflammatory bowel disease, 197, 199
  in lupus erythematosus, 468
  in pneumonia, 173
Bromocriptine
  in hyperprolactinemia, 294, 297, 298, 299, 300
  in premenstrual syndrome, 510
  side effects of, 298
Bronchiectasis, 123

differential diagnosis of, 141
Bronchiolitis obliterans, 166–167
Bronchitis
asthmatic, 141
chronic, 139–153
differential diagnosis of, 123, 140–141
natural history and prognosis in, 149–150
pathogenesis of, 141–142
presentation of, 139–140, 140t
treatment of, 144–149
workup in, 142–144
severe purulent, 141
Bronchodilator drugs
in asthma, 124, 126, 127–130, 128t
in chronic obstructive pulmonary disease, 145–146
Bronchoscopy
in lung cancer, 159
in pneumonia, 165, 172
Bronchospasm in asthma, 119, 120, 123
Brucellosis, chronic, 373, 377
Bruisability, 217
Bruits, 69
Bulge sign, in rheumatoid arthritis of knee, 441
Bulimia, 547, 549–550
Bumetanide in hypertension, 31t
Bupropion in depression, 530t
dosage of, 533–534, 534t
side effects of, 530, 531t
Burns, in sun exposure, 8, 492, 497
Burr cell, 207t
Burrows, in scabies, 484, 485
Buschke-Loewenstein tumor, 318
Buserelin in premenstrual syndrome, 511
Buspirone
in anxiety disorders, 598t
in premenstrual syndrome, 512
Butorphanol in migraine, 394
Bypass surgery in obesity, 288

C
Caffeine
and anxiety, 591
as bronchodilator, 146
and insomnia, 564
in mitral valve prolapse syndrome/dysautonomia, 108, 111, 111f
CAGE questionnaire, 15, 591
Calcification of gallbladder, 186
Calcitonin in osteoporosis, 417
Calcitriol in osteoporosis, 414, 415, 418
Calcium
intake of
in exercise-induced menstrual dysfunction, 551
in hypertension, 30
and malabsorption, 408, 413, 418
in osteoporosis, 414–415, 418, 419
serum levels of
in depression, 522
in hypertension, 27t, 28
in osteoporosis, 407, 408, 413, 414–415
Calcium carbonate in osteoporosis, 414, 415
Calcium channel blockers
in angina pectoris, 88
in heart failure, 97, 99
in hypertension, 33t–34t, 35, 38
in migraine prevention, 395, 395t
side effects of, 38, 88
Calcium pyrophosphate dihydrate crystal deposition disease, 423, 424, 428
differential diagnosis of, 437–438
radiography in, 430f
Calculi
in common bile duct, 183, 183f, 184, 185
management of, 186
in pregnancy, 187
gallstones, 182–187. *See also* Gallstones
Caloric intake and expenditure, 17
in exercise, 16–17
in low calorie diet, 287
in obesity, 280–281, 286–287
and weight loss program, 286–287, 288
in very low calorie diet, 286–287
Calymmatobacterium infections, 340t, 351
Cancer, 7–9
arthritis in, 438
of biliary system, 189–190
of brain
depression in, 522
headache in, 391
of breast, 8
of cervix uteri. *See* Cervix uteri, cancer of
of colon, 78
colonoscopy in, Plate 2
constipation in, 179
in inflammatory bowel disease, 7, 196–197
endometrial, 18
of gallbladder, 186, 189
hirsutism in, 304–305
hypoglycemia in, 275, 276, 277
incidence of, 7, 7t
in inflammatory bowel disease, 7, 189, 196–197
of liver, 189, 190
in hepatitis, 324–325
of lung. *See* Lung, cancer of
mortality rate by site, 7, 7t
in obesity, 282
of ovary, 9, 18
androgen-producing, 304
and papillomavirus infections, 313, 315–317, 316f
of pituitary gland
hyperprolactinemia in, 292–300
hyperthyroidism in, 247
hypothyroidism in, 250
prevention of, 7
risk factors for, 7–8, 9
of skin, 8, 492–499
of thyroid gland, 239, 244, 249, 252
risk factors for, 252
treatment of, 253
Candidiasis
chronic, 373
nasal, 360
vulvovaginal, 343, 344t
Captopril in hypertension, 33t, 38–39
Carbidopa in periodic limb movement disorder, 561
Carbohydrates
intolerance of, 6
in obesity, 281
and weight loss program, 287
in premenstrual syndrome, 510
Carcinoid syndrome, 123
Carcinoma. *See also* Cancer
of bile ducts, 189–190
of lung, 156
of skin, 493–495
basal cell, 493–495
squamous cell, 495
Cardiac output, 91
Frank-Starling curve on, 91–92, 92f, 93
in heart failure, 91–92, 93–94
Cardiomyopathy
hypertension therapy in, 39, 40
peripartum, 99–100
Cardiovascular disorders, 3–4, 23–115
angina pectoris, 83–90
anxiety in, 590t
in diabetes mellitus, 266
heart failure, 91–103
hypertension, 3, 23–43
in hyperthyroidism, 93–94, 244
lipid levels in, 3–4, 44–65
lower extremity edema in, 610, 611
in lupus erythematosus, 456, 457, 458
prognosis in, 468–469
mitral valve prolapse, 104–115
mortality rates in, 29f, 44
in myxedema coma, 260
peripheral vascular disease, 66–82
in rheumatoid arthritis, 443
risk factors for, 3–4, 25, 25t
Carotid artery
atherosclerosis of, 73–77
angioplasty in, 76f, 76–77
endarterectomy in, 75–76
ultrasonography in, 73f, 74
bruits in hypertension, 27
dissection of, headache in, 386, 391
fibromuscular dysplasia of, 77, 77f
Carpal tunnel syndrome in diabetes mellitus, 266, 271
Carteolol in hypertension, 32t
Cartilage degeneration in osteoarthritis, 421–434
factors regulating, 425f
mechanisms of, 424–426
Cataplexy, 559–560
Cathepsin B in osteoarthritis, 426
Catheterization, cardiac, in heart failure, 95
Cefotaxime in pneumonia, 170t, 171t
Ceftriaxone in pneumonia, 170t, 171t
Cefuroxime in pneumonia, 169t, 170t
Celiac artery stenosis, 78, 79f
Central nervous system disorders
Alzheimer's disease in, 4–5, 614–615
brain tumors, 391, 522
constipation in, 179
in lupus erythematosus, 459
in mitral valve prolapse syndrome/dysautonomia, 106
Cephalosporins in pneumonia, 169t, 170t, 171t
in pregnancy, 173
Cerebrovascular disorders, 73–77
in hypertension, 3, 27
stroke in. *See* Stroke
Cervicitis, 345–348
complications of, 347–348
diagnosis of, 345–346, 346t
Cervix uteri
cancer of, 8–9
intraepithelial neoplasia, 8–9, 315, 316, 316f, 318
and papillomavirus infection, 9, 315–317, 316f
risk factors in, 9, 317
screening for, 8, 9, 320
and sexual behavior, 316
cervicitis of, 345–348
collection of specimens from, 343, 346
condylomata of, 318, 319f, 320
treatment of, 322
dysplasia of, 9
and papillomavirus infection, 313, 315, 316f, 320, 322
strawberry, 344, 344t
Chancre in syphilis, 350
Chancroid, genital ulcer disease in, 348, 349t, 350
Charcot joint changes in diabetes mellitus, 266, 271
Charcot-Leyden crystals, 125
Charcot's triad, 184
Chemotherapy
in keratoacanthoma, 496

Chemotherapy (*Continued*)
in lung cancer, 160–161
Chenodeoxycholic acid in gallstones, 186
Chest examination
in chest pain, 86
in chronic obstructive pulmonary disease, 142
in heart failure, 95
in hypertension, 27
in lung cancer, 155
in mitral valve prolapse syndrome/dysautonomia, 107
in pneumonia, 164
Chest pain
in angina pectoris, 83
differential diagnosis of, 84
electrocardiography in, 86, 87t
in esophageal spasm, 84
in lung cancer, 154, 161
physical examination in, 86
in pneumonia, 164
Cheyne-Stokes respirations in heart failure, 95
Children and infants
acne in, 476
bed wetting by, 562
depression in, 525
dermatitis in, seborrheic, 486, 487
hepatitis in, 324, 325–326, 331–332, 333–334
prevention of, 331, 333–334
hyperchylomicronemia syndrome in, 49
hypertension in, 41, 41t
lead poisoning in, 209
lupus erythematosus in, 468
molluscum contagiosum in, 478, 479, 480
nevi in, 497
papillomavirus infection in, 314, 323
pityriasis rosea in, 481
pneumonia in, 163
rhinitis in, allergic, 362
scabies in, 484, 485
sinusitis in, 367, 368
sleep of, 554
and parasomnias, 561, 562
thyroid disorders in, 244, 246, 248, 258
tinea versicolor in, 487
Chlamydia infections, 339, 340t
cervicitis in, 345–346, 346t, 347
and contraceptive methods, 341
diagnosis of, 345–346, 346t, 347
lymphogranuloma venereum in, 350–351
pharyngitis in, 343
pneumonia in, 164, 166, 167, 168
treatment of, 168t, 170, 170t, 171t
screening for, 351
specimen collection in, 343
Chlordiazepoxide in elderly, 609t
Chlorothiazide in hypertension, 31t
Chlorpropamide in diabetes mellitus, 269, 270t
Chlorthalidone in hypertension, 31t
Cholangiocarcinoma, 189–190
Cholangiography, percutaneous transhepatic, 185
Cholangiopancreatography, endoscopic retrograde, 185, 185f
in tumors, 189, 190
Cholangitis, 183
in gallstones, 184, 185
primary sclerosing, 187–189
secondary sclerosing, 188
Cholecystectomy
in gallstones, 185–186
in pregnancy, 187
laparoscopic, 186, 187
and postcholecystectomy syndrome, 187
Cholecystitis
diagnostic evaluation in, 184
in gallstones, 182
in lupus erythematosus, 458
management of, 186
in pregnancy, 186–187
Cholecystography, oral, 184
Choledocholithiasis, 183, 183f, 184, 185
management of, 186
in pregnancy, 187
Cholelithiasis, 182–187. *See also* Gallstones
Cholescintigraphy, nuclear, 184
Cholesterol, 4
in gallstones, 183, 184, 186
serum levels of, 4, 44
in angina pectoris, 86
in autoimmune disorders, 51
in combined hyperlipidemia, familial, 48
and coronary heart disease, 4, 47, 48, 52–53, 61, 89
diet affecting, 4, 5, 54, 55–56, 61, 89
drug-induced disorders of, 52
in elderly, 60–61
in hypercholesterolemia. *See* Hypercholesterolemia
in hypertension, 3, 27t, 28
measurement of, 4, 46, 54
in obesity, 282
therapy lowering, 53, 54, 55–60
in thyroid disease, 50, 51
Cholestyramine in lipid-lowering therapy, 57t, 58–59
in elderly, 61
Chondritis, nasal, 365
Chondrocalcinosis, 428
differential diagnosis of, 437–438
familial, 423
radiography in, 430f
Chronic conditions
fatigue. *See* Fatigue, chronic
obstructive pulmonary disease. *See* Pulmonary disorders, chronic obstructive disease
pain in, 177
in gastrointestinal disorders, 177, 180
in headaches, 389, 395–396
Chylomicrons, 44, 45f
hyperchylomicronemia syndrome, 49
Cigarette smoking. *See* Smoking
Cimetidine
in hirsutism, 306, 307
in mitral valve prolapse syndrome/dysautonomia, 109
Circadian rhythms, 553, 555, 564–565
body temperature in, 555
daylight affecting, 555
in shift work, 565
in time zone change, 564–565
Cirrhosis, 95
in cholangitis, primary sclerosing, 187, 188–189
in hepatitis, 324, 325, 329
and pregnancy, 332
lower extremity edema in, 610, 611
Clarithromycin in pneumonia, 168t
Claudication
intermittent, 67
walking program in, 71–72
and pseudoclaudication, 67
Clindamycin in acne, 477
Clomipramine
in anxiety disorders, 598t
in premenstrual syndrome, 512
Clonazepam
in anxiety disorders, 598t
in mitral valve prolapse syndrome/dysautonomia, 109, 110
in periodic limb movement disorder, 561
Clonidine
in hypertension, 34t, 37
in smoking cessation, 145
Clot formation. *See* Coagulation
Clotting factors. *See* Factors, clotting
Clotting time, 223
prolonged, 224
Cluster headaches, compared to migraine, 386, 386t
Coagulation, 213, 218
disorders of, 213–235. *See also* Bleeding disorders
disseminated intravascular, 219, 231
extrinsic pathway of, 221
laboratory tests of, 221–224
and clinical approach to bleeding disorders, 224–229
mechanisms in, 218, 222f
physiology of, 219–221
regulation of, 218–219
Coarctation of aorta, in hypertension, 27, 28t
Cocaine, 15, 16, 543
Codeine
in headaches, 392t, 394
in lung cancer, 161
Cognitive behavioral therapy, in chronic fatigue, 380
Cognitive symptoms
in dementia, 614
in depression, 520–521
Mini-Mental State Examination of, 615t, 615–616
Cold, common, 357–358
in elderly, 609t
sinusitis in, 365
Colectomy
in inflammatory bowel disease, 193, 200
sexual function in, 200
Colestipol, in lipid-lowering therapy, 57t, 58–59
Colic, biliary, 182, 183, 186
in pregnancy, 186
Colitis
pseudomembranous, 194
ulcerative, 191–201
bile duct cancer in, 189
cholangitis in, primary sclerosing, 188
colon cancer in, 7, 196
compared to Crohn's disease, 193, 194
complications of, 197
diagnosis of, 194
diarrhea in, 178, 194
differential diagnosis of, 193, 194
etiology of, 191–193
evaluation of clinical status in, 194–195
grading severity of, 194
malignancy in, 196–197
and pregnancy, 199–200
and sexual function, 200
symptomatic flares in, 195–196
treatment of, 197–199
Collagen, in osteoarthritis, 424, 426
Collagenase
in osteoarthritis, 425, 426
in rheumatoid arthritis, 439, 439f
Colloid cyst of third ventricle, 391
Colon cancer, 7–8
colonoscopy in, Plate 2
constipation in, 179
in inflammatory bowel disease, 7, 196–197
Colonoscopy
in cancer, Plate 2
normal, Plate 1
Colorectal cancer, 7–8, 179
Coma
in diabetes mellitus, 264
hyperglycemic hyperosmolar, 271, 272–273
myxedema, 259–261

Comedo, 475
Common bile duct stones, 183, 183f, 184, 185
  management of, 186
  in pregnancy, 187
Community-acquired pneumonia, 163–174
Compensatory mechanisms in heart failure, 91–92
Complement levels in lupus erythematosus, 461, 462
Compliance with therapy
  in asthma, 127
  in depression, 519
  in personality disorders, 585
Compression devices in venous insufficiency, 611, 612f
Compulsions, 595
  and obsessive compulsive disorder. *See* Obsessive compulsive disorder
  and obsessive compulsive personality disorder, 581, 582–583
Computed tomography
  in headache, 385–386
  in hepatitis, 330
  in hyperprolactinemia and pituitary tumors, 296–297, 300
  in lung cancer, 159
  in osteoarthritis, 429
  in osteoporosis, bone mass measurements in, 411
  in pneumonia, 172
  in sinusitis, 367f, 367–368, 369
Condoms, 18, 322, 341
Condylomata, 313–323
  anal, 314, 319, 322
  of cervix, 318, 319f, 320, 322
  clinical manifestations of, 317, 317f
  differential diagnosis of, 319
  evaluation of, 319–320
  flat, 318, 320
  histologic features of, 315, 315f
  incidence of, 313, 314
  natural history of, 314
  prevention of, 322–323
  transmission of, 314
  treatment of, 320–322, 321t
  of vulva and vagina, 318, 318f, 320, 322
Confusional state, acute, 590, 614
Congenital disorders
  adrenal hyperplasia in, 305, 305f
  of coagulation, 215
  nevi in, 497
  syphilis in, 359
Connective tissue disorders, autoimmune, nose in, 365
Constipation, 179–180
  in endometriosis, 180
Consumptive coagulopathy, 231
Continuous positive airway pressure, in sleep apnea, 559
  in pregnancy, 556–557
Contraceptive methods, 18, 341
  barrier, 18, 341
  douching in, 341–342
  estrogen in. *See* Estrogen, therapy with
  intrauterine devices in, 341
  in lupus erythematosus, 467
  and sexually transmitted diseases, 17, 18, 340–342
  spermicidal products in, 341
Coomb's test, 210
COPD (chronic obstructive pulmonary disease), 139–153
Copper overload, primary sclerosing cholangitis in, 188
Coronary heart disease, 44
  and alcohol use, 16, 50
  angina pectoris in, 85, 86, 89
    laboratory evaluation of, 87t
  in diabetes mellitus, 61
  in elderly, 61
  and estrogen therapy, 51, 60, 71
  gender differences in, 52–53, 83
  life-style factors in, 16, 56
  lipid levels in, 3–4, 54, 61–62, 89
    in combined hyperlipidemia, familial, 48
    in dyslipidemia, familial, 48
    in elderly, 61
    in familial hypercholesterolemia, 47, 48
    gender differences in, 52–53
    of high density lipoproteins, 4, 46, 52–53, 61
    in hypertriglyceridemia, familial, 48
    in hypoalphalipoproteinemia, familial, 48
    therapy lowering, 53
    in type III hyperlipidemia, 48
  in lupus erythematosus, 458, 468–469
  metabolism of lipoproteins in, 46, 47
  nutrition in, 17, 54, 55–56, 56t, 89
    in elderly, 61
  in obesity, 50, 282
  in peripheral vascular disease, 71
  in renal disorders, 51
  risk factors in, 4, 54, 54t
    and treatment goals, 55t
Corticosteroid therapy
  in asthma, 128t, 129t, 130, 131
    in emergency room care, 136, 137
    nocturnal, 136
    in pregnancy, 133, 134–135
  in chronic obstructive pulmonary disease, 147–148
  and coronary artery disease, 458
  in hirsutism, 306, 307
  in inflammatory bowel disease, 197
    in pregnancy, 199
  lipid levels in, 51, 52
  in lung cancer, 161
  in lupus erythematosus, 454, 459, 465, 466
    and breast-feeding, 468
    and pregnancy, 467, 468
    side effects of, 455, 458
  in osteoarthritis, 432
  osteonecrosis in, 441, 455
  in polymyalgia rheumatica, 437
  in rheumatoid arthritis, 447
  in rhinitis
    allergic, 362–363
    medicamentosa, 364
  side effects of, 130, 148, 362–363
    in lupus erythematosus, 455, 458
  in sinusitis, chronic, 369
Corticotropin-releasing factor in stress, 550
Cost considerations
  in asthma, 119, 127
  in bleeding disorders, 229, 230
  in depression, 518
  in gallstones, 186
  in headaches, 384
  in osteoarthritis, 432
  in osteoporosis, 417, 418
  in personality disorders, 585
  in premenstrual syndrome, 513t
  in smoking, 13–14
Cough
  in asthma, 119, 122
  in chronic obstructive pulmonary disease, 139, 140
  in lung cancer, 154, 161
  in pneumonia, 163, 166
Cradle cap, 486
Cranial nerve disorders
  in lupus erythematosus, 459
  palsy
    in diabetes mellitus, 265
    and headaches, 388t, 389, 391
  trigeminal neuralgia, 390
Creatinine levels in hypertension, 3, 27t, 28
Credé maneuver, 271
Cretinism, 248
Criminal behavior, in antisocial personality disorder, 577, 578
Crohn's disease, 191–201
  bacterial overgrowth in, 195
  colon cancer in, 196–197
  compared to ulcerative colitis, 193, 194
  complications of, 197
  diagnosis of, 193–194
  diarrhea in, 178, 193, 195
  differential diagnosis of, 193–194
  etiology of, 191–193
  fixed obstructions in, 195
  gallstones in, 183
  grading severity of, 194–195
  and irritable bowel syndrome, 195
  and pregnancy, 199–200
  and sexual function, 200
  symptomatic flares in, 195–196
  treatment of, 197–199
Cromolyn
  in allergic rhinitis, 362
  in asthma, 128t, 129t, 130
    exercise-induced, 136
    in pregnancy, 135
Crusted scabies, 484, 485, 485f
Crying, in depression, 522
Cryoprecipitate, 230
Cryotherapy
  in actinic keratoses, 493
  in condylomata, 321t, 321–322
  in osteoarthritis, 431
Culture techniques
  in cervicitis, 346
  in herpes simplex virus infection, 350
  in pneumonia, 167
    of blood, 166, 167
    of sputum, 165, 167
Curschmann's spirals, 125
Cushing's syndrome, hypertension in, 28t
CV205-502 in hyperprolactinemia, 297, 298
Cyclophosphamide in lupus erythematosus, 466–467
Cyclosporin A
  in inflammatory bowel disease, 199
  in rheumatoid arthritis, 449
Cyclothiazide in hypertension, 31t
Cyclothymic depression, 524
Cyproheptadine in migraine prevention, 396
Cyproterone acetate in hirsutism, 306, 307
Cyst
  Baker's, 441
  of breast, 18
    in mitral valve prolapse syndrome/dysautonomia, 106, 108
  of ovary, 304f
    hirsutism in, 304
  popliteal, 441
  of third ventricle, 391
Cystic fibrosis, differential diagnosis of, 141
Cytotoxic mechanisms in hepatitis, 326

D
DaCosta syndrome, 373
Daily living activities, assessment of, 604t, 604–605, 615
Danazol, hirsutism from, 303

Danocrine in premenstrual syndrome, 511, 513, 514
Daytime sleepiness
  in narcolepsy, 559–560
  in restless legs syndrome, 561
  in sleep apnea, 558
De Quervain's thyroiditis, 254–255
Decongestants
  in allergic rhinitis, 362
  rhinitis medicamentosa from, 363
  in sinusitis, 368
    chronic, 369
  in vasomotor rhinitis, 363
Degenerative arthritis. *See* Osteoarthritis
Dehydration, in hyperosmolar hyperglycemic coma, 272, 273
Dehydroepiandrosterone (DHEA) in hirsutism, 302, 305
Dehydroepiandrosterone sulfate (DHEAS) in hirsutism, 302, 303, 304, 305
Dehydrotestosterone in hirsutism, 302
Delirium, 526, 590, 614
Delusional disorder, 575
  anxiety in, 591
Dementia, 590–591, 614–616
  in Alzheimer's disease, 4–5, 614–615
  and depressive pseudodementia, 521
  diagnosis of, 614
  differential diagnosis of, 521, 526
  in elderly, 45, 614–616
  Folstein Mini-Mental State Examination in, 615t, 615–616
  multi-infarct, 614
  sleep disorders in, 566
Densitometry, bone, 410
  indications for, 411–412
  interpretation of, 411–412
Dental disease, headache in, 384
Deoxyribonuclease in chronic obstructive pulmonary disease, 148
Dependency, chemical, 538. *See also* Substance abuse and addiction
Dependent personality disorder, 582
  anxiety in, 582, 592
  differential diagnosis of, 580, 582
Depressant drugs, 544
Depression, 518–537
  adjustment disorder with, 524, 529
  and anxiety disorders, 589–590
  atypical or nonspecific, 524
  bipolar, 524, 529
  with coexisting psychiatric disorders, 526
  cyclothymic, 524
  definition of, 518
  diagnosis of, 526–528
    criteria in, 528, 528t
    medical conditions affecting, 527
  differential diagnosis of, 525–526
  drug-induced, 522, 523, 528
  drug therapy in, 529–534. *See also* Antidepressant drugs
  dysthymic, 524, 529
  etiologies of, 525
  and fatigue, 374–375, 377, 378, 522
    evaluation of, 379
    management of, 380
  gender differences in, 525
  and headaches, 384
    migraine, 386
  major, 523–524
    diagnosis of, 528
  masked, 520
  melancholic, 523
  organic, 522–523, 525
    diagnosis of, 527–528
  in personality disorders, 585
    borderline, 578, 579
    dependent, 582
    narcissistic, 581
    obsessive compulsive, 583
    passive aggressive, 584
    schizotypal, 576, 577
  postpartum, 519, 524, 556
    drug therapy in, 531
  in pregnancy, 519
    drug therapy in, 531, 533
  in premenstrual syndrome, 503, 509f
    proposed etiologies of, 506, 510, 511, 512
    treatment of, 513t, 514
  prevalence of, 518
  psychotic, 523
  recognition of, 520
  referrals in, 526, 534, 535–536
  in rheumatoid arthritis, 449
  seasonal, 523–524
  sleep disorders in, 521, 562, 565
  substance abuse and addiction in, 519, 539, 540, 542
  symptoms of, 520–522
    behavioral, 522
    cognitive, 520–521
    emotional, 520
    vegetative, 521–522
  treatment of, 528–536
    in chronic fatigue, 380
    common mistakes in, 535
    in premenstrual syndrome, 513t, 514
  types of, 522–525
Dermatitis, seborrheic, 485–487
  in infants, 486, 487
Dermatology, 473–499. *See also* Skin disorders
Desipramine
  in anxiety disorders, 598t
  in depression, 530t, 534t
  in migraine prevention, 395, 395t
Desmopressin, 229
  in von Willebrand's disease, 228, 229
Dexamethasone
  in allergic rhinitis, 362
  in hirsutism, 306, 307
  in myxedema coma, 261
  suppression test in depression, 526
  in thyroid storm, 259
DHEA (dehydroepiandrosterone) in hirsutism, 302, 305
DHEAS (dehydroepiandrosterone sulfate) in hirsutism, 302, 303, 304, 305
Diabetes mellitus, 6, 264–277
  angina pectoris in, 85
  atherosclerosis in, 61, 66–67, 265, 274
  cholangitis in, primary sclerosing, 188
  complications of, 6, 265–266
    diagnostic tests in, 271
    treatment of, 271–274
  constipation in, 179
  coronary heart disease in, 61
  diagnosis of, 6, 264–266
    criteria in, 266, 267t
  differential diagnosis of, 264–265
  in elderly, 6, 603–604
  hyperosmolar hyperglycemic coma in, 271, 272–273
  and hypertension, 28, 50
    drug therapy in, 35, 36–37, 39, 40
  hypoglycemia in, 6, 271, 273–274
  insulin-dependent, 50, 264, 266–268
  insulin therapy in, 268t, 268–269, 270
  ketoacidosis in, 265, 266, 271–272
    pathophysiology of, 268
  kidney disorders in, 271, 274
  laboratory tests in, 266
  lipid abnormalities in, 50, 53, 61
  natural history of, 274
  neurologic disorders in, 264, 265, 266, 271
    in hypoglycemia, 273
  non-insulin-dependent, 50, 264, 268, 269
  nutrition in, 269, 269t, 270
    in hypoglycemia, 273
  in obesity, 282
  oral hypoglycemic agents in, 269, 270t
  pathophysiology of, 266–268
  peripheral vascular disease in, 66–67, 265, 271
  physical examination in, 265–266
  pneumonia in, 163, 168
  and pregnancy, 267t, 270, 273
  referrals in, 270–271
  symptoms of, 6, 264
  in syndrome X, 28
  weight in, 264, 282
Diarrhea, 177–179
  causes of, 177–178
  in Crohn's disease, 178, 193, 195
  in diabetes mellitus, 271
  in endometriosis, 180
  evaluation of, 178
  factitious, 178–179
  management of, 178
  in ulcerative colitis, 178, 194
Diazepam in elderly, 609t
Diazoxide in hypoglycemia, 276
Dicyclomine in mitral valve prolapse syndrome/ dysautonomia, 109
Diet. *See* Nutrition
Digitalis
  in heart failure, 96, 98
  in pulmonary edema, 96
Digoxin
  in heart failure, 96, 97, 98
  in pulmonary edema, 96
Dihydroergotamine in headaches, 392t, 393, 394t
  analgesic rebound, 389
  cluster, 386
Dihydropyridines
  in heart failure, 99
  in hypertension, 34t, 38
Diltiazem
  in hypertension, 33t, 38
  in migraine prevention, 395, 395t
  in mitral valve prolapse syndrome/ dysautonomia, 109
Diphenhydramine in elderly, 609t
Diphenoxylate in diarrhea, 178
Diphtheria, 358–359, 607
Disc, intervertebral, degenerative disease of, 427
Discharge, vaginal, 343, 344, 345
Diuretics
  in heart failure, 96, 97–98, 99
  in hypertension, 30–36, 31t–32t
    interaction with other drugs, 35
    lipid abnormalities from, 51
    as second-line therapy, 35
    side effects of, 35–36, 51
    in special populations, 35
  in premenstrual syndrome, 510, 513
  in pulmonary edema, 96
Dizziness
  and falls of elderly, 613
  in mitral valve prolapse syndrome/ dysautonomia, 106, 108, 109
DNA hybridization
  in cervicitis, 346, 347
  in papillomavirus infection, 320
DNA probe test in cervicitis, 346t, 347
Dobutamine in heart failure, 99

Donnatal in mitral valve prolapse syndrome/dysautonomia, 109
Donovanosis, 351
Dopamine, and prolactin secretion, 293, 294
Douching, as contraceptive method, 341–342
Doxazosin in hypertension, 33t, 37
Doxepin in depression, 530, 530t, 534t
Drop attacks, 612–613
Drug abuse and addiction, 15–16, 538–546. *See also* Substance abuse and addiction
Drug-induced disorders
 acne in, 476
 anemia in, 210, 211t
 from antidepressant drugs, 529–531, 531t
 anxiety in, 590t
 bleeding disorders in, 215, 216, 216t, 227, 233, 234
 constipation in, 179
 depression in, 522, 523, 528
 diarrhea in, 177
 dyslipidemia in, 51–52
 in elderly, 609–610
  falls in, 612
 headaches in, 387, 390
  in analgesic rebound, 389
 hirsutism in, 303
 hypertension in, 23, 25, 26
 hypoglycemia in, 274–275, 276
 hypothyroidism in, 250
 inflammatory bowel disease in, 192, 193
 of liver, 330, 432, 446, 448, 449
 lupus syndromes in, 462–463
 in mesalamine intolerance, 195, 198
 of platelets, 216, 227
 in pneumonia, 172
 rhinitis in, 363–364
Drug therapy
 in acne, 477–478
 in angina pectoris, 87–89
 antibiotic. *See* Antibiotics
 anticoagulant, 233–234
 antidepressant. *See* Antidepressant drugs
 in anxiety, 598t
  in pregnancy, 597
 in asthma. *See* Asthma, drug therapy in
 in cholangitis, primary sclerosing, 189
 in chronic obstructive pulmonary disease, 145–148
 in depression, 529–534
 in diarrhea, 178
 in elderly, 61, 608–610
 in gallstones, 186
 in headaches, 392t, 392–396
  combination of drugs in, 394
  in emergency room, 394t, 394–395
  in migraine prevention, 395t, 395–396
 in hyperprolactinemia, 297, 298
 in hypertension. *See* Hypertension, drug therapy in
 in hyperthyroidism, 246
  in pregnancy, 257–258
 in inflammatory bowel disease, 195, 197–199
  and pregnancy, 197, 198
 in insomnia, 563–564
 lipid-lowering, 53, 56–60, 61
  in angina pectoris, 89
 in mitral valve prolapse syndrome/dysautonomia, 108–111, 111f
  sensitivity to, 110
 in obesity, 288–289
 in osteoarthritis, 431–432
 in peripheral vascular disease
  brachiocephalic, 74–75
  lower extremity, 71
 in pneumonia, 168, 168t, 169t, 169–172
  in pregnancy, 173
 in pulmonary edema, 96–97
 in rheumatoid arthritis, 446–449
 in rhinitis, allergic, 361–363
 in sinusitis, 368
 thrombolytic, 233
Dry skin, 488–490
Dual energy absorptiometry, 410–411
Dust mites
 and allergic rhinitis, 361
 and asthma, 121, 126
Dysautonomia, 104–115
 cardiovascular symptoms in, 105
 differential diagnosis of, 107
 drug therapy in, 108–111
  sensitivity to, 110
 history of patient in, 105–106
 hyperadrenergic, 108, 109
 hyperparasympathetic, 109
 hypothesis on, 111–115
 laboratory tests in, 108
 patient education in, 111, 111f
 physical examination in, 106–107
 questionnaire on, 112–113, 113t
 sleep in, 106, 110, 557–558, 566
 spoke-wheel diagram of, 110, 110f
Dysbetalipoproteinemia, familial, 48
Dysfibrinogenemia, 232
Dysfolliculogenesis, 547, 550
Dyslipidemia, 46
 autoimmune, 51
 drug-induced, 51–52
 in elderly, 60–61
 familial, 48
 Frederickson classification of, 47, 47t
 secondary, 49t, 49–52
  identification of, 50t
Dysphoric disorder
 late luteal phase, 503, 505t
 premenstrual, 503
Dysplasia
 cervical, 9, 320
  and papillomavirus infection, 313, 315, 316f, 320, 322
 fibromuscular, 77, 77f
 in nevi, 497
Dyspnea
 in anemia, 205
 in asthma, 119, 125
 in chronic obstructive pulmonary disease, 139, 140
 in heart failure, 94, 98
 in lung cancer, 154, 161
 paroxysmal nocturnal, 94, 98
Dysthymia
 in depression, 524, 529
 in obsessive compulsive personality disorder, 583
 in passive aggressive personality disorder, 584

E
Eating disorders, 547–552
 anorexia nervosa, 547–549
 bulimia, 547, 549–550
Echocardiography
 in angina pectoris, 86–87
 in heart failure, 95
 in mitral valve prolapse, 104
Economic impact. *See* Cost considerations
Eczema
 craquele, 489
 in xerosis, 489, 490
Edema
 brawny, 611
 of lower extremity in elderly, 610–611
 in myxedema coma, 260
 pulmonary
  differential diagnosis of, 95, 96
  in heart failure, 92, 94, 96–97
  treatment of, 96–97
 in venous thromboembolism, 79, 79f
Education of patients
 in antidepressant therapy, 531–532
 in anxiety disorders, 596
 in asthma, 126–127, 131
 in chronic obstructive pulmonary disease, 144
 in diabetes mellitus, 270
 in dysautonomia, 111, 111f
 in hepatitis, 333
 in molluscum contagiosum, 480
 in osteoarthritis, 431
 in premenstrual syndrome, 513
 in rheumatoid arthritis, 446
Effusions
 pericardial, in rheumatoid arthritis, 443
 pleural
  differential diagnosis of, 166
  in heart failure, 95
  in lung cancer, 157f, 157–158
  in pneumonia, 166, 167
  in rheumatoid arthritis, 443
Ehlers-Danlos syndrome, 217
Elbow, rheumatoid arthritis of, 435, 436t, 441
 treatment in, 447, 450
Elderly, 603–617. *See also* Aging
Electrocardiography
 in angina pectoris, 83, 86, 87t
 in heart failure, 95
 in hypertension, 27t, 28
Electrocautery in condylomata, 321t, 322
Electrodesiccation
 in condylomata, 322
 in skin cancer, 494–495, 496
  basal cell, 494–495
  squamous cell, 495, 496
Elevation pallor in atherosclerosis, 69, 69t
Embolism. *See also* Thrombosis and thromboembolism
 atheromatous, 68, 68f
 pulmonary, 86
  chest pain in, 84
  differential diagnosis of, 166, 173
  in pregnancy, 173
  wheezing in, 123
 venous thromboembolism, 66, 78–80, 232, 611
  prevention of, 235
Embryonic development
 in asthma of mother, 132, 133
 of paranasal sinuses, 365, 366
 of thyroid gland, 239, 240
Emergencies, thyroid, 258–261
Emergency room care
 in asthma, 126, 136–137
 in headaches, 394t, 394–395
Emollients, in xerosis, 489
Emotions
 in depression, 520
 in histrionic personality disorder, 579, 580
Emphysema, 139–153
 categories of, 142
 definition of, 142
 differential diagnosis of, 123, 140–141
 natural history and prognosis in, 149–150
 pathogenesis of, 141–142
 presentation of, 139–140, 140t
 treatment of, 144–149
 workup in, 142–144
Empyema, in pneumonia, 166, 171
Enalapril
 in heart failure, 97

Enalapril (*Continued*)
in hypertension, 33t, 38–39
Enalaprilat in pulmonary edema, 97
Encephalopathy, 590
hepatic, 330, 332
portosystemic, 335
Endarterectomy, carotid, 75–76
Endocarditis, and pneumonia, 164
Endocrine disorders, 237–309. *See also specific disorders*
anxiety in, 590t
depression in, 522, 523
diabetes mellitus, 6, 264–277
diarrhea in, 178
hirsutism, 302–309
hyperprolactinemia, 292–301
multiple endocrine neoplasia, 275
obesity, 5–6, 278–291
rheumatoid arthritis in, 440
thyroid, 6, 239–263
Endometrial cancer, 18
Endometriosis, 177, 180
bowel symptoms in, Plate 4, 180
uterosacral ligaments in, Plate 3, 180
Endorphins, in premenstrual syndrome, 511
Endoscopy
cholangiopancreatography in, retrograde, 185, 185f
in tumors, 189, 190
in sinusitis, chronic, 369
Energy intake and expenditure. *See* Caloric intake and expenditure
Enuresis, in sleep, 562
Environmental factors
in antisocial personality disorder, 577
in asthma, 121, 126
in circadian rhythms, 555
in falls of elderly, 612, 613
in hearing loss, 18
in hepatitis, 332
in psychoactive substance use, 539
in rhinitis
allergic, 361
vasomotor, 363
in scabies, 484, 485
in seasonal depression, 523–524
in skin cancer, 8, 492–493, 497
sun exposure in, 8, 492–493
in xerosis, 489
Enzyme immunoassay
in cervicitis, 346t, 347
in lupus erythematosus, 460, 461
Eosinophilia, 123
in asthma, 125
in pneumonia, 167
Epinephrine in chronic obstructive pulmonary disease, 145, 146
Epstein-Barr virus infections, 373, 377
Ergot preparations in headaches, 392t, 393
Ergotism, gangrenous, 298
Erosive osteoarthritis, 423
radiography in, 429, 429f
Erythema
in lupus erythematosus, 455, 465
in rosacea, 482, 483
in seborrheic dermatitis, 485, 486, 487
Erythrocytes
in anemia, 205–206
decreased production of, 205, 210
increased loss or destruction of, 205, 210
morphology of, 205–206, 207t
sedimentation rate in rheumatoid arthritis, 444
Erythromycin
in acne, 477
in diarrhea, 178
in pneumonia, 168t
Erythroplasia of Queyrat, 496
Esophagus
laceration of, in bulimia, 549
spasm of, chest pain in, 84
Estradiol in osteoporosis, 415–416
Estrogen
serum levels of
in osteoporosis, 407
in premenstrual syndrome, 510–511
therapy with
and Alzheimer's disease risk, 5
and atherosclerosis, 51, 60, 71, 73–74
blood pressure in, 23, 25
and cancer risk, 18, 60, 316, 317
coagulation in, 216, 219, 234
in contraception, 18
and coronary heart disease risk, 51, 60, 71
in exercise-induced menstrual dysfunction, 551
headaches in, 387
in hirsutism, 305–306, 308
in hyperprolactinemia, 297, 299, 300
and inflammatory bowel disease, 192, 193
lipid levels in, 51–52, 57t, 60, 66, 71
in osteoporosis, 407, 415–416, 419, 420
in premenstrual syndrome, 511, 514
in sleep disorders, menstrual-associated, 557
in von Willebrand's disease, 229
Ethacrynic acid in hypertension, 31t
Ethinyl estradiol in hirsutism, 306
Ethmoid sinus, 365
infection of, 367, 367f, 368
Etidronate in osteoporosis, 417, 418
Exercise, 12, 13, 16–17
angina pectoris in, 83
asthma in, 135–136
benefits of, 16, 551
calorie consumption in, 16–17
in chronic obstructive pulmonary disease, 149
in heart failure, 97
intolerance of, 94–95
in hypertension, 29–30
lipid levels in, 55, 551
in lupus erythematosus, 465
and menstrual function, 547, 550–551
in mitral valve prolapse syndrome/dysautonomia, 108, 111, 111f
in obesity, 280
in weight loss program, 287–288
in osteoarthritis, 431
in osteoporosis, 415
in prevention, 419
in peripheral vascular disease, 71–72
in premenstrual syndrome, 510, 513
thermic effect of, 280
Extremities
atherosclerosis of, 66–77
lower extremity disease, 66, 67–72
upper extremity disease, 66, 72–77
examination of, in hypertension, 27
lower. *See* Lower extremity
Eyes. *See also* Vision
in diabetes mellitus, 266, 270–271, 274
in glaucoma, 5, 391–392
in Graves' disease, 244
in hypertension, funduscopic examination of, 26
in migraine, 388t
in rheumatoid arthritis, 442–443
in rosacea, 483
in temporal arteritis, 390

F

Face
acne of, 475–478
molluscum contagiosum of, 479, 479f, 480
rosacea of, 482–483
seborrheic dermatitis of, 485, 486, 487
tinea versicolor of, 487
Factitious disorders
diarrhea in, 178–179
hypoglycemia in, 276
purpura in, 217, 227
thyrotoxicosis in, 244, 248
Factors, clotting, 218, 219, 220, 220t
antibodies to, 225, 226
concentrates of, 230
cost of, 230
deficiency of, 215, 217
clinical approach to, 224, 225, 226, 228
hemophilia in, 224, 228
in disseminated intravascular coagulation, 231
in fresh frozen plasma, 230
laboratory assessment of, 221, 223
replacement therapy, 224, 225, 226, 230
Falls of elderly, 408, 420, 611–613
causes of, 613, 613t
frequency of, 408, 611–612
risk factors in, 612
Famotidine in mitral valve prolapse syndrome/dysautonomia, 109
Fat
body, 5
distribution of, 279, 283
measurement of, 278, 279
dietary
and obesity, 280–281, 287
in weight loss program, 287
Fat-free mass, and resting metabolic rate, 280
Fatigue, 374
acute, 374, 375
chronic, 106, 107, 373–383
definition of, 374
diagnostic criteria on, 376t, 377, 377t
incidence of, 373
management of, 380–381
pathogenesis of, 377–378
referrals in, 378–379, 380
transactional meaning of, 375
and depression, 374–375, 377, 378, 522
evaluation of, 379
management of, 380
in diabetes mellitus, 264
differential diagnosis of, 264, 375–377
evaluation of, 375, 378, 379
brief examination in, 378
in depression, 379
in lupus erythematosus, 454, 465
in mitral valve prolapse syndrome/dysautonomia, 105–106, 107
multifactorial, 374, 377
in premenstrual syndrome, 503, 510, 511
Fatty liver of pregnancy, 331
Felodipine
in heart failure, 97, 99
in hypertension, 34t
Felty's syndrome, 443
Femoral artery
atherosclerosis of, 67
pulse of, in hypertension, 27
Femoral osteoporosis
bone mass measurements in, 410, 411
fluoride affecting, 418
hip fractures in, 408, 409
Ferritin levels in anemia, 206
Ferrous sulfate in iron deficiency anemia, 208
Fertility problems, 16
body weight in, 547
in inflammatory bowel disease, 200
Fetus. *See* Embryonic development

Fever
in lupus erythematosus, 454
in pneumonia, 163, 164, 166
rheumatic, 435
in thyroid storm, 258, 259
Fibric acid derivatives in lipid-lowering therapy, 57t, 59–60
Fibrillation, atrial, stroke in, 73, 74
prevention of, 75
Fibrin
degradation products, 223
formation of, 218
defects in, 217
laboratory assessment of, 221, 223
Fibrinogen, 218, 220t, 223
degradation products, 223
in disseminated intravascular coagulation, 231
in fresh frozen plasma, 230
Fibrinolytic therapy, 71, 79, 233
Fibroadenoma of breast, 18
Fibrocystic breast disease, in mitral valve prolapse syndrome/dysautonomia, 106
Fibromuscular dysplasia, 77, 77f
Fibromyalgia, 389, 437
in mitral valve prolapse syndrome/dysautonomia, 106
sleep disorders in, 557
Fibromyositis, 389
Fibrosis, cystic, differential diagnosis of, 141
Fibrositis, 437
sleep disorders in, 557
Fish oil, in hypertriglyceridemia, 60
Fistula, rectovaginal, in inflammatory bowel disease, 197
Flolan in heart failure, 97
Flosequinon in heart failure, 97
Fluids
intake of
in constipation, 179
in diabetic ketoacidosis, 272
in diarrhea, 178
in mitral valve prolapse syndrome/dysautonomia, 108, 111, 111f
retention of, in premenstrual syndrome, 510, 513, 513t
Flunisolide
in allergic rhinitis, 362
in asthma, 128t, 130
in pregnancy, 135
Fluorescent antibody technique, direct, in cervicitis, 346
Fluoride in osteoporosis, 418, 419
5-Fluorouracil
in actinic keratoses, 493
in condylomata, 322
Fluoxetine
in anxiety disorders, 598t
in bulimia, 549
in depression, 530t
dosage of, 534, 534t
side effects of, 530
in mitral valve prolapse syndrome/dysautonomia, 110
in obsessive compulsive disorder, 595
in premenstrual syndrome, 512, 514
Flurazepam in elderly, 609t
Flurohydrocortisone in mitral valve prolapse syndrome/dysautonomia, 109
Flushing, facial, in rosacea, 482, 483
Flutamide in hirsutism, 306, 307
Fluvastatin in lipid-lowering therapy, 57t, 59
Folate deficiency, 211, 212
Follicle-stimulating hormone, 294
in anorexia nervosa, 548
in hirsutism, 304, 305, 307
Follicular occlusion triad, 476
Folstein Mini-Mental State Examination, 615t, 615–616
Food poisoning, diarrhea in, 177
Foot
carcinoma of, squamous cell, Plate 10
in diabetes mellitus, 271
gangrene of, 68, 68f
in peripheral vascular disease, 71
rheumatoid arthritis of, 441–442
radiography in, 445
Forearm, osteoporosis of, 410, 411
Foreign bodies in airway, 123
Forestier's disease, 423
Fosinopril in hypertension, 33t, 39
Fractures
of hip
in falls of elderly, 612
in osteoporosis, 408, 409
nasal, 364
in osteoporosis, 401
bone mass measurements in, 410
clinical presentation of, 408–409
fluoride affecting, 418
pain in, 409
risk for, 406–407
threshold for, 402, 404
Fragility of bones, 406–407
Frank-Starling curve, 91–92, 92f, 93
Frederickson classification of dyslipidemias, 47, 47t
Frontal sinus, 365, 366
infection of, 367, 368
Funduscopic examination in hypertension, 26
Fungal infections
pneumonia in, 163, 165, 167, 168, 169
treatment of, 168t, 169t, 170t, 171t
rhinitis in, 360
sinusitis in, 369–370
tinea versicolor in, 487–488
Furosemide
in heart failure, 96, 98
in hypertension, 31t
in pulmonary edema, 96
Furunculosis, nasal, 358

G
Gait of elderly, and falls, 612, 613
Galactorrhea, in hyperprolactinemia, 292, 295
Gallbladder, 182–190
calcified (porcelain), 186
cancer of, 186, 189
cholecystitis of. *See* Cholecystitis
gallstones of, 182–187
Gallstones, 182–187
asymptomatic, 182, 186
biliary colic in, 182, 183
cancer of gallbladder in, 186, 189
cholecystitis in, 182
in common bile duct, 183, 183f
composition of, 183–184
diagnostic evaluation of, 184–185
differential diagnosis of, 183
laboratory tests in, 184
in obesity, 282, 285
pancreatitis in, 183, 184, 185
in pregnancy, 187
pathogenesis of, 183–184
physical examination in, 184
pigment, 183–184, 186
in pregnancy, 184, 185, 186–187
symptomatic, 182–183
treatment of, 185–186
Gamma globulin therapy in lupus erythematosus, 466
Gangrene, 68, 68f
in ergotism, 298
Gases, arterial blood
in asthma, 125
in pneumonia, 165
in pregnancy, 132
Gastrointestinal disorders, 175–201
abdominal pain in, 180
of biliary tract and gallbladder, 182–190
colon cancer, Plate 2, 7–8, 179, 196–197
constipation, 179–180
in diabetes mellitus, 271
diarrhea, 177–179. *See also* Diarrhea
functional bowel disease, 180
gender differences in, 177, 179
inflammatory bowel disease, 191–201. *See also* Inflammatory bowel disease
in lupus erythematosus, 458–459
in mitral valve prolapse syndrome/dysautonomia, 106, 107, 109
Gastroparesis in diabetes mellitus, 271
Gelatinase in osteoarthritis, 426
Gemfibrozil in lipid-lowering therapy, 57t, 59–60, 61
in diabetes mellitus, 61
in elderly, 61
in hypertriglyceridemia, 61, 62
side effects of, 60
Genetic factors
in antisocial personality disorder, 577
in bleeding disorders, 214, 215, 228
in diabetes mellitus, 267
in hemophilia, 228
in hirsutism, 302
in inflammatory bowel disease, 192
in lung cancer, 156–157
in lupus erythematosus, 454, 462
in melanoma, 497
in obesity, 280, 283
in osteoarthritis, 423
in restless legs syndrome, 561
in rheumatoid arthritis, 440
in substance abuse and addiction, 539, 540
in thalassemia, 209
in thrombosis
arterial, 233
venous, 232
in von Willebrand's disease, 228
Genitalia
Bowenoid papulosis of, 318, 496
Bowen's disease of, 496
molluscum contagiosum of, 479, 480
papillomavirus infections of, 313–323
ulcer disease of, 348–351
Gentamicin in pneumonia, 171t
Genu varus in osteoarthritis, 427
Geriatric medicine, 603–617. *See also* Aging
Giant cell arteritis, 390, 437
headache in, 384, 390, 394
Giant cell thyroiditis, 254–255
Glaucoma, 5
headache in, 391–392
Glipizide in diabetes mellitus, 270t
Glucose
blood levels of
in diabetes mellitus, 6, 266, 267t, 269, 272–274
in hypertension, 3, 27t, 28
in hypoglycemia. *See* Hypoglycemia
in mitral valve prolapse syndrome/dysautonomia, 107, 108
in premenstrual syndrome, 510
tolerance test of, 6, 267t
Glyburide in diabetes mellitus, 270t
Goiter, 241
in Graves' disease, 244
in Hashimoto's thyroiditis, 248, 249

Goiter (*Continued*)
laboratory tests in, 242
multinodular, 254
toxic, 246–247
physical examination in, 241
in pregnancy, 256
sporadic, 254
Goitrogens, 240
Gold compounds in rheumatoid arthritis, 447–448
Gonadotropes, 294
Gonadotropin-releasing hormone, 294
agonists in premenstrual syndrome, 511, 514
analogues in hirsutism therapy, 306, 307
in exercise, 550
in stress, 550
Gonococcal infection, disseminated, 348, 437, 455
Gonorrhea, 339
arthritis in, 348, 437
cervicitis in, 345, 346, 346t
and contraceptive methods, 341
disseminated infection in, 348, 437, 455
epidemiology of, 339–340
physical examination in, 343
screening for, 351
specimen collection in, 343
Gout, 424
differential diagnosis of, 437
and hypertension therapy, 28, 35, 36, 40
in obesity, 282
and pseudogout, 437–438
rheumatic, 435
Grandiose fantasies, in narcissistic personality disorder, 580
Granuloma
annulare, in diabetes mellitus, 266
eosinophilic, 167
inguinale, 348, 351
in sarcoidosis, 364, 365
in thyroiditis, 254–255
vulvar, in inflammatory bowel disease, 197
Granulomatosis, Wegener's, 167
nose in, 365
Graves' disease, 241, 244–246
antithyroid antibodies in, 243
laboratory tests in, 242
physical examination in, 241
in pregnancy, 257
radioiodine therapy in, 246, 250
thyroid storm in, 258
thyroidectomy in, 246, 249
Grief, 525–526
Growth factors
in osteoarthritis, 426
in rheumatoid arthritis, 438
Guanabenz in hypertension, 34t, 37
Guanadrel in hypertension, 34t, 38
Guanethidine in hypertension, 34t, 38
Guanfacine in hypertension, 34t, 37
Guilt feelings, in depression, 520–521
Gumma formation in syphilis, 360

H
Haemophilus infections
ducreyi, 340t, 343
chancroid in, 348, 349t, 350
influenzae, 167, 168, 169
sinusitis in, 368
treatment of, 168t, 169t, 170t, 171t
Hair
age-related changes of, 308
in hirsutism, 302–309
loss in lupus erythematosus, 456
physiology of growth, 302–303
Hallucinations, hypnogogic, 559, 560
Hallucinogens, 545
Hallus valgus in rheumatoid arthritis, 442
Haloperidol in anxiety disorders, 598t
Hand
osteoarthritis of, 6–7, 421, 423, 426, 427f
arthroplasty in, 433
differential diagnosis of, 435
radiography in, 429, 429f
seagull sign in, 429, 429f
rheumatoid arthritis of, 435, 436t, 440–441, 441f
deformities in, 441, 441f
radiography in, 445, 445f
Hashimoto's thyroiditis, 243, 248–249
Headaches, 384–397
analgesic rebound, 389
chronic, 395–396
cluster, compared to migraine, 386, 386t
in dental disease, 384
differential diagnosis of, 384, 390–392
drug therapy in, 392t, 392–396
combination of drugs in, 394
in emergency room, 394t, 394–395
in migraine prevention, 395t, 395–396
emergency room care of, 394t, 394–395
in hemicrania, chronic paroxysmal, 389
history of patient in, 384, 385
laboratory tests in, 385
in lupus erythematosus, 459
in meningitis, 385, 390, 394, 459
migraine. *See* Migraine
in mitral valve prolapse syndrome/dysautonomia, 106, 107
physical examination in, 385
postlumbar puncture, 384, 385t, 386, 389
in pregnancy, 387, 393, 394, 395, 396
in premenstrual syndrome, 503, 509, 510
treatment of, 513
in sleep apnea, 558
in subarachnoid hemorrhage, 385, 385t, 386, 390, 394
in temporal arteritis, 384, 390, 394
tension, 384, 389
chronic, 395
and migraine, 389
treatment of, 392
treatment of, 392t, 392–396
in trigeminal neuralgia, 390
trigger points in, 385, 389
Hearing aids, 5
Hearing loss, 5
in acoustic trauma, 18
Heart
arrhythmias of, 35
stroke in, 73, 74, 75
cardiomyopathy of, 39, 40
peripartum, 99–100
failure of. *See* Heart failure
in hypertension, 27
output of, 91
Frank-Starling curve on, 91–92, 92f, 93
in heart failure, 91–92, 93–94
in rheumatoid arthritis, 443
sounds of. *See* Heart sounds
transplantation of, 99
valvular disease of. *See* Valvular heart disease
Heart failure, 91–103
acute, 94
in anemia, 205
backward, 93
cardiac output in, 91–92, 93–94
high, 93
low, 93
chronic, 94, 97–99
classification of, 94–95
clinical forms of, 93–94
clinical manifestations of, 94–95
compensatory mechanisms in, 91–92
definition of, 91
in diabetic ketoacidosis, 272
in diastolic dysfunction, 92–93, 99
differential diagnosis of, 95–96, 166
etiology of, 91–93
forward, 93
Frank-Starling curve in, 91–92, 92f, 93
in hyperthyroidism, 93–94, 244
incidence of, 91
laboratory tests in, 95
left-sided, 93, 94–95
lower extremity edema in, 610, 611
neurohumoral activation in, 91, 92, 93
in peripartum cardiomyopathy, 99–100
physical examination in, 95
prognosis in, 92, 100
right-sided, 93, 94, 95
in systolic dysfunction, 91–92, 97
transplantation of heart in, 99
treatment of, 96–99
Heart sounds
in heart failure, 95
in mitral valve prolapse syndrome/dysautonomia, 107
in pneumonia, 164
Heat therapy in osteoarthritis, 431
Heberden's nodes, 7, 426, 427f, 435
Height/weight tables, 278–279, 279t
Hemarthrosis, 217
Hematologic disorders, 203–235
anemia, 205–212. *See also* Anemia
coagulation disorders, 213–235
in lupus erythematosus, 459–460, 464t
management of, 466
in rheumatoid arthritis, 443
Hematoma, subdural, headache in, 391
Hematuria in lupus erythematosus, 456, 457
Hemicrania, chronic paroxysmal, 389
Hemiplegic migraine, 388t
Hemoccult examination in endometriosis, 180
Hemoglobin, 209
concentration in anemia, 205
normal adult, 209, 209t
Hemolytic disorders
anemia in, 205, 210, 211t, 459, 466
drug-induced, 211t
in lupus erythematosus, 459, 466
gallstones in, 183–184
in lupus erythematosus, 459, 466
Hemophilia, 215, 224, 228
coagulation test results in, 224, 225
genetic factors in, 228
pregnancy in, 228
treatment of, 229
Hemoptysis in lung cancer, 154, 161
Hemorrhage. *See* Bleeding
Hemostasis. *See* Coagulation
Henderson-Patterson bodies, 479
Heparin, 233–234
in angina pectoris, unstable, 89
in disseminated intravascular coagulation, 231
in hyperosmolar hyperglycemic coma, 273
in pregnancy, 234, 235
side effects of, 233
in venous thromboembolism, 79
Hepatitis
A type, 324, 325, 325t, 326
immune prophylaxis of, 333
laboratory tests in, 328, 328t
in pregnancy, 331
acute, 327, 332
anicteric, 326, 329
autoimmune, 330
B type, 324, 325t, 325–326

carrier state in, 332–333
chronic, 334
immune prophylaxis of, 331, 331t, 333
laboratory tests in, 328t, 328–329
in pregnancy, 331
treatment of, 332–333, 334, 334t
biopsy of liver in, 330
C type, 324, 325t, 325–326
chronic, 334–335
laboratory tests in, 328, 328t, 329
in pregnancy, 331
prevention and treatment of, 332, 333, 334t, 334–335
chronic, 327
complications in, 335
treatment and prevention of, 332–333, 334–335
course of, 329
D type, 324, 325t, 325–326
laboratory tests in, 328t, 329
in pregnancy, 332
prevention and treatment of, 332, 335
diagnostic algorithm in, 327f
differential diagnosis of, 188, 329–330
in pregnancy, 330–331
E type, 324, 325, 325t, 326
laboratory tests in, 328t, 329
in pregnancy, 324, 331
epidemiology of, 324–326
fulminant, 330, 335
household contacts in, 332
icteric, 326
immune prophylaxis of, 331, 331t, 332, 333–334
interferon therapy in, 326, 334t, 334–335
laboratory tests in, 328t, 328–329
liver transplantation in, 324, 335
in lupus erythematosus, 458–459
in needle stick injury, 332, 333–334
pathogenesis of, 326
in pregnancy, 330–332, 333–334
transmission to child in, 324, 325–326, 331–332, 333–334
prevention of, 331, 331t, 332
in neonate, 331, 333–334
reporting of, 332
signs and symptoms of, 326–327
transmission of, 325t, 325–326, 332, 333
blood-borne, 325–326
in needle stick injury, 332, 333–334
in pregnancy, 324, 325–326, 331–332, 333–334
waterborne, 325
types of viruses in, 324, 325t
Hepatotoxicity of drugs, 330
of anti-inflammatory drugs, 432, 446
in rheumatoid arthritis, 448, 449
Herald patch in pityriasis rosea, 481, 481f
Herpes simplex virus infections
and contraceptive methods, 341
diagnosis of, 349t, 350
genital ulcer disease in, 348, 349t, 349–350
Hip
fractures of
in falls of elderly, 612
in osteoporosis, 408, 409
osteoarthritis of, 6, 421, 423, 426, 435
radiography in, 430f
treatment of, 431, 432, 433
osteonecrosis of, 441
rheumatoid arthritis of, 435, 440, 441, 450
Hirschsprung's disease, 179
Hirsutism, 302–309
and acne, 477
causes of, 303–305
idiopathic, 303–304
long-term follow-up in, 308
physiology of hair growth in, 302–303
scoring system on, 302, 303f
therapy in, 305–308
Histamine H_1-receptor antagonists in allergic rhinitis, 361–362
Histiocytosis X, 167
Histocompatibility complex, major, in rheumatoid arthritis, 438, 440
Histoplasmosis, 360
History of patient
in anemia, 205, 206t
in angina pectoris, 84, 85, 85t
in asthma, 121–122
in coagulation disorders, 213, 214
in diarrhea, 178
in hypertension, 25–26
in lung cancer, 154, 156
in mitral valve prolapse syndrome/dysautonomia, 105–106, 108
in obesity, 283, 284
in papillomavirus infections, 319–320
in peripheral vascular disease, 68
in pneumonia, 163–164
Histrionic personality disorder, 579–580
differential diagnosis of, 579, 580, 581, 582, 584
HIV infection and AIDS, 17, 18, 339, 341
dermatitis in, seborrheic, 486, 487
hepatitis in, 330
molluscum contagiosum in, 478, 479, 479f, 480
nasal disorders in, 358, 360
papillomavirus infection in, 314, 320
physical examination in, 342, 343
screening for, 351
sinusitis in, 366, 369
HLA gene in rheumatoid arthritis, 438, 440
HMG CoA reductase inhibitors in lipid-lowering therapy, 57t, 59
Hoover's sign, 142
Horner's syndrome, in headaches, 388, 391
Hospitalization
in asthma, 137
in pneumonia, 168–169, 170t
House dust mites
and allergic rhinitis, 361
and asthma, 121, 126
Huntington's disease, 614
Hutchinson's sign, Plate 15, 497
Hydralazine
in heart failure, 97
in hypertension, 34t
Hydrochlorothiazide in hypertension, 31t, 32t
Hydrocortisone
in dermatitis, seborrheic, 487
in myxedema coma, 261
in thyroid storm, 259
Hydroflumethiazide in hypertension, 31t
α-Hydroxy acid preparations in xerosis, 489, 490
Hydroxychloroquine
in lupus erythematosus, 466, 469
and breast-feeding, 468
and pregnancy, 468
in rheumatoid arthritis, 447
side effects of, 447, 466
21-Hydroxylase deficiency, 305
Hydroxymethylglutaryl (HMG) CoA reductase inhibitors in lipid-lowering therapy, 57t, 59
17-Hydroxyprogesterone serum levels, 305, 305f
Hydroxyzine in anxiety disorders, 598t
Hyperactive airway disease, 119–138. *See also* Asthma
Hypercholesterolemia, 44
coronary heart disease in, 47, 48
gender differences in, 52–53
screening for, 54
in elderly, 60–61
familial, 47–48
polygenic, 47–48
nutrition in, 54, 55–56, 56t
secondary causes of, 49t
in thyroid disease, 50, 51
Hyperchylomicronemia syndrome, 49
Hyperglycemic hyperosmolar coma, in diabetes mellitus, 271, 272–273
Hyperlipidemia, 4, 44–65
drug therapy in, 53, 56–60
familial combined, 48
secondary causes of, 49t, 49–52
type III, 48
Hyperosmolar hyperglycemic coma, in diabetes mellitus, 271, 272–273
Hyperostosis, diffuse idiopathic skeletal, 423–424
Hyperparathyroidism, secondary, osteoporosis in, 408, 413
Hyperplasia, adrenal congenital, 305, 305f
Hyperprolactinemia, 292–301
evaluation of, 295–297
natural history of, 292–295
treatment of, 297–300
long-term, 299f, 299–300, 300f
Hypersomnia, 553
in depression, 521
Hypertension, 3, 23–43
age of onset, 25
alcohol use in, 26, 30
angina pectoris in, 85
and coarctation of aorta, 27, 28t
definition of, 23
and diabetes mellitus, 28, 50
drug therapy in, 35, 36–37, 39, 40
diagnosis of, 3, 23–24
drug-induced, 23, 25, 26
drug therapy in, 30–41
angiotensin-converting enzyme inhibitors, 33t, 38–39
calcium channel blockers, 33t–34t, 35, 38
diuretics, 30–36, 31t–32t
dyslipidemia in, 51
general guidelines on, 39–40
in special populations, 40–41
in stepped care approach, 30
sympatholytic agents, 32t–33t, 34t, 36–38
in elderly, 3, 35, 40
drug therapy in, 38, 39, 40
in estrogen use, 23, 25
exogenous factors in, 25–26
headache in, 385, 390–391
history in, 25–26
intracranial, headache in, 390–391
laboratory tests in, 3, 27t, 27–28
life-style factors in, 15, 16
modification of, 29t, 29–30, 39
low renin, 35, 38, 39
nutrition in, 25–26, 30, 38
and obesity, 28, 50, 282
physical examination in, 26t, 26–27
in renal disorders, 27, 28t
in renovascular disorders, 27, 28t
as risk factor, 3, 4, 25, 25t
screening for, 3, 23–24, 24t
secondary, 28, 28t
stages of, 23, 24t
stroke in, 74, 75
in syndrome X, 28, 282
target organ damage in, 25
treatment of, 29–41
algorithm on, 40f
weight loss and exercise in, 29–30
Hyperthecosis, ovarian, hirsutism in, 304

Hyperthyroidism, 239, 244–248
  causes of, 244, 245
  clinical presentation of, 244, 245
  in goiter, 254
    toxic multinodular, 246–247
  in Graves' disease, 244–246
  heart failure in, 93–94, 244
  hypertension in, 27
  laboratory tests in, 241, 242, 244
  in neonate, 244
  physical examination in, 241
  in pituitary adenoma, 247
  in postpartum thyroiditis, 256
  in pregnancy, 257–258
  in silent thyroiditis, 255
  in subacute thyroiditis, 254, 255
  in thyroid nodules, 246–247, 252
    autonomously functioning, 247
  thyroid storm in, 258–259
  in thyrotoxicosis factitia, 244, 248
Hypertriglyceridemia, 61–62
  in alcohol use, 50
  coronary heart disease in, 61–62
  in diabetes mellitus, 50
  familial, 48–49
  in obesity, 50
  secondary causes of, 49t
Hypnogogic hallucinations, 559, 560
Hypoalphalipoproteinemia, familial, 48
Hypocalcemia, depression in, 522
Hypochondriasis, 583, 591
Hypochromic anemia, 206
  microcytic, 206–210, 207f
Hypoestrogenic states, osteoporosis in, 407
Hypoglycemia, 273, 274–277
  in diabetes mellitus, 6, 271, 273–274
  differential diagnosis of, 274–275
  drug-induced, 274–275, 276
  laboratory tests in, 275
  in mitral valve prolapse syndrome/dysautonomia, 107, 108
  natural history of, 277
  nutrition in, 273, 276
  pathophysiology of, 275–276
  physical examination in, 275
  in premenstrual syndrome, 510
  reactive, 274, 276, 277
  referrals in, 276
  symptoms of, 274
Hypoglycemic agents, oral, in diabetes mellitus, 269, 270t
Hypokalemia in diabetic ketoacidosis, 272
Hyponatremia in myxedema coma, 260
Hypotension, orthostatic
  in diabetes mellitus, 266
  in mitral valve prolapse syndrome/dysautonomia, 109
Hypothermia in myxedema coma, 259, 260
Hypothyroidism, 6, 239, 248–251
  causes of, 248, 249
  central, 248, 250–251
  constipation in, 179
  depression in, 522, 523, 529
  drug-induced, 250
  hormone replacement therapy in, 249, 250, 251–252
  laboratory tests in, 241, 242
  lipid abnormalities in, 50–51
  myxedema coma in, 259–260
  in neonate, 244, 258
  in postpartum thyroiditis, 256
  in pregnancy, 256–257
  primary, 248
  in radioiodine therapy, 246, 250
  signs and symptoms of, 6, 248, 249
  in silent thyroiditis, 255
  in subacute thyroiditis, 254, 255
  in thyroidectomy, 246, 249
  treatment of, 6, 249
Hypoventilation syndrome in obesity, 282

I
Ibuprofen
  in headaches, 392t, 393
  in lupus erythematosus, 468
Ileoanal anastomosis, sexual function in, 200
Ileostomy, sexual function in, 200
Iliac artery atherosclerosis, 67, 71f
Imidazole in hirsutism, 306, 307
Imipenem-cilastatin in pneumonia, 171t
Imipramine
  in anxiety disorders, 598t
  in cataplexy, 560
  in depression, 530, 530t, 534t
Immune mechanisms
  in dermatitis, seborrheic, 486
  in fatigue, chronic, 377
  in hepatitis, 326
  in lupus erythematosus, 462, 464t
  in rheumatoid arthritis, 438–439, 439f
Immunizations. *See* Vaccinations
Immunoassay
  in cervicitis, 346t, 347
  in lupus erythematosus, 460, 461
  of thyroid hormones, 241
  of thyroid-stimulating hormone, 242
Immunocompromised patients
  molluscum contagiosum in, 478, 479, 480
  pneumonia in, 163, 170
  scabies in, 484
Immunodeficiency syndrome, acquired. *See* HIV infection and AIDS
Immunoglobulins
  in hepatitis prophylaxis, 331, 331t, 333
  IgC, in chronic fatigue, 381
  IgE
    in allergic rhinitis, 360, 361
    in asthma, 125
  thyroid-stimulating, 243–244
Immunoprophylaxis of hepatitis, 331, 331t
Immunosorbent assay, enzyme-linked, in lupus erythematosus, 460, 461
Immunosuppressive therapy
  in cholangitis, primary sclerosing, 189
  in inflammatory bowel disease, 199
  lipid levels in, 51, 52
  papillomavirus infection in, 314
Immunotherapy
  in asthma, 126
  in condylomata, 321t, 322
Impulse control disorders, 591
Indapamide
  in heart failure, 98
  in hypertension, 31t
Indomethacin in chronic paroxysmal hemicrania, 389
Infants. *See* Children and infants
Infarction
  myocardial, in lupus erythematosus, 458
  pulmonary, differential diagnosis of, 166
Infections, 311–353
  cholangitis in, primary sclerosing, 188
  in diabetes mellitus, 264, 265
  diarrhea in, 177, 178
  hepatitis, 324–338
  inflammatory bowel disease in, 191, 198
  myxedema coma in, 261
  papillomavirus, 313–323
  pneumonia in, 163–174
  rhinitis in, 357–360
  sexually transmitted, 17, 18, 339–353
  sinusitis in, 365, 366–370
Infertility, 16
  body weight in, 547
  in inflammatory bowel disease, 200
Inflammation
  in acne, 475, 476
  in asthma, 119
  in lupus erythematosus, 461–462
  in osteoarthritis, 423, 429
  in rheumatoid arthritis, 438–439
Inflammatory bowel disease, 191–201
  arthritis in, 438
  cancer in, 7, 189, 196–197
  cholangitis in, primary sclerosing, 188
  complications of, 197
  Crohn's disease. *See* Crohn's disease
  diagnosis of, 193–194
  diarrhea in, 178
    in Crohn's disease, 178, 193, 195
    in ulcerative colitis, 178, 194
  etiology of, 191–193
  evaluation of clinical status in, 194–195
  and irritable bowel syndrome, 195
  and pregnancy, 199–200
    drug therapy in, 197, 198, 199–200
  and sexual function, 200
  symptomatic flares in, 195–196
  treatment of, 197–199
    in pregnancy, 197, 198, 199–200
  ulcerative colitis. *See* Colitis, ulcerative
Influenza, 358, 605–607
  amantadine or rimantidine in, 149, 605–607
  clinical presentation of, 605
  vaccination for, 149, 358, 605, 606t
    adverse reactions to, 605
    in chronic obstructive pulmonary disease, 149
    in elderly, 605
Inotropic agents in heart failure, 98, 99
Insomnia, 553, 562–564
  in alcohol use, 562, 566
  in anxiety, 562, 566
  in depression, 521, 562
  misperception of, 563
Insulin
  in diabetes mellitus, 266–267, 268
    and hypoglycemia, 273
    and ketoacidosis, 272
    methods of administration, 268–269
    and oral hypoglycemic agents, 270
    preparations of, 268, 268t
  resistance to, 28, 50
    in obesity, 282, 286
    in syndrome X, 28, 282
  secretion in hypoglycemia, 275–276
Insulinomas, 275, 276, 277
Interferons
  role in rheumatoid arthritis, 438, 439f
  therapy with
    in condylomata, 321t, 322
    in hepatitis, 326, 334t, 334–335
Interleukins
  in osteoarthritis, 426
  in rheumatoid arthritis, 438, 439f, 449
Intervertebral disc disease, degenerative, 427
Intrauterine contraceptive devices, 341
Iodide, 240
  hypothyroidism from, 250
Iodine, 240
  intake of, 240, 242
    in pregnancy, 256
  radioactive. *See* Radioiodine
Ipratropium bromide
  in asthma, 128t, 130
    nocturnal, 136

in pregnancy, 135
in chronic obstructive pulmonary disease, 146
in lung cancer, 161
in vasomotor rhinitis, 363
Iron deficiency, 206, 207–209
causes of, 208
differential diagnosis of, 209
laboratory values in, 206, 208, 208t
in rheumatoid arthritis, 443
Irritable bowel syndrome
abdominal pain in, 180
constipation in, 179
diarrhea in, 178
differential diagnosis of, 193
and endometriosis, 180
and inflammatory bowel disease, 195
Ischemia
mesenteric, 78, 79f
myocardial, angina pectoris in, 83, 84–85
optic neuropathy in, 390
ulcerations in, 68
Ischemic attacks, transient, 74
Islet cells of pancreas
in diabetes mellitus, 266–268
tumors of, 277
Isorbide dinitrate in heart failure, 97, 98
Isotretinoin therapy
in acne, 478
lipid levels in, 52
Isradipine in hypertension, 34t

J
Jaundice
in cholangiocarcinoma, 189
in cholangitis, primary sclerosing, 187
in gallbladder cancer, 189
in gallstones, 184
in pregnancy, 187
in hepatitis, 324, 326–327
in pregnancy, 331
Jet lag, 564–565

K
Katz Index of Activities of Daily Living, 604, 604t
Keratoacanthoma, 496
volcano appearance of, Plate 13, 496
Keratoconjunctivitis sicca in rheumatoid arthritis, 442–443
Keratoses, actinic, 493
Ketoacidosis, diabetic, 265, 266, 271–272
pathophysiology of, 268
Ketoconazole
in dermatitis, seborrheic, 487
in hirsutism, 306, 307
in tinea versicolor, 488
Kidney disorders
biopsy in, 457
bleeding disorders in, 215, 216, 227–228
in diabetes mellitus, 271, 274
in hepatitis, 327
hypertension in, 27, 28t
lipid abnormalities in, 51
lower extremity edema in, 610, 611
in lupus erythematosus, 456–457, 464t
management of, 466–467
and pregnancy, 467
prognosis in, 468
pneumonia in, 164, 168, 170
Kindling, in premenstrual syndrome, 503
Klebsiella infections, rhinoscleroma in, 359
Knee
osteoarthritis of, 6, 421, 423, 426–427, 435
treatment of, 431, 432, 433
rheumatoid arthritis of, 435, 436t, 441
treatment of, 447, 450
Koilocytes in papillomavirus infection, 313, 315, 315f, 316
Kussmaul's respirations, 265
Kveim test in sarcoidosis, 364
Kyphoscoliosis in mitral valve prolapse syndrome/dysautonomia, 107

L
Labetalol in hypertension, 33t
Lactation, 292
in hyperprolactinemia, 292
Lactotropes, 293, 294
Laparoscopy
cholecystectomy in, 186
in pregnancy, 187
in pelvic inflammatory disease, 347
Laryngeal disorders
differential diagnosis of, 122–123, 140
flow-volume loop in, 123f
wheezing in, 122–123
Laser therapy in condylomata, 321t, 322
Lassitude, 374
Lead poisoning, 209
Learning theory on substance abuse and addiction, 540
Leg. *See also* Lower extremity
in periodic limb movement disorder, 560–561, 563
in restless legs syndrome, 561, 563
Legionella infections, pneumonia in, 165, 168, 169, 172
treatment of, 168t, 169t, 170, 170t, 171t
Lentigo maligna melanoma, Plate 16, 497–498
Leptospirosis, 330
Leukemia, nose in, 365
Leukopenia, 210
in lupus erythematosus, 460, 466
Leuprolide acetate in hirsutism, 306
Levodopa in periodic limb movement disorder, 561
Levothyroxine, 251
metabolism of, 251
in thyroid nodules, 254
Libido in depression, 522
Libman-Sacks lesions, 458
Lidocaine in cluster headaches, 386
Life expectancy, 12–13
Life-style, 12–19
and cancer, 7
and coronary heart disease, 16, 56
exercise in, 16–17
and fatigue, 374, 375, 380
and headaches, 384, 392
and hypertension, 15, 16
modification of risk factors, 29t, 29–30, 39
and longevity, 12–13
nutrition in, 17
and obesity, 283, 285, 287–288
sexuality and contraception in, 17–18
and sexually transmitted diseases, 340
smoking in, 13–15
substance abuse in, 15–16, 541
support network in, 18–19
work environment in, 18
Light-headedness, in mitral valve prolapse syndrome/dysautonomia, 106, 108, 109
Lindane in scabies, 485
Linoleic acid in premenstrual syndrome, 509
Liothyronine, 251
Liotrix, 251
Lip carcinoma, squamous cell, Plate 8
Lipase levels in pancreatitis, 184
Lipid levels, 3–4, 44–65
in alcohol use, 50
in angina pectoris, 85, 86, 89
in atherosclerosis, 61–62, 71, 89
gender differences in, 3, 52–53
measurement of, 4, 54
as risk factor, 4, 52–53, 54
in autoimmune disorders, 51
in combined hyperlipidemia, familial, 48
in coronary heart disease. *See* Coronary heart disease, lipid levels in
in diabetes mellitus, 50, 53, 61
diet affecting, 4, 54, 55–56, 56t, 61, 89
drug-induced disorders of, 51–52
drugs lowering, 53, 56–60, 61, 89
in dyslipidemia, familial, 48
in elderly, 60–61
in estrogen therapy, 51–52, 57t, 60, 66, 71
in exercise, 55, 551
in hypercholesterolemia, familial, 47–48
in hyperchylomicronemia syndrome, 49
in hypertension, 3, 27t, 28
in hypertriglyceridemia, familial, 48
in hypoalphalipoproteinemia, familial, 48
in liver disease, 50
measurement of, 4, 46–47, 54
and metabolism, 44–46
in obesity, 49t, 50, 282, 286
phenotypic classification of disorders, 46–47, 47t
and choice of drug therapy, 58t
in pregnancy, 46, 53
primary disorders of, 47–49
in renal disorders, 51
screening of, 3–4, 54
secondary disorders of, 49t, 49–52
in syndrome X, 28, 282
therapy lowering, 53, 54, 55–60, 89
in thyroid disease, 50–51
in type III hyperlipidemia, 48
Lipodermatosclerosis, 611
Lipoprotein a, 46, 66
Lipoprotein lipase, 44
deficiency of, 49
Lipoproteins, 4, 44–65
in alcohol use, 50
in angina pectoris, 86, 89
characteristics of, 44, 45t
in combined hyperlipidemia, familial, 48
composition of, 44, 45f
in diabetes mellitus, 50, 61
drug-induced disorders of, 51–52
drug therapy lowering levels of, 56–60, 61
in dyslipidemia, familial, 48
in elderly, 60–61
in estrogen therapy, 51–52, 57t, 60, 66, 71
gender differences in, 52–53
high density, 4
in coronary heart disease, 46, 52–53, 61
isolated low levels of, 61
in hypercholesterolemia, familial, 47
in hyperchylomicronemia syndrome, 49
in hypertriglyceridemia, familial, 48
in hypoalphalipoproteinemia, familial, 48
low density, 4
measurement of, 4, 46–47, 54
metabolism of, 44–46, 50
nutrition affecting, 55–56, 61, 89
in obesity, 50, 282
in renal disorders, 51
in thyroid disease, 50–51
in type III hyperlipidemia, 48
very low density, 4
Lisinopril in hypertension, 33t, 39
Lithiasis. *See* Calculi
Lithium therapy
hypothyroidism in, 250
in premenstrual syndrome, 512

Lithotripsy, extracorporeal shock wave, 186
Livedo reticularis, 68, 456
Liver
  biopsy of, 330
  cancer of, 189, 190
    in hepatitis, 324–325
  chronic disease of, 335
  disorders of
    bleeding disorders in, 215, 216, 219
    differential diagnosis of, 188
    drug-induced, 330, 432, 446, 448, 449
    hypoglycemia in, 276
    lipid abnormalities in, 50
    lower extremity edema in, 610, 611
    in lupus erythematosus, 458–459
    pneumonia in, 164, 168, 170
  in drug metabolism, 608
  fatty, of pregnancy, 331
  fulminant failure of, 335
  function tests of, 329, 330
  hepatitis of, 324–338. *See also* Hepatitis
  hepatotoxicity of drugs, 330
    of anti-inflammatory drugs, 432, 446
    in rheumatoid arthritis, 448, 449
  in lipoprotein metabolism, 44, 50
  transplantation of, 324, 335
Longevity, and life-style, 12–13
Loop diuretics
  in heart failure, 98
  in hypertension, 31t, 35
Loperamide in diarrhea, 178
Lorazepam
  in anxiety disorders, 598t
  in mitral valve prolapse syndrome/dysautonomia, 109, 110
Lovastatin in lipid-lowering therapy, 57t, 59, 61
Lower extremity
  edema in elderly, 610–611
  in periodic limb movement disorder, 560–561, 563
  peripheral vascular disease of, 66, 67–72
  in restless legs syndrome, 561, 563
  venous thromboembolism of, 78–79, 79f
Lugol's solution in thyroid storm, 259
Lumbar canal stenosis, pseudoclaudication in, 67
Lumbar puncture
  headache in, 384, 385t, 386, 389
  in headaches, 390, 391
Lung
  abscess of, differential diagnosis of, 166
  in asthma, 119–138
  cancer of, 7, 154–162
    differential diagnosis of, 166
    early evaluation in, 157–159
    mortality rate in, 7, 7t, 154, 155f
    non-small cell, 156, 159–160
    pathogenesis of, 156–157
    physical examination in, 154–155
    risk factors in, 154, 156
    screening for, 155–156
    signs and symptoms of, 154, 156
    small cell, 156, 159
    staging and diagnosis of, 159, 160t
    treatment of, 159–162
    types of, 156
  edema of. *See* Edema, pulmonary
  embolism in, 84, 86, 123, 166, 173
  function tests of
    in asthma, 124f, 124–125, 125f, 126
    in chronic obstructive disease, 143, 144
    in lung cancer, 158–159
    in lupus erythematosus, 458
    in pregnancy, 132
    in rheumatoid arthritis, 443
  in hypertension, 27
  in lupus erythematosus, 457–458
  parenchymal abnormalities of, 158, 158f
  pneumonia of, 163–174
  rheumatoid nodules in, 442, 443
  transplantation of, 148
Lupus anticoagulant, 223, 225, 226, 232, 460
  and pregnancy, 234–235
Lupus erythematosus, 454–471
  autoantibodies in, 460–461, 461t, 462
  breast-feeding in, 468
  cardiovascular disorders in, 456, 457, 458
    prognosis in, 468–469
  clinical features of, 454–461
  constitutional symptoms of, 454
  coronary heart disease in, 458, 468–469
  diagnosis and assessment of, 463–465
    criteria in, 463, 464t
  differential diagnosis of, 437
  etiology and pathogenesis of, 461–463
  gastrointestinal disorders in, 458–459
  genetic factors in, 454, 462
  hematologic disorders in, 459–460, 464t, 466
  kidney disorders in, 456–457, 464t, 466–467
    in pregnancy, 467
    prognosis in, 468
  laboratory tests in, 460–461, 463, 465
  lung disease in, 457–458
  management of, 465–468
  musculoskeletal disorders in, 454–455, 466
  neonatal, 468
  neuropsychiatric disorders in, 459
  nose in, 365
  oral ulcers in, 456, 463, 464t, 466
  pleuropericardial disease in, 457, 466
  pregnancy in, 462, 467–468
  prevalence of, 454
  profundus, 456
  prognosis in, 468–469
  radiography in, 429
  skin in, 455–456, 463, 464t
    management of, 465–466
Lupus syndromes, drug-induced, 462–463
Lupus vulgaris, 359
Luteal phase of menstrual cycle
  dysphoric disorder in, 503, 505t
  premenstrual syndrome in, 503–517
  short, 547
Luteinizing hormone, 294
  in anorexia nervosa, 548, 549
  in exercise, 550
  in hirsutism, 304, 305, 306, 307
Lyme disease, 438
Lymphadenopathy, in sexually transmitted diseases, 343
Lymphangioleiomyomatosis, 141
Lymphocytic thyroiditis, 255
Lymphogranuloma venereum, 345, 348, 350–351
Lymphoma of thyroid gland, 249, 253

M

Macrocytic anemia, 205, 207t, 210–212, 212f
Magnetic resonance imaging
  angiographic, in peripheral vascular disease, 70, 71f, 74
  in headache, 385–386
  in hyperprolactinemia and pituitary tumors, 296f, 296–297, 297f, 300
  in osteoarthritis, 429
Malabsorption
  of calcium, osteoporosis in, 408, 413, 418
  diarrhea in, 178
  of iron, 209
Mallory-Weiss tear in bulimia, 549
Mammography in breast cancer screening, 8
Manic-depressive disorder, 524
Marfan's syndrome, 217
Marijuana, 15, 16, 545
Masoprocol in actinic keratoses, 493
Mastitis, cystic, in mitral valve prolapse syndrome/dysautonomia, 106, 108
Mastocytosis, 123
Maxillary sinus, 365–366
  infection of, 367, 367f
  purulent drainage from, Plate 5
Meclizine in mitral valve prolapse syndrome/dysautonomia, 110
Medroxyprogesterone
  in hirsutism, 306
  in osteoporosis, 417
  in premenstrual syndrome, 511, 514
Mefenamic acid in premenstrual syndrome, 509, 513
Megaloblastic anemia, 211
Melanoma, 8, 497–499
  ABCDs of diagnosis, Plate 14, 497, 498
  acral-lentiginous, Plate 15, 497
  lentigo maligna, Plate 16, 497–498
  mitosis in, 498–499
  nodular, 497
  regression of, 498
  site of, 498
  staging of, 498
  in sun exposure, 8, 493
  superficial spreading, 497
Melatonin in circadian rhythms, 555
Memory
  in aging, 614
  in depression, 521
Meningitis
  headache in, 385, 390, 394, 459
  in lupus erythematosus, 459, 466
Menopause
  bone mass in, 402, 403f
  coronary heart disease in, 53
  osteoporosis in, 407
  sleep disorders in, 557
Menstrual function
  in anorexia nervosa, 548, 549
  body weight affecting, 547, 550
  exercise affecting, 547, 550–551
  in hyperprolactinemia, 292, 295
  and premenstrual syndrome, 503–517
  stress affecting, 547, 550
Meperidine in headaches, 392t, 394, 394t
6-Mercaptopurine in inflammatory bowel disease, 199
Mesalamine in inflammatory bowel disease, 197–198
  intolerance of, 195, 198
  in pregnancy, 199
Mesenchymoid transformation in rheumatoid arthritis, 439
Mesenteric ischemia, 78, 79f
Metabolic syndrome, 282–283
Metabolism, 5–6
  disorders of
    anxiety in, 590t
    constipation in, 179
    hypertension therapy in, 35, 36, 40
  of drugs, age-related changes in, 608
  of lipoproteins, 44–46
  in obesity, 5–6, 279, 280, 282–283
  resting rate of, 280
Metalloproteinases, 424–426
  tissue inhibitors of, 426
Metaproterenol in asthma, 127, 128t
  in pregnancy, 134
Metastases
  of biliary system, 189–190
  of skin cancer, 495, 499

Methacholine challenge test in asthma, 124–125, 125f
Methimazole, 240
in hyperthyroidism, 246
in pregnancy, 257
side effects of, 246
Methotrexate in rheumatoid arthritis, 448
Methyclothiazide in hypertension, 31t
Methyldopa in hypertension, 34t, 37
Methylprednisolone
in asthma, 128t, 130
in pregnancy, 135
in lupus erythematosus, 466
Methylxanthines
in asthma, 128t
in pregnancy, 135
in chronic obstructive pulmonary disease, 146–147
Methysergide in migraine prevention, 396
Metoclopramide
in headaches, 392t, 393, 394t
in mitral valve prolapse syndrome/ dysautonomia, 109
in pregnancy, 393
Metolazone
in heart failure, 98
in hypertension, 31t, 36
Metoprolol in hypertension, 32t, 36
Metronidazole
in diarrhea, 178
in inflammatory bowel disease, 198–199
in pregnancy, 199–200
Microcytic anemia, 205, 207t
hypochromic, 206–210, 207f
Migraine, 384, 386–388
aura in, 387, 388
compared to cluster headaches, 386, 386t
equivalent, 386, 388t
headache phase in, 387–388
and hypertension therapy, 37
in mitral valve prolapse syndrome/ dysautonomia, 106, 107
onset and causes of, 386–387
pain in, 386
prevention of, 395t, 395–396
spreading depression hypothesis on, 387
and stroke, 388
and tension headaches, 389
treatment of, 392, 393, 394
vascular hypothesis on, 387, 388
Mikulicz's cells, 359
Milrinone in heart failure, 98
Mini-Mental State Examination, 615t, 615–616
Minoxidil in hypertension, 34t
Miscarriage, recurrent, in lupus erythematosus, 468
Mites
and allergic rhinitis, 361
and asthma, 121, 126
and rosacea, 482
and scabies, 483–485
Mitosis in melanoma, 498–499
Mitral valve prolapse and dysautonomia syndrome, 104–115. *See also* Dysautonomia
Mohs' microscopic surgery in skin cancer, 494, 495, 496
Molds, indoor, 126
Molluscum contagiosum, 319, 478–480
giant atypical lesions in, 479, 479f
Monoamine oxidase inhibitors
in anxiety disorders, 598t
in depression, 529, 530t
in migraine prevention, 396
Mononeuritis multiplex in lupus erythematosus, 459
Mononucleosis, 330, 373
Mood changes, 503
differential diagnosis of, 525
in premenstrual syndrome, 503
treatment of, 513–514
Moraxella infections, pneumonia in, 169t, 170t, 171t
Morphine in pulmonary edema, 96
Mortality rates
in asthma, 120, 120f
blood pressure affecting, 29, 29f
in cancer, 7, 7t
of lung, 7, 7t, 154, 155f
in cardiovascular disorders, 29f, 44
in chronic obstructive pulmonary disease, 139
in gallstones and pregnancy, 187
life-style factors affecting, 12–13
in pneumonia, 163, 164, 164t, 168–169
Mouth
headache in dental disease, 384
squamous cell of lip, Plate 8
ulcers of, in lupus erythematosus, 456, 463, 464t
management of, 466
Mucolytics
in chronic obstructive pulmonary disease, 148
in sinusitis, 368
Mucormycosis, 360
Multinodular goiter, 254
toxic, 246–247
Multiple endocrine neoplasia, 275
Multiple sclerosis, depression in, 522, 523
Munchausen's syndrome, 178–179
Murmurs. *See* Heart sounds
Murphy's sign, 184
Musculoskeletal disorders
in diabetes mellitus, 266, 271
in lupus erythematosus, 454–455, 466
in obesity, 282
in osteoarthritis, 421–434. *See also* Osteoarthritis
in osteopenia, 401
in osteoporosis, 401–420. *See also* Osteoporosis
in rheumatoid arthritis, 435–453. *See also* Rheumatoid arthritis
tension headache in, 389
Myalgia
fibromyalgia, 389, 437
in mitral valve prolapse syndrome/ dysautonomia, 106
sleep disorders in, 557
polymyalgia rheumatica, 437
tension, 389
Mycobacterial infections
inflammatory bowel disease in, 191
pneumonia in, 163, 165, 168, 172
treatment of, 168t, 169t, 170t, 171t
tuberculosis in, 359
Mycoplasma infections, pneumonia in, 163, 168, 169
history of patient in, 164
pathophysiology in, 167
radiography in, 166
treatment of, 168t, 170, 170t, 171t
Myelitis in lupus erythematosus, 459, 466
Myeloma, multiple, nose in, 365
Myocardial disorders
angina pectoris in, 83, 84–85
in lupus erythematosus, 458
Myoclonus, nocturnal, 560
Myositis
fibromyositis, 389
polymyositis, 460
Myxedema, 244, 248
coma in, 259–261
precipitating factors in, 259, 260

N
Nadolol
in hypertension, 32t, 36
in migraine prevention, 395, 395t
in mitral valve prolapse syndrome/ dysautonomia, 109
Naltrexone in premenstrual syndrome, 512
Nandrolone decanoate in osteoporosis, 417
Naproxen
in migraine prevention, 395t, 396
in premenstrual syndrome, 509, 513
in rebound headaches, 389
Narcissistic personality disorder, 580–581
differential diagnosis of, 580, 581
Narcolepsy, 553, 559–560
Narcotic drugs
abuse of, 544–545
in elderly, 609t, 610
in headaches, 392t, 394
Nasal disorders, 357–365. *See also* Nose
Nausea and vomiting
antiemetic drugs in
in elderly, 609t
in migraine, 392t, 393
in diabetes mellitus, 264–265, 272
differential diagnosis of, 264–265
Neck
examination in hypertension, 27
pain in, and headache, 385, 386, 389
rheumatoid arthritis of, 442
radiography in, 445–446
treatment in, 450
Necrosis
osteonecrosis
of hip, 441
in lupus erythematosus, 455
of pituitary gland, postpartum, 250
Nedocromil sodium in asthma, 128t, 129t, 130
Needle stick injury, hepatitis in, 332, 333–334
Neisseria infections, 340t
arthritis in, 348, 437
cervicitis in, 345, 346, 346t
disseminated, 348, 437, 455
gonorrhea in. *See* Gonorrhea
Neonates. *See also* Children and infants
acne in, 476
hepatitis in, 324, 325–326, 331–332, 333–334
prevention of, 331, 333–334
hypothyroidism in, 244, 258
lupus erythematosus in, 468
nevi in, 497
sleep of, 554
Neoplasms. *See* Cancer
Nephritis, in lupus erythematosus, 456–457, 462
management of, 466–467
and pregnancy, 467
Nephrotic syndrome
lipid abnormalities in, 51
lower extremity edema in, 610, 611
in lupus erythematosus, 457
Nesidioblastosis, hypoglycemia in, 275, 276
Neuralgia, trigeminal, 390
Neurasthenia, 373
Neurohumoral mechanisms in heart failure, 91, 92, 93
Neurologic disorders, 371–397
Alzheimer's disease in, 4–5, 614–615
anxiety in, 590t
constipation in, 179
depression in, 522, 523
dermatitis in, seborrheic, 486
in diabetes mellitus, 264, 265, 266, 271
and hypoglycemia, 273

Neurologic disorders (*Continued*)
  fatigue in, chronic, 373–383
  headaches in, 384–397
  in hypertension, 27
  in lupus erythematosus, 459, 464t
  in mitral valve prolapse syndrome/dysautonomia, 106
  in osteoarthritis of spine, 427
  in rheumatoid arthritis, 442
  in syphilis, 614
Neuroretinopathy of hypertension, 26
Neurosyphilis, 614
Neurotransmitters
  in depression, 525
  in premenstrual syndrome, 503, 512
Nevus, 497
Niacin, in lipid-lowering therapy, 57t, 59, 61
Nicardipine in hypertension, 34t
Nicotine replacement therapy in smoking cessation, 14, 15, 145
Nicotinic acid, in lipid-lowering therapy, 57t, 59, 61
Nifedipine
  in angina pectoris, 88
  in hypertension, 34t, 38
Nitrates
  in angina pectoris, 83, 87–88
  in heart failure, 96, 97, 98–99
  in pulmonary edema, 96
Nitroglycerin
  in angina pectoris, 83, 87, 88
  in heart failure, 96, 99
  in pulmonary edema, 96
Nitroprusside in pulmonary edema, 96
Nizatidine in mitral valve prolapse syndrome/dysautonomia, 109
Nodules
  in acne, 475, 476, 476f
  apple jelly, 359
  in lupus erythematosus, 456
  in melanoma, 497
  rheumatoid, 442, 443
  in scabies, 484, 485
  of thyroid gland. *See* Thyroid gland, nodules of
Nonoxynol-9, 341
Norepinephrine
  in depression, 525
  in mitral valve prolapse syndrome/dysautonomia, 114
  reuptake inhibitors, 529, 529t, 531t
Norethindrone
  in hirsutism, 306
  in osteoporosis, 417
Nortriptyline
  in anxiety disorders, 598t
  in depression, 530t, 533, 534t
  in migraine prevention, 395, 395t
Norwegian scabies, 484, 485f
Nose, 357–365
  in allergies, 360–363
  anatomy of, 357
  in autoimmune connective tissue disorders, 365
  bacterial infections of, 358–360
  blood supply of, 357
  drug-induced disorders of, 363–364
  external, 357
  fungal infections of, 360
  lateral wall of, 357
  in leukemia, 365
  nerve supply of, 357
  polyps of, Plate 6, 364, 367
    sinusitis in, 367, 369, 370
  rhinitis of, 357–364
  rhinoscleroma of, 359
  in sarcoidosis, 364–365
  septum of, 357
  trauma of, 364
  viral infections of, 357–358
  in Wegener's granulomatosis, 365
Nutrition, 12, 13, 17
  in anorexia nervosa, 548, 549
  in atherosclerosis, 71
  in bulimia, 549
  caloric intake in, 17, 280–281, 286–287
    in low calorie diet, 287
    in very low calorie diet, 286–287
  in cholangitis, primary sclerosing, 187, 188
  and cholesterol levels, 4, 5, 54, 55–56, 89
    in elderly, 61
  in chronic obstructive pulmonary disease, 149
  and colorectal cancer, 7
  in constipation, 179
  in coronary heart disease, 17, 54, 55–56, 56t, 89
    in elderly, 61
  in depression, 521–522
  in diabetes mellitus, 269, 269t, 270
    and hypoglycemia, 273
  in gallstones, 183
  and headaches, 387
  in hypertension, 25–26, 30, 38
  in hypoglycemia, 273, 276
  in inflammatory bowel disease, 192, 195, 199
  in insomnia, 564
  in iron deficiency, 207
  in irritable bowel syndrome, 180
  in lipid disorders, 4, 54, 55–56, 56t, 89
    in elderly, 61
  and menstrual function, 547, 550
  in mitral valve prolapse syndrome/dysautonomia, 106, 108, 111, 111f
  and mortality rates, 12
  in obesity, 17, 280–281, 286–287, 288
    and weight loss program, 285, 286–287
  in osteoporosis, 407, 408, 419
  in premenstrual syndrome, 510
  and prolactin levels, 295, 295f
  in rheumatoid arthritis, 449
  and thermic effect of food, 280
  vitamin deficiencies in, 212, 216, 225, 408

O

Obesity, 5–6, 12, 17, 278–291
  abdominal, 282–283, 286
  behavioral modification in, 286, 287
  clinical presentation of, 278–279
  complications of, 281–283
  definition of, 5–6, 278, 279
  differential diagnosis of, 279–280
  etiology of, 280–281
  fatigue in, 375
  heart failure in, 97
  history of patient in, 283, 284
  and hypertension, 28, 50, 282
  hypoventilation syndrome in, 282
  incidence of, 5, 278
  laboratory studies in, 285
  lipid levels in, 49t, 50, 282
    in weight loss, 286
  metabolism in, 5–6, 279, 280, 282–283
  nutrition in, 17, 280–281, 288
    in weight loss program, 285, 286–287
  osteoarthritis in, 282, 421
  physical examination in, 283, 284
  pregnancy in, 283, 288
  risk factors in, 6, 281
  sleep apnea in, 282, 285, 558
  in syndrome X, 28, 282
  weight loss in, 285–289
    benefits of, 286
    measures of success, 289
    risks of, 285–286
Obsessions, 594, 595
Obsessive compulsive disorder, 591, 593t, 594–595
  compared to obsessive compulsive personality disorder, 583
  prevalence of, 586, 587t
  treatment of, 593t, 595, 597
Obsessive compulsive personality disorder, 582–583
  compared to obsessive compulsive disorder, 583
  differential diagnosis of, 581, 583
Obstructive pulmonary disease, chronic, 139–153. *See also* Pulmonary disorders, chronic obstructive disease
Occupation. *See* Work
Occupational therapy in rheumatoid arthritis, 449
Olsalazine in inflammatory bowel disease, 198
Oncogenes in lung cancer, 156–157
Ophthalmopathy, in Graves' disease, 244
Ophthalmoplegic migraine, 388t
Opiates
  abuse of, 544–545
  endogenous, in premenstrual syndrome, 511–512
  therapy with, in headaches, 392t, 394
Optic neuropathy, ischemic, 390
Oral cavity. *See* Mouth
Organic brain syndrome, in lupus erythematosus, 459, 466
Orthopnea in heart failure, 94
Orthostatic hypotension
  in diabetes mellitus, 266
  in mitral valve prolapse syndrome/dysautonomia, 109
Osteoarthritis, 6–7, 421–434
  bone density in, 422–423
  classification of, 423t, 423–424
  clinical features of, 6–7, 426–428, 427f, 427t
  differential diagnosis of, 435–437
  drug therapy in, 7, 431–432
  erosive, 423, 429, 429f
  etiopathogenesis of, 6, 422f, 424–426
  gender differences in, 6, 421
  generalized, 423, 429
  genetic factors in, 423
  inflammatory, 423, 429
  laboratory tests in, 428, 428t
  in obesity, 282, 421
  pathology of, 424
  physical therapy in, 431
  prevalence of, 6, 421
  primary, 423t, 423–424, 429
  radiography in, 428t, 428–431, 429f, 430f
  seagull sign in, 429, 429f
  secondary, 423, 423t, 424, 429
  surgery in, 432–433
Osteoblasts, declining function of, 408
Osteomyelitis, in sinusitis, 368
Osteonecrosis
  of hip, 441
  in lupus erythematosus, 455
Osteopenia, 401, 429
Osteoporosis, 401–420
  antiresorptive agents in, 415, 416f
  bone turnover in, 406, 406f
    assessment of, 412–413
  clinical presentation of, 408–410
  definition of, 401
  diagnosis of, 410f, 410–414
  estrogen therapy in, 407, 415–416, 420
  etiology of, 407–408
  exercise in, 415, 419
  fluoride in, 418, 419
  fragility of bones in, 406–407
  hip fractures in, 408, 409

involutional, 401, 402, 403t
management of, 414–420
measurement of bone mass in, 410–412
pain in, 409–410, 414
parathyroid hormone in, 408, 413, 418–419
pathogenesis of changes in, 402–406, 403f
prevention of changes in, 419–420
primary, 401
progestins in, 416–417
risk for fractures in, 406–407
secondary, 401, 402t
differential diagnosis of, 413–414
of spine. *See* Spine, osteoporosis of
threshold for fractures in, 402, 404
trabecular disconnectivity in, 405f, 407
type I, 401, 403t, 407
type II, 401, 403t, 408
vertebral compression deformity in, 408–409, 409f, 410, 410f
Osteotomy, in osteoarthritis, 432–433
Otolaryngology, 355–370
nasal disorders, 357–365
sinus disorders, 365–370
Ovary
cancer of, 9, 18
androgen-producing, 304
hyperthecosis of, hirsutism in, 304
polycystic, 304f
hirsutism in, 304
Overweight, definition of, 278
Oximetry, transcutaneous, in peripheral vascular disease, 70
Oxygen therapy
in chronic obstructive pulmonary disease, 148
in cluster headaches, 386
in pneumonia, 170
in pregnancy, 172–173
in pulmonary edema, 96

P
Pain
abdominal. *See* Abdominal pain
in angina pectoris, 83, 84
in biliary colic, 182
in chest. *See* Chest pain
in cholangitis, primary sclerosing, 187
in cholelithiasis, 182, 184
chronic, 177
in gastrointestinal disorders, 177, 180
headaches in, 389, 395–396
in claudication, intermittent, 67
in Crohn's disease, 193
in headaches, 384–397
chronic, 389, 395–396
in irritable bowel syndrome, 180
in lung cancer, 154, 161
in lupus erythematosus, 457, 458
in mesenteric ischemia, 78
in osteoarthritis, 6
management of, 431, 432, 433
in osteoporosis, 409–410, 414
pleuritic, 457
in pneumonia, 164
in premenstrual syndrome, 503, 509, 513, 513t
psychoactive substance use in, 542, 544
in rheumatoid arthritis, 435, 446–447, 449
in thyroiditis, 255
subacute, 254
in trigeminal neuralgia, 390
in ulcerative colitis, 194
in venous thromboembolism, 78, 79
Palate disorders in lupus erythematosus, 456
Palsy, cranial nerve
in diabetes mellitus, 265
and headache, 388t, 389, 391
Pancreatic islet cells
in diabetes mellitus, 266–268
tumors of, 277
Pancreatitis
differential diagnosis of, 183
gallstone, 183, 184, 185
in pregnancy, 187
in hyperchylomicronemia syndrome, 49
in hypertriglyceridemia, 61
in lupus erythematosus, 459
Panic attacks, 592, 596
and agoraphobia, 594
and depression, 590
Panic disorders, 592–594, 593t
in mitral valve prolapse syndrome/dysautonomia, 105, 109
in pregnancy, 597
prevalence of, 586, 587t
in primary care setting, 587
screening for, 587
treatment of, 592–594, 593t, 596, 597
Panniculitis, nodular, in lupus erythematosus, 456
Pannus, in rheumatoid arthritis, 439
Pap smear, 351
in cervical cancer, 8, 9
in papillomavirus infection, 313, 315, 320
Papillomatosis, respiratory, in infants and children, 314, 323
Papillomavirus infections, 313–323
Bowenoid papulosis in, 318, 496
and cancer, 313, 315–317, 316f
clinical manifestations of, 317–319
and contraceptive methods, 322, 341
differential diagnosis of, 319
epidemiology of, 313–314
evaluation of, 319–320
in infants and children, 314, 323
latent, 318
natural history of, 314
pathogenesis and pathology of, 314–317
prevention of, 322–323
transmission of, 314, 323
treatment of, 320–322, 321t
types of, 313, 314t
of vulva and vagina, 318, 318f
Papules
Bowenoid, 318, 496
in rosacea, 482, 482f, 483
in scabies, 484, 484f
Papulosis, Bowenoid, 318, 496
Parafollicular cells, 239
Paralysis, sleep, 559, 560
Paranasal sinuses, 365–370
anatomy of, 365–366
infections of, 365, 366–370
pain over, 386
Paranoid personality disorder, 575, 576
Parasitic infections, sexually transmitted, 340t, 344
Parasomnias, 561–562
Parathyroid disorders, osteoporosis in, 408, 413
Parathyroid hormone in osteoporosis, 408, 413, 418–419
Parkinson's disease
constipation in, 179
drug therapy in, 298
Paroxetine
in anxiety disorders, 598t
in depression, 530, 530t, 533, 534t
Passive aggressive personality disorder, 583–584
Peer group influence in psychoactive substance use, 539
Pelvic examination, 343
Pelvic inflammatory disease, 341, 342, 347–348, 348t
diagnosis of, 347–348, 348t
risk factors in, 347
Pemphigus erythematosus, 487
Penbutolol in hypertension, 32t
D-Penicillamine in rheumatoid arthritis, 448–449
Penicillin
in pneumonia, 169t
in pregnancy, 173
in sinusitis, 368
in syphilis, 359, 360
Pentoxiphylline in peripheral vascular disease, 71
Pergolide mesylate in hyperprolactinemia, 297, 298
Pericarditis, 86
chest pain in, 84
in lupus erythematosus, 457
Periodic limb movement disorder, 560–561, 563
Peripartum cardiomyopathy, 99–100
Peripheral vascular disease, 66–82
abdominal aortic, 77–78
arterial atherosclerosis, 66–78
brachiocephalic, 72–77
in diabetes mellitus, 66–67, 265, 271
lower extremity, 66, 67–72
physical examination in, 68–69
venous thromboembolism, 66, 78–80
Permethrin in scabies, 485
Personality disorders, 573–585
antisocial, 577–578
differential diagnosis of, 577–578, 580, 581
anxiety in, 585, 592
in avoidant disorder, 581, 582, 592
in borderline disorder, 578, 592
in dependent disorder, 582, 592
in schizotypal disorder, 576, 577
avoidant, 581–582, 592
differential diagnosis of, 576, 577, 581–582
borderline. *See* Borderline personality disorder
causes of, 574
cluster A, 574–577
cluster B, 574, 577–581
cluster C, 574, 581–584
definition of, 573–574
dependent, 580, 582, 592
histrionic, 579–580
differential diagnosis of, 579, 580, 581, 582, 584
narcissistic, 580–581
obsessive compulsive, 581, 582–583
paranoid, 575, 576
passive aggressive, 583–584
referrals in, 584–585
schizoid, 575–576
differential diagnosis of, 576, 577, 581–582, 583
schizotypal, 576–577
and sleep disorders, 558, 566
substance abuse and addiction in, 539, 577–578, 579, 584–585
temperament and character in, 574
Personality traits, 573
Petechiae, 217
Pharyngitis
chlamydial, 343
in gonorrhea, 345
Phencyclidine, 543
Phenelzine
in anxiety disorders, 598t
in migraine prevention, 396
Phenobarbital in mitral valve prolapse syndrome/dysautonomia, 109
Phenothiazine therapy, lipid levels in, 52
Phenotypes, in lipid disorders, 46–47, 47t
and choice of drug therapy, 58t
Phenylpropanolamine hydrochloride in allergic rhinitis, 362
Pheochromocytoma, hypertension in, 28t

Phobias, 596
  agoraphobia, 582, 593t, 594, 596
    prevalence of, 586, 587t
  simple, 593t, 594
    prevalence of, 586, 587t
  social, 582, 593t, 594
    prevalence of, 586, 587t
  treatment of, 596, 597
Photodamage, skin cancer in, 8, 492–493
  basal cell, 493–494
  squamous cell, 495
Photoprotection, 493
  sunscreens in, 8, 493
Photosensitivity in lupus erythematosus, 455, 463, 464t, 465
Physical therapy
  in falls of elderly, 613
  in osteoarthritis, 431
  in rheumatoid arthritis, 449
Pigmentation
  in basal cell carcinoma of skin, 494
  of gallstones, 183–184, 186
  in melanoma, 497, 498
  in tinea versicolor, 487, 487f
Pindolol in hypertension, 32t, 36
Pink puffers, 139, 142
Pirbuterol in asthma, 127, 128t
Pituitary gland
  adenoma of
    hyperprolactinemia in, 292–300
    hyperthyroidism in, 247
    hypothyroidism in, 250
    long-term management in, 299f, 299–300, 300f
    pregnancy in, 299
    radiography in, 296–297
    surgery in, 297–298
    visual fields in, 296, 296f
  postpartum necrosis of, 250
  prolactin secretion of, 292–295
  in thyroid regulation, 240
Pityriasis rosea, 480–482
  herald patch in, 481, 481f
Pityrosporum infection
  seborrheic dermatitis in, 486
  tinea versicolor in, 487, 488
Plasma, fresh frozen, 230
Plasminogen, 219, 220
  deficiency of, 232
Plasminogen activator, tissue, 219, 426
Platelets, 218
  adhesion and aggregation of, 218
  count of, 223
    normal, bleeding in, 226, 227
  disorders of, 217t, 227–228
    acquired, 215–216, 227–228
    congenital, 215
    drug-induced, 216, 227
    signs of, 217
    treatment of, 229
  storage pool diseases, 215, 227
  transfusion of, 230–231
Pleural effusions. *See* Effusions, pleural
Pleuropericardial disease in lupus erythematosus, 457, 466
Pneumococcal disease, 607
  vaccination for, 149, 607
Pneumocystis infections, pneumonia in, 165, 172
Pneumonia, 163–174
  atypical, 163
  community-acquired, 163–174
  differential diagnosis of, 166–167
    in pregnancy, 173
  eosinophilic, 167
  history of patient in, 163–164
  hospitalization in, 168–169, 170t
  laboratory tests in, 165–166
  in lung cancer, 154
  mortality rate in, 163, 164, 164t, 168–169
  organizing, and bronchiolitis obliterans, 166–167
  pathophysiology of, 167–168
  physical examination in, 164–165
  pneumococcal, 607
  in pregnancy, 172–173
  presentation of, 163–164
  radiography in, 166
    resolution of abnormalities, 171–172
  risk factors in, 164, 164t, 165
  severe, 169
  treatment of, 168t, 169t, 169–172
    duration of therapy in, 170–171
    in pregnancy, 172–173
  typical, 163
Pneumonitis, in lupus erythematosus, 457–458, 466
Podophyllin in condylomata, 321, 321t, 322
Podophyllotoxin in condylomata, 321, 321t
Poisoning. *See* Toxicity
Polychondritis, relapsing, nose in, 365
Polycystic ovary syndrome, 304f
  hirsutism in, 304
Polymerase chain reaction techniques
  in cervicitis, 347
  in papillomavirus infections, 320
Polymyalgia rheumatica, 437
Polymyositis, 460
Polyps, nasal, Plate 6, 364, 367
  sinusitis in, 367, 369, 370
Polysomnography
  in narcolepsy, 560
  in sleep apnea, 558, 559
Polythiazide in hypertension, 31t
Popliteal artery atherosclerosis, 67
Popliteal cyst, 441
Postcholecystectomy syndrome, 187
Postoperative disorders
  in cholecystectomy, 187
  in chronic obstructive pulmonary disease, 143, 144
  in lung cancer, 161–162
Postpartum period
  depression in, 519, 524, 556
    drug therapy in, 531
  pituitary necrosis in, 250
  sleep in, 556
  thyroiditis in, 255–256
Post-traumatic stress disorder, 593t, 595, 596
  treatment of, 593t, 595, 596, 597
Postural hypotension
  in diabetes mellitus, 266
  in mitral valve prolapse syndrome/dysautonomia, 109
Potassium
  dietary, in hypertension, 30
  diuretics sparing, in hypertension, 31t–32t, 35, 36
  serum levels of
    in arrhythmias, 35
    in diabetic ketoacidosis, 272
    in diuretic therapy, 35, 36, 97–98
    in hyperosmolar hyperglycemic coma, 273
    in hypertension, 3, 27t, 28, 35, 36
  supplementation of, in diuretic therapy, 32t, 35, 36
Pravastatin in lipid-lowering therapy, 57t, 59
Prazosin
  in heart failure, 97
  in hypertension, 33t, 37
Prednisolone in asthma, 128t, 130
  in pregnancy, 135
Prednisone
  in asthma, 128t, 130
    in pregnancy, 135
  in chronic obstructive pulmonary disease, 148
  in hirsutism, 306, 307
  in inflammatory bowel disease, 197
  in lung cancer, 161
  in lupus anticoagulant and pregnancy, 234
  in lupus erythematosus, 465, 466
    and pregnancy, 467, 468
  in polymyalgia rheumatica, 437
  in rheumatoid arthritis, 447
  in rhinitis
    allergic, 362
    medicamentosa, 364
Pre-eclampsia in lupus erythematosus, 467
Pregnancy, 17, 18
  acne in, 477, 478
  airway responsiveness in, 132, 132f
  in anorexia nervosa, 548
  anticoagulant therapy in, 234, 235
  anxiety disorders in, 597
  asthma in, 131–135
  cardiomyopathy in, peripartum, 99–100
  coagulation in, 219
    disorders of, 216, 218, 229, 230
    disseminated intravascular, 231
  and contraceptive methods, 18, 341, 342
  and coronary heart disease risk, 53
  depression in, 519
    drug therapy in, 531, 533
  and diabetes mellitus, 267t, 270, 273
  fatty liver of, 331
  gallstones in, 184, 185, 186–187
  gonococcal infection in, disseminated, 348
  headaches in, 387, 393, 394, 395, 396
  in hemophilia, 228
  in hepatitis, 324, 325–326, 330–332, 333–334
  in hyperprolactinemia, 299
  and inflammatory bowel disease, 199–200
    drug therapy in, 197, 198, 199–200
  lipid levels in, 46, 53
  in lupus anticoagulant, 234–235
  in lupus erythematosus, 462, 467–468
    recurrent miscarriage in, 468
  in obesity, 283
    bypass surgery affecting, 288
  and papillomavirus infection, 314, 318, 321, 323
  pneumonia in, 172–173
  rhinitis in, 363
  scabies in, 484f, 485
  screening for sexually transmitted diseases in, 351
  sleep in, 555–557
    and apnea, 556–557
  thrombosis in, 233, 234
  thyroid gland in, 256–258
    fetal, 239, 240
    nodules of, 243, 253
    and thyroid storm, 259
  in von Willebrand's disease, 228, 229
  weight gain in, 17, 281, 283
Premenstrual syndrome, 503–517
  androgens in, 511
  diagnosis of, 505–506
    criteria in, 505t
  differential diagnosis of, 504–505
  estrogen and progesterone levels in, 510–511, 514
  etiologies of, 506–512
  evaluation of, 504, 505
  exercise in, 510, 513
  fluid retention and bloating in, 503, 510, 513, 513t

glucose levels in, 510
gonadotropin-releasing hormone agonists in, 511, 514
in mitral valve prolapse syndrome/ dysautonomia, 106, 107
natural history of, 514
nutrition in, 510
opiate levels in, 511–512
prolactin levels in, 510
prostaglandins in, 509
psychiatric theories and treatment in, 512, 513–514
pyridoxine in, 506
referrals in, 514
risk factors in, 506
serotonin deficiency in, 512
symptoms of, 503–504
daily log of, 506, 507f
graphic representation of, 509f
self-rating scale on, 506, 508f
treatment of, 512–514, 513t
cost of, 513t
long-term, 514
Preoperative assessment
in chronic obstructive pulmonary disease, 143–144
in lung cancer, 158–159
Prethrombotic conditions, 231–235
Primary care setting, anxiety disorders in, 586–588
PRIME-MD, 587
Prinzmetal's angina, 83, 86, 88
Probucol in lipid-lowering therapy, 57t, 60
Prochlorperazine in headaches, 389, 394t
Progesterone
deficiency of, premenstrual syndrome in, 510–511
therapy with
lipid levels in, 66
in premenstrual syndrome, 511
Progestin therapy
lipid levels in, 51–52
in menstrual-associated sleep disorder, 557
in osteoporosis, 416–417
Progestogen therapy in hirsutism, 305–306
Prolactin secretion
biology of, 292–295
breast examination affecting, 295, 295f
evaluation of, 295–297
food intake affecting, 295, 295f
in hyperprolactinemia, 292–301
in premenstrual syndrome, 510
Prolactinomas, 294–295
drug therapy in, 298
radiation therapy in, 298–299
radiography in, 296–297
Promethazine
in headaches, 392t, 393, 394t
in pregnancy, 393
Propionibacterium acnes, 475, 477
Propoxyphene in elderly, 609t
Propranolol
in anxiety disorders, 598t
in hypertension, 32t, 36
in hyperthyroidism, 245, 257, 259
in migraine prevention, 395, 395t
in pregnancy, 257, 395
in social phobia, 594
Proprioception, and falls in elderly, 612
Propylene glycol in tinea versicolor, 488
Propylthiouracil
actions of, 240
in hyperthyroidism, 246
in pregnancy, 257
and thyroid storm, 259
Prostaglandins, in premenstrual syndrome, 509
Protein C, 219, 220, 220t
deficiency of, 232
Protein S, 219, 220, 220t
deficiency of, 232
Proteinuria
in diabetes mellitus, 271
in lupus erythematosus, 456, 457
and pregnancy, 467
Proteoglycans in osteoarthritis, 424, 426
Prothrombin, 220, 220t
Prothrombin time, 221
normal, bleeding in, 226, 227
prolonged, 224–225, 226
Proto-oncogenes in lung cancer, 156–157
Protozoan infections, sexually transmitted, 340t
Protriptyline, in sleep apnea and pregnancy, 556
Protrusio acetabuli, 441
Pruritus
in cholangitis, primary sclerosing, 187, 188
in pityriasis rosea, 480, 481–482
in scabies, 483, 484, 485
in seborrheic dermatitis, 485, 486
in tinea versicolor, 487
in xerosis, 489
Pseudoclaudication, 67
Pseudodementia, depressive, 521
Pseudoephedrine hydrochloride in allergic rhinitis, 362
Pseudogout, 437–438
Pseudotumor cerebri, headache in, 390–391
Psoriasis
arthritis in, 429, 438
differential diagnosis of, 486–487
Psychiatry, 501–600
Psychoactive substances, 538. *See also* Substance abuse and addiction
Psychogenic amenorrhea, 547
Psychological factors, 501–600
in anxiety and anxiety disorders, 586–600. *See also* Anxiety and anxiety disorders
in chronic fatigue, 373–374, 375–376, 377, 378
evaluation of, 379–380
in depression, 518–537. *See also* Depression
in eating disorders, 547–552
in headaches, 384, 392
migraine, 386–387
in hypoglycemia, 276
in irritable bowel syndrome, 180
in lupus erythematosus, 459
in mitral valve prolapse syndrome/ dysautonomia, 104, 105, 106
management of, 109, 110
in narcolepsy, 560
in obesity, 283, 286
in personality disorders, 573–585. *See also* Personality disorders
in premenstrual syndrome, 512, 513–514
in rheumatoid arthritis, 449
in sleep disorders, 553–572
in substance abuse and addiction, 538–546
Psychotic depression, 523
Psychotropic drugs in premenstrual syndrome, 503, 512
Psyllium in constipation, 179
Puberty, acne in, 475, 476
Pulmonary disorders, 119–174
anxiety in, 590t
asthma, 119–138
chronic obstructive disease, 139–153
differential diagnosis of, 123, 140–141
natural history and prognosis in, 149–150
pathogenesis of, 141–142
physical examination in, 142
pneumonia in, 163, 168
presentation of, 139–140, 140t
treatment of, 144–149
workup in, 142–144
in heart failure, 94, 95
in hypertension, 27
lung cancer, 154–162
in lupus erythematosus, 457–458
in mitral valve prolapse syndrome/ dysautonomia, 106
in myxedema coma, 260
in obesity, 282, 285
pneumonia, 163–174
postoperative, 143, 144
preoperative assessment in, 143–144
in rheumatoid arthritis, 443
Pulsus paradoxus in asthma, 124
Purpura, 217
self-induced, 217, 227
Pustules, facial, in rosacea, 482, 482f, 483
Pyridoxine in premenstrual syndrome, 506

Q
Quinapril in hypertension, 33t, 39
Quinethazone in hypertension, 31t

R
Radiation therapy
in lung cancer, 160
in pituitary adenoma and hyperprolactinemia, 297, 298–299
in skin cancer, 495, 496
Radioactive iodine. *See* Radioiodine
Radioallergosorbent test (RAST), in rhinitis, 361, 363
Radiography
in asthma, 125
in chronic obstructive pulmonary disease, 142–143
in gallstones, 184–185
in heart failure, 95
in hyperprolactinemia, 296–297
in hypertension, 27t, 28
in lung cancer, 155, 157, 158
in osteoarthritis, 428t, 428–431, 429f, 430f
in pneumonia, 166
resolution of abnormalities, 171–172
in rheumatoid arthritis, 429, 435, 441, 445f, 445–446
Radioimmunoassay
in lupus erythematosus, 460, 461
of thyroid hormones, 241
Radioiodine
therapy with
in hyperthyroidism, 245, 246, 247, 250
hypothyroidism in, 246, 250
in thyroid cancer, 253
in thyroid scan, 242–243
uptake test, 242
factors affecting, 242, 243
Radionuclide scans
in angina pectoris, 86, 87t
in cholecystitis, 184
in heart failure, 95
in osteoporosis, 413
in thyroid disorders, 242–243
Raloxifene, 416
Ramipril in hypertension, 33t, 39
Ranitidine in mitral valve prolapse syndrome/ dysautonomia, 109
Rash, in lupus erythematosus, 455, 463, 464t
management of, 465
RAST (radioallergosorbent test), in rhinitis, 361, 363
Rauwolfia alkaloids in hypertension, 34t
Rebound headaches, 389

Rectovaginal fistula in inflammatory bowel disease, 197
Rectum
cancer of, 7–8
constipation in, 179
fistula in inflammatory bowel disease, 197
Red blood cells. *See* Erythrocytes
Referrals
in angina pectoris, 89
in anxiety disorders, 595, 596, 597
in chronic obstructive pulmonary disease, 149–150
in constipation, 180
in depression, 526, 534, 535–536
in diabetes mellitus, 270–271
in falls of elderly, 613
in fatigue, chronic, 378–379, 380
in hepatitis, 330
in hypoglycemia, 276
in lung cancer, 159
in obesity, 285
in osteoporosis, 413
to otolaryngologist, 370
in post-traumatic stress disorder, 595
in premenstrual syndrome, 514
in pseudotumor cerebri, 391
in rheumatoid arthritis, 450–451
in skin cancer, 494
in temporal arteritis, 390
in thyroid nodules, 252
Referred pain, headaches in, 385, 389
Rehabilitation
in chronic obstructive pulmonary disease, 149
in rheumatoid arthritis, 449
Reid index, 142
Reiter syndrome, 438
Remodeling of bone, 404f, 404–406, 406f
antiresorptive agents affecting, 415, 416f
Renin activity in hypertension, 35, 38, 39
Repetitive behaviors, 594, 595
Repetitive stress, osteoarthritis in, 421–422
Reserpine in hypertension, 34t, 38
Respirations
Kussmaul's, 265
rate of, in asthma, 124
Respiratory disorders, 119–174. *See also* Pulmonary disorders
Restless legs syndrome, 561, 563
Reticulocyte count in anemia, 206, 210
Retinal migraine, 388t
Retinoic acid. *See* Tretinoin
Retinopathy
diabetic, 266, 270–271, 274
in hypertension, 26
Rheumatic fever, 435
Rheumatoid arthritis, 435–453
clinical manifestations of, 440–443
extra-articular, 442–443
diagnosis of, 435
criteria in, 435, 436t
differential diagnosis of, 435–438
drug therapy in, 446–449
etiology and pathogenesis of, 438–440
genetic factors in, 440
incidence of, 435
joints involved in, 436t
laboratory tests in, 443–445, 460
neuroendocrine system in, 440
nutrition in, 449
physical and occupational therapy in, 449
prognosis in, 450
psychosocial issues in, 449
radiography in, 429, 435, 441, 445f, 445–446
referrals in, 450–451
and silicone breast implants, 440
surgery in, 449–450
synovial pathology in, 439
treatment of, 446–450
unconventional, 450
Rheumatoid factor, 439, 443–444, 444t
Rheumatology, 399–471
lupus erythematosus, 454–471
osteoarthritis, 421–434
osteoporosis, 401–420
rheumatoid arthritis, 435–453
Rhinitis, 357–364
allergic, 360–363
bacterial, 358–360
fungal, 360
medicamentosa, 363–364
in pregnancy, 363
vasomotor, 363
viral, 357–358
Rhinophyma in rosacea, 482, 483
Rhinoscleroma, 359
Rhinosporidium infections, 360
Rimantidine in influenza prophylaxis, 605–607
Risk factors, 3–9
in Alzheimer's disease, 5
in asthma, 120
in atherosclerosis, 66–67, 73–74
modification of, 70–71
in cancer, 7–8, 9
of cervix uteri, 9, 317
of lung, 7, 154, 156
of skin, 8, 497
of thyroid, 252
in cardiovascular disorders, 3–4, 25, 25t, 54, 54t
in coronary heart disease, 4, 54, 54t
and treatment goals, 55t
in diabetes mellitus, 6
in falls of elderly, 612
in hypertension, 3, 4, 25, 25t
lipid levels as, 4, 52–53, 54
longevity, 12–13
modification of, 12–13, 70–71
in obesity, 6, 281
in papillomavirus infection, 314
in pneumonia, 164, 164t, 165
in premenstrual syndrome, 506
in psychoactive substance use, 539
in sexually transmitted diseases, 17, 340
in stroke, 75
in thrombosis
arterial, 232–233
venous, 232
Rosacea, 482–483
differential diagnosis of, 476

S
Salicylic acid preparations in tinea versicolor, 488
Salmeterol in asthma, 127, 128t
nocturnal, 136
Sarcoidosis, nose in, 364–365
Sarcoptes scabiei infestation, 483–485
Scabies, 483–485
crusted, 484, 485, 485f
Scale, in xerosis, 489, 489f
Scalp, seborrheic dermatitis of, 485, 486, 487
Scarring in acne, 476, 477, 478
Schistocytes, 207t, 231
Schizoid personality disorder, 575–576
differential diagnosis of, 576, 577, 581–582, 583
Schizophrenia, 526
anxiety in, 591
differential diagnosis of, 575, 576, 577
Schizophreniform disorder, anxiety in, 591
Schizotypal personality disorder, 576–577
Schmidt's syndrome, 260, 261
Scleritis, in rheumatoid arthritis, 443
Scleroderma, 460, 465
Scleromalacia perforans, 443
Sclerosis, multiple, depression in, 522, 523
Scoliosis, in mitral valve prolapse syndrome/dysautonomia, 107
Screening, 3–9
for anxiety disorders, 587–588
blood pressure measurements in, 3, 23–24, 24t
for breast cancer, 8
for cervical cancer, 8, 9, 320
for colorectal cancer, 8
for diabetes mellitus, 6
lipid profile in, 3–4, 54
for lung cancer, 155–156
for ovarian cancer, 9
for sexually transmitted diseases, 351
vision assessment in, 5
weight measurements in, 6
Sebaceous gland activity
in acne, 475
in seborrheic dermatitis, 486
in tinea versicolor, 487
Seborrheic dermatitis, 485–487
in infants, 486, 487
Sebum production
in acne, 475, 477
in seborrheic dermatitis, 486
Selenium sulfide in tinea versicolor, 488
Self-examination
of breast, 8
of skin, 8
Self-image
in borderline personality disorder, 578
in depression, 521
in narcissistic personality disorder, 580, 581
in substance abuse and addiction, 539
Sepsis syndrome in pneumonia, 172
Septic arthritis, 435, 437
Septum, nasal, 357
Serositis in lupus erythematosus, 457, 463, 464t
management of, 466
Serotonin
in depression, 525
in migraine, 388
in premenstrual syndrome, 512
reuptake inhibitors, 529, 529t, 531t
in anxiety disorders, 598t
side effects of, 530, 531t
Sertraline
in anxiety disorders, 598t
in depression, 530, 530t, 534, 534t
in mitral valve prolapse syndrome/dysautonomia, 110
Sex hormone therapy, lipid levels in, 51–52, 60
Sexual abuse
and borderline personality disorder, 579
molluscum contagiosum in, 479
Sexual behavior, 17–18
in antisocial personality disorder, 577
in borderline personality disorder, 578
and cervical cancer, 9, 316
in depression, 522
history of, 342, 342t
in histrionic personality disorder, 579
in inflammatory bowel disease, 200
psychoactive substance use affecting, 543–544
in rheumatoid arthritis, 449
Sexually transmitted diseases, 17, 18, 339–353
cervical, 345–348
and contraceptive methods, 17, 18, 340–342
diarrhea in, 177
epidemiology of, 339–340
genital ulcer disease in, 348–351
history of patient in, 342, 342t
molluscum contagiosum in, 319, 478–480
papillomavirus infections in, 313–323
pathogens in, 340t
physical examination in, 342–343

prevention of, 322–323
reporting of, 340
risk factors in, 17, 340
screening for, 351
specimen collection in, 343, 346
vaginal, 343–345
Shampoos
in seborrheic dermatitis, 487
in tinea versicolor, 488
Sheehan's syndrome, 250, 547
Shift work sleep disorder, 565
Shoulder
osteoarthritis of, 432, 433
rheumatoid arthritis of, 435, 436t, 441
treatment of, 447, 450
Sick role in irritable bowel syndrome, 180
Sigmoidoscopy
in diarrhea, 178
in ulcerative colitis, 194
Silent thyroiditis, 255
Silicone breast implants, and rheumatoid arthritis, 440
Simvastatin in lipid-lowering therapy, 57t, 59
Sinuses, paranasal, 365–370
anatomy of, 365–366
infections of, 365, 366–370
pain over, 386
Sinusitis, 365, 366–370
acute, 366–368
bacteriology of, 368, 369
chronic, 366, 369
complications of, 368
fungal, 369–370
management of, 368, 369
pathophysiology of, 366, 369
physical examination in, 367–368, 369
subacute, 366
symptoms of, 367, 369
Sjögren's syndrome, 457, 460, 465
secondary, 443
Skin disorders, 473–499
acne, 475–478
actinic keratoses, 493
Bowenoid papulosis, 318, 496
Bowen's disease, Plate 12, 496
cancer, 8, 492–499
basal cell, 493–495
melanoma. *See* Melanoma
squamous cell, 495
in sun exposure, 8, 492–493
in diabetes mellitus, 265, 266
in Graves' disease, 244
in hepatitis, 326–327
in hypothyroidism, 248
keratoacanthoma, 496
in lupus erythematosus, 455–456, 463, 464t
management of, 465–466
molluscum contagiosum, 319, 478–480
in peripheral vascular disease, 71
pityriasis rosea, 480–482
rosacea, 476, 482–483
scabies, 483–485
seborrheic dermatitis, 485–487
self-examination of, 8
in sexually transmitted diseases, 343
tinea versicolor, 487–488
in tuberculous infection, 359
xerosis, 488–490
Skin testing in allergic rhinitis, 361
Sleep, 553–572
in adjustment disorder, 562
age-related changes in, 554, 561
in menopause, 557
in anxiety and anxiety disorders, 562, 565–566, 591
apnea in, 553, 558–559. *See also* Apnea, sleep
and circadian rhythms, 553, 555, 564–565
in dementia, 566
in depression, 521, 562, 565
deprivation of, effects of, 554–555
in dysautonomia, 106, 110, 557–558, 566
enuresis in, 562
in fibromyalgia syndrome, 557
individual needs for, 554, 563
and insomnia, 553, 562–564, 566
in depression, 521, 562
latency test, 560
and narcolepsy, 553, 559–560
neurologic mechanisms in, 554
non-rapid eye movement, 553–554
stages of, 553, 554
paradoxical, 553
paralysis in, 559, 560
periodic leg movements of, 560–561, 563
and personality disorders, 558, 566
in pregnancy, 555–557
rapid eye movement, 553, 554
behavior disorder in, 561, 562
restless legs syndrome in, 561, 563
in shift work, 565
stages and cycles in, 553, 554
in substance abuse and addiction, 562, 564, 566
in time zone change, 564–565
Sleep terrors, 561, 562
Sleepiness, daytime
in narcolepsy, 559–560
in restless legs syndrome, 561
in sleep apnea, 558
Sleeptalking, 561
Sleepwalking, 561, 562
Small cell lung cancer, 156, 159, 160–161
Smoking, 12, 13–15
angina pectoris in, 85
in asthma, 127
in pregnancy, 133
atherosclerosis in, 67, 71
and cervical cancer, 316, 317
cessation of, 14–15
in asthma, 127, 133
in atherosclerosis, 71
in chronic obstructive pulmonary disease, 144–145
clonidine in, 37
materials available on, 14–15
nicotine replacement therapy in, 14, 15, 145
role of physician in, 145
steps in, 14, 145
weight gain in, 281
chronic obstructive pulmonary disease in, 139, 149
cessation of, 144–145
pathogenesis of, 141–142
and preoperative assessment, 143, 144
economic costs of, 13–14
infertility in, 16
inflammatory bowel disease in, 192
lung cancer in, 7, 154, 161
social impact of, 14
Snoring, sleep apnea in, 558
Social activities
in depression, 518, 522
phobia or anxiety disorder in, 582, 593t, 594
prevalence of, 586, 587t
Social support, 18–19
and psychoactive substance use, 542, 546
Sociocultural factors
in depression, 525
in eating disorders, 547, 549
in fatigue, chronic, 373–374
in substance abuse and addiction, 539, 542, 545, 546
Sodium
dietary, in hypertension, 25–26, 30, 38
serum levels of
in heart failure, 95
in myxedema coma, 260
Somatization disorder, 580
chronic fatigue in, 376, 379–380
differential diagnosis of, 591
Somatostatin in hypoglycemia, 276
Somnambulism, 561, 562
Spasm
bronchial, in asthma, 119, 120, 123
esophageal, chest pain in, 84
in vasospastic angina, 83, 86, 88
Specimen collection in sexually transmitted diseases, 343, 346
Spermicidal contraceptives, 341
Sphenoid sinus, 365, 366
infection of, 367
Spherocytosis, 207t
Sphincter
esophageal, 84
of Oddi, disorders of, 187
Spine
osteoarthritis of, 423–424, 427–428, 435
radiography in, 429
osteoporosis of
bone mass measurements in, 410, 411
fluoride affecting, 418
pain in, 410, 414
parathyroid hormone affecting, 419
secondary events in, 409, 410f
vertebral compression deformity in, 408–409, 409f, 410, 410f
rheumatoid arthritis of, 440, 442
radiography in, 445–446
treatment in, 450
Spirometry
in asthma, 124, 124f
in chronic obstructive pulmonary disease, 144
Spironolactone
in heart failure, 98
in hirsutism, 306, 307, 308
in hypertension, 31t, 35
in premenstrual syndrome, 510
Spleen disorders, anemia in, 210
Spondylitis, ankylosing, 423, 438
Sputum
in asthma, 125
in chronic obstructive pulmonary disease, 139
in lung cancer, 154, 155
in pneumonia, 165, 167
Squamous cell carcinoma of skin, 495
of foot, Plate 10
in situ, Plate 12, 496
large, with ulcerated surface, Plate 11
of lip, Plate 8
of pinna, Plate 9
Stage fright, 594
Stanozolol in osteoporosis, 417
Staphylococcal infections
nasal, 358
pneumonia in, 168, 169
treatment of, 168t, 169t, 170t, 171t
septic arthritis in, 437
Steal, vertebral artery, 72
Steatorrhea in primary sclerosing cholangitis, 187, 188
Stents
in aortic stenosis, 78, 78f
in carotid stenosis, 76f, 76–77
in lower extremity peripheral vascular disease, 72, 72f
Steroid therapy. *See* Corticosteroid therapy
Stimulant drugs, 543–544
in depression, 529, 530t
Straight back syndrome, 107

Strawberry cervix, 344, 344t
Streptococcal infections
pneumococcal disease in, 149, 607
pneumonia in, 163, 166, 167, 168, 169
radiography in, 171
treatment of, 168t, 169t, 170, 170t, 171t
sinusitis in, 368
Streptokinase, 220
Stress
anxiety symptoms in, 589
fatigue in, chronic, 374, 375, 378
headaches in, 384, 392
migraine, 386–387
menstrual function in, 547, 550
and mitral valve prolapse syndrome/ dysautonomia, 104, 105, 106, 109, 110
and post-traumatic stress disorder, 593t, 595, 596, 597
psychoactive substance use in, 542
Stridor, 122
Stroke, 73–74
embolic, 75
hemorrhagic, 75
in hypertension, 3
in migraine, 388
prevention of, 74–75
risk factors in, 3, 75
Stromelysin
in osteoarthritis, 425, 426
in rheumatoid arthritis, 439, 439f
Subarachnoid hemorrhage, headache in, 385, 385t, 386, 390, 394
Subclavian artery stenosis, 72f, 72–77, 73f
Subdural hematoma, headache in, 391
Substance abuse and addiction, 15–16, 538–546
of alcohol. *See* Alcohol use and alcoholism
in anxiety, 539, 540, 542, 591
availability of drugs in, 539, 541
in bulimia, 549
CAGE questionnaire on, 15, 591
classification of psychoactive substances in, 543–545
clinical presentation of, 541–543
dependency in, 538
in depression, 519, 539, 540, 542
endocarditis and pneumonia in, 164
etiology of, 538–539
gender differences in, 544, 545, 546
incidence of, 539–540
interaction of drugs in, 543, 544
in personality disorders, 539, 584–585
antisocial, 577–578
borderline, 578, 579
passive aggressive, 584
sleep disorders in, 562, 564, 566
theories on, 539–541
treatment of, 545–546
barriers to, 545
Suicide, 518, 521, 522, 584
assessment of risk for, 527
in bipolar depression, 524
in borderline personality disorder, 578
in dysthymic depression, 524
in major depression, 523
in overdose of antidepressant drugs, 531
Sulfasalazine
in inflammatory bowel disease, 197–198
in pregnancy, 199
in rheumatoid arthritis, 448
Sulfonylurea therapy in diabetes mellitus, 269–270
Sumatriptan in headaches, 392t, 393–394, 394t
Sun exposure
actinic keratoses in, 493
avoidance of, 8, 493
burns in, 8, 492, 497
in lupus erythematosus, 455, 463, 464t, 465
skin cancer in, 8, 492–493
basal cell, 493–494
keratoacanthoma, 496
melanoma, 8, 497
squamous cell, 495
Sundowning syndrome, 566
Sunscreens, 8, 493
Support network, 18–19
and psychoactive substance use, 542, 546
Surgery
carotid endarterectomy, 75–76
in cholangiocarcinoma, 189
in chronic obstructive pulmonary disease, 143–144
lung transplantation in, 148
in condylomata, 321t, 322
diarrhea after, 178
in gallbladder cancer, 189
in gallstones, 185–186
in pregnancy, 187
in heart failure, cardiac transplantation in, 99
in hyperthyroidism, 246, 247
in pregnancy, 257
hypothyroidism in, postoperative, 246, 249
in inflammatory bowel disease, 193, 195, 200
liver transplantation in, 335
in lung cancer, 159–160
postoperative care in, 161–162
preoperative assessment in, 158–159
in nasal polyposis, 364
in obesity, 288
in osteoarthritis, 432–433
in pituitary tumors, 247, 297–298
postcholecystectomy syndrome in, 187
in rheumatoid arthritis, 449–450
in rhinitis, vasomotor, 363
in sinusitis, 368, 369
in skin cancer, 494, 495, 496
melanoma, 499
in sleep apnea, 559
in thrombosis, arterial, 233
in thyroid cancer, 253
Swan neck deformity in rheumatoid arthritis, 441, 441f
Sympatholytic agents in hypertension, 32t–33t, 34t, 36–38
Sympathomimetic agents in chronic obstructive pulmonary disease, 145–146
Syndrome X, 28, 85, 282–283
Synovectomy in rheumatoid arthritis, 449–450
Synovial fluid analysis
in osteoarthritis, 428
in rheumatoid arthritis, 444–445
Synovial tissue in rheumatoid arthritis, 439
Syphilis, 339, 614
condylomata in, 319
congenital, 359
diagnosis of, 349t, 350
epidemiology of, 339, 340
genital ulcer disease in, 348, 349t, 350
nasal disorders in, 359–360
physical examination in, 342, 343
primary, 359
screening for, 351
secondary, 359
tertiary, 360
Systolic dysfunction, heart failure in, 91–92

T
Tachypnea in pneumonia, 164
Tacrine in Alzheimer's disease, 614–615
Takayasu's disease, nose in, 365
Tamoxifen, 416
Tanning booths, 8, 493
Technetium scans
of bone, 413
of thyroid gland, 243
Telangiectasia in rosacea, 482–483
Temporal arteritis, 437
headache in, 384, 390, 394
Temporomandibular joint syndrome, 107
Tenosynovitis
in disseminated gonococcal infection, 437, 455
in lupus erythematosus, 455
Tension headaches, 384, 389
chronic, 395
and migraine, 389
treatment of, 392
Terazosin in hypertension, 33t, 37
Terbutaline in asthma, 127, 128t
nocturnal, 136
in pregnancy, 134, 135
Testosterone in hirsutism, 302, 303, 304
Tetanus, 607
Tetracycline
in acne, 477–478
in diarrhea, 178
in inflammatory bowel disease and pregnancy, 200
in pneumonia, 168t
in rosacea, 483
Thalassemia, 209
Theophylline
in asthma, 128t, 129, 129t, 130
exercise-induced, 136
nocturnal, 136
in pregnancy, 133, 135
in chronic obstructive pulmonary disease, 146–147
in lung cancer, 161
serum levels of, 129, 147
side effects of, 129, 147
Thiazide diuretics
in heart failure, 97–98
in hypertension, 31t, 35
lipid abnormalities from, 51
Thirst in diabetes mellitus, 264
Thrombectomy, 233
Thrombin, 218, 219
in clotting time test, 223
Thrombocytopenia, 210, 215, 223
antifibrinolytic agents in, 229
in lupus erythematosus, 460, 466
Thrombocytosis in rheumatoid arthritis, 443
Thromboembolism. *See* Thrombosis and thromboembolism
Thrombolytic therapy, 233
in lower extremity peripheral vascular disease, 71
in venous thromboembolism, 79
Thromboplastin time, partial, 221–223
in lupus erythematosus, 460
normal, bleeding in, 226, 227
prolonged, 224–225, 225f, 226
Thrombosis and thromboembolism
arterial, 232–233
prevention of, 235
in disseminated intravascular coagulation, 231
in hyperosmolar hyperglycemic coma, 273
in lupus erythematosus, 458
and prethrombotic conditions, 231–235
pulmonary, 84, 86, 123, 166, 173
treatment of, 233–234
venous, 66, 78–80, 232, 611
deep, 233
physical examination in, 78–79
prevention of, 235
risk factors for, 232
treatment of, 233, 234

Thromboxane, 218
Thrombus formation, 218
Thyroglobulin, 239
  measurement of, 244
Thyroid-binding globulin, 241–242
  in pregnancy, 256, 257
Thyroid gland
  anatomy of, 239
  antibodies to, 243–244
  aspiration of, fine needle, 244, 247, 252–253, 254
  cancer of, 239, 244, 249, 252
    risk factors for, 252
    treatment of, 253
  disorders of, 6, 239–263
    bleeding in, 228
    constipation in, 179
    depression in, 522, 523, 529
    in diabetes mellitus, 266
    heart failure in, 93–94, 244
    hypertension in, 27
    lipid abnormalities in, 50–51
    myxedema coma in, 259–261
    thyroid storm in, 258–259
  embryology of, 239, 240
  enlargement of, 241
    in Hashimoto's thyroiditis, 249
  hyperthyroidism, 244–248. *See also* Hyperthyroidism
  hypothyroidism, 248–251. *See also* Hypothyroidism
  laboratory tests of, 241–244
  nodules of, 241, 243, 252–254
    autonomously functioning, 247
    benign, 253–254
    evaluation of, 252, 253f
    hyperthyroidism in, 246–247, 252
    in multinodular goiter, 246–247, 254
    radiation-induced, 254
    solitary, 252–254
  physical examination of, 241
  physiology of, 239–240
  in pregnancy, 256–258
    nodules of, 243, 253
    and thyroid storm, 259
  radionuclide scans of, 242–243
  thyroiditis of, 254–256. *See also* Thyroiditis
  ultrasonography of, 243
Thyroid hormones, 239–241
  in anorexia nervosa, 548
  deficiency of, 248–251
  drugs affecting, 240
  excess of, 244–248
  free, 241
  functions of, 240
  immunoassay of, 241
  measurement of serum levels, 241–242
  in myxedema coma, 261
  in postpartum thyroiditis, 256
  in pregnancy, 256, 257, 258
  regulation of, 240–241
  replacement therapy, 249, 250, 251–252
    in pregnancy, 257
  resin uptake, 241–242
  secretive use of, 248
  in silent thyroiditis, 255
  in sporadic goiter, 254
  in subacute thyroiditis, 255
  synthesis and secretion of, 240
  in thyroid cancer, 253
  in thyroid nodules, 253, 254
  in thyroid storm, 258–259
  total, 241
Thyroid storm, 258–259
Thyroidectomy
  in Graves' disease, 246, 249
  hypothyroidism in, 246, 249
Thyroiditis, 254–256
  autoimmune, 248–249, 254, 255–256
  Hashimoto's, 243, 248–249
  laboratory tests in, 242
  postpartum, 255–256
  silent, 255
  subacute, 254–255
Thyroid-stimulating hormone, 239, 240
  antibodies to, 243–244
  deficiency of, 250
  measurement of serum levels, 242
  in myxedema coma, 260
  pituitary secretion of, 240
    in adenoma, 247
  in postpartum thyroiditis, 256
  in pregnancy, 256, 257
  and prolactin secretion, 293
  in sporadic goiter, 254
  in thyroid cancer, 253
  in thyroid nodules, 253
Thyroid-stimulating immunoglobulin, 243–244
Thyrotoxicosis. *See* Hyperthyroidism
Thyrotropin-releasing hormone, 240
  deficiency of, 248, 250
  and prolactin secretion, 293
Thyroxine, 239–241. *See also* Thyroid hormones
Tic douloureux, 390
Ticarcillin-clavulanate, in pneumonia, 170t
Ticlopidine, 74–75, 235
  in stroke prevention, 74–75
Time zone change, circadian rhythm disorders in, 564–565
Timolol in hypertension, 32t, 36
Tinea versicolor, 487–488
Tobacco use, 13–15. *See also* Smoking
Tobramycin in pneumonia, 171t
Tolazamide in diabetes mellitus, 270t
Tolbutamide in diabetes mellitus, 270t
Tophi, gouty, 442
Toxic multinodular goiter, 246–247
Toxicity
  food poisoning, 177
  hepatotoxicity of drugs, 330
    of anti-inflammatory drugs, 432, 446
    in rheumatoid arthritis, 448, 449
  of lead, 209
Toxoid, tetanus, 607
Tracheal disorders
  differential diagnosis of, 122–123, 140
  flow-volume loop in, 123f
  wheezing in, 122–123
Tracheostomy in sleep apnea, 559
Tranexamic acid, 229
Transactional meaning in chronic fatigue, 375
Transforming growth factor
  in osteoarthritis, 426
  in rheumatoid arthritis, 438
Transfusion of platelets, 230–231
Transplantation
  of heart, 99
  of liver, 324, 335
  of lung, 148
Tranylcypromine in anxiety disorders, 598t
Trauma
  acoustic, hearing loss in, 18
  in falls of elderly, 612, 613
  headaches in, 386
  nasal, 364
  osteoarthritis in, 421–422, 424
  and post-traumatic stress disorder, 593t, 595, 596, 597
Travel, time zone change and circadian rhythm disorders in, 564–565
Trazodone
  in anxiety disorders, 598t
  in depression, 530t
    dosage of, 533, 534t
    side effects of, 530, 531t
Treponema pallidum infections, 340t. *See also* Syphilis
Tretinoin
  in acne, 477
  in rosacea, 483
  in tinea versicolor, 488
Triamcinolone in asthma, 128t, 130
  in pregnancy, 135
Triamterene in hypertension, 31t, 32t, 35
Trichlormethiazide in hypertension, 31t
Trichloroacetic acid
  in actinic keratoses, 493
  in condylomata, 321, 321t, 322
Trichomonas infection, 340t, 341, 343
  of vagina, 343, 344, 344t
Trichotillomania, 591
Trigeminal neuralgia, 390
Trigger factors
  in asthma, 121, 122
    avoidance of, 126
  in migraine, 386–387
Trigger points in headaches, 385, 389
Triglycerides, 61–62
  in alcohol use, 50
  in autoimmune disorders, 51
  in combined hyperlipidemia, familial, 48
  and coronary heart disease, 52–53, 61–62
  in diabetes mellitus, 50, 61
  drugs affecting, 52
  in dyslipidemia, familial, 48
  in hyperchylomicronemia syndrome, 49
  in hypertriglyceridemia. *See* Hypertriglyceridemia
  measurement of, 54
  in obesity, 50
  in renal disorders, 51
  secondary causes of disorders, 49t
  in thyroid disease, 50, 51
Triiodothyronine, 239–241. *See also* Thyroid hormones
Trimethoprim-sulfamethoxazole
  in diarrhea, 178
  in pneumonia, 169t
Truelove and Witts scale on ulcerative colitis, 194
Tuberculosis, 359
Tumor necrosis factor
  in osteoarthritis, 426
  in rheumatoid arthritis, 438, 439f, 449
Tumors. *See* Cancer

U
Ulcer(s)
  genital, 348–351
  ischemic, 68
  in lupus erythematosus, 456, 458, 463, 464t
    management of, 466
  in skin carcinoma, Plate 11, 495
  in venous insufficiency, 611
Ulcerative colitis, 191–201. *See also* Colitis, ulcerative
Ultrasonography
  in carotid artery atherosclerosis, 73f, 74
  in gallstones, 184
  in hepatitis, 330
  in osteoporosis, bone mass measurements in, 411
  of thyroid gland, 243
Ultraviolet radiation exposure. *See* Sun exposure
Upper extremity atherosclerosis, 66, 72–77
Urea cream in xerosis, 489

Urea nitrogen, blood, in hypertension, 27t, 28
Uremia, bleeding disorders in, 215, 223, 227
Uric acid levels in hypertension, 3, 27t, 28
Urinalysis in hypertension, 3, 27t, 28
Urokinase, 220
 in lower extremity peripheral vascular disease, 71
Ursodeoxycholic acid
 in cholangitis, primary sclerosing, 189
 in gallstones, 186
Uterosacral ligaments in endometriosis, Plate 3, 180

V
Vaccinations
 in chronic obstructive pulmonary disease, 149
 in elderly, 605-607, 606t
 in hepatitis, 331, 331t, 332, 333-334
 influenza, 149, 358, 605, 606t
 in lupus erythematosus, 465
 pneumococcal, 149, 607
 tetanus, 607
Vagina, 343-345
 candidiasis of, 343, 344t
 collection of specimens from, 343
 discharge from, 343, 344, 345
 fistula in inflammatory bowel disease, 197
 horizontal, 200
 papillomavirus infection of, 318, 318f, 320
  treatment of, 322
 signs and symptoms in diseases of, 344t
Vaginitis, 343, 344, 344t
Vaginosis, bacterial, 343, 344t, 344-345
Valproic acid in migraine prevention, 396
Valvular heart disease
 angina pectoris in, 85
 in lupus erythematosus, 458
 mitral prolapse, 104-115
 stroke in, 73, 74
  prevention of, 75
Varicosities
 bleeding, 335, 611
 venous, 80, 611
Vasculitis
 leukocytoclastic, 442
 in lupus erythematosus, 456, 458, 459, 460
  management of, 466
 rheumatoid, 442
Vasoactive intestinal peptide, and prolactin secretion, 293, 294
Vasodilators
 in heart failure, 97
 in hypertension, 34t
Vasomotor rhinitis, 363
Vegetarian diet, 12
Veins
 insufficiency of, 610, 611
 thrombosis and thromboembolism of. *See* Thrombosis and thromboembolism, venous
 varicosities of, 80, 611
Venlafaxine in depression, 530t
 dosage of, 534, 534t
 side effects of, 530-531, 531t
Ventricles, cardiac
 diastolic dysfunction of, 92-93
 hypertrophy of
  angina pectoris in, 85
  in hypertension, 27, 28
 in left-sided heart failure, 93
 in right-sided heart failure, 93
 systolic dysfunction of, 91-92
Ventricles, cerebral, colloid cyst of, 391
Verapamil
 in angina pectoris, 88
 in hypertension, 33t-34t, 38
 in migraine prevention, 395, 395t
Vertebral compression deformity in osteoporosis, 408-409, 409f, 410, 410f
Vertigo, benign paroxysmal, 388t
Vesnarinone in heart failure, 98
Vestibulitis, nasal, 358
Vincristine in lupus erythematosus, 466
Viral infections, 339, 340t
 Bowenoid papulosis in, 318, 496
 diarrhea in, 177
 hepatitis in, 324-338
 herpes simplex. *See* Herpes simplex virus infections
 HIV infection and AIDS in. *See* HIV infection and AIDS
 influenza in, 149, 358, 605-607
 molluscum contagiosum in, 319, 478-480
 papillomavirus, 313-323. *See also* Papillomavirus infections
 pneumonia in, 163, 165, 167, 168, 169
  secondary infections in, 172
  treatment of, 168t, 169t, 170t, 171t
 rhinitis in, 357-358
 sinusitis in, 365, 368
Vision
 assessment of, 5
 in diabetes mellitus, 264, 265, 266
 in glaucoma, 5
  acute narrow-angle, 391-392
 in migraine, 387
 in pituitary adenoma, 296, 296f
 in pseudotumor cerebri, 390-391
 in temporal arteritis, 390
Vitamin B_6 in premenstrual syndrome, 506
Vitamin B_{12} deficiency, 211, 212, 614
Vitamin C, and coronary heart disease risk, 60
Vitamin D in osteoporosis
 deficiency of, 408, 413, 414-415
 supplementation of, 414-415
Vitamin E, and coronary heart disease risk, 60
Vitamin K, 215, 216
 administration of, 229
 coagulation factors dependent on, 215, 220, 224
  laboratory assessment of, 221
 deficiency of, 216, 224, 225, 229
  osteoporosis in, 408
 dietary requirement for, 220
Vitamins, deficiency of, 216, 224, 225, 229
 anemia in, 211
 causes of, 212
 in cholangitis, primary sclerosing, 187, 188
 dementia in, 614
 osteoporosis in, 408, 413, 414-415
Von Willebrand's disease, 215, 217, 223-224, 228-229
 acquired, 228
 pregnancy in, 228, 229
 treatment of, 228-229
Von Willebrand factor, 215, 218, 219, 228-229
 deficiency of, 228-229
 required for hemostasis, 220t
Vulva
 Bowenoid papulosis of, 318, 496
 candidiasis of, 343, 344t
 granulomatous disease of, in inflammatory bowel disease, 197
 papillomavirus infection of, 318, 318f

W
Waist-to-hip ratio, 279, 282, 283
Walking program in peripheral vascular disease, 71-72
Warfarin, 233, 234
 in pregnancy, 234
 side effects of, 234
 in stroke prevention, 75
Warts, anogenital, 313-323. *See also* Condylomata
Weakness, 374
Wegener's granulomatosis, 167
 nose in, 365
Weight, 5-6, 12
 in anorexia nervosa, 548, 549
 and body fat distribution, 279, 282, 283
 and body mass index, 6, 278, 282
 in bulimia, 549
 in depression, 522
 in diabetes mellitus, 264, 282
 in heart failure, 97
 and height tables, 278-279, 279t
 in hypertension, 26, 28, 29, 50, 282
 ideal, 17, 278-279, 279t
 in lupus erythematosus, 454
 and menstrual function, 547, 550
 in mitral valve prolapse syndrome/dysautonomia, 107
 and nutrition, 17, 280-281, 286-287, 288
 in obesity, 56, 278-291. *See also* Obesity
 in pregnancy, 17, 281, 283
 in smoking cessation, 281
 and waist-to-hip ratio, 279, 282, 283
Wheezing
 in asthma, 122-123, 124
  severity of, 125, 126
 in chronic obstructive pulmonary disease, 139, 140
 differential diagnosis of, 122-123, 139
Whipple's triad, 274, 275
Wilson's disease, 330
Withdrawal from drugs, psychoactive, 544, 545
Withdrawal from social activities, in depression, 522
Wolff-Chaikoff effect, 240
Wolfram's syndrome, 266
Work, 18
 and acne, 476
 and hearing loss, 18
 and occupational therapy in rheumatoid arthritis, 449
 in personality disorders
  antisocial, 577, 578, 581
  avoidant, 581
  dependent, 582
  narcissistic, 580
  obsessive compulsive, 583
  paranoid, 575
  passive aggressive, 583, 584
  schizoid, 576
 psychoactive substance use affecting, 542
 repetitive stress in, and osteoarthritis, 421-422
 rotating shifts in, 565
 and xerosis, 489
Wrist
 fractures in osteoporosis, 408
 rheumatoid arthritis of, 436t, 440, 441, 445, 445f
  treatment in, 447, 450

X
Xanthelasma in angina pectoris, 86
Xanthomas, 47, 48, 49
 in diabetes mellitus, 266
Xerosis, 488-490, 489f
Xerostomia in rheumatoid arthritis, 442-443

Z
Z deformity in rheumatoid arthritis, 441
Zinc pyrithione in tinea versicolor, 488
Zolpidem tartrate in insomnia, 563